INTRODUCTORY

Clinical

Pharmacology

TWELFTH EDITION

INTRODUCTORY

Clinical Pharmacology

Susan M. Ford, MN, RN, CNE Ret

Professor Emeritus, Former Associate Dean for Nursing
Tacoma Community College
Tacoma, Washington

TWELFTH EDITION

. Wolters Kluwer

Philadelphia • Baltimore • New York • London
Buenos Aires • Hong Kong • Sydney • Tokyo

Vice President, Nursing Segment: Julie K. Stegman
Director, Nursing Education and Practice Content: Jamie Blum
Senior Acquisitions Editor: Jonathan Joyce
Senior Development Editor: Julie M. Vitale
Editorial Coordinator: Vino Varadharajalu
Marketing Manager: Brittany Riney
Editorial Assistant: Molly Kennedy
Production Project Manager: David Saltzberg
Manager, Graphic Arts & Design: Stephen Druding
Art Director: Jennifer Clements
Manufacturing Coordinator: Margie Orzech-Zeranko
Prepress Vendor: TNQ Technologies

12th Edition

9 8 7 6 5 4 3 2 1

Printed in China

Library of Congress Cataloging-in-Publication Data

ISBN-13: 978-1-975163-73-0

Cataloging in Publication data available on request from publisher.

LWW.com

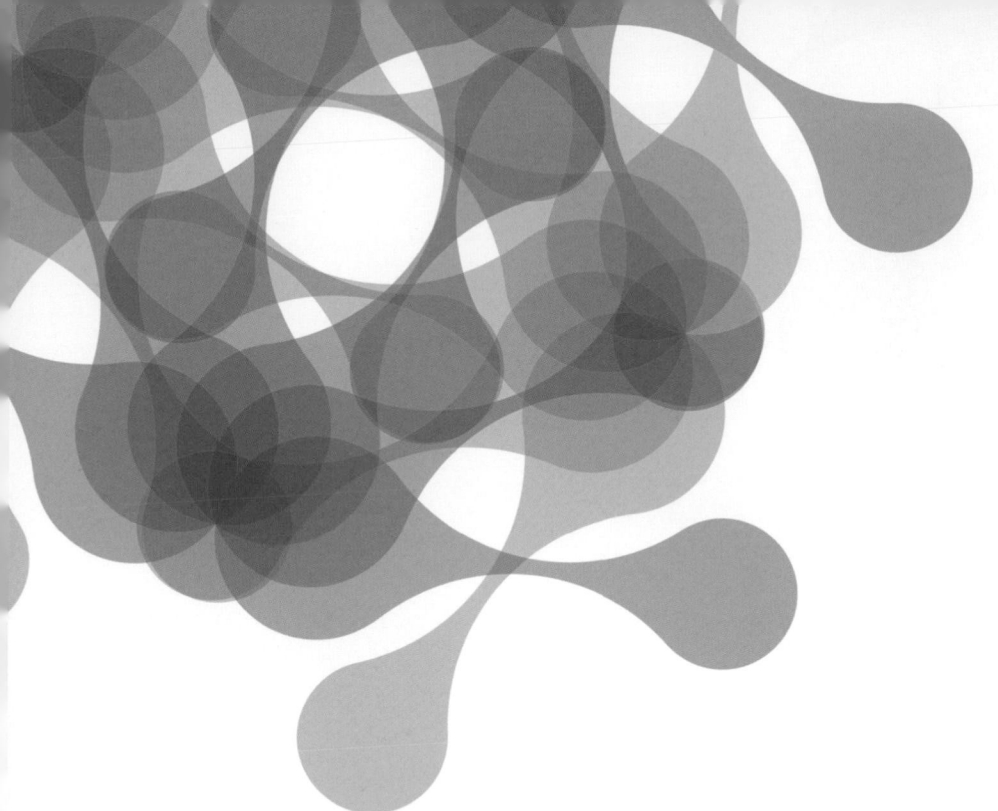

I dedicate the 12th edition to three young women, my grandchildren.

My future—Pyrola Grothford, Rory Ford, and Leighton Ford, my granddaughters;
who I hope may see health care in their lifetimes become a right for all,
not just a privilege for those who can pay.

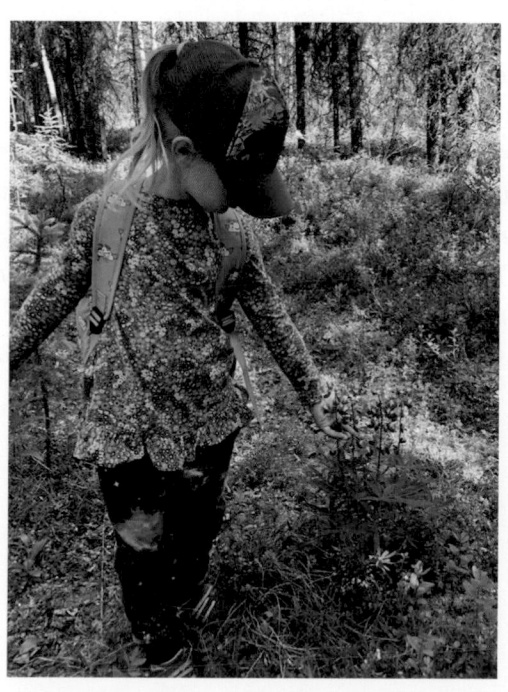

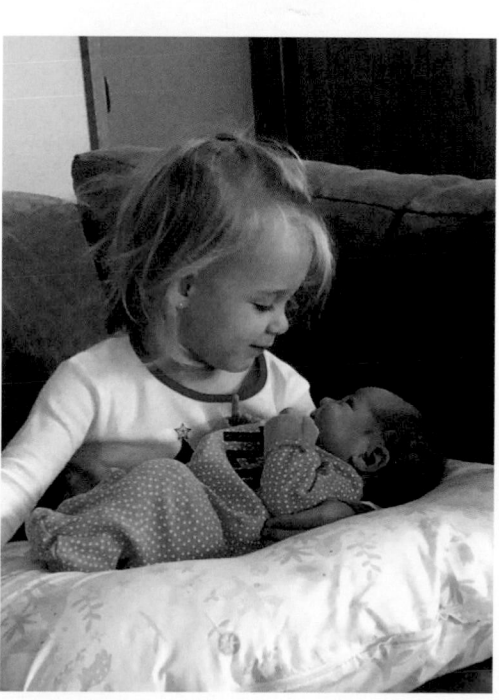

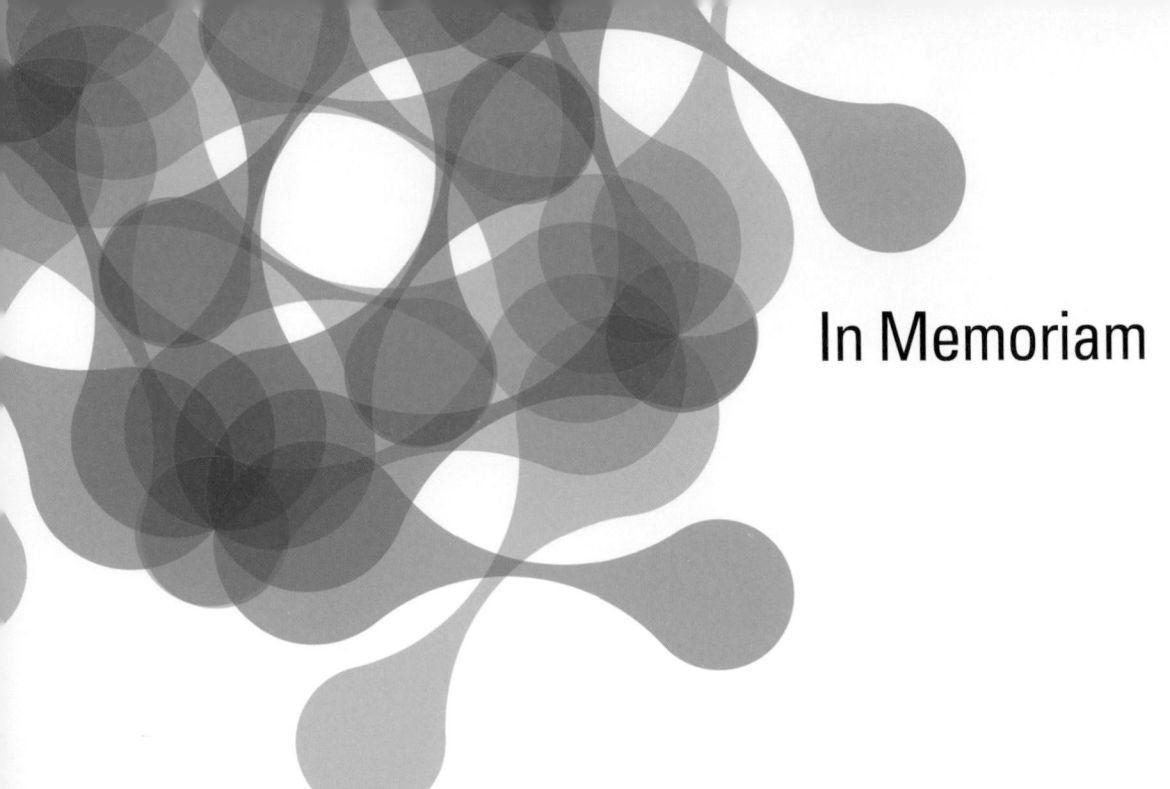

In Memoriam

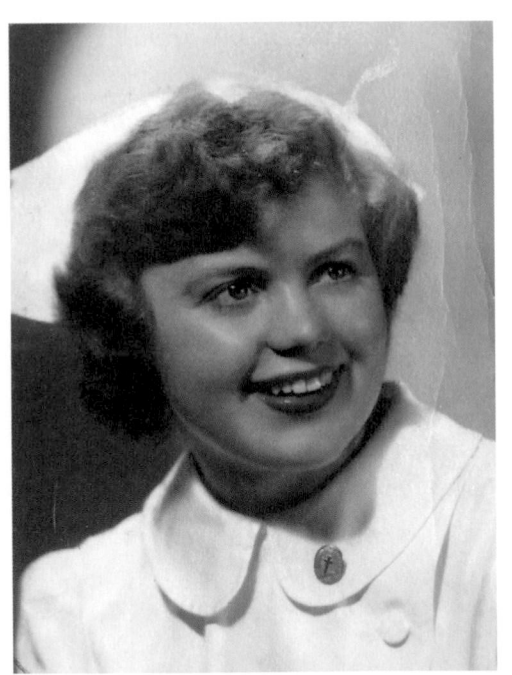

In loving memory—Sylvia Jones, my mother and the nurse who suggest I follow her into the nursing profession as a career. We lost this wonderful woman in the year of COVID; not due to it, but because of it. Her own mother orphaned during the 1918 Influenza Pandemic, she started nursing school at the age of 17, during WWII. She was a delivery room nurse for some, school nurse to the neighborhood, and psych counselor to many friends and family. She was the strength we all hold in our hearts. Her dedication to thinking of others first and altruistic helping resulted in a number of health providers and educators in our family. Teaching us to think of others first, she spent her last day on earth personally hauling out the garbage canisters to the farm gate. Living to be 92 years old, I know she is proud of us, may we all carry on in her spunk and spirit!

Reviewers

Danette Ver Woert, MN, BSN, RN
Assistant Professor of Nursing
Buntain College of Nursing, Northwest University
Kirkland, Washington

Ruth A Lopes RN, MN
Nursing Professor
Tacoma Community College
Tacoma, Washington

MaryAnn D'Alesandro, DNP, RN, MSN, CNOR, BC
Associate Professor, Nursing
The University of Tampa
Tampa, Florida

Preface

*I*ntroductory Clinical Pharmacology is one in a series of texts designed to assist beginning nursing students in acquiring a foundation of basic nursing theory and for developing clinical skills. Many publishers present a choice of texts offering information on drug action and activity. Yet, this text is uniquely written *by* nurses *for* nurses in an easy-to-read language, not only to teach the novice provider about the drugs but also to role model how to relay this information to clients.

Here are the key features new to the 12th edition across the entire text:

Learning objectives set the tone for students on what to find in a chapter. The language of learning objectives has been clarified and both learners and instructors know what level of understanding to expect from the information provided.

NEW Tall man lettering is now featured in Summary Drug Tables as well as Appendix B. Visual cueing to name differences helps bolster safety in drug administration.

Two new alerts are featured across chapters, LASA and PIP. Look-alike, Sound-alike (LASA) boxes list many of the drug names which, when spoken such as between providers, can be mistaken for other agents. Chapter displays alert providers to possible drug misinterpretation. Practice considerations (PIP) provide information about select drugs or actions that might not be critical, yet relevant to the drugs in the select chapters.

Nursing assessment is displayed as bulleted items. Providers need quick and organized presentation of information. By bullet listing key assessments, learners see the data needed for quick and succinct assessment. This helps learners to develop clinical reasoning skills by the delineation of crucial versus minor data.

Summary Drug Tables illustrate pronunciation of generic drug terms in an easier, learnable format.

Pharmacology in Practice discussion questions are threaded through every chapter to give the learner the opportunity to check knowledge and the instructor the means to stimulate discussion with learners.

TEXT ORGANIZATION

The 12th edition of *Introductory Clinical Pharmacology* is organized into 14 units. The unit expansion allows for more information on immunotherapy in general and cancer specifically. Changes and additions from the last edition are *italicized* below in addition to a brief explanation of unit information:

- **Unit 1: Nursing Foundation of Clinical Pharmacology**—is the basis of understanding drug therapy in order to better learn about pharmacology in general. Basic concepts include pharmacological concepts, techniques of administration and the math needed to provide safe dosing, how the nursing process and pharmacology work in tandem, and interacting with clients for best outcomes. *New to 12th edition—greater emphasis on clarifying examples (e.g. FDA drug approval process), in-depth information on enteral and topical drug administration, the inclusion of TALLman lettering explanation (for later chapters), and viewing client problems in an expanded context of nursing.*
- **Unit 2: Drugs Used to Fight Infections**—The infection chapter begins with bacterial microorganisms, moves on to viral, and the unit ends with fungi and protozoa. Antibacterial chapters (Chapters 6–9) group the drugs according to interaction with bacterial cells. This presentation helps in understanding how the different classes are similar and what to look for in terms of similar actions or adverse reactions. *Antibiotic stewardship is emphasized in these chapters.* Highlight of

combination drugs used with diseases such as TB or HIV (Chapters 10 and 11) emphasizes methods to increase adherence to drug therapy and improving quality of life. Chapter 11 includes the expanding number of drugs to treat once acute illness (such as HIV and Hep C) shifting care to that of chronic conditions. Chapter 12 views drug therapy both in treating infections at home or those severe enough for hospitalization.

- **Unit 3: Drugs Used to Manage Pain**—Pain-assessment strategies, as well as the drugs for pain relief, are threaded through Chapters 13–15. *A deeper look at chronic pain management includes a new pain relief ladder and information on the opiate crisis. Because of this, Chapter 15 now includes information on opiate antagonists, eliminating that chapter from this edition.* As nurses, we need to acknowledge that many of our clients will have used marijuana for medical or recreational purposes. Therefore, it is important to provide knowledge of this drug and its uses as well as its effects and interactions. Inclusion of medical marijuana, written with neither the intent to support nor dismiss its use, is featured in Chapter 15. Many nurses never enter the operating room suites; therefore, Chapter 16 is now about anesthetic drugs *with inclusion of conscious sedation.*

- **Unit 4: Drugs That Affect the Central Nervous System**—When clients become stressed, mental health issues may surface. This can be a surprising experience for providers in nonpsychiatric settings such as acute med-surg floors or intensive care units. The chapters of this unit provide explanation and information to help reduce the stigma associated with clients labeled with a psychiatric diagnosis and see the benefit of drugs in helping care for those with mental health issues. *The name change of Chapter 18 to Antidementia Drugs allows one to see it includes all drugs used beside the category of cholinesterase inhibitors; additionally, Alzheimer disease stages are explained according to the pathological stages of the disease to better correspond with different types of drugs used for different behaviors and pathology.*

- **Unit 5: Drugs That Affect the Peripheral Nervous System**—Repetition and clarification of terminology in all chapters in this unit help students understand the importance of the neurologic system in many facets of drug therapy.

- **Unit 6: Drugs That Affect the Neuromuscular System**—Drug reclassification of *anticonvulsant* to *antiepileptic* terminology provides consistency in antiepileptic drug understanding and treatment.

- **Unit 7: Drugs That Affect the Respiratory System**—Over-the-counter products make self-treatment for respiratory conditions a growing concern. Both drugs and strategies for client teaching are updated in these chapters. *Abuse of over-the-counter respiratory meds by adolescents is featured in this unit as well as new guidelines for Asthma Action Plans.*

- **Unit 8: Drugs That Affect the Cardiovascular System**—*National guideline updates are included in multiple chapters leading to the combination of cardiotonic and antiarrhythmic drugs into one chapter (Chapter 37).* Encouraging students to use their skills at using clinical judgment with Pharmacology in Practice Case Studies in each chapter and linkages to the ancillary products will help the student to discover the polypharmacology issues when cardiac medications are prescribed in tandem with most any other category of drug.

- **Unit 9: Drugs That Affect the Gastrointestinal System**—Biologics used to treat inflammatory bowel diseases are now *connected to information in Unit 12.* These chapters focus on strategies for self-treatment of both upper and lower gastrointestinal issues.

- **Unit 10: Drugs That Affect the Endocrine System**—Antidiabetic medications in addition to insulin are provided in Chapter 40, which corresponds with the rise of clients being diagnosed with diabetes.

- **Unit 11: Drugs That Affect the Urinary System**—Clarity of information to help clients remain safe while using medications supporting healthy aging is highlighted in this unit.

- **NEW Unit 12: Drugs That Affect the Immune System**—*Removing two earlier chapters allows for expansion into immunological agents. Vaccines are pulled out separately (Chapter 47) and new information is provided on immunostimulant and immunomodulating (or blocking) agents in Chapters 48 and 49.* Information on biologic therapies for multiple chronic conditions as well as updated immunization schedules in easy-to-read versions makes information suitable to share with clients.

- **NEW Unit 13: Drugs that Fight Cancer**—*With the addition of many biologic agents used in the treatment of cancers, another chapter exclusive to these agents was added to the text.*

Chapter 50 includes drug categories known as the traditional chemotherapy agents, and Chapter 51 includes immunotherapy and target agents used in the treatment of cancers.

- **Unit 14: Drugs That Affect Other Body Systems**—Topicals are featured in Chapter 52, drugs for ear and eye disorders in Chapter 53, and Chapter 54 includes elements and parenteral therapy.

FEATURES

Written with client outcomes in mind, complex concepts are introduced in simplified language, helping learners to grasp concepts quicker and to use client teaching information right from the text leading to better understanding on the part of the client and adherence to treatment strategies.

Benefit to the Instructor

The basic explanations presented in the text are *not* intended to suggest that pharmacology is an easy subject. As we know it, drug therapy is one of the most important and complicated treatment modalities in modern health care. This text is written to help you *teach* the latest pharmacologic information available by including:

- Clear, concise language to introduce learners to the basics of pharmacology.
- Presentation of drugs in a way to make integration of this text into concept-based curricula seamless and effortless.
- Learning objectives are leveled to make your expectations of knowledge retention clear to the learner.
- Comprehensive bibliography entries that link the text to the latest evidence-based information and practice.

The new, or improved, features that make this the best pharmacology text for teaching your students include the following:

- Nursing process planning language makes client problem recognition understandable to an array of health care disciplines as well as nursing.
- Special features such as *Alerts* and *Considerations,* which include information to care for a more diverse client population.
- Removal of old drug brand names that have lost their exclusive patents and confuse learners when used.
- New to this edition are highlighted questions embedded in the text, to make the learner stop, ponder, and examine learning retention. All skills need to develop clinical judgment in the field.

Benefit to the Learner

As a novice provider, this text gives you the introduction and foundation you need to begin developing your own clinical judgment skills. This text is written to help you *learn* the latest pharmacologic information available by including:

- Drug therapy explained uniquely from a nursing perspective.
- Connection of drug therapy to the basic nursing theory you are learning in your nursing curriculum.
- Presentation in an easy-to-read and follow format that helps you understand the drugs and their effects on the human body, which in turn motivates you to continue to learn more about this subject independently and helps you to provide better care, educate clients, and improve outcomes.
- A nursing process section in each chapter that uses a familiar step-by-step method to show how medications are used in the care of clients. Elements of the nursing process—assessment, analysis, planning, intervention, and evaluation—illustrate basic and practical nursing skills to help develop clinical reasoning in order for you to help clients meet their health care needs, and to improve adherence to treatment, all designed for better client outcomes.
- Medication calculation using principles of safe practice rather than mathematical formulas used in traditional math classes. Learning focuses on reducing medication errors that result from mathematical mistakes rather than on the traditional arithmetic exercises.
- Seven clients introduced in Chapter 5, whose health issues are woven into subsequent chapters in order to build a story of how drugs impact real people. Your ability to use outcome strategies and communicate what you do to support client and family confidence in learning self-management

skills of medication administration is highlighted using health literacy principles and appreciation of cultural diversity using one of these seven clients individually featured in each chapter.
- Specific quiz review items that are directly linked to the latest NCLEX test plan.
- A list of abbreviations on the inside back cover for easy reference.
- Informational data to construct mind mapping visuals of the case study clients when used in conjunction with the suite of product ancillaries or for those who prefer—the *Study Guide to Accompany Introductory Clinical Pharmacology,* 12th Edition, with either product, it provides you with multiple opportunities to identify potential drug–drug interactions, once again helping you as you build your skills of reasoning and clinical judgement.

Building Clinical Judgment

Pharmacology courses are typically taught preprogram or as a preclinical course in nursing programs. Therefore, the focus of concepts in this text are to prepare the learner with a good foundation of lower layers of clinical judgment skill building for when learners begin clinical and lab courses where they are able to connect the foundations of pharmacology with clinical situations.

This title provides repetition of concepts, introduction to case studies, and mind mapping tools for learning to help provide a base for clinical judgment development, and subsequent nursing competency.

Specifics found in this text to develop clinical judgment include the following:

- Chapter 4 discusses Nursing Process within the context of medication administration. Each subsequent drug chapter has a *Nursing Process—Steps to Build Clinical Judgment* section to help learners understand how select drug categories impact clients.
- Chapter 5 introduces learner to seven clients, who are randomly featured in case study situations in each subsequent drug chapter helping learners examine medications in a client context.
- LASA (look alike, sound alike) and Nursing Alerts in addition to health-related considerations are highlighted in each chapter to help learners recognize and attend to cues which may vary from routine.
- Case studies with visual mind mapping exercises are offered in the ancillary package. Learners can layer and build scenarios in order to understand how and begin to anticipate how drugs interact with each other and the disease processes involved resulting in positive outcomes, bothersome side effects, or serious adverse reactions.

What My Nursing Experiences Offer in This Text

To learn skills one needs repetitive practice, and nurses gain this in the clinical setting. This means as elders we must step aside so that new nurses may gain that experience. Retiring from paid clinical positions does not mean we stop learning; I continued to gain teaching experience as a volunteer scripted/standardized client in the Nursing Simulation Center at Swedish RN Residency Program and learn about client experiences as a volunteer facilitator in chronic illness workshops at Kaiser Foundation Health Plan of Washington. COVID changed all that, being isolated at home and privileged to have good resources I had the time to study, research drug interactions, and speak to nurses regarding the clinical decision making happening for both critical and what we now think of as routine care. I listen to what new nurses and clients need in our ever-changing health care systems. Participating as a healthcare volunteer in COVID-19 vaccination clinics; I witnessed the exhaustion of providers, and both the fear and jubilation of those getting the vaccine. These experiences help me to appreciate what novice nurses need in their pharmacologic education and how clients understand what we say as we communicate about drugs in our interventions and teaching. Where we have to be expedient, yet demonstrate a high degree of caring in our interactions with every client. This text is a blending of this newly gained insight with well over 40 years of nursing practice and teaching experience in mental health, acute care, operating room, ambulatory care, home health, and hospice settings, as well as holding nursing certification in areas such as oncology, medical-surgical clinical nurse specialist, and as a certified nurse educator.

As You Learn and Enter Practice

You may find that certain drugs or drug dosages described in this publication may no longer be available. Likewise, there may be new drugs on the market that were not approved by the U.S. Food and Drug Administration (FDA) at the time of publication. With the availability of computers, smart phones, and other Internet resources, current information is always there for verification of any drug question and should be checked when you do have a question before administering a drug. Do not forget that your colleagues, clinical pharmacists, and primary health care providers are also resources for information concerning a specific drug including dosage, adverse reactions, contraindications, precautions, interactions, or administration. Check out my pharmacology blog - things I can't get to press in this book, you will see there - https://icp-ford.blogspot.com/

TEACHING AND LEARNING RESOURCES

To facilitate mastery of this text's content, a comprehensive teaching and learning package has been developed to assist faculty and students.

Resources for Instructors
Tools to assist you with teaching your course are available upon adoption of this text at http://thepoint.lww.com/Ford12e

- A **Test Generator** lets you put together exclusive new tests from a bank containing hundreds of questions to help you in assessing your students' understanding of the material. Test questions link to chapter learning objectives.
- **PowerPoint Presentations** have been totally revised to provide greater flexibility to the instructor for use in-class, as online study, or for a completely self-paced course. These provided an easy way for you to integrate the textbook with your students' classroom experience, either via slide shows or handouts. Multiple-choice and true/false questions are integrated into the presentations to promote class participation and allow you to use iClicker technology.
- An **Image Bank** lets you use the photographs and illustrations from this textbook in your PowerPoint slides or as you see fit in your course.
- **Case Studies** with related questions (and suggested answers) give students an opportunity to apply their knowledge to a client case similar to one they might encounter in practice.
- **Pre-Lecture Quizzes** (and answers) are quick, knowledge-based assessments that allow you to check students' reading and are written in the Next-Generation NCLEX style offering additional practice in this new format.
- **Guided Lecture Notes** walk you through the chapters to help you present information in an informative and educational manner.
- **Discussion Topics** (and suggested answers) are based off of the Pharmacology in Practice questions of the text. Helping students connect information from the book with situations in the clinical setting, they can be used as conversation starters or in online discussion boards.
- Plus **Syllabi (including an online self-paced course), Lesson Plans, QSEN Competency Maps,** and **Assignments** (for discussion or mind mapping exercises).

Resources for Students
An exciting set of free resources is available to help students review material and become even more familiar with vital concepts. Students can access all these resources at http://thePoint.lww.com/Ford12e using the codes printed in the front of their textbooks.

- **NCLEX-Style Review Questions** for each chapter help students review important concepts and practice for the NCLEX.
- **Concepts in Action Animations** bring pharmacology concepts to life.
- **Watch & Learn Videos** explain how to prepare unit dose-packaged medications as well as administering oral medication, subcutaneous injections, and intramuscular injections. (Icons in the textbook direct readers to relevant videos.)
- **Journal Articles** provided for each chapter offer access to current research available in Wolters Kluwer journals.
- Plus **Learning Objectives, Drug Monographs, Dosage Calculation Quizzes,** and an **Audio Glossary.**

Study Guide

The *Study Guide to Accompany Introductory Pharmacology,* 12th Edition, offers exercises, puzzles, and multiple-choice questions to quiz your pharmacologic knowledge. In the 12th edition, the same seven clients as the text are included to continue the real-life case studies connected to situations in the text. Mind mapping templates are provided to help you learn visually as you go. These maps, which correlate to each of the text case study clients, give you a visual method to see drug–drug interactions, and anticipate problems of polypharmacy as you follow the stories of these seven clients in the text and study guide.

A FULLY INTEGRATED COURSE EXPERIENCE

We are pleased to offer an expanded suite of digital solutions and ancillaries to support instructors and students using *Introductory Clinical Pharmacology,* 12th Edition. To learn more about any solution, please contact your local Wolters Kluwer representative.

Lippincott CoursePoint+

Lippincott® CoursePoint is an integrated, digital curriculum solution for nursing education that provides a completely interactive experience geared to help students understand, retain, and apply their course knowledge and be prepared for practice. The time-tested, easy-to-use, and trusted solution includes engaging learning tools, evidence-based practice, case studies, and in-depth reporting to meet students where they are in their learning, combined with the most trusted nursing education content on the market to help prepare students for practice. This easy-to-use digital learning solution of *Lippincott® CoursePoint+,* combined with unmatched support, gives instructors and students everything they need for course and curriculum success!

Lippincott® CoursePoint+ includes:

- Leading content provides a variety of learning tools to engage students of all learning styles.
- A personalized learning approach gives students the content and tools they need at the moment they need it, giving them data for more focused remediation and helping to boost their confidence and competence.
- Powerful tools, including varying levels of case studies, interactive learning activities, and adaptive learning powered by PrepU, help students learn the critical thinking and clinical judgment skills to help them become practice-ready nurses.
- Preparation for Practice improves student competence, confidence, and success in transitioning to practice.
  - *vSim®* for Nursing: Codeveloped by Laerdal Medical and Wolters Kluwer, *vSim®* for Nursing simulates real nursing scenarios and allows students to interact with virtual patients in a safe, online environment.
  - *Lippincott®* Advisor for Education: With over 8500 entries covering the latest evidence-based content and drug information, Lippincott® Advisor for Education provides students with the most up-to-date information possible, while giving them valuable experience with the same point-of-care content they will encounter in practice.
- Unparalleled reporting provides in-depth dashboards with several data points to track student progress and help identify strengths and weaknesses.
- Unmatched support includes training coaches, product trainers, and nursing education consultants to help educators and students implement *CoursePoint* with ease.

Acknowledgments

MY SINCERE APPRECIATION

Few people besides textbook writers really know how these books are made. They start on a computer in a home or office, materials take flight electronically to travel cross country, and return to the writers. Documents are sent to places around the world I have never traveled and are edited and processed by people I will never physically meet. Then the finished book makes it to you, the reader. You may find some mistakes - and with all the hands these pages have passed through, I'm not surprised. But, drop me an email and let me know so we can correct them - ford10icp@gmail.com. I might send you a nice Thank-you! I would like to extend a special thanks to the employees of TNQ Technologies - thank you for your dedication during cyclones that hit India, destruction of homes, caring for you loved ones with COVID, having to find electricity to power your computers and so much more to produce this book - from the other side of the world. It does take a global village - to make the world function properly - Thank-you!

To my literary team at Wolters Kluwer—writing a text during a pandemic might sound easy; sit at home by yourself and type away. Living that experience—proves different. The motivation to do the conceptualizing, research, and editing does not just happen. That creativity is grown out of interactions, and when those routine interactions cease—two specific people stepped up their game.

Thank you—Julie Vitale and Jonathan Joyce—my editorial team. You two got me through unanticipated divots in the publishing process, COVID isolation, family illness, deaths, and births—keeping me on track. You connected with me when I needed it most. Think of me when you hear the following words…

To Julie—Iditarod, Taylor's ham, the Farm, Formula 1, and Rory's antics.

To Jonathan—No summer camp, da Bears, Go Hawks, who gets Wilson, let's talk about baseball instead.

To the many others involved at WK, it is impossible to single out the importance of one person over another—thank you for making every edition better than the one before.

To my extended family, friends, colleagues, and students-turned fellow nurses: thank you for being there with ideas and stories to share.

To my sister, Nancy Rauch, iBest college faculty member, thank you for helping make math skills real to these students. To Madison Hjelmeland, LPN and Finnly Jones, LPN (my nieces) thanks for keeping me connected to the student experience and continuing the tradition of nursing in the family. To Dr. Tiffany Zyniewicz of Northwest University, stepping in to help develop a contemporary and useful ancillary package for nurse educators. To my friends, Pam and Marion, thank you for keeping connected and willing to listen—keeping me motivated to the end of this project.

Most importantly, to my family—Jerry, Stephanie, Eric, Peter, Lexy, and those darling granddaughters—who inspire me on a daily basis to be the best person and nurse possible!

—S. F. (87ord)

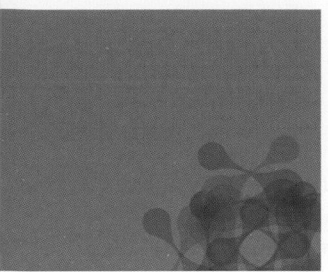

User's Guide

UNIT STRUCTURE AND ORGANIZATION

Learners are more successful when they know *how* to use the text as well as what is in the text. Here are some quick tips on how to use your text more effectively. Fourteen units offer 54 chapters providing information in learnable segments that are not overwhelming to the learner. Organization of the text in this manner allows you to move about the chapters easily when these specific areas of content are covered in your program curriculum.

The text starts with the basic fundamentals of drug therapy. Then units about infection and pain, followed by units about drugs related to different body systems. These units are written in a head-to-toe sequence, making the specific drugs easier to find.

Learning about drug therapy is easier when you can connect the information with life-like clinical experiences. In Chapter 5, you will be introduced to a group of clients in the clinic setting. Their stories establish for you a context in which to begin learning about the selected drugs and their real-world application.

I—Nursing Foundation of Clinical Pharmacology	Basics first, followed by infection and pain. Then Units IV to XIV are organized and presented in a head-to-toe fashion. This gives you an easier way to find information as well as to organize understanding of how drugs affect the human body.
The Drug Units	
II—Infection Fighters	
III—Pain Management	
IV—Central Nervous System	
V—Peripheral Nervous System	
VI—Neuromuscular System	
VII—Respiratory System	
VIII—Cardiovascular System	
IX—Gastrointestinal System	
X—Endocrine System	
XI—Urinary System	
XII—Immune System	
XIII—Cancer	
XIV—Other Body Systems	

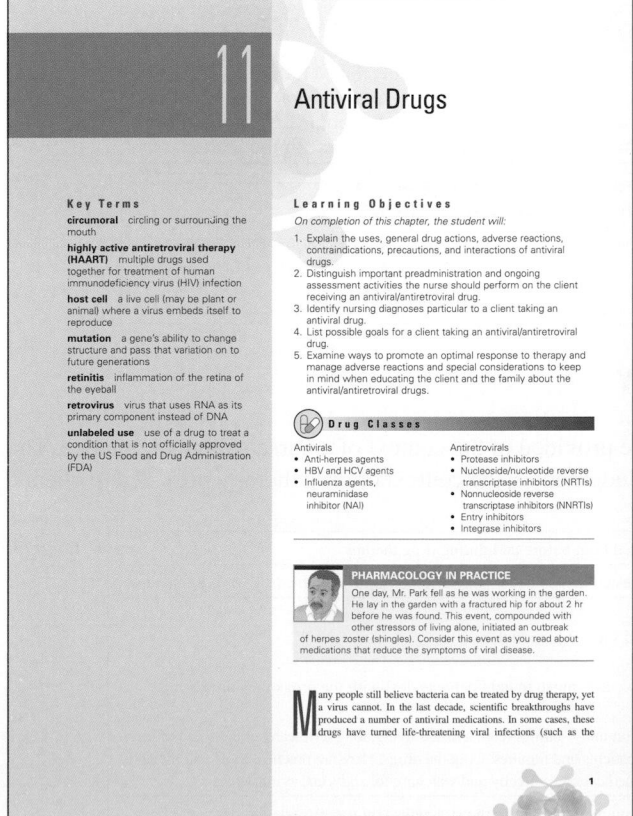

BEGINNING OF THE CHAPTER

The chapter opening page is designed to guide you, the learner, in organizing your study routine as you learn the essential elements of drug therapy in each chapter.

Learning Objectives
These define what you will learn in a specific chapter. Review the objectives first to help you understand what you need to learn after reading the chapter.

Key Terms
With accompanying definitions, the Key Terms help you build your vocabulary. Look for **bold type** in the text at first mention of the word in the chapter to remind you of the definition.

Drug Classes
This gives you a sense of how drugs are grouped according to similar properties. Learning these groupings helps you identify potential errors and safety concerns.

Pharmacology in Practice
Each chapter features a case study individual dealing with an issue related to drugs featured in the chapter. Scenarios focus on assessment, administration, or teaching issues that have an impact on real-life patients. Their stories help you to focus your attention on the concepts important to patient care.

DRUG INFORMATION

Consistent Framework

Each chapter presents the drugs in such a way that you learn to recognize and respond to client questions quickly and accurately. Illustrated concepts guide you as each chapter features information about the drug class in a logical and sequential order as **Action, Uses, and Adverse Reactions**—the concepts you, the nurse, deal with on a consistent basis. This is followed by **Contraindications, Precautions, LASA alerts, and Interactions**—all items typically reviewed earlier and considered by other health care providers, yet at the same time important for you to know to provide safe drug administration to your clients.

Special Features

Special features are sprinkled throughout the text to direct you to priority information about the drugs or individuals who will receive the drugs.

Nursing Alerts
Quickly identify urgent nursing actions in the management of the patient receiving a specific drug or drug category.

Lifespan Considerations
Draw your attention to specific populations at risk or needing specific administration considerations (e.g., gerontology and pediatric). Because texts are written dealing specifically with obstetrical and pediatric patients, the primary focus of these alerts is for geriatric patients, or when specific populations (e.g., women of childbearing age or transgender persons) take a medication that will interact differently than the general population.

Drug Interaction Tables
A quick visual scan of these tables can tell you if a patient is likely to have a problem when multiple drugs are given. Using these tables as you construct concept maps on the case study patients in each chapter will help you identify harmful interactions, before you see them happen in practice.

Herbal Considerations
Provide information on herbs and complementary and alternative remedies used by patients under your care. Additional information is provided in Appendix D where examples of a number of natural products are provided.

Practice Considerations
Provide information about select drugs or actions that might not be critical, yet relevant to the drugs in the select chapters.

! NURSING ALERT

Clients receiving antiretroviral drugs for HIV infection may continue to contract opportunistic infections and other complications of HIV disease. Monitor all clients closely for signs of infection such as fever (even low-grade fever), malaise, sore throat, or lethargy. All caregivers are reminded to use good hand hygiene technique.

 Lifespan Considerations

Pediatrics
Severely ill children infected with influenza show significant improvement and decreased mortality when treated within 48 hr of flu symptom recognition with NAI drugs.

Interacting Drug	Common Use	Effect of Interaction
probenecid	Gout treatment	Increased serum levels of the antivirals
cimetidine	Gastric upset, heartburn	Increased serum level of the antiviral valacyclovir

---

 Herbal Considerations

Individuals use St. John's wort (Fig. 11.3) for antibacterial, antidepressive, and antiviral effects of the supplement. This herbal supplement is one of the most commonly purchased herbal products in the United

---

PRACTICE CONSIDERATIONS

Owing to the high rates of viral resistance the drugs rimantadine and amantadine are no longer recommended for treatment of influenza type A.

NURSING PROCESS AND DRUG THERAPY

Uniquely presented, nursing actions regarding drug information are provided in the context of a nurse's clinical practice. The nursing process is featured as a practical guide to building clinical judgment in the context of drug therapy provided to clients.

Assessment	Here are the questions to ask for the information needed both before and during drug therapy.
Analysis and Planning	Frequently seen **Nursing Problems** are listed and suggested outcomes for patient responses to specific drugs or drug therapy.
Implementation	**Promoting an Optimal Response** Gives you specific information to use for effective and safe administration. **Monitoring and Managing Patient Needs** Gives you a number of strategies to use in your practice as a nurse to help patients deal with the drugs they are taking. **Educating the Patient and Family** LPN/LVNs are the first and often primary contacts in community settings (e.g., assisted living, long-term care, clinics, and offices). You will be the one to teach and provide information to patients and families about the drugs. Here are practical tools and methods to help you work with people to be sure they are taking medications correctly and watching for signs and symptoms.
Evaluation	Bulleted lists highlight important measures and help you decide whether the strategies you use provide the best outcomes while building confidence in your patient's abilities to adhere to medication plans.

END OF THE CHAPTER

Here is where you determine what you have learned from reading each chapter. Information is summarized in an easy-to-read format, giving you the opportunity to demonstrate your growing clinical reasoning skills by applying information in the chapter case study. Once you review the chapter, use the review questions to demonstrate your skill as you would when you take the NCLEX examination.

Pharmacology In Practice: Clinical Reasoning

Each chapter ends with a return to the case study patient. Realistic patient care situations help learners apply the material contained in the chapter by exploring options and making clinical judgments related to the administration of drugs. The case histories of seven patients are used, and different aspects of care are presented in different chapters like puzzle pieces, making connections for learners to appreciate the complex issues in providing care to both individuals and families. Coupled with information from the *Study Guide to Accompany Roach's Introductory Clinical Pharmacology* the learner is encouraged to map out patient problems discovering potential complications or areas for improved patient care.

Key Points

Key points are summarized and the important concepts of the chapter are listed to help you determine if you have mastered the learning objectives.

Summary Drug Tables

Conveniently placed, these tables provide a list of drugs from the classes discussed in each chapter. Current names (generic and, when appropriate, brand names), uses, frequent adverse reactions, and general dosing information are given in an accessible, easy-to-read format.

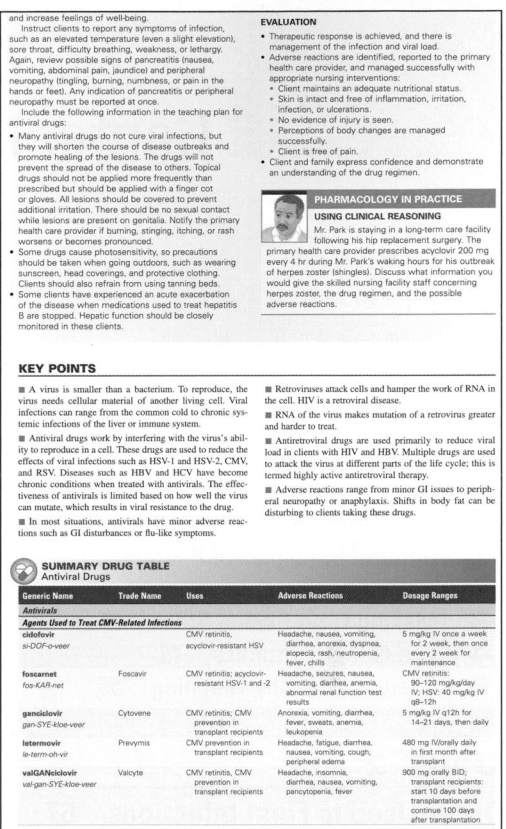

CHAPTER REVIEW

Know Your Drugs

Use the matching exercise to identify drug names and connect generic with brand names to help you recognize the potential for and prevention against using the wrong drug.

Calculate Medication Dosages

Practice the math skills to learn accurate drug dosing and recognize the potential for error, thus ensuring that you give the correct dose.

Prepare for the NCLEX

At the end of each chapter, you'll find questions to test your knowledge base and retention of pharmacology information. Here questions allow you to test your knowledge of the material.

1. **Recall the facts** provides questions about information and content retention.

2. **Analyze the facts** provides analysis and application questions.

3. **Alternate-Format Questions** provide you experience in applying what you've learned in a different manner.

Special Features Questions are structured like the NCLEX examination. The design helps you become familiar with the language and format of NCLEX testing.

Numbered (1, 2, 3, 4) Distractors The NCLEX provides a single question on a computer screen. The options you are given are listed as numbers. Distractor options in these questions are labeled 1, 2, 3, 4 instead of A, B, C, D—again, to simulate the NCLEX examination.

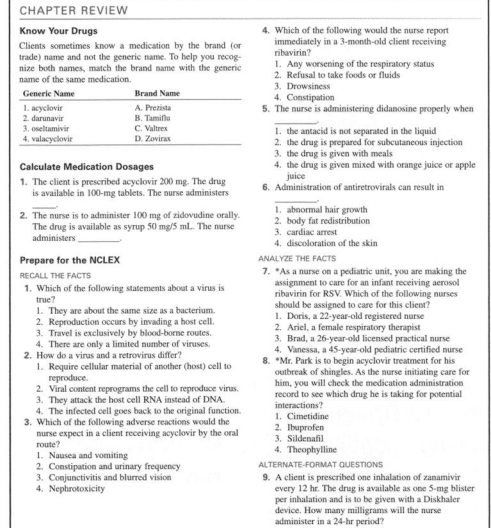

Contents

UNIT 1
Nursing Foundation of Clinical Pharmacology

Becoming a nurse means medication administration and management are possibly the most significant tasks of your nursing practice. In an institutional setting, the clients rely on nurses to accurately administer and monitor medications to keep them safe and promote health. Although clients at home and in the clinic setting are more independent, they rely heavily on the knowledge and instruction given by nurses to learn how to become good managers of their own health care needs (Bonsall, 2016). Both situations require a competent nursing professional who has a strong foundation of clinical pharmacology.

Unit 1 provides you with the foundation for understanding pharmacology in the context of nursing clinical practice. Three of the five chapters in this unit specifically discuss concepts focal to nursing: drug administration, nursing process, and client teaching. In addition, the general principles of pharmacology and the mathematics involved in dosage calculation are concepts used by all providers. These concepts are included in their own chapters. The following is a brief summary of the content in each chapter of Unit 1.

Basic principles are covered in Chapter 1, beginning with how drugs are derived from natural sources, such as plants, or made synthetically. Other key concepts include facts about drug categories and the differences between a prescription drug (those given under the supervision of a licensed health care provider) and a nonprescription drug (those obtained over the counter and designated as safe when taken as directed). Finally, you will gain an understanding of how drugs undergo a series of steps to be processed, utilized, and eliminated by the body—this is the basis for the study of pharmacology for health care providers.

Administration of a drug is primarily the responsibility of the nurse and is discussed in Chapter 2. Nurses have the duty to safely provide client care by correctly administering the medication prescribed by the primary health care provider. This is achieved by learning and following the principles of drug administration, proper technique, and using medication systems correctly.

Chapter 3 provides both the opportunity to practice drug dosage calculations and an overview of the tasks that you will undertake to be sure drug doses are correct *before* administration. Your ability to correctly calculate mathematical problems is one of the most important steps

in providing safe care to clients. Mastering steps in drug administration and delivery help to ensure accuracy in those math calculations.

Nursing process concepts are covered in Chapter 4. Most clients experience problems of anxiety or a lack of knowledge regarding new medication routines. The nursing process is used by the nurse to develop an individualized care and teaching plan for use when medications are ordered. This process is used to help members of the health care team provide effective and efficient client care.

To complete the first unit components needed for successful client teaching are described in Chapter 5. It is crucial that the client understands basic information about the medication prescribed, including the dosage, how to take the medication, the expected effect, and adverse reactions. In the textbook many examples are given using the case study method. In this chapter, the group of individuals receiving nursing care in an ambulatory setting are introduced. Their stories are designed to help you understand how all this information is used in the nursing care of clients receiving drug therapy. You will learn how concepts are put into practice using these case study individuals throughout the textbook.

By understanding the basic principles of pharmacology, you can build a sound knowledge base of the drugs used to help clients maintain their highest levels of wellness.

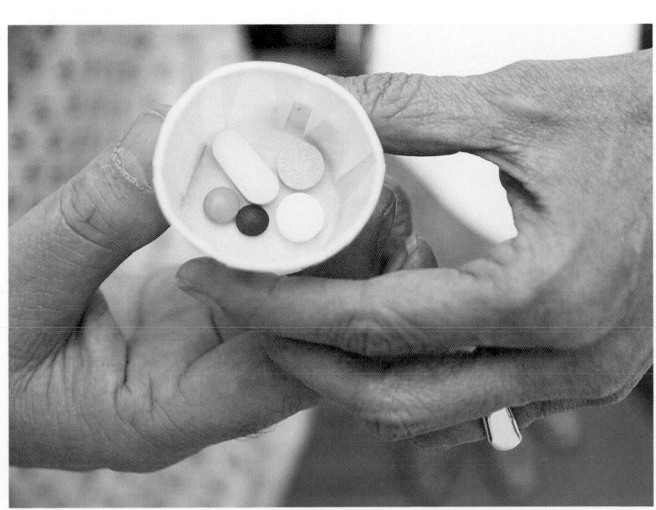

1

General Principles of Pharmacology

Key Terms

absorption a drug is moved from the site of administration to body fluids; first process during pharmacokinetics

adverse reaction undesirable drug effect

allergic reaction hypersensitive reaction by the immune system; it presents as itching, hives, swelling, and difficulty breathing

anaphylactic shock sudden, severe hypersensitivity reaction with symptoms that progress rapidly and may result in death if not treated; also called *anaphylactic reaction* or *anaphylactoid reaction*

angioedema localized wheals or swellings in subcutaneous tissues or mucous membranes, which may be caused by an allergic response; also called *angioneurotic edema*

bioavailability the proportion of a drug available to body tissues when it reaches the circulatory system

controlled substances drugs that have the potential for abuse and dependency, both physical and psychological

cumulative drug effect when the body is unable to metabolize and excrete one dose of a drug before the next is given

complementary/alternative medicine (CAM) group of diverse medical practices or products not presently part of conventional medicine

distribution drug moves from circulation to body tissue or a target site

drug idiosyncrasy any unusual or abnormal response that differs from the response normally expected to a specific drug and dosage

drug tolerance decreased response to a drug, requiring an increase in dosage to achieve the desired effect

(continued)

Learning Objectives

On completion of this chapter, the student will:

1. Define the term *pharmacology.*
2. Compare and contrast the different names assigned to drugs.
3. Distinguish between prescription drugs, nonprescription drugs, and controlled substances.
4. Discuss drug development in the United States.
5. Compare and contrast the various types of drug activity and reactions produced in the body.
6. Identify factors that influence drug action.
7. Explain drug tolerance, cumulative drug effect, and drug idiosyncrasy.
8. Discuss the types of drug interactions that may be seen with drug administration.
9. Examine the nursing implications associated with drug actions, interactions, and effects.
10. Discuss the use of herbal medicines.

Pharmacology is the study of drugs and their action on living organisms. For nurses, a sound knowledge of basic pharmacologic principles is essential in administering medications safely and monitoring clients who receive these medications. This chapter presents a basic overview of the pharmacologic principles needed to understand medication administration. Finally, **herbal medicines** as they relate to pharmacology are discussed.

Over the last century, drugs have changed the way health care providers treat clients. In the early 1900s, individuals died from infections and surgical complications partly because of a lack of sanitary conditions and the fact that medicines used to combat infection did not exist at the time. One example is the discovery of drug substances (antibiotics), which changed an infection that meant certain death to now a diagnosis of a treatable acute and typically short-lived health condition. Drug therapy also means that clients lacking certain substances in their bodies, such as insulin, or those diagnosed with cancerous tumors can now live long and productive lives.

Medications are substances derived from natural sources, such as plants and minerals, or they are synthetically produced in a laboratory. An example of a drug derived from a natural source is digitalis, which is an extract from the foxglove plant that acts as a potent heart medication. Mipomersen (brand name Kynamro) is a chemically engineered drug designed to target specific cell components in people with high cholesterol.

excretion elimination of a drug from the body

first-pass effect action by which an oral drug is absorbed and carried directly to the liver, where it is inactivated by enzymes before it enters the general bloodstream

half-life time required for the body to eliminate 50% of a drug

herbal medicine type of complementary/alternative therapy that uses plants or herbs to treat various disorders; also called *herbalism*

hypersensitive undesirable reaction produced by a normal immune system

metabolism drug is changed to a form that can be excreted

metabolite inactive form of the original drug

nonprescription drugs drugs designated by the US Food and Drug Administration (FDA) to be safe (if taken as directed) and obtainable without a prescription; also called *over-the-counter* (OTC) drugs

pharmaceutic pertaining to the phase during which a drug dissolves in the body

pharmacodynamics study of the drug mechanisms that produce biochemical or physiologic changes in the body

pharmacokinetics study of drug transit (or activity) after administration

physical dependency habitual use of a drug, where negative physical withdrawal symptoms result from abrupt discontinuation

prescription drugs drugs the federal government has designated

as potentially harmful unless their use is supervised by a licensed health care provider, such as a nurse practitioner, physician, or dentist

psychological dependency compulsion or craving to use a substance to obtain a pleasurable experience

receptor *in pharmacology,* a reactive site on the surface of a cell; when a drug binds to and interacts with the receptor, a pharmacologic response occurs

risk evaluation and mitigation strategies (REMS) program of the FDA, designed to monitor drugs that have a high risk compared with benefit ratio

teratogen drug or substance that causes abnormal development of the fetus, leading to deformities

toxic poisonous or harmful

DRUG NAMES

To begin understanding the principles of pharmacology, let us start with learning about how drugs are named. Once you understand this concept, it will be easier to understand classes and categories of drugs, as well as federal regulations pertaining to drugs and how they are developed. Throughout the process of development, drugs may have several names assigned to them. These different names can be confusing. Therefore, if you have a clear understanding of the different names used, you can promote client safety by reducing errors.

A drug may have three different names:

- Chemical name—a scientific term that describes the molecular structure of a drug; it typically is the chemical component of the drug.

- Generic name—considered the official name of a drug and is the name given to a drug that can be made or marketed by any company; it is nonproprietary, meaning it is not owned by any specific agency.

- Trade name—selected by a specific company producing the drug for marketing purposes. When a drug name is followed by a trademark symbol ™ or a registered trademark symbol ®, this signifies that it is the trade or brand name.

Table 1.1 identifies the various chemical, generic, and trade names and provides an example and explanation for each name.

The generic name is the official name that is given to a drug by the US Food and Drug Administration (FDA). It also is the name found in the *National Formulary* or the *US Pharmacopeia* for an approved drug. To avoid confusion, it is best to use the generic name. One safety practice is the

TABLE 1.1 Drug Names

DRUG NAME	EXAMPLE	EXPLANATION
Chemical name (scientific name)	Example: ethyl 4-(8-chloro-5,6-dihydro-11*H*-benzo[5,6] cyclohepta[1,2-*b*]-pyridin-11-ylidene)-1-piperidinecarboxylate	Gives the exact chemical structure of the drug and placing of the atoms or molecules; the chemical name is not capitalized
Generic name (official or nonproprietary name)	Example: loratadine	Name given to a drug before it becomes official; may be used in any country, by all manufacturers; the generic name is typically not capitalized
Trade name (brand name)	Example: Claritin®	Name that is registered by the manufacturer and is followed by the trademark symbol; the name can be used only by the manufacturer; a drug may have several trade names, depending on the number of manufacturers; the first letter of the trade name is capitalized

use of Tall man lettering for drugs that look or sound alike. Using capital letters within the name of a drug helps health care providers to distinguish different drugs that have similar or confusing names. You will find examples in the chapter Drug Summary Tables, LASA alerts, and in Appendix B.

DRUG CLASSES AND CATEGORIES

Different organizations classify drugs for different reasons. Medicare and Insurance companies classify drugs in a tier system for cost and coverage purposes. The Drug Enforcement Agency (DEA) defines drugs according to legality. In our study of pharmacology, we are going to look at how drugs are developed by pharmaceutical companies, named, and then classified.

Drugs are organized into different classes and categories to help people better understand how they work in the body. A drug may be classified by the chemical type of the active ingredient or by the way it is used to treat a particular condition. Each drug can be classified into one or more drug classes. For instance, in Unit 2, drugs that retard or destroy pathogens are classified as anti-infectives. In each chapter, these drugs are further categorized by the way they work (such as antivirals) or their chemical structure (e.g., penicillins). In addition, once a drug is approved for use, the FDA assigns it to one of the following categories: prescription, nonprescription, or controlled substance. This method of assignment helps you to understand the ease of accessibility of a drug to the client. To help you learn these classes, a list is included at the start of each chapter.

! NURSING ALERT

Study the patterns used in the naming of drugs. This may help you to identify names and prevent medication errors. Certain portions of the drug name may be similar in specific drug classes or categories. For example, beta-adrenergic (β-adrenergic) blocking drug names end with "lol." *Atenolol, metoprolol,* and *propranolol* are all antihypertensive drugs from the same category.

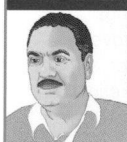

PHARMACOLOGY IN PRACTICE

DRUG RECOGNITION

Mr. Garcia is prescribed the drug metoprolol. Use your drug resources to identify the three names for this drug and the drug's category and class.

Prescription Drugs

Prescription drugs, also called *legend drugs,* are the largest category of drugs. **Prescription drugs** are prescribed by a licensed health care provider. The prescription (Fig. 1.1) contains the name of the drug, the dosage, the method and times of administration, and the electronic signature of the licensed health care provider prescribing the drug. Typically, the health care provider writes the prescription electronically and it is transmitted to the pharmacy. A paper copy

---

```
            XYZ PHARMACY SYSTEM
     Electronically Transmitted to Smith Pharmacy
                 1234 Broad Street
               Anytown, State, Zip

    Date: 10/20/20yy
    Rx # 9876543        ID # 11223344

                Patient Information
    Last Name:    Jones
    First Name:   Mary
    DOB:          10/18/YY
    Sex:          F
    Address:      567 King Street
                  Anytown, State, Zip
    Phone:        (XXX)-888-7777

            Drug, SIG, and Refill Information
    Drug Name: Gabapentin
    Strength:     100 mg
    Quantity:     60        Dose Form: capsules
    SIG:          Take 1 capsule at bedtime
    Refills:      6
    Label:        yes

    Prescriber Information
    Last Name: Brown
    First Name: James M
    Address:    100 Main Street
                Anytown, State, Zip
    DEA:        CB1234XXX
    NPI:        9876543XXX
```

FIGURE 1.1 Example of an electronically transmitted prescription form.

may be printed for a client if a pharmacy outside the health care system will be used to obtain the medication.

Drugs requiring prescription are designated as such by the federal government because they are potentially harmful unless their use is supervised by a licensed health care provider, such as a nurse practitioner, physician, or dentist. Supervision is important because, although these drugs have been tested for safety and therapeutic effect, prescription drugs may cause different reactions in some individuals.

In institutional settings, the nurse administers the drug and monitors the client for therapeutic effect and **adverse reactions** (undesirable effect). Some drugs have the potential to be **toxic** (harmful). As a nurse, you will play a critical role in evaluating the client for toxic effects. When these drugs are prescribed to be taken at home, you will provide client and family education about the drug.

Nonprescription Drugs

Nonprescription drug designation is made by the FDA when the drug is safe (taken as directed) and obtainable without a prescription. These drugs are frequently called over-the-counter (OTC) drugs and may be purchased without a prescription in a variety of settings, such as a drugstore, local supermarket, or a large warehouse retailer (e.g., Costco or Sam's Club). OTC drugs include those given for symptoms of the common cold, minor aches and pains, constipation, diarrhea, heartburn, and minor fungal infections.

Labeling requirements give the consumer important information regarding the drug, dosage, contraindications, precautions, and adverse reactions. Consumers are urged to read the directions carefully before taking OTC drugs. Yet, these drugs are not without risk. For example, acetaminophen, commonly used for pain relief, is also found in many OTC products, such as cough and cold remedies. When taken for both pain and in a cold remedy, this accumulative amount of the drug can potentially harm a person's liver.

Controlled Substances

Controlled substances are the most carefully monitored class of drugs. These drugs have a high potential for abuse and may cause physical or psychological dependency. **Physical dependency** is defined as the habitual use of a drug in which negative physical withdrawal symptoms result from abrupt discontinuation; it is the body's dependence on repeated administration of a drug. **Psychological dependency** is a compulsion or craving to use a substance to obtain a pleasurable experience. It is the mind's desire for the repeated administration of a drug. Physical and psychological dependence do not always occur together, yet one type of dependency may lead to the other.

The Controlled Substances Act of 1970 established a classification system for drugs with abuse potential. The act regulates the manufacture, distribution, and dispensing of these drugs. The Controlled Substances Act divides drugs into five groups, called schedules, which are based on the substance's potential for abuse and physical and psychological dependence. Appendix A describes the five schedules.

Prescription practices of the primary health care provider for controlled substances are monitored by the DEA. Under federal law, limited quantities of certain schedule V drugs may be purchased without a prescription, with the purchase recorded by the dispensing pharmacist. In some cases, state laws are more restrictive than federal laws and impose additional requirements for the sale and distribution of controlled substances. In hospitals or other agencies that dispense controlled substances, the scheduled drugs are counted every 8–12 hr to account for each injectable, tablet, or other form of the drug. Any discrepancy in the number of drugs must be investigated and explained immediately.

DRUG DEVELOPMENT

Drug development is a long and arduous process that can take from 7–12 years, and sometimes longer. The FDA has the responsibility for approving new drugs and monitoring drugs currently in use for adverse or toxic reactions. The development of a new drug is divided into the pre-FDA phase and the FDA phase. During the pre-FDA phase, a manufacturer conducts in vitro testing (testing in an artificial environment, such as a test tube) using animal and human cells to discover new drug compounds. This testing is followed by studies in live animals. The manufacturer then makes application to the FDA for Investigational New Drug (IND) status.

During the FDA phase, clinical (i.e., human) testing of the new drug begins. Clinical testing consists of three phases, with each phase involving a larger number of people (Fig. 1.2). In all phases the effects, both pharmacologic and

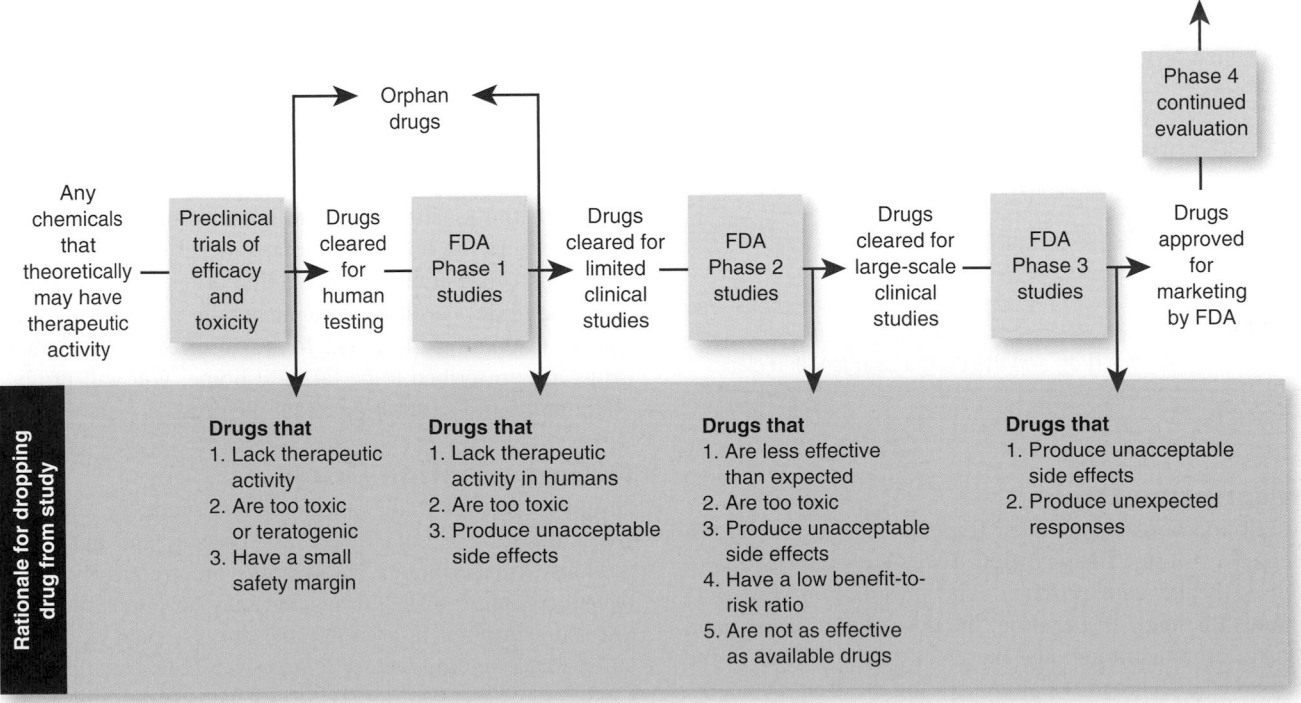

FIGURE 1.2 Phases of drug development.

biologic, are studied. *Phase 1* involves 20–100 individuals who are healthy volunteers. This phase of testing is designed to see what the drug substance does to healthy tissue. If Phase 1 studies are successful, the testing moves to *Phase 2,* where the drug is given to people who have the disease or condition for which the drug is thought to be effective. If those results are positive for helping to reduce or eliminate the problem and adverse reactions are not too great, the testing progresses to *Phase 3,* in which the drug is given to large numbers of clients in medical research centers to provide information about adverse reactions. Phase 3 studies offer additional information on dosing and safety. Because of this extensive process, clinical trial studies can extend for many years.

 Concept Mastery Alert

> A reason for a drug to enter a Phase 2 study would be to test the potential drug on clients with the disease the drug is designed to treat. A reason for a drug to enter a Phase 3 study is to determine any unanticipated effects.

A New Drug Application (NDA) is submitted after the investigation of the drug in Phases 1, 2, and 3 is complete and the drug is found to be safe and effective. With the NDA, the manufacturer submits all data collected concerning the drug during the clinical trials. A panel of experts, including pharmacologists, chemists, physicians, and other professionals, reviews the application and makes a recommendation to the FDA. The FDA then either approves or denies approval of the drug for use. This process can cost well over a billion dollars for a successful drug and take up to 12 years to be ready for marketing to the public (Lim, 2019). Although the cost of drugs is not covered in this textbook, it is of primary concern to many of the clients you will come into contact with during your career as a nurse.

After FDA approval, the company making the drug will give the new drug a brand name. This allows the company to sell the specific drug using this name for a limited time. The hope is that some of the research and development cost will be defrayed by the sales of this brand name drug. After the specified time, other companies may sell the drug using the generic name. The brand name is reserved for the company that first produced the specific drug substance.

After FDA approval, continued surveillance is done to ensure safety. Postmarketing surveillance (*Phase 4*) occurs after the manufacturer places the drug on the market. During this surveillance, an ongoing review of the drug occurs with particular attention given to adverse reactions. Health care providers are encouraged to help with this surveillance by reporting adverse effects of drugs to the FDA by using MedWatch (Box 1.1) or the Institute for Safe Medication Practices Medication Errors Reporting System.

BOX 1.1   MedWatch and Reporting Adverse Events

- The FDA established a program called MedWatch for reporting safety and adverse events. Nurses or other health care providers can report observations of serious adverse drug effects or find safety information. Anyone can access the website (https://www.fda.gov/safety/medwatch-fda-safety-information-and-adverse-event-reporting-program) to obtain safety alerts on drugs, devices, or dietary supplements.
- The website provides a standardized form for reporting, which can be submitted electronically or downloaded, filled out, and mailed/faxed in to the program. Nurses play an important role in monitoring for adverse reactions. Therefore, it is important to submit reports, even if there is uncertainty about the cause–effect relationship. The FDA protects the identity of those who voluntarily report adverse reactions.
- The FDA considers serious adverse reactions those that may result in death, life-threatening illness, hospitalization, or disability or those that may require medical or surgical intervention. This form also is used to report an undesirable experience associated with the use of medical products (e.g., latex gloves, pacemakers, infusion pumps, anaphylaxis, blood, blood components).

SPECIAL FOOD AND DRUG ADMINISTRATION PROGRAMS

Although it takes considerable time for most drugs to get FDA approval, the FDA has special programs to meet different needs. Examples of these special programs include:

- Orphan drug program
- Accelerated programs for urgent needs
- Risk Evaluation and Mitigation Strategies (REMS) program

Orphan Drug Program

The Orphan Drug Act of 1983 was passed to encourage the development and marketing of products used to treat rare diseases. The act defines a rare disease as a condition affecting fewer than 200,000 individuals in the United States or a condition affecting more than 200,000 persons in the United States but for which the cost of producing and marketing a drug to treat the condition would not be recovered by sales of the drug.

The National Organization of Rare Disorders reports (2019) that there are more than 7000 rare disorders that affect approximately 30 million individuals. Examples of rare disorders include amyloidosis, Gaucher disease, and phenylketonuria.

The act provides for incentives such as research grants, protocol assistance by the FDA, and special tax credits to encourage manufacturers to develop orphan drugs. If the drug is approved, the manufacturer has 7 years of exclusive marketing rights. More than 1,700 new drugs and biologics have received FDA approval since the law was passed. Examples of orphan drugs include Velcade for multiple myeloma, Cerezyme—enzyme replacement therapy for Gaucher disease, and Valstar for the treatment of bladder cancer.

Accelerated Programs

Accelerated approval of drugs is offered by the FDA as a means to make promising products for life-threatening diseases available on the market, based on preliminary evidence and before formal demonstration of client benefit. The approval that is granted is considered a "provisional approval," with a written commitment from the pharmaceutical company to complete clinical studies that formally demonstrate client benefit. If the drug continues to prove beneficial, the process of approval is accelerated.

Acquired immunodeficiency syndrome (AIDS) is an example of a disease that qualified as posing a significant health threat, and finding new drugs qualified for the accelerated program. When first discovered, AIDS was very devastating to the individuals affected and health agencies feared the danger the disease posed to public health. Therefore, the FDA and pharmaceutical companies worked together to shorten the IND approval process for drugs that showed promise in treating AIDS. This accelerated process allowed primary health care providers to administer medications that indicated positive results in early Phase 1 and 2 clinical trials, rather than wait until final approval was granted. HIV is now viewed as a chronic disease, partly because of the efforts of accelerating the clinical trial process for drugs to treat AIDS.

The COVID-19 vaccine development is another example. Emergency use authorization was granted to two organizations (Pfizer-BioNTech and Moderna) within less than 1 year (Solis-Moreira, 2020). Owing to the pandemic nature of the SARS-CoV-2 pathogen, research and clinical trials were carried out in tandem and not sequentially, reducing the time needed to prepare the vaccines for market when international research and funding was provided (Solis-Moreira, 2020).

Risk Evaluation and Mitigation Strategies

The **Risk Evaluation and Mitigation Strategies** (REMS) program is designed to monitor drugs that have higher risk to the client compared with benefit. To use a drug included in this program, there are specific educational requirements of the health care providers (prescribing and administering techniques) and education and monitoring for clients taking the drug. Therefore, only HCP-trained, enrolled, and certified providers may prescribe drugs with REMS restrictions. You can see the restrictions placed upon these drugs in a REMS program by visiting the brand name drug's website.

HOW DRUGS WORK WITHIN THE BODY

Having learned about the naming and development of drugs, we turn to how drugs work. Once in the body, drugs act in certain ways or phases. Oral drugs go through three phases: the *pharmaceutic* phase, *pharmacokinetic* phase, and the *pharmacodynamic* phase (Fig. 1.3). Because liquid and parenteral drugs (drugs given by injection) are already in a fluid form they only go through the latter two phases, bypassing phase one entirely.

Pharmaceutic Phase

In the **pharmaceutic phase**, the drug is dissolved. Drugs must be a soluble liquid to be absorbed by the body. Drugs that are liquid or drugs given by injection (parenteral drugs) are already dissolved and are absorbed quickly. A tablet or capsule (solid forms of a drug) goes through this phase in the gastrointestinal (GI) tract as it disintegrates into small particles and dissolves into the body fluids. Tablets that have an enteric coating and time-release capsules do not disintegrate until they reach the alkaline environment of the small intestine.

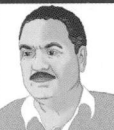

PHARMACOLOGY IN PRACTICE

INTERVENTIONS
A client wants to know why their primary health care provider prescribes a liquid medication for an illness. How should the nurse best explain the process to the client?
1. Easier to swallow
2. Is absorbed faster by the body system
3. Delays absorption until the liquid reaches the small intestine
4. Disintegrates into small pieces

Pharmacokinetic Phase

Pharmacokinetics refers to the transportation activity of drugs in the body after administration. These activities include absorption, distribution, metabolism, and excretion. These phases can be broken down into subphases such as transport, first-pass effect during absorption, and half-life during excretion of the drug.

Absorption

Absorption is the process by which a drug is made available for use in the body. This process involves moving the drug from the site of administration into the body fluids. It occurs after the solid form (e.g., a pill or tablet) of the drug dissolves or after the administration of an oral liquid or parenteral drug. During this process, the drug particles in the GI tract are moved into the body fluids. This movement can be accomplished in several ways:

- Active transport—cellular energy is used to move the drug from an area of low concentration to one of high concentration.

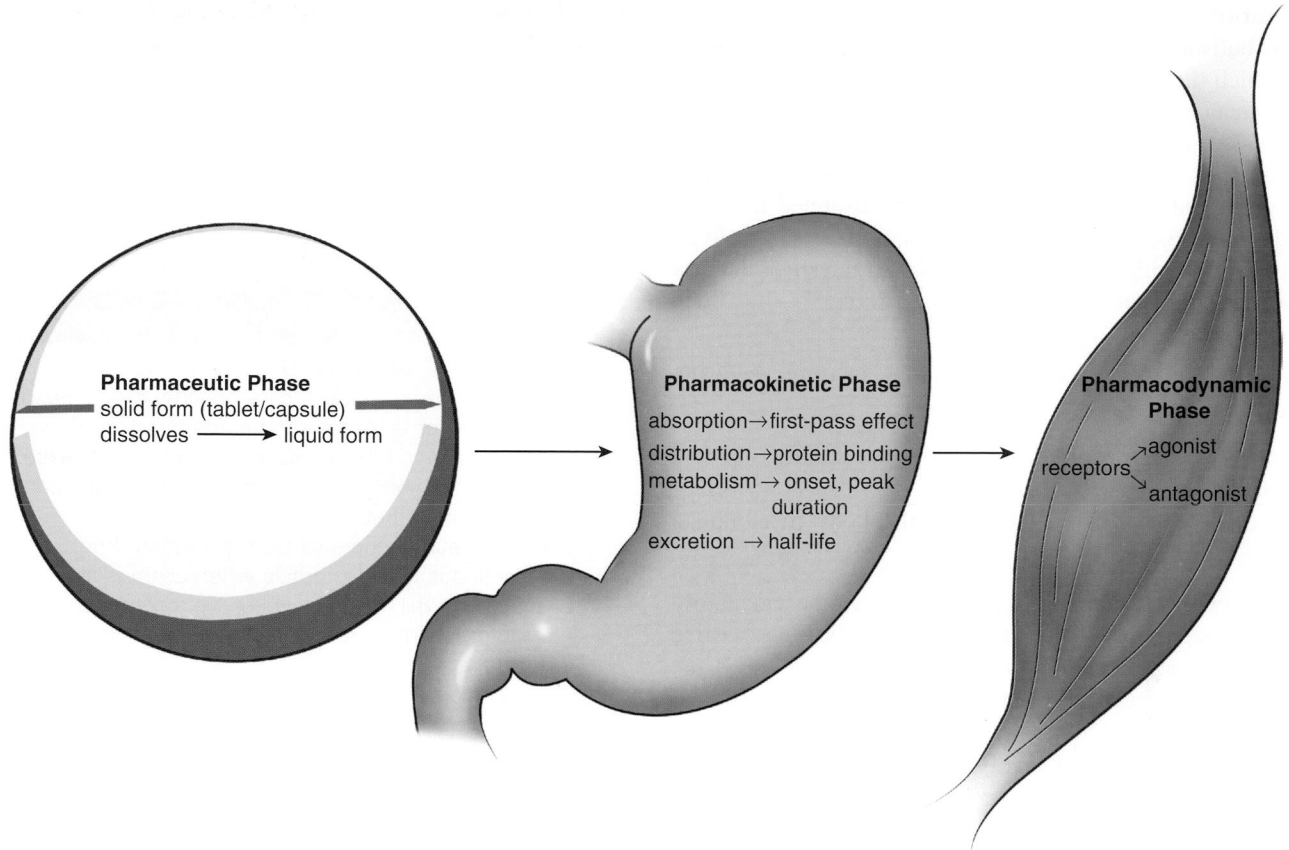

FIGURE 1.3 Drug activity within the body: pharmaceutic, pharmacokinetic, and pharmacodynamic phases.

- Passive transport—no cellular energy is used as the drug moves from an area of high concentration to an area of low concentration (small molecules diffuse across the cell membrane).
- Pinocytosis—cells engulf the drug particle (the cell forms a vesicle to transport the drug across the cell membrane and into the cell).

Several factors influence the rate of absorption, including the route of administration, the solubility of the drug, and specific conditions of the body's tissues. The most rapid route of drug absorption occurs when the drug is given by the intravenous (IV) route. When 100% of the drug given is available to the cells of the body, this is called **bioavailability**. Absorption occurs more slowly when the drug is administered orally, intramuscularly, or subcutaneously. This is because the complex membranes of the GI mucosal layers, muscle, and skin delay drug passage. Conditions in the body, such as *lipodystrophy* (the atrophy of subcutaneous tissue from repeated subcutaneous injections) inhibit absorption of a drug given in the affected site. This can occur when clients have to administer drugs repeatedly into the skin tissue, such as insulin administration for diabetes.

Another factor effecting absorption is the **first-pass effect**. When a drug is absorbed by the small intestine, it passes first into the liver before being released to circulate within the rest of the body. The liver metabolizes (or filters out) a significant amount of the drug before releasing it into the body. When the drug is released into the circulation from the liver, the remaining amount of active (or available) drug may not be enough to produce a therapeutic effect, and the client will need a higher dosage.

Distribution

Once in the systemic circulation a drug is transported and distributed to various body tissues or target sites. **Distribution** of an absorbed drug in the body depends on:

- Blood flow—a drug is distributed quickly to areas with a large blood supply, such as the heart, liver, and kidneys. In other areas, such as the internal organs, skin, and muscle, distribution of the drug occurs more slowly.
- Solubility—the drug's ability to cross the cell membrane affects its distribution. Lipid-soluble drugs easily cross the cell membrane, whereas water-soluble drugs do not.
- Protein binding—when a drug travels through the blood, it comes into contact with proteins such as the plasma protein *albumin.* The drug can remain free in the circulation or bind to the protein. Only free drugs can produce a therapeutic effect. Drugs bound to protein are pharmacologically inactive. Only when the protein molecules release the drug can the drug diffuse into the tissues, interact with receptors, and produce a therapeutic effect. A drug is said to be highly protein bound when more than 80% of the circulating drug is bound to protein.

Metabolism

Metabolism, also called *biotransformation,* is the process by which the body changes a drug to a more or less active form that can be excreted. A **metabolite** is the inactive form of the original drug. In some drugs, one or more of the metabolites may have some drug activity. Metabolites may undergo further metabolism or may be excreted from the body unchanged. Most drugs are metabolized by the liver, although the kidneys, lungs, plasma, and intestinal mucosa also aid in the metabolism of drugs.

Excretion

Two important elements of elimination of drugs from the body are:

- Excretion—removal of drugs by the kidneys or the intestine.
- Half-life—the time required for the body to eliminate 50% of a drug.

After the liver renders drugs inactive, the circulatory system takes these products to the kidney where the inactive compounds are excreted from the body. Other drugs are eliminated in sweat, in breast milk, or by breath or by the GI tract through feces. Some drugs are excreted unchanged by the kidney without liver involvement; because this happens it can put undue stress on the kidney. Clients with kidney disease may require a dosage reduction and careful monitoring of kidney function. Children have immature kidney function and may require dosage reduction and kidney function tests during drug therapy. Similarly, older adults have diminished kidney function and require careful monitoring and lower dosages.

Half-life refers to the time required for the body to eliminate 50% of the drug. Knowledge of the half-life of a drug is important in planning the frequency of dosing. Drugs with a short half-life (2–4 hr) need to be administered frequently, whereas drugs with a long half-life (21–24 hr) require less frequent administration. For example, digoxin (Lanoxin) has a long half-life (36 hr) and requires once-daily dosing. However, aspirin has a short half-life and requires frequent dosing. It takes five to six half-lives to eliminate approximately 98% of a drug from the body. Although half-life is fairly stable, clients with liver or kidney disease may have problems excreting a drug. Difficulty in excreting a drug increases the half-life and the risk of toxicity, because these organs do not remove the substances and the drug remains in the body longer. Older clients or clients with impaired kidney or liver function require frequent diagnostic tests measuring renal or hepatic function.

Onset, Peak, and Duration—Drug Actions

Three additional factors influence the therapeutic action of a drug and in turn determine the timing of drug administration. These factors are important when considering how a drug acts in the body:

- Onset of action—time between administration of the drug and onset of its therapeutic effect.

- Peak concentration—when absorption rate equals the elimination rate (not always the time of peak response).
- Duration of action—length of time the drug produces a therapeutic effect.

These factors are taken into consideration when determining the dose schedule of a specific drug. This ensures that proper blood levels are maintained in the body for the drug to work properly.

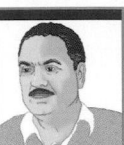

PHARMACOLOGY IN PRACTICE

INTERVENTIONS

A primary health care provider prescribes a lower drug dose to be administered every 6 hr instead of every 4 hr to a client with kidney disease. Which of the following are reasons for such a prescriptive change? Select all that apply.
1. Disease prevents kidneys from excreting drug.
2. Drug action is more effective when client is ill.
3. Client could exhibit blood level above therapeutic range.
4. Altered prescription reduces chance of accumulation of the drug.
5. Client could become drug dependent.

Pharmacodynamic Phase

Pharmacodynamics is the study of the drug mechanisms that produce biochemical or physiologic changes in the body. **Pharmacodynamics** deals with the drug's action and effect in the body. After administration, most drugs enter the systemic circulation and expose almost all body tissues to possible effects of the drug. This exposure in all tissue causes the drug to produce more than one effect in the body.

- Primary effect—the desired or therapeutic effect on targeted tissue or organ.
- Secondary effects—all other effects, desirable or undesirable, produced by the drug.

Most drugs have an affinity for certain organs or tissues and exert their greatest action at the cellular level on those specific areas, which are called *target sites.* A drug exerts its action by one of two main mechanisms:

- Alteration in cellular function
- Alteration in cellular environment

Alteration in Cellular Function

Most drugs act on the body by altering cellular function. A drug cannot completely change the function of a cell, but it can alter the cell's function. A drug that alters cellular function can increase or decrease certain physiologic functions, such as increasing heart rate, decreasing blood pressure, or increasing urine output.

Receptor-Mediated Drug Action

Many drugs act through drug–receptor interaction. The function of a cell is altered when a drug interacts with a receptor. This occurs when a drug molecule selectively joins with a reactive site—the receptor—on the surface of a cell. When a drug binds to and interacts with the receptor, a pharmacologic response occurs. This process is explained in greater depth in Units 4 and 5.

An *agonist* is a drug that binds with a receptor and stimulates the receptor to produce a therapeutic response; antidepressants are drugs that work this way. An *antagonist* is a drug that joins with receptors but does not stimulate the receptors. The therapeutic action in this case consists of blocking the receptor's function, an opioid reversal drug works in this way.

Receptor-Mediated Drug Effects

The number of available receptor sites influences the effects of a drug. When only a few receptor sites are occupied, although many sites are available, the response will be small. When the drug dose is increased, more receptor sites are used, and the response increases. When only a few receptor sites are available, and once all the receptor sites are used, the response does not increase when more of the drug is administered. However, not all receptors on a cell need to be occupied for a drug to be effective. Some extremely potent drugs are effective even when the drug occupies few receptor sites.

Alteration in Cellular Environment

Some drugs act on the body by changing the cellular environment, either physically or chemically. Physical changes in the cellular environment include changes in osmotic pressure, lubrication, absorption, or the conditions on the surface of the cell membrane.

An example of a drug that changes osmotic pressure is *mannitol,* which produces a change in the osmotic pressure in brain cells, causing a reduction in cerebral edema. A drug that acts by altering the cellular environment by lubrication is sunscreen. An example of a drug that acts by altering absorption is activated charcoal, which is administered orally to absorb a toxic chemical ingested into the GI tract. The stool softener docusate is an example of a drug that acts by altering the surface of the cellular membrane. Docusate has emulsifying and lubricating activity that lowers the surface tension in the cells of the bowel, permitting water and fats to enter the stool. This softens the fecal mass, allowing easier passage of the stool.

Chemical changes in the cellular environment include inactivation of cellular functions or alteration of the chemical components of body fluid, such as a change in the pH. For example, antacids neutralize gastric acidity in clients with peptic ulcers.

Other drugs, such as some anticancer drugs and some antibiotics, have as their main site of action the cell membrane and various cellular processes. They incorporate themselves into the normal metabolic processes of the cell and cause the formation of a defect, such as a weakened cell wall, which results in cell death, or reduces a needed energy substrate that leads to cell starvation and death.

Pharmacogenomics

Most pharmacodynamic mechanisms deal with principles that affect each cell in the same way, whereas *pharmacogenomics* is the study of how people's responses to medications are variable because of individual genetic variation. The genetic makeup of a person can affect the pharmacodynamics of a drug. This discovery was made during the Human Genome Project when many scientists were able to determine the different components of the human genetic code. One example is the way some individuals respond to the drug warfarin. This is a drug taken to reduce the chance of blood clots and is a blood thinner. Clients with a specific gene duplication who take warfarin are more likely to bleed when taking the average dose of the drug. This pharmacological response to a genetic variation is discussed in Chapter 36.

Pharmacogenetics (a subcategory of the above) is the study of differences in body function due to genetic differences and how that impacts the creation of individualized drug therapy that allows for the best choice and dose of drugs (Saini et al., 2010).

DRUG USE, PREGNANCY, AND LACTATION

With the abundance of self-help information on the Internet, women of childbearing age are bombarded with a large amount of information regarding drug use, pregnancy, and lactation. In general, most drugs are contraindicated during pregnancy and lactation unless the potential benefits of taking the drug outweigh the risks to the fetus or the infant. Pregnant woman should not take any drug, legal or illegal, prescription or nonprescription, unless the drug is prescribed or recommended by the primary health care provider. Children born of mothers using addictive drugs, such as methamphetamine or oxycontin, often are born with a dependency to the drug used by the mother. Although promoted as a natural substance, herbal supplements can act like drugs, too. Women should not take an herbal supplement without discussing it first with the primary health care provider.

Smoking tobacco or drinking any type of alcoholic beverage carries risks and should be eliminated for the duration of pregnancy. Drinking alcohol is associated with risks of low birth weight, premature birth, and fetal alcohol syndrome. Inhalation of substances other than tobacco, such as electronic cigarettes or marijuana, have not been studied to the extent of making recommendations, yet most health care providers do not recommend use because of potential effects on the fetus.

Both expectant mothers and drug manufactures are concerned about the risk of causing birth defects in the developing fetus. The use of any medication (prescription or nonprescription) carries this risk, particularly during the first trimester (3 months), when the drug may have teratogenic effects. A **teratogen** is any substance that causes abnormal development of the fetus, often leading to severe deformation or fetal death. Drugs known to cause fetal abnormalities are classified as teratogens.

In 2015, requirements for prescribing information to health care professionals by manufacturers changed. Subheadings within the Pregnancy and Lactation subsections of drug labels such as *risk summary, clinical considerations,* and *data* were now required. The old system to assign a drug's risk during pregnancy and breastfeeding used the letter categories of A, B, C, D, and X to classify the amount of risk to the developing fetus; to date, the new classification system is still transitioning into place and in many monographs you will see both the old letter system and the new informational system used. Therefore, the older letter-based system is provided as reference for you in Appendix A.

The letter categories for drug labeling have been in use since the 1970s and were often misinterpreted as a grading system of risk. The new method provides explanations, based on available information, about the potential benefits and risks for the mother, the fetus, children who are breastfeeding, and women and men of reproductive age. The new system will be used as new drugs are introduced to the market and as older drugs are reviewed by the FDA; therefore, you will see the old system in this text and in drug information resources as well as the new categories as they are developed.

A number of drugs are excreted in breast milk. Therefore, if a mother is lactating (breastfeeding), some of the drug she is taking will travel through her to the infant or child via the breast milk to be ingested and absorbed. It is important for both mothers and nurses to know the potential of exposure to a breastfeeding child when the mother is taking a drug.

The National Library of Medicine provides a free online database with information on drugs and lactation called LactMed (http://www.ncbi.nlm.nih.gov/books/NBK501922/). This website is geared to the health care practitioner and nursing mother and contains over 1,100 drug records. It includes information such as maternal levels in breast milk, infant levels in blood, and potential effects in breastfeeding infants. A pharmacist, Dr. Thomas Hale, from Texas Tech University has developed a system of lactation risk categories similar to that of the FDA pregnancy risk categories for drugs. Drugs are assigned an L1 to L5 risk according to the drug's transmission in breast milk and the effect it may have on the child. Hale's listing of certain drugs may differ from those published by organizations such as the American Academy of Pediatrics, yet it is a good starting point for discussion with mothers who are breastfeeding.

DRUG REACTIONS

Drugs produce many reactions in the body beyond the intended reaction. The following sections discuss adverse drug reactions, allergic drug reactions, drug idiosyncrasy, drug tolerance, cumulative drug effect, and toxic reactions.

Adverse Drug Reactions

Clients may experience one or more adverse reactions or side effects when they are given a drug. Adverse reactions are undesirable drug effects. **Adverse reactions** may be common or may occur infrequently. They may be mild, severe, or life-threatening. They may occur after the first dose, after a few doses, or after many doses. Often, an adverse reaction is unpredictable, although some drugs are known to cause certain adverse reactions in many clients. Often these reactions affect the GI system. For example, drugs used in treating cancer are very toxic and are known to produce adverse reactions in many clients receiving them. Other drugs produce adverse reactions in fewer clients. Some adverse reactions are predictable, but many adverse drug reactions occur without warning.

! NURSING ALERT

There are some adverse reactions that you will see with each client you care for in your role as a nurse. Other adverse reactions are so infrequent you may never see one. In this text we list both the common and unusual adverse reactions, because as a nurse you see many clients and the likelihood that you will care for a person experiencing a severe adverse reaction is much greater than it is for other types of health care providers. If you could avert a lasting complication or even a death through your knowledge of adverse reactions, it would be a wonderful accomplishment in your career.

Some texts use both the terms *side effects* and *adverse reactions,* using *side effects* to explain mild, common, and nontoxic reactions and *adverse reactions* to describe more severe and life-threatening reactions. For the purposes of this text and to avoid confusion, only the term *adverse reaction* is used, with the understanding that these reactions may be mild, severe, or life-threatening and will be defined as such.

Allergic Drug Reactions

An **allergic reaction** is a **hypersensitive** response of the immune system. Allergy to a drug usually begins to occur when more than one dose of the drug has been given. On occasion, the nurse may observe an allergic reaction the first time a drug is given, because the client has been exposed to the drug in the past.

A drug allergy occurs because the individual's immune system responds to the drug as a foreign substance called an *antigen.* When the body responds to the drug as an antigen, a series of events occurs in an attempt to render the invader harmless. Lymphocytes respond by forming *antibodies* (protein substances that protect against antigens). Common allergic reactions occur when the individual's immune system responds aggressively to the antigen. Chemical mediators released during the allergic reaction produce symptoms ranging from mild to life-threatening.

Even a mild allergic reaction produces serious effects if it goes unnoticed and the drug is given again. Any indication of an allergic reaction is reported to the primary health care provider before the next dose of the drug is given. Serious allergic reactions require contacting the primary health care provider immediately, because emergency treatment may be necessary.

Some allergic reactions occur within minutes (even seconds) after the drug is given; others may be delayed for hours or days. Allergic reactions that occur immediately often are the most serious.

Allergic reactions are manifested by a variety of signs and symptoms observed by the nurse or reported by the client. Examples of some allergic symptoms include itching, various types of skin rashes, and hives (urticaria). Other symptoms include difficulty breathing, wheezing, cyanosis, a sudden loss of consciousness, and swelling of the eyes, lips, or tongue.

Anaphylactic shock is an extremely serious allergic drug reaction that usually occurs shortly after the administration of a drug to which the individual is sensitive. This type of allergic reaction requires immediate medical attention. Symptoms of anaphylactic shock are listed in Table 1.2.

An anaphylactic reaction should be considered if all or only some of these symptoms are present. Anaphylactic shock can be fatal if the symptoms are not identified and treated immediately. The treatment goal is to raise the blood pressure, improve breathing, restore cardiac function, and treat other symptoms as they occur. Epinephrine (adrenalin) may be given by subcutaneous injection in the upper extremity or thigh and may be followed by a continuous IV infusion. Hypotension and shock may be treated with fluids and vasopressors. Bronchodilators are given to relax the smooth muscles of the bronchial tubes. Antihistamines and corticosteroids may also be given to treat urticaria and angioedema (swelling). These are all drugs you will learn about in subsequent chapters of this book.

TABLE 1.2 Symptoms of Anaphylactic Shock

BODY SYSTEM	SYMPTOMS
Respiratory	Bronchospasm Dyspnea (difficult breathing) Feeling of fullness in the throat Cough Wheezing
Cardiovascular	Extremely low blood pressure Tachycardia (heart rate >100 bpm) Palpitations Syncope (fainting) Cardiac arrest
Integumentary	Urticaria (hives) Angioedema Pruritus (itching) Sweating
Gastrointestinal	Nausea Vomiting Abdominal pain

Angioedema (angioneurotic edema) is another type of allergic drug reaction. It is manifested by the collection of fluid in subcutaneous tissues. Areas that are most commonly affected are the eyelids, lips, mouth, and throat, although other areas also may be affected. Angioedema can be dangerous when the mouth and throat are affected because the swelling may block the airway and asphyxia may occur. Difficulty in breathing and swelling in any area of the body are reported immediately to the primary health care provider.

Drug Idiosyncrasy

Drug idiosyncrasy is a term used to describe any unusual or atypical reaction to a drug. It is any reaction that is different from the one normally expected from a specific drug and dose. For example, a client may be given a drug to help them sleep (e.g., a hypnotic). Instead of falling asleep, the client remains wide awake and shows signs of nervousness or excitement. This response is idiosyncratic because it is different from what one expects from this type of drug. Another client may receive the same drug and dose, fall asleep, and after 8 hr be difficult to awaken. This, too, is abnormal and describes an overresponse to the drug.

The cause of drug idiosyncrasy is not clear, although study in the science of genetics can give us insight into possible explanations. The inability to tolerate certain chemicals and drugs is believed to be because of a genetic deficiency. Pharmacogenetics, the study of ways that specific genes can enhance sensitivity or resistance to certain drugs, helps to explain some drug idiosyncrasies. A pharmacogenetic disorder is a genetically determined abnormal response to normal doses of a drug. This abnormal response occurs because of inherited traits that cause abnormal metabolism of drugs. For example, individuals with glucose-6-phosphate dehydrogenase (G6PD) deficiency have abnormal reactions to a number of drugs. These clients exhibit varying degrees of hemolysis (destruction of red blood cells) when these drugs are administered. More than 100 million people are affected by this disorder. Examples of drugs that cause hemolysis in clients with a G6PD deficiency include aspirin, nonsteroidal anti-inflammatory drugs (NSAIDs), and the sulfonamides.

Drug Tolerance

Drug tolerance is a term used to describe a decreased response to a drug, requiring an increase in dosage to achieve the desired effect. Drug tolerance may develop when a client takes certain drugs, such as opioids and anti-anxiety drugs, for a long time. The individual who takes these drugs at home increases the dose when the expected drug effect does not occur. The development of drug tolerance is a sign of physical drug dependence. Drug tolerance may also occur in the hospitalized client. When the client begins to ask for the drug at more frequent intervals, the nurse needs to assess whether the dose is not adequate based on the disease process or whether the client is building a tolerance to the drug's effects.

Cumulative Drug Effect

A **cumulative drug effect** may be seen especially in those people with liver or kidney disease because these organs are the major sites for the breakdown and excretion of most drugs. This drug effect occurs when the body is unable to metabolize and excrete one (normal) dose of a drug before the next dose is given. Thus, if a second dose of the drug is given, some drug from the first dose remains in the body. A cumulative drug effect can be serious because too much of the drug can accumulate in the body and lead to toxicity.

Clients with liver or kidney disease are usually given drugs with caution because a cumulative effect may occur. When the client is unable to excrete the drug at a normal rate, the drug accumulates in the body, causing a toxic reaction. Sometimes, the primary health care provider lowers the dose of the drug to prevent a toxic drug reaction.

Toxic Reactions

Most drugs can produce toxic or harmful reactions if administered in large dosages or when blood concentration levels exceed the therapeutic level. Toxic levels build up when a drug is administered in doses that exceed the normal level or if the client's kidneys are not functioning properly and cannot excrete the drug. Some toxic effects are immediately visible; others may not be seen for weeks or months. Some drugs, such as lithium or digoxin, have a narrow margin of safety, even when given in recommended dosages. It is important to monitor these drugs closely to detect and avoid toxicity.

Drug toxicity can be reversible or irreversible, depending on the organs involved. Damage to the liver may be reversible because liver cells can regenerate. However, the anti-infective drug, streptomycin, may cause permanent hearing loss due to its toxic effect on the eighth cranial nerve. Sometimes drug toxicity can be reversed by administering another drug that acts as an antidote. For example, when too much opiate is taken, the drug naloxone (Narcan) may be given to counteract the effect.

When testing, carefully monitor the client's blood level of drug to ensure that the level remains within the therapeutic range. Any deviation should be reported to the primary health care provider. Because some drugs can cause toxic reactions even in recommended doses, you should be aware of the signs and symptoms of toxicity of commonly prescribed drugs.

Minimizing Drug Reactions Through Pharmacogenomics

Drug developers are researching ways to target cell structures and selected cells to minimize reactions in other body tissues, thereby reducing or eliminating adverse reactions. Genetic specialists search for genetic variations associated with drug efficiency. One of the goals of pharmacogenomics is the creation of drugs that can be tailor-made for individuals, target specific cells in the body, and adapt to each person's own individual genetic makeup.

DRUG INTERACTIONS

It is important when administering medications to be aware of the various drug interactions that can occur, especially *drug–drug interactions* and *drug–food interactions.* This section gives a brief overview of drug interactions. Specific drug–drug and drug–food interactions are discussed in subsequent drug specific chapters.

Drug–Drug Interactions

A drug–drug interaction occurs when one drug interacts with or interferes with the action of another drug. For example, taking an antacid with oral tetracycline causes a decrease in the effectiveness of the tetracycline. The antacid chemically interacts with the tetracycline and impairs its absorption into the bloodstream, thus reducing the effectiveness of the tetracycline. Drug categories known to cause interactions with other drugs include oral anticoagulants, oral hypoglycemics, anti-infectives, antiarrhythmics, cardiac glycosides, and alcohol. Drug–drug interactions can produce effects that are additive, synergistic, or antagonistic; these reactions are explained below.

Additive Drug Reaction

An *additive drug reaction* occurs when the combined effect of two drugs is equal to the sum of each drug given alone. The equation $1 + 1 = 2$ is sometimes used to illustrate the additive effect of drugs.

- Example—taking the drug heparin with alcohol will increase bleeding.

Synergistic Drug Reaction

Drug *synergism* occurs when drugs interact with each other and produce an effect that is greater than the sum of their separate actions. The equation $1 + 1 = 3$ may be used to illustrate synergism.

- Example—when a person takes both a hypnotic and alcohol. When alcohol is taken shortly before or after the hypnotic drug, the action of the hypnotic increases considerably. The individual experiences a drug effect that is greater than each drug taken alone. On occasion, the occurrence of a synergistic drug effect is serious and even fatal.

Antagonistic Drug Reaction

An *antagonistic* drug reaction occurs when one drug interferes with the action of another, causing neutralization or a decrease in the effect of one of the drugs. The equation $1 - 1 = 0$ may be used to illustrate antagonistic reactions.

- Example—protamine is a heparin antagonist. This means that the administration of protamine completely neutralizes the effects of heparin in the body and blood clotting will happen in the body.

Drug–Food Interactions

When a drug is given orally, food may impair or enhance its absorption. A drug taken on an empty stomach is absorbed into the bloodstream more quickly than when the drug is taken with food in the stomach. Some drugs (e.g., captopril) must be taken on an empty stomach to achieve an optimal effect. Drugs that should be taken on an empty stomach are administered 1 hr before or 2 hr after meals.

Other drugs, especially drugs that irritate the stomach, result in nausea or vomiting, or cause epigastric distress, are best given with food or meals. This minimizes gastric irritation. The NSAIDs and salicylates are examples of drugs that are given with food to decrease epigastric distress.

Still other drugs combine with a food and may form an insoluble food–drug mixture. For example, when tetracycline is administered with dairy products, a drug–food mixture is formed that is not absorbable by the body. When a drug cannot be absorbed by the body, no pharmacologic effect occurs.

Components in foods may also prevent the medication from working. An enzyme in the human body that breaks down many drugs is prevented from working when people eat grapefruit.

FACTORS INFLUENCING DRUG RESPONSE

Certain factors may influence drug response and are considered when the primary health care provider prescribes and the nurse administers a drug. These factors include age, weight, sex, disease, and route of administration.

Age

The age of the client may influence the effects of a drug. Infants and children usually require smaller doses of a drug than adults. Immature organ function, particularly of the liver and kidneys, can affect the ability of infants and young children to metabolize drugs. An infant's immature kidneys impair the elimination of drugs in the urine. Liver function is not yet fully developed in infants and young children. Drugs metabolized by the liver may produce more intense effects for longer periods. Parents must be taught the potential problems associated with administering drugs to their children. For example, a safe dose of a nonprescription drug for a 4-year-old child may be dangerous for a 6-month-old infant.

Elderly clients may also require smaller doses, although this may depend on the type of drug administered. For example, the elderly client may be given the same dose of an antibiotic as a younger adult. However, the same older adult may require a smaller dose of a drug that depresses the central nervous system, such as an opioid. Changes that occur with aging affect the pharmacokinetics (absorption, distribution, metabolism, and excretion) of a drug. Any of these processes may be altered because of the physiologic changes that occur with aging. Table 1.3 summarizes the changes that occur with aging and their possible pharmacokinetic effects.

Polypharmacy is the taking of numerous drugs that can potentially react with one another. This is seen particularly in elderly clients who may have multiple chronic diseases; polypharmacy leads to an increase in the number of potential adverse reactions. Although multiple drug therapy is necessary to treat certain disease states, it always increases the possibility of adverse reactions. You need good assessment skills to detect any problems when monitoring the geriatric client's response to drug therapy.

Weight

In general, standard dosages are based on a weight of approximately 77 kg (170 lb), which is calculated to be the average weight of men and women. A drug dose may sometimes be increased or decreased because the client's weight is significantly higher or lower than this average. With opioids, for example, higher- or lower-than-average dosages may be necessary, depending on the client's weight, to produce relief of pain.

TABLE 1.3 Factors Altering Drug Response in Children and Older Adults

BODY SYSTEM CHANGES	CHILDREN/INFANTS	OLDER ADULTS
Gastric acidity	Higher pH—slower gastric emptying resulting in delayed absorption	Higher pH—slower gastric emptying resulting in delayed absorption
Skin changes	Less cutaneous fat, yet greater surface area—faster absorption of topical drugs	Decreased fat content—decreased absorption of transdermal drugs
Body water content	Increased body water content—greater dilution of drug in tissues	Decreased body water content—greater concentration of drug in tissues
Serum protein	Less protein—less protein binding creating more circulating drug	Less protein—less protein binding creating more circulating drug
Liver function	Immature function—increased half-life of drugs and less first-pass effect	Decreased blood flow to liver—delayed and decreased metabolism of drug
Kidney function	Immature kidney function—decreased elimination, potential for toxicity at lower drug levels	Decreased renal mass and glomerular filtration rate—increased serum levels of drugs

Sex

The sex of an individual may influence the action of some drugs. Women may require a smaller dose of some drugs than men. This is because many women are smaller and have a different body fat-to-water ratio than men.

Disease

The presence of disease may influence the action of some drugs. Sometimes disease is an indication for not prescribing a drug or for reducing the dose of a certain drug. Both hepatic (liver) and renal (kidney) diseases can greatly affect drug response.

In liver disease, for example, the ability to metabolize or detoxify a specific type of drug may be impaired. If the average or normal dose of the drug is given, the liver may be unable to metabolize the drug at a normal rate. Consequently, the drug may be excreted from the body at a much slower rate than normal. The primary health care provider may then decide to prescribe a lower dose and lengthen the time between doses because liver function is abnormal.

Clients with kidney disease may exhibit drug toxicity and a longer duration of drug action. The dosage of drugs may be reduced to prevent the accumulation of toxic levels in the blood or further injury to the kidney.

Route of Administration

The method used to get the drug into a person's body will affect the drug response. IV administration of a drug produces the most rapid drug action because the GI tract is completely bypassed. Next in order of time of action is the intramuscular (IM) route, followed by the subcutaneous (Subcut) route. Giving a drug orally usually produces the slowest drug action.

Some drugs can be given only by one route; for example, antacids are only given orally. Other drugs are available in oral and parenteral (IV, IM, Subcut) forms. The primary health care provider selects the route of administration based on many factors, including the desired rate of action. For example, the client with a severe cardiac problem may require IV administration of a drug that affects the heart. Another client with a mild cardiac problem may experience a good response to oral administration of the same drug.

NURSING IMPLICATIONS WITH DRUG ACTIONS

Many factors can influence drug action. Consult appropriate references or the clinical pharmacist if there is any question about the dosage of a drug, whether other drugs the client is receiving will interfere with the drug being given, or whether the oral drug should or should not be given with food.

Drug reactions are potentially serious. Observe all clients for adverse drug reactions, drug idiosyncrasy, and evidence of drug tolerance (when applicable). It is important to report all drug reactions or any unusual drug effect to the primary health care provider.

Use good judgment when reporting adverse drug reactions to the primary health care provider. Accurate observation and evaluation of the circumstances are essential; record all observations in the client's record. If there is any question regarding the events that are occurring, withhold the drug and immediately contact the primary health care provider.

HERBAL MEDICINE AND HEALTH CARE

Herbal medicine, herbalism, and herbal therapy are all names used for complementary/alternative therapies that use plants or herbs to treat various disorders. Individuals worldwide use herbal therapy and dietary supplements extensively. According to the World Health Organization, 80% of the world's population relies on herbs for a substantial part of their health care. Herbs have been used by virtually every culture in the world throughout history. For example, Hippocrates prescribed St. John's wort, currently a popular herbal remedy for depression. Native Americans use plants such as coneflower, ginseng, and ginger for therapeutic purposes. Herbal therapy is part of the group of nontraditional therapies commonly known as complementary and alternative medicine (CAM).

Complementary and Alternative Medicine

The National Center for Complementary and Integrative Health (NCCIH) is one of the 27 institutes and centers that make up the National Institutes of Health. The NCCIH explores complementary and alternative (or also called integrative) healing practices through scientific research. It also trains CAM scientists and disseminates the information gleaned from the research it conducts. Among the various purposes of the NCCIH is to evaluate the safety and efficacy of widely used natural products, such as herbal remedies and dietary and food supplements. The NCCIH is dedicated to developing programs and encouraging scientists to investigate CAM treatments that show promise. The NCCIH budget has steadily grown, reflecting the public's interest and need for CAM information that is based on rigorous scientific research.

The NCCIH defines CAM as a "group of diverse medical and health care systems, practices, and products that are not presently considered to be part of conventional medicine." Examples of complementary therapies are relaxation techniques, massage, aromatherapy, and healing touch. Complementary therapies are often used with traditional health care to "complement" conventional medicine. Alternative therapies, on the other hand, are therapies used in place of or instead of conventional or Western medicine. The term *complementary/alternative therapy* often is used as an umbrella term for many therapies from all over the world.

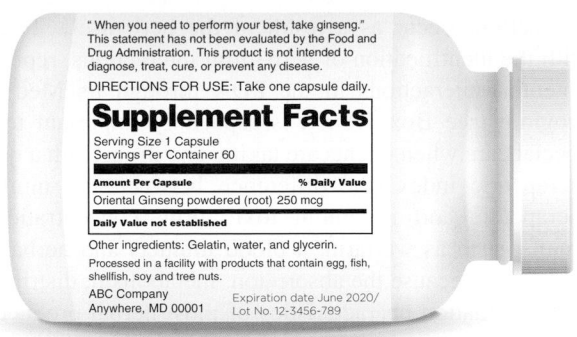

FIGURE 1.4 Example of herbal supplement labeling.

Dietary Supplement Health and Education Act

In addition to vitamins and minerals, herbs are classified as dietary or nutritional supplements. *Nutritional* or *dietary substances* are terms used by the federal government to identify substances that are not regulated by the FDA but are purported to be effective in promoting health. Herbs are not sold and promoted in the United States as drugs. Therefore, they do not have to meet the same standards as drug and OTC medications for proof of safety and effectiveness and what the FDA calls "good manufacturing practices."

Because natural products cannot be patented in the United States, it is not profitable for drug manufacturers to spend the millions of dollars and the 7–12 years needed to study and develop these products as drugs. In 1994, the US government passed the Dietary Supplement Health and Education Act (DSHEA). This act defines substances such as herbs, vitamins, minerals, amino acids, and other natural substances as "dietary supplements." The act permits general health claims such as "improves memory" or "promotes regularity" as long as the label also has a disclaimer stating that the supplements are not approved by the FDA and are not intended to diagnose, treat, cure, or prevent any disease (Fig. 1.4). The claims must be truthful and not misleading and supported by scientific evidence. Some manufacturers have abused the law by making exaggerated claims, but the FDA has the power to enforce the law, which it has done, and these claims have decreased.

Educating Clients About Herbs and Dietary Supplements

The use of herbs and dietary supplements to treat various disorders is common. At least 76% of the adult population in the United States use dietary supplements on a daily basis (CRN Survey, 2017). Herbs are used for various effects, such as boosting the immune system, treating depression, and promoting relaxation. Individuals are becoming more aware of the benefits of herbal therapies and dietary supplements. Advertisements, books, magazines, and Internet sites concerning these topics are prolific. People eager to cure or control various disorders take herbs, teas, megadoses of vitamins, and various other natural products. Although much information is available on dietary supplements and

herbal therapy, obtaining the correct information can be difficult at times. Medicinal herbs and dietary substances are available at supermarkets, pharmacies, health food stores, and specialty herb stores and through the Internet. The potential for misinformation abounds.

Because these substances are "natural products," many individuals incorrectly assume that they are without adverse effects. When any herbal remedy or dietary supplement is used, it should be reported to the nurse and the primary health care provider. Many of these natural substances have

---

BOX 1.2 Teaching Points When Discussing Herbal Therapy

- *Herbal preparations are not necessarily safe just because they are natural.* Unlike prescription and OTC medicines, herbal products and supplements do not have to be tested to prove they work well and are safe before they are sold. Also, they may not be pure. They might contain other ingredients, such as plant pollen, that could make you sick. Sometimes they contain drugs that are not listed on the label, such as steroids or estrogens.
- *If you have health problems, there may be an increased danger in taking herbal preparations.* These conditions include blood-clotting problems, cancer, diabetes, an enlarged prostate gland, epilepsy, glaucoma, heart disease, high blood pressure, immune system problems, psychiatric problems, Parkinson disease, liver problems, stroke, and thyroid problems.
- *If you are going to have surgery, be sure to tell your doctor if you use herbal products.* Herbal products can cause problems with surgery, including bleeding and problems with anesthesia. Stop using herbal products at least 2 weeks before surgery, or sooner if your doctor recommends it.
- *Herbal products can change the way prescription and OTC drugs work.* Herbal health products or supplements can affect the way the body processes drugs. When this happens, your medicine may not work the way it should. This may mean the drugs are not absorbed at high-enough levels to help the conditions for which they are prescribed. This can cause serious problems. You should be especially cautious about using herbal health products or supplements if you take a drug in one of the following categories.

  If you take any of these drugs, talk to your doctor before taking any type of herbal product or supplement.
  - Drugs to treat depression, anxiety, or other psychiatric problems
  - Antiseizure drugs
  - Blood thinners
  - Blood pressure medicine
  - Heart medicine
  - Drugs to treat diabetes
  - Cancer drugs
- *Herbal products can cause other problems, too.* You should not take more than the recommended dose of any herbal health product or supplement. The problems that these products can cause are much more likely to occur if you take too much or take them for too long.

(Karch's focus on nursing pharmacology (5th ed.). 2011, Figure 1.3, p. 9.)

strong pharmacologic activity, and some may interact with prescription drugs or be toxic in the body. For example, *comfrey,* an herb that was once widely used to promote digestion, can cause liver damage. Although it may still be available in some areas, it is a dangerous herb and is not recommended for use as a supplement.

When obtaining the drug history, always question the client about the use of herbs, teas, vitamins, or other dietary supplements. Many clients consider herbs as natural and therefore safe. Some also neglect to report the use of an herbal tea as part of the health care regimen because they do not think of it as such. Explain to the client that just because an herbal supplement is labeled "natural," it does not mean the supplement is safe or without harmful effects. Herbal supplements can act the same way as drugs and can cause medical problems if not used correctly or if taken in large amounts. Box 1.2 identifies teaching points to consider when discussing the use of herbs and dietary supplements with clients.

Because herbal supplements are not regulated by the FDA, products lack standardization with regard to purity and potency. In addition, multiple ingredients in products and batch-to-batch variation make it difficult to determine

if reactions occur as a result of the herb itself. To assist with the identification of herb–drug interactions, report any potential interactions to the FDA through its MedWatch program (see Box 1.1). It is especially important to take special care when clients are taking any drugs with a narrow therapeutic index (the difference between the minimum therapeutic and minimum toxic drug concentrations is small—such as warfarin, a blood thinner) and herbal supplements. Because the absorption, metabolism, distribution, and elimination characteristics of most herbal products are poorly understood, much of the information on herb–drug interactions is speculative. Herb–drug interactions are sporadically reported and difficult to determine.

Although a complete discussion about the use of herbs is beyond the scope of this book, it is important to remember that the use of herbs and dietary supplements is commonplace in many areas of the country. To help you become more aware of herbal therapy and dietary supplements, Appendix D gives an overview of selected common herbs and dietary supplements featured in select chapters. In addition, "alerts" related to herbs and dietary supplements appear throughout this text to alert the learner to valuable information and precautions.

KEY POINTS

■ Pharmacology is the study of drugs and their action on living organisms.

■ Each drug has several names: a chemical name (chemical structure), a generic (nonproprietary, official—any company can use) name, and a trade (or brand) name.

■ Drugs are classified by use (such as anti-infectives) and categorized by their potential to be harmful (prescription, nonprescription, and controlled substances).

■ Controlled substances are restricted by a schedule system (C-I to V) and monitored by the DEA because they have higher abuse potential that can result in physical and/or psychological dependency.

■ The FDA has revised how drugs are categorized for potential benefits and risks for the mother, the fetus, children who are breastfeeding, and women and men of reproductive age.

■ The FDA has strict controls for research, study, and production of drug substances; these processes can take many years between substance discovery and actual marketing of a drug. There are special programs to speed this process for rare diseases or life-threatening conditions and provide for greater benefit than detriment from drug therapy.

■ The three main phases of drug activity are pharmaceutic, pharmacokinetic, and pharmacodynamic.

■ Principles involved in pharmacokinetics include the following: absorption involves moving the drug from the site of administration; the drug is then distributed to tissues via the body circulation; metabolism changes the drug for use; and the drug is finally eliminated by the kidneys or made inactive by the liver and eliminated via the GI system.

■ Principles of pharmacodynamics involve the biochemical movement of drugs into a cell; by the receptors on cells; by altering the environment around the cell to gain entry.

■ Adverse reactions to drugs can range from minor GI distress to anaphylactic shock.

■ Drugs interact with many foods or other drugs, resulting in reactions less than or greater than when given alone.

■ Age, weight, sex, disease, and route of administration all influence a person's response to drug therapy.

■ Herbal preparations are not considered drugs, yet they should be considered part of a medical routine.

CHAPTER REVIEW

Prepare for the NCLEX

RECALL THE FACTS

1. The best definition of *pharmacology* would be:
   1. the study of plants and living organisms
   2. making of chemical compounds for illnesses
   3. the study of drugs and their action on living organisms
   4. monitoring and accounting for substances used to make people well

2. A client tells the nurse that he is taking Claritin. Which type of drug name is this?
   1. chemical
   2. official
   3. brand
   4. generic

3. A new drug will be given to healthy volunteers to see what happens. In what phase of clinical trial is the drug being currently tested?
   1. Preclinical
   2. Phase 1
   3. Phase 2
   4. Phase 3

4. A newly admitted client has a history of liver disease. In planning care, the nurse must consider that liver disease may result in a(n) _____.
   1. increase in the excretion rate of a drug
   2. impaired ability to metabolize or detoxify a drug
   3. need to increase the dosage of a drug
   4. decrease in the rate of drug absorption

5. A client asks the nurse to define a hypersensitivity reaction. The nurse begins by telling the client that a hypersensitivity reaction is also called a(n) _____.
   1. synergistic reaction
   2. antagonistic reaction
   3. drug idiosyncrasy
   4. allergic reaction

6. In monitoring drug therapy, the nurse is aware that a synergistic drug effect may be defined as _____.
   1. an effect greater than the sum of the separate actions of two or more drugs
   2. an increase in the action of one of the two drugs being given
   3. a neutralizing drug effect
   4. a comprehensive drug effect

ANALYZE THE FACTS

7. *A client has a rash and pruritus (itching). As the nurse, you suspect an allergic reaction and immediately assess him for other more serious symptoms. What question would be most important to ask the client?
   1. Are you having any difficulty breathing?
   2. Have you noticed any blood in your stool?
   3. Do you have a headache?
   4. Are you having difficulty with your vision?

8. *Under the Controlled Substances Act, schedule II to V drugs are typically accounted for in the health care setting. Which of the following drugs would the nurse least expect to be counted during change-of-shift duties?
   1. opioids
   2. antidiarrheals with codeine
   3. anabolic steroids
   4. heroin

ALTERNATE-FORMAT QUESTIONS

9. Arrange the following steps of pharmacokinetics correctly:
   1. absorption
   2. distribution
   3. elimination
   4. metabolism

10. Identify the drug responses seen in children. **Select all that apply.**
    1. pH of gastric acid is higher
    2. decreased body water
    3. less protein, less binding of drug
    4. greater amount of circulating drug

To check your answers, see Appendix F.

———————

*Indicates the question is directly linked to the NCLEX-PN test plan in Appendix G.

WANT TO KNOW MORE? A wide variety of resources are available to enhance your learning and understanding of this chapter.
- Visit for thePoint resources such as:
  - NCLEX-Style Student Review Questions
  - Journal Articles
  - Dosage Calculations
  - Drug Monographs
  - Watch and Learn Videos
  - Concepts in Action Animations
- The *Study Guide to Accompany Introductory Clinical Pharmacology*, 12th edition, sold separately, will help you review and apply essential content.
- ✓PrepU is available to help students prepare for the NCLEX-PN examination.

2
Administration of Drugs

Key Terms

buccal mouth cavity between jaw and cheek

enteral entry by way of the gastrointestinal system

inhalation drug administration route in which the client inhales the drug orally or nasally

intradermal pertaining to the dermis area within the upper layers of the skin

intramuscular (IM) area within a muscle

intravenous (IV) area within a vein

medication errors any preventable event or activity that can cause inappropriate medication use or client harm

parenteral administration of a substance, such as a drug, by any route other than through the gastrointestinal system (e.g., oral or rectal route)

Personal protective equipment (PPE) items worn when touching blood or body fluid, or having the potential of splashing on the provider, such as gloves, gowns, masks, eye protection or facial and/or foot coverings

Standard Precautions recommendation that gloves and/or other protective gear be worn when touching any blood or body fluids, mucous membranes, or any broken skin area; also termed *Universal Precautions*

subcutaneous (subcut) under the skin or dermis layer in the fatty tissue layer

sublingual in the mouth, under the tongue

transdermal through the skin

unit dose system of drug delivery by which a drug order is filled and medication dispensed to fill each medication order(s) for a 24-hr period; each drug dose (unit) is dispensed in a package labeled with the drug name and dosage

Learning Objectives

On completion of this chapter, the student will:

1. Describe the five + 1 rights of drug administration.
2. Examine general principles of drug administration.
3. Identify the different types of medication orders.
4. Designate general guidelines that should be followed when preparing a drug for administration.
5. Describe methods used to help nurses reduce medication-related errors.
6. Define the various types of medication-dispensing systems.
7. Distinguish the administration of enteral and parenteral drugs.
8. Discuss the administration of drugs through the skin and mucous membranes.
9. Explain nursing responsibilities before, during, and after a drug is administered.

Drug administration is a fundamental nursing responsibility. By understanding the basic concepts of administering drugs you will master this task safely and accurately. In addition to administering the drug, your monitoring of the therapeutic response (desired response) and reporting adverse reactions is critical. Additionally, in the ambulatory setting, you are responsible for teaching the client and family members the information needed to self-administer drugs safely in the home.

THE (FIVE + 1) RIGHTS OF DRUG ADMINISTRATION

The nurse who administers a drug assumes a degree of responsibility for accuracy in the preparation of the medication. Accuracy in preparation is provided by a procedure termed the five "rights" of drug administration:

1. Right client
2. Right drug
3. Right dose
4. Right route
5. Right time

   In recent years, the concern for increasing medication errors has produced a sixth right:
6. Right documentation

Right Client

When administering a drug, you must be certain that the client receiving the drug is the client for whom the drug has been ordered. It is important to use two methods to identify the client before administering the

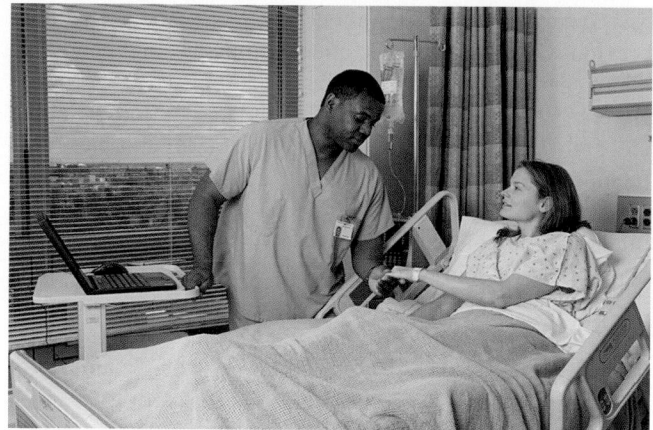

FIGURE 2.1 Always verify that the "right client" is receiving the medication by using two identifiers, one of which is checking the client's identification bracelet.

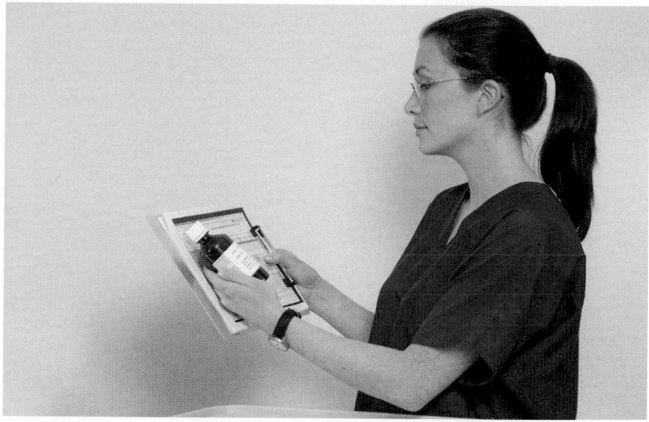

FIGURE 2.2 Before administering the medication, compare the medication, the container label, and the medication record to ensure that the client receives the "right drug" and the "right dose."

medication. Identifiers can include visual as well as verbal methods. A visual identifier may include checking the client's name on their wristband (Fig. 2.1). If the client is institutionalized and there is no written identification verifying the client's name, you should obtain a wristband or other form of identification before administering the drug. When in the clinic setting, you may also ask the client to identify themselves and request another unique identifier such as date of birth. However, do not ask, "Are you Mr. Jones?" Some clients, particularly those who are confused or have difficulty hearing, may respond by answering "yes," even though that is not their name. Some long-term care or rehabilitation care facilities have pictures of the client available, which allow the nurse to verify the correct client. If pictures are used to identify clients, it is critical that they are recent and bear a good likeness of the individual.

Right Drug

Similarity in spelling or sound can make drug names confusing. Hurriedly preparing a drug for administration or failing to look up questionable drugs can put you at increased risk for administering the wrong drug. Tall man letters used to focus on name differences of drugs are demonstrated in the drug chapter Summary Drug Tables and Appendix B. These examples help to remove the confusion of drugs that look similar in name. Error in drug name or amount can be prevented when you compare the medication administration record (MAR) (1) with the container label, (2) as the item is removed from the cart, and (3) before the actual administration of the drug (Fig. 2.2).

Right Dose, Right Route, and Right Time

Written orders are obtained from a primary health care provider for the administration of all drugs. The primary health care provider's order must include the client's name, the drug name, the dosage form and route, the dosage to be administered, and the frequency of administration. The primary health care provider's signature must follow the drug order. In an emergency situation, you may administer a drug with a verbal order from the primary health care provider. However, the primary health care provider must write and sign the order as soon as the emergency is over.

If a verbal order is given over the telephone, write down the order, repeat back the information exactly as written, and then ask for a verbal confirmation that it is correct. Any order that is unclear should be questioned, particularly unclear directions for the administration of the drug or a drug dose that is higher or lower than the dosages given in approved references.

Right Documentation

When medication administration is incorporated into electronic health records, the computer program typically requires the nurse to scan in their identification as they access the MAR. The medication is then scanned as it is removed from the medication station, which provides both documentation and charging of the item.

Further recording of medication specifics after the administration of a drug may be necessary (Fig. 2.3). Additional documentation is particularly important when drugs are given on an as-needed (PRN) basis. For example, recording why an analgesic was given and knowing it requires 20–30 min before the drug begins to relieve pain can prevent duplication of dosing. A client may forget that they received a drug for pain, may not understand that the administered drug was for pain, or may not know that pain relief is not immediate, and may ask another nurse for the drug again. If the administration of the analgesic was not recorded, the client might receive a second dose of the analgesic shortly after the first dose. This type of situation can be extremely serious, especially when opioids or other central nervous system depressants are administered. Immediate documentation prevents accidental administration of a drug by another individual. It also indicates when the client should be evaluated for success of the medication given for relief of the pain. Proper documentation is essential to the process of administering drugs correctly.

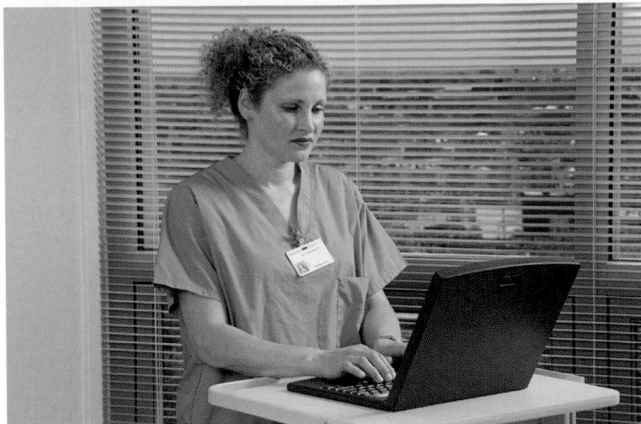

FIGURE 2.3 Always document the medication immediately after the drug is administered.

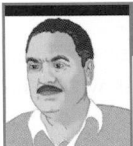

PHARMACOLOGY IN PRACTICE

CORRECT DRUG ADMINISTRATION
A nurse administers a drug on an as-needed (PRN) basis. Which of the following tasks should the nurse perform after administering the drug to the client? Select all that apply.

1. Record administration of the drug
2. Evaluate client's response to the drug
3. Record the site used for parenteral administration
4. Inform physician about the drugs administered

GENERAL PRINCIPLES OF DRUG ADMINISTRATION

Considerations in Drug Administration

Always have factual knowledge of each drug, the reasons for use of the drug, the drug's general action, the more common adverse reactions associated with the drug, special precautions in administration (if any), and the normal dose ranges before you administer the drug to a client.

When drugs are given frequently, you will become familiar with their pharmacologic information. Yet, when drugs are given less frequently or when a new drug is introduced, you should obtain information from reliable sources before preparing and giving the drug. Good sources for information include items such as the drug package insert, Internet sources, or the clinical pharmacist in the hospital department of pharmacy. Many health care providers download free drug information apps to their smartphones for quick access when needed. It is important to check current and approved references for all drug information. To remind yourself how important it is to understand the drugs you are preparing to give, always be sure a current drug handbook or other resource is easily accessible to the work area. Make it a habit to never give a medication without knowing the drug's action and anticipated client response.

Take client considerations, such as allergy history, previous adverse reactions, client comments, and change in client condition, into account before administering the drug. Before giving any drug for the first time, ask the client about any known allergies and any family history of allergies. This includes allergies not only to drugs but also to food, pollen, animals, and so on. Clients with a personal or family history of allergies are more likely to experience additional allergies and must be monitored closely.

If the client makes any statement about the drug or if there is any change in the client, these situations are carefully considered before the drug is given. Examples of situations that require consideration before a drug is given include:

- Problems that may be associated with the drug, such as nausea, dizziness, ringing in the ears, and difficulty walking. Any comments made by the client indicating the occurrence of a previous adverse reaction. Withhold the drug until references are consulted and the primary caregiver is contacted. The decision to withhold the drug must have a sound rationale and be based on knowledge of pharmacology.
- Client or family comments stating that the drug looks different from the one previously received, that the drug was just given by another nurse, or that the client thought the primary health care provider discontinued the drug therapy.
- A change in the client's condition, a change in one or more vital signs, or the appearance of new symptoms. Depending on the drug being administered and the client's diagnosis, these changes may indicate that the drug should be withheld and the primary health care provider contacted.

The Medication Order

Before a medication can be administered in a hospital or other agency, you must have an order. Medications are ordered by the primary health care provider, such as a physician, dentist, or, in some cases, an advanced nurse practitioner. Common orders include the standing order, the single order, the PRN order, and the STAT order. See Box 2.1 for an explanation of each.

Most health care facilities have converted medication ordering—and in some cases the entire client record—to computerized systems. As primary health care providers enter the drug prescription in the electronic record, it is sent to the pharmacy for preparation. This removes the transcription step and potential for error.

The medication is then added to the medication database of the electronic record. Built-in safeguards are a feature of the electronic MAR, such as data entry screens that require the entry of specific data before the drug administration screen can be viewed. This is designed to ensure that vital assessments such as blood pressure and pulse or blood glucose levels are taken and reviewed before

BOX 2.1 Types of Medication Orders

Standing order: This type of order is pre-established and approved for use by nurses and other health care providers under specific conditions in the absence of the primary or attending health care provider. They may be drug orders for presurgical/procedure or postsurgical/procedure nursing care. *Example:* Cefotetan 1 g IV 30 min preoperatively.

Single order: An order to administer the drug one time only. *Example:* Valium 10 mg IM at 10:00 A.M.

PRN order: An order to administer the drug as needed. *Example:* Percocet 1–2 tablets orally every 4 hr PRN for pain.

STAT order: A one-time order given as soon as possible. *Example:* Morphine 10 mg IV STAT for cardiac pain.

administering specific drugs, such as heart medication or insulin. This extra step alerts the nurse and reduces the chance of serious consequences of incorrect medication administration.

Preparing a Drug for Administration

When preparing a drug for administration, observe the following guidelines:

- Validate that the health care provider's original orders were checked and verify any questions with the primary health care provider before preparing the medication.
- Be alert for drugs with similar names. Some drugs have names that sound alike but are very different (see Summary Drug Tables and Appendix B). To give one drug when another is ordered could have serious consequences.
- Never give a drug that someone else has prepared. The individual preparing the drug must administer the drug.
- Perform hand hygiene immediately before preparing a drug for administration. Do not let your hands touch medication, especially topical preparations that you may absorb through the tissue of your hands. Use gloves as personal protective equipment (PPE) when possible contact with medication is anticipated.
- Always check and compare the label of the drug with the MAR three times:
  1. when the drug is taken from its storage area,
  2. immediately before removing the drug from the container, and
  3. before administering the drug to the client.

This pattern is called the "three checks" of medication administration.

- Never remove a drug from an unlabeled container or from a package whose label is illegible. Do not remove the wrappings of the unit dose until the drug reaches the bedside of the client who is to receive it. After administering the drug, document immediately on the MAR drug record.
- Never crush tablets or open capsules without first checking with the clinical pharmacist. Some tablets can be

crushed or capsules can be opened and the contents added to water or a tube feeding when the client cannot swallow a whole tablet or capsule. Some tablets have a special coating that delays the absorption of the drug. Crushing the tablet may destroy the drug's properties and result in problems such as improper absorption of the drug or gastric irritation. Capsules are gelatin and dissolve on contact with a liquid. The contents of some capsules do not mix well with water and therefore are best left in the capsule. If the client cannot take an oral tablet or capsule, consult the primary health care provider because the drug may be available in liquid form.

- Place drugs requiring special storage in the storage area immediately after they are prepared for administration. This rule applies mainly to drugs that need refrigeration but may also apply to drugs that must be protected from exposure to light or heat.

Preventing Medication Errors

Medication errors include any event or activity that can cause a client to receive the wrong dose, the wrong drug, an incorrect dosage of the drug, a drug by the wrong route, or a drug given at the incorrect time. Errors may occur in transcribing medication orders, when the drug is dispensed, or in administration of the drug. As a nurse and the medication administrator, you serve as the last defense against medication errors. When a medication error occurs, report it immediately so that any necessary steps to counteract the action of the drug or any observation can be made as soon as possible. In most institutions, if you made the error or discovered the error you must complete an unusual occurrence report and notify the primary care provider. It is important to report errors even when the client suffers no harm.

Medication errors occur when one or more of the five + 1 rights have not been followed. Each time a drug is prepared and administered, the five + 1 rights must be a part of the procedure. In addition to consistently practicing the five + 1 rights, you should adhere to the following precautions to help prevent drug errors:

- Confirm any questionable orders.
- When calculations are necessary, verify them with another nurse.
- Listen to the client when they question a drug, the dosage, or the drug regimen.
- Never administer the drug until the client's questions have been adequately researched.
- Avoid distractions and concentrate on only one task at a time.

A significant number of errors can be made during administration of a drug. Errors most commonly occur because of a failure to administer a drug that has been ordered, administration of the wrong dose or strength of a drug, or administration of a drug at the wrong time. Two drugs often associated with errors are insulin and heparin.

Innovative nurses are using various methods to study and reduce medication errors in cost-effective ways. Workplace distractions are one of the biggest issues being addressed by these nurses. Bright vests, mats on the floor, and "Do Not Disturb" signs are used to help lessen the number of people who interrupt the nurse as medications are being prepared and given to clients. An example is illustrated in Figure 2.4.

A number of agencies have instituted policies and practices to help in the reporting and reduction of errors. These practices (termed *Just Culture*) focus on finding the system problem, not punishing the person who made the error. Therefore, it is even more important for you and other nurses to report errors and omissions so problems can be discovered and changed.

National Patient Safety Goals

To evaluate the safety and quality of care provided by various accredited health care organizations, the Joint Commission establishes National Patient Safety Goals (NPSGs) on a yearly basis. These goals are established to help accredited organizations address specific areas of concern with regard to client safety. Facilities accredited by the Joint Commission are required to be in compliance with the National Patient Safety Standards. Several of these goals directly affect medication administration. For example, one of the first goals written that affects medication

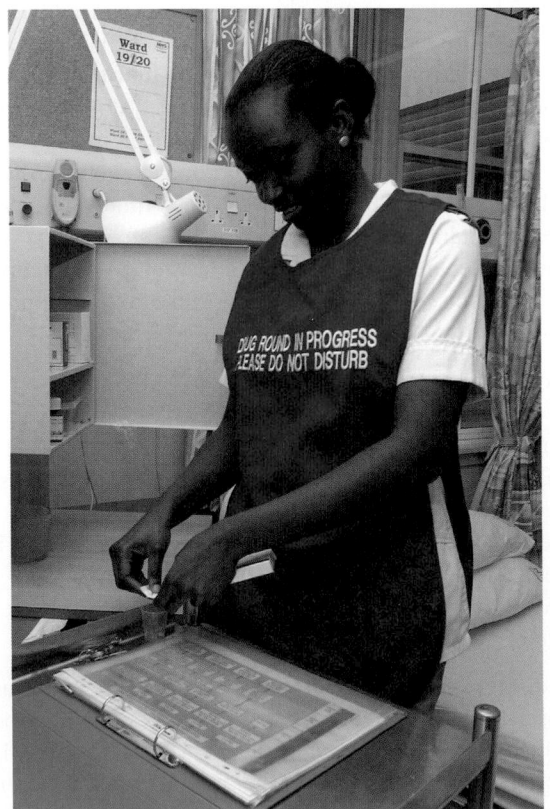

FIGURE 2.4 Reducing interruptions by wearing "Do Not Disturb" apparel is a cost-effective way to reduce drug errors.

safety was the 2009 NPSGs requiring improvement in the accuracy of client identification. To meet this goal, institutions were required to use the two-identifier rule, where two methods had to be used to identify the client (other than the client's room number) when administering medication or blood products. Another important standard that institutions desiring accreditation must follow is to compile a list of abbreviations, symbols, and acronyms *not* to be used throughout the institution. The Joint Commission has developed its own list of abbreviations that may no longer be used in any written medical documents (e.g., care plans, medical orders, nurses' notes). This list is referred to as the "minimum list." See Table 2.1 for the official "Do Not Use" list. Current information on these standards can be found at the Joint Commission website (http://www.jointcommission.org/standards_information/npsgs.aspx).

The list of error-prone abbreviations shown in Table 2.2 includes more abbreviations that are easily misinterpreted; therefore, providers are attempting to standardize terminology to reduce error.

The Institute for Safe Medication Practices

The Institute for Safe Medication Practices is a nonprofit organization devoted to the study of medication errors and their prevention. In addition to offering safety and educational information, it contains a section called the Medication Errors Reporting Program. This program is designed to identify the number and type of drug errors occurring around the country. This program is similar to the MedWatch program of the U.S. Food and Drug Administration (FDA). The goal of this voluntary reporting system is to collect data and disseminate information that will prevent such errors in the future. A link to the report form may be found online at http://www.ismp.org/. You are urged to participate in this important program as a means of protecting the public by identifying ways to make drug administration safer.

Drug Distribution Systems

The process of drug administration is standard in most facilities. Drugs are ordered by primary or specialty providers for administration. Pharmacists dispense the medications, and nurses carry out the actual administration. What may differ is the distribution system of the facility. Several drug distribution systems are available to be used to carry out the process. A brief description of three methods follows.

Unit Dose System

The **unit dose** system is a method in which drug orders are filled and medications dispensed to satisfy each client's medication orders for at least a 24-hr period. The pharmacist dispenses each dose (unit) in a package that is typically labeled by the manufacturer and contains one tablet or capsule, a premeasured amount of a liquid drug, a prefilled syringe, or

TABLE 2.1 Joint Commission Official "Do Not Use" List[a]

ABBREVIATION	POTENTIAL PROBLEM	USE INSTEAD
U (unit)	Mistaken as 0 (zero), 4 (four), or "cc"	Write "unit"
IU (international unit)	Mistaken as IV (intravenous) or 10 (ten)	Write "international unit"
Q.D., QD, q.d., qd (daily)	Mistaken for each other	Write "daily" and "every other day"
Q.O.D., QOD, q.o.d., qod (every other day)	The period after the "Q" can be mistaken for an "I" and the "O" can be mistaken for "I"	
Trailing zero (X.0 mg)[b]	Decimal point is missed	Write X mg
Lack of leading zero (.X mg)		Write 0.X mg
MS	Can mean morphine sulfate or magnesium sulfate	Write "morphine sulfate" or "magnesium sulfate"
MSO_4 and $MgSO_4$	Confused for one another	

[a]Applies to all orders and medication-related documentation that is handwritten (including free-test computer entry) or on preprinted forms.
[b]Exception: A "trailing zero" may be used only where required to demonstrate the level of precision of the value being reported, such as for laboratory results, imaging studies that report size of lesions, or catheter/tube sizes. It may not be used in medication orders or other medication-related documentation.
© The Joint Commission, 2020, reprinted with permission.

one suppository. Enough packaged drug for a select number of days is placed in drawers in a special portable medication cart with a drawer for each client. If the drug does not come individually packaged, a clinical pharmacist also may prepare unit doses. The pharmacy restocks the cart with the drugs needed. If the cart is portable, you take the drug cart to each client's room, preparing medications immediately outside the doorway. Before entering the client room, medications are locked in the cart and the electronic MAR is covered so others walking by cannot look at the client record.

In facilities where clients may stay for a long time, such as long-term care, the drug may be packaged using a multiunit dose method. With this system, single doses are "bubble" packed onto a card that may hold up to 60 single doses (Fig. 2.5). Cards are labeled for individual clients and may hold 1 to 2 months' supply of a drug. These cards are then stored in slots for individual clients in a locked medication cart. When administering a drug, the client's drug card is selected and the single dose is "popped" out of the card. The card with its remaining doses is returned to the medication cart.

Automated Medication Management System

Automated or computerized management systems (Fig. 2.6) are used in most hospitals or agencies distributing drugs.

Drug orders are managed in the pharmacy from physician orders that are sent electronically as they are written by the provider from the individual rooms or units. Each floor or unit has a medication station in which medications are placed in specific drawers. Medications are individually packaged as in the unit dose system. The difference is that there are more drugs in the tray if a number of clients are prescribed the same medication. Once the order is entered into the system, you may select the client's name and the drug to be administered at the unit's automated medication station. The drawer with the specific drug opens for you to remove the drug, and then using a computer touch screen, the dose is automatically recorded into the computerized system.

Bar-Coded Point-of-Care Medication System

Some hospitals use a bar-code scanner in the administration of drugs. This system is the most effective way to reduce medication administration errors. To use this system, a bar code is placed on the client's hospital identification band when the client is admitted to the hospital (Fig. 2.7). The bar codes, along with bar codes on the drug unit dose packages, are used to identify the client and to record and charge routine and PRN drugs. In addition, provider identification badges are scanned during the procedure, thus identifying

TABLE 2.2 Error-Prone Abbreviations

> (greater than) < (less than)	Misinterpreted as the number "7" or the letter "L"; confused with one another	Write "greater than" or "less than"
Abbreviations for drug names	Misinterpreted because of similar abbreviations for multiple drugs	Write drug names in full
Apothecary units	Unfamiliar to many practitioners; confused with metric units	Use metric units
@	Mistaken for the number "2" (two)	Write "at"
cc (cubic centimeter)	Mistaken for U (units) when poorly written	Write "mL" for milliliters
µg (microgram)	Mistaken for mg (milligrams), resulting in 1000-fold overdose	Write "mcg" or "micrograms"

the nurse giving the medication. The scanner also keeps an ongoing inventory of controlled substances, which eliminates the need for manual controlled substance counts at the end of each shift.

Because of the serious consequences of administering the wrong drug, newer and more sophisticated automated systems to administer drugs are being constantly researched to provide the best safety to clients.

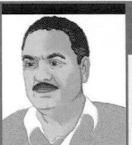

PHARMACOLOGY IN PRACTICE

SAFE DRUG ADMINISTRATION
Which is the safest drug distribution system?

1. Automated medication management system
2. Bar-coded point-of-care medication systems
3. Unit dose system
4. Multidose system

ADMINISTRATION OF DRUGS BY THE ORAL ROUTE

The oral route is the most frequent route of drug administration and rarely causes physical discomfort to clients. Oral drug forms include tablets, capsules, and liquids. Some capsules and tablets contain sustained-release drugs, which dissolve over an extended period. Administration of oral drugs is relatively easy for clients who are alert and can swallow.

Nursing Responsibilities
Observe the following points when giving an oral drug:

- Verify that the client is able to swallow and is not nauseated or vomiting. Place the client in an upright position. It is difficult, as well as dangerous, to swallow a solid or liquid when lying down.

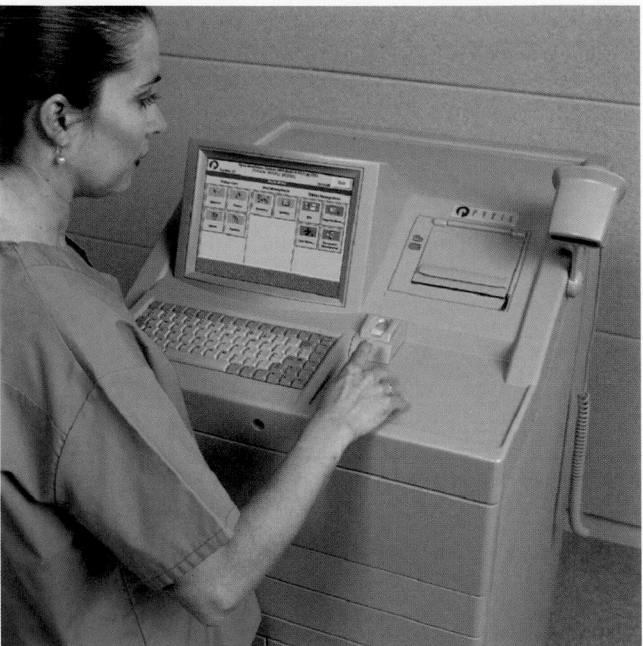

FIGURE 2.6 An automated medication system.

- Assess the client's need for assistance in holding the tablet or capsule or holding a glass of water. Some clients with physical disabilities cannot handle or hold these objects and may require assistance.
- Make sure that a full glass of water is readily available. Advise the client to take a few sips of water before placing a tablet or capsule in the mouth.
- Instruct the client to place the pill or capsule on the back of the tongue and tilt the head back to swallow a tablet or slightly forward to swallow a capsule. Encourage the client first to take a few sips of water to move the drug down the esophagus and into the stomach and then to finish the whole glass.
- Give the client any special instructions, such as drinking extra fluids or remaining in bed, that are pertinent to the drug being administered.
- Never leave a drug at the client's bedside to be taken later unless there is a specific order by the primary care

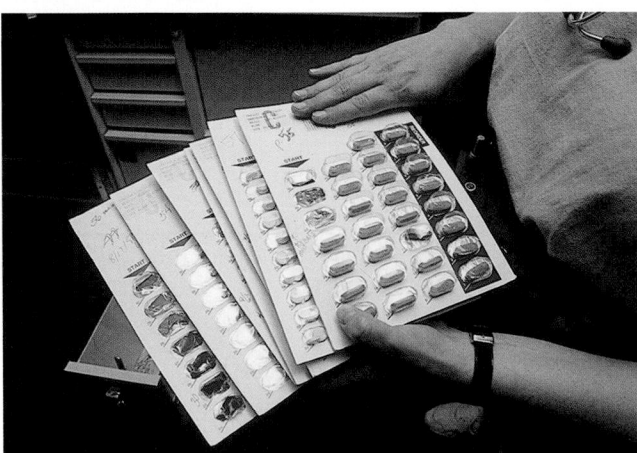

FIGURE 2.5 Multiunit dose packs, frequently used for medication administration in long-term care settings.

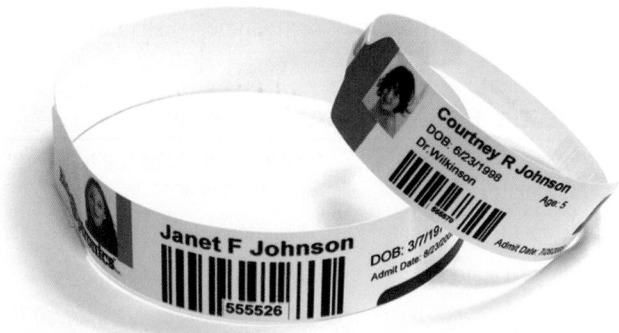

FIGURE 2.7 Bar-coded, point-of-care client wrist bands used for medication administration.

provider to do so. Some units, such as postpartum, may offer self-administered medications. A few drugs (e.g., antacids) may be ordered to be left at the bedside.

- Instruct the client to place **buccal** drugs in the mouth against the mucous membranes of the cheek in either the upper or lower jaw. They are absorbed slowly from the mucous membranes of the mouth. Examples of drugs given buccally are lozenges and troches.
- Certain drugs are also given by the **sublingual** (placed under the tongue) route. These drugs must not be swallowed or chewed and must be dissolved completely before the client eats or drinks. Nitroglycerin is commonly given sublingually.

ADMINISTRATION OF DRUGS BY THE NON-ORAL ENTERAL ROUTE

The term **enteral** refers to the gastrointestinal (GI) system. When used in a health care context, it often refers to feedings or medications entering the GI system via a tube, either nasally or directly into the stomach or small intestine. Roughly 450,000 individuals in the United States have swallowing/digestion issues requiring the use of feedings using a tube (Esposito, 2016). When using the tube equipment for medication administration, oral forms of drug are used and need to be crushed or provided in liquid form before administering in the tube.

Nursing Responsibilities

Observe the following points when giving a drug via tube used for enteral feedings:

- Place the client in an upright position; this reduces the risk of aspiration of the medication.
- Before administration, check the tube for placement.
- Never try to put a tablet or capsule in a tube.
- Use syringes meant only for oral liquids to avoid the accidental parenteral administration of an oral preparation (Fig. 2.8).
- Tablets are crushed and dissolved in water before administering them through the tube.
- Flush the tube with 30 mL of water after each drug is injected in the tube to clear the tubing completely.
- Never crush extended- or timed-release medications for enteral tube administration; it could cause an overdose of the drug.
- Medications to be taken on an empty stomach may require pausing of a tube feeding before and after administration.

! NURSING ALERT

Sorbitol, an inactive ingredient, is used as a sweetener for oral liquid medications. In large amounts, such as multiple medications administered via enteral tube, sorbitol acts as an osmotic laxative. Tablets crushed and mixed with water may reduce diarrhea if it occurs.

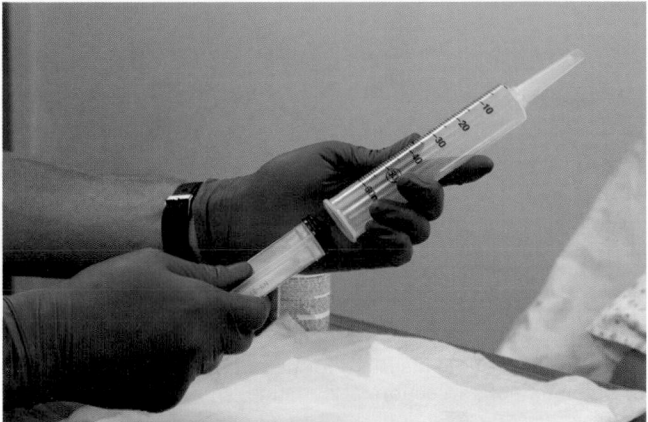

FIGURE 2.8 Specially designed syringes for enteral feedings should be used exclusively for tube feeding or medication administration to prevent parenteral (IV) administration. (From Springhouse. *Lippincott's visual encyclopedia of clinical skills.* Wolters Kluwer Health, 2009.)

Infrequent Dosing of Drugs

Many drugs are available for once-a-week, or even once-a-year, administration. The doses are designed to replace daily doses of drugs. One of the first was alendronate (Fosamax), a drug used to treat osteoporosis (see Chapter 29). In 2001, the FDA approved two strengths for this drug to be given once a week. In clinical trials, once-a-week dosing showed no greater adverse reactions than the once-daily regimen. Since that time, other drugs have been developed for dosing infrequently. A similar product, ibandronate (Boniva), is administered once a month for the treatment of osteoporosis. Infrequent dosing is beneficial for those experiencing mild adverse reactions in that the reactions would be experienced less frequently than every day, and adherence in taking the drug is improved. These are both examples of once oral drugs now given in less frequent parenteral administration form for better client outcomes.

ADMINISTRATION OF DRUGS BY THE PARENTERAL ROUTE

Parenteral drug administration entails giving a drug by the **intradermal**, **subcutaneous** (subcut), **intramuscular** (IM), or **intravenous** (IV) route (Fig. 2.9). Other routes of parenteral administration that may be used by the primary health care provider are intradural (into the dural space of the spine), intra-arterial (into an artery), intracardiac (into the heart), and intra-articular (into a joint). In some instances, intra-arterial drugs are administered by a nurse. However, administration is not by direct arterial injection but by means of a catheter that has been placed in an artery.

! NURSING ALERT

More active drug will be in the circulation when given parenterally over enteral delivery. Since the drug is not filtered or partially removed by the liver, both the intended and adverse reactions can be more pronounced. Clients, particularly children and older adults, should be monitored closely for drug reactions.

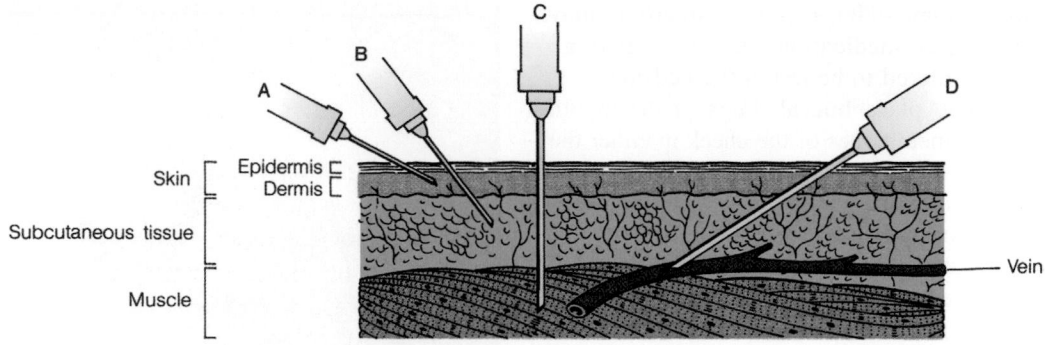

FIGURE 2.9 Needle insertion for parenteral drug. **A.** Intradermal injection: a 26-gauge, 3/8-in.-long needle is inserted at a 10° angle. **B.** Subcutaneous injection: a 25-gauge, 1/2-in.-long needle is inserted at an angle (45°–90°) that depends on the size of the client. **C.** Intramuscular injection: a 20- to 23-gauge, 1- to 3-in.-long needle is inserted into the relaxed muscle at a 90° angle with a quick (dart-throwing) type of hand movement. **D.** Intravenous injection: the diameter (18–26 gauge) of the needle used depends on the substance to be injected and on the size of the vein. (From Timby, B. K. (2017). *Fundamental nursing skills and concepts* (11th ed.). Wolters Kluwer, Lippincott Williams & Wilkins.)

Nursing Responsibilities

Observe the following points when giving a drug by the parenteral route:

- Wear gloves for protection from the potential of a blood spill when giving parenteral drugs. The risk of exposure to infected blood is increasing for all health care workers. The Centers for Disease Control and Prevention recommends that gloves (**personal protective equipment–PPE**) be worn when touching blood or body fluids, mucous membranes, or any broken skin area. This recommendation is referred to as **Standard Precautions**, which combine the Universal Precautions for Blood and Body Fluids with Body Substance Isolation guidelines.
- After selecting the site for injection, cleanse the skin. Most hospitals have a policy regarding the type of skin antiseptic used for cleansing the skin before parenteral drug administration. Cleanse the skin with a circular motion, starting at an inner point and moving outward.
- After removing the needle from an IM, subcut, or IV injection site, place pressure on the area. Clients with bleeding tendencies often require prolonged pressure on the area.
- Most hospitals use needles designed to prevent needle-stick injuries. This needle has a plastic guard that slips over the needle and locks in place as it is withdrawn from the injection site.
- Do not recap syringes, and dispose of them according to agency policy. Discard needles and syringes into clearly marked, appropriate containers to prevent needle-stick injuries. Most agencies have a "sharps" container located in each room for immediate disposal of needles and syringes after use. Proper disposal protects the nurse and others from injury and contamination.

Administration of Drugs by the Intradermal Route

Drugs given by the intradermal route are usually those for sensitivity tests (e.g., the tuberculin test or allergy skin testing; see Fig. 2.9A). Absorption is slow and allows for good results when testing for allergies.

Nursing Responsibilities

Observe the following points when administering drugs by the intradermal route:

- The inner part of the forearm and the upper back may be used for intradermal injections. The area should be hairless; avoid areas near moles or scars or pigmented skin areas. Cleanse the area in the same manner as for subcut and IM injections.
- A 1-mL syringe with a 25- to 27-gauge needle that is 1/4–5/8 in. long is best suited for intradermal injections. Small volumes (usually smaller than 0.1 mL) are used for intradermal injections and administered with the bevel up.
- Insert the needle at a 15° angle between the upper layers of the skin. Do not aspirate the syringe or massage the area. Injection produces a small wheal (raised area) on the outer surface of the skin. If a wheal does not appear on the outer surface of the skin, there is a good possibility that the drug entered the subcut tissue, and any test results would be inaccurate.

Administration of Drugs by the Subcutaneous Route

A subcut injection places the drug into the tissues between the skin and the muscle (see Fig. 2.9B). Drugs administered in this manner are absorbed more slowly than IM injections. Drugs for blood thinning and diabetes are commonly given by the subcut route.

Nursing Responsibilities

Observe the following points when giving a drug by the subcut route:

- A volume of 0.5–1 mL is used for subcut injection. Larger volumes (e.g., more than 1 mL) are best given as IM injections. If a volume larger than 1 mL is ordered through the subcut route, the injection is given in two sites, with separate needles and syringes.
- Medications are absorbed at a more consistent rate if injections are rotated within a general area, such as

consistently use the abdomen for subcut heparin injections.

- Absorption is fastest when the abdomen is used. If the abdomen cannot be used, use the upper arm; thigh absorption is the third option; lastly, the buttocks has the slowest rate of subcut absorption (Fig. 2.10).

- When giving a drug by the subcut route, insert the needle at a 45° angle. However, to place the drug in the subcut tissue, select the needle length and angle of insertion based on the client's body weight. Clients experiencing obesity have excess subcut tissue, and it may be necessary to give the injection at a 90° angle. If the client is thin or cachectic, there usually is less subcut tissue. For such clients, the upper abdomen is the best site for injection. Generally, a syringe with a 23- to 25-gauge needle that is 3/8–5/8 in. in length is most suitable for a subcut injection.

- Should blood appear in the syringe, withdraw the needle, discard the syringe, and prepare a new injection.

Administration of Drugs by the Intramuscular Route

An IM injection is the administration of a drug into a muscle (see Fig. 2.9C). Drugs that are irritating to subcut tissue can be given by IM injection. Drugs given by this route are absorbed more rapidly than drugs given by the subcut route because of the rich blood supply in the muscle. In addition, a larger volume (1–3 mL) can be given at one site.

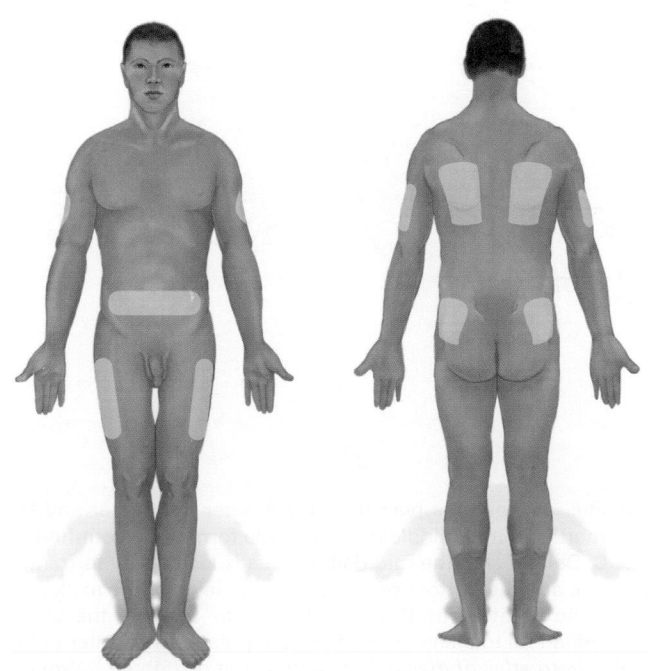

FIGURE 2.10 Sites on the body at which subcutaneous injections can be given. (From Timby, B. K. (2017). *Fundamental nursing skills and concepts* (11th ed.). Wolters Kluwer, Lippincott Williams & Wilkins.)

Nursing Responsibilities

The nurse should observe the following points when giving a drug by the IM route:

- If an injection is more than 3 mL, divide the drug and give it as two separate injections. Volumes larger than 3 mL will not be absorbed properly.

- A 22-gauge needle that is 1½ in. in length is most often used for IM injections.

- The sites for IM administration are the deltoid muscle (upper arm), the ventrogluteal or dorsogluteal sites (hip), and the vastus lateralis (thigh). See Figure 2.11 for IM injection sites. The vastus lateralis site is frequently used for infants and small children because it is more developed than the gluteal or deltoid sites. In children who have been ambulating for more than 2 years, the ventrogluteal site may be used.

- When giving a drug by the IM route, insert the needle at a 90° angle. When injecting a drug into the ventrogluteal or dorsogluteal muscles, it is a good idea to place the client in a comfortable position, preferably in a prone position with the toes pointing inward. When injecting the drug into the deltoid, a sitting or lying-down position may be used. Place the client in a recumbent position for injection of a drug into the vastus lateralis.

- Aspiration is not necessary when giving vaccines, most injectable IM, subcut or intradermal injections.

- When administering viscous medications such as penicillin, aspirate before injecting. After inserting the needle for IM administration, pull back the syringe barrel to aspirate the drug. Aspirate for 5–10 seconds. If blood is in a small vessel, it takes time for the blood to appear. If blood appears in the syringe, remove the needle so the drug is not injected. Discard the drug, needle, and syringe and prepare another injection. If no blood appears in the syringe, inject the drug.

Z-Track Technique

The **Z-track** technique of IM injection is used when a drug is highly irritating to tissues or has the ability permanently to stain the skin. The nurse should adhere to the following procedure when using the Z-track technique (Fig. 2.12):

- Draw the drug up into the syringe.

- Discard the needle and place a new needle on the syringe. This prevents any solution that may remain in the needle (that was used to draw the drug into the syringe) from contacting tissues as the needle is put into the muscle.

- Pull the plunger down to draw approximately 0.1–0.2 mL of air into the syringe. The air bubble in the syringe follows the drug into the tissues and seals off the area where the drug was injected, thereby preventing oozing of the drug up through the extremely small pathway created by the needle.

- Place the client in the correct position for administration of an IM injection.

- Cleanse the skin.

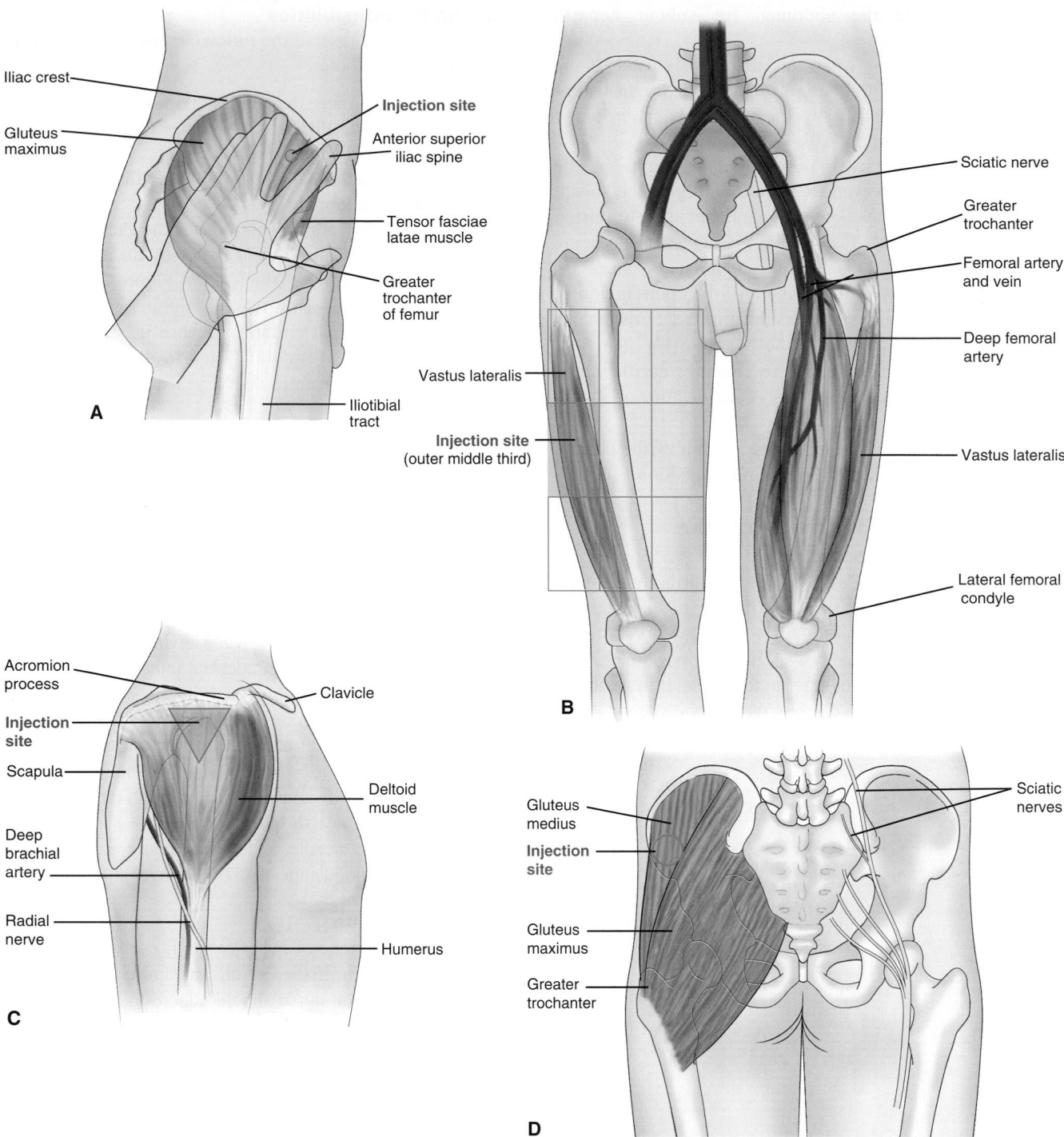

FIGURE 2.11 Sites for intramuscular administration. **A.** Ventrogluteal site: your palm is placed on the greater trochanter and the index finger is placed on the anterior superior iliac spine; the injection is made into the middle of the triangle formed by your fingers and the iliac crest. **B.** Vastus lateralis site: the client is supine or sitting. **C.** Deltoid site: the mid-deltoid area is located by forming a rectangle, the top of which is at the level of the lower edge of the acromion, and the bottom of which is at the level of the axilla; the sites are one-third and two-thirds of the way around the outer aspect of the client's arm. **D.** Dorsogluteal site: to avoid the sciatic nerve and accompanying blood vessels, choose an injection site above and lateral to a line drawn from the greater trochanter to the posterior superior iliac spine. (Adapted from Lynn, P. (2015). *Lippincott's photo atlas of medication administration* (5th ed.). Wolters Kluwer.)

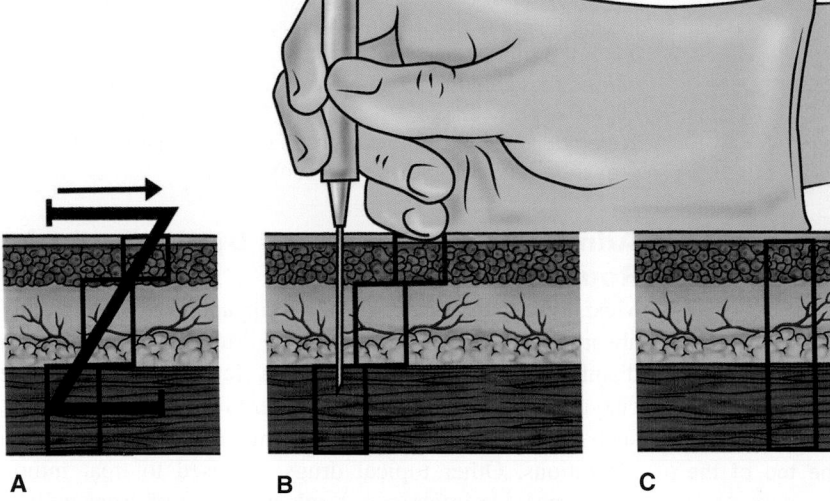

FIGURE 2.12 Z-track injection. **A.** The tissue is tensed laterally at the injection site before the needle is inserted. This pulls the skin, subcutaneous tissue, and fat planes into a "Z" formation. **B.** After the tissue has been displaced, the needle is thrust straight into the muscular tissue. **C.** After injection, tissues are released while the needle is withdrawn. As each tissue plane slides by the other, the track is sealed.

A   B   C

- Pull the skin, subcut tissues, and fat (that lie over the injection site) laterally, displacing the tissue to the side (approximately 1 in.).
- While holding the tissues in the lateral position, insert the needle at a 90° angle and inject the drug.
- After the drug is injected, wait 10 seconds to permit the medication to disperse into the muscle tissue, and then while withdrawing the needle, release the tissue. This technique prevents the backflow of drug into the subcut tissue.

Administration of Drugs by the Intravenous Route

A drug administered by the IV route is injected directly into the blood by a needle inserted into a vein (see Fig. 2.9D). Drug action occurs almost immediately. Drugs administered by the IV route may be given:

- Slowly, over 1 or more minutes
- Rapidly (IV push)
- By piggyback/syringe pump infusions (drugs are mixed with 50–100 mL of compatible IV fluid and administered during a period of 30–60 min piggybacked onto the primary IV line)
- Into an existing IV line (the IV port)
- Into an intermittent venous access device called a *saline lock* (a small IV catheter in the client's vein; the catheter is connected to a small fluid reservoir with a rubber cap through which the needle is inserted to administer the drug). In specific situations, a weak heparin solution may be used in the lock device instead of saline (Goossens, 2015)
- By being added to an IV solution and allowed to infuse into the vein over a longer period

For explanation of the procedure and nursing responsibilities, see Chapter 54.

Other Parenteral Routes of Drug Administration

The primary care provider may administer a drug by the intracardial, intra-arterial, or intra-articular routes. You may be responsible for preparing the drug for administration. If so, ask the primary health care provider what special materials will be required for administration.

Venous access ports are totally implanted ports with a self-sealing septum that is attached to a catheter leading to a large vessel, usually the vena cava. These devices are most commonly used for chemotherapy or other long-term therapy and require surgical insertion and removal. Drugs are administered through injections made into the portal through the skin using specialized (Huber) point needles. These drugs are administered by the primary health care provider or a registered nurse.

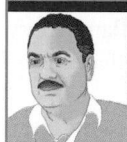

PHARMACOLOGY IN PRACTICE

DRUG ROUTE ADMINISTRATION
The primary health care provider has asked a nurse to administer a subcutaneous injection to a client. The nurse observes that the client is very thin. Which of the following sites should the nurse select to administer the injection to this client?

1. Upper arm
2. Lower back
3. Upper abdomen
4. Thigh muscle

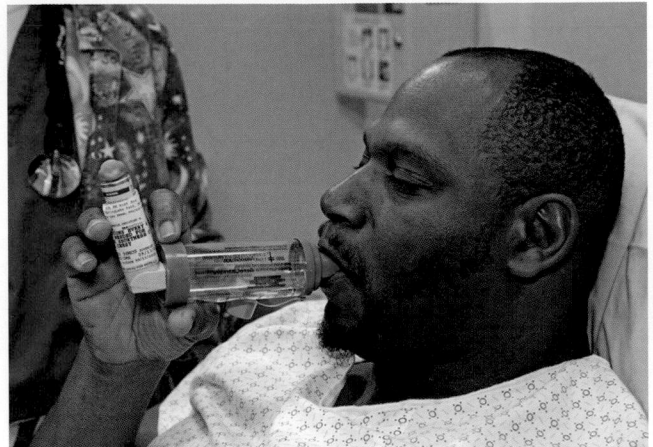

FIGURE 2.13 A respiratory inhalant is used to deliver a drug directly into the lungs. To deliver a dose of the drug, the client takes a slow, deep breath while depressing the top of the inhaler's canister. (Photo by Rick Brady.)

ADMINISTRATION OF DRUGS THROUGH THE SKIN AND MUCOUS MEMBRANES

Drugs may be applied to the skin and mucous membranes using several routes: inhaled through the membranes of the upper respiratory tract, topically (on the outer layers of skin), or transdermally through a patch on which the drug has been implanted.

Administration of Drugs Through Inhalation

Drug droplets, vapor, and gas are administered through the mucous membranes of the respiratory tract using a face mask, nebulizer, or positive-pressure breathing machine. Examples of drugs administered through **inhalation** include bronchodilators, mucolytics, and some anti-inflammatory drugs. These drugs primarily produce a local effect in the lungs.

Nursing Responsibilities

The primary nursing responsibility with drugs administered by inhalation is to provide the client with proper instructions for administering the drug. For example, many clients with asthma use a metered-dose inhaler to dilate the bronchi and make breathing easier. Without proper instruction on how to use the inhaler, much of the drug can be deposited on the tongue rather than in the respiratory tract. This decreases the therapeutic effect of the drug. Instructions may vary with each inhaler. To be certain that the inhaler is used correctly, refer the client to the instructions accompanying each device. Figure 2.13 illustrates the proper use of one type of inhaler.

! NURSING ALERT

A number of inhaled drugs end with the name Ellipta. Ellipta is the inhaler delivery system trademark; it is not a medication. Be aware of the following drug names that could be confused with each other: Anoro Ellipta, Arnuity Ellipta, Breo Ellipta, Incruse Ellipta, and Trelegy Ellipta. These drugs are in different classes and are prescribed for completely different reasons.

Administration of Drugs by the Topical Route

Most topical drugs act on the skin and are not typically absorbed into the circulation. These drugs are used to soften, disinfect, or lubricate the skin. A few topical drugs are enzymes that have the ability to remove superficial debris, such as the dead skin and purulent matter present in skin ulcerations. Other topical drugs are used to treat minor, superficial skin infections. A select number of drugs may be applied topically for slow systemic absorption such as some testosterone creams. The various forms of topical applications and locations of use are described in Box 2.2.

Nursing Responsibilities

Consider the following points when administering drugs by the topical route:

- The primary care provider may write special instructions for the application of a topical drug, for example, to apply the drug in a thin, even layer or to cover the area after application of the drug to the skin.
- Other drugs may have special instructions provided by the manufacturer, such as to apply the drug to a clean, hairless

BOX 2.2 | Topical Applications and Locations of Use

- Creams, lotions, or ointments applied to the skin with a tongue blade, gloved fingers, or gauze
- Sprays applied to the skin or into the nose or oral cavity
- Liquids inserted into body cavities, such as fistulas
- Liquids inserted into the bladder or urethra
- Solids (e.g., suppositories) or jellies inserted into the urethra
- Liquids dropped into the eyes, ears, or nose
- Ophthalmic ointments applied to the eyelids or dropped into the lower conjunctival sac
- Solids (e.g., suppositories, tablets), foams, liquids, and creams inserted into the vagina
- Continuous or intermittent wet dressings applied to skin surfaces
- Solids (e.g., tablets, lozenges) dissolved in the mouth
- Sprays or mists inhaled into the lungs
- Liquids, creams, or ointments applied to the scalp
- Solids (e.g., suppositories), liquids, or foams inserted into the rectum

TABLE 2.3 Examples of Medications Delivered Percutaneously in Patch Form

TRANSDERMAL PATCH (FOR SYSTEMIC ABSORPTION)	SKIN PATCH (LOCAL ABSORPTION)
Fentanyl—pain relief	Lidocaine—local pain relief
Estrogen—menopause	Diclofenac—local pain relief
Estrogen alone or with progesterone—birth control	Salonpas—local pain relief
Nicotine—smoking cessation	
Nitroglycerine—dilate coronary arteries	
Rotigotine—Parkinson disease	
Scopolamine—motion sickness	
Testosterone—hormonal replacement	

area or to let the drug dissolve slowly in the mouth. All of these instructions are important because drug action may depend on correct administration of the drug.

- Ointments are sometimes used and come with a special paper marked in inches. Measure the correct length (onto the paper), place the paper with the drug ointment side down on the skin, and secure it with tape. Before the next dose, remove the paper and tape and cleanse the skin.

Administration of Drugs by the Transdermal Route

When slow, consistent absorption of a drug is indicated, the **transdermal** route may be used. Drugs administered by the transdermal route are readily absorbed from the skin and provide systemic effects. This type of administration is called a *transdermal drug delivery system* (Fig. 2.14). The drug dosages are implanted in a small, patch-type bandage, and the drug is gradually absorbed into the systemic circulation. This type of drug system maintains a relatively constant blood concentration and reduces the possibility of toxicity. In addition, the administration of drugs transdermally causes fewer adverse reactions, and administration is less frequent than when the drugs are given by another route. Table 2.3 lists examples of drugs delivered topically using patches. Duragesic (used to treat severe pain) and Ortho Evra (used as birth control) are two drugs given frequently by the transdermal route. See Figure 2.14 for the application of transdermal medications.

Nursing Responsibilities

Observe the following points when administering drugs by the transdermal route:

- Wear gloves to prevent accidental exposure to the medication.

- Remove all old patches to prevent added dosing of the drug, fold sticky sides together, and discard in sharp container (if not available, flush down a toilet)—do not place in waste container.
- Choose a dry, hairless area of intact skin, large enough for the patch to fit smoothly.
- Rotate sites for transdermal patches to prevent skin irritation. The chest, abdomen, buttocks, and upper arm are the most commonly used sites. Do not shave the area to apply the patch; shaving may cause skin irritation.
- Use the back between the shoulder blades for clients with dementia who are likely to remove the patch by themselves.

NURSING RESPONSIBILITIES AFTER DRUG ADMINISTRATION

After the administration of any type of drug, you are responsible for the following:

- Immediately record the administration of the drug. This is particularly important when PRN drugs (especially opioids) are given to prevent duplication of drug application.
- Record (when necessary) any information concerning the administration of the drug, including information such as IV flow rate, the site used for parenteral administration, problems with administration (if any), and vital signs taken immediately before administration.
- Evaluate and record the client's response to the drug. Evaluation may include such facts as relief of pain, decrease in body temperature, relief of itching, and decrease in the number of stools passed.
- Observe for adverse reactions. The frequency of these observations depends on the drug administered. Record all suspected adverse reactions and report them to the primary care provider. Immediately report serious adverse reactions to the primary care provider.

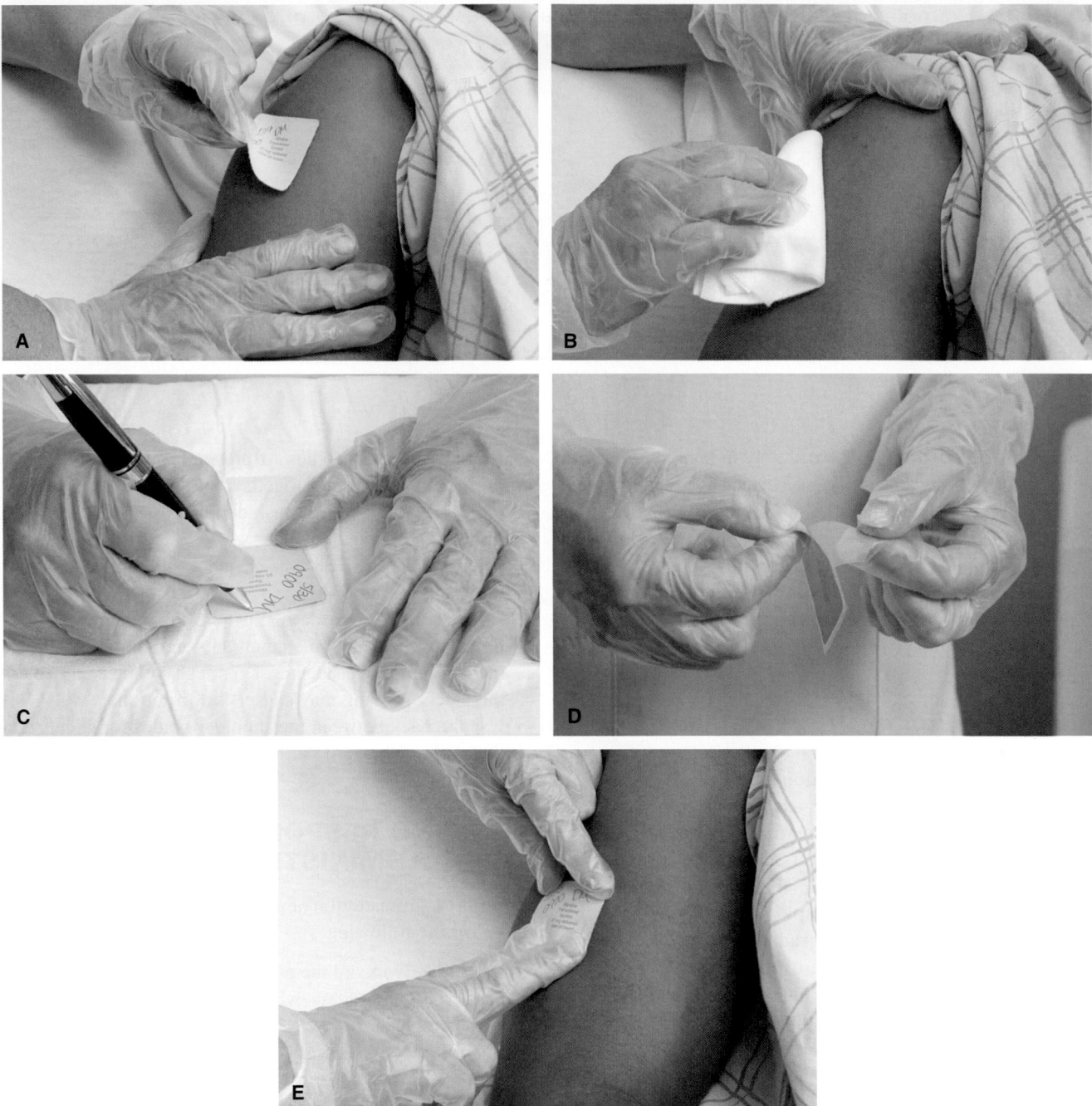

FIGURE 2.14 Transdermal drug delivery system. **A.** Find and remove a previously placed patch. **B.** Cleanse application site. **C.** Record date, time, and initials on the new patch. **D.** Remove protective covering. **E.** Apply new patch to hairless area of skin.

ADMINISTRATION OF DRUGS IN THE HOME

Often, drugs are not administered by the nurse in the home setting, but rather by the client or family members serving as caregivers. When this is the case, it is important that the client or caregivers understand the treatment regimen and are given an opportunity to ask questions concerning the drug therapy, such as why the drug was prescribed, how to administer the drug, and adverse reactions of the drug (see Chapter 5 for information concerning client and family education). When a client is taking a drug at home, special equipment or items may be needed in the home to administer the drug. Client Teaching for Improved Outcomes: Assessing the Home for Safe Drug Use gives some guidelines to follow when drugs are administered in the home by the client or caregiver, rather than by the nurse.

Client Teaching for Improved Outcomes

Assessing the Home for Safe Drug Use
For most clients, drugs will be prescribed after discharge to be taken at home. Because the home is not a controlled environment like a health care facility, you should assess the client's home environment carefully to ensure complete safety. It is important to keep in mind the following when making a home safety assessment:

✔ Does the home have a space for medicines that is relatively free of clutter and easily accessible to the client or a caregiver?
✔ Is there a cool, dry area that is not in direct sunlight for medication storage? Avoid humid areas such as a bathroom.
✔ Do small children live in or visit the home? If so, is there a place where drugs can be stored safely out of their reach?
✔ Does the drug require refrigeration? If so, does the refrigerator work?
✔ If the client needs several drugs, can the client or caregiver identify which drugs are used and when?
✔ Do they know how to use them and why?
✔ Does the client need special equipment, such as needles and syringes? If so, where and how can the equipment be stored for safety and convenience?
✔ Does the client have an appropriate disposal container? Will the refuse be safe from children and pets?
  • Suggest using plastic storage containers with snap-on lids made especially for home syringe disposal.
  • Advise the client to use an impervious container with a properly fitting lid, such as a plastic milk jug, for safe disposal of needles.
  • Advise the client of Sharps Disposal Programs in the area. These may be at local pharmacies, police and fire stations, or local health care centers.

KEY POINTS

■ The nurse administering the drug is responsible for all steps in preparing the drug including the right (correct) client, drug, dose, route, and time (the five rights). Document the administration immediately upon giving the drug to prevent inadvertent drug errors.

■ Standard practice is to use two identifiers (means to identify who the client is) before administering a medication. The client room number should never be used as one of the client identifiers.

■ Be aware that drug names may look or sound alike.

■ When taking medication orders, confirm verbal orders with a "read back" confirmation and make efforts to get the orders in writing before the drug is administered. Always question unclear orders before administration.

■ Nurses are the last defense in preventing medication errors before the drug is administered. Using methods to reduce distraction and better identify clients and drugs helps to reduce errors.

■ Automation and use of bar coding in the administration of medications helps reduce drug errors.

■ Medications are given orally, via tube into the GI system, parenterally, through the skin, or by inhalation. Many drugs can be given by multiple routes to best meet client needs. Each method has specific steps associated with it to ensure the best absorption of the medication.

CHAPTER REVIEW

Prepare for the NCLEX

RECALL THE FACTS

1. The nurse correctly documents administration of a drug
   _____.
   1. at the beginning of the shift
   2. when preparing to give the drug
   3. immediately after giving the drug
   4. at the end of the shift

2. The nurse is to administer aspirin 325 mg now. This is an example of what type of order?
   1. standing order
   2. single order
   3. PRN order
   4. STAT order

3. An IM injection is correctly administered by _____.
   1. displacing the skin to the side before making the injection
   2. using a 1-in. needle
   3. inserting the needle at a 90° angle
   4. using a 25-gauge needle
4. When preparing a drug for subcutaneous administration, the nurse should be aware that the usual volume of a drug injected by the subcutaneous route is _____.
   1. less than 0.5 mL
   2. 0.5–1 mL
   3. 2–5 mL
   4. 3–4 mL
5. The nurse explains to a client receiving an IV injection that the action of the drug occurs _____.
   1. in 5–10 min
   2. in 15–20 min
   3. within 30 min
   4. almost immediately
6. The best placement of a transdermal patch for a client with dementia is the _____.
   1. abdomen
   2. back
   3. chest
   4. upper arm

ANALYZE THE FACTS

7. *A new long-term care center is being built, and the nurse is requested to help in planning the medication administration system. Which is the most cost-effective system to use to prevent errors in this facility?
   1. automated dispensing medication carts
   2. bar-code identification bracelets
   3. "Do Not Disturb" apparel
   4. two-identifier client system
8. *When administering a drug, the nurse _____.
   1. should check the drug label two times before administration
   2. ask the client to identify themselves
   3. may administer a drug prepared by another nurse
   4. may crush any tablet that the client is unable to swallow

ALTERNATE-FORMAT QUESTIONS

9. Identify selected items the nurse uses as part of the "five rights" of medication administration. **Select all that apply.**
   1. right language
   2. right route
   3. right client
   4. right time
10. Identify which items you can use for client identification before giving a medication. **Select all that apply.**
    1. client room number
    2. medical record number
    3. date of birth
    4. maiden name of client

To check your answers, see Appendix F.

_____

*Indicates the question is directly linked to the NCLEX-PN test plan in Appendix G.

WANT TO KNOW MORE? A wide variety of resources are available to enhance your learning and understanding of this chapter.
- Visit for the**Point** resources such as:
  - NCLEX-Style Student Review Questions
  - Journal Articles
  - Dosage Calculations
  - Drug Monographs
  - Watch and Learn Videos
  - Concepts in Action Animations
- The *Study Guide to Accompany Introductory Clinical Pharmacology,* 12th edition, sold separately, will help you review and apply essential content.
- ✓*PrepU* is available to help students prepare for the NCLEX-PN examination.

3

Making Drug Dosing Safer

Key Terms

denominator part of a fraction representing the total number of parts (the number under the line)

dimensional analysis newer method of calculating drug dosages based on fractions

dosage strength amount of drug in the given form, such as tablet or capsule

gram mass metric measure equivalent to one thousandth of a kilogram

liter metric measure of volume, roughly equivalent to a quart in household measure

manual redundancy system process of medication prescription and delivery in which each person checks the drug dosage for accuracy

meter metric measure of distance

metric system system of measurement based on units of 10

numerator part of a fraction representing the number of parts taken (the number above the line)

parenteral administered in the body without using the mouth or gastrointestinal system

solvent fluid in which a solid dissolves; also called the diluent

Learning Objectives

On completion of this chapter, the student will:

1. Explain how safety is provided by the use of systematic processes in drug administration.
2. Identify information on a drug label used for calculating drug dosages.
3. Describe the importance of labeling numbers during the calculation process.
4. Accurately perform mathematical calculations when they are necessary to compute drug dosages.

Accurate dosage calculations are critical to the health of a client who is receiving medications. When drugs are administered, it is important that the numbers used and the answers obtained are correct. Unlike an error on a math test in school, there is no partial credit for simple arithmetic errors or incomplete answers in dosage conversions and calculations. Harm, and even death, can result from an error in a drug dosage calculation.

Information about the process of drug preparation for administration and calculation is examined in this chapter. Many textbooks are designed to teach the methodology of dosage calculations; this chapter is meant to teach the process involved in obtaining and preparing the dose of the drug and includes math as a review and supplement to that instruction. Examples of drug dose calculations are provided throughout the ensuing chapters to test your ability to properly complete the math.

SYSTEMATICALLY CHECKING ACCURACY

It has been estimated that 1 in 10,000 hospital deaths occur each year in the United States owing to mistakes made *specifically when calculating a drug dosage.* Human error is often the blame for these miscalculations. Fatigue, distraction, and stress all may contribute to errors made by health care providers (Carlton & Blegen, 2006). Factors in the work environment often contribute to errors made by people. These factors include poor lighting, noise, interruptions, and a taxing workload (Shahrokhi et al., 2013). We should be aware of all of these elements of our environment when preparing or calculating any drug regardless of how minor the dose or type of drug.

To reduce errors, technological changes such as computerized order entry and bar-coding systems can detect errors made by health care providers. However, the best method of error detection is the **manual redundancy system**. This is a system in which each person in the process of medication prescription and delivery checks the drug dosage for accuracy. Nurses use this system when they perform the

"5 rights and 3 checks" to catch a potential error in drug administration. Although nurses may not be responsible for the initial mixing, packaging, or delivery of a medication, 95% of potential dose calculation errors are found during manual redundancy checks. When a nurse checks the dose calculation of a drug, during preparation or at the bedside, a serious error can be detected before it reaches the client.

CALCULATING DRUG DOSES SAFELY

You should always systematically look at the process of drug delivery to calculate drug doses safely by doing the following:

1. Recognize the way drugs are packaged and how to look for the information on the labels needed to calculate drug doses.
2. Look at the orders and how these are presented on the medication administration record (MAR).

The focus of this chapter is to help you learn to recognize essential information from drug labels. Basic mathematical calculations are provided in Appendix E if you need to review them.

Reading Drug Labels

Drug labels give important information used to obtain the correct dosage. Although labels contain a great amount of information about the drug being given, three specific items are needed to administer a drug: the name, form, and dosage strength.

Drug labels may contain two names: the trade (brand) name and the generic name (see Chapter 1). The trade name is usually capitalized, written first on the label, and identified by the registration symbol. The generic name is written in smaller print, often in parentheses, and usually located under the trade name. Drugs may be prescribed by either the trade name or the generic name. Often the generic drug is less expensive than the brand-name drug (companies that make generic-only drugs do not include a trade name on the label). If the primary health care provider does not specify that a substitution *cannot* be made, it is likely that a generic version of the drug will be dispensed to reduce the cost to the client. Problems can arise if a client recognizes the brand name of a drug but does not know the generic name and refuses the medication. Therefore, it is important to know the generic name of drugs and always check for brand-name versions if the client questions the prescription.

Question #1

Use the label in Figure 3.1 to identify the brand and generic names for this drug. (*See* Appendix F *for answer.*)

The unit dose is the most common type of labeling seen in hospitals. The unit dose is a method of dispensing drugs in which each capsule or tablet is packaged separately. On the label, the type of preparation will be specified; in other words, it will list the drug as a capsule, tablet, or other form of the drug.

At times the drug will come to the nursing unit in a container with a number of capsules or tablets or as a solution. The nurse must then determine the number of capsules/tablets or the amount of solution to administer. Therefore, the nurse must know the amount of drug in each tablet or capsule (**dosage strength**). The dosage strength is also given on the container. The dosage strength is used to calculate the number of tablets or the amount of solution to administer.

Question #2

Use the label in Figure 3.1 to identify the form of the drug and the dosage strength. (*See* Appendix F *for answer.*)

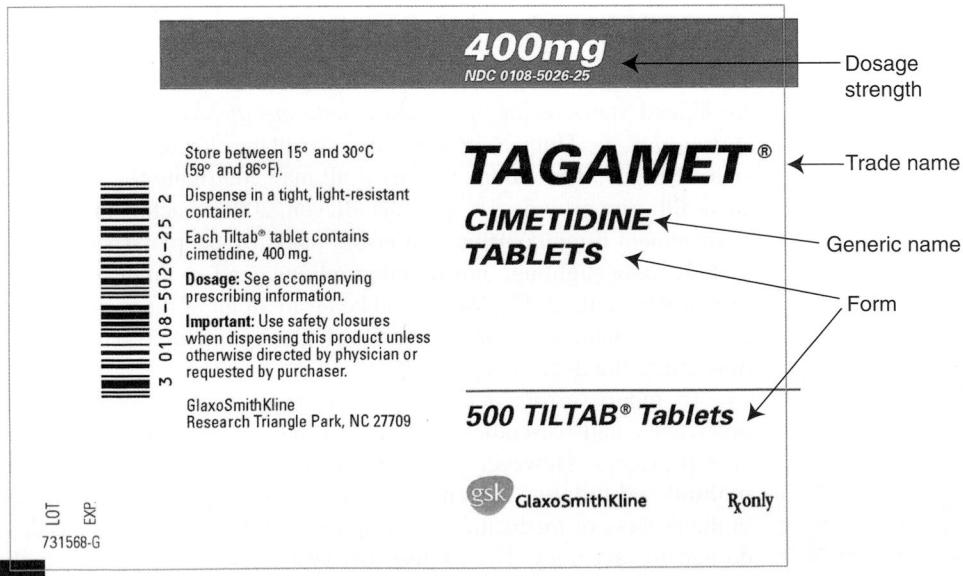

FIGURE 3.1 Standard drug label. (Courtesy of GlaxoSmithKline.)

Mathematical Ability

Nurses find that mathematical calculations are performed using various methods to prepare drugs for administration. Sometimes the math is relatively simple, and a calculation can be done quickly in one's head. When distractions are present or if conversions are involved, the nurse may use a pen and paper to handwrite out the mathematical equations needed to determine the correct dose. A nurse may use a number of steps in the calculation of a medication and find that a calculator is helpful to hasten the process. When using any of these methods, it is important for the nurse to understand the basic concepts of the dose calculation to ensure the right answer is obtained.

In the remainder of this chapter a variety of calculation methods are presented. Try the calculations with the different formulas to discover the best way for you to calculate drug doses. See Appendix E for a review of basic mathematical concepts if you have difficulty understanding the math involved with the calculations.

Basic Formula Method of Dosage Calculation

Once the nurse has identified the basic information about the drug, the calculation can be performed to prepare the drug.

Calculation #1

Looking at the label in Figure 3.1, use this information to solve the following dose problem:

The primary health care provider orders: 400 mg of cimetidine after each meal. How many tablets will the nurse administer following breakfast? (*See Appendix F for answer.*)

Although most hospital pharmacies dispense drugs as single doses or in a unit dose system, on occasion you must compute a drug dosage because it differs from the dose of the drug that is available. This is particularly true of long-term care facilities, of outpatient clinics, and in the home where the dose may be changed periodically or in situations in which having multiple dosage strengths of a particular drug for the client would be costly.

Calculation #2

Looking at the label in Figure 3.1, use this information to solve the following dose problem:

The primary health care provider changes the order after late morning rounds: 800 mg of cimetidine after each meal. How many tablets will the nurse now administer after meals? (*See Appendix F for answer.*)

Some nurses can do this type of calculation in their heads; others find it helpful to do the problem by hand on paper. This is especially helpful when the dosage ordered by the primary health care provider may not be available.

Basic Formula Method by Hand

To find the correct dosage of a solid oral preparation, such as a tablet, the following formula may be used:

$$\frac{\text{dose desired}}{\text{dose on hand}} = \text{dose administered}\left(\text{the unknown or X}\right)$$

This formula may be abbreviated as:

$$\frac{\text{D}}{\text{H}} = \text{X}$$

When the dose ordered by the primary health care provider (dose desired) is written in the same *measurement* as the dose on the drug container (dose on hand) (e.g., they are both milligrams), then these two figures may be inserted into the formula without changes.

Example

The primary health care provider orders cimetidine 800 mg (milligrams). The drug is available as cimetidine 400 mg (milligrams). We put numbers in place of letters in the above equation.

$$\frac{800\,\text{mg}\left(\text{dose desired}\right)}{400\,\text{mg}\left(\text{dose on hand}\right)} = 2 \text{ tablets of 400 mg cimetidine}$$

Question #3

Try a different dose problem, using the label in Figure 3.2 solve the following problem.

Looking at the label, find the drug name, form, and dosage strength. (*See for Appendix F answer.*)

When looking up drug names, you will see the use of capital or TALLman letters on the label of medications that may be easily confused with names of other drugs. Confusion with drug name can result in errors, such as the example below where an antipsychotic drug could be confused with a hay fever relief medication. The TALLman letters are used to spell out the portion of the drug name that distinguishes the difference in the drug names. In Figure 3.2 the end of the drug Zy**PREXA** is in TALLman letters to prevent confusion with another drug named ZyRTEC. Drug Summary Tables in each chapter will identify drugs that may look like other drugs. In addition, in the text some drugs that sound alike and may be confused with drugs of different categories will be listed, as LASA Alerts, to help you learn the differences. Appendix B, additionally, has a listing of drugs that use TALLman letters because the drug names look alike.

Calculation #3

Looking at the label in Figure 3.2, use this information to solve the following dose problem:

The primary health care provider orders: 10 mg ZyPREXA daily. How many tablets will the nurse administer? (*See Appendix F for answer.*)

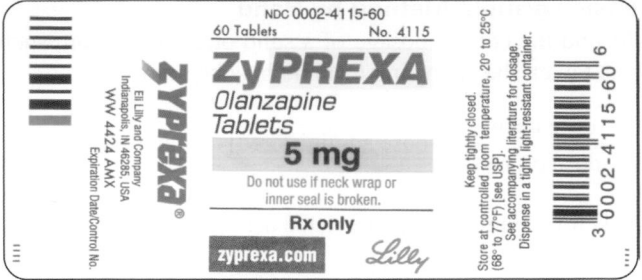

FIGURE 3.2 Drug label with TALLman lettering. (Courtesy of Lilly Company.)

UNDERSTANDING THE METRIC SYSTEM OF MEASUREMENT

Since the majority of medications are prepared using the **metric system**, it is important for the nurse to understand this system of measurement. To review, there are three systems of measurement sometimes associated with drug dosing: (1) the metric system, (2) the apothecary system, and (3) household measurements. The metric system is covered here with reference to the other two systems.

The metric system is the most commonly used system of measurement in medicine. In the metric system, the **gram** is the unit of weight, the **liter** the unit of volume, and the **meter** the unit of length. Box 3.1 lists the measurements used in the metric system. The acceptable abbreviations for the measurements are given in parentheses in Box 3.1.

At one time, the apothecary system was used for medical weight measurement. In 1994, recommendations made by the Institute for Safe Medication Practices (ISMP) eliminated this system because of the high rate of medication errors it produced, yet still today we continue to see mention of this system (information about this system can be found in Appendix E). The household system is rarely used in a hospital setting but may be used to measure drug dosages in the home.

BOX 3.1   Metric Measurements

Weight
The unit of weight is the gram.
    1 kilogram (kg) = 1000 grams (g)
    1 gram (g) = 1000 milligrams (mg)
    1 milligram (mg) = 1000 micrograms (mcg)

Volume
The unit of volume is the liter.
    1 deciliter (dL) = 10 liters (L)
    1 liter (L) = 1000 milliliters (mL)
    1 milliliter (mL) = 0.001 liter (L)

Length
The unit of length is the meter.
    1 meter (m) = 100 centimeters (cm)
    1 centimeter (cm) = 0.01 meters (m)
    1 millimeter (mm) = 0.001 meters (m)

Ratio and Proportion Method of Dosage Calculation
Converting Units for Calculation

When using this basic formula, calculations are solved using fractions. What is important to remember is that the **numerator** and the **denominator** must be of like terms—for example, milligrams over milligrams NOT milligrams over grams. Therefore, the first step to setting up a problem is to check and see if both parts of the fraction are in *like terms*.

> **! NURSING ALERT**
>
> Errors made by nurses in using this and other drug formulas will be reduced if the entire dose is labeled rather than just writing the numbers.

$$\frac{0.5\,g}{250\,mg} \text{ rather than } \frac{0.5}{250}$$

This will eliminate the possibility of using unlike terms in the fraction.

Instead of looking at a drug label for this example, use this information about a drug order to learn the following method of dosage calculation and conversion.

Example

The primary health care provider orders ascorbic acid (vitamin C) 0.5 g, and the drug container label reads ascorbic acid 250 mg per tablet.

As you can see, the order reads ascorbic acid 0.5 g and the drug container is labeled ascorbic acid 250 mg, a conversion of grams to milligrams is necessary to perform the dose calculation. A nurse may be able to perform this calculation without writing it down. If it is done by hand, the proportion and a known equivalent are set up in a ratio and used for this type of conversion.

Ratio and Proportion Method by Hand

Example

Convert 0.5 gram (g) to milligrams (mg); using proportion and the known equivalent 1000 mg = 1 g. Set up the ratio:

$$\frac{1000\,mg}{1\,g} = \frac{X\,mg}{0.5\,g}$$
$$X = 1000 \times 0.5$$
$$X = 500\,mg$$

Therefore, 0.5 gram (g) equals 500 milligrams (mg). After changing 0.5 g–500 mg, use the basic method formula:

$$\frac{D}{H} = X$$

Now replace the letters with numbers in the equation.

$$\frac{500\,mg}{250\,mg} = 2 \text{ tablets of 250 mg ascorbic acid}$$

Safeguard in Preventing Errors

To prevent dose calculation errors, many manufacturers include both levels of measurement (grams and milligrams) on the label if the drug is frequently ordered in doses different from the size dispensed (Fig. 3.3). This is very important when doses are in small amounts such as micrograms (mcg). Again, manufacturers typically include the dose strength in both units of measurement (milligrams and micrograms). Even when both are included, the nurse should perform the calculation to double check that the dose is correct.

Errors are a frequent problem when zeros (0) are involved. When there is no number to the left of the decimal, a zero is written, for example, 0.25. Although in general mathematics the zero may not be required, it should be used in the writing of all drug doses. *Use of the zero lessens the chance of drug errors,* especially when the dose of a drug is hurriedly written and the decimal point is indistinct.

For example, if a drug order is written as digoxin (Lanoxin) **.25 mg** instead of digoxin **0.25 mg**, the order might be interpreted as **25 mg**, which is 100 times the prescribed dose.

Question #4

Use the label in Figure 3.3 to understand the following example.

Looking at the label, find the drug name, form, and dosage strength in both units of measurement. (*See Appendix F for answer.*)

Calculation #4

Looking at the label in Figure 3.3, use this information to solve the following dose problem:

The primary health care provider orders: 0.50 mg of digoxin daily. How many tablets will the nurse administer? (*See Appendix F for answer.*)

If this calculation is confusing, return to the Ratio and Proportion Method of Dosage Calculation section. Substitute the digoxin values for the ascorbic acid numbers. Does this help you understand the dosage calculation?

DRUGS IN LIQUID FORM

Drugs may be ordered in liquid form for many reasons: The client is a child, the drug is to be put in a feeding tube or injected directly into the tissues or intravenous (IV) line (**parenteral**), or the client is too ill to swallow a solid form of the drug like a tablet. In these situations, the drug is made in a solution form.

Solutions

A solution is made by dissolving a solute into a **solvent**. Usually, water is used as the solvent for preparing a solution unless another liquid is specified. Today, most solutions are prepared by a clinical pharmacist or the manufacturer and not by the nurse. It is important for the nurse to understand how the solutions are prepared and labeled.

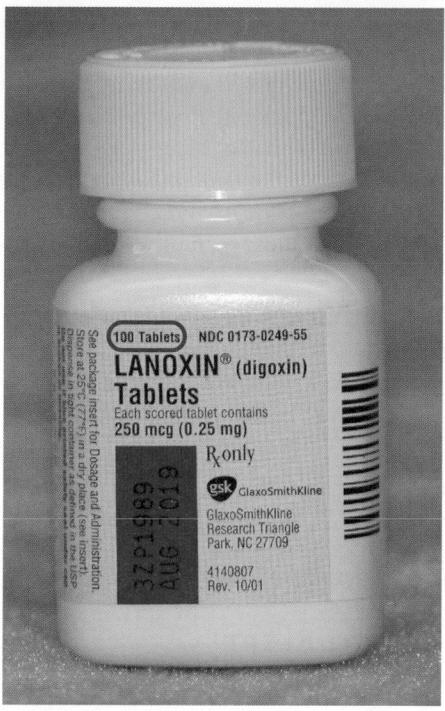

FIGURE 3.3 Drug label with dose equivalent noted (both mcg and mg). (From Kronenberger, J., & Ledbetter, J. (2016). *Lippincott Williams & Wilkins' comprehensive medical assisting* (5th ed). Wolters Kluwer.)

Examples of how solutions may be labeled include:

- 10 mg/mL—10 mg of the drug in each milliliter
- 1:1000—a solution strength of 1 part of the drug per 1000 parts of solvent
- 5 mg/teaspoon—5 mg of the drug in each teaspoon of solution (home use)

Parenteral Drug Dosage Forms

Drugs for parenteral use must be in liquid form before they are administered. Parenteral drugs may be available in the following forms (Fig. 3.4):

1. As liquids in disposable cartridges or syringes that contain a specific amount of a drug in a specific volume, for example, meperidine 50 mg/mL. *After administration, the cartridge or syringe is discarded.*

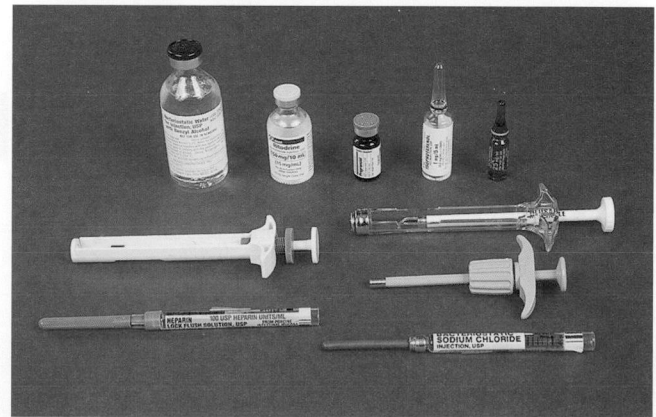

FIGURE 3.4 Drug preparations in solution form: (top row) vials and ampules; (middle/bottom rows) prefilled cartridges and holders.

2. In ampules or vials that contain a specific amount of the liquid form of the drug in a specific volume. The vials may be single-dose vials or multidose vials. *A multidose vial contains more than one dose of the drug.*

3. In ampules or vials that contain powder or crystals, to which *a liquid (called a diluent) must be added before the drug can be removed from the vial* and administered. Vials may be single-dose or multidose vials.

Dose Calculations With Liquids

With drugs in liquid form, there is a specific amount of drug in a given volume of solution. In Figure 3.5, for example, the dosage strength of Augmentin is 125 mg in 5 mL of solution (typically written as 125 mg/5 mL). Instead of labeling the drug in one unit of measure (tablet or capsule), the drug is written as a specific amount of drug in a specific *quantity* of solution. For example, if the label states that there is 125 mg/5 mL, 5 mL is the *quantity* (or volume) in which there is 125 mg of this drug.

> ## ⓘ NURSING ALERT
>
> Use "mL" instead of "ml" when writing the abbreviation for milliliters. This prevents the error of ml being misread as m 1 or meter 1.

The basic formula for computing the dosage of liquids is:

$$\frac{\text{dose desired}}{\text{dose on hand}} \times \text{quantity} = \text{volume administered}$$

This may be abbreviated as

$$\frac{D}{H} \times Q = X$$

The quantity (or Q) in this formula is the amount of liquid in which the available drug is contained.

Question #5

Use the label in Figure 3.5 to understand the following example. **Looking at the label, find the drug name, form, and dosage strength.** (*See Appendix F for answer.*)

Calculation #5

Looking at the label in Figure 3.5, use this information to solve the following dose problem:

The primary health care provider orders: Augmentin 125 mg 4 times daily. How many mL (milliliters) will the nurse administer in each dose? (*See Appendix F for answer.*)

As with the other example using tablets and capsules, the prescribed dose of the drug may not be the same as what is on hand (or available). For example, the primary health care provider may order 500 mg Augmentin and the drug is labeled as 125 mg/5 mL.

$$\frac{D}{H} \times Q = X \left(\text{the liquid amount to be given}\right)$$

Now fill in the numbers to this equation. You desire (D) 500 mg of Augmentin and have (H) 125 mg. The 5 mL is the amount (quantity or Q) that contains 125 mg of the drug.

$$\frac{500 \text{ mg}}{125 \text{ mg}} \times 5 \text{ mL} = X$$

Reduce the fractions and multiply, here is the answer.

$$\frac{4 \text{ mg}}{1 \text{ mg}} \times 5 \text{ mL} = 20 \text{ mL}$$

Therefore, 20 mL contains the desired dose of 500 mg of Augmentin.

Wasting Parenteral Drugs From Disposable Syringes or Cartridges

In some instances, the specific dosage strength is not available and it will be necessary to administer less than the amount contained in the syringe.

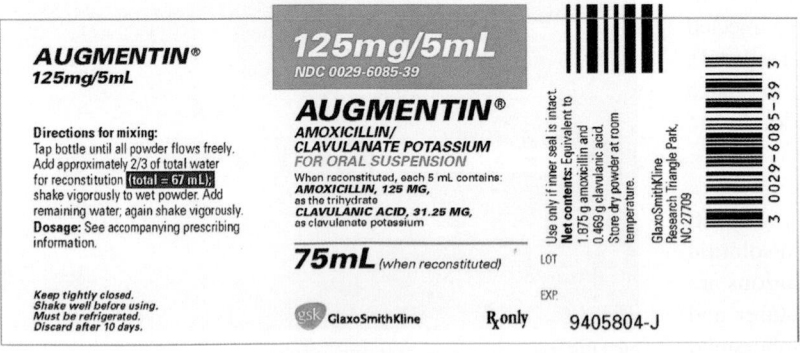

FIGURE 3.5 Drug label in solution. (Courtesy of GlaxoSmithKline.)

Example

The physician orders diazepam 5 mg IM. The drug is available as a 2-mL disposable syringe labeled 5 mg/mL. Set up the equation then replace the letters with the appropriate numbers.

$$\frac{D}{H} \times Q = X$$

$$\frac{5 \text{ mg}}{10 \text{ mg}} \times 2 \text{ mL} = X$$

Reduce the fractions and multiply, here is the answer.

$$X = \frac{1}{2} \times 2 = 1 \text{ mL}$$

Note in this example the syringe contains 2 mL of the solution with a total of 10 mg of the drug in the syringe and because *each* mL contains 5 mg of the drug, there is more than the client needs in the disposable syringe Therefore, half of the liquid in the syringe (1 mL) is discarded, and the remaining half (1 mL) is administered to the client as the prescribed dose of 5 mg.

Parenteral Drugs in Ampules and Vials

If the drug is in liquid form in the ampule or vial, the desired amount is withdrawn from the ampule or vial. In some instances, the entire amount is used; in others, only part of the total amount is withdrawn from the ampule or vial and administered.

Whenever the dose to be administered is different from that listed on the label, the volume to be administered must be calculated. To determine the volume to be administered, the formula for liquid preparations is used. The calculations are the same as those given in the preceding section for parenteral drugs in disposable syringes or cartridges.

Example

The physician orders chlorpromazine 12.5 mg IM. Use the equation from the previous example and substitute these number values in place of the letters in the equation. Reduce the fractions and multiply, here are the calculations leading up to your answer.

The drug is available as chlorpromazine 25 mg/1 mL in a 1-mL ampule.

$$\frac{D}{H} \times Q = X$$

$$\frac{12.5 \text{ mg}}{25 \text{ mg}} \times 1 \text{ mL} = X$$

Reduce the fraction and multiply, here is the answer.

$$\frac{1}{2} \times 1 \text{ mL} = \frac{1}{2} \text{mL} \left(\text{or } 0.5 \text{ mL} \right) \text{volume to be administered}$$

In this example, 0.5 mL is the amount of solution that contains the dose 12.5 mg of the drug. Using a syringe, 0.5 mL of the solution is withdrawn. Because you cannot store medications once an ampule has been opened, the remainder of the drug is discarded.

Example

The physician orders hydroxyzine 12.5 mg. The drug is available as hydroxyzine 25 mg/mL in 10-mL vials. In this calculation, set up the equation from the previous example and see if you can start by using only the number values in place of the letters in the basic equation.

$$\frac{12.5 \text{ mg}}{25 \text{ mg}} \times 1 \text{ mL} = \frac{1}{2} \text{mL} \left(\text{or } 0.5 \text{ mL} \right)$$

Using a syringe, 0.5 mL is withdrawn from the 10-mL multidose vial and administered. The amount in this or any multidose vial is *not* entered into the equation. What is entered into the equation as quantity (Q) is the amount of the available drug that is contained in a specific volume.

Parenteral Drugs in Dry Form

Some parenteral drugs are not available in solution, but instead as a crystal or a powder, because they are not stable in liquid form. They come in ampules or vials in dry form (for longer storage) and are then made into a solution (reconstituted) shortly before they are removed and administered. Often the drug is in a container with both the powder and liquid separated by a barrier that is broken right before mixing and administering. If the drug is not dispensed in this form, the product directions for reconstitution on the label or on the enclosed package insert should be included with the drug. The manufacturer may give the following information for reconstitution: (1) the name of the diluent(s) that must be used with the drug or (2) the amount of diluent that must be added to the drug.

In some instances, the manufacturer supplies a diluent with the drug. If a diluent is supplied, no other stock diluent should be used. Before a drug is reconstituted, the label is carefully checked for instructions.

Reconstitution

Use the label in Figure 3.5 to understand how dry powder drugs are reconstituted. To make the Augmentin into a solution 67 mL of sterile water is added to the powder and mixed. When reconstituted 5 mL contains approximately 25 mg of amoxicillin and 31.25 mg of clavulanate potassium (the components of the drug Augmentin). If there is any doubt about the reconstitution of the dry form of a drug, and there are no manufacturer's directions, the clinical pharmacist should be consulted.

Once a diluent is added, the volume to be administered is determined. In some cases, the entire amount is given; in others, a part (or fraction) of the total amount contained in the vial or ampule is given.

After reconstitution of any multidose vial, the following information *must* be added to the label:

- Amount of diluent added
- Dose of drug in mL (500 mg/mL, 10 mg/2 mL, etc.)
- Date of reconstitution
- Expiration date (the date after which any unused solution is discarded)

DOSAGE CALCULATION USING DIMENSIONAL ANALYSIS

Dimensional analysis (DA) is a method to perform calculations where the focus is on the elimination of units of measure, thereby eliminating the need to memorize equations. Because the units are set up in a specific order, it eliminates the need to be concerned about setting up proportions correctly. When using DA to calculate dosage problems, dosages are written as common fractions. For example:

$$\frac{1\ mL}{4\ mg}\ \frac{5\ mL}{10\ mg}\ \frac{1\ tablet}{100\ mg}$$

When written as common fractions, the numerator is the top number. In the example above, 1 mL, 5 mL, and 1 tablet are the numerators.

The numbers on the bottom are called denominators. In the example above, 4, 10, and 100 mg are denominators.

Example

The primary health care provider orders 10 mg of diazepam. The drug comes in a dosage strength of 5 mg/mL. How many milliliters would the nurse administer?

Step 1. To work this problem using DA, always begin by **identifying the unit of measure** to be calculated. The unit to be calculated will be milliliters if the drug is to be administered parenterally. Another drug form is the solid, and the unit of measure would be a tablet or capsule. In this problem, the **unit of measure to be calculated is milliliters**.

Step 2. Write the identified unit of measure to be calculated, followed by an equal sign. In this problem, milliliter is the unit to be calculated, so the nurse writes:

$$mL =$$

Step 3. Next, the dosage strength is written with the numerator **always expressed in the same unit that was identified before the equal sign.** For example:

$$mL = \frac{1\ mL}{5\ mg}$$

Step 4. Continue by writing the next fraction with the numerator having the same unit of measure as the denominator in the previous fraction. For example, our problem continues:

$$mL = \frac{1\ mL}{5\ mg} \times \frac{10\ mg}{X\ mL}$$

In this step, the "mg" cancel each other out and can be eliminated.

Step 5. The problem is solved by multiplication of the two fractions.

$$mL = \frac{1\ mL}{5\ mg} \times \frac{10\ mg}{X\ mL}\ or\ \frac{1\ mL \times 10}{5}\ reduce\ to\ \frac{2}{1} = 2\ mL$$

NOTE: Each alternate denominator and numerator cancel, with only the final unit remaining.

Here is another example of dosage calculation using the DA method.

Example

Ordered: 200,000 Units
On hand: Drug labeled 400,000 Units/mL

$$mL = \frac{1\ mL}{400,000\ U} \times \frac{200,000\ U}{X\ mL} = \frac{1}{2}\ mL\ or\ 0.5\ mL$$

Metric Conversions Using Dimensional Analysis

Occasionally, the primary health care provider may order a drug in one unit of measure, whereas the drug is available in another unit of measure.

Example

The physician orders 0.4 mg of atropine. The drug label reads 400 mcg per 1 mL. This dosage problem is solved by expanding the DA equation, repeating two steps to the equation.

Step 1. As above, begin by writing the unit of measure to be calculated, followed by an equal sign.

Step 2. Next, express the dosage strength as a fraction with the numerator having the same unit of measure as the number before the equal sign.

$$mL = \frac{1\ mL}{400\ mcg}$$

Step 3. Continue by writing the next fraction with the numerator having the same unit of measure as the denominator in the previous fraction.

$$mL = \frac{1\ mL}{400\ mcg} \times \frac{mcg}{mg}$$

Step 4. Expand the equation by filling in the missing numbers using the appropriate equivalent. In this problem, the equivalent would be 1000 mcg = 1 mg. This will convert micrograms to milligrams.

$$mL = \frac{1\ mL}{400\ mcg} \times \frac{1000\ mcg}{1\ mg}$$

Repeat steps 3 and 4. Continue with the equation by placing the next fraction, beginning with the unit of measure of the denominator of the previous fraction.

$$mL = \frac{1\ mL}{400\ mcg} \times \frac{1000\ mcg}{1\ mg} \times \frac{0.4\ mg}{X\ mL}$$

When possible, cancel out the units, leaving only mL.

Step 5. Solve the problem by multiplication. Cancel out the numbers when possible.

$$mL = \frac{1\ mL}{400\ mcg} \times \frac{1000\ mcg}{1\ mg} \times \frac{0.4\ mg}{X\ mL} = \frac{400}{400X} = 1\ mL$$

Solve the following problems using DA. Refer to the equivalents table if necessary (see Box 3.1).

Again, follow this example.

Example

Ordered: 250 mg
On hand: Drug labeled 1 g per 1 mL

$$mL = \frac{1\ mL}{1\ g} \times \frac{1\ mcg}{1000\ mg} \times \frac{250\ mg}{X\ mL} = \frac{1\ mL}{4} = 0.25\ mL$$

ADDITIONAL METHODS USED IN CALCULATION OF DRUG DOSAGES

Pediatric Dosages

The dosages of drugs given to children are usually less than those given to adults. The dosage may be based on age, weight, or body surface area (BSA). Today, most pediatric dosages are clearly given by the manufacturer, thus eliminating the need for formulas, except for determining the dosage of some drugs based on the child's weight or BSA.

Drug Dosages Based on Weight

The dosage of an oral or parenteral drug may be based on the client's weight. In many instances, references give the dosage based on the weight in kilograms (kg) rather than pounds (lb) (to convert pounds to kilograms you need to know the conversion equivalent, 2.2 lb = 1 kg). Knowing this kilogram to pound conversion will be helpful when you teach parents to administer medications to their children based on weight.

When the dosage of a drug is based on weight, the primary health care provider or clinical pharmacist, in most instances, computes and orders the dosage to be given. However, errors can occur for any number of reasons. The nurse should be able to calculate a drug dosage based on weight to detect any type of error that may have been made in the prescribing or dispensing of a drug whose dosage is based on weight.

Example

To convert a known weight in pounds to kilograms, divide the known weight by 2.2.
Client's weight in pounds is 135:

$$\frac{135}{2.2} = 61.36\ (\text{or}\ 61.4)\ kg$$

Calculation #6

Determine the client's weight in kilograms when the client weighs 142 lb. (*See Appendix F for answer.*)
Determine the child's weight in kilograms when the child weighs 43 lb. (*See Appendix F for answer.*)

Once the weight is converted to pounds or kilograms, this information is used to determine drug dosage.

Example

A drug dosage is 5 mg/kg/day. The client weighs 135 lb, which is converted to 61.4 kg.

$$61.4\ kg \times 5\ mg = 307\ mg$$

DA also can be used:

$$mg = \frac{5\ mg}{1\ kg} \times \frac{61.4\ kg}{X\ mg} = 307\ mg$$

Here is another drug problem to try. A drug dosage is 60 mg/kg/day in three equally divided doses. In this case, the client weighs 143 lb, which is converted to 65 kg.

$$65\ kg \times 60\ mg = \frac{3900\ mg}{day}$$

$$3900\ mg \div 3\ (\text{doses per day}) = 1300\ mg\ \text{each dose}$$

Body Surface Area

If the drug dosage is based on BSA (m^2), the same method of calculation may be used.

Charts (called nomograms, see Appendix E) are used to determine the BSA in square meters according to the child's height and weight. Once the BSA is determined, the following formula is used:

$$\frac{\text{surface area of the child in square meters}}{\text{surface area of an adult in square meters}}$$
$$\times\ \text{usual adult dose} = \text{pediatric dose}$$

Example

A drug dosage is 60 mg/m^2 as a single IV injection.
The BSA of a client is determined by means of a nomogram for estimating BSA and is found to be 1.8 m^2. The physician orders 60 mg/m^2.

$$60\ mg \times 1.8\ m^2 = 108\ mg$$

DA can also be used:

$$mg = \frac{60\ mg}{1\ m^2} \times \frac{1.8\ m^2}{X\ mg} = 108\ mg$$

Temperatures

Two scales used in the measuring of temperatures are Fahrenheit (F) and Celsius (C) (also known as centigrade). On the Fahrenheit scale, the freezing point of water is 32 °F, and the boiling point of water is 212 °F. On the Celsius scale, 0 °C is the freezing point of water and 100 °C is the boiling point of water.

To convert from Celsius to Fahrenheit, the following formula may be used: F = 9/5 C + 32 (9/5 times the temperature in Celsius, then add 32).

Example

Convert 38 °C to Fahrenheit:

$$F = \frac{9}{5} \times 38° + 32$$

$$F = 68.4° + 32$$

$$F = 100.4°$$

To convert from Fahrenheit to Celsius, the following formula may be used: C = 5/9(F − 32) (5/9 times the temperature in Fahrenheit minus 32).

Example

Convert 100 °F to Celsius:

$$C = \frac{5}{9} \times (100 - 32)$$

$$C = \frac{5}{9} \times 68$$

$$F = 37.78° \text{ or } 37.8°$$

Household Measurements

When used, household measurements are for liquids or powders to make solutions. In the hospital, household measurements are rarely used because they are less accurate when used to measure drug dosages. On occasion, the nurse may use the pint, quart, or gallon when ordering, irrigating, or sterilizing solutions. For the ease of a client taking a drug at home, the physician may order a drug dosage in household measurements. Box 3.2 lists the more common household measurements.

BOX 3.2 Household Measurements

3 teaspoons = 1 tablespoon
2 tablespoons = 1 ounce
2 pints = 1 quart
4 quarts = 1 gallon

KEY POINTS

■ One in every 10,000 hospital deaths is a result of a drug calculation error.

■ Nurses systematically and repeatedly check for drug accuracy by performing the 5 rights and 3 checks when preparing to administer drugs to clients. Ninety-five percent of the time, an error will be found before the medication is given to the client.

■ Drug labels should always contain the name, form, and strength of a drug.

■ The metric system is the preferred dose system. Household measures may be used to simplify administration by family members in the home, and the apothecary system is rarely seen because of the higher rate of drug errors when used.

■ Nurses use basic, DA, and ratio/proportion formulas to calculate drug doses.

■ Numbers are always labeled (0.25 mg) when doing a calculation, especially if conversion between units is done. For safety purposes zeros before decimal points (0.25) should be used, as well as "mL" for milliliters.

■ Use specified diluents to make powders into solutions when needed, and always discard unused ampules. Vials should be dated when opened and solutions specified if mixed by the nurse.

CHAPTER REVIEW

Prepare for the NCLEX

RECALL THE FACTS

1. Manual redundancy activities help the nurse provide:
   1. control over dangerous drugs.
   2. safety by recognizing error.
   3. reassurance to the client.
   4. feedback to other providers.

2. What percentage of potential drug errors is found when nurses check medication calculations for accuracy?
   1. 25%
   2. 49%
   3. 67%
   4. 95%

3. Identify the portion of this drug label in **bold:**
   LANOXIN (digoxin) **Tablets**, 250 mcg (0.25 mg).
   1. Dose strength
   2. Trade name
   3. Generic name
   4. Form
4. Knowing both trade and generic drug names is important because:
   1. cost is reduced using generic drugs.
   2. only one name is provided on the drug label.
   3. primary health care providers do not know the differences.
   4. clients may think the drug is incorrect.
5. The ISMP discourages use of which measurement system?
   1. household
   2. metric
   3. apothecary
   4. BSA
6. Which of the following is the correct abbreviation for milligram?
   1. mg
   2. gm
   3. mL
   4. mcg
7. If the nurse has 2 mL remaining in an ampule. It should be _____.
   1. labeled and dated
   2. placed in the refrigerator
   3. thrown in a sharps container
   4. returned to client medication storage

ANALYZE THE FACTS

8. *Which of the following drug doses is written correctly?
   1. Lanoxin .25 mg orally
   2. Lanoxin .250 mg orally
   3. Lanoxin 0.25 mg orally
   4. Lanoxin 0.250 mg orally
9. *One gram of ascorbic acid (vitamin C) is equivalent to:
   1. 10,000 mg of ascorbic acid
   2. 1000 mg of ascorbic acid
   3. 100 mg of ascorbic acid
   4. 10 mg of ascorbic acid
10. *A child weighs 53 lb. How many kilograms would the child weigh? (Round to the nearest whole number.)
    1. 0.23 kg
    2. 24 kg
    3. 54 kg
    4. 117 kg

To check your answers, see Appendix F.

---

*Indicates the question is directly linked to the NCLEX-PN test plan in Appendix G.

WANT TO KNOW MORE? A wide variety of resources are available to enhance your learning and understanding of this chapter.
- Visit thePoint for resources such as:
  - NCLEX-Style Student Review Questions
  - Journal Articles
  - Dosage Calculations
  - Drug Monographs
  - Watch and Learn Videos
  - Concepts in Action Animations
- The *Study Guide to Accompany Introductory Clinical Pharmacology,* 12th edition, sold separately, will help you review and apply essential content.
- ✓*PrepU* is available to help students prepare for the NCLEX-PN examination.

4

The Nursing Process

Key Terms

analysis using data to determine client need or nursing diagnosis

assessment collection of subjective and objective data

evaluation decision-making process determining the effectiveness of nursing actions or interventions

expected outcome expected behavior and physical and mental state of the client after a therapeutic intervention

implementation carrying out of a plan of action

independent nursing actions actions that do not require a physician's orders

initial assessment gathering of baseline data

nursing diagnosis description of a client problem

nursing process framework for nursing action, consisting of a series of problem-solving steps, which helps members of the health care team provide effective and consistent client care

objective data information obtained through a physical assessment or physical examination, laboratory tests, or scans

ongoing assessment continuing assessment activities that proceed from the initial nursing assessment

planning design of steps to carry out nursing actions

subjective data information supplied by the client or family

Learning Objectives

On completion of this chapter, the student will:

1. List the five phases of the nursing process.
2. Discuss assessment, analysis, nursing diagnosis, planning, implementation, and evaluation as they apply to the administration of drugs.
3. Differentiate between objective and subjective data.
4. Identify common nursing diagnoses used in the administration of drugs and nursing interventions related to each diagnosis.

The **nursing process** is a framework for nursing action consisting of problem-solving steps that help members of the health care team provide effective client care. It is a specific and orderly plan used to gather data, identify client problems from the data, develop outcomes and implement a plan of action, and then evaluate the results of nursing activities, including the administration of drugs.

The five phases of the process are used not only in nursing but also in daily life. For example, when buying a computer, first think about what type of device is needed, shop in several different stores to find out more about computer types and brands (**assessment**), and then determine what each store has to offer (**analysis**). At this point, decide exactly what computer to buy and how to pay for the computer (**planning**); then purchase the computer (**implementation**). After purchase and use, make the decision to keep or upgrade the computer (**evaluation**).

Using the nursing process requires practice, experience, and a constant updating of knowledge. It is not within the scope of this textbook to list all of the assessments, nursing diagnoses, plans, implementations, and evaluations for the vast number of nursing problems associated with an illness that requires the administration of a specific drug. The nursing process is used in this text specifically as it applies to drug administration.

THE FIVE PHASES OF THE NURSING PROCESS

Although the nursing process can be described in various ways, it generally consists of five phases: assessment, analysis (or formation of the **nursing diagnosis** or problem), planning, implementation, and evaluation. Each part is applicable, with modification, to the administration of medications. Figure 4.1 illustrates the nursing process in the administration of medications.

Assessment

Assessment involves collecting objective and subjective data. **Objective data** are facts obtained by means of a physical assessment or physical

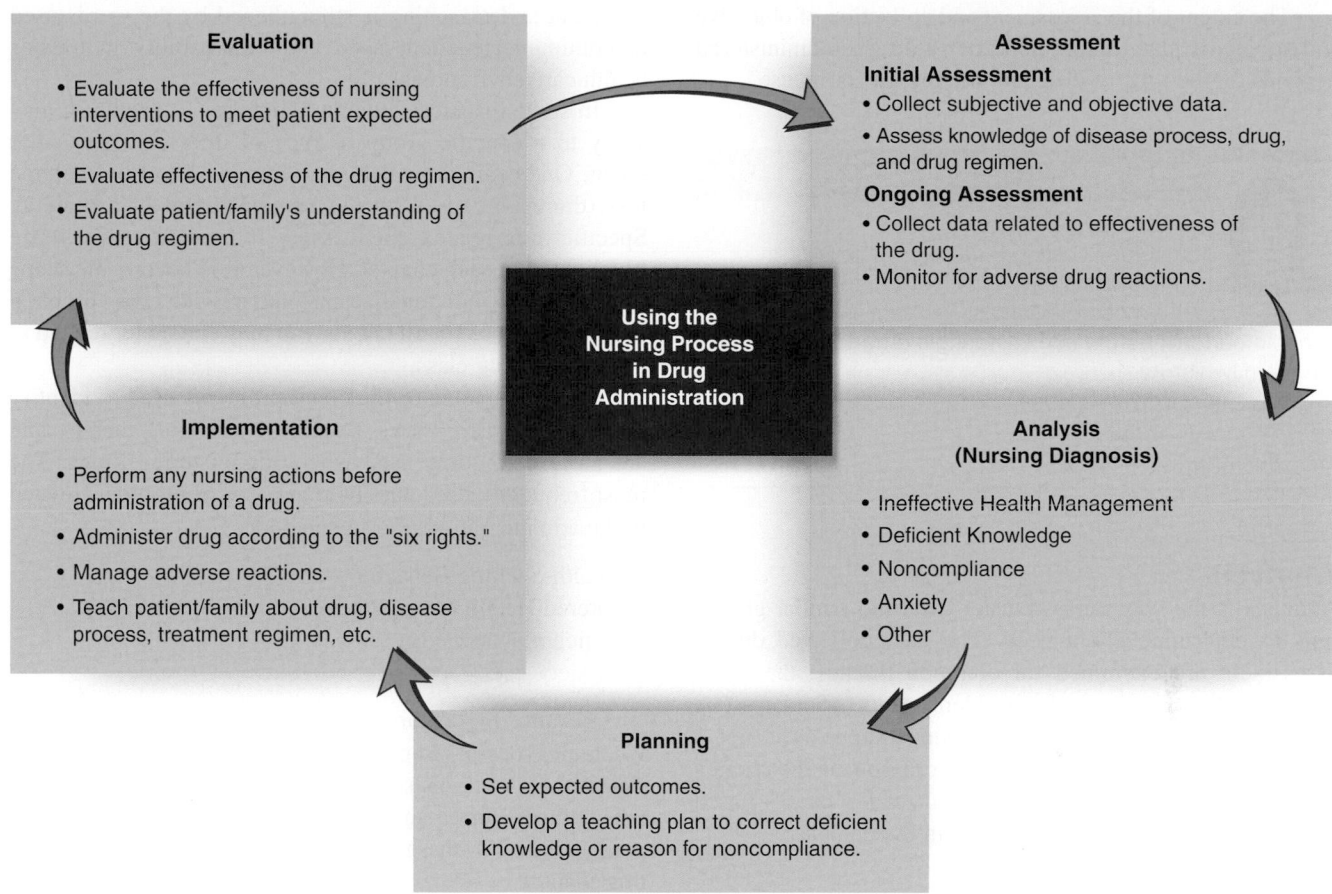

Evaluation

- Evaluate the effectiveness of nursing interventions to meet patient expected outcomes.
- Evaluate effectiveness of the drug regimen.
- Evaluate patient/family's understanding of the drug regimen.

Assessment

Initial Assessment
- Collect subjective and objective data.
- Assess knowledge of disease process, drug, and drug regimen.

Ongoing Assessment
- Collect data related to effectiveness of the drug.
- Monitor for adverse drug reactions.

Using the Nursing Process in Drug Administration

Implementation

- Perform any nursing actions before administration of a drug.
- Administer drug according to the "six rights."
- Manage adverse reactions.
- Teach patient/family about drug, disease process, treatment regimen, etc.

Analysis (Nursing Diagnosis)

- Ineffective Health Management
- Deficient Knowledge
- Noncompliance
- Anxiety
- Other

Planning

- Set expected outcomes.
- Develop a teaching plan to correct deficient knowledge or reason for noncompliance.

FIGURE 4.1 The nursing process as it relates to administration of medication.

examination. **Subjective data** are facts supplied by the client or the client's family.

Assessments are both initial and ongoing. An **initial assessment** is made based on objective and subjective data collected when the client is first seen in a hospital, ambulatory setting (clinic or health care provider's office), or long-term care facility. The initial assessment usually is more thorough and provides a database (sometimes called a *baseline*) against which later data can be compared and decisions made. The initial assessment provides information that is analyzed to identify problems that can be resolved or alleviated by nursing actions.

Objective data are obtained during an initial assessment through activities such as examining the skin, obtaining vital signs, palpating a lump, and auscultating the lungs. A review of the results of any recent laboratory tests and diagnostic studies also is part of the initial physical assessment. Subjective data are acquired during an initial assessment by obtaining information from the client, such as a family history of disease, an allergy history, an occupational history, a description (in the client's own words) of the current illness or chief complaint, a medical history, and a drug history. In addition to the prescription drugs that the client may be taking, it is important to know the over-the-counter drugs, vitamins, or health supplements that the client uses.

For women of childbearing age, ask about the woman's pregnancy status and whether or not she is breastfeeding.

An **ongoing assessment** is one that is made at the time of each client contact and may include the collection of objective data, subjective data, or both. The scope of an ongoing assessment depends on many factors, such as the client's diagnosis, the severity of illness, the response to treatment, and the prescribed medical or surgical treatment.

The assessment phase (including the initial and ongoing assessment) of the nursing process can be applied to the administration of drugs, with objective and subjective data collected before and after to obtain a thorough baseline or initial assessment. This allows subsequent assessments to be compared with the baseline information. This comparison helps to evaluate the effectiveness of the drug and the presence of any adverse reactions. Ongoing assessments of objective and subjective data are equally important when administering drugs. Important objective data include blood pressure, pulse, respiratory rate, temperature, weight, appearance of the skin, appearance of an intravenous infusion site, and pulmonary status as assessed by auscultation of the lungs. Important subjective data include any statements made by the client about relief or nonrelief of pain or other symptoms before administration of a drug (note: evaluation is the term used for data gathering after the intervention).

The extent of the assessment and collection of objective and subjective data before and after a drug is administered depends on the type of drug and the reason for its use.

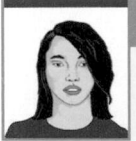

PHARMACOLOGY IN PRACTICE

DRUG ASSESSMENT
A nurse is caring for a client who is of childbearing age. Which of the following is the most relevant assessment that the nurse should perform before administering a drug to this patient?
1. Family history
2. Relationship with spouse
3. Pregnancy status
4. Menstruation history

Analysis

Analysis is the way nurses cluster data into similar groupings to determine client need. The data collected during assessment are examined for common threads; the nurse identifies the client's needs (problems) and formulates one or more nursing diagnoses. A nursing diagnosis is not a medical diagnosis; rather, it is a description of the client's problems and their probable or actual related causes based on the subjective and objective data in the database.

Nursing Diagnosis

A nursing diagnosis is a method using clinical judgment to identify problems that can be solved or prevented by **independent nursing actions**—actions that do not require a physician's order and may be legally performed by a nurse. Nursing diagnoses provide the framework and consistent language for selection of nursing interventions to achieve **expected outcomes**.

One organization who has attempted to provide consistent language and meaning to the nursing diagnostic process is the North American Nursing Diagnosis Association International (NANDA-I). This group formed to standardize the terminology used for nursing diagnoses. NANDA-I continues to define, explain, classify, and research summary statements about health problems related to nursing. NANDA-I has approved a list of diagnostic categories to be used in formulating a nursing diagnosis. This list of diagnostic categories is periodically revised and updated.

As nurses work in a multidisciplinary health care environment, there has been question regarding whether these diagnostic problems are solely of nursing or are client issues addressed by other disciplines, too (Beyea, 1999)? Other organizations such as the International Council of Nurses (ICN) may identify lists of nursing-specific diagnoses as client or care planning problems. The ICN publishes the *Nursing Diagnosis and Outcome Statements International Classification for Nursing Practice* (ICNP) catalog. This is an excellent resource for learners and instructors to explore together, in the use of terminology and how clinical judgment and reasoning is strengthened by the words used to communicate client need and vulnerability in today's health care environment.

In some instances, nursing diagnoses or problems may apply to a specific group or type of drug or a particular client. One example is dehydration related to fluid volume loss (diuresis) caused by the administration of a diuretic. Specific drug-related client issues (nursing diagnoses) are highlighted in each chapter. However, it is beyond the scope of this book to individualize care and provide every problem that you may use for all clients you may encounter related to a drug or a drug class.

Listed are some of the client problems used to identify nursing diagnostic issues associated with drug therapy and are more commonly used when administering drugs. The most frequently used nursing diagnoses or problems related to the administration of drugs include:

- Health-Seeking Behavior
- Altered Health Management
- Deficient Knowledge
- Anxiety

Because these nursing diagnoses are commonly used when all types of drugs are administered, they will not be repeated for each chapter. Keep these client issues in mind when administering any drug. Expansion of nursing actions corresponding to these nursing diagnoses is featured later in this chapter.

Planning

After the nursing diagnoses are formulated, a client-oriented goal and expected outcomes are developed for each client problem. The goal statement is a broad expectation that will indicate the problem is resolved. An **expected outcome** is a direct statement of how client goals are to be achieved. The expected outcome describes the maximum level of health promotion that is reasonably attainable for the client. For example, common expected client outcomes related to drug administration, in general, include the following:

- The client will effectively manage the drug regimen.
- The client will understand the drug regimen.
- The client will comply with the drug regimen.

The expected outcomes define the behavior of the client or family that indicates the problem is being resolved or that progress toward resolution is occurring.

 Concept Mastery Alert

Nurses in the planning phase of the nursing process describe the steps for carrying out nursing activities that will assist in achieving client goals. Nurses in this phase describe what will be done and plan care.

Selecting the appropriate interventions is based on the expected outcomes that help to develop a plan of action or client care plan. Planning for nursing actions specific to the drug to be administered can result in greater accuracy in drug administration, enhanced client understanding of the drug regimen, and improved client adherence to the prescribed drug therapy after discharge from the hospital. For example, during the initial assessment interview, the client may report an allergy to penicillin. This information is important, and you must now plan the best methods of informing all members of the health care team of the client's allergy to penicillin.

The planning phase describes the steps for carrying out nursing activities or interventions that are specific and that will meet the expected outcomes. Planning anticipates the actions to use during the implementation phase or the carrying out of nursing actions that are specific to the drug being administered. If, for example, the client is to receive a drug by the intravenous route, you must plan for the materials needed and the client instruction for administration of the drug by this route. In this instance, the planning phase occurs immediately before the implementation phase and is necessary to carry out the technique of intravenous administration correctly. Failing to plan effectively may result in forgetting to obtain all of the materials necessary for drug administration.

Implementation

Implementation is the carrying out of a plan of action and is a natural outgrowth of the assessment and planning phases of the nursing process. When related to the administration of drugs, implementation refers to the preparation and administration of one or more drugs to a specific client. Before administering a drug, review the subjective and objective data obtained on assessment and consider any additional data, such as blood pressure, pulse, or statements made by the client. The decision of whether to administer the drug is based on an analysis of all information. For example, a client is hypertensive and is supposed to receive a drug to lower the blood pressure. Objective data obtained at the time of admission (baseline) included a blood pressure of 188/110. Additional objective data obtained immediately before the administration of the drug (ongoing) included a blood pressure of 182/110. A decision is made by the nurse to administer the drug because the change in the client's blood pressure is minimal. However, if the client's blood pressure is suddenly 132/84, and this is only the second dose of the drug, the nurse could decide to withhold the drug and contact the prescribing health care provider regarding this swift drop in blood pressure. Giving or withholding a drug and contacting the client's health care provider are nursing activities related to the implementation phase of the nursing process.

Nursing Actions Based Upon Nursing Diagnoses

The more common nursing diagnoses used when administering drugs are Health-Seeking Behavior, Altered Health Maintenance, Deficient Knowledge, and Anxiety. Nursing interventions applicable to each of these nursing diagnoses are discussed in the following sections. However, each client is an individual and nursing care must be planned on an individual basis after a careful collection and analysis of the data. In addition, each drug is different and may have various effects in the body. (For drugs discussed in subsequent chapters, some possible nursing diagnoses related to that specific drug are featured.)

Health-Seeking Behavior

This nursing diagnosis takes into consideration that the client is seeking to promote their own well-being by their willingness to participate and integrate into daily living the treatment of an illness, such as the self-administration of medications. The significant assessment here is that the client verbalizes the desire to self-manage the medication schedule.

When the client is willing and able to manage the treatment activities, they may simply need:

- Information concerning the drug.
- Instruction on method of administration.
- Information on type of reactions to expect.
- Information concerning what to report to the primary health care provider.

A client willing to take responsibility for Health Management may need:

- Development of a teaching plan.
- Information needed to manage the treatment activities properly (see Chapter 5 for more information on educating clients).

Altered Health Management

Altered Health Management involves the inability of the client to integrate into daily living a program for treatment of illness and the effects of the illness owing to issue they cannot readily control. In the case of medication administration, the client may not be taking the medication correctly because something hampers their ability to do so or because of the inability to follow the medication schedule prescribed by the primary health care provider because a barrier to learning or understanding exists.

The reasons for not following the drug routine vary (Box 4.1). For example, some people do not fill their prescriptions because they do not have enough money to pay for them. Other clients skip doses, take the drug at the wrong times, or take an incorrect dose. Some may simply forget to take the drug; others take a drug for a few days, see no therapeutic effect, and quit.

When working with a client who is not managing the drug routine correctly, nursing actions include:

- Further assessment of the client's level of health literacy (see Chapter 5).
- Observation of the client as they self-administer the drug before discharge from the health care facility.
- Instruction on anticipated effects both positive and negative for this drug.
- Determine if adequate funds are available to obtain the drug and any necessary supplies.

For example, when a bronchodilator is administered by inhalation, a spacer or extender may be required for

BOX 4.1 Possible Causes of Ineffective Health Management

When clients perceive there is little help or assistance in managing the following:

Ongoing therapy for chronic illness, with the inability to go back to pre-illness state

Adverse reactions experienced that are worse than the illness itself

Health literacy issues regarding the drugs prescribed

Depression, forgetfulness, apathy, impaired cognition

Poor provider -client relationships

Monetary issues regarding payment/not understanding reimbursement

Inability to get drugs/supplies due to dependence or mobility

True or perceived lack of family support

Impairments such as visual or hearing

(Reprinted with permission from Carpenito-Moyet, L. (2010). *Handbook of nursing diagnosis* (13 ed., pp. 424-425). Lippincott Williams & Wilkins.)

proper administration. This device is an additional expense. A referral to the social services department of the institution may help the client when finances are a problem.

For those who need help to remember to take the drug, you may suggest the use of small compartmentalized boxes marked with the day of the week or time the drug is to be taken (Fig. 4.2). These containers can be obtained from the local pharmacy.

It is important to discuss the drug schedule with the client, including the reason the drug is to be taken, the times, the amount, adverse reactions to expect, and reactions that should be reported. The client needs a thorough understanding of the desired or expected therapeutic effect and the approximate time expected to attain that effect. For example, a client may become discouraged after taking an antidepressant for 5–7 days and seeing no response. An explanation that 2–3 weeks is required before the depression begins to lift will, in many cases, promote adherence to the drug schedule.

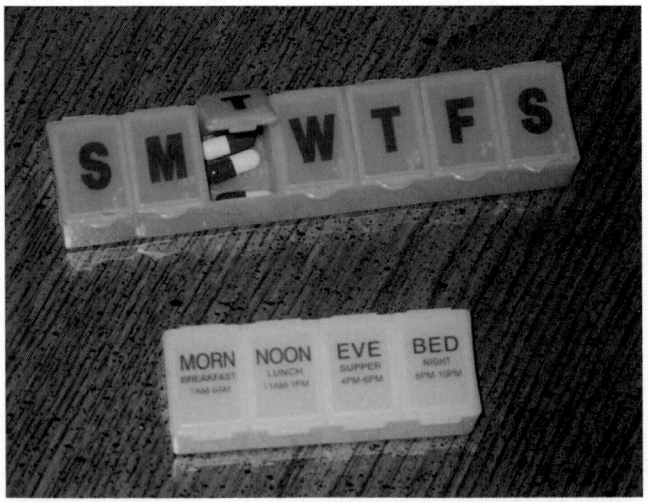

FIGURE 4.2 Various types of drug containers may be used to help individuals remember to take their medication at the correct time.

It is important to provide ways to minimize adverse reactions if possible. For example, many anticholinergic drugs cause dry mouth. Instruct the client to take frequent sips of water or suck on hard candy to help minimize the discomfort of a dry mouth.

Frequent follow-up sessions are needed to determine adherence to the drug schedule. If a follow-up visit is not feasible, consider a telephone call or home visit. It is vital that you strive to develop a caring and nurturing relationship with the client. Adherence to the drug schedule is enhanced when a client trusts you and feels comfortable confiding any problem encountered during drug therapy.

Deficient Knowledge

Deficient knowledge is the absence or deficiency of cognitive information on a specific subject. In the case of self-administration of drugs, the client lacks sufficient knowledge to administer the drug regimen correctly. It may also relate to a lack of interest in learning, cognitive limitation, or inability to remember.

Most clients, at least in the initial treatment stages, lack knowledge about the drug, its possible adverse reactions, and the times and method of administration. At times, the client may lack knowledge about the disease condition. In these situations, address the specific knowledge deficit (e.g., adverse reactions, disease process, method of administration) in words that the client can understand.

When addressing a deficit in knowledge, it is important to:

- Determine what information the client is lacking.
- Plan a teaching session that directly pertains to the specific area of need (see Chapter 5 for more information on client education).
- Special note: If the client lacks the cognitive ability to understand the information concerning self-administration of drugs, then one or more of the caregivers should be taught to administer the proper treatment regimen.

Anxiety

Anxiety is a vague uneasiness or apprehension that manifests itself in varying degrees, from expressions of concern regarding drug regimen to total lack of adherence to the drug routine. The anxiety experienced during drug administration depends on the severity of the illness, the occurrence of adverse reactions, and the knowledge level of the client. When anxiety is high, the ability to focus on details is reduced. If the client or caregiver is given information concerning the medication regimen during a high-anxiety state, the client may not remember the information. This could lead to nonadherence to the regimen. Anxiety usually decreases with understanding of the treatment plan. To decrease anxiety before discussing the treatment plan with the client, take time to talk with and actively listen to the client. This helps to build a caring relationship and decrease client anxiety. It is critical to allow time for a thorough explanation and to answer all questions and concerns in a language the client can understand (see Chapter 5).

Nursing actions to mitigate anxiety include:

- Identify and address the specific fear.
- Reassure the client that the drug will alleviate the symptoms or, if possible, cure the disorder.
- Thoroughly explain any procedure.
- Actively listen and provide encouragement as the client expresses fears and concerns.

Reassurance and understanding on your part are required; the amount of reassurance and understanding depends on the individual client.

PHARMACOLOGY IN PRACTICE

NURSING PROCESS

A nurse is caring for a patient who has to continue with the drug regimen on an outpatient basis. Ongoing assessments of the patient reveal that the patient is not adhering to the medication regimen. What is the first task the nurse should perform to support the patient's adherence?

1. Prepare a fixed schedule for the patient to take the drug.
2. Find out the reason for nonadherence if possible.
3. Teach the patient the importance of following a drug regimen.
4. Frequently monitor the patient's condition to identify a relapse.

Evaluation

Evaluation is a decision-making process that involves determining the effectiveness of the nursing interventions in meeting the expected outcomes. When related to the administration of a drug, this phase of the nursing process is used to evaluate the client's response to drug therapy. Expected outcomes define the behavior of the client or family that indicates that the problem is being resolved or that progress toward resolution is occurring. Expected outcomes serve as

---

BOX 4.2 Setting Up Nursing Interventions Based on Expected Outcomes

Goal: Baseline blood pressure is maintained.
Expected Outcome: The client experiences no further elevation in blood pressure.
Nursing Interventions:
- Give medications as ordered.
- Monitor the blood pressure every hour.
- Reduce environmental stressors.
Evaluation: Blood pressure at or below baseline assessment.

---

a basis for evaluating the effectiveness of nursing interventions. Box 4.2 illustrates this process.

The evaluation is complete if the expected outcomes are accomplished or if progress occurs. If the outcomes are not accomplished, different interventions are needed. During the administration of the drug, the expected response is alleviation of specific symptoms or the presence of a therapeutic effect. Evaluation also may be used to determine if the client or family member understands the drug schedule.

To evaluate the client's response to therapy, and depending on the drug administered, you may do activities such as check the client's blood pressure every hour, inquire whether pain has been relieved, or monitor the client's pulse every 15 min. After evaluation, certain other decisions may need to be made and plans of action implemented. For example, you may need to notify the primary health care provider of a marked change in a client's pulse and respiratory rate after a drug was administered, or you may need to change the bed linen because sweating occurred after a drug used to lower the client's elevated temperature was administered.

You can evaluate the client's or family's understanding of the drug regimen by noting if one or both appear to understand the material that has been presented. Facial expression may indicate that one or both do or do not understand what has been explained. You also may ask questions about the information that has been given to evaluate further the client's or family's understanding.

KEY POINTS

■ Nursing process is the method of problem solving used in the nursing discipline. It consists of five phases: assessment, analysis, planning, implementation, and evaluation.

■ Assessment involves the collection of client data. The initial assessment provides baseline information for comparison later. It can be objective, that is, facts obtained from information sources such as the examination, laboratory tests, or other findings. It can also be subjective, data that are told to the nurse from the client or the family. Ongoing assessment helps to update information about the client's progress.

■ Analysis involves the grouping of assessment data into like threads. Review of the data determines the client needs and is described using consistent language, termed a *nursing diagnosis*. A nursing diagnosis is different from a medical

diagnosis because interventions carried out are independent nursing actions, that is, those not requiring a health care provider's order.

■ The planning phase is the formulation of the goals and expected outcomes to assist the client to return to the maximum level of wellness. These should be reasonably attainable and client oriented. The outcomes help to formulate the plan of action to be used during implementation and help to measure success during the evaluation phase.

■ With most drug therapy routines, there are typical client problems to address: Altered Health Management, Deficient Knowledge, and Anxiety. Other specific problems depend on the illness type, drugs ordered, and client knowledge and experience with the treatment routine.

CHAPTER REVIEW

Prepare for the NCLEX-PN

RECALL THE FACTS

1. When the nurse enters subjective data in the client's record, this information is obtained from _____.
   1. the primary health care provider
   2. other members of the health care team
   3. the client or family
   4. laboratory and x-ray reports
2. What is the name of one of the organizations that approves and standardizes nursing diagnoses?
   1. ANA
   2. NLN
   3. NCSBN
   4. NANDA-I
3. A client states that they do not understand why a specific medication has to be taken. The most accurate nursing diagnosis for this client would be _____.
   1. Altered Health Management
   2. Anxiety
   3. Deficient Knowledge
4. Which of the following would be an appropriate expected outcome related to drug administration?
   1. The client will verbalize three ways to use crutches.
   2. The client will take an antibiotic pill daily.
   3. The client will understand the use of blood pressure medications.
   4. The client will demonstrate ways to prevent having to use insulin.
5. Which of the following is an independent nursing action?
   1. Administering insulin
   2. Withholding a drug according to physician standing orders
   3. Client teaching about drug therapy
   4. Asking respiratory care to come do an inhalation treatment
6. During the evaluation phase of the nursing process, the nurse _____.
   1. makes decisions regarding the effectiveness of nursing interventions based on the outcome
   2. ensures nursing procedures have been performed correctly
   3. makes notations regarding the client's response to medical treatment
   4. makes a list of all adverse reactions the client may experience while taking the drug

ANALYZE THE FACTS

7. *Which of the following is an example of objective client data?
   1. Adult child states, "Mom's BP is always 150/90."
   2. "My pain is about 7 out of 10 right now."
   3. "I think the doctor said my blood sugar was 105."
   4. The nurse's aide reports a BP of 132/78.
8. *The nurse makes a note in the chart that the client's pain has lessened following a 14-day course of antibiotics. This is an example of which phase of the nursing process?
   1. Assessment
   2. Analysis
   3. Implementation
   4. Evaluation

ALTERNATE-FORMAT QUESTIONS

9. Arrange the following steps of the nursing process correctly:
   1. Analysis
   2. Assessment
   3. Evaluation
   4. Implementation
   5. Planning
10. The nurse greets the new clinic client, saying, "Tell me about the pain you are having." This is an example of gathering data. Describe the type of data. **Select all that apply.**
    1. Baseline assessment
    2. Objective data
    3. Ongoing assessment
    4. Subjective data

To check your answers, see Appendix F.

_____

*Indicates the question is directly linked to the NCLEX-PN test plan in Appendix G

WANT TO KNOW MORE? A wide variety of resources are available to enhance your learning and understanding of this chapter.
- Visit thePoint for resources such as:
  - NCLEX-Style Student Review Questions
  - Journal Articles
  - Dosage Calculations
  - Drug Monographs
  - Watch and Learn Videos
  - Concepts in Action Animations
- The *Study Guide to Accompany Introductory Clinical Pharmacology*, 12th edition, sold separately, will help you review and apply essential content.
- ✓*PrepU* is available to help students prepare for the NCLEX-PN examination.

5

Client and Family Teaching

Key Terms

client-centered care ability of client to have autonomy in directing care and services rendered to them

cultural competency the ability to understand, appreciate, and interact with persons from cultures different from our own

health communication the use of communication strategies to inform and influence individual and community decisions that enhance health

health literacy the ability to understand information about health and disease, then use the information to make decisions about health care

learning acquisition of new knowledge or skills; outcome of learning is change in behavior, thinking, or both

motivation desire for action or recognition of need

teach back method confirmation that a client understands what is being explained by teaching back the information to the provider

teaching interactive process that promotes learning

Learning Objectives

On completion of this chapter, the student will:

1. Describe the steps of client teaching about drug therapy.
2. Identify important aspects of the client–nurse relationship.
3. Describe the three components of good health communication.
4. Identify important aspects of the teaching/learning process.
5. Describe how to use information about relationship and communication with the nursing process.
6. Discuss suggestions to make to the client for adapting drug administration in the home.

Client **teaching** is an integral part of nursing. When drugs are ordered by the primary health care provider, you are responsible for supplying the client with accurate and up-to-date information about the drugs prescribed. The client is educated about the drugs they have taken while in the hospital and any drugs to be taken after being discharged. By understanding the reason for the prescribed medications, the client is more likely to be adherent to the treatment plan and get better.

Described as a sequential plan, client teaching can logically be viewed as an essential nursing task. To best accomplish the task of client teaching, you need to optimize the relationship between the client and yourself as well as use principles of **learning**.

CLIENT–NURSE RELATIONSHIP

The relationship between a nurse and a client is built upon trust and respect. Different factors can either support or block the ability to form positive relationships. Nurses use their knowledge of understanding changes in the health care system and the emphasis on better health communication to build strong relationships. This relationship makes the client the focal point and is referred to as **Client-Centered Care** (Fig. 5.1).

Evolution in Health Care

In the United States, we are undergoing health care reform on a yearly basis. These changes are on a level equal to or greater than the advent of Medicare more than 50 years ago. The Health Care and Education Reconciliation Act, passed in 2010 has changed health care as we have known it. This legislation changed laws wherein all people were required to have health insurance. Under the Affordable Care Act (ACA), all citizens were assured basic health coverage, with no denials for existing conditions.

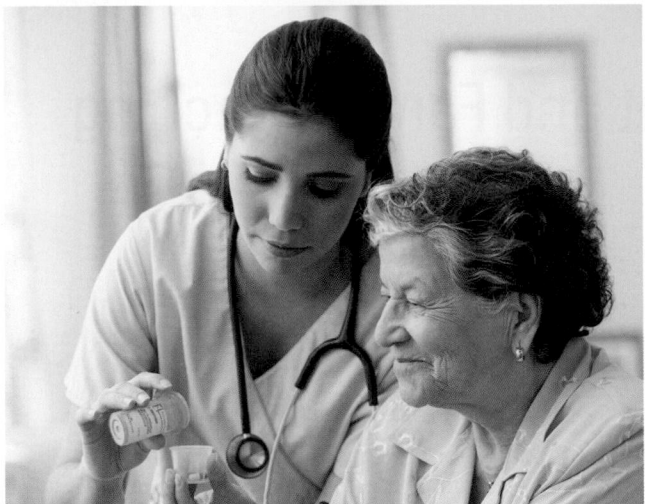

FIGURE 5.1 Client-centered care is built from the mutual respect of the client and the provider for each other.

The election in 2016 saw portions of the ACA removed, and the following changes took place:

- The mandate for individual health insurance was repealed, resulting in private premiums rising as high as 32% in a single year.
- States can require Medicaid recipients to work or go to school.
- Incentives for insurance companies was eliminated, resulting in some states with only one company offering ACA insurance.
- Plans with low premiums and high deductibles can be offered.
- ACA navigator program to help people understand the changes was eliminated.

These changes dramatically affected the ability to fund medications for some individuals; as a result the ability to use medications to treat diseases was impacted. With the changes in president and majority party in the 2020 national election, health insurance may be affected once again.

What is known is that the ease with which this next transition happens is dependent on how well change is received by the client. An example of this is the roll-out of the COVID-19 vaccine program. After health providers, one of the target populations for vaccination are those who are 65 years of age and older. Requirements for checking eligibility and signing up for vaccine appointments involves technology and the Internet. For many in this age group, the ability to pull up and sign up for appointments can be challenging. Some health providers are calling clients to make those appointments because they understand the difficulty, making the process manageable.

By learning about health care funding and coverage, health care providers and nurses specifically can educate clients in navigating the complexities of change and the understanding of health promotion and illness concerns. Important factors that influence clients and their willingness to change include attitudes, the aging population, and chronic illness.

Attitudes

Less than a decade ago, traditional health care was practiced differently than care today. It was a *patriarchal relationship,* meaning the doctor gave the nurse an order, and then the nurse carried out the treatment on the patient. Previously, people were hospitalized for long periods and not responsible for schedules and treatments—everything was done to them. Relating to patients was very different. Doctors told patients what to do and they followed the instructions. If the patient questioned care, they were seen as "bad patients."

At present, depending on the setting, we call individuals different titles—patient, client, or consumer. The title change indicates a different relationship between the health care provider and receiver. Clients are frequently cared for on an outpatient basis or even at home. Treatments once done only in a hospital may be assumed by the client or family members in the home. Despite the name we choose or the setting of care they are all persons with a deviation of their health caused by an acute disease, accident, genetic affliction, or chronic condition worsening over time.

Aging Population

Older individuals grew up in the traditional health care system. They regard the doctor as an authoritative expert. This attitude is seen especially when a client has an acute medical problem. Again, the patient waits for direction from the doctor and allows nurses to do the treatments to them.

This presents a problem because older people use more health care resources than others. People aged 65 years and older presently make up 15.6% of the population, but they account for over 30% of the medications, hospital stays, and emergency responses. By 2040, it is estimated that 21.6% of our population will be over 65 years (Fig. 5.2). If costs rise at the same rate, health care will be unaffordable to those individuals. You can help older people take a greater role in their own care by finding ways to empower them to help cut costs. One option is to help educate clients to direct their own care rather than rely on their health care providers.

Chronic Illness

As people with medical conditions live longer and our population ages, there will be increasing rates of chronic illnesses. This group of clients is thought to be the best group to handle the change from provider-directed care to client-centered care. According to some researchers, clients with chronic illnesses exercise a great deal of control. No matter what health care providers do or say, when clients leave the hospital or clinic, it is the client who determines what to do. Clients decide what they are going to eat, whether they will exercise, and to what extent they will take prescribed medications.

It is imperative that clients make wise and cost-conscious decisions in managing their own health care. You can support this by practicing good **health communication** with clients.

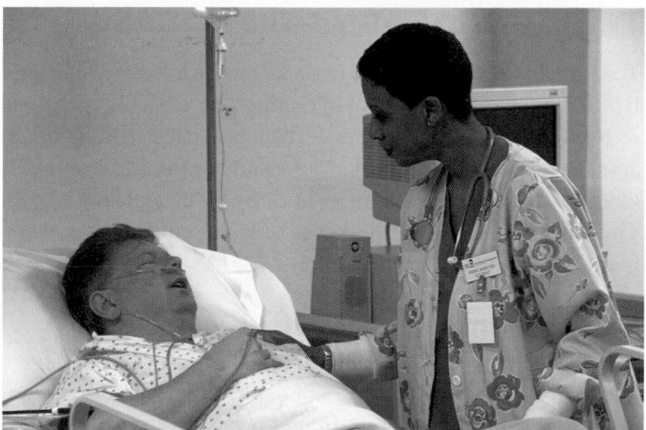

FIGURE 5.2 By 2060, the number of older adults served by the health care system will double in size to almost 100 million people.

Health Communication

The quality of health communication has an impact on the outcome of client–nurse interactions. Clients' ability to follow instructions is heavily influenced by your communication style.

Results of effective health communication include better medication adherence. Rates of client adherence to prescribed treatments increase when health care providers deliver clear and concise instructions. Poor health communication results in the inability to follow medication instructions.

To practice effective health communication, remember that it involves understanding clients as well as talking to them. Three important factors include **health literacy**, **cultural competency**, and identifying limited English proficiency (LEP).

Health Literacy

Health literacy is the ability to understand information about health and disease and then use the information to make decisions about health care. Assessment is required to determine a client's ability to understand health concepts and carry out health care instructions. Clients with limited health literacy can be difficult to identify. For example, a person may speak well and appear well educated, yet fail to grasp disease concepts or understand how to follow medication dosage instructions properly.

 Lifespan Considerations

Health literacy is not the same thing as language or skill ability. One-third of the adult population in the United States has limited health literacy.

Identifying Limited Health Literacy

Clients with limited health literacy often try to hide their literacy issues. Box 5.1 describes populations at risk or behaviors that may alert nurses to suspect limited health literacy. Identify potential limited health literacy by understanding which

---

| **BOX 5.1** | **Identifying Limited Health Literacy** |

Groups with higher rates of limited health literacy include:
- Older adults
- Individuals experiencing low income
- US born but speak English as a second language
- Deaf or hard of hearing
- People who do not have a high school diploma or equivalent
- Learning disabilities
- Immigrants who do not speak English
- Individuals experiencing unemployment

Behaviors that may indicate a client has limited health literacy include:
- Medical forms incomplete or inaccurately completed
- Frequently missed appointments
- Not following medication directions
- Inability to name or give purpose of medications
- Inability to describe how to take medications
- Laboratory test results do not change when clients say they are taking their medication.

population groups are at higher risk for limited health literacy skills. Once identified you can be alert for certain behaviors that may indicate a limited health literacy problem exists.

Improving Health Literacy

Using simple and clear language helps clients understand and follow instructions. People who are highly literate can have problems understanding language used in health care. Here is an example, the word *negative* is a positive finding when discussing an infection or cancer. This can be confusing to those who use negative in a different context. Use everyday language instead of medical terms; for example, say "pain killer" instead of "analgesic" when talking to clients. Other examples include "wound" instead of "lesion" or "tumor" instead of "carcinoma."

Limit the amount of information at each interaction with a client. Clients remember small pieces of information that are relevant to current needs or situations. This does not mean withholding information. Rather, focus communication on the one or two most important things the client needs to know at that time.

 Lifespan Considerations

Up to 80% of clients forget instructions spoken to them. Of those who say they remember the instruction, 50% recall the instruction incorrectly.

Cultural Competency

Cultural competency is the ability to interact with people from different cultures. Many people fail to realize that the United States is a nation of immigrants and we have people from almost every country or culture of the world within our borders. There are many things that you need to take into account when working with a wide array of different people from different cultures. This may make you feel overwhelmed to think you must know everything about any culture you may encounter. This is not the case. A way to start becoming culturally competent is to care for different people, by respecting their traditions, norms, and other traits.

To become respectful, the first thing you should learn is, at your institution, who are the people and from what different cultures and backgrounds do they come? Learning about some of the cultural norms of the people served will help you to identify certain behaviors that are acceptable. Health care providers gain the trust from clients and family members when their customs are respected or advocated for in the care setting.

Taking care not to stereotype clients because of their culture is another important concept. For example, when caring for an Asian client, you may know that rice is a basic staple in many Asian diets. Do not assume that the client would prefer rice for a meal. Instead, ask what the client's preference is for diet choices. The important concept is to acknowledge cultural differences and to ask if the individual practices these traditions.

Limited English Proficiency

In recent years, the United States has become increasingly multilingual. During the past decade, the number of Spanish- and Asian-language speakers has grown by 50%. Almost 62 million people in the United States speak a language other than English; additionally, 20% of the nation's population speak a language other than English at home. Many individuals also speak or understand English, yet 25 million people in this country are considered limited English proficient (Scamman, 2018).

With the growing complexity of treatments and medication instructions, it is important to provide teaching resources for clients with LEP. Use written instructions that have been translated into the familiar language when teaching LEP clients. During conversations, use the service of professional interpreters to relay oral interactions. Avoid using family and friends for interpretation. Sometimes family members or friends will paraphrase communication, losing some important parts of the interaction. Do not rely on children for interpretation as this puts an unfair burden on them, because they may feel they have to tell bad news or may be embarrassed by the conversation.

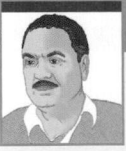

PHARMACOLOGY IN PRACTICE

CLIENT-CENTERED CARE
An 86-year-old client is seen at an urgent care center for sudden heartburn. Which of the following statements made by the assigned nurse demonstrates the use of client-centered care concepts?
1. "Did you try to fix this at home first?"
2. "The doctor will be in soon to give you a recommendation"
3. "Why didn't you just go see your own doctor in the morning?"
4. "You can treat this with over-the-counter medications"

TEACHING/LEARNING PROCESS

Teaching is an interactive process that promotes learning. Both the client and the nurse must be actively involved if teaching is to be effective. You are better prepared to actively engage clients when you understand the principles of motivation, adult learning, and different learning styles. The client's behavior, thinking, or both can change when learning occurs.

Motivation

A client must be motivated (having a desire or seeing a need) to learn. **Motivation** depends on the client's perception of the need to learn. Educating the client about the disease process improves the client's motivation to learn tasks to stay healthy. Encouraging client participation in planning realistic and attainable goals also promotes motivation. Creating an accepting and positive atmosphere also enhances learning. If the client has little or no motivation, they are likely to be nonadherent to therapy.

Adult Learning

Generally, adults learn only what they feel they need to learn. Adults learn best when they have a strong inner motivation to acquire a new skill or new knowledge. They will learn less if they are passive recipients of "canned" educational content. Adults have a vast array of experiences and knowledge to bring to a new learning experience. Nurses who use this experience will bring about the greatest behavior change. Most adults retain the information taught if they are able to "do" something with that new knowledge immediately. For example, in teaching a client how to administer their own insulin, demonstrate the technique, allow time for supervised practice, and, as soon as they appear ready, allow the client to prepare and inject the insulin. Most adults prefer an informal learning environment in which mutual exchange and freedom of expression prevail.

Learning Styles and Domains of Learning

Learning styles involve preferred ways to learn a concept and are frequently grouped as visual, auditory, or kinesthetic. Assessing a client's learning style helps you to discover the best methods to use when providing client teaching.

 Lifespan Considerations

Remember that 83% of adults are visual learners and only 11% learn by listening (auditory learners). When instructing clients, use props and visual materials as much as possible.

Learning occurs in what is known as three domains: cognitive, affective, and psychomotor. When developing a teaching plan for the client, consider how a client learns and what they are to learn. Box 5.2 describes both learning styles and domains of learning.

COMBINING TEACHING SKILLS AND THE NURSING PROCESS

Nurses are in the unique position of delivering health care and educating clients. Using the above concepts, nurses teach clients to master skills and to assume self-care responsibilities. The empowered client feels confident that they are part of a client-centered relationship with you, and positive outcomes will occur.

A Framework for Client Teaching

The nursing process is a systematic method of identifying client health needs, devising a plan of care to meet the identified needs, initiating the plan, and evaluating its effectiveness. This process provides the necessary framework to develop an effective teaching plan. However, the teaching plan differs from the nursing process in that the nursing process encompasses all of the client's health care needs, whereas the teaching plan focuses primarily on the client's learning needs. The use of the nursing process as the framework and the concepts of relationships, health communication, and the learning process demonstrate ways to teach

BOX 5.2	Learning Styles and Domains of Learning

Learning Styles
Visual learners: learn by seeing or watching
Auditory learners: learn by listening (actually only a small percentage of people learn best this way)
Kinesthetic learners: learn by moving, touching, and doing
Domains of Learning.
Cognitive domain: intellectual activities such as thought, recall, decision making, and drawing conclusions. In this domain, the client uses previous experiences, prior knowledge, and perceptions to give meaning to new information or to modify previous thinking.
Affective domain: includes the attitudes, feelings, beliefs, and opinions of the client or caregiver
Psychomotor domain: involves learning physical skills (such as injection of insulin) or tasks (such as performing a dressing change)

clients about taking drugs, the possibility of adverse reactions, and the signs and symptoms of toxicity (if applicable).

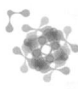

NURSING PROCESS
Client Teaching for Medication Information

ASSESSMENT

Assessment is the data-gathering phase of the nursing process. Assessment assists you in choosing the best teaching methods and individualizing the teaching plan. To develop an effective teaching plan, first determine the client's needs. Needs stem from three areas:

- Information the client or family needs to know about a particular drug
- Client's or family member's ability to learn, accept, and use information
- Barriers or obstacles to learning.

Some drugs have simple uses and, therefore, relatively little client teaching is needed. For example, applying a nonprescription ointment to the skin requires minimal teaching. Other drugs, such as insulin, require detailed information that may need to be given over several days.

Assessing an individual's ability to learn may be difficult. Using the concept of good *health communication,* you may find that not all adults have the same *health literacy* level.

- Information should be geared to the client's level of understanding. Carefully assess the client's ability to communicate, language preference, and health literacy skills. You may find that some clients do not read well. If the client has a learning impairment, a family member or friend should be included in the teaching process.
- People may readily understand what is being taught, but some cannot. For example, a visually impaired client may be unable to read a label or printed directions supplied by the primary health care provider, pharmacist, or nurse.

- Because clients can mimic instructions does not mean they understand them. Provide the opportunity for a teach back to assess. Box 5.3 illustrates use of the "Brown Bag Method" to assess medication use and understanding.

Through assessment, you can determine what barriers or obstacles (if any) may prevent the client or family member from fully understanding the material being presented. Use your skills of *cultural competency* to consider the client's cultural background when planning a teaching session. For example, for some clients, an interpreter is needed. In other cultures, a certain individual (e.g., mother or grandmother) is the decision maker in the family. In such cases, it is important to include the decision maker and/or an interpreter with the client in the teaching session.

NURSING DIAGNOSES (ANALYSIS)

The nursing diagnosis is formulated after analyzing the information obtained during the assessment phase. Examples of nursing diagnoses related to the administration of drugs are listed in the Nursing Diagnosis Checklist.

Nursing Diagnosis Checklist
- Readiness for Enhanced Health Management
- Ineffective Health Management related to lack of knowledge
- Deficient Knowledge related to the drug regimen, possible adverse reactions, disease process, or other factors

---

BOX 5.3 Performing a Brown-Bag Medication Review

This is a simple method to identify clients with limited health literacy.

1. **Ask the client to bring all medications to the clinic or appointment.**

   "Please bag up and bring in any medications that you use—prescription, over the counter, nutritional supplements, and preparations others may have given you."

2. **Ask the client to name each medication and explain its purpose and how it is taken.**

   Note whether they identify medications by reading the label or by opening the bottle, pouring out the pills, and identifying the medication by looking at the pills.

3. **Listen to how the client responds to questions about how to take the medication.**

   It is important to listen nonjudgmentally, being aware of your body language to make sure you are not sending subtle signs of disapproval.

4. **Reframe the question if it sounds like the client may have memorized instructions.**

   When the client says, "Take one pill three times per day," try asking, "When was the last time you took one of these pills?" and "When was the time before that?"

   You may find out that the client does not understand the directions but is merely able to repeat them.

The nursing diagnosis *Readiness for Enhanced Health Management* generally describes a client who is successfully managing the medication regimen. Use this nursing diagnosis to enhance the client's management by teaching the client possible adverse reactions that could affect their health and how to manage them or reduce the potential harmful effects.

The nursing diagnosis *Ineffective Health Management* is useful for discharging teaching, especially when you must teach the client how to manage the medication tasks and schedules. Often, chronic illness or a variety of health problems may mean that the client is taking as many as eight or more medications and may have difficulty managing a complicated medication regimen. This diagnosis describes individuals who are having difficulty achieving positive results.

Deficient Knowledge is a nursing diagnosis that may be used when the client has a deficit in cognitive knowledge or psychomotor skills necessary to administer a medication properly. The defining characteristic would be that the client would report deficient knowledge or request information, or the client does not correctly perform a prescribed skill necessary to the medication task. It is sometimes difficult to know exactly when to use the nursing diagnosis of Deficient Knowledge because all nursing diagnoses have related client teaching as part of their nursing interventions. If teaching is related directly to a nursing diagnosis, then incorporate the teaching into the plan.

PLANNING

Planning begins with the development of a goal and the expected outcomes that the nurse will use to measure

---

BOX 5.4 Important Information to Include in Any Medication Teaching Plan

1. Therapeutic response expected from the drug
2. Adverse reactions to expect when taking the drug
3. Adverse reactions to report to the nurse or primary health care provider
4. Dosage and route
5. Any special considerations or precautions associated with the particular drug prescribed
6. Additional education regarding special considerations for certain drugs, such as techniques for giving injections, applying topical patches, or instilling eye drops

---

attainment of the goal. Developing strategies to be used in the teaching plan and the selection of information to be taught is the next step. Box 5.4 identifies important basic information about any drug to include in any teaching plan.

 Concept Mastery Alert

Nurses who are developing a teaching plan for a client should first determine the goal of the teaching plan. An effective plan starts with a goal, and the remaining options—such as who the teaching plan is for, the education level of the client, and who the caregivers will be—are addressed in light of this goal.

Developing an Individualized Teaching Plan

Teaching plans are individualized because clients' needs are unique. Make use of the client's cognitive abilities when information is given to the client or caregivers about the disease process, medication regimen, and adverse reactions. The client uses the *cognitive domain* to process the information, ask questions, and make decisions.

Areas covered in an individualized teaching plan vary depending on the drug prescribed, the primary health care provider's preference for including or excluding specific facts about the drug, and what the client needs to know to take the drug correctly. Teaching strategies will reflect your knowledge of *LEP* of the client. For example, a client who speaks and reads only Spanish should be given materials prepared in Spanish and not discharge instructions written in English. If needed, ask for assistance in communicating through another nurse who is fluent in Spanish.

Develop strategies for the individualized teaching plan based on information gained during the assessment. For example, if during the assessment you discover that the client is a *kinesthetic learner*, the teaching plan may focus on learning using the *psychomotor domain*. Plan to teach a task or skill using a step-by-step method. The client will have hands-on practice under your supervision. Plan for a return demonstration (**teach back**) by the client to show mastery of the skill.

Selecting Relevant Information

Use concepts of *health literacy* to develop an individualized teaching plan for clients and their families by selecting information relevant to a specific drug, adapting teaching to the individual's level of understanding, and avoiding medical terminology unless terms are explained or defined.

It is important to remember that repetition enhances learning. Repeated teaching sessions help you to assess better what the client is actually learning and provide time for clarification. Encourage the client to ask questions and express feelings to build confidence in the care provided or the ability to engage in self-health strategies.

When individualized written material is provided, if the client has *LEP,* be sure the material includes the basic information that a client would receive in English. Box 5.5 identifies basic drug information for all clients regardless of language.

BOX 5.5 Basic Considerations When Developing a Drug Teaching Plan

General information to consider when developing a teaching plan includes information on the dosage regimen and adverse reactions, issues relating to family members, and basic information about drugs, drug containers, and drug storage.

All clients should understand the following information before discharge:

- **Take with a full (8-ounce) glass of water:** capsules or tablets should be taken with water unless the primary health care provider or clinical pharmacist directs otherwise (e.g., take with food, milk, or an antacid). Some liquids, such as coffee, tea, fruit juice, and carbonated beverages, may interfere with the action of certain drugs.
- **Do not crush or chew:** it is important not to chew capsules before swallowing; they must be swallowed whole. The client also should not chew tablets unless they are labeled "chewable." This is because some tablets have special coatings that are required for specific purposes, such as proper absorption of the drug or prevention of irritation of the lining of the stomach.
- **Same dose, same time:** the dose (amount) of a drug or the time between doses is never increased or decreased unless directed by the primary health care provider.
- **Take all of it:** a prescription drug or nonprescription drug course of therapy recommended by a primary health care provider is not stopped or omitted except on the advice of the primary health care provider.
- **Call your primary health care provider if:** the symptoms for which a drug was prescribed do not improve or become worse; the primary health care provider must be contacted as soon as possible, because a change in dosage or a different drug may be necessary.
- **Do not change or add a dose:** if a dose of a drug is omitted or forgotten, the next dose must not be doubled or the drug taken at more frequent intervals unless advised to do so by the primary health care provider.
- **Tell all your providers:** all health care providers, including physicians, dentists, nurses, and health personnel must always be informed of all drugs (prescription and nonprescription) currently being taken on a regular or occasional basis.
- **Keep a list:** the exact names of all prescription and nonprescription drugs currently being taken should be kept in a wallet or purse for instant reference when seeing a physician, dentist, or other health care provider.
- **Report differences:** check prescriptions carefully when obtaining refills from the pharmacy and report any changes in the prescribed drug (e.g., changes in color, size, shape) to the clinical pharmacist or primary health care provider before taking the drug, because an error may have occurred.

- **Resources to learn more:** the Internet (or World Wide Web) is one of the most frequently used resources when taking responsibility to understand your care and medications. Be sure your sources are true and accurate by looking at who posts the site. As a general rule, sites ending with .gov, .edu, or .org are reputable. Commercial sites end with .com; remember anyone can put those sites on the Internet. When in doubt, ask your health care provider about the source.
- **Wear a MedicAlert bracelet** or other type of medical identification when taking a drug for a long time. This is especially important for drugs such as anticoagulants, steroids, oral hypoglycemic agents, insulin, or digitalis. In case of an emergency, the bracelet ensures that medical personnel are aware of health problems and current drug therapy.

Adverse Drug Effects

- **All drugs cause adverse reactions** (side effects). Examples of some of the more common adverse reactions are nausea, vomiting, diarrhea, constipation, skin rash, dizziness, drowsiness, and dry mouth. Some effects may be mild and subside with time or when the primary health care provider adjusts the dosage. In some instances, mild reactions, such as dry mouth, may have to be tolerated. Some adverse reactions, however, are potentially serious and even life-threatening.
- **Report adverse reactions** to the primary health care provider as soon as possible.
- **Report drug allergies:** medical personnel must be informed of all drug allergies before any treatment or drug is given.

Family Members

Consider the following points concerning family members when developing a teaching plan:

- **Never take another person's drugs:** a drug prescribed for one family member is never given to another family member, relative, or friend unless directed to do so by the primary health care provider.
- **Tell your family:** make sure that all family members or relatives are aware of all drugs, prescription and nonprescription, that are currently being taken by the client.

Drugs, Drug Containers, and Drug Storage/Disposal

- **A drug must be kept in the container in which it was dispensed or purchased:** some drugs require special containers, such as light-resistant (brown) bottles, to prevent deterioration that may occur on exposure to light.
- **Keep the original label on the drug container:** do not remove directions on the label (e.g., "shake well before using," "keep refrigerated," "take before meals"), as these must be followed to ensure drug effectiveness.

- **Never mix different drugs in one container,** even for a brief time, because one drug may chemically affect another. Mixing drugs can also lead to mistaking one drug for another, especially when the size and color are similar.
- **All drugs must be kept out of the reach of children and pets.**
- **Do not expose a drug** to excessive sunlight, heat, cold, or moisture, because deterioration may occur.

- **When traveling, always carry drugs in their original containers with proper labeling.**
- **Never save a prescription for later use** unless the primary health care provider so advises.
- **Dispose of unused drugs properly:** use containers provided, or plastic containers for sharp objects. Never flush unused drugs down a toilet; return them to your primary health care provider or an accepted disposal area.

IMPLEMENTATION

Implementation is the actual performance of the interventions identified in the teaching plan—putting the plan into action. Using knowledge of the *affective domain of learning,* develop a therapeutic relationship with the client (a relationship that is based on trust and caring). When you take the time to develop a therapeutic relationship, the client/family has confidence in you and more confidence in the information conveyed. As shown in Figure 5.3, approach the client and caregivers with respect and encourage the expression of thoughts and feelings. Exploring the client's beliefs about health and illness enhances your understanding of the client's behavior.

Teaching at an appropriate time for each client fosters learning. Plans for teaching should begin when a client comes to the hospital, and sessions can begin at a time when the client is alone, alert, and free of distractions. For example, do not perform client teaching when there are visitors (unless they are to be involved in the administration of the client's drugs), immediately before discharge from the hospital, or if the client is sedated or in pain. Understand the principle of *motivation* and realize that physical discomfort negatively affects the client's concentration and, thus, the ability to learn. A client in pain is motivated to be pain-free, not educated about a medication.

Gear teaching to the client's level of understanding and, when necessary, provide written as well as oral instructions. If a lot of information is given, it is often best to present the material in two or more sessions. Drug administration modifications may be necessary once the client is at home (see Client Teaching to Improved Client Outcomes: Preparing the Client and Family for Drug Administration in the Home). Keep these modifications in mind when teaching the client.

EVALUATION

To determine the effectiveness of client teaching, evaluate the client's confidence in understanding the knowledge of the material presented. Evaluation can occur in several ways, depending on the nature of the information. For example, if the client is being taught to administer insulin, a return demonstration by the client with you observing the client's technique is an evaluation method. This is also known as *teach-back,* when the client using their own words teaches the information or procedure back to the nurse (London, 2016).

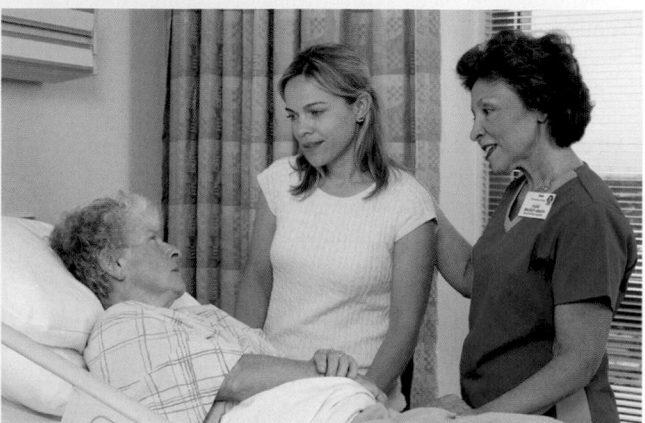

FIGURE 5.3 The nurse uses communication skills to build a therapeutic relationship to enhance learning.

Be knowledgeable about limited health literacy so you will know that questions such as "Do you understand?" or "Is there anything you don't understand?" should be avoided because the client may feel uncomfortable admitting a lack of understanding. Or, the client may not feel well enough to be aware of what they do not know. When factual material is being evaluated, periodically ask the client to list or repeat some of the information presented.

Client Teaching for Improved Outcomes

Preparing the Client and Family for Drug Administration in the Home

Once the client is at home, some modifications may be necessary to ensure safe drug administration. Provide written instructions using words that the client and caregiver can understand. It is important to modify your teaching by using the following suggestions.

When you teach, make sure your client understands the following:

✔ For clients taking more than one drug, develop a clear, easy-to-read drug schedule for the client or caregiver to consult.

✔ Try using a daily calendar as an inexpensive, yet effective, means for scheduling.

✔ If the client or caregiver has a problem with drug names, refer to the drug by shape or color only if other teaching has been unsuccessful. Another idea is to number bottles and use this number on the drug chart.

✔ Suggest the use of commercially available drug organizers.
✔ If your client finds it helpful to keep all drugs together, suggest using a small box (fishing tackle box) to hold all the containers and keep it away from children and pets.
✔ Suggest conducting an inventory of medications early each week to ensure supply for weekends and holidays.
✔ If temporary refrigeration is necessary, suggest the use of a small cooler or insulated bag.
✔ If equipment items, such as needles and syringes, are used, suggest keeping all the supplies in one area. If the supplies come in a delivery box, suggest that the client use it for storage.
✔ Advise the client to use an approved container with a properly fitting lid for safe disposal of needles

and syringes. Return used supplies to the hospital, pharmacy, or local health facility.
✔ Explain the importance of disposing any unused medication in the proper facility and not to flush items into the water supply through a toilet.

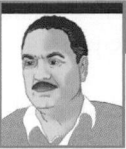

PHARMACOLOGY IN PRACTICE

USING CLINICAL REASONING
A client must have which of the following to learn?
1. Reading skills
2. Ability to write
3. Motivation
4. Good eyesight

KEY POINTS

■ Client teaching is an essential task in nursing. It involves both an established relationship and the use of teaching/learning principles. It involves supplying the client with information and evaluating that understanding.

■ Client–nurse relationships are built upon mutual trust and respect. Nurses who understand the changing health care system and practice good health communication skills can empower clients, resulting in better outcomes.

■ Good health communication includes assessment and interventions to enhance health literacy, having cultural competency, and providing resources for those with LEP.

■ For learning to occur, one needs to be motivated. Adults learn best when they have an inner motivation. Most adults are visual learners, others learn hands-on, while only a few

learn best by listening. You will use cognitive, affective, and psychomotor learning strategies to enhance learning by clients and families. All three domains of learning help to evaluate teaching effectiveness.

■ As you assess health literacy, know that basic language literacy and understanding about health and disease are not the same thing. Analysis of data may indicate how motivated a client is to learn. Learning style preferences help plan the best methods of client teaching. Cultural competency and knowing if clients have LEP guide the choice of interventions used for client teaching.

■ Adapt basic drug information for the home setting to ensure safety of both the client and other family members.

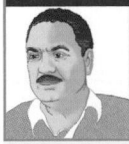

PHARMACOLOGY IN PRACTICE

THINK CRITICALLY
Adults learn best by applying familiar concepts to new situations with information presented multiple times. To support your learning, this book uses a case study approach to help you learn drug information.

Rather than introduce a different client with each new case study, you will be presented with a group of seven clients presenting to a local ambulatory clinic who appear throughout the various chapters across the many pharmacology concepts. Therefore, you can become familiar with their health care situations and needs, leading to a better understanding of how pharmacology and your nursing skills work hand in hand.

In each subsequent unit, information related to specific types of drugs is discussed. The case study presented at the beginning of each chapter will make you think about a client with either an acute or chronic medical

problem. Each selected client in the introduction of the chapter will challenge you to think critically about nursing interventions as you read the information in the chapter. At the end of each chapter, the section Pharmacology in Practice: Think Critically gives more information about the client scenario presented earlier for discussion and reflection to explore the best way to meet client needs.

More information can be gained in the *Study Guide to Accompany Introductory Clinical Pharmacology, 12th edition,* which builds upon each case study client. In the Study Guide, concept-mapping exercises using the clients and situations illustrated in the text help you learn how medication actions reduce symptoms, interact with one another, or complicate client problems.

Now visualize yourself as the nurse obtaining vital signs in the clinic. Given the information you learned in this chapter, review the list of clients, identify any clients who may have limited health literacy, and prepare a list of questions you would want to ask to help you determine who has limited health literacy.

MEET THE CLIENTS

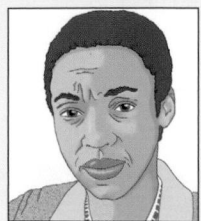

Lillian Chase is a 36-year-old woman who has had asthma for most of her childhood and adult life. After an accident, she suffered seizures and injuries to both her head and her leg; she now needs knee replacement surgery. In addition, she is a smoker who has hypertension.

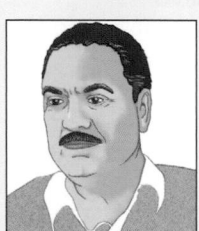

Alfredo Garcia speaks little English. He is seen for an upper respiratory infection, and, upon examination, we discover he lives with hypertension.

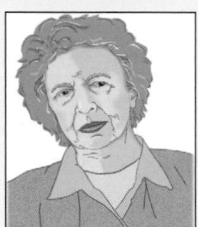

Mrs. Agnes Moore is 85 years of age and seems forgetful and confused at times. She was able to manage her heart failure until she had a urinary tract infection. Her chest pain is now worse, and she has lots of medications to manage.

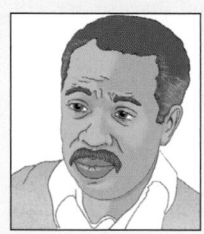

Mr. Bernard Park, aged 77 years, is staying in a long-term care facility following hip replacement surgery. The stress of the procedure has caused an outbreak of herpes zoster (shingles).

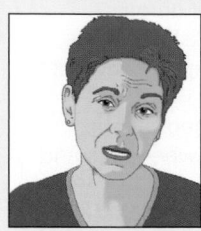

Betty Peterson lives in an apartment. She suffers from aches, pains, and depression.

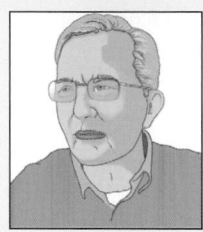

Mr. Rodger Phillip is a 72-year-old widower, and he lives alone. He has both diabetes and early-stage chronic kidney disease. His children do not live close; therefore, in addition to managing his own health care issues, he must learn to live alone and manage a household.

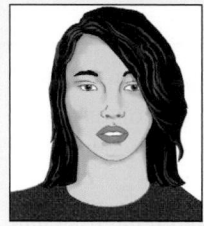

Janna Wong is a 16-year-old high school gymnast. We learn from Janna's mother that she was recovering from mononucleosis before the school year. They both attribute her increased fatigue level to Janna's busy extracurricular schedule.

CHAPTER REVIEW

Prepare for the NCLEX

RECALL THE FACTS

1. An interactive process that promotes learning is defined as:
   1. motivation.
   2. cognitive ability.
   3. psychomotor domain.
   4. teaching.
2. The client–nurse relationship is built upon:
   1. communication.
   2. cultural competency.
   3. health literacy.
   4. respect.

3. Typically, what percentage of people remember instructions given by the primary health care provider?
   1. 80%
   2. 65%
   3. 20%
   4. 10%
4. When developing a teaching plan, the nurse assesses the affective learning domain, which means that the nurse considers the client's:
   1. attitudes, feelings, beliefs, and opinions.
   2. ability to perform a return demonstration.
   3. intellectual ability.
   4. home environment.

5. Development of the strategies to be used in the teaching plan and selection of the information to be taught occur in this phase of the nursing process.
   1. Assessment
   2. Planning
   3. Implementation
   4. Evaluation

ANALYZE THE FACTS

6. A client is preparing for discharge from the hospital tomorrow. She tells you that she has some questions about the medications that she will be taking at home. She explains that the regimen is complicated, and she is afraid she will not be able to remember when to take her medications. Which of the following nursing diagnoses would be most appropriate for this client?
   1. Readiness for Enhanced Health Management
   2. Ineffective Health Management
   3. Deficient Knowledge
   4. Risk for Impaired Home Maintenance

7. *Unless the primary health care provider or clinical pharmacist directs otherwise, the nurse informs the client to take oral medications with:
   1. fruit juice
   2. milk
   3. water
   4. food

8. *The nurse is teaching a mother of twin toddlers to give self-injections. She says, "I will see if we have anything at home to put needles in when I get there." The best action for the nurse to do is:
   1. compliment the woman for planning ahead.
   2. obtain a sharps container from the pharmacy.
   3. note her answer in the medical record.
   4. request that she demonstrate the technique before going home.

ALTERNATE-FORMAT QUESTIONS

9. Arrange the following steps of client teaching correctly.
   1. Provide drug information sheets in the preferred language.
   2. Call for an interpreter to attend the teaching session.
   3. Assess for health literacy and LEP.
   4. Have the client demonstrate how to give the medication.

10. Identify high-risk populations for limited health literacy. **Select all that apply.**
    1. Older persons
    2. High income
    3. Unemployed
    4. Hard of hearing

To check your answers, see Appendix F.

_____

*Indicates the question is directly linked to the NCLX-PN test plan in Appendix G.

WANT TO KNOW MORE? A wide variety of resources are available to enhance your learning and understanding of this chapter.
- Visit for thePoint resources such as:
  - NCLEX-Style Student Review Questions
  - Journal Articles
  - Dosage Calculations
  - Drug Monographs
  - Watch and Learn Videos
  - Concepts in Action Animations
- The *Study Guide to Accompany Introductory Clinical Pharmacology,* 12th edition, sold separately, will help you review and apply essential content.
- ✓*PrepU* is available to help students prepare for the NCLEX-PN examination.

UNIT 2
Drugs Used to Fight Infections

The majority of units in this book use body systems to discuss drug therapy. In this unit, drugs used to fight infections are grouped together because they do not focus on one body system but rather because they work in similar ways through the entire body. Infective organisms are all around us. Some are beneficial, others are not.

To protect ourselves, the body is equipped with a natural defense system, our skin and bodily secretions. An infection occurs when a pathogenic microorganism (which can cause a disease) breaches the body's defense system. Microbes breach our bodily defenses and enter in different ways; this can happen through a break in the skin or by ingestion, breathing, or contact with the mucous membranes of the body. Unit 2 discusses drugs used to kill or retard the growth of microorganisms that invade the body. These drugs are classed together as anti-infective drugs. They include drugs used to treat infections caused by bacteria, viruses, fungi, and protozoans.

Anti-bacterial drugs are a difficult group of drugs to learn; therefore, the unit is broken up into chapters that make learning the material easier. This unit begins with Chapter 6 (sulfa-based drugs), which discusses the first antibacterials developed and used as early as the 1930s. Since that time, scientists have learned the complexity of the bacterial cell and drugs have been developed to target different parts of the cell. Therefore, Chapters 7–9 are uniquely divided up according to what part of the bacterial cell the drugs target. Dividing chapters this way will help you better understand why certain antibacterial agents are used and why others are not. What common adverse reactions of like classes of drugs are and why some drugs produce severe allergic reactions while others do not are better explained with this chapter format. Bacterial pathogens have select components that differ from human cells, such as specific enzymes and a cell wall instead of a cell membrane. Drugs, known as antibiotics, target these bacterial cell differences. You will learn about the mechanisms of action of the antibacterial drugs and how they inhibit the following bacterial cell activities: cell wall synthesis (Chapter 7), DNA or RNA synthesis (Chapter 8), and protein synthesis (Chapter 9). Drugs used to treat the bacterial infections associated with tuberculosis are included in Chapter 10.

In addition to learning about the bacterial infections and drugs, strategies to fight infections effectively are presented. Bacterial resistance is an important issue in the use of anti-infective drugs. Each chapter highlights a concept about the use or misuse of anti-infectives in addition to providing information about selected drug categories. This aides in both your understanding of the drugs and ability to teach clients about anti-infectives. Specific steps are presented in the Client Teaching for Improved Outcomes box in Chapters 7–10 and are designed to build upon each other as you learn about bacterial infections.

These concepts include:

- Basics about infection detection and diagnosis as you are introduced to the sulfonamides (Chapter 6).
- How appropriate drugs are selected along with a discussion about the first antibiotic drugs developed to effectively treat bacterial infections (Chapter 7).
- How foods and drugs together can reduce effectiveness (Chapter 8).
- How fighting a pathogen can cause a superinfection of another pathogen (Chapter 9).
- Why bacteria can become resistant to drugs (Chapter 10).

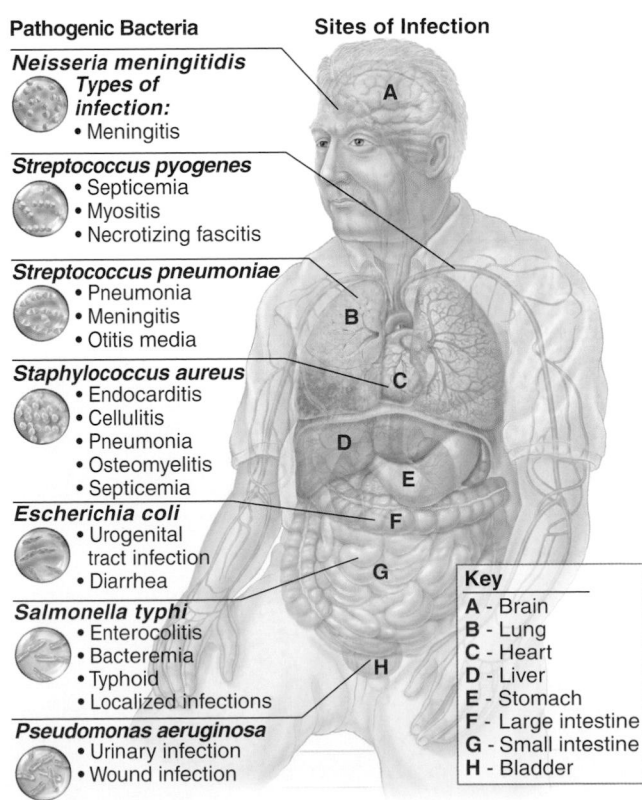

Pathogenic Bacteria **Sites of Infection**

Neisseria meningitidis
Types of infection:
- Meningitis

Streptococcus pyogenes
- Septicemia
- Myositis
- Necrotizing fascitis

Streptococcus pneumoniae
- Pneumonia
- Meningitis
- Otitis media

Staphylococcus aureus
- Endocarditis
- Cellulitis
- Pneumonia
- Osteomyelitis
- Septicemia

Escherichia coli
- Urogenital tract infection
- Diarrhea

Salmonella typhi
- Enterocolitis
- Bacteremia
- Typhoid
- Localized infections

Pseudomonas aeruginosa
- Urinary infection
- Wound infection

Key
A - Brain
B - Lung
C - Heart
D - Liver
E - Stomach
F - Large intestine
G - Small intestine
H - Bladder

Chapter 11 covers drugs that are used to treat viral infections. Unlike bacteria, viruses are organisms that do not have a typical cell structure and use host cells to grow and divide. Because viruses use the DNA or RNA of other cells, their ability to constantly change has posed problems in making drugs to treat viral infections. Unlocking those issues has led to scientific discoveries and an increased production of a number of effective antiviral drugs.

The last chapter of this unit focuses on fungal and protozoal infections. These infections have surfaced to play a more prominent role in health issues in recent years because of advances in medical treatments that cause a condition called immunosuppression (a reduction in white blood cells). Infections that are minor in a healthy body have become life-threatening to immunosuppressed clients because they have low numbers of infection-fighting white blood cells leaving the body, unable to resist the infection. These drugs are covered in Chapter 12.

By understanding the basics of infective processes and the drugs used to treat them, you can help clients deal with fighting infections and promoting healthy lifestyles.

6

Antibacterial Drugs: Sulfonamides

Key Terms

anorexia loss of appetite

antibacterial active against bacteria

antibiotic term used synonymously with antibacterial

aplastic anemia blood disorder caused by damage to the bone marrow resulting in a marked reduction in the number of red blood cells and some white blood cells

bactericidal drug or agent that destroys or kills bacteria

bacteriostatic drug or agent that slows or retards the multiplication of bacteria

crystalluria formation of crystals in the urine

leukopenia decrease in the number of leukocytes (white blood cells)

pruritus itching

Stevens–Johnson syndrome (SJS) fever, cough, muscular aches and pains, headache, and lesions of the skin, mucous membranes, and eyes; the lesions appear as red wheals or blisters, often starting on the face, in the mouth, or on the lips, neck, and extremities

stomatitis inflammation of a cavity opening, such as the oral cavity

thrombocytopenia decreased number of platelets in the blood

toxic epidermal necrolysis (TEN) toxic skin reaction with sloughing of skin and mucous membranes

urticaria hives; itchy wheals on the skin resulting from contact with or ingestion of an allergenic substance or food

Learning Objectives

On completion of this chapter, the student will:

1. Describe the concept of bacterial sensitivity.
2. Explain the uses, general drug actions, and general adverse reactions, contraindications, precautions, and interactions for the sulfonamides.
3. Distinguish important preadministration and ongoing assessment activities the nurse should perform on the client taking sulfonamides.
4. List nursing diagnoses particular to a client taking sulfonamides.
5. Examine ways to promote an optimal response to therapy, how to manage adverse reactions, and important points to keep in mind when educating clients about the use of the sulfonamides.
6. Identify the rationale for increasing fluid intake when taking sulfonamides.
7. Describe the objective signs indicating that a severe skin reaction, such as Stevens–Johnson syndrome, is present.

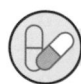 **Drug Classes**

Single sulfonamide agents
Urinary anti-infective combinations
Topical preparations

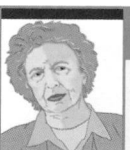
PHARMACOLOGY IN PRACTICE

Each chapter features a specific case study corresponding to the drug therapy in each chapter. In this chapter, the client featured is Mrs. Agnes Moore. She is 85 years old and has been prescribed a sulfonamide for a urinary tract infection (UTI). She is to take the drug for 10 days. Mrs. Agnes Moore seems forgetful and a bit confused as you talk with her. Use your preassessment interview skills and look for the *Pharmacology in Practice* guideposts as you read to see if this is the best medication choice for her.

When learning about antibacterial drug therapy, you need to understand how these drugs interact with bacteria. Drugs that are used against bacteria are either **bacteriostatic** (they slow or retard the multiplication of bacteria) or **bactericidal** (they destroy the bacteria). To choose the appropriate drug, the primary health care provider needs to know if the bacteria will react to the drugs. This response is called sensitivity.

ANTIBIOTIC STEWARDSHIP: CULTURE AND SENSITIVITY TESTING

To determine if a specific type of bacteria is sensitive to an **antibiotic** drug, culture and sensitivity tests are performed. A culture is performed by placing infectious material obtained from areas such as the skin, respiratory tract, and blood on a culture plate that contains a special growing medium. This growing medium is "food" for the bacteria. After a specified time, the bacteria are examined under a microscope and identified. The sensitivity test involves placing the infectious material on a separate culture plate and then placing small disks impregnated with various antibiotics over the area. After a specified time, the culture plate is examined. If there is little or no growth around a disk, the bacteria are considered sensitive to that particular antibiotic. Therefore, the infection will be controlled by the antibiotic. If there is considerable growth around the disk, then the bacteria are considered resistant to that particular antibiotic, and the infection will not be controlled by the antibiotic (Fig. 6.1).

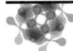 # SULFONAMIDES

Sulfonamides (commonly called sulfa drugs) are **antibacterial** agents, meaning they are active against bacteria. Sulfadiazine and sulfamethizole are examples of sulfonamide preparations. Important for the treatment of certain types of infections, the use of sulfonamides declined significantly after the introduction of more effective anti-infectives such as the penicillins and other antibiotics. Frequently, sulfa drugs are used in combination with other drugs to treat infections (this concept is explained in depth in Chapter 46).

ACTIONS

The sulfonamides are primarily *bacteriostatic* (slows growth) because the drug only inhibits the activity of folic acid in bacterial cell metabolism. Once the rate of bacterial multiplication is slowed, the body's own defense mechanisms (white blood cells) are able to rid the body of the invading microorganisms and therefore control the infection. The sulfonamides are well absorbed by the gastrointestinal (GI) system and excreted by the kidneys (see Chapter 46). They are often used to control infections caused by both gram-positive and gram-negative bacteria, such as *Escherichia coli, Staphylococcus aureus,* and *Klebsiella,* and *Enterobacter* species. Additionally, when sulfasalazine interacts with intestinal bacteria, it helps to inhibit the inflammatory process, which is how the drug works to treat ulcerative colitis.

 Concept Mastery Alert

Sulfonamides are classified as bacteriostatic because they inhibit the action of folic acid in bacterial cell metabolism. This slows the multiplication of the bacteria.

USES

The sulfonamides are often used in the treatment of infections, such as:

- Urinary tract infections (UTIs).
- Acute otitis media.
- Ulcerative colitis.
- Bacterial skin and eye infections.
- Mafenide (Sulfamylon) and silver sulfadiazine (Silvadene) are topical sulfonamides used in the treatment and prevention of infections in second- and third-degree burns.

Additional uses of the sulfonamides are given in the Summary Drug Table: Sulfonamides.

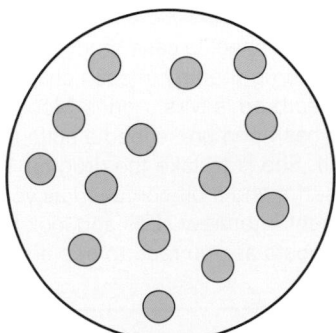 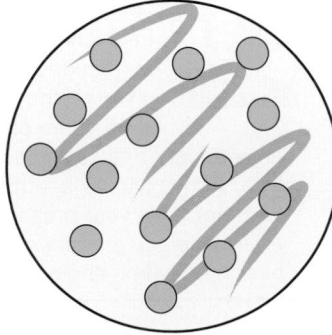 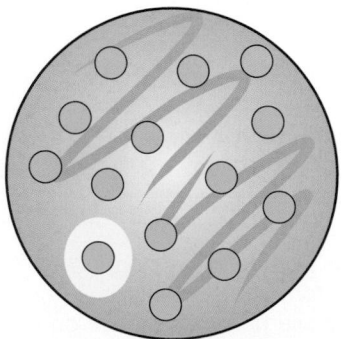

A Culture plate with small disks containing various antibiotics.

B Infectious material is spread on the culture plate.

C After a specific time, the culture plate is inspected. If there is little or no growth around a disk, the bacteria is said to be sensitive to that antibiotic.

FIGURE 6.1 **A–C.** Culture and sensitivity tests indicate which drug is most effective against the bacteria on the culture plate.

ADVERSE REACTIONS

The sulfonamides are capable of causing a variety of adverse reactions. Some of these are serious or potentially serious; others are mild. **Anorexia** (loss of appetite) is an example of a mild adverse reaction. An example of a serious reaction, Stevens–Johnson syndrome, is explained in the Nursing Alert.

Gastrointestinal System Reactions
- Nausea, vomiting, anorexia
- Diarrhea, abdominal pain
- **Stomatitis** (inflammation of the mouth)

In some instances, these reactions may be mild. At other times, they may cause serious problems, such as pronounced weight loss, requiring discontinuation of the drug.

Other Reactions
- Chills, fever
- **Crystalluria** (crystals in the urine)
- Photosensitivity

Various types of hypersensitivity (allergic) reaction may be seen during sulfonamide therapy, including **urticaria** (hives), **pruritus** (itching), generalized skin eruptions, or severe reactions leading to potentially lethal conditions such as **toxic epidermal necrolysis (TEN) or Stevens–Johnson syndrome (SJS)**.

> ### ! NURSING ALERT
>
> TEN and SJS are serious and sometimes fatal hypersensitivity reactions. Widespread sloughing of both the skin and mucous membranes can occur. If internal organs are involved, death may occur. Clients with SJS may complain of fever, cough, muscular aches and pains, and headache, all of which are signs and symptoms of many other disorders. Be alert for the additional signs of lesions on the skin and mucous membranes, eyes, and other organs, a diagnostically important indicator of these problems. The lesions appear as red wheals or blisters, often starting on the face, in the mouth, or on the lips, neck, and extremities. These conditions may also occur with the administration of other types of drugs. Notify the primary health care provider and withhold the next dose of the drug. In addition, exercise care to prevent injury to the involved areas.

The most frequent adverse reaction seen with the topical application of a sulfonamide is a burning sensation or pain when the drug is applied to the skin. Other possible allergic reactions include rash, itching, edema, and urticaria. It may be difficult to distinguish between adverse reactions caused by the use of mafenide or silver sulfadiazine and those that occur from a severe burn injury or from other agents used for the management of burns.

The following hematologic changes may occur during prolonged sulfonamide therapy:

- **Leukopenia**—decrease in the number of white blood cells
- **Thrombocytopenia**—decrease in the number of platelets.
- **Aplastic anemia**—deficient red blood cell production in the bone marrow.

These changes are examples of serious adverse reactions. If any of these occur, discontinuation of sulfonamide therapy may be required.

CONTRAINDICATIONS

The sulfonamides are contraindicated in clients with hypersensitivity to the sulfonamides, during lactation, and in children younger than 2 years. The sulfonamides are not used near the end (at term) of pregnancy (pregnancy category D). If the sulfonamides are given near the end of pregnancy, significantly high blood levels of the drug may occur, causing jaundice or hemolytic anemia in the neonate. In addition, the sulfonamides are not used for infections caused by group A beta-hemolytic (β-hemolytic) streptococci because the sulfonamides have *not* been shown to be effective in *preventing* the complications of rheumatic fever or glomerulonephritis.

PRECAUTIONS

The sulfonamides are used with caution in clients with renal impairment, hepatic impairment, or bronchial asthma.

These drugs are given with caution to clients with allergies. When used in pregnant women to treat *Toxoplasmosis gondii* infections, be aware the drug can cross the placenta. Safety for use during pregnancy has not been established (pregnancy category C, except at term; see above).

INTERACTIONS

The following interactions may occur when a sulfonamide is administered with another agent:

Interacting Drug	Common Use	Effect of Interaction
Oral anticoagulants	Blood thinner; prevent clot formation	Increased action of the anticoagulant
Methotrexate	Immunosuppression and chemotherapy	Increased bone marrow suppression
Hydantoins	Anticonvulsants	Increased serum hydantoin level

 Chronic Care Considerations

When diabetic clients are prescribed sulfonamides, assess for a possible hypoglycemic reaction. Sulfonamides may disrupt the (hepatic) metabolism of the oral hypoglycemic drugs and the parenteral drugs which enhance insulin production.

Herbal Considerations

Cranberries and cranberry juice are commonly used folk remedies for preventing and relieving symptoms of UTIs. The use of cranberries in combination with antibiotics has been recommended by physicians for the long-term suppression of UTIs. Cranberries are thought to prevent bacteria from attaching to the walls of the urinary tract. The suggested dose is 6 ounces of juice twice daily. Cranberry capsules are not recommended because the juice's fluid for hydration may be as helpful as the berries (Brown, 2012). Extremely large doses can produce GI disturbances, such as diarrhea or abdominal cramping. Although cranberries may relieve symptoms or prevent the occurrence of a UTI, their use will not cure a UTI. If an individual suspects a UTI, medical attention is necessary.

NURSING PROCESS—STEPS TO BUILDING CLINICAL JUDGMENT
Client Receiving a Sulfonamide

ASSESSMENT

Preadministration Assessment

Data gathering suggestions before the initial administration of the drug include the following:

Objective data

- Description of general appearance, especially affect and orientation of elderly.
- Vital signs (temperature, pulse, respirations and blood pressure).
- Urine collection for urinalysis.

Subjective data

- Type and duration of symptoms (genitourinary and other systems).
- Remedies attempted before seeking care.

Signs of a UTI are not limited to the genitourinary system. If an elderly client appears distracted or the family notes sudden confusion, these may be signs of a genitourinary infection. Many infections are diagnosed and treated in ambulatory settings; therefore, it is important to ask about self-remedies the client may have tried before seeing a primary health care provider. Depending on the type and location of the infection or disease, review the results of tests such as a urine culture, urinalysis, complete blood count, intravenous pyelogram, renal function tests, and examination of the stool.

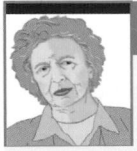

PHARMACOLOGY IN PRACTICE

DATA COLLECTION

In Mrs. Moore's situation, information from the preassessment can help you determine whether her confusion is an ongoing problem or caused by her current illness. Which data item makes you think this is acute confusion caused by infection?

1. She has trouble telling you what day it is today.
2. Her urine is amber and cloudy.
3. She smells of urine.
4. Urinalysis shows 3+ bacteria and white blood cells.

Ongoing Assessment

During the course of therapy, evaluate the client at periodic intervals for response to the drug—that is, a relief of symptoms and a decrease in temperature (if it was elevated before therapy started), as well as the occurrence of any adverse reactions.

If fever is present and the client's temperature suddenly increases or if the temperature was normal and suddenly increases, instruct the client to contact the primary health care provider immediately.

The ongoing assessment for clients receiving sulfasalazine for ulcerative colitis includes observation for evidence of the relief or intensification of the symptoms of the disease. Ask the client to monitor when using the bathroom for changes in number or appearance of the stool. The client should contact the primary health care provider regarding changes.

When administering a sulfonamide for a burn, inspect the burned areas every 1 to 2 hr, because some treatment regimens require keeping the affected areas covered with the mafenide or silver sulfadiazine ointment at all times. Any adverse reactions should be reported immediately to the primary health care provider.

NURSING DIAGNOSES

Drug-specific nursing diagnoses include the following:

- **Altered urinary elimination** related to effect on the bladder from sulfonamides.
- **Altered skin integrity** related to burns.
- **Altered skin integrity** related to photosensitivity or severe allergic reaction to the sulfonamides.
- **Infection (secondary) Risk** related to lowered white blood cell count resulting from sulfonamide therapy.

Nursing diagnoses related to drug administration are discussed in Chapter 4.

PLANNING

The expected client outcomes depend on the reason for administration of the sulfonamide but may include an optimal response to drug therapy, meeting client needs related to the management of adverse drug reactions, and confidence in an understanding of the medication regimen.

IMPLEMENTATION

Promoting an Optimal Response to Therapy

The client receiving a sulfonamide drug almost always has an active infection. Some clients may be receiving one of these drugs to prevent an infection (prophylaxis) or as part of the management of a disease such as ulcerative colitis.

Unless the primary health care provider orders otherwise, give sulfonamides to the client whose stomach is empty—that is, 1 hr before or 2 hr after meals. If GI irritation occurs, give sulfasalazine with food or immediately after meals.

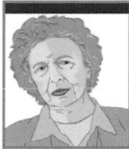

PHARMACOLOGY IN PRACTICE

DOSAGE CALCULATION

The primary health care provider wants to give a loading dose and has prescribed sulfamethoxazole–trimethoprim tablets 2 g to be given while in the clinic. The drug is available in 400 mg tablets. How many tablets should the nurse administer to the client in this initial dose?

Sulfasalazine may cause the urine and skin to take on an orange-yellow color; this is normal. Crystalluria may occur during administration of a sulfonamide. Often, this potentially serious problem can be prevented by increasing fluid intake during sulfonamide therapy. It is important to instruct the client to drink a full glass (8 ounces) of water when taking an oral sulfonamide and to drink at least eight more large glasses of water throughout the day until therapy is finished.

Monitoring and Managing Client Needs

Observe the client for adverse reactions, especially an allergic reaction (see Chapter 1). If one or more adverse reactions should occur, withhold the next dose of the drug and notify the primary health care provider.

Altered Urinary Elimination

One adverse effect of the sulfonamide drugs is altered elimination patterns. Therefore, it is important to help the client maintain adequate fluid intake and output. Encourage clients to increase fluid intake to 2,000 mL (68 ounces) or more per day to prevent crystalluria and stones (calculi) forming in the genitourinary tract, as well as to aid in removing microorganisms from the urinary tract. It is important to measure and record the client's intake and output every 8 to 12 hr and notify the primary health care provider if the urinary output decreases or the client fails to increase their oral intake (Fig. 6.2).

 Lifespan Considerations

Gerontology

Because renal function diminishes normally as people age, administer the sulfonamides with great caution to the older client. There is an increased danger of

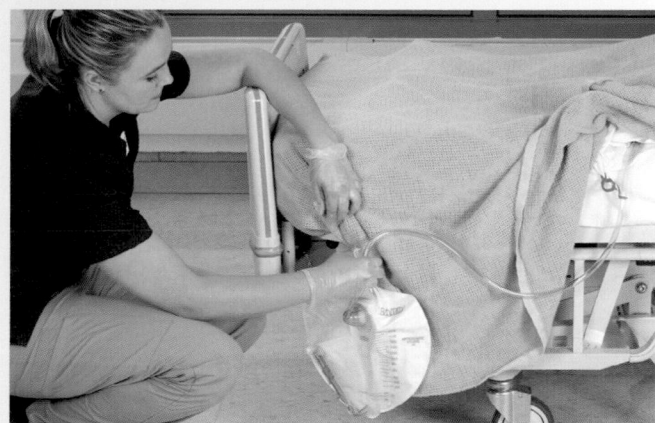

FIGURE 6.2 Nurses monitor for decreased urinary output and possible crystal formation in the client receiving sulfonamides.

the sulfonamides causing additional renal damage when renal impairment is already present. An increase of fluid intake up to 2,000 mL (if the older adult can tolerate this amount) decreases the risk of crystals and stones forming in the urinary tract. The older adult may be hesitant to increase oral fluid intake because of fear of incontinence. It is important to assess for this fear and teach the client when to take fluids to maintain continence and reduce the risk of crystal formation.

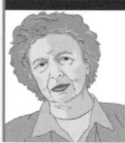

PHARMACOLOGY IN PRACTICE

INTERVENTIONS

Mrs. Agnes Moore is hesitant to increase her fluid intake. Which of the following reasons should the nurse give her to improve fluid intake? Select all that apply.
1. Removes microorganisms from urinary system.
2. Allows for easy absorption of the drug in the GI system.
3. Prevents formation of crystals in the urine.
4. Allows for easy excretion by the kidneys.

Altered Skin Integrity: Burn Injury

When mafenide or silver sulfadiazine is used in treating burns, the treatment regimen is outlined by the primary health care provider or the personnel in the burn treatment unit. There are various burn treatment regimens, such as débridement (removal of burned or dead tissue from the burned site), special dressings, and cleansing of the burned area (Box 6.1). The use of a specific treatment regimen often depends on the extent of the burned area, the degree of the burns, and the physical condition and age of the client. Other concurrent problems, such as lung damage from smoke or heat or physical injuries that occurred at the time of the burn injury, also may influence the treatment regimen.

BOX 6.1 Steps in Applying Topical Preparations to Burns

1. Clean and remove debris present on the surface of the skin.
2. Apply drug in a layer approximately 1/16 in. thick; thicker application is not recommended.
3. While wound is exposed, minimize air draft because it can cause pain.
4. Warn the client that stinging or burning may be felt during and for a short time after application.

Altered Skin Integrity: Photosensitivity

The skin can become more sensitive to sunlight during sulfonamide therapy. Even where the climate is overcast, solar glare and indirect sunshine can cause a sunburn reaction. Clients should be cautioned to wear protective clothing and sunscreen whenever outside. When in a facility, the skin should be inspected, each shift when treatment is started, for signs of sores or blisters indicating the possibility of a severe allergic reaction. When taken on an outpatient basis, the skin should be inspected frequently. The skin and mucous membranes should be inspected for up to 14 days after the end of therapy, the period of time during which reactions can still occur.

Infection (secondary) Risk

Scan laboratory results to monitor the client for leukopenia and thrombocytopenia. Leukopenia may also present with physical signs and symptoms of an infection, such as fever, sore throat, and cough. Protect the client with leukopenia from individuals who have an infection.

Thrombocytopenia is manifested by easy bruising and unusual bleeding after moderate to slight trauma to the skin or mucous membranes. The extremities of the client with thrombocytopenia are handled with care to prevent bruising. Care is taken to prevent trauma when moving the client. Inspect the skin daily for the extent of bruising and evidence of exacerbation of existing ecchymotic areas. It is important to encourage the client to use a soft-bristled toothbrush to prevent any trauma to the mucous membranes of the oral cavity. Report any signs of leukopenia or thrombocytopenia immediately because these are indications to stop drug therapy.

Educating the Client and Family

Carefully planned client and family education is important to foster adherence to the therapy, relieve anxiety, and promote a therapeutic effect. When a sulfonamide is prescribed for an infection, symptoms may diminish quickly and some clients have a tendency to discontinue the drug once symptoms are gone. When teaching the client and family, emphasize the importance of completing the prescribed course of therapy to ensure all microorganisms causing the infection are eradicated. Help clients to understand that failure to complete a course of therapy may result in a recurrence of the infection. To increase adherence to the treatment recommendations, a teaching plan is developed to include the information that appears in the Client Teaching for Improved Outcomes: Taking Anti-Infectives.

Client Teaching for Improved Outcomes

Taking Anti-Infectives

When you teach, make sure your client understands the following:

✔ Take the drug at the prescribed time intervals. These time intervals are important because a certain amount of the drug must be in the body at all times for the infection to be controlled.

✔ Drink six to eight 8-ounce glasses of fluid while taking these drugs, and take each dose with a full glass of water.

✔ Do not increase or omit the dose unless advised to do so by the primary health care provider.

✔ Complete the entire course of treatment. Do not stop the drug, except on the advice of a primary health care provider, before the course of treatment is completed, even if symptoms improve or disappear. Failure to complete the prescribed course of treatment may result in a return of the infection.

✔ Follow the directions supplied with the prescription regarding taking the drugs with meals or on an empty stomach. Take drugs that must be taken on an empty stomach 1 hr before or 2 hr after a meal.

✔ Distinguish between immediate- and extended-release medications. Do not break, chew, or crush extended-release medications.

✔ Notify the primary health care provider if symptoms of the infection become worse or if original symptoms do not improve after 5 to 7 days of drug therapy.

✔ Avoid any exposure to sunlight or ultraviolet light (tanning beds, sunlamps) while taking these drugs and for several weeks after completing the course of therapy. Wear sunblock, sunglasses, and protective clothing when exposed to sunlight.

✔ Avoid tasks requiring mental alertness until response to the drug is known.

Specific Instructions Regarding Sulfonamides

✔ Take sulfasalazine with food or immediately after a meal.

✔ When taking sulfasalazine, the skin or urine may turn orange-yellow; this is *normal*. Soft contact lenses may acquire a permanent yellow stain. It is a good idea to seek the advice of an ophthalmologist regarding disposable lenses while taking this drug.

EVALUATION

- Therapeutic response is achieved, and there is no evidence of infection.
- Adverse reactions are identified, reported to the primary health care provider, and managed successfully with appropriate nursing interventions:
  - Client maintains an adequate fluid intake for proper urinary elimination.

- Skin is intact and free of inflammation, irritation, infection, or ulcerations.
- No evidence of infection is seen.
- Client and family express confidence and demonstrate an understanding of the drug regimen.

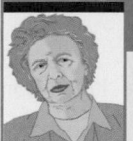

PHARMACOLOGY IN PRACTICE

USING CLINICAL REASONING
Mrs. Agnes Moore returns to the clinic for a 2-week follow-up appointment. When her urinalysis comes back from the laboratory showing 3+ for bacteria, how does that influence your assessment?

KEY POINTS

■ Infections occur when pathogenic microorganisms breach our natural defenses, such as the skin.

■ Culture and sensitivity testing helps to identify the best drug for eradicating the bacterial infection.

■ Sulfonamides are primarily bacteriostatic; they slow or retard the multiplication of bacteria, not destroy it.

■ Sulfonamides are used primarily for UTIs and as topical preparations.

■ Persons taking sulfonamides need to increase fluid intake to at least 2,000 mL to prevent genitourinary problems caused by the drug. Because kidney function diminishes as we age, there is an increased danger of renal damage and fluid increase is even more important with the elderly.

■ Photosensitivity is an adverse reaction of sulfonamides; people taking these drugs should lessen outdoor activities or take care to protect their skin while outdoors.

SUMMARY DRUG TABLE SULFONAMIDES

Generic Name	Trade Name	Uses	Adverse Reactions	Dosage Ranges
Single Agents				
⊘ **sulfADIAZINE** sul-fa-DYE-a-zeen		UTIs, chancroid, acute otitis media, *Haemophilus influenzae*, and rheumatic fever	Vomiting, headache, diarrhea, chills, fever, anorexia, crystalluria, stomatitis, urticaria, pruritus, hematologic changes, Stevens–Johnson syndrome, nausea	Loading dose: 2–4 g orally; maintenance dose: 2–4 g/day orally in 4–6 divided doses
sulfaSALAzine sul-fa-SAL-a-zeen		UTI, acute otitis media, *H. influenzae*	Same as sulfadiazine; may cause skin and urine to turn orange-yellow	Initial therapy: 1–4 g/day orally in divided doses; maintenance dose: 2 g/day orally in evenly spaced doses (500 mg QID)
Urinary Anti-Infective Combinations				
trimethoprim (TMP) and sulfamethoxazole (SMZ) trye-METH-oh-prim sul-fa-meth-OKS-a-zole	Bactrim, Bactrim DS, Septra, Septra DS	Acute bacterial UTI, acute otitis media, traveler's diarrhea caused by *E. coli*	Headache, GI disturbances, allergic skin reactions, hematologic changes, Stevens–Johnson syndrome, anorexia, glossitis	160 mg TMP/800 mg SMZ orally every 12 hr; 8–10 mg/kg/day (based on TMP) IV in 2–4 divided doses
Topical Sulfonamide Preparations				
mafenide MA-fe-nide	Sulfamylon	Second- and third-degree burns	Pain or burning sensation, rash, itching, facial edema	Apply to burned area 1–2 times/day
silver sulfadiazine SIL-ver sul-fa-DYE-a-zeen	Silvadene, Thermazene, SSD (cream)	Same as mafenide	Leukopenia, skin necrosis, skin discoloration, burning sensation	Same as mafenide

 This drug should be administered at least 1 hr before or 2 hr after a meal.
See Chapters 52 and 53 for topical and eye preparation drugs.

CHAPTER REVIEW

Know Your Drugs

Clients sometimes know a medication by the brand (or trade) name and not the generic name. To help you recognize both names, match the brand name with the generic name of the same medication.

Generic Name	Brand Name
1. silver sulfadiazine	A. Bactrim
2. sulfamethoxazole/ trimethoprim	B. Silvadene

Calculate Medication Dosages

1. The primary health care provider prescribed sulfasalazine oral suspension 500 mg every 8 hr. The nurse has sulfasalazine oral suspension 250 mg/5 mL on hand. What dosage should the nurse give?
2. The primary health care provider orders sulfamethoxazole 2 g orally initially, followed by 1 g orally two times a day. The nurse has 1,000-mg tablets on hand. How many tablets should the nurse give for the initial dose?

Prepare for the NCLEX

RECALL THE FACTS

1. A nurse working in the clinic asks how the sulfonamides control an infection. The most accurate answer is that these drugs _____.
   1. encourage the production of antibodies
   2. inhibit folic acid metabolism
   3. reduce urine output
   4. make the urine alkaline, which eliminates bacteria
2. Clients receiving sulfasalazine for ulcerative colitis are told that the drug _____.
   1. is not to be taken with food
   2. rarely causes adverse effects
   3. may cause hair loss
   4. may turn the urine an orange-yellow color
3. On an overcast day, the nurse instructs the client taking sulfonamides to _____.
   1. wear sunscreen
   2. sunbathe without fear of skin reaction
   3. stay indoors with blinds shut
   4. protect feet from harm
4. A client with diabetes who takes oral medications is receiving a sulfonamide for a UTI. The client is taught that compared to what the usual reading has been, the blood glucose level will be:
   1. higher
   2. the same
   3. lower
   4. unreadable because of the medication

5. The nurse observes a client receiving a sulfonamide for Stevens–Johnson syndrome. The signs and symptoms that might indicate this syndrome include _____.
   1. swelling of the extremities
   2. increased blood pressure and pulse rate
   3. lesions on the skin or mucous membranes
   4. pain in the joints
6. The nurse can evaluate the client's response to therapy by asking them if _____.
   1. they completed the entire course of therapy
   2. have symptoms been relieved
   3. any evidence of blood in the urine
   4. they have experienced any constipation

ANALYZE THE FACTS

7. *The nurse instructs a client to drink at least 2,000 mL of fluid while taking a sulfa drug. The client states they cannot drink that much. The nurse should ask questions to assess which body system?
   1. respiratory
   2. genitourinary
   3. neurologic
   4. cardiac
8. *When mafenide (Sulfamylon) is applied to a burned area, the nurse _____.
   1. first covers the burned area with a sterile compress
   2. irrigates the area with normal saline solution
   3. warns the client that stinging or burning may be felt
   4. instructs the client to drink two to three extra glasses of water each day

ALTERNATE-FORMAT QUESTIONS

9. *Arrange the following steps of caring for a burn with Silvadene correctly:
   1. apply dressing material
   2. cleanse and remove debris on surface
   3. apply drug according to directions
   4. remove dressing
10. Identify the correct properties of sulfonamide drugs. **Select all that apply.**
    1. bactericidal
    2. reduces inflammation in colon
    3. inhibits folic acid in bacterial cells
    4. antibacterial

To check your answers, see Appendix F.

---

*Indicates the question is directly linked to the NCLEX-PN test plan in Appendix G.

WANT TO KNOW MORE? A wide variety of resources are available to enhance your learning and understanding of this chapter.

■ Visit for the Point resources such as:
  • NCLEX-Style Student Review Questions
  • Journal Articles
  • Dosage Calculations
  • Drug Monographs
  • Watch and Learn Videos
  • Concepts in Action Animations

■ The *Study Guide to Accompany Introductory Clinical Pharmacology*, 12th edition, sold separately, will help you review and apply essential content.

■ ✓*PrepU* is available to help students prepare for the NCLEX-PN examination.

7

Antibacterial Drugs That Disrupt the Bacterial Cell Wall

Key Terms

anaphylactic reactions unusual or exaggerated allergic reactions; see anaphylactic shock (Chapter 1)

angioedema localized wheals or swellings in subcutaneous tissues or mucous membranes, which may be caused by an allergic response

bacterial resistance phenomenon by which a bacteria-produced substance inactivates or destroys an antibiotic drug

beta-lactam (β-lactam) ring portion of the penicillin drug molecule that can break a bacterial cell wall

cross-sensitivity allergy to drugs in the same or related groups

culture and sensitivity test culture of bacteria to determine to which antibiotic the microorganism is sensitive

glossitis inflammation of the tongue

malaise discomfort, uneasiness

methicillin-resistant *Staphylococcus aureus* (MRSA) bacterium that is resistant to methicillin

nephrotoxicity damage to the kidneys by a toxic substance

otitis media infection of the middle ear

pathogens disease-producing microorganisms

penicillinase enzyme produced by bacteria that deactivates penicillin

perioperative pertaining to the preoperative, intraoperative, or postoperative period

phlebitis inflammation of a vein

prophylaxis prevention

pseudomembranous colitis severe, life-threatening form of diarrhea that occurs when normal flora of the bowel is eliminated and replaced with *Clostridium difficile (C. diff)* bacteria

(continued)

Learning Objectives

On completion of this chapter, the student will:

1. Explain the uses, general drug actions, and general adverse reactions, contraindications, precautions, and interactions of antibacterial drugs that disrupt bacterial cell walls.
2. Distinguish important preadministration and ongoing assessment activities the nurse should perform on the client taking an antibacterial drug that disrupts bacterial cell walls.
3. List nursing diagnoses particular to a client taking an antibacterial drug that disrupts bacterial cell walls.
4. Discuss hypersensitivity reactions as they relate to antibiotic therapy.
5. Examine ways to promote optimal response to therapy, nursing actions to minimize adverse effects, and important points to keep in mind when educating clients about the use of antibacterial drugs that disrupt bacterial cell walls.

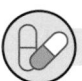 **Drug Classes**

Penicillins	Cephalosporins	Carbapenems
• Natural penicillins • Aminopenicillins • Extended-spectrum penicillins	• First generation • Second generation • Third generation • Fourth generation • Fifth generation	Miscellaneous drugs that break the bacterial cell wall

PHARMACOLOGY IN PRACTICE

Alfredo Garcia is seen in the outpatient clinic for an upper respiratory infection. The primary health care provider prescribes a cephalosporin and asks you to give the client instructions for taking the drug. You note that Mr. Garcia appears to understand very little English. You are concerned about his ability to take the medication as directed. Think about why this is important as you read this chapter.

The cellular contents in a human being are contained by a cell membrane. Unlike the human cell, the structure of a bacterial cell is different. A bacterial cell has a wall, not a membrane. The drugs in this chapter, penicillins, cephalosporins, carbapenems, and vancomycin, all inhibit bacterial cell wall **synthesis** (growth and repair). The classes of drugs in this chapter are effective against bacteria because they target

the bacterial cell wall. When the drug breaks down the cell wall, the bacteria die.

Enzymes known as penicillin-binding proteins are involved in bacterial cell wall synthesis and cell division. Antibiotics, which interfere with these processes, inhibit cell wall synthesis, causing rapid destruction of the bacterial cell. When penicillin was first used, these drugs worked very well because bacteria have a receptor on the cell wall that attracts the penicillin molecule. That is, when the drug attaches to the cell, a portion of the drug molecule (the **beta-lactam [β-lactam] ring**) breaks the cell wall and the cell dies (bactericidal action). Figure 7.1 illustrates how the drug breaks down the bacteria's cell wall. Unfortunately, after many years of use of the penicillins, drug-resistant strains of microorganisms developed, making the penicillins less effective than some of the new antibiotics in treating a broad range of infections.

Cephalosporins are a more commonly used group of drugs and are structurally and chemically related to penicillin. The cephalosporins are a valuable group of drugs that are effective in the treatment of infection with almost all of the strains of bacteria affected by the penicillins, as well as some strains of bacteria that have become resistant to penicillin. Carbapenems are a relatively new class of bactericidal drugs that have the largest spectrum of any antibiotic.

ANTIBIOTIC STEWARDSHIP: IDENTIFYING THE APPROPRIATE ANTI-INFECTIVE

Selection of Drugs

Typically, a person sees a primary care provider with complaints that are identified as a possible infection. A broad-spectrum antibacterial may be ordered at the same time a swab of the infected area is taken and sent to the laboratory for a **culture and sensitivity (C&S)** test (see Chapter 6). After a C&S test report is received, the strain of microorganisms causing the infection is identified as well as which antibiotics will or will not kill the microorganisms. The primary health care provider then selects the antibiotic to which the microorganism is sensitive, because that is the antibiotic that will be effective in the treatment of the infection. This is why it is important to view the C&S report as a drug may need to be changed.

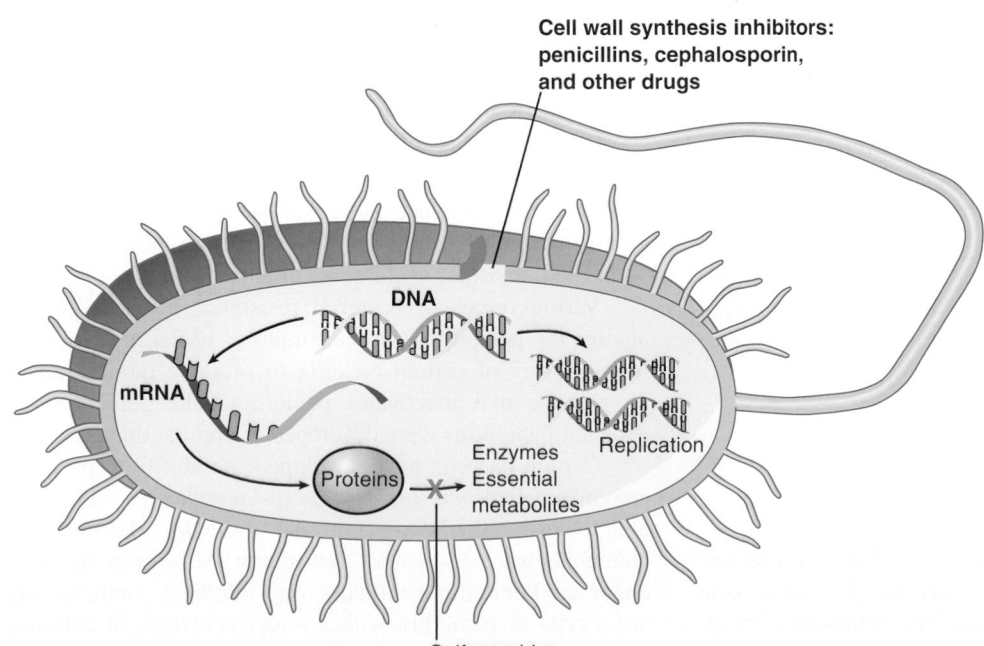

Cell wall synthesis inhibitors: penicillins, cephalosporin, and other drugs

DNA

mRNA

Replication

Proteins

Enzymes
Essential
metabolites

Sulfonamides

FIGURE 7.1 Bacterial cell. Sites of action of penicillins, cephalosporins, and other drugs are noted, which is together termed cell wall synthesis inhibition.

Resistance to Drugs

Bacterial resistance is the ability of bacteria to produce substances that inactivate or destroy the antibiotic. Because bacteria have this ability, many more drugs have been developed in addition to the sulfonamides and penicillins to fight bacterial infections. They include cephalosporins, the tetracycline group, and various other drugs.

When antibiotics are used by one person over time, or by a group of people who live in close proximity (as in a long-term care facility), drug resistance becomes an issue. Some bacteria may be naturally resistant to an antibiotic, or they may acquire a resistance to the drug. When the susceptible bacteria are destroyed, what remains are the resistant bacteria. As a result, strains of drug-resistant bacteria multiply. These can range from the penicillinase enzyme–producing bacteria to **methicillin-resistant *Staphylococcus aureus* (MRSA)**.

MRSA is a type of bacteria that is resistant to certain antibiotics. These antibiotics include methicillin and other more common antibiotics, such as oxacillin, penicillin, and amoxicillin. According to the Centers for Disease Control and Prevention (CDC), staphylococcal infections, including MRSA, occur most frequently among persons who are in hospitals and health care facilities (such as skilled nursing facilities and dialysis centers) and who have weakened immune systems. In recent years, outbreaks in the community have heightened the public's awareness of MRSA. Also emerging are newer resistant bacteria. An example is vancomycin-resistant enterococci. This drug resistance is affecting severely ill, immunocompromised clients in intensive care, transplant, and some cancer treatment units. It is estimated that 1 of every 31 hospitalized clients has at least one health facility–associated infection (CDC, 2019).

Dealing with efforts to educate providers regarding bacterial resistance and the appropriate use of antibiotics resulted in the publishing of the "Ten Commandments of Antibiotic Use" (Levy-Hara et al., 2011). This was a way to use empirical data and communication/education of clients to provide better antibiotic prescribing (Box 7.1). Since that time, the Antibiotic Stewardship program has evolved with standards of practice for different care delivery systems.

Client education to increase behaviors that will prevent or diminish resistance is important when antibiotics are prescribed (see Client Teaching for Improved Outcomes: Preventing Anti-Infective Resistance at the end of this chapter). You will recognize concepts from the Ten Commandments of Antibiotic Use here and the importance of your role in Antibiotic Stewardship.

PENICILLINS

Historically, the sulfonamides were the first anti-infective drugs and the natural penicillins were the first large-scale antibiotics used to combat infection. The antibacterial properties of natural penicillins were discovered in 1928 and used clinically to treat infections by 1941. Used for almost

BOX 7.1	**Ten Commandments of Antibiotic Use**

1. Teach clients nondrug ways to manage nonbacterial infections
2. Know the bacteria, treat it specifically
3. Treat for effectiveness and shorten the course, if appropriate
4. Communicate with clients to increase adherence
5. Use a combination of drugs only in specific situations
6. Substitute only when equivalent product is available
7. Educate to prevent self-prescription
8. Follow evidence-based guidelines
9. Use laboratory results correctly to prescribe
10. Research and understand your local trends and limits

Adapted from Levy-Hara, G., et al. (2011). Ten commandments for the appropriate use of antibiotics by the practicing physician in an outpatient setting. *Front Microbiology*, 2, 230.

80 years, the penicillins are still an important and effective group of antibiotics for the treatment of susceptible **pathogens** (disease-causing microorganisms).

ACTIONS

There are four groups of penicillins: (1) natural penicillins, (2) penicillinase-resistant penicillins, (3) aminopenicillins, and (4) extended-spectrum penicillins, all of which work to inhibit the integrity of the bacterial cell wall. See the Summary Drug Table: Antibacterial Drugs That Disrupt Cell Wall Synthesis for a more complete listing of the penicillins.

The natural penicillins have a fairly narrow spectrum of activity, which means that they are effective against only a few strains of bacteria. Chemically modified aminopenicillins were developed to combat this problem. Because of their chemical modifications, they are more slowly excreted by the kidneys and thus have a somewhat wider spectrum of antibacterial activity.

Drugs are bactericidal when there is an adequate concentration of the drug in the body. The concentration of any drug in the body is referred to as the *blood level*. An inadequate concentration (or inadequate blood level) of an antibiotic may produce bacteriostatic activity, which may or may not control the infection. When the infection is not controlled, resistant bacteria are able to grow.

Various types of bacterial resistance have developed against the penicillins. One example of bacterial resistance is the ability of certain bacteria to produce **penicillinase**, an enzyme that inactivates penicillin. The penicillinase-resistant penicillins were developed to combat this problem.

Certain bacteria have developed the ability to produce enzymes called *beta-lactamases* (β-*lactamases*), which are able to destroy the beta-lactam ring of the drug. Fortunately, chemicals were discovered that inhibit the activity of these enzymes. Penicillin–beta-lactamase inhibitor combinations are a type of penicillin with a wider spectrum of antibacterial activity. Examples of these beta-lactamase inhibitors are clavulanic acid, sulbactam, and tazobactam. When these

BOX 7.2	Penicillin–Beta-Lactamase Inhibitor Combinations

- Augmentin—combination of amoxicillin and clavulanic acid
- Unasyn—combination of ampicillin and sulbactam
- Zosyn—combination of piperacillin and tazobactam

chemicals are used alone, they have little antimicrobial activity. However, when combined with certain penicillins, they extend the spectrum of the penicillin's antibacterial activity. The beta-lactamase inhibitors bind with the penicillin and protect the penicillin from destruction. Examples of combinations of penicillins with beta-lactamase inhibitors are given in Box 7.2; also see the Summary Drug Table: Antibacterial Drugs That Disrupt Cell Wall Synthesis for more information on these combinations.

Extended-spectrum penicillins are effective against an even wider range of bacteria than the broad-spectrum penicillins. These penicillins are used to destroy bacteria such as *Pseudomonas.*

USES

Infectious Disease
The natural and semisynthetic penicillins are used in the treatment of moderate to mildly severe bacterial infections. Penicillins may be used to treat infections such as:

- Urinary tract infections (UTIs)
- Septicemia
- Meningitis
- Intra-abdominal infections
- Sexually transmitted infections (syphilis)
- Pneumonia and other respiratory infections
- Soft tissue infections and injuries

Examples of infectious microorganisms (bacteria) that may respond to penicillin therapy include pneumococci and group A beta-hemolytic (β-hemolytic) streptococci. Because of the increasing resistance of staphylococci to penicillin G, the penicillinase-resistant penicillins are used as initial therapy for any suspected staphylococcal infection until C&S results are known.

Prophylaxis
Because penicillin targets bacterial cells, it is of no value in treating viral or fungal infections. However, the primary health care provider occasionally prescribes penicillin as **prophylaxis** (prevention) against a potential secondary bacterial infection that can occur in a client with a viral infection. In these situations, the viral infection has weakened the body's defenses and the person is susceptible to other infections, particularly a bacterial infection.

Again, antibiotics such as penicillin have been historically prescribed as prophylaxis for a potential infection in high-risk individuals undergoing a procedure that will break the skin defense system (see Chapter 6), such as

those with a history of rheumatic fever about to have a dental procedure. In this case, penicillin is taken several hours or, in some instances, days before and after an operative procedure, such as dental, oral, or upper respiratory tract procedures, that can result in bacteria entering the bloodstream. Researchers believe this practice in non–high-risk clients is another reason many bacteria have become resistant to drugs. Penicillin also may be given prophylactically on a continuing basis to those with rheumatic fever or chronic ear infections.

ADVERSE REACTIONS

Gastrointestinal System Reactions
- **Glossitis** (inflammation of the tongue) when given orally
- **Stomatitis** (inflammation of the mouth), dry mouth
- Gastritis
- Nausea, vomiting
- Diarrhea, abdominal pain

Administration route reactions include pain at the injection site when given intramuscularly (IM) and irritation of the vein and phlebitis (inflammation of a vein) when given intravenously (IV).

Hypersensitivity Reactions
A hypersensitivity (or allergic) reaction to a drug occurs in some individuals, especially those with a history of allergy to many substances. Signs and symptoms of a hypersensitivity to penicillin are highlighted in Box 7.3.

An **anaphylactic reaction,** which is a severe form of hypersensitivity, also can occur (see Chapter 1). Anaphylactic reactions occur more frequently after parenteral administration but can occur with oral use. This reaction is likely to be immediate and severe in susceptible individuals. Signs of anaphylactic reaction or shock include severe hypotension, loss of consciousness, and acute respiratory distress. If not immediately treated, anaphylactic shock can be fatal.

Once an individual is allergic to one penicillin, they are usually allergic to all of the penicillins. Those allergic to

BOX 7.3	Signs and Symptoms of Hypersensitivity to Penicillin and Other Antibiotics

- Skin rash
- Urticaria (hives)
- Sneezing
- Wheezing
- Pruritus (itching)
- Bronchospasm (spasm of the bronchi)
- Laryngospasm (spasm of the larynx)
- Angioedema (also called angioneurotic edema)—swelling of the skin and mucous membranes, especially around and in the mouth and throat
- Hypotension—can progress to shock
- Signs and symptoms resembling serum sickness—chills, fever, edema, joint and muscle pain, and malaise

penicillin also have a higher incidence of allergy to the cephalosporins. Allergy to drugs in the same or related groups is called **cross-sensitivity**. For example, a person allergic to penicillin may also be sensitive to the cephalosporins.

Other Reactions

Other more severe adverse reactions associated with penicillin include hematopoietic (blood cell) changes:

• Anemia (low red blood cell count)
• Thrombocytopenia (low platelet count)
• Leukopenia (low white blood cell count)
• Bone marrow depression

CONTRAINDICATIONS AND PRECAUTIONS

Penicillins are contraindicated in clients with a history of hypersensitivity to penicillin or the cephalosporins.

Penicillins should be used cautiously in clients with renal disease, asthma, bleeding disorders, gastrointestinal (GI) disease, pregnancy (pregnancy category C) or lactation (may cause diarrhea or candidiasis in the infant), and history of allergies. Any indication of sensitivity is reason for caution.

LASA ALERT

The following drugs may sound alike; be sure to clarify when they are ordered:

Drug Name	Sounds Like
Amoxil	amoxapine
ampicillin	Aminophylline
penicillin	Penicillamine
Zosyn	Zofran or Zyvox

Drugs that look alike are noted in the Summary Drug Tables of each chapter.

INTERACTIONS

The following interactions may occur when a penicillin is administered with another agent.

Interacting Agent	Common Use	Effect of Interaction
Oral contraceptives (with estrogen)	Contraception	Decreased effectiveness of contraceptive agent (with ampicillin, penicillin V)
Tetracyclines	Anti-infective	Decreased effectiveness of penicillins
Anticoagulants	Prevent blood clots	Increased bleeding risks (with large doses of penicillins)
Beta-adrenergic blocking (β-adrenergic blocking) drugs	Blood pressure control and heart problems	May increase the risk for an anaphylactic reaction

 Herbal Considerations

Goldenseal (*Hydrastis canadensis*) is an herb found growing in certain areas of the northeastern United States, particularly the Ohio River valley. Goldenseal has been used to wash inflamed or infected eyes and in making yellow dye. There are many more traditional uses of the herb, including as an antiseptic for the skin, as a mouthwash for canker sores, and in the treatment of sinus infections and digestive problems such as peptic ulcers and gastritis. Goldenseal is touted as an "herbal antibiotic" for treating gonorrhea and UTIs. Its effect may occur due to the component berberine. The chemical berberine is somewhat effective against bacteria and fungi and has been used in *Escherichia coli* infections of the urinary tract. A myth surrounding goldenseal's increase in popularity is that taking the herb masks the presence of illicit drugs in urine testing—this does not happen (DerMarderosian, 2003). Evidence does support the use of goldenseal to treat diarrhea caused by bacteria or intestinal parasites, such as *Giardia*. The herb is contraindicated during pregnancy and in clients with hypertension. Adverse reactions are rare when the herb is used as directed. However, this herb should not be taken for more than a few days to 1 week (Gurley, 2012).

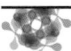 # CEPHALOSPORINS

The cephalosporins are divided into first-, second-, third-, fourth-, and fifth-generation drugs. In general, progression from the first-generation to the fourth-generation drugs shows an increase in the sensitivity of gram-negative microorganisms and a decrease in the sensitivity of gram-positive microorganisms. For example, a first-generation cephalosporin would be more useful against gram-positive microorganisms than would a third-generation cephalosporin. This scheme of classification is becoming less clearly defined as newer drugs are introduced. The fourth generation of cephalosporins has a broader spectrum and longer duration of resistance to beta-lactamase. These drugs are used to treat urinary tract and skin infections and hospital-acquired pneumonias. As bacteria have become resistant to anti-bacterial drugs (i.e., *S. aureus*) a newer group of cephalosporins has emerged, which is called by some as fifth-generation drugs (Duplessis and Crum-Cianflone, 2011). Their unique property is effectiveness against MRSA and other resistant bacteria. Examples of first-, second-, third-, fourth-, and fifth-generation cephalosporins are listed in Box 7.4. For a complete listing, see the Summary Drug Table: Antibacterial Drugs That Inhibit Cell Wall Synthesis.

ACTIONS

Cephalosporins have a beta-lactam ring and target the bacterial cell wall, making it defective and unstable, ultimately killing the bacteria. This action is similar to the action of penicillin. The cephalosporins are usually bactericidal.

BOX 7.4	**Examples of First-, Second-, Third-, Fourth-, and Fifth-Generation Cephalosporins**

- First generation—cephalexin
- Second generation—cefaclor
- Third generation—cefoperazone
- Fourth generation—cefepime
- Fifth generation—ceftaroline

USES

The cephalosporins are used in the treatment of infections caused by bacteria, including:

- Respiratory infections
- **Otitis media** (ear infection)
- Bone/joint infections
- Complicated intra-abdominal or genitourinary tract infections

Cephalosporins are used prophylactically to prevent infection when victims are treated following a sexual assault. The most frequent infections diagnosed following an assault include trichomoniasis, bacterial vaginitis, gonorrhea, and chlamydia.

This class of drugs also may be used throughout the **perioperative** period—that is, during the preoperative, intraoperative, and postoperative periods—to prevent infection in clients having surgery on a contaminated or potentially contaminated area, such as the GI tract or vagina. In some instances, a specific drug may be recommended for postoperative prophylactic use only.

ADVERSE REACTIONS

Gastrointestinal System Reactions
- Nausea
- Vomiting
- Diarrhea

Other Reactions
- Headache
- Dizziness
- **Malaise** (general discomfort)
- Heartburn
- Fever
- **Nephrotoxicity** (toxic to kidneys)
- Hypersensitivity (allergic) reactions—may occur with administration of the cephalosporins and may range from mild to life-threatening. Mild hypersensitivity reactions include pruritus, urticaria, and skin rashes; the more serious reactions include **Stevens–Johnson syndrome** and hepatic and renal dysfunction
- Aplastic anemia (deficient red blood cell production)
- Toxic epidermal necrolysis (death of the epidermal layer of the skin)
- Positive direct Coombs test (cefepime)

NURSING ALERT

Because of the close relationship of the cephalosporins to penicillin, a client who is allergic to penicillin also may be allergic to the cephalosporins. Approximately 10% of the people allergic to a penicillin drug are also allergic to a cephalosporin drug.

Administration route reactions include pain, tenderness, and inflammation at the injection site when given IM, and **phlebitis** or **thrombophlebitis** along the vein when given IV. Therapy with cephalosporins may result in a bacterial or fungal superinfection. Diarrhea may be an indication of **pseudomembranous colitis**, which is one type of bacterial superinfection (see Chapter 9).

CONTRAINDICATIONS AND PRECAUTIONS

Do not administer cephalosporins if the client has a history of allergies to cephalosporins.

Cephalosporins should be used cautiously in clients with renal disease (seizures may occur), hepatic impairment, bleeding disorder, pregnancy (pregnancy category B), and known penicillin allergy.

LASA ALERT

All the cephalosporins may sound like another drug in the same category. The following drugs may also sound alike; be sure to clarify when they are ordered:

Drug Name	*Sounds Like*
Suprax	Sporanox
Ceftin	Cipro
Zinacef	Zithromax

Drugs that look alike are noted in the Summary Drug Tables of each chapter.

INTERACTIONS

The following interactions may occur when a cephalosporin is administered with another agent:

Interacting Drug	Common Use	Effect of Interaction
Aminoglycosides	Anti-infective	Increased risk for nephrotoxicity
Oral anticoagulants	Blood thinner	Increased risk for bleeding
Loop diuretics	Hypertension, reduce edema	Increased cephalosporin blood level

Probenecid (used for gout pain) will increase the levels of most cephalosporins (*except* cefoperazone, ceftazidime, and ceftriaxone).

CARBAPENEMS AND MISCELLANEOUS DRUGS THAT INHIBIT CELL WALL SYNTHESIS

The carbapenems, vancomycin, and monobactam drugs all play a role in the inhibition of bacterial cell wall synthesis.

ACTIONS

Carbapenems inhibit synthesis of the bacterial cell wall and cause the death of susceptible cells. Vancomycin and its synthetic derivative drug (telavancin) and the drug oritavancin (Orbactiv) all act against susceptible gram-positive bacteria by inhibiting bacterial cell wall synthesis and increasing cell wall permeability. Aztreonam has a beta-lactam nucleus and therefore is called a *monobactam*. This is structurally different from the beta-lactam ring of the penicillins, yet it still functions to inhibit bacterial cell wall synthesis.

USES

Meropenem (Merrem IV) is used for intra-abdominal infections and bacterial meningitis. Imipenem-cilastatin (Primaxin) is used to treat serious infections, endocarditis, and septicemia. Doripenem is used to treat intra-abdominal and complicated UTIs caused by bacteria. Telavancin (Vibativ) and oritavancin (Orbactiv) are used to treat complicated skin and skin structure infections because they are effective against many strains of *Staph* and *Strep* infections including the methicillin-resistant organisms. Vancomycin (Vancocin) is used in the treatment of serious gram-positive infections that do not respond to treatment with other anti-infectives. It also may be used in treating anti-infective–associated pseudomembranous colitis caused by *C. difficile*. The monobactams have bactericidal action and are used to treat gram-negative microorganisms.

ADVERSE REACTIONS

The most common adverse reactions with these drugs include nausea, vomiting, diarrhea, and rash. As with many other anti-infectives, there is a risk of pseudomembranous colitis (see Chapter 9). Assess stools for blood when the client has diarrhea.

Carbapenems also can cause an abscess or phlebitis at the injection site. An abscess is suspected if the injection site appears red or is tender and warm to the touch. Tissue sloughing at the injection site also may occur.

Nephrotoxicity (damage to the kidneys) and ototoxicity (damage to the organs of hearing) may be seen with the administration of vancomycin especially in clients with pre-existing kidney disease. Additional adverse reactions include chills, fever, urticaria, and sudden fall in blood pressure with parenteral administration. For more information, see Summary Drug Table: Anti-infective Drugs That Inhibit Cell Wall Synthesis.

CONTRAINDICATIONS, PRECAUTIONS, AND INTERACTIONS

Carbapenems, aztreonam, and telavancin are contraindicated in clients who are allergic to cephalosporins and penicillins and in clients with renal failure. These drugs are not recommended in children younger than 3 months or for women during pregnancy (pregnancy category B) or lactation. Carbapenems are used cautiously in clients with central nervous system (CNS) disorders, seizure disorders, or renal or hepatic failure. The excretion of carbapenems is inhibited when the drug is administered to a client also taking probenecid. Aztreonam should be used cautiously in clients with renal or hepatic impairment.

Vancomycin should not be used in clients with a known hypersensitivity to the drug and is used cautiously in clients with renal or hearing impairment and during pregnancy (pregnancy category C) and lactation. When administered with other ototoxic and nephrotoxic drugs, additive effects may occur. In other words, one drug alone may not cause the hearing or kidney problem, but when another drug with similar adverse effects is given with vancomycin, the client is more likely to experience a problem. These drugs should be used with caution in clients undergoing anticoagulant therapy because of an increased risk of bleeding.

> **LASA ALERT**
>
> The following drugs may sound alike; be sure to clarify when they are ordered:
>
> | Drug Name | Sounds Like |
> |-----------|-------------|
> | doripenem | Ertapenem |
> | INVanz | AVINza, IV vancomycin |
> | aztreonam | azidothymidine |
>
> Drugs that look alike are noted in the Summary Drug Tables of each chapter.

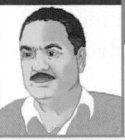

> **PHARMACOLOGY IN PRACTICE**
>
> **DRUG RECOGNITION**
>
> Cephalosporins are structurally and chemically related to which classes of antibiotics?
>
> 1. Fluoroquinolones
> 2. Aminoglycosides
> 3. Tetracyclines
> 4. Penicillins

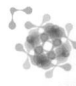

NURSING PROCESS—STEPS TO BUILDING CLINICAL JUDGMENT
Client Receiving Penicillin, Cephalosporin, Carbapenems, or Miscellaneous Cell Wall Inhibitors

ASSESSMENT

Preadministration Assessment

Data gathering suggestions before administering the first dose of penicillin or a cephalosporin include:

Objective data

- General client appearance (paleness, flushing)
- Vital signs (temperature, pulse, respiration, and blood pressure)
- Description of the infection, such as site, color, and type of drainage from a wound; pain; redness and inflammation; color of sputum; or presence of an odor
- C&S culture results, liver or kidney function results depending upon drug ordered

Subjective data

- Current symptoms of the infection (malaise, fatigue, pain)
- Allergy history, particularly a drug allergy—be sure to explore this area to ensure the client is not allergic to penicillin or a cephalosporin
- Drug history, particularly other anti-infectives or home remedies used for this infection
- History of all medical and surgical treatment

 NURSING ALERT

Is the reaction really an allergy? Approximately 30 million people report having an allergy to penicillin. Is the reaction a true allergy response or did the person experience a nonallergy reaction such as contact dermatitis? Research in skin testing has found that about 95% of individuals who self-define as being allergic to a drug are not, which creates greater health care costs when more expensive drugs are used to treat a response that is not really an allergy and that can create longer hospital stays (Macy & Contreras, 2013). Any report of drug allergy should be thoroughly investigated.

Ongoing Assessment

An ongoing assessment is important in evaluating the client's response to therapy, such as a decrease in temperature, the relief of symptoms caused by the infection (e.g., pain or discomfort), an increase in appetite, and a change in the appearance or amount of drainage (when originally present). Notify the primary health care provider if signs of the infection appear to worsen.

Additional C&S tests may be performed during therapy because microorganisms causing the infection may become resistant to the antibiotic, or a superinfection may occur. Check laboratory reports within 3–7 days of the initial treatment, verify that the infection being treated is susceptible to the drug given, and notify the primary health provider. Check the client's skin regularly for rash and be alert for any loose stools or diarrhea. A urinalysis, complete blood count, and renal and hepatic function tests also may be performed at intervals during therapy.

 NURSING ALERT

Observe the client closely for a hypersensitivity reaction, which may occur any time during therapy with the penicillins. If it does occur, it is important to contact the primary health care provider immediately and withhold the drug. The interventions mentioned below outline supportive care measures for hypersensitivity reactions while awaiting primary health care provider orders.

NURSING DIAGNOSES

Drug-specific nursing diagnoses include the following:

- **Altered skin integrity** related to hypersensitivity to the drug
- **Altered gas exchange risk** related to an allergic reaction to the drug
- **Altered urinary elimination** related to nephrotoxic effects of cephalosporin
- **Diarrhea** related to a bacterial secondary infection or superinfection
- **Altered oral mucous membranes** related to a secondary bacterial or fungal infection
- **Altered comfort: increased fever** related to ineffectiveness of antibiotic against the infection

Nursing diagnoses related to drug administration are discussed in Chapter 4.

PLANNING

The expected outcomes for the client depend on the reason for administering the antibiotic but may include an optimal response to drug therapy, meeting client needs related to management of common adverse reactions, and confidence in an understanding of the medication regimen.

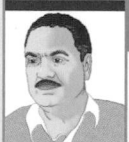 **PHARMACOLOGY IN PRACTICE**

PLANNING

Given below, in random order, are important interventions when caring for a client receiving antibiotics for an infection. Arrange the interventions in the order they most likely occur in most situations.

1. Identify the appropriate penicillin or cephalosporin
2. Order a **culture and sensitivity test**
3. Document improvement on client's chart
4. Administer penicillin or cephalosporin to client
5. Obtain general history of client

IMPLEMENTATION

Promoting Optimal Response to Therapy: Proper Administration

The results of a C&S test may take up to 3 days, because time must be allowed for the bacteria to grow on the culture media. Note some sputum results may take up to 2 months. However, infections are treated as soon as possible. The primary health care provider determines the treatment of choice until the results of the C&S tests are known. In many instances, the primary health care provider selects a broad-spectrum antibiotic for initial treatment because of the many penicillin-resistant strains of microorganisms.

 NURSING ALERT

Be sure to question the client about allergy to penicillin or cephalosporins before administering the first dose, even when an accurate drug history has been taken. It is important to tell clients what drug they are receiving because information regarding a drug allergy may have been forgotten at the time the initial drug history was obtained. If a client states they are allergic to penicillin or a cephalosporin, withhold the drug and contact the primary health care provider.

Oral Administration

Adequate blood levels of the drug must be maintained for the agent to be effective. Accidental omission or delay of a dose results in decreased blood levels, which will reduce the effectiveness of the antibiotic. It is best to give oral penicillins on an empty stomach, 1 hr before or 2 hr after a meal. Penicillin V and amoxicillin may be given with meals. Most cephalosporins may be taken on an empty stomach, especially ceftibuten (Cedax). However, if the client experiences GI upset, you can administer the drugs with food. The absorption of oral cefuroxime and cefpodoxime is increased when given with food.

Some antibiotics are available as powder for a suspension and are reconstituted by a pharmacist or a nurse. Shake oral suspensions well before administering them. It is important to keep this form of the drug refrigerated until it is used.

 Chronic Care Considerations

People with phenylketonuria (PKU) need to be aware that the oral suspension cefprozil (Cefzil) contains phenylalanine, a substance that people with PKU cannot process. In addition, diabetic clients who use urine testing for determining diabetic medicine dosing and who are prescribed cephalosporins need to be aware that this drug may interfere with accurate test results. The primary care provider should be consulted before diet and drug changes are made.

Parenteral Administration

In most health care facilities, the drug is prepared in the pharmacy and delivered to the nurse for administration. When this service is not available in preparing a parenteral form of antibiotics, you should read the manufacturer's package insert for each drug for instructions regarding reconstitution of powder for injection, storage of unused portions, life of the drug after it is reconstituted, methods

of IV administration, and precautions to be taken when the drug is administered.

 NURSING ALERT

Administer each IV dose of vancomycin or telavancin over 60 min (oritavancin is infused over 3 hr). Too rapid an infusion may result in a sudden and profound fall in blood pressure and shock.

When giving vancomycin, telavancin, or oritavancin IV, closely monitor the infusion rate and the client's blood pressure. Report any decrease in blood pressure or occurrence of throbbing neck or back pain. These symptoms could indicate a severe adverse reaction referred to as red neck or red man syndrome. Other symptoms of red man syndrome include fever, chills, paresthesias, and erythema (redness) of the neck and back.

It is important to note that penicillin is often ordered in units; milligram equivalency may or may not be included. The exact equivalency usually is stated on the container or package insert. If there is any question regarding the reconstitution of any drug, consult with a clinical pharmacist.

 Lifespan Considerations

Gerontology

When a penicillin or cephalosporin is given IM, inject the drug into a large muscle mass, such as the gluteus muscle or lateral aspect of the thigh. If the client has been nonambulatory for any length of time or has paralysis, assess the muscle carefully because the large muscle may be atrophied. It is important to rotate injection sites. Warn the client that at the time the drug is injected into the muscle, there may be a stinging or burning sensation and the area may be sore for a short time. Inform the primary health care provider if previously used areas for injection appear red or if the client reports continued pain in the area.

Monitoring and Managing Client Needs

Altered Skin Integrity

Dermatologic reactions such as hives, rashes, and skin lesions can occur with the administration of penicillin or cephalosporin. Treatment of minor hypersensitivity reactions may include administration of an antihistamine such as diphenhydramine (Benadryl) for a rash or itching. In mild cases, or where the benefit of the drug outweighs the discomfort of skin lesions, administer frequent skin care. Emollients, antipyretic creams, or a topical corticosteroid may be prescribed to promote comfort. Harsh soaps and perfumed lotions are avoided. Instruct the client to avoid rubbing the area and to wear clothing that is not rough or irritating. It is important to report a rash or hives to the primary health care provider because this may be a precursor to a severe anaphylactic reaction (see section on Hypersensitivity Reactions). In severe cases, the primary health care provider may discontinue the drug therapy.

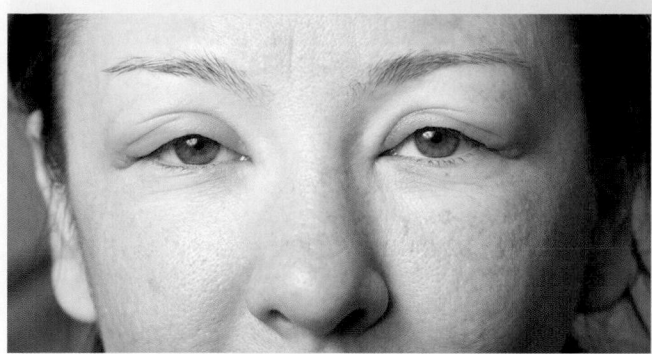

FIGURE 7.2 Example of person with an angioedema reaction to a drug.

Risk for Altered Gas Exchange

Major hypersensitivity reactions, such as bronchospasm, laryngospasm, hypotension, and **angioedema** (Fig. 7.2), require immediate treatment with drugs such as epinephrine, cortisone, or an IV antihistamine. If respiratory occlusion occurs, a tracheostomy may need to be performed.

 NURSING ALERT

After administering penicillin IM in the outpatient setting, ask the client to wait in the area for at least 30 min. Anaphylactic reactions are most likely to occur within 30 min after injection.

Altered Urinary Elimination

Nephrotoxicity may occur with the administration of cephalosporins. An early sign of this adverse reaction may be a decrease in urine output. Measure and record the fluid intake and output and notify the primary health care provider if the output is less than 500 mL daily. Any changes in the fluid intake–output ratio or in the appearance of the urine also may indicate nephrotoxicity. It is important that you report these findings to the primary health care provider promptly.

Lifespan Considerations

Gerontology

The older adult is more susceptible to the nephrotoxic effects of the cephalosporins, particularly if renal function is already diminished because of aging or disease. If renal impairment is present, a lower dosage and monitoring of blood creatinine levels are indicated. Blood creatinine levels greater than 4 mg/dL indicate serious renal impairment. In older clients with decreased renal function, a dosage adjustment may be necessary.

Diarrhea

Diarrhea may be an indication of a superinfection of the GI tract or pseudomembranous colitis (see Chapter 9). Inspect all stools and notify the primary health care provider if diarrhea occurs, because it may be necessary to stop the drug. If diarrhea does occur and there appears to be blood and mucus in the stool, it is important to save a sample of the stool, which should be sent to the laboratory to rule out *C. difficile*. You should also collect a sample for occult blood using a test on the nursing unit such as Hemoccult. If the stool tests positive for blood, save the sample for possible further laboratory analysis. To reduce the spread of infection to other clients, good hand hygiene is critical when dealing with bodily excrement.

Observe the client for other symptoms of a bacterial or fungal superinfection in the vaginal or anal area, such as pain or itching. It is important to report any signs and symptoms of a superinfection to the primary health care provider before administering the next dose of the drug. When symptoms are severe, additional treatment measures may be necessary, such as administration of an antipyretic drug for fever or an antifungal drug.

Altered Oral Mucous Membranes

The administration of oral penicillin may result in a fungal superinfection in the oral cavity. This condition is characterized by varying degrees of oral mucous membrane inflammation, swollen and red tongue, swollen gums, and pain in the mouth and throat. To detect this problem early, inspect the client's mouth daily for evidence of glossitis, sore tongue, ulceration, or a black, furry tongue. You may explain that if the diet permits, yogurt, buttermilk, or *Acidophilus* capsules may be taken to reduce the risk of fungal superinfection.

 Concept Mastery Alert

Taking cephalosporins can lead to a fungal superinfection. It may be characterized by a client reporting a "funny" feeling in the mouth and seeing white patches on the tongue. Fungal superinfections occur when an antibiotic kills off the good bacteria that keep the fungus under control and is not technically an adverse drug reaction.

Inspect the mouth and gums often and give frequent mouth care with a nonirritating solution. A soft-bristled toothbrush is used when brushing is needed. A nonirritating soft diet may be required. Monitor the dietary intake to ensure that the client is receiving adequate nutrition. Antifungal agents or local anesthetics are sometimes recommended to soothe the irritated membranes.

Altered Comfort: Increased Fever

An increase in body temperature several days after the start of therapy may indicate a secondary bacterial infection or failure of the drug to control the original infection. Take vital signs every 4 hr, or more often if necessary. It is important to report any increase in temperature to the primary health care provider, because additional treatment measures, such as administration of an antipyretic drug or change in the drug or dosage, may be necessary. On occasion, the fever may be caused by an adverse reaction to the penicillin. In these cases, the fever can usually be managed by using an antipyretic drug.

Educating the Client and Family

Any time a drug is prescribed for a client, you are responsible for ensuring that the client has a thorough understanding of the drug, the treatment regimen, and

PHARMACOLOGY IN PRACTICE

INTERVENTIONS

Mr. Garcia has developed a rash after the administration of cephalexin. The primary health care provider has diagnosed it as a mild hypersensitivity reaction. Which of the following interventions should the nurse perform to reduce the client's skin condition?

1. Reduce the dosage to provide relief to the client
2. Instruct the client to avoid taking baths
3. Tell the client to avoid contact of clothing with the affected area
4. Teach the client to do frequent skin care to the affected area

adverse reactions. Some clients do not adhere to the prescribed drug regimen for a variety of reasons, such as failure to comprehend the prescribed regimen or failure to understand the importance of continued and uninterrupted therapy. Describing the drug regimen and stressing the importance of continued and uninterrupted therapy when teaching the client who is prescribed an antibiotic will help prevent drug resistance caused by stopping the medication too early.

Provide the following information to clients who are prescribed an antibiotic:

- Prophylaxis: Take the drug as prescribed until the primary health care provider discontinues therapy.
- Infection: Complete the full course of therapy. Do not stop taking the drug, even if the symptoms have disappeared, unless directed to do so by the primary health care provider.
- Take the drug at the prescribed times of day because it is important to keep an adequate amount of drug in the body throughout the entire 24 hr of each day.
- Penicillin (oral): Take the drug on an empty stomach either 1 hr before or 2 hr after meals (exceptions: penicillin V and amoxicillin).
- Take each dose with a full 8-ounce glass of water.
- Oral suspensions: Keep the container refrigerated (if so labeled), shake the drug well before pouring (if so labeled), and return the drug to the refrigerator immediately after pouring the dose. Drugs that require refrigeration lose their potency when kept at room temperature. A small amount of the drug may be left

Client Teaching for Improved Outcomes

Preventing Anti-infective Resistance
When you teach, make sure your client understands the following:

✔ Review the reason for the drug and the prescribed drug regimen, including drug name, correct dose, and frequency of administration. Have the client or family member tell you about the reason and drug in their own terms. Use the services of an interpreter if the client has limited English proficiency.
✔ Stress the importance of continued and uninterrupted therapy, even if the client feels better after a few doses and symptoms have disappeared.
✔ Give written materials to take home; find language-appropriate items if the client has limited English proficiency.
✔ Instruct the client to continue taking the drug until the drug is finished or the prescriber discontinues therapy.
✔ Urge the client and family to discard any unused drug once therapy is discontinued or completed.
✔ Warn the client not to use any leftover antibiotic or to take another family member's antibiotic as self-treatment for a suspected infection.
✔ Review the possible adverse reactions and the signs and symptoms of a new infection or of a worsening infection, both verbally and in writing.
✔ Instruct the client and family to notify the health care provider at once should the client experience any adverse reactions or signs and symptoms of infection.

after the last dose is taken. Discard any remaining drug, because the drug (in suspension form) begins to lose its potency after a few weeks.

- Avoid drinking alcoholic beverages when taking the cephalosporins and for 3 days after completing the course of therapy, because severe reactions may occur.
- To reduce the risk of superinfection during antibiotic therapy, eat yogurt, buttermilk, or *Acidophilus* capsules.
- If you are a woman who has been prescribed ampicillin and penicillin V and who takes birth control pills containing estrogen, use additional contraception measures.
- Notify the primary health care provider immediately should one or more of the following occur: skin rash; hives (urticaria); severe diarrhea; vaginal or anal itching; black, furry tongue; sores in the mouth; swelling around the mouth or eyes; breathing difficulty; or GI disturbances such as nausea, vomiting, and diarrhea. Do not take the next dose of the drug until the problem has been discussed with the primary health care provider.

- Never give this drug to another individual, even though their symptoms appear to be the same as yours.
- Notify the primary health care provider if the symptoms of the infection do not improve or if the condition becomes worse.
- Never skip doses or stop therapy unless told to do so by the primary health care provider (see Client Teaching for Improved Client Outcomes: Preventing Anti-infective Resistance). When a penicillin is to be taken for a long time for prophylaxis, you may feel well despite the need for long-term antibiotic therapy. There may be a tendency to omit one or more doses or even neglect to take the drug for an extended time.

EVALUATION

- Therapeutic response is achieved, and there is no evidence of infection.
- Adverse reactions are identified, reported to the primary health care provider, and managed successfully with appropriate nursing interventions:
  - Skin is intact and free of infection.
  - Client maintains adequate gas exchange.

- Client maintains an adequate fluid intake for proper urinary elimination.
- Client reports adequate bowel movements.
- Mucous membranes are moist and intact.
- Client reports comfort without fever.
- Client and family express confidence and demonstrate understanding of the drug regimen.

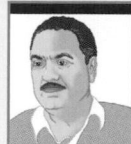

PHARMACOLOGY IN PRACTICE

USING CLINICAL REASONING

Mrs. Garcia also came to the clinic visit. She has been telling the staff members about the party they are giving this weekend and hopes that Mr. Garcia is well enough to be the bartender for the event. As you prepare to assess and teach Mr. Garcia, what do you know about limited health literacy? What teaching points should you emphasize after your discussion with Mrs. Garcia? What tools can you use to help you with his limited English proficiency?

KEY POINTS

■ Penicillin, cephalosporin, carbapenem, and vancomycin-type drugs are primarily bactericidal; they work by breaking or inhibiting the growth of the cell walls found in bacterial cells. Categories of penicillin drugs are defined by modifications for resistance, and cephalosporin generations tend to define the sensitivity of the drugs to microorganisms.

■ These drugs are used to treat bacterial infections such as UTIs or otitis media, or prophylactically to prevent secondary bacterial infections.

■ People allergic to penicillin may also have an allergy to cephalosporins because they are structurally and chemically related drugs.

■ Bacteria can become resistant to certain drugs. Drugs with modifications are created to combat resistance. One of the best methods to prevent resistance is to teach the client to take the medication as instructed: take on time, no omissions, and for the length of the prescription.

■ Adverse reactions are often GI, and superinfections can occur when normal flora is also killed by the drugs. Chronic use of cephalosporins may result in damage to the kidneys. Older clients using these drugs should be monitored closely for kidney function.

SUMMARY DRUG TABLE
Antibacterial Drugs That Disrupt Bacterial Cell Wall Synthesis

Generic Name	Trade Name	Uses	Adverse Reactions	Dosage Ranges
Penicillins				
Narrow-Spectrum Penicillins				
penicillin G (aqueous) *pen-i-SIL-in*	Pfizerpen	Streptococcal infections, syphilis meningococcal meningitis, septicemia	Glossitis, stomatitis, gastritis, furry tongue, nausea, vomiting, diarrhea, rash, fever, pain at injection site, hypersensitivity reactions, hematopoietic changes	Up to 20–30 million units/day IV or IM; dosage may also be based on weight
penicillin G benzathine	Bicillin L-A	Streptococcal infections (respiratory), syphilis; prophylaxis of rheumatic fever	Same as penicillin G	Up to 2.4 million units/day IM

Continued

SUMMARY DRUG TABLE (continued)
Antibacterial Drugs That Disrupt Bacterial Cell Wall Synthesis

Generic Name	Trade Name	Uses	Adverse Reactions	Dosage Ranges
penicillin G procaine		Streptococcal infections, soft tissue injuries	Same as penicillin G	600,000–2.4 million units/day IM
penicillin V		Streptococcal infections, soft tissue injuries	Same as penicillin G	125–500 mg orally every 6 hr or every 8 hr
Semisynthetic Penicillins				
Penicillinase-Resistant Penicillins (Narrow Spectrum)				
dicloxacillin *dye-kloks-a-SIL-in*		Staphylococcal infections	Same as penicillin G	125–250 mg orally every 6 hr
nafcillin *naf-SIL-in*		Staphylococcal infections	Same as penicillin G	500 mg IV every 4 hr
oxacillin *oks-a-SIL-in*	Bactocill	Cath-related *Staph A* infections	Same as penicillin G	500 mg–1 g orally every 4–6 hr; 250 mg–1 g every 4–6 hr IM, IV
Aminopenicillins (Broad Spectrum)				
amoxic illin *a-moks-i-SIL-in*	Amoxil	Acute otitis media (children), Strep soft tissue infections (SSTI), *Helicobacter pylori*	Same as penicillin G	500–875 mg orally every 12 hr or 250 mg orally every 8 hr
ampicillin *am-pi-SIL-in*		EENT, respiratory, GU infections, endocarditis	Same as penicillin G	250–500 mg orally every 6 hr; 1–12 g/day IM, IV in divided doses every 4–6 hr
amoxicillin and clavulanate *a-moks-i-SIL-in/klav-yoo-LAN-ate*	Augmentin	Otitis media, pneumonia, SSTI	Same as penicillin G	250 mg orally every 8 hr or 500 mg orally every 12 hr; for severe infections: up to 875 mg every 12 hr
ampicillin/sulbactam *am-pi-SIL-in/SUL-bak-tam*	Unasyn	SSTI	Same as penicillin G	1.5–3 g every 6 hr IM or IV
Extended-Spectrum Penicillins				
piperacillin and tazobactam *pi-PER-a-sil-in/ta-zoe-BAK-tam*	Zosyn	Pneumonia, GI infections, SSTI	Same as penicillin G	3.375–4.5 g every 6 hr IV
Cephalosporins				
First-Generation Cephalosporins				
cefadroxil *sef-a-DROKS-il*		Strep EENT, urinary infections, SSTI	Nausea, diarrhea	1–2 g/day orally in divided doses
ceFAZolin *sef-A-zoe-lin*	Ancef	Multiple bacterial infections perioperative prophylaxis	Same as cefadroxil	250 mg–1 g IM, IV every 6–12 hr; perioperative: 0.5–1 g IM, IV
cephalexin *sef-a-LEKS-in*	Keflex	Same as cefadroxil	Same as cefadroxil	1–4 g/day orally in divided doses
Second-Generation Cephalosporins				
cefaclor *SEF-a-klor*		Respiratory, EENT, SSTI Infections	Nausea, diarrhea, headache, rhinitis, vaginitis	250 mg orally every 8 hr
cefoTEtan *SEF-oh-tee-tan*		Bone/joint, CNS infections, GU/GI infections, SSTI, perioperative prophylaxis	Same as cefaclor	1–2 g IM, IV every 12 hr for 5–10 days; perioperative: 1–2 g in a single dose IV
cefOXitin *se-FOKS-i-tin*	Mefoxin	Same as cefaclor; perioperative prophylaxis	Same as cefaclor	1–2 g IV every 6–8 hr

Generic Name	Trade Name	Uses	Adverse Reactions	Dosage Ranges
cefprozil *sef-PROE-zil*		Same as cefaclor	Same as cefaclor	250–500 mg orally every 12 hr
cefuroxime *se-fyoor-OKS-eem*	Zinacef	Respiratory, EENT, GU, SSTI infections, Lyme disease	Nausea, vomiting, diarrhea	250 mg orally BID; 750 mg–1.5 g IM or IV every 8 hr
Third-Generation Cephalosporins				
cefdinir *SEF-di-ner*		Respiratory, EENT, SSTI infections	Nausea, diarrhea, headache, vaginitis	300 mg orally every 12 hr or 600 mg orally every 24 hr
cefditoren *sef-de-TOR-en*		Same as cefdinir	Nausea, vomiting, dyspepsia, diarrhea, headache, vaginitis	200–400 mg orally BID
cefixime *sef-IKS-eem*	Suprax	Same as cefdinir	Nausea, gas pains, dyspepsia, diarrhea	400 mg/day orally
cefotaxime *sef-oh-TAKS-eem*		Bone/joint, CNS infections, GU/GI infections, SSTI; perioperative prophylaxis	Injection phlebitis, skin reactions	2–8 g/day IM, IV in equally divided doses every 6–8 hr; maximum 12 g/day
cefpodoxime *sef-pode-OKS-eem*		Respiratory, SSTI; sexually transmitted infection treatment	Nausea, diarrhea	100–400 mg/day orally in equally divided doses
cefTAZidime *SEF-tay-zi-deem*	Tazicef, Avycaz	Bone/joint, CNS infections, GU/GI infections, SSTI	Rash, pruritus	250 mg–2g IV, IM every 8–12 hr
cefTRIAXone *sef-trye-AKS-one*		Bone/joint, CNS infections, GU/GI infections, SSTI, perioperative prophylaxis	Injection phlebitis	1–2 g/day IM, IV every 12 hr, maximum 4 g/day; perioperative: 1 g IV; gonorrhea: 250 mg IM as a single dose
Fourth-Generation Cephalosporins				
cefepime *SEF-e-pim*	Maxipime	UTI, SSTI, febrile neutropenia	Injection phlebitis	0.5–2 g IV, IM every 12 hr
Fifth-Generation Cephalosporins				
ceftaroline *sef-TAR-oh-leen*	Teflaro	MRSA, acute bacterial skin/soft tissue infections, pneumonia	Nausea, diarrhea, rash, pruritus	600 mg IV, every 12 hr
ceftobiprole *sef-toe-bBI-prol*	Zeftera, Zevtera	MRSA, penicillin-resistant skin/soft tissue infections	Nausea, taste changes, vomiting, diarrhea, headache	500 mg IV, every 8 hr
ceftolozane/ taxobactam *sef-TOL-oh-zane/taz-oh-BAK-tam*	Zerbaxa	Complicated intra-abdominal or urinary tract infections, pneumonia	Nausea, diarrhea, headache, fever	1.5 g IV, every 8 hr
Carbapenems				
doripenem *dore-i-PEN-em*		Complicated intra-abdominal or urinary tract infections	Headache, nausea, diarrhea, and anemia	500 mg IV every 8 hr
ertapenem *er-ta-PEN-em*	INVanz	Complicated intra-abdominal or urinary tract infections	Headache, nausea, diarrhea, and liver dysfunction	1 g IV daily, 3–14 days
imipenem-cilastatin *i-mi-PEN-em/sye-la-STAT-in*	Primaxin	Serious infections caused by *Staphylococcus* spp., *Streptococcus* spp., and *Escherichia coli*	Nausea, diarrhea, pancytopenia, liver dysfunction	250 mg–1 g every 6 hr, not to exceed 4 g/day
imipenem-cilastatin-relebactam *i-mi-PEN-em/sye-la-STAT-in/REL-e-BAK-tam*	Recarbrio	Complicated intra-abdominalor urinary tract infections, pyelonephritis	Nausea, diarrhea, local phlebitis	1.25 g IV every 6 hr

Continued

SUMMARY DRUG TABLE (continued)
Antibacterial Drugs That Disrupt Bacterial Cell Wall Synthesis

Generic Name	Trade Name	Uses	Adverse Reactions	Dosage Ranges
meropenem *mer-oh-PEN-em*	Merrem IV	Intra-abdominal and soft tissue infections caused by multiresistant gram-negative organisms	Headache, diarrhea, abdominal pain, nausea, pain and inflammation at injection site, pseudomembranous colitis	500 mg–1 g IV every 8 hr
meropenem/ vaborbactam *mer-oh-PEN-em/va-bor-BAK-tam*	Vabomere	Complicated UTIs, pyelonephritis	Same as meropenem	4 g IV every 8 hr
Miscellaneous Drugs That Inhibit Bacterial Cell Wall Synthesis				
aztreonam *AZ-tree-oh-nam*	Azactam, Cayston	*E. coli* (and related bacteria) infections of urinary, respiratory, and GI tract, skin and soft tissue	Nausea, vomiting, diarrhea, rash	1–2 g every 8–12 hr, not to exceed 8 g/day
dalbavancin *dal-ba-VAN-sin*	Dalvance	Acute bacterial skin/soft tissue infections	Nausea, vomiting, and headache	1000 mg IV, follow in 1 week with 500 mg IV
oritavancin *or-it-a-VAN-sin*	Orbactiv	Acute bacterial skin/soft tissue infections	Nausea, vomiting, and headache	Single dose of 1200 mg IV
telavancin *tel-a-VAN-sin*	Vibativ	Complicated skin infections	Nausea, vomiting, and altered taste	10 mg/kg IV daily, 4–7 days
vancomycin *van-koe-MYE-sin*	Vancocin	Serious susceptible gram-positive infections not responding to treatment with other antibiotics	Nausea; chills; fever; urticaria; sudden fall in blood pressure, with redness on face, neck, arms, and back; nephrotoxicity; ototoxicity	500 mg–2 g/day orally in divided doses; 500 mg IV every 6 hr or 1 g IV every 12 hr

 This drug should be administered at least 1 hr before or 2 hr after a meal.

CHAPTER REVIEW

Know Your Drugs

Clients sometimes know a medication by the brand (or trade) name and not the generic name. To help you recognize both names, match the brand name with the generic name of the same medication.

Generic Name	Brand Name
1. ceftriaxone	A. Augmentin
2. telavancin	B. Vancocin
3. amoxicillin/clavulanic acid	C. Rocephin
4. vancomycin	D. Vibativ

Calculate Medication Dosages

1. A client is prescribed amoxicillin in oral suspension. The drug is reconstituted to a solution of 250 mg/5 mL. The primary health care provider prescribes 500 mg of the amoxicillin. The caregiver insists on using a spoon to administer the drug. Answer the following questions: How much amoxicillin will 1 teaspoon contain? How many milliliters (mL) were ordered, and what is the conversion to teaspoons (how much should the nurse teach the caregiver to administer)?

2. The health care provider at the Sexual Assault Clinic prescribes 1 g of cefoxitin (Mefoxin) for parenteral administration. Cefoxitin is available in a solution of 250 mg/1 mL. What amount of cefoxitin would the nurse prepare? Could this be given in one IM injection?

Prepare for the NCLEX

RECALL THE FACTS

1. Bacterial cells are different from human cells because they:
   1. have a cell wall
   2. synthesize DNA and RNA
   3. contain a beta-lactam ring
   4. contain proteins
2. Cephalosporins are divided into "generations" according to:
   1. when they were discovered
   2. their administration method
   3. manufacturer's preference
   4. sensitivity to microorganisms

3. A client taking oral penicillin reports a sore mouth. On inspection, the nurse notes a black, furry tongue and bright red oral mucous membranes. The primary care provider is notified immediately, because these symptoms may be caused by:
   1. a vitamin C deficiency
   2. a superinfection
   3. an allergic reaction
   4. poor oral hygiene

4. The nurse correctly administers penicillin V:
   1. 1 hr before or 2 hr after meals
   2. without regard to meals
   3. with meals to prevent GI upset
   4. every 3 hr around the clock

5. When giving a cephalosporin by the IM route, the nurse tells the client that _____.
   1. a stinging or burning sensation and soreness at the site may be experienced
   2. the injection site will be red for several days
   3. all injections will be given in the same area
   4. the injection will not cause any discomfort

6. The nurse observes a client taking a cephalosporin for common adverse reactions, which include _____.
   1. hypotension, dizziness, urticaria
   2. nausea, vomiting, diarrhea
   3. skin rash, constipation, headache
   4. bradycardia, pruritus, insomnia

7. After administering penicillin in an outpatient setting, the nurse:
   1. asks the client to wait 10–15 min before leaving the clinic
   2. instructs the client to report any numbness or tingling of the extremities
   3. keeps pressure on the injection site for 10 min
   4. asks the client to wait in the area for at least 30 min

ANALYZE THE FACTS

8. *When reviewing a client's culture and sensitivity test results, the nurse learns that the bacteria causing the infection are sensitive to penicillin. The nurse interprets this result to mean that:
   1. the client is allergic to penicillin
   2. penicillin will be effective in treating the infection
   3. penicillin will not be effective in treating the infection
   4. the test must be repeated to obtain accurate results

9. *A nurse asks if the client is allergic to penicillin before the first dose of the cephalosporin is given. The rationale for this question is that persons allergic to penicillin _____.
   1. are usually allergic to most antibiotics
   2. respond poorly to antibiotic therapy
   3. require higher doses of other antibiotics
   4. have a higher incidence of allergy to the cephalosporins

ALTERNATE-FORMAT QUESTIONS

10. *Which of the following are signs and symptoms of a drug hypersensitivity reaction? **Select all that apply.**
    1. skin rash
    2. wheezing
    3. hypertension
    4. angioedema
    5. urinary incontinence

To check your answers, see Appendix F.

---

*Indicates the question is directly linked to the NCLEX-PN test plan in Appendix G.

WANT TO KNOW MORE? A wide variety of resources are available to enhance your learning and understanding of this chapter.
- Visit for the**Point** resources such as:
  - NCLEX-Style Student Review Questions
  - Journal Articles
  - Dosage Calculations
  - Drug Monographs
  - Watch and Learn Videos
  - Concepts in Action Animations
- The *Study Guide to Accompany Introductory Clinical Pharmacology*, 12th edition, sold separately, will help you review and apply essential content.
- ✓**PrepU** is available to help students prepare for the NCLEX-PN examination.

8

Antibacterial Drugs That Interfere With Protein Synthesis

Key Terms

adjunctive treatment therapy used in addition to the primary treatment

blood dyscrasias abnormality of blood cell structure

bowel preparation treatment protocol to cleanse the bowel of bacteria before surgery or other procedures; also known as *bowel prep*

circumoral encircling the mouth

enteric coated special coating on drug that prevents absorption until drug reaches the small bowel

Helicobacter pylori stomach bacterium that causes peptic ulcer; also known as *H. pylori*

hematuria blood in the urine

hepatic coma coma induced by liver disease

nephrotoxicity damage to the kidneys by a toxic substance

neuromuscular blockade acute muscle paralysis and apnea (absence of breathing)

neurotoxicity damage to the nervous system by a toxic substance

ototoxicity damage to the organs of hearing by a toxic substance

phenylketonuria (PKU) a genetic birth defect causing the amino acid phenylalanine to build up to toxic levels in the body

proteinuria protein in the urine

tinnitus ringing or buzzing sound in the ears

vancomycin-resistant *Enterococcus faecium* (VREF) bacteria resistant to the drug vancomycin

Learning Objectives

On completion of this chapter, the student will:

1. Explain the uses, general drug actions, adverse reactions, contraindications, precautions, and interactions of antibacterial drugs that interfere with protein synthesis.
2. Distinguish important preadministration and ongoing assessment activities the nurse should perform on the client taking an antibacterial drug that interferes with protein synthesis.
3. List nursing diagnoses particular to a client taking an antibacterial drug that interferes with protein synthesis.
4. Examine ways to promote an optimal response to therapy, how to manage adverse reactions, and important points to keep in mind when educating clients about the use of antibacterial drugs that interfere with protein synthesis.

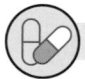 **Drug Classes**

Tetracycline
  • Glycylcycline
Aminoglycosides
Macrolides
  • Ketolide
Lincosamides
Miscellaneous agents
  • Oxazolidinone

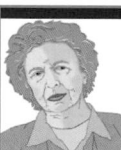 **PHARMACOLOGY IN PRACTICE**

In the morning, you check Mrs. Agnes Moore's C&S report to see "**RESISTANT**" next to the drug she is taking for a urinary tract infection (UTI). She is called back into the outpatient clinic and the tetracycline drug, minocycline (Minocin) is ordered. When taking her drug history you note that she has been taking 0.25 mg digoxin and one baby aspirin each day. As you read this chapter, think about possible drug interactions.

The drugs in this chapter are antibacterial agents that interfere with the development of protein (*synthesis*) in the bacterial cell, which in turn kills the bacterial cell. Here is how this death occurs: to make protein, a message is made by messenger RNA (mRNA) that tells the cell how to build amino acids. The message is translated by the ribosomes to make the string of amino acids that becomes a protein. These drugs act on different areas of the cell, interfering with the process of

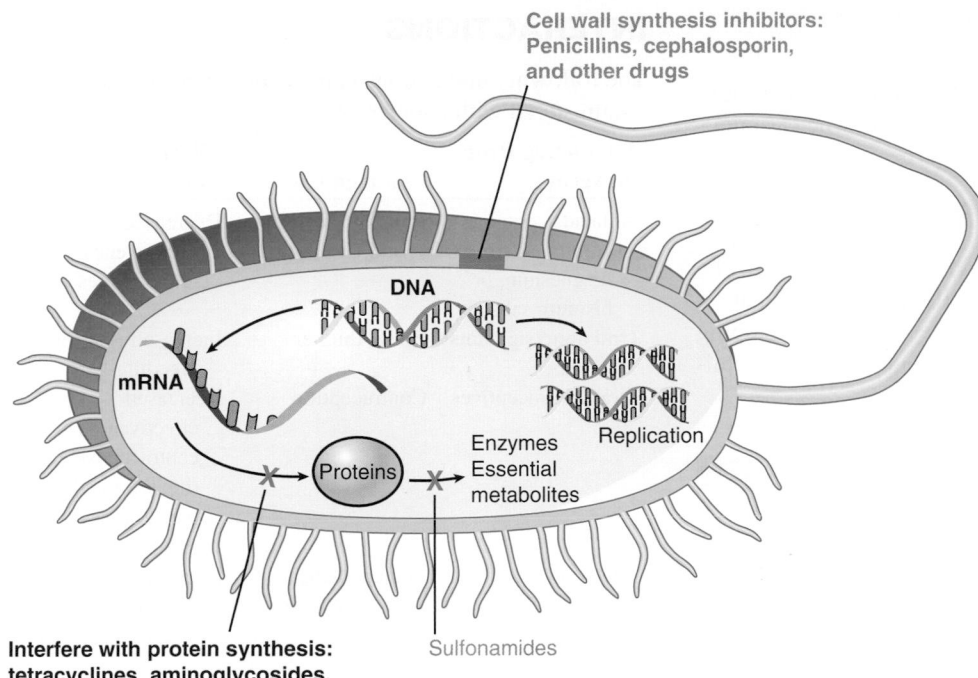

Cell wall synthesis inhibitors:
Penicillins, cephalosporin,
and other drugs

DNA

mRNA

Proteins

Enzymes
Essential
metabolites

Replication

Interfere with protein synthesis:
tetracyclines, aminoglycosides,
macrolides, and lincosamides

Sulfonamides

FIGURE 8.1 Bacterial cell. Sites of action of drugs such as tetracycline, aminoglycosides, macrolides, and lincosamides. This is called protein synthesis inhibition.

protein synthesis (Fig. 8.1), and the amino acids do not link together to make the protein and eventually the cell dies.

This chapter discusses four classes of broad-spectrum antibiotics: the tetracyclines, the aminoglycosides, the macrolides, and the lincosamides. There are a number of newer antibacterial drugs that are a single drug in a class, and these are grouped as miscellaneous drugs. The Summary Drug Table: Antibacterial Drugs That Interfere With Protein Synthesis describes the broad-spectrum antibiotics discussed in this chapter.

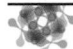 # TETRACYCLINES

The tetracyclines are a group of antibacterial drugs composed of natural and semisynthetic compounds. They are useful in select infections when the organism shows sensitivity (see Chapter 6) to the tetracyclines, such as *E. coli,* gonorrhea, respiratory, and skin and skin structure infections caused by *Staphylococcus aureus.* Gastrointestinal (GI) upset, discoloration of teeth, and sun sensitivity make other drug classes more acceptable. These drugs are also useful when a client is allergic to the penicillins or cephalosporins.

ACTIONS

The tetracyclines are bacteriostatic and exert their effect by inhibiting bacterial protein synthesis, which is a process necessary for reproduction of the microorganism. Growing bacterial resistance to the drugs is a problem with the

tetracyclines. Tigecycline (Tygacil) is the first drug in the glycylcycline class of tetracycline-like drugs that is more bacteria resistant.

USES

These antibiotics are effective in the treatment of infections caused by a wide range of gram-negative and gram-positive microorganisms. Tetracyclines are used as broad-spectrum antibiotics when penicillin is contraindicated and also to treat the following infections:

- *E. coli* infections
- Respiratory infections
- Rickettsia diseases (Rocky Mountain spotted fever, typhus fever, and tick fevers)
- Intestinal amebiasis
- Some skin and soft tissue infections
- Uncomplicated urethral, endocervical, or rectal infections caused by *Chlamydia trachomatis*
- Severe acne as an **adjunctive treatment**
- Infection with **Helicobacter pylori** in combination with metronidazole and bismuth subsalicylate

ADVERSE REACTIONS

Gastrointestinal System Reactions
- Nausea or vomiting
- Diarrhea
- Epigastric distress
- Stomatitis
- Sore throat

Other Reactions

- Skin rashes
- Photosensitivity reaction (demeclocycline seems to cause the most serious photosensitivity reaction, whereas minocycline is least likely to cause this type of reaction)

CONTRAINDICATIONS

Tetracyclines are contraindicated in the client known to be hypersensitive to any of the tetracyclines; during pregnancy, because of the possibility of toxic effects to the developing fetus (pregnancy category D); during lactation; and in children younger than 9 years.

 Lifespan Considerations

Pediatric
Tetracyclines are not given to children younger than 9 years unless their use is absolutely necessary. This is because these drugs may cause permanent yellow-gray-brown discoloration of the teeth. The use of tetracyclines, especially prolonged or repeated therapy, may result in overgrowth of nonsusceptible bacterial or fungal organisms.

PRECAUTIONS

Tetracyclines should be used cautiously in clients with impaired renal function (when degradation of the tetracyclines occurs, the agents are highly toxic to the kidneys) and those with liver impairment (doses greater than 2 g/day can be extremely damaging to the liver).

 Chronic Care Considerations

Tetracyclines may reduce insulin requirements in clients with diabetes. Blood glucose levels should be monitored frequently during tetracycline therapy.

LASA ALERT

The following drugs may sound alike; be sure to clarify when they are ordered:

Drug Name	Sounds Like
doxycycline	dicyclomine, doxepin, doxylamine
Doxy100	Doxil
Oracea	Orencia
Tetracycline	tetradecyl
Vibramycin	vancomycin, Vibativ

Drugs that look like a similar drug are noted in the Summary Drug Tables of each chapter.

INTERACTIONS

The following interactions may occur when a tetracycline is administered with another agent:

Interacting Drug or Agent	Common Use	Effect of Interaction
Antacids containing aluminum, zinc, magnesium, or bismuth salts	Relief of heartburn and GI upset	Decreased effectiveness of tetracyclines
Oral anticoagulants	Blood thinner	Increased risk for bleeding
Oral contraceptives	Contraception	Decreased effectiveness of contraceptive agent (breakthrough bleeding or pregnancy)
Digoxin	Management of heart disease	Increased risk for digitalis toxicity (see Chapter 37)

 Lifespan Considerations

Women
Women of childbearing age should be assessed for oral contraception use whenever tetracyclines are prescribed. The contraception effectiveness is decreased, and women should always be taught and feel confident in the use of other forms of birth control during and after tetracycline treatment.

 AMINOGLYCOSIDES

The aminoglycosides primarily act against gram-negative bacilli and partially against gram-positive bacilli, too. Because these drugs may easily produce toxic reactions (neuro-, oto-, and nephrotoxicities) clients should be monitored carefully during administration.

ACTIONS

The aminoglycosides exert their bactericidal effect by blocking the ribosome from reading the mRNA, one of the steps in protein synthesis necessary for bacterial multiplication.

USES

Aminoglycosides are used primarily in the treatment of infections caused by gram-negative microorganisms. In addition, the drugs may be used to reduce bacteria (normal flora) in the bowel when clients are having abdominal surgery or when a client is in a **hepatic coma**. Oral aminoglycosides are poorly absorbed, and for this reason they are useful in suppressing GI bacteria because they stay in the gut and kill the normal flora. For example, neomycin is used before surgery to reduce intestinal bacteria. It is thought this reduces the possibility of abdominal infection that may occur after surgery on the bowel. This drug treatment protocol is referred to as a portion of the surgical **bowel preparation** (bowel prep). By destroying bacteria in the gut and washing it out with laxatives or enemas, the surgical area becomes as clean as possible before the operation.

Neomycin and paromomycin are used orally in the management of hepatic coma. In this disorder, liver failure results in an elevation of blood ammonia levels. By reducing the number of ammonia-forming bacteria in the intestines, blood ammonia levels may be lowered, thereby temporarily reducing some of the symptoms associated with this disorder.

ADVERSE REACTIONS

General system reactions include the following:

- Nausea
- Vomiting
- Anorexia
- Rash
- Urticaria

More serious adverse reactions may lead to discontinuation of the drug. These reactions include:

- **Nephrotoxicity**
- **Ototoxicity**
- **Neurotoxicity**

All these toxicities are more likely to occur if the client has impaired renal function. Signs and symptoms of nephrotoxicity may include **proteinuria** (protein in the urine), **hematuria** (blood in the urine), an increase in the blood urea nitrogen (BUN) level, a decrease in urine output, and an increase in the serum creatinine concentration. Nephrotoxicity is usually reversible once the drug is discontinued.

Signs and symptoms of ototoxicity include **tinnitus** (ringing in the ears), dizziness, roaring in the ears, vertigo, and a mild to severe loss of hearing. If hearing loss occurs, it is usually permanent. Ototoxicity may occur during drug therapy or even after therapy is discontinued. The short-term administration of neomycin as a preparation for bowel surgery rarely causes these two adverse reactions (ototoxicity and nephrotoxicity).

Signs and symptoms of neurotoxicity include numbness, skin tingling, **circumoral** (around the mouth) paresthesia, peripheral paresthesia, tremors, muscle twitching, convulsions, muscle weakness, and **neuromuscular blockade** (acute muscular paralysis and apnea).

The administration of the aminoglycosides may result in a hypersensitivity reaction, which can range from mild to severe and, in some cases, be life-threatening. Mild hypersensitivity reactions may require only discontinuing the drug, whereas the more serious reactions require immediate treatment. When aminoglycosides are given, individual drug references, such as the cell phone app for your drug handbook or the package insert, should be consulted for more specific adverse reactions. As with other anti-infectives, bacterial or fungal superinfections and pseudomembranous colitis (see Chapter 9) may occur with the use of these drugs.

CONTRAINDICATIONS

The aminoglycosides are contraindicated in clients with hypersensitivity to aminoglycosides, preexisting hearing loss, myasthenia gravis, and Parkinson disease. They are also contraindicated during lactation or pregnancy (pregnancy category C, except for neomycin, amikacin, gentamicin, and tobramycin, which are in pregnancy category D). Aminoglycosides are also contraindicated for long-term therapy, because of the potential for ototoxicity and nephrotoxicity.

PRECAUTIONS

The aminoglycosides are used cautiously in older clients and clients with renal failure (dosage adjustments may be necessary) and neuromuscular disorders.

LASA ALERT

The following drugs may sound alike; be sure to clarify when they are ordered:

Drug Name	Sounds Like
Gentamicin	gentian violet, kanamycin, vancomycin

Drugs that look like a similar drug are noted in the Summary Drug Tables of each chapter.

INTERACTIONS

The following interactions may occur when an aminoglycoside is administered with another agent:

Interacting Drug	Common Use	Effect of Interaction
Cephalosporins	Anti-infective agent	Increased risk of nephrotoxicity
Loop diuretics (water pills)	Management of edema and water retention	Increased risk of ototoxicity
Pavulon or Anectine (general anesthetics)	Anesthesia (e.g., for surgery)	Increased risk of neuromuscular blockade

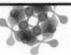 MACROLIDES

The macrolides are effective against a variety of pathogenic organisms, particularly infections of the respiratory and genitourinary tract. Macrolides are less commonly used in skin and soft tissue infections because of the high rate of bacterial resistance to this class.

ACTIONS

The macrolides are bacteriostatic or bactericidal in susceptible bacteria. The drugs act by causing changes in protein function and synthesis.

USES

These antibiotics are effective as prophylaxis before dental or other procedures in high-risk clients allergic to penicillin and in the treatment of:

- A wide range of gram-negative and gram-positive infections
- Acne vulgaris and skin infections
- Upper respiratory infections caused by *Haemophilus influenzae* (with sulfonamides)

ADVERSE REACTIONS

GI reactions include the following:

- Nausea
- Vomiting
- Diarrhea
- Abdominal pain or cramping

As with almost all antibacterial drugs, pseudomembranous colitis may occur, ranging in severity from mild to life-threatening.

CONTRAINDICATIONS

These drugs are contraindicated in clients with hypersensitivity to the macrolides and in clients with preexisting liver disease.

PRECAUTIONS

Macrolides should be used cautiously in clients who have liver dysfunction or myasthenia gravis (a disease that affects the myoneural junction in nerves and is manifested by extreme weakness and exhaustion of the muscles). Azithromycin may cause abnormal change in the electrical activity of the heart (QT interval prolongation), which could cause a fatal arrhythmia. Caution should also be taken with women who are pregnant or lactating (azithromycin and erythromycin are in pregnancy category B; clarithromycin and telithromycin are in pregnancy category C).

LASA ALERT

The following drugs may sound alike; be sure to clarify when they are ordered:

Drug Name	Sounds Like
azithromycin	azathioprine, erythromycin
Zithromax	Fosamax, Zinacef, Zovirax
clarithromycin	Claritin, clindamycin, erythromycin
Eryc	Emcyt, Ery-Tab

Drugs that look like a similar drug are noted in the Summary Drug Tables of each chapter.

INTERACTIONS

The following interactions may occur when a macrolide is administered with another agent:

Interacting Drug	Common Use	Effect of Interaction
Antacids (kaolin, aluminum salts, or magaldrate)	Relief of GI upset, such as diarrhea	Decreased absorption and effectiveness of the macrolides
Digoxin	Management of cardiac disorders	Increased serum levels
Anticoagulants	Blood thinner	Increased risk of bleeding
Clindamycin, lincomycin, or chloramphenicol	Anti-infective agent	Decreased therapeutic activity of the macrolides
Theophylline	Management of respiratory problems, such as asthma	Increased serum theophylline level

---

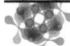 LINCOSAMIDES

The lincosamides, another group of antibacterial drugs with a high potential for toxicity, are usually used only for treating serious infections in which penicillin or erythromycin (a macrolide) is not effective.

ACTIONS

The lincosamides act by inhibiting protein synthesis in susceptible bacteria, causing cell death. They disrupt the functional ability of the ribosomes (which assemble amino acids in the cell), causing cell death.

USES

These antibiotics are effective in the treatment of infections caused by a range of gram-negative and gram-positive microorganisms. Lincosamides are used for the more serious infections and may be used in conjunction with other antibiotics.

ADVERSE REACTIONS

Gastrointestinal System Reactions
- Abdominal pain
- Esophagitis
- Nausea
- Vomiting
- Diarrhea

Other Reactions
- Skin rash
- **Blood dyscrasias**

These drugs also can cause pseudomembranous colitis, which may range from mild to very severe. Discontinuing the drug may relieve mild symptoms of pseudomembranous colitis.

CONTRAINDICATIONS

The lincosamides are contraindicated in infants younger than 1 month and in clients

- Hypersensitive to the lincosamides
- With minor bacterial or viral infections

PRECAUTIONS

These drugs should be used cautiously in clients with a history of GI disorders, renal disease, liver impairment, or myasthenia gravis (lincosamides have neuromuscular blocking action).

LASA ALERT

The following drugs may sound alike; be sure to clarify when they are ordered:

Drug Name	Sounds Like
Cleocin clindamycin	bleomycin, Clinoril, Cubicin, Lincocin clarithromycin, Claritin, vancomycin, lincomycin
Lincocin	Cleocin, Indocin, Minocin

Drugs that look like a similar drug are noted in the Summary Drug Tables of each chapter.

INTERACTIONS

The following interactions may occur when a lincosamide is administered with another agent:

Interacting Drug	Common Use	Effect of Interaction
Kaolin- or aluminum-based antacids	Relief of stomach upset	Decreased absorption of the lincosamides
Neuromuscular blocking drugs	Anesthesia	Increased action of neuromuscular blocking drug, possibly leading to severe and profound respiratory depression

MISCELLANEOUS DRUGS INHIBITING PROTEIN SYNTHESIS

ACTIONS

These drugs are unique and individually in their own classes, yet they all interfere with protein synthesis in the bacterial cell. Daptomycin is a member of a new category of antibacterial agents called *cyclic lipopeptides*. Linezolid (Zyvox) is the first drug in a new drug class, the oxazolidinones. Quinupristin/dalfopristin has bactericidal action against both methicillin-susceptible and methicillin-resistant staphylococci.

USES

Daptomycin is used to treat complicated skin and skin structure bacterial infections as well as *S. aureus* infections of the blood. Linezolid is the drug of choice for skin and skin structure infections caused by methicillin-resistant *S. aureus* (MRSA). It is also used in the treatment of **vancomycin-resistant *Enterococcus faecium* (VREF)**, health care–acquired and community-acquired pneumonias. Quinupristin/dalfopristin is a bacteriostatic agent also used in the treatment of VREF.

ADVERSE REACTIONS

The most common adverse reactions include the following:

- Nausea
- Vomiting
- Diarrhea or constipation
- Headache and dizziness
- Insomnia
- Rash
- Chills

Less common adverse reactions include:

- Fatigue
- Depression
- Nervousness
- Photosensitivity

Pseudomembranous colitis and thrombocytopenia are the most serious adverse reactions caused by linezolid.

NURSING ALERT

Quinupristin/dalfopristin is irritating to the vein. After peripheral infusion, the vein should be flushed with 5% dextrose in water (D_5W), because the drug is incompatible with saline or heparin flush solutions.

CONTRAINDICATIONS AND PRECAUTIONS

Linezolid is contraindicated in clients who are allergic to the drug or who are pregnant (pregnancy category C) or lactating and in clients with **phenylketonuria**. Daptomycin and quinupristin/dalfopristin are contraindicated in clients with a known hypersensitivity to the drug, and it should not be used during pregnancy (pregnancy category B) or lactation.

Linezolid is used cautiously in clients with bone marrow depression, hepatic dysfunction, renal impairment, hypertension, and hyperthyroidism. If another sexually transmitted infection is present with gonorrhea, anti-infectives (in addition to spectinomycin) may be needed to eradicate the infectious processes. Because prolonged use of anti-infectives can disrupt normal flora, the client should be monitored for secondary bacterial or fungal infections.

LASA ALERT

The following drugs may sound alike; be sure to clarify when they are ordered:

Drug Name	Sounds Like
Cubicin	Cleocin
Zyvox	Zosyn, Zovirax

Drugs that look like a similar drug are noted in the Summary Drug Tables of each chapter.

INTERACTIONS

The following interactions may occur when linezolid is administered with another agent:

- Antiplatelet drugs (aspirin or the nonsteroidal anti-inflammatory drugs)—increased risk of bleeding and thrombocytopenia
- Monamine oxidase inhibitor antidepressants—decreased effectiveness
- Large amounts of food containing tyramine (e.g., aged cheese, caffeinated beverages, yogurt, chocolate, red wine, beer, pepperoni)—risk of severe hypertension

Myopathy with elevated creatine phosphokinase levels may occur if daptomycin is administered with statin drugs (cholesterol reduction). Daptomycin should be used cautiously in clients taking warfarin. When taking quinupristin/dalfopristin, the serum levels of the following drugs may increase: antiretrovirals, antineoplastic and immunosuppressant agents, calcium channel blockers, benzodiazepines, and cisapride.

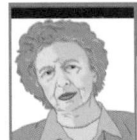

PHARMACOLOGY IN PRACTICE

CELLULAR ACTION

Mrs. Moore has been prescribed a drug from the class of tetracyclines. Infections are treated by inhibiting which of the following cellular actions?
1. Protein synthesis
2. Bacterial cell wall synthesis
3. Inhibiting bacterial DNA gyrase
4. Depolarizing the bacterial cell wall

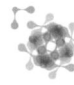

NURSING PROCESS—STEPS TO BUILDING CLINICAL JUDGMENT
Client Receiving an Antibacterial Interfering With Protein Synthesis

ASSESSMENT

Preadministration Assessment

Signs and symptoms may vary and often depend on the organ or system involved and whether the infection is external or internal.

Data gathering suggestions before the initial administration of the drug include:
Objective data

- Description of external signs of infection, such as drainage, redness, changes in the appearance of sputum, cough, and swelling
- Vital signs (temperature, pulse, respirations, and blood pressure)
- Infection culture results
- Renal and hepatic function tests, complete blood count, and urinalysis if client has impaired function in any of these body systems
- Hearing test results, when client has impaired hearing or at risk for hearing loss
- When using for hepatic coma, level of consciousness, ability to swallow orally

Subjective data

- Client's description of infection, including pain, general malaise, chills, and fever
- Type and duration of symptoms (genitourinary and other systems)
- Allergy history, especially a history of drug allergies
- Remedies attempted before seeking care

Some antibiotics have a higher incidence of hypersensitivity reactions in those with a history of allergy to drugs or other substances. If the client has a history of drug allergies and has not told the primary health care provider, do not administer the first dose of the drug; instead, immediately contact the primary health care provider to discuss the allergy history.

Ongoing Assessment

An ongoing assessment is important during therapy with antibacterials that interfere with protein synthesis. When institutionalized, take vital signs every 4 hr or as ordered by the primary health care provider. Notify the primary health care provider if there are changes in the vital signs, such as a significant drop in blood pressure, an increase in the pulse or respiratory rate, or a sudden increase in temperature. When an aminoglycoside is being administered, it is important to monitor the client's respiratory rate because neuromuscular blockade (which can affect breathing) has been reported with the administration of these drugs. Report any changes in the respiratory rate or rhythm to the primary health care provider because immediate treatment may be necessary. When neomycin is given for hepatic coma, assess and record the client's general condition and changes in mentation daily.

Each day, compare current signs and symptoms of the infection against the initial signs and symptoms and record any specific findings in the client's chart.

When an antibiotic is ordered for prevention of a secondary infection (prophylaxis), observe the client for signs and symptoms that may indicate the beginning of an infection despite the prophylactic use of the antibiotic. If signs and symptoms of an infection occur, report them to the primary health care provider.

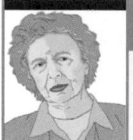

PHARMACOLOGY IN PRACTICE

ASSESSMENT

Mrs. Moore has been administered a tetracycline drug. Which of the following should the nurse immediately report to the primary health care provider during the ongoing assessment of the client? Select all that apply.
1. Drop in blood pressure
2. Regular urine output
3. Increase in pulse rate
4. Normal blood sugar level
5. Increase in temperature

NURSING DIAGNOSES

Drug-specific nursing diagnoses include the following:

- **Impaired comfort: increased fever** related to ineffectiveness of anti-infective therapy
- **Acute confusion** related to increased ammonia blood levels
- **Ineffective tissue perfusion: renal** related to adverse drug reactions to aminoglycosides
- **Injury risk** related to paresthesia secondary to neurotoxicity, or auditory damage from aminoglycosides
- **Diarrhea** related to superinfection secondary to anti-infective therapy, adverse drug reaction

Nursing diagnoses related to drug administration are discussed in Chapter 4.

PLANNING

The expected outcomes for the client may include an optimal response to therapy, which includes control of the infectious process or prophylaxis of bacterial infection, meeting of client needs related to the management of adverse drug effects, and confidence in an understanding of the medication regimen.

IMPLEMENTATION

Promoting an Optimal Response to Therapy

These drugs are of no value in the treatment of infections caused by a virus or fungus. There may be times when a secondary bacterial infection has occurred or may occur when the client has a fungal or viral infection. The primary health care provider may then order one of the broad-spectrum antibiotics, but its purpose is for preventing (prophylaxis) or treating a secondary bacterial infection that could potentially develop after the primary fungal or viral infection.

Oral Administration

Adverse reactions to most anti-infective drugs include nausea, vomiting, or abdominal pain. Clients may want to eat foods when these drugs are administered to reduce GI problems. It is important for you to know how medications will be affected if taken with foods.

TETRACYCLINES. It is important to give tetracyclines on an empty stomach. The exceptions are minocycline (Minocin) and tigecycline (Tygacil), which may be taken with food. All tetracyclines should be given with a full glass of water (8 ounces).

! NURSING ALERT

Do not give tetracyclines along with dairy products (milk or cheese), antacids, laxatives, or products containing iron. When the aforementioned drugs are prescribed, make sure they are given 2 hr before or after the administration of a tetracycline. Food or drugs containing calcium, magnesium, aluminum, or iron prevent the absorption of the tetracyclines if ingested concurrently.

AMINOGLYCOSIDES. When neomycin is given to suppress intestinal bacteria before surgery, the primary health care provider's orders regarding the timing of the administration of the drug are extremely important. Omission of a dose or failure to give the drug at the specified time may result in inadequate suppression of intestinal bacteria. When neomycin is given, **enteric-coated** erythromycin may be given at the same time as part of surgical bowel preparation. Enteric-coated tablets have a special coating that prevents the drug from being absorbed in the stomach. Absorption takes place lower in the GI tract after the coating has dissolved.

MACROLIDES. Clarithromycin and fidaxomicin may be taken with meals, and clarithromycin may be taken with milk if desired. Azithromycin is given 1 hr or more before a meal or 2 hr or more after a meal. Erythromycin is given on an empty stomach (1 hr before or 2 hr after meals) and with 180–240 mL of water.

LINCOSAMIDES. Food impairs the absorption of lincomycin. The client should take nothing by mouth (except water) for 1–2 hr before and after taking lincomycin. Clindamycin may be taken with food or a full glass of water.

Parenteral Administration

When these drugs are given intramuscularly, inspect previous injection sites for signs of pain or tenderness, redness, and swelling. Some antibiotics may cause temporary local reactions, but persistence of a localized reaction should be reported to the primary health care provider. It is important to rotate injection sites and record the site used for injection in the client's chart.

When these drugs are given intravenously (IV), inspect the needle site and area around the needle site for signs of extravasation of the IV fluid or signs of tenderness, pain, and redness (which may indicate *phlebitis* or *thrombophlebitis*). If these symptoms are apparent, restart the IV in another vein and bring the problem to the attention of the primary health care provider.

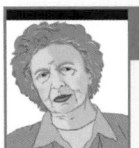

PHARMACOLOGY IN PRACTICE

ADMINISTRATION

Mrs. Moore appears confused as the nurse is discussing tetracycline administration with her. Which of the following is a priority concept for the nurse to include in the client teaching plan?
1. Take the drug on an empty stomach
2. Take the drug just before a meal
3. Take the drug with milk
4. Take the drug only at bedtime

Monitoring and Managing Client Needs

Observe the client at frequent intervals, especially during the first 48 hr of therapy. It is important to report to the primary health care provider the occurrence of any adverse reaction before the next dose of the drug is due.

! NURSING ALERT

Always report serious adverse reactions, such as a severe hypersensitivity reaction, respiratory difficulty, severe diarrhea, or a decided drop in blood pressure, to the primary health care provider immediately, because a serious adverse reaction may require emergency intervention.

Impaired Comfort: Increased Fever

Monitor the temperature at frequent intervals, usually every 4 hr unless the client has an elevated temperature. When the client has an elevated temperature, check the temperature, pulse, and respirations every hour until the temperature returns to normal and administer an antipyretic medication if prescribed by the primary health care provider.

Acute Confusion: Hepatic Coma

Exercise care when the aminoglycosides, such as neomycin, are administered orally as treatment for hepatic coma. During the early stages of this disorder, various changes in the level of consciousness may be seen. At times, the client may appear lethargic and respond poorly to commands. Because of these changes in the level of consciousness, the client may have difficulty swallowing and a danger of aspiration is present. If the client appears to have difficulty taking an oral drug, withhold the drug and contact the primary health care provider.

Ineffective Tissue Perfusion: Renal

The client taking an aminoglycoside is at risk for nephrotoxicity. Measure and record the intake and output and notify the primary health care provider if the output is less than 750 mL/day. It is important to keep a record of the fluid intake and output as well as the client's daily weight to assess hydration and renal function. Encourage fluid intake to 2000 mL/day (if the client's condition permits). Any changes in the intake–output ratio or in the appearance of the urine may indicate nephrotoxicity. Report these types of changes to the primary health care provider promptly. In turn, the primary health care provider may order daily laboratory tests (e.g., serum creatinine and BUN) to monitor renal function. Report elevations in the creatinine or BUN level to the primary health care provider because elevation may indicate renal dysfunction.

Injury Risk

Be alert for symptoms such as numbness or tingling of the skin, circumoral paresthesia, peripheral paresthesia (numbness or tingling in the extremities), tremors, and muscle twitching or weakness. The nurse reports any symptom of neurotoxicity immediately to the primary health care provider. Convulsions can occur if the drug is not discontinued.

! NURSING ALERT

Neuromuscular blockade or respiratory paralysis may occur after administration of the aminoglycosides. Therefore, it is extremely important that any symptoms of respiratory difficulty be reported immediately. If neuromuscular blockade occurs, it may be reversed by the administration of calcium salts, but mechanical ventilation may be required.

The client taking a prolonged course of aminoglycosides is at risk for ototoxicity. Instruct the client to report any ringing in the ears, difficulty hearing, or dizziness to the primary health care provider. Changes in hearing may not be noticed initially by the client, but when changes occur they usually progress from difficulty in hearing high-pitched sounds to problems hearing low-pitched sounds. Auditory changes are irreversible, usually bilateral, and may be partial or total. The risk is greater in clients with renal impairment or those with preexisting hearing loss.

! NURSING ALERT

To detect ototoxicity, carefully evaluate the client's complaints or comments related to hearing, such as a ringing or buzzing in the ears. The client may report a sensation of stuffiness in the ears or difficulty hearing. If hearing problems do occur, report this problem to the primary health care provider immediately. To monitor for damage to the eighth cranial nerve, an evaluation of hearing may be done by audiometry before and throughout the course of therapy.

Diarrhea

Diarrhea may be an indication of a superinfection or pseudomembranous colitis, both of which can be serious. Inspect all stools for blood or mucus. If diarrhea is dark or there is mucus in the stool, save enough material for two tests: one sample should be sent to rule out *C. difficile* (*C. diff*) and one to test for occult blood using a test on the nursing unit such as Hemoccult. If the stool tests positive for blood, save a sample of the stool for possible further laboratory analysis. To reduce the spread of infection to other clients, good hand hygiene is critical when dealing with bodily excrement.

Encourage the client to drink fluids to replace those lost with the diarrhea. It is also important to maintain an accurate intake and output record to help determine fluid balance.

Observe the client for other signs and symptoms of a bacterial or fungal superinfection, such as vaginal or anal itching, sores in the mouth, diarrhea, fever, chills, and sore throat. It is important to report any new signs and symptoms occurring during antibiotic therapy to the primary health care provider, who determines if these problems are part of the original infection or if a superinfection is occurring.

Educating the Client and Family

The client and family should feel confident in their understanding of the prescribed drug regimen. It is not uncommon for clients to stop taking a prescribed drug because they feel better. A detailed plan of teaching helps to reduce the incidence of this problem.

Use principles to support health literacy and easy-to-understand terms when teaching about the adverse reactions associated with the specific prescribed antibiotic. Advise the client to contact the primary health care provider if any potentially serious adverse reactions, such as hypersensitivity reactions, moderate to severe diarrhea, sudden onset of chills and fever, sore throat, or sores in the mouth, occur.

Develop a teaching plan that includes the following information:

- Take the drug at the prescribed time intervals. These intervals are important because a certain amount of the drug must be in the body at all times for the infection to be controlled.
- Do not increase or omit the dose unless advised to do so by the primary health care provider.
- Complete the entire course of treatment. Never stop the drug, except on the advice of a primary health care provider, before the course of treatment is completed even if symptoms improve or disappear. Failure to complete the prescribed course of treatment may result in a return of the infection.
- Take each dose with a full (8-ounce) glass of water. Follow the directions given by the clinical pharmacist regarding taking the drug on an empty stomach or with food (see Client Teaching for Improved Client Outcomes: Avoiding Drug–Food Interactions).
- Notify the primary health care provider if symptoms of the infection become worse or there is no improvement in the original symptoms after about 5 days.
- When a tetracycline has been prescribed, avoid exposure to the sun or any type of tanning lamp or bed. When exposure to direct sunlight is unavoidable, completely cover the arms and legs and wear a wide-brimmed hat

to protect the face and neck. Application of a sunscreen may or may not be effective. Therefore, consult the primary health care provider before using a sunscreen to prevent a photosensitivity reaction.

Client Teaching for Improved Outcomes

Avoiding Drug–Food Interactions
When you teach, make sure your client understands the following:
- ✔ Drugs may be taken with food or milk to minimize the risk for GI upset. However, most tetracyclines, when given with foods containing calcium, such as dairy products, are not absorbed as well as when they are taken on an empty stomach. So, if the client is to receive tetracycline at home, it is important to be sure they know to take the drug on an empty stomach, 1 hr before or 2 hr after a meal.
- ✔ Demonstrate to the client how to read labels in the grocery store and to beware of items (e.g., cereals) that may be fortified with calcium.
- ✔ In addition, teach the client to avoid the following dairy products before or after taking tetracycline:
  - Milk (whole, low fat, skim, condensed, or evaporated) and milkshakes
  - Cream (half-and-half, heavy, light), sour cream, coffee creamers, and creamy salad dressings
  - Eggnog
  - Cheese (natural and processed) and cottage cheese
  - Yogurt and frozen yogurt
  - Ice cream, ice milk, and frozen custard

EVALUATION

- Therapeutic response is achieved, and there is no evidence of infection.
- Adverse reactions are identified, reported to the primary health care provider, and managed successfully with appropriate nursing interventions:
  - Client reports comfort without fever.
  - Orientation and mentation remain intact.
  - Client has adequate renal tissue perfusion.
  - No evidence of injury is seen because of visual or auditory disturbances.
  - Client does not experience or is able to manage diarrhea.
- Client and family express confidence and demonstrate an understanding of the drug regimen.

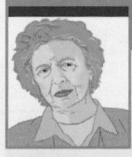

PHARMACOLOGY IN PRACTICE

USING CLINICAL REASONING

Based on your knowledge of the tetracyclines, determine whether there is any reason to be concerned about Mrs. Moore's drug regimen. Given her confusion, how will you teach her about potential interactions of the drugs?

KEY POINTS

■ Tetracyclines are primarily bacteriostatic and are often used when the client is allergic to penicillin or a cephalosporin.

■ A larger number of bacteria are becoming resistant to this class of drug. A newer class, glycylcycline, is more resistant to bacteria. Aminoglycosides, macrolides, and lincosamides are primarily bactericidal; they work by preventing the bacterial cell from making protein (synthesis), causing cell death.

■ These drugs are used to treat a wide range of both gram-negative and gram-positive microorganisms. Many of these drugs are used to remove bacteria from the bowel as part of preparing the GI tract for surgical procedures. When used for other infections and indications, these drugs may still cause bowel issues, ranging from diarrhea to pseudomembranous colitis.

■ These drugs can have serious toxicities to neurological (including hearing) and renal systems; therefore, they are typically not the first-line antibacterial drugs prescribed if possible.

■ Although some drugs can be taken with food, many have interactions with foods and fluids. Dairy and calcium products inhibit the absorption of the tetracyclines. Therefore, take these drugs at least 1 hr before or 2 hr after a meal.

■ Hearing, neurologic status, and contraception should all be monitored when these drugs are taken.

SUMMARY DRUG TABLE
Antibacterial Drugs That Interfere With Protein Synthesis

Generic Name	Trade Name	Uses	Adverse Reactions	Dosage Ranges
Tetracyclines				
demeclocycline *dem-e-kloe-SYE-kleen*		Infrequently used for antibacterial treatment of infections, sometimes as an adjuvant	Nausea, vomiting, diarrhea, dizziness, headache, hypersensitivity reactions, photosensitivity reactions, pseudomembranous colitis, hematologic changes, discoloration of teeth in fetus and young children	150 mg orally QID or 300 mg orally BID; gonorrhea: 600 mg orally initially then 300 mg orally every 12 hr for 4 days
doxycycline *doks-i-SYE-kleen*	Atridox, Doryx, Oracea, Vibramycin	Early Lyme disease, gram-negative infections, suspected anthrax exposure	Same as demeclocycline	100 mg orally every 12 hr first day then 100 mg/day orally. Severe infections: 100 mg every 12 hr
eravacycline *ER-a-va-SYE-kleen*	Xerava	Complicated intra-abdominal infections	Nausea, vomiting, diarrhea, infusion site irritation, hypersensitivity, photosensitivity reactions	1mg/kg IV every 12 hr
minocycline *mi-noe-SYE-kleen*	Arestin, Dynacin, Minocin, Solodyn, Ximino	Acne, gram-negative infections	Dizziness, fatigue, malaise, pruritus	200 mg orally initially then 100 mg orally every 12 hr
omadacycline *oh-MAD-a-SYE-kleen*	Nuzyra	Pneumonia, soft tissue infections	Nausea, vomiting, infusion site irritation	300 mg IV daily
sarecycline *Sar-e-SYE-kleen*	Seysara	Acne	Nausea	Orally based on body weight
tetracycline *tet-ra-SYE-kleen*		Same as demeclocycline	Same as demeclocycline	1–2 g/day orally in 2–4 divided doses
tigecycline *tiye-ge-SYE-kleen* (glycylcycline class similar to tetracycline)	Tygacil	Complicated skin structures and complicated intra-abdominal infections	Nausea, vomiting, diarrhea	100 mg IV initially then 50 mg IV every 12 hr
Aminoglycosides				
amikacin *am-i-KAY-sin*	Arikayce	Treatment of nontuberculous mycobacterium	Hoarseness, cough, fatigue, headache, nausea, diarrhea, ototoxicity, muscle pains nephrotoxicity	590 mg/inhaler daily

Generic Name	Trade Name	Uses	Adverse Reactions	Dosage Ranges
Aminoglycosides (continued)				
gentamicin jen-ta-MYE-sin		Serious bacterial infections	Nephrotoxicity, ototoxicity	3 mg/kg/day in 3 divided doses IM or IV. For life-threatening infection: 5 mg/kg/day in divided doses
neomycin nee-oh-MYE-sin		Hepatic coma, suppress intestinal bacteria	Nausea, vomiting, diarrhea	Hepatic coma: 4–12 g/day in divided doses. Preoperative prophylaxis: 1 g/day orally for 3 days
paromomycin pa-ra-mo-MYE-sin		Hepatic coma, intestinal amebiasis	Same as neomycin	25–35 mg/kg/day
plazomicin Pla-zoe-MYE-sin	Zemdri	Complicated UTI, pyelonephritis	Nausea, vomiting, diarrhea	15 mg/kg/day
streptomycin strep-toe-MYE-sin		Serious bacterial infections, treatment of tuberculosis	Same as neomycin	15 mg/kg/day IM or 25–30 mg/kg IM 2–3 times/week
tobramycin toe-bra-MYE-sin		Serious bacterial infections	Same as neomycin	3–5 mg/kg/day IM, IV in 3 equal doses
Macrolides				
⊘ **azithromycin** az-ith-roe-MYE-sin	Zithromax, Zmax	Pneumonia	Nausea, vomiting, diarrhea, abdominal pain, hypersensitivity reactions, pseudomembranous colitis, heart arrhythmias	500 mg orally first day then 250 mg/day orally
clarithromycin kla-RITH-roe-mye-sin		Pneumonia, H. pylori therapy	Same as azithromycin	250–500 mg orally every 12 hr
⊘ **erythromycin** er-ith-roe-MYE-sin	Emcyt, Ery-Tab, Eryc, EryPed, E.E.S.	Pneumonia	Same as azithromycin	250 mg orally every 6 hr or 333 mg every 8 hr up to 4 g/day
fidaxomicin fye-DAX-oh-mye-sin	Dificid	Treatment of diarrhea from C. diff	Nausea, vomiting, stomach pain, rash	200 mg orally every 24 hr
Lincosamides				
clindamycin klin-da-MYE-sin	Cleocin	Systemic and skin, soft tissue infections	Abdominal pain, esophagitis, nausea, vomiting, diarrhea, skin rash, pseudomembranous colitis, hypersensitivity reactions	Serious infection: 150–450 mg orally every 6 hr; severe infection: 600–2700 mg/day in 2–4 equal doses; life-threatening infection: up to 4.8 g/day IV, IM
⊘ **lincomycin** lin-koe-MYE-sin	Lincocin	Serious bacterial infections	Same as clindamycin	500 mg orally every 6–8 hr; 600 mg IM every 12–24 hr; up to 8 g/day IV in life-threatening situations
Miscellaneous Drugs That Interfere With Protein Synthesis				
⊘ **DAPTOmycin** dap-toe-mye'-sin	Cubicin	Complicated skin and skin structure infections, S. aureus blood infections	Nausea, diarrhea, constipation, rash, vein irritation	4 mg/kg IV daily for 7–14 days
linezolid li-NE-zoh-lid	Zyvox	Infections with VREF and MRSA; pneumonia from S. aureus and penicillin-susceptible Streptococcus pneumoniae; skin and skin structure infections	Nausea, diarrhea, headache, insomnia, pseudomembranous colitis	600 mg orally or IV every 12 hr

Continued

SUMMARY DRUG TABLE (continued)
Antibacterial Drugs That Interfere With Protein Synthesis

Generic Name	Trade Name	Uses	Adverse Reactions	Dosage Ranges
quinupristin/ dalfopristin *kwi-NYOO-pris-tin/dal-FOE-pris-tin*	Synercid	VREF, *Staph.* skin/soft tissue infections	Vein inflammation, nausea, vomiting, diarrhea	7.5 mg/kg IV every 8 hr
tedizolid *ted-eye-ZOE-lid*	Sivextro	Acute bacterial skin/soft tissue infections	Diarrhea, headache, heartburn	200 mg orally/IV daily
Helicobactor pylori treatment combinations				
tetracycline/bismuth/ metronidazole	Pylera	*H. pylori* treatment	See individual drugs	3 capsules 4 times daily
clarithromycin/ amoxicillin/ omeprazole	Omeclamox-Pak	*H. pylori* treatment	See individual drugs	Pill combination twice daily
rifabutin/amoxicillin/ omeprazole	Talicia	*H. pylori* treatment	See individual drugs	

 This drug should be administered at least 1 hr before or 2 hr after a meal.

CHAPTER REVIEW

Know Your Drugs

Clients sometimes know a medication by the brand (or trade) name and not the generic name. To help you recognize both names, match the brand name with the generic name of the same medication.

Generic Name	Brand Name
1. doxycycline	A. Cubicin
2. tigecycline	B. Dificid
3. fidaxomicin	C. Tygacil
4. DAPTOmycin	D. Vibramycin

Calculate Medication Dosages

1. A client is prescribed 600 mg of lincomycin every 12 hr IM. The drug is available as 300 mg/mL. How many milliliters does the nurse administer?
2. A client is prescribed 200 mg of minocycline oral suspension now, followed by 100 mg orally every 12 hr. The minocycline is available as an oral suspension of 50 mg/5 mL. How many milliliters does the nurse administer as the initial dose?

Prepare for the NCLEX

RECALL THE FACTS

1. A client asks the nurse why the primary health care provider prescribed an antibiotic when they are told that they had a viral infection. The correct response by the nurse is that the antibiotic may be used for a suspected _____.
   1. primary fungal infection
   2. repeat viral infection
   3. secondary bacterial infection
   4. breakdown of the immune system

2. A client is receiving erythromycin for an infection. The client's response to therapy is best evaluated by _____.
   1. monitoring vital signs every 4 hr
   2. comparing initial and current signs and symptoms
   3. monitoring fluid intake and output
   4. asking the client if he is feeling better

3. When asked to describe a photosensitivity reaction, the nurse correctly states that this reaction may be described as a(n) _____.
   1. tearing of the eyes on exposure to bright light
   2. aversion to bright lights and sunlight
   3. sensitivity to products in the environment
   4. exaggerated sunburn reaction when the skin is exposed to sunlight

4. When giving doxycycline for gonorrhea, the nurse advises the client to _____.
   1. return for a follow-up examination
   2. limit fluid intake to 1200 mL/day while taking the drug
   3. return the next day for a second injection
   4. avoid drinking alcohol for the next 10 days

5. Which of the following complaints by a client taking tetracycline would be most indicative that they are experiencing ototoxicity?
   1. Tingling of the extremities
   2. Inability to hear the television
   3. Changes in mental status
   4. Short periods of dizziness

ANALYZE THE FACTS

6. When giving one of the macrolide antibiotics, the nurse assesses the client for the most common adverse reactions, which are _____.
1. related to the GI tract
2. skin rash and urinary retention
3. sores in the mouth and hypertension
4. related to the nervous system

7. Which of the following urinary output measurements should be reported to the primary health care provider immediately?
1. 2400 mL in 24 hr
2. 30 mL in 1 hr
3. 750 mL in 1 hr
4. 1000 mL in 1 day

8. Which of the following medications may be taken with food?
1. Erythromycin
2. Doxycycline
3. Demeclocycline
4. Tigecycline

ALTERNATE-FORMAT QUESTIONS

9. *When a client is instructed not to take a drug with dairy products, what can the client drink when swallowing the medication? **Select all that apply.**
1. Water
2. Yogurt fruit smoothie
3. Iced tea
4. Cranberry juice
5. Milk

10. A client with limited health literacy is prescribed azithromycin for a lower respiratory tract infection. Azithromycin is available in 250 mg tablets. The primary health care provider has ordered 500 mg on the first day, followed by 250 mg on days 2 through 5. The nurse shows the client how many tablets to be taken on the first day? _____. On the last day of therapy? _____

To check your answers, see Appendix F.

_____

*Indicates the question is directly linked to the NCLEX-PN test plan in Appendix G.

WANT TO KNOW MORE? A wide variety of resources are available to enhance your learning and understanding of this chapter.
- Visit for thePoint resources such as:
  • NCLEX-Style Student Review Questions
  • Journal Articles
  • Dosage Calculations
  • Drug Monographs
  • Watch and Learn Videos
  • Concepts in Action Animations
- The *Study Guide to Accompany Introductory Clinical Pharmacology,* 12th edition, sold separately, will help you review and apply essential content.
- ✓PrepU is available to help students prepare for the NCLEX-PN examination.

9

Antibacterial Drugs That Interfere With DNA/RNA Synthesis

Key Terms

extended release   formulation in which drug is released over time

extravasation   escape of fluid from a blood vessel into surrounding tissue

normal flora   nonpathogenic microorganisms in the body

photosensitivity   exaggerated sunburn reaction when the skin is exposed to sunlight or ultraviolet light

pseudomembranous colitis   severe, life-threatening form of diarrhea that occurs when normal flora of the bowel is eliminated and replaced with *Clostridium difficile* (*C. diff*) bacteria

superinfection   overgrowth of bacterial or fungal microorganisms not affected by the antibiotic being administered

Learning Objectives

On completion of this chapter, the student will:

1. Explain the uses, general drug actions, contraindications, precautions, interactions, and adverse reactions of antibacterial drugs that interfere with DNA/RNA synthesis.
2. Distinguish preadministration and ongoing assessment activities the nurse should perform on the client taking an antibacterial drug that interferes with DNA/RNA synthesis.
3. List nursing diagnoses particular to a client receiving an antibacterial drug that interferes with DNA/RNA synthesis.
4. Examine ways to promote an optimal response to therapy, how to manage adverse reactions, and important points to keep in mind when educating clients about the use of antibacterial drugs that interfere with DNA/RNA synthesis.

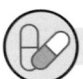 **Drug Classes**

Fluoroquinolones

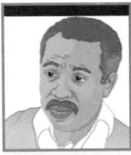 **PHARMACOLOGY IN PRACTICE**

Mr. Bernard Park, 77 years old, is a client in a skilled nursing facility receiving gemifloxacin for a lower respiratory tract infection over the last 9 days. Think about the adverse reactions experienced by clients as they end a course of antibacterial drug therapy.

As microorganisms become resistant to various antibiotics, researchers develop drugs that affect different portions of the bacterial cell. In Chapters 7 and 8 you read about how the cell wall and protein-building capabilities of the bacteria are targeted by antibacterial drugs. In this chapter, you will read about drugs that kill bacteria by interfering with the synthesis of DNA or RNA. When these processes are interrupted, the bacterial cell cannot reproduce and it dies (Fig. 9.1). Some of these drugs are used to treat a broad spectrum of infections, others only for the treatment of one type of infection, and still others may be limited to the treatment of serious infections not treatable by other anti-infectives. The Summary Drug Table: Antibacterial Drugs That Interfere With DNA/RNA Synthesis lists the drugs discussed in this chapter.

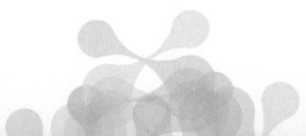

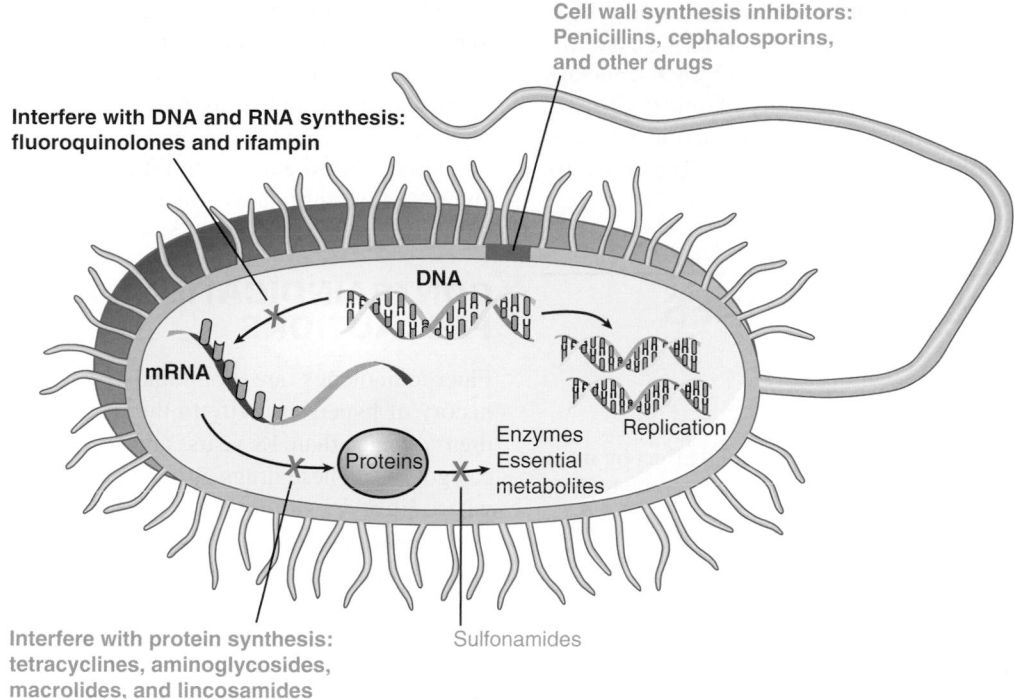

Cell wall synthesis inhibitors:
Penicillins, cephalosporins,
and other drugs

Interfere with DNA and RNA synthesis:
fluoroquinolones and rifampin

DNA

mRNA

Proteins

Enzymes
Essential
metabolites

Replication

Interfere with protein synthesis:
tetracyclines, aminoglycosides,
macrolides, and lincosamides

Sulfonamides

FIGURE 9.1 Action of bacterial DNA/RNA synthesis inhibitors such as the fluoroquinolones.

ANTIBIOTIC STEWARDSHIP: SUPERINFECTIONS

Dellit et al. (2007) reported on drug use in long-term care (LTC), finding that 40%–75% of antibiotics prescribed were unnecessary. This is when problems of antibiotic overuse in the LTC setting was identified, thus leading to the initiation of the Antibiotic Stewardship for Nursing Homes program in 2015 in response to *C. diff* infection (the most common cause of antibiotic-related acute diarrhea in LTC facilities). The intention was to reduce the inappropriate and unnecessary prescription of antibiotics in LTC.

Superinfections

A **superinfection** can develop rapidly and is potentially serious and even life-threatening. Antibiotics can disrupt the **normal flora** (nonpathogenic bacteria in the bowel), causing a secondary infection or superinfection. This new infection is "superimposed" on the original infection. The destruction of large numbers of nonpathogenic bacteria (normal flora) by the antibiotic alters the chemical environment. This allows uncontrolled growth of bacteria or fungal microorganisms that are not affected by the antibiotic being administered. A superinfection may occur with the use of any antibiotic, especially when these drugs are given for a long time or when repeated courses of therapy are necessary.

 Lifespan Considerations

Gerontology

Older adults who are debilitated, chronically ill, or taking oral antibiotics for an extended period are more likely to develop a superinfection.

Symptoms of bacterial superinfection of the bowel include diarrhea or bloody diarrhea, rectal bleeding, fever, and abdominal cramping. **Pseudomembranous colitis** is one type of a bacterial superinfection. This potentially life-threatening problem develops because of an overgrowth of the microorganism *Clostridium difficile (C. diff)* in the bowel. This organism produces a toxin that affects the lining of the colon. Signs and symptoms include severe diarrhea with visible blood and mucus, fever, and abdominal cramps. This adverse reaction usually requires immediate discontinuation of the antibiotic. Mild cases may respond to drug discontinuation. Moderate to severe cases may require treatment with intravenous (IV) fluids and electrolytes, protein supplementation, and treatment with drugs such as fidaxomicin (Dificid) to eliminate the microorganism.

Candidiasis or moniliasis is a common type of fungal superinfection. Fungal superinfections commonly occur throughout the gastrointestinal (GI) and reproductive systems. Symptoms include lesions of the mouth or tongue, vaginal discharge, and anal or vaginal itching.

Vaginal yeast infections are frequent because a yeast-like fungus normally exists in small numbers in the vagina.

The multiplication rate of these microorganisms is normally slowed and kept under control by a strain of bacteria (*Döderlein bacillus*) in the vagina. If anti-infective therapy destroys these normal microorganisms of the vagina, the fungi become uncontrolled, multiply at a rapid rate, and cause symptoms of the fungal infection candidiasis (or moniliasis).

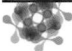 # FLUOROQUINOLONES

ACTIONS

The fluoroquinolones exert their bactericidal effect by interfering with the synthesis of bacterial enzymes, which in turn prevent the making of bacterial DNA. This interference prevents cell reproduction, causing death of the bacterial cell (Fig. 9.1).

USES

The fluoroquinolones are effective in treating infections caused by gram-positive and gram-negative microorganisms. They are primarily used in the treatment of the following:

- Lower respiratory tract infections
- Bone and joint infections
- Urinary tract infections
- Infections of the skin
- Sexually transmitted infections

Ciprofloxacin and ofloxacin are available in ophthalmic forms for infections in the eyes.

ADVERSE REACTIONS

Common adverse effects include the following:

- Nausea
- Diarrhea
- Headache
- Abdominal pain or discomfort
- Dizziness
- **Photosensitivity** (exaggerated skin reaction to sun exposure), which is a more serious adverse reaction seen with the administration of the fluoroquinolones, especially ofloxacin.

The risk for aortic dissection or rupture when using fluoroquinolones is of concern. Therefore, these antibacterial drugs should not be used with clients diagnosed with an existing aortic aneurysm, hypertension, peripheral atherosclerosis, or genetic blood vessel disorders.

The administration of any drug may result in a hypersensitivity reaction, which can range from mild to severe and, in some cases, be life-threatening. Mild hypersensitivity reactions may require only discontinuing the drug, whereas the more serious reactions require immediate treatment. Bacterial or fungal superinfections and pseudomembranous colitis may occur with the use of these drugs.

CONTRAINDICATIONS AND PRECAUTIONS

Fluoroquinolones are contraindicated in clients with a history of hypersensitivity to the fluoroquinolones, in children younger than 18 years, and in pregnancy (pregnancy category C). These drugs also are contraindicated in clients whose lifestyles do not allow for adherence to the precautions regarding photosensitivity.

Tendonitis and tendon rupture risk increase when taking a fluoroquinolone. For this reason, gemifloxacin is reserved for use in clients with chronic bronchitis only when all other alternatives are exhausted. Although this can happen at any age, those older than 60 years who also take corticosteroids are at greater risk.

Fluoroquinolones are used cautiously in clients with diabetes, renal impairment, or a history of seizures; older clients; and clients on dialysis.

INTERACTIONS

The following interactions may occur when a fluoroquinolone is administered with another agent:

Interacting Drug	Common Use	Effect of Interaction
Theophylline	Management of respiratory problems, such as asthma	Increased serum theophylline level
Cimetidine	Management of GI upset	Interferes with elimination of the antibiotic
Oral anticoagulants	Blood thinner	Increased risk of bleeding
Antacids, iron salts, or zinc	Relief of heartburn and GI upset	Decreased absorption of the antibiotic
Nonsteroidal anti-inflammatory drugs (NSAIDs)	Relief of pain and inflammation	Risk of seizure activity

There is also a risk of severe cardiac arrhythmias when the fluoroquinolones—moxifloxacin are administered with drugs that increase the QT interval (e.g., quinidine, procainamide, amiodarone, sotalol).

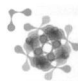

NURSING PROCESS—STEPS TO BUILDING CLINICAL JUDGMENT
Client Receiving a Fluoroquinolone or Miscellaneous Anti-infective

ASSESSMENT

Preadministration Assessment
Data gathering suggestions before the initial administration of a fluoroquinolone or miscellaneous DNA/RNA inhibitor include:

Objective data

- Description of external signs of infection, such as drainage, redness, changes in the appearance of sputum, cough, and swelling
- Vital signs (temperature, pulse, respirations, and blood pressure)
- Infection culture and sensitivity results
- Renal and hepatic function tests, complete blood count, and urinalysis if client has impaired function in any of these body systems

Subjective data

- Current symptoms of the infection (malaise, fatigue, pain)
- Allergy history, particularly a drug allergy
- History of heart, renal, or hepatic disease, any previous seizure activity
- All medical and surgical treatment

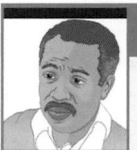

PHARMACOLOGY IN PRACTICE

DRUG HISTORY
Mr. Park is being treated with a fluoroquinolone for an infection. Tendon rupture occurs more frequently in the older adult when taking which of the following drugs with the fluoroquinolones?
1. Antianginal drugs
2. Corticosteroids
3. Oral antidiabetic drugs
4. Respiratory bronchodilators

Ongoing Assessment
During drug therapy with the miscellaneous DNA/RNA inhibitors, it is important for you to perform an ongoing assessment. In general, compare the initial signs and symptoms of the infection, which were recorded during the initial assessment, with the current signs and symptoms. Document these findings in the client's chart. When in an institution, monitor the client's vital signs every 4 hr or as ordered by the primary health care provider. Notify the primary health care provider if there are changes in the vital signs, such as a significant drop in blood pressure, an increase in the pulse or respiratory rate, or a sudden increase in temperature.

NURSING DIAGNOSES

Drug-specific nursing diagnoses include the following:

- **Impaired comfort** related to fever
- **Altered skin integrity** related to photosensitivity
- **Acute pain** related to tissue injury during drug therapy
- **Diarrhea** related to superinfection secondary to antibiotic therapy, adverse drug reaction

Nursing diagnoses related to drug administration are discussed in Chapter 4.

PLANNING

The expected outcomes for the client may include an optimal response to therapy, which includes control of the infectious process, meeting of client needs related to the management of adverse drug reactions, and confidence in an understanding of the medication regimen.

IMPLEMENTATION

Promoting an Optimal Response to Therapy
A variety of adverse reactions can be seen with the administration of the fluoroquinolones. You should observe the client, especially during the first 48 hr of therapy. It is important to report the occurrence of any adverse reaction to the primary health care provider before the next dose of the drug is due. If a serious adverse reaction, such as a hypersensitivity reaction, respiratory difficulty, severe diarrhea, or a decided drop in blood pressure occurs, then contact the primary health care provider immediately. These adverse reactions can be distressing for the client, so be sure to offer comfort measures, such as a warm blanket or gentle touch, while awaiting a response from the primary health care provider.

Always listen to, evaluate, and report any complaints the client may have; certain complaints may be an early sign of an adverse drug reaction. Report all changes in the client's condition and any new problems that occur (e.g., nausea or diarrhea) as soon as possible. The primary health care provider will determine if these changes or problems are a part of the client's infectious process or the result of an adverse drug reaction.

Encourage clients who receive the fluoroquinolones to increase their fluid intake. Norfloxacin is given on an empty stomach (e.g., 1 hr before or 2 hr after meals). Some drugs are made so that they release the drug over time in the body; these formulations are known as **extended-release** (XR), sustained-release, or controlled-release drugs. Because the amount of drug would be too great if released in the body at once, it is important to swallow these medications whole. Clients should not crush, chew, or break prolonged-release medications. If the client is taking an antacid, ciprofloxacin and moxifloxacin should be administered 2–4 hr before or 6–8 hr after the antacid.

PHARMACOLOGY IN PRACTICE

DOSAGE CALCULATION
Mr. Park was prescribed 320 mg of gemifloxacin per day for 5 days. Today is Thursday and the first day the patient will take the drug. What will be the last day to take this prescription?

Intravenous Administration

When these drugs are administered intravenously, inspect the needle site and area around the needle at frequent intervals for signs of **extravasation**, or leakage into the soft tissue, of the IV fluid. More frequent assessments are performed if the client is restless or uncooperative. Many of the miscellaneous anti-infectives irritate the vein when administered by the IV route.

The rate of infusion is checked every 15 minutes and adjusted as needed. Inspect the vein used for the IV infusion every 4–8 hr for signs of tenderness, pain, and redness (which may indicate phlebitis or thrombophlebitis). If these symptoms are apparent, the IV infusion is restarted in another vein and the problem is brought to the attention of the primary health care provider.

Monitoring and Managing Client Needs

Although the drugs in this chapter are different, many of the client problems are similar. Consider the commonalities of the drugs to look for common problems.

Impaired Comfort: Increased Fever

The infectious process is accompanied by an elevation in temperature. Monitor the vital signs, particularly the body temperature, when clients have an infection. As the anti-infective works to rid the body of the infectious organism, the body temperature should return to normal. Monitoring the vital signs (temperature, pulse, and respiration) frequently aids in assessing the drug's effectiveness in eradicating the infection. Promptly notify the primary health care provider if a temperature rises over 101 °F.

Altered Skin Integrity

The fluoroquinolone drugs cause severe photosensitivity reactions. Clients may experience "sunburn" reactions even when they use sunscreen or sunblock products. Caution clients to wear cover-up clothing with long sleeves and wide-brimmed hats when outside in addition to sunblock preparations. Remind clients that sunscreen needs to be applied repeatedly throughout the day or when going into water. Clients should be aware that glare during hazy or cloudy days can cause skin reactions as readily as direct sunlight on a clear day.

Acute Pain: Tissue Injury

Many of these antibacterial drugs are irritating to the vein when administered IV. You should read instructions carefully for infusion rates. For intravenously administered fluoroquinolones, as with other caustic drugs, inspect the needle site and the area around the needle every hour for signs of extravasation of the IV fluid while the drug is infused. Inspect the vein used for the IV infusion every 4 hr for signs of tenderness, pain, and redness (which may indicate phlebitis or thrombophlebitis). Perform these assessments more frequently if the client is restless or

uncooperative. Be sure the proper flush solution is used after the infusion to keep the vein open and minimize irritation. If tissue or vein injury is apparent, the IV is stopped and restarted in another vein and the problem brought to the attention of the primary health care provider.

ⓘ NURSING ALERT

There is a risk with all fluoroquinolone drugs of causing pain, inflammation, or rupture of a tendon. The Achilles tendon is particularly vulnerable. Those 60 years and older who take corticosteroids are at greatest risk for tendon rupture.

Diarrhea

Frequent liquid stools may be an indication of a superinfection or pseudomembranous colitis. If pseudomembranous colitis occurs, it is usually seen 4 to 10 days after treatment is started.

Teach the client or family to feel confident in the ability to check bowel movements and immediately report to the primary health care provider the occurrence of diarrhea or loose stools containing blood and mucus. It may be necessary to discontinue drug therapy and institute treatment for diarrhea, a superinfection, or pseudomembranous colitis.

Client Teaching for Improved Outcomes

Superinfections

Antibiotics are one of the most commonly administered types of drug therapy in the home. Any client taking antibacterial drugs is susceptible to superinfection. Make sure the client knows the signs and symptoms of superinfection. A bacterial superinfection commonly occurs in the bowel.

When you teach, make sure your client understands the following:
Report any of the following:

✔ Fever
✔ Burning sensation in the mouth or throat
✔ Localized redness, inflammation, and excoriation, particularly inside the mouth, in the groin, or in skin folds of the anogenital area
✔ Abdominal cramps
✔ Scaly, reddened, papular rash commonly in the breast folds, axillae, groin, or umbilicus
✔ Diarrhea, possibly severe with visible blood and mucus

A fungal superinfection commonly occurs in the mouth, vagina, and anogenital areas. Teach the client to report any of the following:

✔ Creamy white, lace-like patches on the tongue, mouth, or throat
✔ White or yellow vaginal discharge
✔ Anal or vaginal itching, increased perianal redness

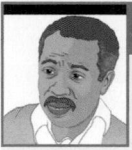

PHARMACOLOGY IN PRACTICE

MANAGING NEEDS

A superinfection can develop rapidly and is potentially serious. Identify how antibacterial drug therapy can lead to a superinfection. Arrange the following steps as they relate to developing a superinfection during anti-infective therapy.

1. Secondary infection is superimposed on the original infection
2. Uncontrolled growth of bacteria
3. Antibiotics disrupt the normal flora of the bowel
4. Patient experiences cramping, diarrhea, and bleeding
5. Microorganism produces toxins

If diarrhea is bloody or there is mucus in the stool, save enough material for two tests: one sample should be sent to rule out *C. diff* and the other sample to test for occult blood using a test on the nursing unit such as Hemoccult. If the stool tests positive for blood, save a sample of the stool for possible further laboratory analysis. To reduce the spread of infection to other clients, good hand hygiene is critical when dealing with bodily excrement.

Educating the Client and Family

When you teach the client and family members, explain all adverse reactions associated with the specific prescribed antibiotic. Use written materials in the language of preference to describe the signs and symptoms of potentially serious adverse reactions, such as hypersensitivity reactions, moderate to severe diarrhea, and sudden onset of chills and fever. The client should feel confident about when to contact the primary health care provider if such symptoms occur. Instruct the client not to take the next dose of the drug until the problem is discussed with the primary health care provider (see Client Teaching for Improved Outcomes: Superinfections).

EVALUATION

- Therapeutic response is achieved, and there is no evidence of infection.
- Adverse reactions are identified, reported to the primary health care provider, and managed successfully with appropriate nursing interventions:
  - Client reports comfort without fever.
  - Skin is intact and free of inflammation, irritation, infection, or ulcerations.
  - Client reports no pain or injury.
  - Client does not experience diarrhea.
- Client and family express confidence and demonstrate an understanding of the drug regimen.

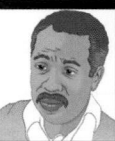

PHARMACOLOGY IN PRACTICE

USING CLINICAL REASONING

Mr. Park complains about gas pains in his stomach and lots of "rumbling feelings." The nursing assistant reports that he has made multiple trips to the bathroom because of diarrhea for the past 2 days. He gets upset and says he cannot wait for ambulation assistance; the nursing assistant is concerned he will get up at night by himself and fall. Analyze whether this matter should be investigated.

KEY POINTS

■ Fluoroquinolones are the primary class of bactericidal drugs affecting the bacterial cell by interfering with the synthesis of DNA. These drugs are used to treat a wide range of both gram-negative and gram-positive microorganisms. Some drugs of this class come in ophthalmic solutions to treat infections of the eye.

■ Some of these drugs are given in an oral form (XR form) so the drug is released into the body over time. When given IV, the vein needs to be monitored frequently because the medications can be irritating to the tissue.

■ Photosensitivity can be a severe adverse reaction of this class of drugs. Sunscreen and lightweight clothing should be worn at all times when outdoors, even on overcast days.

■ Tendon rupture has been noted, especially in those older than 60 years, when taking these drugs.

■ When taking any antibacterial drug, overgrowth of other bacteria or elimination of normal flora can result in superinfection. Drugs may be stopped and supportive care with IV fluids, dietary supplement, and a different antibacterial drug can help.

SUMMARY DRUG TABLE
Antibacterial Drugs That Interfere With DNA/RNA Synthesis

Generic Name	Trade Name	Uses	Adverse Reactions	Dosage Ranges
Fluoroquinolones				
ciprofloxacin *sip-roe-FLOKS-a-sin*	Cipro	Treatment of bone, joint, GI, GU infections caused by susceptible microorganisms	Nausea, diarrhea, headache, abdominal discomfort, photosensitivity, superinfections, hypersensitivity reactions	250–750 mg orally q12h; 200–400 mg IV q12h
delafloxacin *del-a-FLOKS-a-sin*	Baxdela	Bronchitis and community-acquired pneumonia, soft tissue infections	Nausea, diarrhea	450 mg orally every 12 hr
gemifloxacin *je-mi-FLOKS-a-sin*		Bronchitis and community-acquired pneumonia	Vomiting, diarrhea, stomach pain, restlessness, dizziness, confusion, taste changes, sleep disturbances	320 mg/day orally
levoFLOXacin *lee-voe-FLOKS-a-sin*		Same as ciprofloxacin	Same as ciprofloxacin	250–750 mg/day orally, IV
moxifloxacin *mox-i-FLOKS-a-sin*	Avelox	Same as ciprofloxacin	Same as ciprofloxacin	400 mg/day orally
ofloxacin *oh-FLOKS-a-sin*		Same as ciprofloxacin	Same as ciprofloxacin	200–400 mg orally, IV q12h
Miscellaneous Drugs That Inhibit RNA/DNA Synthesis				
metroNIDAZOLE *met-roe-NYE-da-zole*	Flagyl	Treatment of anaerobic microorganisms in bone, skin, central nervous system, internal body cavity, respiratory system	Headache, nausea, peripheral neuropathy, disulfiram-like interaction with alcohol	Loading dose 15 mg/kg, then 7.5 mg/kg
rifAXimin *rif-AX-i-min*	Xifaxan	Hepatic encephalopathy, irritable bowel syndrome, *C. diff* infection	Gas pains, headache	400–550 mg orally, 2–3 times daily

This drug should be administered at least 1 hr before or 2 hr after a meal.

CHAPTER REVIEW

Know Your Drugs

Clients sometimes know a medication by the brand (or trade) name and not the generic name. To help you recognize both names, match the brand name with the generic name of the same medication.

Generic Name	Brand Name
1. ciprofloxacin	A. Baxdela
2. delafloxacin	B. Cipro
3. metronidazole	C. Flagyl

Calculate Medication Dosages

1. A client is prescribed 500 mg of ciprofloxacin orally every 12 hr for an acute sinus infection. The drug is available in 500 mg tablets. The nurse teaches the client to administer _____.
2. Metronidazole is available in 250 mg tablets. The client is instructed to take 750 mg once daily. How many tablets will the client take with each dose? _____

Prepare for the NCLEX

RECALL THE FACTS

1. Fluoroquinolones kill bacterial cells by _____.
   1. inhibiting protein synthesis
   2. destroying the bacterial cell wall
   3. eliminating oxygen from the ribosome
   4. prohibiting DNA synthesis
2. Clients taking a fluoroquinolone are encouraged to _____.
   1. nap 1 to 2 hr daily while taking the drug
   2. eat a high-protein diet
   3. increase their fluid intake
   4. avoid foods high in carbohydrates
3. When taking levofloxacin the client is taught to _____.
   1. wear sun protection whenever outside
   2. assess for hearing loss
   3. carry an EpiPen at all times
   4. eat more fruits and vegetables

4. When monitoring the IV infusion of levofloxacin, the nurse makes sure the needle is in the vein because if not it can result in _____.
   1. irritation of the surrounding tissue
   2. a blood clot in the arm
   3. fluid deficit and dehydration
   4. a sudden and severe rise in blood pressure
5. To avoid a superinfection when taking fluoroquinolones, instruct the client to _____.
   1. eat a high-fiber diet
   2. wash with antibacterial soaps
   3. monitor for diarrhea
   4. use over-the-counter (OTC) creams on skin rashes

ANALYZE THE FACTS

6. *A client is prescribed moxifloxacin. The nurse notes that the client is also taking an antacid. The nurse correctly administers moxifloxacin _____.
   1. once daily orally, 4 hr before the antacid
   2. twice daily orally, immediately after the antacid
   3. once daily IM, without regard to the administration of the antacid
   4. every 12 hr IV, without regard to the administration of the antacid
7. The client taking a fluoroquinolone plans to enter a marathon after treatment. The nurse is concerned about _____.
   1. prolonged QT interval cardiac changes
   2. spontaneous tendon rupture
   3. phlebitis at the IV site
   4. pseudomembranous colitis symptoms
8. *Which of the following statements if made by the client would indicate that they understand to take the entire course of an antibacterial medication?
   1. "If it gets red, stop taking the medicine that is not working."
   2. "When the pain stops, stop the medicine."
   3. "Take this until you get diarrhea."
   4. "Take all the medicine in the bottle."

ALTERNATE-FORMAT QUESTIONS

9. Levofloxacin 500 mg IV is ordered for a client hospitalized with pneumonia. The drug is mixed in a syringe for an IV pump as a solution of 250 mg/15 mL. How many mL should be in the syringe?
10. Identify the interventions to use when taking drugs with photosensitive reactions. **Select all that apply.**
    1. Wash the skin frequently.
    2. Use high SPF value sunscreen.
    3. Wear head coverings on overcast days.
    4. Clothing should be long sleeved.

To check your answers, see Appendix F.

_____

*Indicates the question is directly linked to the NCLEX-PN test plan in Appendix G.

WANT TO KNOW MORE? A wide variety of resources are available to enhance your learning and understanding of this chapter.
- Visit for thePoint resources such as:
  - NCLEX-Style Student Review Questions
  - Journal Articles
  - Dosage Calculations
  - Drug Monographs
  - Watch and Learn Videos
  - Concepts in Action Animations
- The *Study Guide to Accompany Introductory Clinical Pharmacology*, 12th edition, sold separately, will help you review and apply essential content.
- ✓*PrepU* is available to help students prepare for the NCLEX-PN examination.

Antitubercular Drugs

Key Terms

directly observed therapy (DOT) drug dose taken in front of the administrator

extrapulmonary occurring outside of the lungs in the respiratory system

gout a metabolic disorder resulting in increased levels of uric acid and causing severe joint pain

latent TB inactive *Mycobacterium tuberculosis* bacterium in the body, which is alive but noninfectious and can become active later

Multidrug-resistant *M. tuberculosis* (MDR-TB) bacterium that is resistant to a number of different drugs; becomes costly to treat

Mycobacterium leprae bacterium that causes leprosy (Hansen disease), which is a chronic, communicable disease infrequently seen in the United States

Mycobacterium tuberculosis bacterium that causes TB

optic neuritis inflammation of the optic nerve, causing a decrease in visual acuity and changes in color perception

peripheral neuropathy numbness and tingling of the extremities

vertigo feeling of a spinning or rotational motion; dizziness

Learning Objectives

On completion of this chapter, the student will:

1. Discuss the drugs used in the treatment of mycobacteria for tuberculosis (TB).
2. Explain the uses, general drug actions, contraindications, precautions, interactions, and general adverse reactions associated with the administration of the antitubercular drugs.
3. Distinguish important preadministration and ongoing assessment activities the nurse should perform on the client taking an antitubercular drug.
4. List nursing diagnoses particular to a client taking an antitubercular drug.
5. Describe directly observed therapy (DOT).
6. Examine ways to promote an optimal response to therapy, how to manage adverse reactions, and important points to keep in mind when educating clients about the use of the antitubercular drugs.

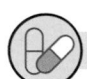 **Drug Classes**

Primary antitubercular	Secondary antitubercular

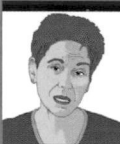

PHARMACOLOGY IN PRACTICE

Betty Peterson has come into the clinic with complaints of a chronic cough. Ms. Peterson requests that a TB skin test be performed as well as a chest x-ray. She is concerned that she will be diagnosed with TB, telling you that she watched a TV show about the rise in TB in crowded areas. When questioned, she states that "a lot of people" live in the apartment next door. Should Betty Peterson be assessed for TB?

Hospitals full of clients with tuberculosis (TB) are a historical item of US medical history, yet TB remains a major health problem throughout the rest of the world. It is especially prevalent in Asia and Sub-Saharan Africa where almost 1.5 million deaths each year are caused by TB. In addition, TB has become the leading cause of death for individuals with human immunodeficiency virus (HIV) (CDC, 2019). The World Health Organization (WHO) predicts that 10 million people worldwide will contract this disease each year despite the fact that the TB death rate has fallen by 38% over the past 20 years (WHO, 2019). Individuals living in crowded conditions, those with compromised immune systems, and those with debilitative conditions are especially susceptible to TB.

Approximately 9000 cases of TB are reported yearly in the United States (CDC, 2019). Although this seems like a small number of cases, the issue is important for two reasons: (1) individuals travel globally with greater frequency and can possibly become infected with **latent TB**, and (2) the bacterium is becoming more and more resistant to drug therapy.

TB is an infectious disease caused by the *Mycobacterium tuberculosis* bacterium. The pathogen is also referred to as the tubercle bacillus. The disease is transmitted from one person to another by droplets dispersed in the air when an infected person coughs or sneezes. These droplets are then inhaled by noninfected persons. Although TB primarily affects the lungs, other organs may be involved.

! NURSING ALERT

TB in clients infected with HIV can be difficult to diagnose. TB skin tests (TSTs) require activation of the immune system to show a reaction. Because the immune systems of clients with HIV are deficient, the test may be negative even when the disease is present. X-ray studies, gene-specific blood testing, sputum analyses, or physical examinations may be needed to diagnose *M. tuberculosis* infection accurately in clients with HIV infection (Padmapriyadarsini, 2011).

Drugs to treat TB are classified as two tiers: primary (first-line) and secondary (second-line) drugs. Primary drugs provide the foundation for treatment. TB responds well to long-term treatment with a combination of three or more antitubercular drugs. Antitubercular drugs are also used as prophylactic therapy to prevent the spreading of TB. Secondary drugs are used for **multidrug-resistant TB (MDR-TB)**, which are more costly and toxic than primary drugs.

Extrapulmonary (outside of the lungs) TB is the term used to distinguish TB affecting other organs of the body from the infection located only in the lungs. Organs that can be affected include the liver, bones, spleen, and adrenal glands. Figure 10.1 illustrates the areas affected by TB and the drugs used in treatment.

Secondary drugs are also used to treat extrapulmonary TB. The primary antitubercular drugs are discussed in this chapter. Both primary and secondary antitubercular drugs are listed in the Summary Drug Table: Antitubercular Drugs. Certain fluoroquinolones such as ciprofloxacin, ofloxacin, and levofloxacin have proven effective against TB and are considered secondary drugs; toxic adverse reactions may be weighed against benefit when these drugs are considered (see Chapter 9).

ACTIONS

Antitubercular drugs are both bacteriostatic and bactericidal against the *M. tuberculosis* bacillus. These drugs usually act to inhibit bacterial cell wall synthesis, slowing the multiplication rate of the bacteria. Isoniazid (INH) is bactericidal, with rifampin and streptomycin having some bactericidal activity.

USES

Antitubercular drugs are used in a protocol called *Standard Treatment* to treat active TB. INH, however, may be used alone in **latent TB** therapy (prophylaxis). Box 10.1 describes the signs of latent TB infection.

Latent TB Treatment

Latent treatment is used for those infected with *M. tuberculosis* but do not have the active disease TB. These individuals have a positive skin/blood test yet are not infectious and cannot spread the disease to others. If not treated, 5%–10% of these individuals will eventually present with active disease during their lifetime. Therefore, selected client populations are typically treated for 6–9 months with INH with a daily or biweekly dosing schedule. To increase adherence and prevent drug resistance, less frequent protocols are being used, such as a rifapentine/INH combination taken weekly for 12 weeks. Box 10.2 lists the individuals identified as high risk for activation of the *M. tuberculosis* bacteria and should be considered for treatment of Latent TB (LTB).

Standard Treatment Protocol

Standard treatment is the term used for treatment of clients with active TB and is divided into two phases: the *initial* phase, followed by a *continuing* phase. During the initial

---

BOX 10.1 **Identifying the Individual With Latent TB Infection**

- Does not feel sick or have symptoms of the disease
- PPD skin test or blood test is positive for TB infection
- Normal chest x-ray and negative sputum test
- Has alive TB bacteria, but it is inactive
- Cannot spread the TB bacteria to others
- *Needs treatment* for the disease to prevent active disease at a later time

---

BOX 10.2 **High-Risk Individuals for LTB**

- Positive IGRA TB blood test
- TST greater than 5 mm in clients who are:
  - HIV positive
  - Recent contact with active TB cases
  - X-ray shows old TB
  - Organ transplant clients
  - Selected immunosuppressed clients
- TST greater than 10 mm in clients who are:
  - Traveling from countries where TB is prevalent
  - IV drug users
  - Residents/employees of high-risk living settings, e.g., long-term care, hospitals
  - Laboratory personnel working with *Mycobacteria*
  - Children under 4 years up to adolescents exposed to high-risk adults

IGRA, interferon-gamma release assay; TST, tuberculin skin test.

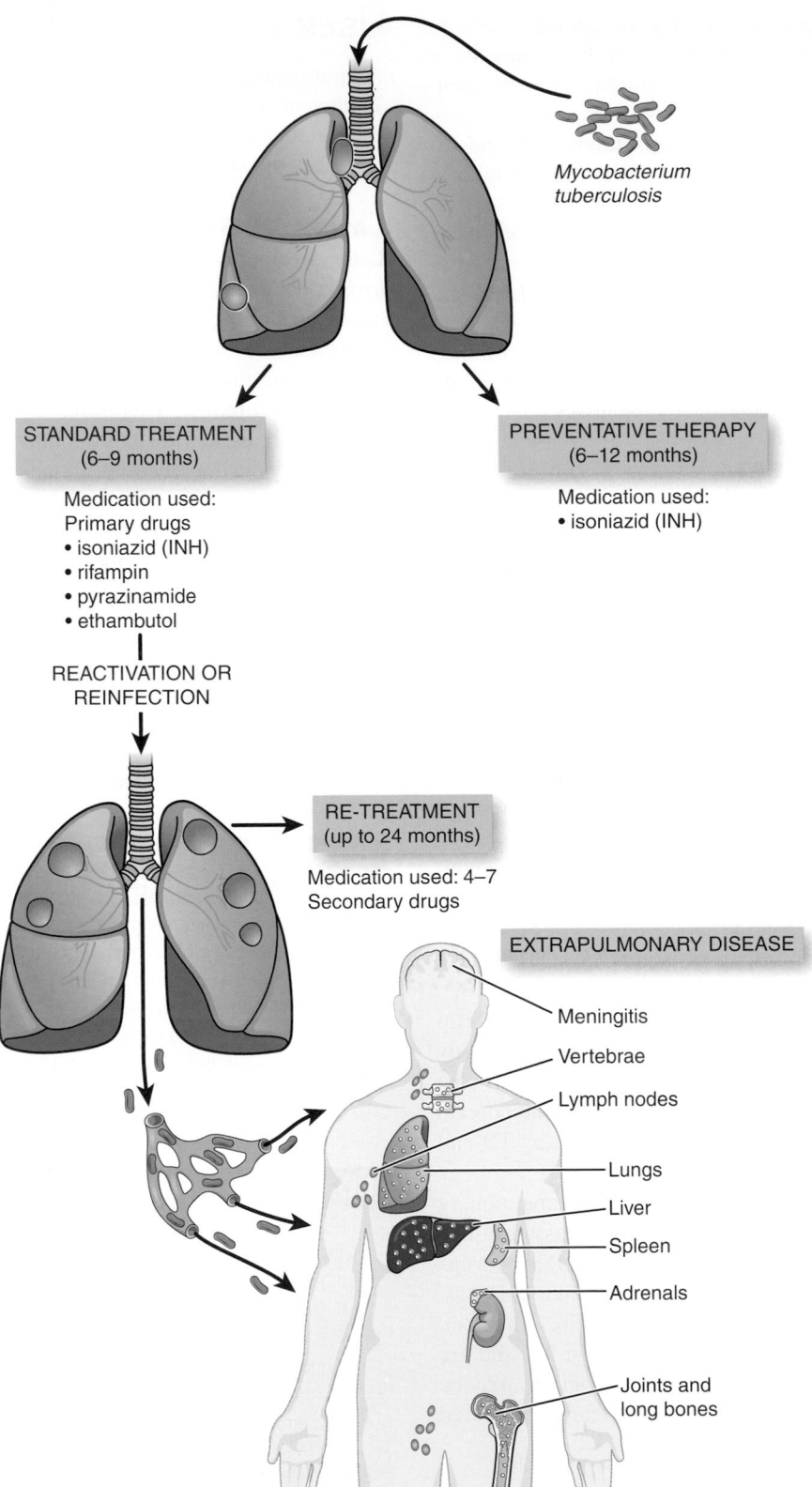

FIGURE 10.1 Sites of tuberculosis infection and treatment options. (Adapted from Rubin, E., & Farber, J. L. (1999). *Pathology* (3rd ed.). Lippincott Williams & Wilkins.)

phase, drugs are used to kill the rapidly multiplying *M. tuberculosis* and to prevent drug resistance. The initial phase lasts approximately 2 months and the continuing phase approximately 4 months, with the total treatment regimen lasting for 6–9 months, depending on the client's response to therapy.

The Centers for Disease Control and Prevention (CDC) recommends that treatment begin as soon as possible after the diagnosis of TB. The recommended treatment regimen is for the administration of the primary drugs—rifampin (Rifadin), INH, pyrazinamide, and ethambutol (Myambutol)—for a minimum of 2 months. The second or continuation phase includes only the drugs rifampin and INH. The CDC recommends this phase for 4 months or up to 7 months in special populations. These special circumstances include the following:

- Positive sputum culture after completion of initial treatment
- Cavitary (hole or pocket of) disease and positive sputum culture after initial treatment
- When pyrazinamide was not included in the initial treatment
- Positive sputum culture after initial treatment in a client with previously diagnosed HIV infection

Retreatment Protocol

At times, treatment fails because of inadequate initial drug treatment or noncompliance with the drug regimen. When treatment fails, retreatment is necessary using the secondary drugs. Retreatment generally includes the use of four or more antitubercular drugs. Retreatment drug regimens most often consist of ethionamide (Trecator), aminosalicylic acid (Paser), cycloserine, and capreomycin (Capastat). Ofloxacin and ciprofloxacin (Cipro) may also be used in retreatment. Sometimes during retreatment, seven or more drugs may be used, with the ineffective drugs discontinued when susceptibility test results are available. Treatment is individualized based on the susceptibility of the microorganism. Up to 24 months of continued treatment after sputum cultures are no longer positive for TB can be part of the plan.

Resistance to the Antitubercular Drugs

Of increasing concern is multidrug resistant TB (**MDR-TB**). Bacterial resistance develops, sometimes rapidly, primarily owing to a lack of adherence to lengthy drug dosing schedules. Individualized treatment is based on laboratory studies that identify the drugs to which the organism is susceptible. The CDC recommends using three or more drugs with initial therapy, as well as in retreatment, because using a combination of drugs slows the development of bacterial resistance. TB caused by drug-resistant organisms should be considered in clients who have no response to therapy and in clients who have been treated in the past. A couple of newer drugs, pretomanid and bedaquiline (Sirturo) were developed to specifically treat MDR-TB.

These drugs work by interfering with bacterial enzymes. Both drugs were fast-tracked through the US Food and Drug Administration approval process (see Chapter 1) to treat the resistant bacterium because of the public health dangers associated with MDR-TB. They must be used in combination with the drug linezolid. Unfortunately, they come with harsh adverse reactions—hepatic, myelosuppression, and peripheral neuropathy. Bedaquiline comes with an increased risk of cardiac death, and clients should be monitored at frequent intervals for prolonged QT intervals on ECG.

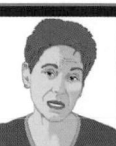

PHARMACOLOGY IN PRACTICE

PATHOPHYSIOLOGY
A nurse is assigned to care for a client with extrapulmonary TB in a long-term care facility. Which of the following organs are frequently affected by extrapulmonary TB? Select all that apply.
1. Heart
2. Liver
3. Spleen
4. Brain
5. Kidneys

This chapter focuses on the following primary antitubercular drugs: ethambutol, INH, pyrazinamide, and rifampin. Other primary and secondary drugs are listed in the Summary Drug Table: Antitubercular Drugs.

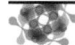 # ETHAMBUTOL

ADVERSE REACTIONS

Generalized Reactions
- Dermatitis and pruritus (itching)
- Joint pain
- Anorexia
- Nausea and vomiting

Severe Reactions
- Anaphylactoid reactions (unusual or exaggerated allergic reactions)
- **Optic neuritis** (a decrease in visual acuity and changes in color perception); optic neuritis is dose related.

CONTRAINDICATIONS, PRECAUTIONS, AND INTERACTIONS

Ethambutol is not recommended for clients with a history of hypersensitivity to the drug or children younger than 13 years. The drug is used with caution during pregnancy (category B), in clients with hepatic or renal impairment, and in clients with diabetic retinopathy or cataracts.

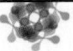
ISONIAZID

ADVERSE REACTIONS

The incidence of adverse reactions appears to be higher when larger doses of INH are prescribed.

Generalized Reactions
- Nausea and vomiting
- Epigastric distress
- Fever
- Skin eruptions
- Hematologic changes
- Jaundice
- Hypersensitivity

Toxicity
- **Peripheral neuropathy** (numbness and tingling of the extremities) is the most common symptom of toxicity.
- Severe hepatitis has been associated with INH therapy and may appear after many months of treatment and be fatal.

CONTRAINDICATIONS AND PRECAUTIONS

INH is contraindicated in clients with a history of hypersensitivity to the drug. The drug is used with caution during pregnancy (category C) or lactation and in clients with hepatic and renal impairment.

INTERACTIONS

The following interactions may occur when INH is administered with another agent:

Interacting Drug	Common Use	Effect of Interaction
Antacids containing aluminum salts	Relief of heartburn and gastrointestinal upset	Reduced absorption of isoniazid
Anticoagulants	Blood thinner	Increased risk for bleeding
Phenytoin	Antiseizure drug	Increased serum levels of phenytoin
Alcohol (in beverages)	Social situations	Higher incidence of drug-related hepatitis

When INH is taken with foods containing tyramine, such as aged cheese and meats, bananas, yeast products, and alcohol, an exaggerated sympathetic nerve-type response can occur (i.e., hypertension, increased heart rate, and palpitations).

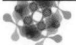
PYRAZINAMIDE

ADVERSE REACTIONS

Generalized Reactions
- Nausea and vomiting
- Diarrhea
- Myalgia (aches)
- Rashes

Hepatotoxicity
Hepatotoxicity is the principal adverse reaction seen with pyrazinamide use. Symptoms of hepatotoxicity may range from none (except for slightly abnormal hepatic function test results) to a more severe reaction such as jaundice.

CONTRAINDICATIONS AND PRECAUTIONS

Pyrazinamide is contraindicated in clients with a history of hypersensitivity to the drug, acute **gout** (a metabolic disorder resulting in increased levels of uric acid and causing severe joint pain), or severe hepatic damage.

Pyrazinamide should be used cautiously in clients during pregnancy (category C) and lactation and in clients with hepatic and renal impairment, HIV infection, and diabetes mellitus.

INTERACTIONS

When pyrazinamide is administered with the antigout medications allopurinol (Zyloprim), colchicine, or probenecid, its effectiveness decreases.

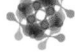
RIFAMPIN

ADVERSE REACTIONS

Generalized reactions include the following:

- Nausea and vomiting
- Epigastric distress, heartburn, fatigue
- **Vertigo** (dizziness)
- Rash
- Reddish-orange discoloration of body fluids (urine, tears, saliva, sweat, and sputum)
- Hematologic changes, renal insufficiency

CONTRAINDICATIONS AND PRECAUTIONS

Rifampin is contraindicated in clients with a history of hypersensitivity to the drug. The drug is used with caution during pregnancy (category C) and lactation and in clients with hepatic or renal impairment.

LASA ALERT

The following drugs may sound alike; be sure to clarify when they are ordered:

Drug Name	Sounds Like
Capastat	Cepastat
cycloSERINE	cyclobenzaprine, cyclosporine
dapsone	Diprosone
myambutol	Nembutal
rifabutin	rifAMPin, rifapentine
Rifadin	Rifater, Ritalin
rifAMPin	ribavirin, rifabutin, Rifamate, rifapentine, rifaximin
streptomycin	streptozocin

Drugs that look alike are noted in the Summary Drug Tables of each chapter.

INTERACTIONS

The following interactions may occur when rifampin is administered with another agent:

Interacting Drug	Common Use	Effect of Interaction
Antiretrovirals (efavirenz, nevirapine)	HIV infection	Decreased serum levels of antiretrovirals
Digoxin	Management of cardiac problems	Decreased serum levels of digoxin
Oral contraceptives	Contraception	Decreased contraceptive effectiveness
Isoniazid	Antitubercular agent	Higher risk of hepatotoxicity
Oral anticoagulants	Blood thinner	Increased risk for bleeding

Interacting Drug	Common Use	Effect of Interaction
Oral hypoglycemics	Antidiabetic agent	Decreased effectiveness of oral hypoglycemic agent
Chloramphenicol	Anti-infective agent	Increased risk for seizures
Phenytoin	Antiseizure agent	Decreased effectiveness of phenytoin
Verapamil	Management of cardiac problems and blood pressure	Decreased effectiveness of verapamil

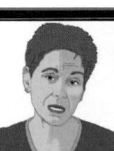

PHARMACOLOGY IN PRACTICE

DRUG ASSESSMENT

A nurse will be following a client being treated prophylactically with the drug, INH, for latent TB. The treatment lasts for many months, and ongoing assessment reveals that the client drinks alcohol frequently. The nurse should monitor specifically for which of the following adverse reactions in this person?
1. Peripheral neuropathy
2. Anaphylactoid reactions
3. Severe hepatitis
4. Epigastric distress

Another condition of the *Mycobacterium* family is **leprosy** *Mycobacterium leprae* (*M. leprae*), also referred to as *Hansen disease*. Leprosy is a chronic, communicable disease that is not easily spread and has a long incubation period. Since 1985, the prevalence of leprosy has dropped by 90%. About 100 new cases are diagnosed yearly in the United States (primarily the southern states, Hawaii, and US possessions).

Peripheral nerves are affected, causing sensory loss and muscle weakness. The traditional fear of leprosy relates to skin involvement, which may present with lesions confined to a few isolated areas or may be fairly widespread over the entire body. Dapsone, rifampin (Rifadin), and ethionamide (Trecator) are drugs currently used to treat leprosy. The leprostatic drugs are listed in the Summary Drug Table: Antitubercular Drugs.

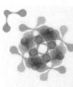
NURSING PROCESS STEPS TO BUILDING CLINICAL JUDGMENT
Client Receiving an Antitubercular Drug

ASSESSMENT

Preadministration Assessment
Typically, TB is diagnosed with either a positive skin test (Mantoux or purified protein derivative—PPD) or the currently used (QuantiFERON-TB Gold In-Tube) blood test. Although

the skin test requires the client to return in 48–72 hr for a reading, it is a cheaper test than the one-visit blood test. Once the diagnosis of TB is confirmed, the primary health care provider selects the drugs that will best control the spread of the disease and make the client noninfectious to others.

Additional data gathering suggestions before starting antitubercular therapy include:

Objective data

- General client appearance (weight loss, sweating)
- Vital signs (temperature—especially fever, pulse, respirations, and blood pressure)
- Description of the infection—cough, color of sputum if productive
- Results of radiographic studies, sputum culture, and sensitivity tests
- Laboratory results—complete blood count, hepatic/kidney function tests

Subjective data

- Current symptoms of the infection (malaise, fatigue, chills, loss of appetite)
- Drug history, particularly if treated before for TB
- Social history, association with those who might have had TB
- Travel history to areas where the disease is prevalent

Depending on the severity of the disease, clients may be treated initially in the hospital and then discharged for supervised follow-up care or they may have all treatment instituted on an outpatient basis.

Ongoing Assessment

When performing the ongoing assessment, teach the client or caregiver to observe daily for the appearance of adverse reactions. These observations are especially important when a drug is known to be toxic to nerves or eyes. It is important to report any adverse reactions to the primary health care provider. In addition, carefully monitor vital signs daily or as frequently as every 4 hr when the client is hospitalized.

NURSING DIAGNOSES

Drug administration-specific nursing diagnoses are the following:

- **Injury Risk** related to extremity numbness caused by neurotoxicity
- **Malnutrition: less than body requirements** related to gastric upset and general poor health status
- **Risk for altered health maintenance** related to indifference, lack of knowledge, long-term treatment regimen, and other factors

The nursing diagnosis of Altered Health Maintenance may be especially important with clients considering the long-term therapy required to treat TB. Refer to interventions discussed in Chapter 4 to deal with client needs.

PLANNING

The expected outcomes for the client may include an optimal response to antitubercular therapy, meeting client needs related to the management of common adverse reactions, and confidence in an understanding of and adherence with the prescribed medication regimen.

IMPLEMENTATION

Promoting an Optimal Response to Therapy

The diagnosis of TB, along with the necessity of long-term treatment and follow-up, is often distressing to the client. Clients with a diagnosis of TB may have many questions about the disease and its treatment. TB infection is of concern in communities where immigrants from areas of the world with high TB rates have settled. Health literacy may be low; clients may be unfamiliar with medical terms and treatment strategies. Try asking clients what they think is causing the illness. Cultural beliefs may play a role in the client's understanding about the disease cause and treatment. Clients may have limited English proficiency, and education is important for the client to remain compliant with long-term therapy. Use interpretative services and translated client education tools in teaching sessions. Allow ample time for the client and family members to ask questions. In some instances, it may be necessary to refer the client to other health care professionals, such as a social service worker or a registered dietitian.

Monitoring and Managing Client Needs

Managing adverse reactions in clients taking antitubercular drugs is an important nursing responsibility. Continuously observe for signs of adverse reactions and immediately report them to the primary health care provider.

Injury Risk

INH inhibits the activation of pyridoxine (vitamin B_6), which results in neurologic symptoms of numbness and tingling in the extremities. For this reason, clients are typically prescribed vitamin B_6. Since it is an OTC medication, clients may choose to stop taking the vitamin if they are tired of prolonged therapy. Therefore, when vitamin supplementation is ordered, the following teaching points are important to emphasize to ensure adherence:

- *The reason for taking the vitamin.* It is being given to prevent neurologic problems, not just as a nutritional supplement for dietary reasons.
- *Immediately report any strange sensations experienced.* For example, a sensation like a glove is over the hand or a feeling of sensory loss and paralysis. Clients are more likely to experience an extremity injury with these different sensations.

Malnutrition: Less Than Body Requirements

When TB affects clients who live in crowded and impoverished conditions, malnutrition may be prevalent. In some cases, alcoholism may compound the client's difficulties. This complicates the administration of drugs and compromises the general condition of the client's gastrointestinal tract. Ethambutol should be given at the same time daily and may be given with food. Pyrazinamide may also be given with food. Other antitubercular drugs are given by the oral route and on an empty stomach, unless epigastric upset occurs. If gastric upset occurs, it is important to notify the primary health care provider before the next dose is given. If a dose is missed, tell the client *not* to double the dose the next day.

An alternative, twice-weekly dosing regimen has been developed to promote adherence on an outpatient basis. This may improve client nutrition by decreasing the gastric upset of frequent dosing. Combination drugs (e.g., Rifater, which contains isoniazid, rifampin, and pyrazinamide) are being manufactured to promote adherence to medication regimens and reduce the need to take multiple drugs that produce gastric upset.

Teach the client the importance of reducing alcohol consumption because of the increased risk of hepatitis. Again, the inclusion of pyridoxine (vitamin B$_6$) is recommended to promote nutrition and prevent neuropathy.

It is helpful to explain to clients that their bodily fluids (urine, feces, saliva, sputum, sweat, and tears) may be colored reddish-orange from the different drugs and that this is expected. It is even more important to teach the client that this is different from the skin and eye color changes that could indicate hepatic dysfunction (jaundice). Carefully monitor all clients at least monthly for any evidence of liver dysfunction. It is important to instruct clients to report any of the following symptoms: anorexia, nausea, vomiting, fatigue, weakness, yellowing of the skin or eyes, darkening of the urine, or numbness in the hands and feet.

Lifespan Considerations

Women of Color

INH is broken down by the liver into a potent liver toxin. Because of the lengthy duration of therapy, 1 in 100 clients treated acquires hepatitis. It is typically seen in the first 3 months of treatment, in older adults, and in those who consume alcohol daily. African American and Hispanic women are particularly susceptible to a potentially fatal hepatitis when taking INH, especially if they consume alcohol on a regular basis. Two other antitubercular drugs, rifampin and pyrazinamide, can cause liver dysfunction in the older adult as well. Careful observation and monitoring for signs of liver impairment are necessary (e.g., increased serum aspartate aminotransferase [AST], alanine aminotransferase [ALT], and bilirubin levels and jaundice).

Altered Health Maintenance

Because the antitubercular drugs must be taken for prolonged periods, adherence to the treatment regimen becomes a problem and increases the risk for development of MDR-TB. To help prevent the problem of nonadherence, better combinations and less frequent dosing schedules are continually researched. Still, the most successful method is **directly observed therapy (DOT).** With DOT, the client makes periodic visits to the office of the primary care provider or the health clinic; here the drug is taken in the presence of the nurse. Nurses watch the client swallow each dose of the medication. In some cases, the nurse may travel to the client's home, place of employment,

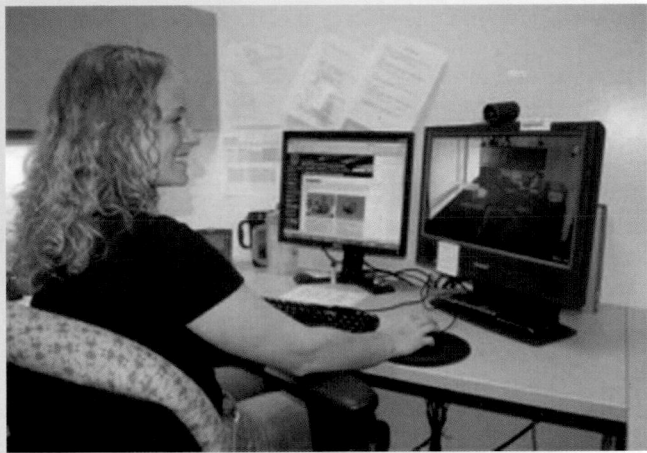

FIGURE 10.2 Nurse shown using of video monitoring for DOT observation of tuberculosis medication adherence. (From Allendar, J. A., Rector, C., & Warner, K. D. (2014). *Community & public health nursing: Promoting the public's health* (8th ed.). Wolters Kluwer Health, Lippincott Williams & Wilkins.)

or school to observe or administer medication. When a client lives a great distance away and/or nurses have large caseloads of clients to observe, technology is employed. Nurses may use video monitoring, such as Skype or FaceTime, to watch on the monitor as a client prepares and takes the medications (see Fig. 10.2).

DOT may occur daily or two to three times weekly, depending on the client's health care regimen. Studies indicate that taking the drugs intermittently does not cause a drop in the therapeutic blood levels of antitubercular drugs, even if the drugs are given only two or three times a week (Munsiff, 2006).

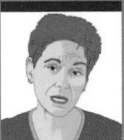

PHARMACOLOGY IN PRACTICE

TEACHING AND LEARNING

A nurse is caring for a client with TB on an outpatient basis who has been prescribed antitubercular drugs. Which of the following is an important teaching point for the nurse to emphasize to prevent the risk of hepatitis in the client with TB?
1. Take the new multidrug tablets
2. Use DOT to take drugs on outpatient basis
3. Take vitamin B$_6$ according to prescription
4. Minimize alcohol consumption

Educating the Client and Family

Antitubercular drugs are given for a long time, and careful client and family education and close medical supervision are necessary. Nonadherence to the medication regimen can be a problem whenever a disease or disorder requires long-term treatment. For this reason, the DOT method of administration is preferred. The client and family must understand that short-term therapy is of no value in treating this disease. Remain alert for statements made by the client or family that may indicate future nonadherence to the drug regimen necessary in controlling the disease. See Client Teaching for Improved Outcomes: Increasing Medication Adherence to Tubercular Drug Treatment Program for more information.

Increasing Medication Adherence to Tubercular Drug Treatment Program

When you teach, make sure your client understands the following:

✔ Ask the client what they think causes the symptoms; promote health literacy by integrating the client's beliefs and fears into how the bacteria invade the body and how the drugs work to kill it.

✔ Discuss TB, its causes and communicability, and the need for long-term therapy for disease control using simple, nonmedical terms.

✔ Use visual props or educational materials to help emphasize that short-term treatment is ineffective.

✔ Review the drug therapy regimen, including the prescribed drugs, doses, and frequency of administration.

✔ Reassure the client that various combinations of drugs are effective in treating TB.

✔ Urge the client to take the drugs exactly as prescribed and not to omit, increase, or decrease the dosage unless directed to do so by the health care provider.

✔ Instruct the client about possible adverse reactions and the need to notify the prescriber should any occur.

✔ Arrange for direct observation therapy with the client and family.

✔ Instruct the client in measures to minimize gastrointestinal upset.

✔ Advise the client to avoid alcohol and the use of nonprescription drugs, especially those containing aspirin, unless use is approved by the health care provider.

✔ Reassure the client and family that the results of therapy will be monitored by periodic laboratory and diagnostic tests and follow-up visits with the health care provider.

EVALUATION

- Therapeutic response is achieved, and there is no evidence of infection.
- Adverse reactions are identified, reported to the primary health care provider, and managed successfully with appropriate nursing interventions:
  - No evidence of injury is seen because of neurosensory changes.
  - Client maintains an adequate nutritional status.
  - Client manages the therapeutic regimen effectively.
- Client and family express confidence and demonstrate an understanding of the drug regimen.

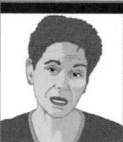

PHARMACOLOGY IN PRACTICE

USING CLINICAL REASONING

After reading this chapter, what data would help you decide if Betty Peterson is at risk for TB? Determine what rationale and information to use in teaching Ms. Peterson about risks for TB.

KEY POINTS

■ TB is an infectious disease that continues to be a major health problem throughout the world. Crowded living conditions, especially where immune-compromised or debilitated people live, are sites of concern.

■ TB typically involves the lungs and other structures of the respiratory system. Other organs, such as the liver, bones, spleen, and even adrenal glands, can be affected by the bacterium.

■ Clients with latent TB disease cannot spread the disease, yet need treatment to prevent active disease in the future. This treatment involves one drug taken for 6 months to 1 year.

■ Treatment for active TB involves many months of multidrug therapy. The standard treatment protocol includes two phases, initial (about 2 months) and continuing (approximately 4 months). At least four different drugs are involved. Treatment failure may result in an additional four- to seven-drug course for 2 years. Bacterial resistance may occur, which is why multiple drugs are used. Combination drugs are being developed to include multiple drugs and to be given less frequently to increase adherence to continuing the entire course of treatment.

■ DOT involves a client being directly watched when taking the antitubercular drugs by a health provider.

■ Body fluids may become orange in color; client teaching needs to include the ability to differentiate this from liver involvement (hepatitis). Both gastrointestinal upset and hepatitis are adverse reactions to the antitubercular drugs.

SUMMARY DRUG TABLE
Antitubercular Drugs

Generic Name	Trade Name	Uses	Adverse Reactions	Dosage Ranges
Primary (First-Line) Drugs				
ethambutol *e-THAM-byoo-tole*	Myambutol	Pulmonary TB	Optic neuritis, fever, pruritus, headache, nausea, anorexia, dermatitis, hypersensitivity, psychic disturbances	15–25 mg/kg/day orally
isoniazid (INH) *eye-soe-NYE-a-zid*		Active TB; prophylaxis for TB	Peripheral neuropathy, nausea, vomiting, epigastric distress, jaundice, hepatitis, pyridoxine deficiency, skin eruptions, hypersensitivity	*Active TB:* 5 mg/kg (up to 300 mg/day) orally or 15 mg/kg 2–3 times weekly *TB prophylaxis:* 300 mg/day orally
pyrazinamide *peer-a-ZIN-a-mide*		Active TB	Hepatotoxicity, nausea, vomiting, diarrhea, myalgia, rashes	15–30 mg/kg/day orally, maximum 3 g/day orally; 50–70 mg/kg twice weekly orally
rifabutin *rif-a-BYOO-tin*	Mycobutin	*Mycobacterium avium*	Nausea, vomiting, diarrhea, rash, discolored urine	300 mg/day orally or 150 mg orally BID
rifAMPin *rif-AM-pin*	Rifadin, Rimactane	Active TB, Hansen disease	Heartburn, drowsiness, fatigue, dizziness, epigastric distress, hematologic changes, renal insufficiency, rash, body fluid discoloration	10 mg/kg (up to 600 mg/day) orally, IV
rifapentine *rif-a-PEN-teen*	Priftin	Active TB	Hyperuricemia, proteinuria, hematuria, rash, lymphopenia	600 mg twice weekly orally
Combination Primary Drugs				
isoniazid 150 mg and rifAMPin 300 mg	Rifamate	TB	See individual drugs	1–2 tablets daily orally
isoniazid 50 mg, rifAMPin 120 mg, and pyrazinamide 300 mg	Rifater	TB	See individual drugs	1–2 tablets daily orally
Secondary (Second-Line) Drugs				
aminosalicylate *a-mee-noe-sal-i-SIL-ik-AS-id (p-aminosalicylic acid; 4-aminosalicylic acid)*	Paser	MDR-TB	Nausea, vomiting, diarrhea, abdominal pain, hypersensitivity reactions	4 g (1 packet) orally TID
bedaquiline *bed-AK-wi-leen*	Sirturo	MDR-TB	Nausea, headache, arthralgia, chest pain, hemoptysis	Only use in DOT setting: 400 mg daily (2 weeks), 200 mg (3 times weekly)
capreomycin *kap-ree-oh-MYE-sin*	Capastat	TB	Hypersensitivity reactions, nephrotoxicity, hepatic impairment, pain and induration at injection site, ototoxicity	1 g/day (maximum 20 mg/kg/day) IM
cycloSERINE *sye-kloe-SER-een*		TB	Convulsions, somnolence, confusion, renal impairment, sudden development of congestive heart failure, psychoses	500 mg–1 g orally in divided doses
ethionamide *e-thye-on-AM-ide*	Trecator	TB, Hansen disease	Nausea, vomiting, diarrhea, headache	15–20 mg/kg/day orally
pretomanid *pre-TOE-ma-nid*		MDR-TB	Nausea, vomiting, headache, peripheral neuropath, skin rash, acne, muscle/abdominal pain, fatigue	200 mg daily orally
streptomycin *strep-toe-MYE-sin* (although still available, this drug is seldom used)		TB, infections caused by susceptible microorganisms	Nephrotoxicity, ototoxicity, numbness, tingling, paresthesia of the face, nausea, dizziness	15 mg/kg but no more than 1 g IM daily (120 g therapeutic maximum)

Continued

SUMMARY DRUG TABLE (continued)
Antitubercular Drugs

Generic Name	Trade Name	Uses	Adverse Reactions	Dosage Ranges
Drugs to Treat M. leprae				
dapsone *DAP-sone*		Hansen disease, dermatitis herpetiformis, *Pneumocystis carinii* pneumonia, rheumatic disorders (rheumatic arthritis, systemic lupus erythematosus), brown recluse spider bite	Hemolytic anemia, headache, insomnia, phototoxicity, nausea, vomiting, anorexia, rash, fever, jaundice, toxic epidermal necrolysis	50–300 mg/day orally

This drug should be administered at least 1 hr before or 2 hr after a meal.

CHAPTER REVIEW

Know Your Drugs

Clients sometimes know a medication by the brand (or trade) name and not the generic name. To help you recognize both names, match the brand name with the generic name of the same medication.

Generic Name	Brand Name
1. ethambutol	A. Myambutol
2. rifabutin	B. Mycobutin
3. rifampin	C. Priftin
4. rifapentine	D. Rifadin

Calculate Medication Dosages

1. A client is prescribed isoniazid syrup 300 mg. The isoniazid is available as 50 mg/mL. The nurse should administer _____.
2. Oral rifampin 600 mg is prescribed. The drug is available in 150-mg tablets. The nurse should administer_____.

Prepare for the NCLEX

RECALL THE FACTS

1. Which of the following drugs is the only antitubercular drug to be prescribed alone?
   1. Rifampin
   2. Pyrazinamide
   3. Streptomycin
   4. Isoniazid

2. The nurse monitors the client taking isoniazid for toxic symptoms. The most common symptom of toxicity is _____.
   1. peripheral edema
   2. circumoral edema
   3. peripheral neuropathy
   4. jaundice

3. Which of the following is a dose-related adverse reaction to ethambutol?
   1. Peripheral neuropathy
   2. Optic neuritis
   3. Hyperglycemia
   4. Fatal hepatitis

4. Which of the following antitubercular drugs is contraindicated in clients with gout?
   1. Rifampin
   2. Streptomycin
   3. Isoniazid
   4. Pyrazinamide

5. Hansen disease (leprosy) is caused by which of the following bacteria?
   1. *Mycobacterium leprae*
   2. *Clostridium difficile*
   3. *Mycobacterium tuberculosis*
   4. *Pneumocystis carinii*

ANALYZE THE FACTS

6. *A client reports orange stains on paper tissues when she urinates. Which of the following interventions should the nurse do first?
   1. Notify the primary health care provider.
   2. Ask the client what she thinks is happening.
   3. Explain that this is an anticipated adverse reaction.
   4. Obtain a urine sample for laboratory studies.

7. The nurse explains to the client that to prevent multidrug resistance to the antitubercular drugs, the primary health care provider may prescribe

   _____.

   1. at least three antitubercular drugs
   2. an antibiotic to be given with the drug
   3. vitamin B_6
   4. that the drug be given only once a week

8. *Which of the following best describes DOT in the care of clients with TB?
   1. The client takes at least four drugs daily.
   2. The client calls the clinic once a week to describe adverse reactions.
   3. The nurse involves family in client teaching activities.
   4. The nurse observes the client swallow the TB drugs.

ALTERNATE-FORMAT QUESTIONS

9. Identify which drugs are included in primary (first-line) treatment for TB. Select all that apply.
   1. Ethambutol
   2. Isoniazid
   3. Ofloxacin
   4. Pyrazinamide
   5. Rifampin

10. Identify which culture plate (from culture and sensitivity testing) indicates the bacterium is resistant to all the drugs tested on the plate.
    1.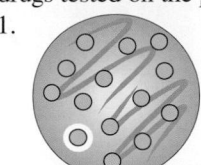

    2.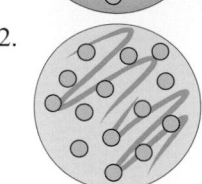

    3.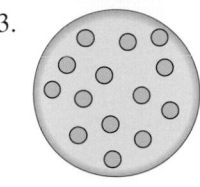

To check your answers, see Appendix F.

_____

*Indicates the question is directly linked to the NCLEX-PN test plan in Appendix G.

WANT TO KNOW MORE? A wide variety of resources are available to enhance your learning and understanding of this chapter.

■ Visit for thePoint resources such as:
  • NCLEX-Style Student Review Questions
  • Journal Articles
  • Dosage Calculations
  • Drug Monographs
  • Watch and Learn Videos
  • Concepts in Action Animations
■ The *Study Guide to Accompany Introductory Clinical Pharmacology*, 12th edition, sold separately, will help you review and apply essential content.
■ ✓**PrepU** is available to help students prepare for the NCLEX-PN examination.

Antiviral Drugs

Key Terms

circumoral   circling or surrounding the mouth

highly active antiretroviral therapy (HAART)   multiple drugs used together for treatment of human immunodeficiency virus (HIV) infection

host cell   a live cell (may be plant or animal) where a virus embeds itself to reproduce

mutation   a gene's ability to change structure and pass that variation on to future generations

retinitis   inflammation of the retina of the eyeball

retrovirus   virus that uses RNA as its primary component instead of DNA

unlabeled use   use of a drug to treat a condition that is not officially approved by the US Food and Drug Administration (FDA)

Learning Objectives

On completion of this chapter, the student will:

1. Explain the uses, general drug actions, adverse reactions, contraindications, precautions, and interactions of antiviral drugs.
2. Distinguish important preadministration and ongoing assessment activities the nurse should perform on the client receiving an antiviral/antiretroviral drug.
3. Identify nursing diagnoses particular to a client taking an antiviral drug.
4. List possible goals for a client taking an antiviral/antiretroviral drug.
5. Examine ways to promote an optimal response to therapy and manage adverse reactions and special considerations to keep in mind when educating the client and the family about the antiviral/antiretroviral drugs.

 Drug Classes

Antivirals
- Anti-herpes agents
- HBV and HCV agents
- Influenza agents, neuraminidase inhibitor (NAI)

Antiretrovirals
- Protease inhibitors
- Nucleoside/nucleotide reverse transcriptase inhibitors (NRTIs)
- Nonnucleoside reverse transcriptase inhibitors (NNRTIs)
- Entry inhibitors
- Integrase inhibitors

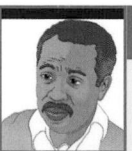 **PHARMACOLOGY IN PRACTICE**

One day, Mr. Park fell as he was working in the garden. He lay in the garden with a fractured hip for about 2 hr before he was found. This event, compounded with other stressors of living alone, initiated an outbreak of herpes zoster (shingles). Consider this event as you read about medications that reduce the symptoms of viral disease.

Many people still believe bacteria can be treated by drug therapy, yet a virus cannot. In the last decade, scientific breakthroughs have produced a number of antiviral medications. In some cases, these drugs have turned life-threatening viral infections (such as the

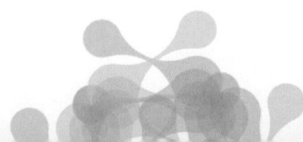

human immunodeficiency virus [HIV] or hepatitis C virus [HCV]) into chronic conditions. These drugs can also make less life-threatening viral infections manageable as well.

Compared with a fungus or bacterium, a virus is a very tiny infectious organism that enters the body through various routes. It can be swallowed, inhaled, injected with a contaminated needle, or transmitted through the bite of an insect. Unlike a bacterium that is its own cell, a virus needs the cellular material of another living cell (the **host cell**) to replicate. The virus attaches to a host cell, enters it, and releases its DNA or RNA inside the cell. The viral material takes control of the host cell and forces it to replicate the virus. The host cell releases new viruses, which go on to infect other cells. The infected host cell usually dies, because the virus keeps it from performing its normal functions. The HIV is called a retrovirus (uses RNA in place of DNA), and its replication process is illustrated in Figure 11.1.

More than 200 viruses have been identified as capable of producing disease. Commonly seen viral infections are those of the nose, throat, and respiratory system. An example is the common cold or influenza. A wart on the skin also comes from a common virus. Other common viral infections we see include those caused by the herpes viruses, such as a lip cold sore. Eight different herpes viruses alone infect people. Many of these common viruses are localized, meaning they infect a selected site or body system. On the other hand, systemic viral infections attack entire structures inside the body like the nervous system (West Nile), liver (hepatitis C), or white blood cells (immunodeficiency diseases).

The drugs used to treat viral infection are split into two categories: antiviral and antiretroviral agents. For a more complete listing, see the Summary Drug Table: Antiviral Drugs, where drugs are clustered according to the infection they treat.

ANTIVIRALS

Drugs that combat viral infections are called *antiviral drugs.* Antiviral drugs work by interfering with the virus's ability to reproduce in a cell. A virus consists of genetic material and some enzymes encased in a protein capsule. This capsule is located inside a lipid envelope. A virus itself cannot reproduce; instead it "slips" the envelope into a living cell to multiply. Therefore, to be effective, the drugs need to be able to target specific events that happen in the viral replication cycle.

ACTIONS

Antiviral drugs attempt to disable the protein part of the virus. An example is inhibition of the "uncoating" of viral content of the influenza A virus by a drug, such

as rimantadine (Flumadine). The antiviral drug attempts to prevent the virus from removing the protein capsule, which keeps the genetic material from spilling out into the host cell. Difficulty with this process occurs because viruses can develop resistance to antiviral drugs making the development of antiviral drugs difficult and expensive.

USES

Labeled Uses

Although infections caused by viruses are common, antiviral drugs have limited use because they are effective against only a small number of specific viral infections (Box 11.1). Antiviral drugs are used in the treatment or prevention of infections caused by:

- Cytomegalovirus (CMV), such as **retinitis** (inflammation of the retina)
- CMV prevention in transplant recipients
- Hepatitis B and C virus (HBV) and (HCV)
- Herpes simplex virus (HSV) 1 and 2 (genital) and herpes zoster
- Human immunodeficiency virus (HIV)
- Influenza A and B (respiratory tract illness)
- Respiratory syncytial virus (RSV; severe lower respiratory tract infection primarily affecting children)

Lifespan Considerations

Pediatrics
Severely ill children infected with influenza show significant improvement and decreased mortality when treated within 48 hr of flu symptom recognition with neuraminidase inhibitor (NAI) drugs.

Unlabeled Use of Antiviral Drugs

With a limited number of antiviral drugs and more than 200 viral diseases, antivirals are one of the drug categories where the primary health care provider may decide to prescribe a drug for an **unlabeled use**, even though its effectiveness for that use is not well documented. Approval by the US Food and Drug Administration (FDA) is necessary for a drug to be prescribed. On occasion, the use of a drug for a specific disorder or condition may be under investigation, or it may be approved for use in another country. In this instance, the drug may be prescribed by the primary health care provider for the condition under investigation. The use of the drug for a specific disorder or condition that is not officially approved by the FDA is called an *unlabeled use.* Examples of unlabeled uses of the antiviral drugs include prevention of CMV and HSV infections after transplantation procedures and varicella pneumonia.

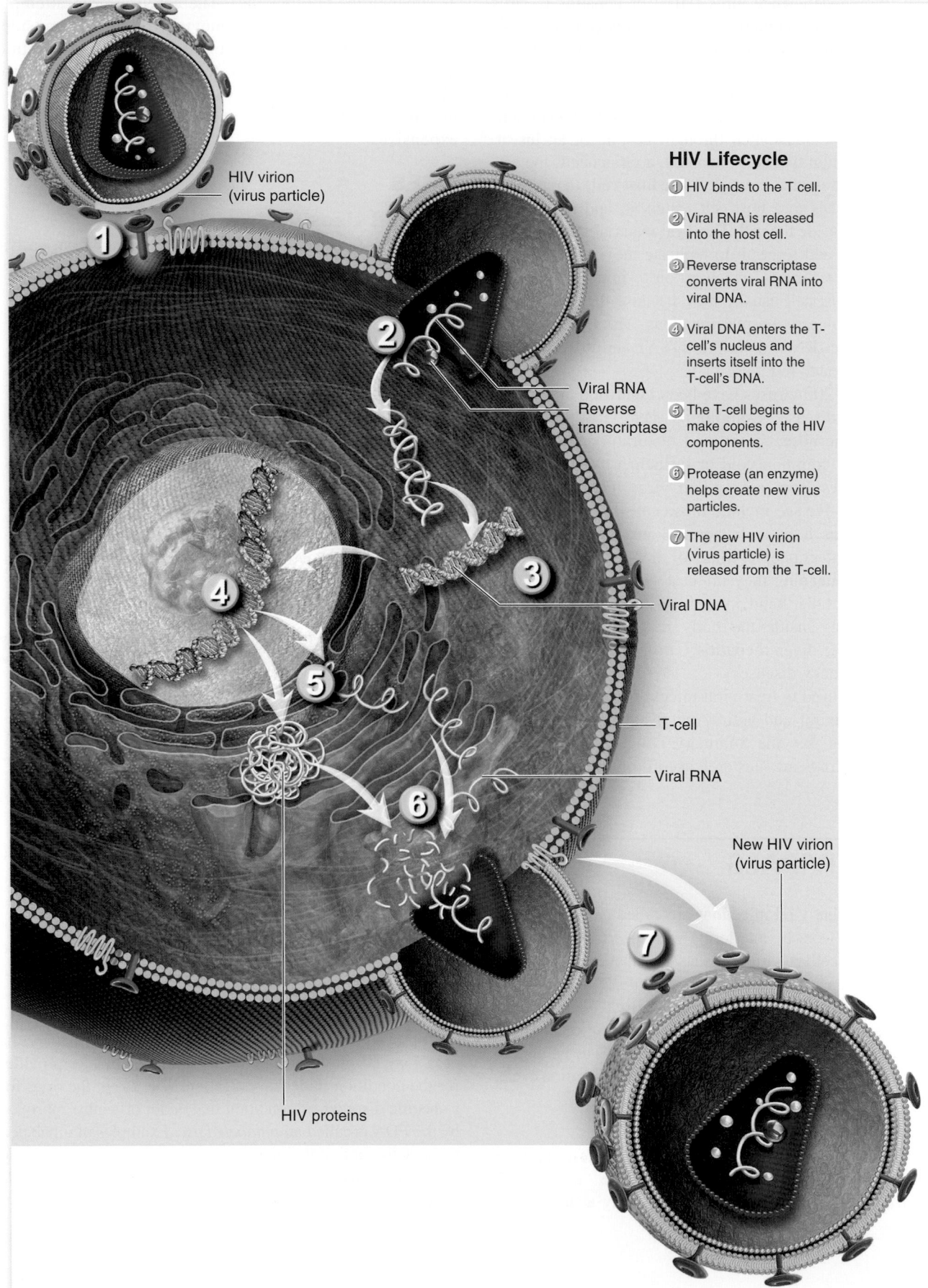

HIV virion (virus particle)

HIV Lifecycle

① HIV binds to the T cell.

② Viral RNA is released into the host cell.

③ Reverse transcriptase converts viral RNA into viral DNA.

④ Viral DNA enters the T-cell's nucleus and inserts itself into the T-cell's DNA.

⑤ The T-cell begins to make copies of the HIV components.

⑥ Protease (an enzyme) helps create new virus particles.

⑦ The new HIV virion (virus particle) is released from the T-cell.

Viral RNA
Reverse transcriptase

Viral DNA

T-cell

Viral RNA

New HIV virion (virus particle)

HIV proteins

FIGURE 11.1 Viral (HIV) replication cycle. (Courtesy of Anatomical Chart Co.)

BOX 11.1 Description of Viral Infections

Cytomegalovirus

CMV, a virus of the herpes family, is a common viral infection. Healthy individuals may become infected yet have no symptoms. However, immunocompromised clients (such as those with HIV or cancer) may have the infection. Symptoms include malaise, fever, pneumonia, and superinfection. Infants may acquire the virus from the mother while in the uterus, resulting in learning disabilities and mental retardation. CMV can infect the eye, causing retinitis. Symptoms of CMV retinitis are blurred vision and decreased visual acuity. Visual impairment is irreversible and can lead to blindness if untreated.

Human Papillomavirus

HPV is the most common sexually transmitted infection. There are over 40 different HPV types that infect the genitals, mouth, and throat. However, symptoms can be minor enough that most people do not even know they are infected. HPV infection can lead to genital warts, cervical cancer, and rare forms of throat warts or cancers. Warts can appear weeks to months after contact with an infected partner. Cervical symptoms do not appear until late in the disease. Treatment includes removal of warts, yet HPV is best treated by prevention with vaccine (see Chapter 47).

Hepatitis B and Hepatitis C Virus

Hepatitis is an inflammation of the liver. HBV is spread by infected blood or body fluids. Sexual contact is the most frequent mode of transmission, followed by use of contaminated needles. Symptoms of infection include fever and joint pains. Acute HBV typically resolves; chronic HBV is treated to boost the immune system. HCV is related to the yellow fever and West Nile virus and is primarily spread by exposure to infected blood. Most people show no signs or symptoms of HCV until the infection becomes chronic and laboratory results show persistent liver inflammation. Treatment with antivirals can offer cure in 60%–90% of the infected cases. Late-stage cirrhosis caused by HCV is currently the primary reason for liver transplant.

Herpes Simplex Virus

HSV is divided into HSV-1, which causes oral, ocular, or facial infections, and HSV-2, which causes genital infection. However, either type can cause disease at either body site. HSV-1 causes painful vesicular lesions in the oral mucosa, on the face, or around the eyes. HSV-2 or genital herpes is usually transmitted by sexual contact and causes painful vesicular lesions on the mucous membranes of the genitalia.

Vaginal lesions may appear as mucous patches with grayish ulcerations. The client may appear irritable, lethargic, and jaundiced and may have difficulty breathing or experience seizures. The lesions usually heal within 2 weeks. Immunosuppressed clients may develop a severe systemic disease.

Varicella Zoster Virus

Herpes zoster (shingles) is caused by the varicella zoster (chickenpox) virus. It is highly contagious. The virus causes chickenpox in the child and is easily spread via the respiratory system. Recovery from childhood chickenpox results in the infection lying dormant in the nerve cells. The virus may become reactivated later in life as the older adult's immune system weakens or the individual becomes ill with other disorders. The lesions of herpes zoster appear as pustules along a sensory nerve route. Pain often continues for several months after the lesions have healed.

Human Immunodeficiency Virus

HIV or AIDS is a type of viral infection transmitted through an infected person's bodily secretions, such as blood or semen. HIV destroys the immune system, causing the body to develop opportunistic infections such as Kaposi sarcoma, *Pneumocystis carinii* pneumonia, or tuberculosis. Symptoms include chills and fever, night sweats, dry productive cough, dyspnea, lethargy, malaise, fatigue, weight loss, and diarrhea.

Influenza (flu)

Influenza, commonly called the "flu," is an acute respiratory illness caused by influenza viruses A and B. Symptoms include fever, cough, sore throat, runny or stuffy nose, headache, muscle aches, and extreme fatigue. Most people recover within 1–2 weeks. Influenza may cause severe complications such as pneumonia in children, the elderly, and other vulnerable groups. The viruses causing influenza continually change over time, which enables them to evade the immune system of the host. These rapid changes in the most commonly circulating types of influenza virus necessitate annual changes in the composition of the flu vaccine.

Respiratory Syncytial Virus

RSV infection is highly contagious and affects mostly children, causing bronchiolitis and pneumonia. Infants younger than 6 months are the most severely affected. In adults, RSV causes colds and bronchitis, with fever, cough, and nasal congestion. When RSV affects immunocompromised clients, the consequences can be severe and sometimes fatal.

ADVERSE REACTIONS

Gastrointestinal System Reactions
- Nausea, vomiting
- Diarrhea

Other Reactions
- Headache
- Rash
- Fever
- Insomnia

CONTRAINDICATIONS

Do not administer antivirals if the client has a history of allergies to the drug or other antivirals. Cidofovir should not be given to clients who have renal impairment or in combination with medications that are nephrotoxic, such as aminoglycosides. Ribavirin should not be used in clients with unstable cardiac disease. Zanamivir (Relenza) is not recommended for use in clients with chronic obstructive pulmonary disease. Most antivirals should be used during pregnancy (pregnancy categories B and C) and lactation only when the benefit outweighs the risk to the fetus or child. Ribavirin is a pregnancy category X; any HCV therapy using this drug requires two forms of nonhormone birth control during and up to 6 months following treatment.

 Lifespan Considerations

Childbearing Women
Influenza (the flu) is likely to cause severe illness in pregnant women because of the body changes of pregnancy. Flu *vaccine injections* (in comparison with drugs used to treat the flu) are safe and recommended for women who are or may become pregnant.

PRECAUTIONS

Antivirals should be used cautiously in clients with renal impairment, low blood cell counts, history of epilepsy (rimantadine), and history of respiratory disease (zanamivir). Clients are known to suffer electrolyte depletion when taking foscarnet. Ganciclovir is associated with reduced fertility in both males and females and has the potential of birth defects when pregnant women take the drug. Clients treated for HBV may experience an exacerbation of hepatitis after discontinuation of adefovir dipivoxil (Hepsera) or entecavir (Baraclude).

INTERACTIONS

The following interactions may occur when an antiviral is administered with another agent:

Interacting Drug	Common Use	Effect of Interaction
probenecid	Gout treatment	Increased serum levels of the antivirals
cimetidine	Gastric upset, heartburn	Increased serum level of the antiviral valacyclovir
ibuprofen	Pain relief	Increased serum level of the antiviral adefovir
imipenem–cilastatin	Anti-infective agent	With ganciclovir only, increased risk of seizures
anticholinergic agents	Management of bladder spasms	Increased adverse reactions of anticholinergic agent
theophylline	Management of respiratory problems	With acyclovir only, increased serum level of theophylline

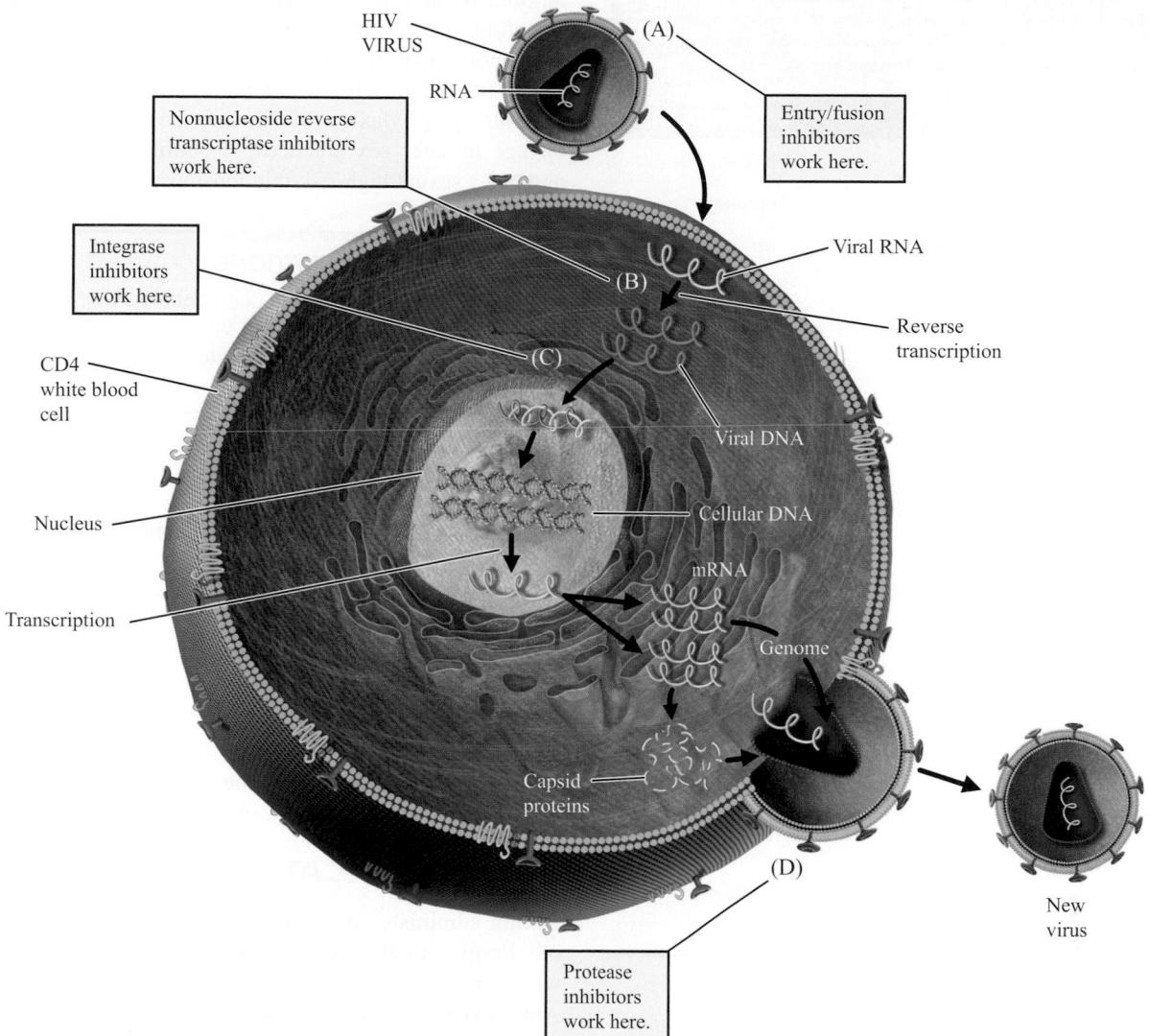

HIV VIRUS

RNA

Nonnucleoside reverse transcriptase inhibitors work here.

Entry/fusion inhibitors work here.

(A)

Integrase inhibitors work here.

Viral RNA

(B)

Reverse transcription

CD4 white blood cell

(C)

Viral DNA

Nucleus

Cellular DNA

mRNA

Transcription

Genome

Capsid proteins

(D)

New virus

Protease inhibitors work here.

FIGURE 11.2 Example of drug targeting during HIV replication. **A.** Entry/fusion inhibitors work to prevent the HIV from shedding its protective coating and inserting its genetic material into the cell. **B.** NNRTIs prevent unlinking of the viral RNA so it cannot be transcribed. **C.** Integrase inhibitors prevent viral genetic material from getting into nucleus. **D.** Protease inhibitors prevent the newly assembled HIV from leaving the cell to infect other CD4 cells. (Courtesy of Anatomical Chart Co.)

ANTIRETROVIRALS

ACTIONS

Retroviruses attack the host cell just like a virus; the difference is that RNA is the primary component of the virus instead of DNA. Retroviruses also contain an enzyme called *reverse transcriptase* that is used to turn the RNA of the virus into DNA, helping to reproduce more of the virus. An example of a **retrovirus** is the HIV. Left untreated this viral infection can progress to acquired immunodeficiency syndrome (AIDS).

Because the viral material of a retrovirus is RNA rather than DNA, retrovirus **mutation** is greater. When HIV was first treated, providers found that the virus had the ability to become resistant to medication when a single drug was used owing to mutation. Research on antiretroviral drugs has found that this occurred less when multidrug regimens were used. Using multiple antiretroviral drugs in therapy is termed **highly active antiretroviral therapy (HAART)**. Figure 11.2 illustrates where the antiretroviral drug action occurs during HIV replication within the host cell. The following types of drugs are used in HAART (for more information see the Summary Drug Table: Antiviral Drugs):

- Entry inhibitors, which prevent the attachment or fusion of HIV to a host cell for initial entry
- Nonnucleoside reverse transcriptase inhibitors (NNRTIs), which latch on to the reverse transcriptase molecule to block the ability to make viral DNA
- Integrase inhibitors, which prevent enzymes from inserting HIV genetic material into the cell's DNA

TABLE 11.1 Antiretroviral Drug Combinations

ALL THESE DRUG COMBINATIONS ARE TAKEN AS ONE PILL, ONCE DAILY. EXCEPTION WHERE ONE PILL IS TAKEN TWICE DAILY (BID) ARE NOTED WITH (*) AN ASTERISK	
GENERIC DRUGS	**COMBINATION DRUG TRADE NAME**
abacavir/lamivudine	Epzicom
abacavir/lamivudine/dolutegravir	Triumeq
abacavir/lamivudine/zidovudine	Trizivir*
atazanavir/cobicistat	Evotaz
bictegravir/emtricitabine/tenofovir alafenamide	Biktarvy
darunavir/cobicistat	Prezcobix
darunavir/cobicistat/emtricitabine/tenofovir alafenamide	Symtuza
dolutegravir/lamivudine	Dovato
dolutegravir/rilpivirine	Juluca
doravirine/lamivudine/tenofovir disoproxil	Delstrigo
efavirenz/emtricitabine/tenofovir disoproxil	Atripla
elvitegravir/cobicistat/emtricitabine/tenofovir alafenamide	Genvoya
elvitegravir/cobicistat/emtricitabine/tenofovir disoproxil	Stribild
emtricitabine/rilpivirine/tenofovir disoproxil	Complera
emtricitabine/tenofovir disoproxil	Truvada*, Descovy
lamivudine/zidovudine	Combivir*
lopinavir/ritonavir	Kaletra*

- Reverse transcriptase inhibitors, which block the reverse transcriptase enzyme so the HIV material cannot change into DNA in the new cell, preventing new HIV copies from being created
- Protease inhibitors, which block the protease enzyme so the new viral particles cannot mature

Successful treatment outcomes rely on adherence to multiple drug regimens. As discussed in Chapter 10, having to take a number of pills daily is problematic for clients and their caregivers. Drug manufactures attempt to solve this issue by providing a number of drug combinations to promote adherence. Table 11.1 provides a listing of many of these antiretroviral drug combinations. These combination drugs have reduced the administration number and times dramatically. The drug cobicistat (Tybost) is an antiretroviral boosting agent used in combination with antiretrovirals. This agent inhibits liver enzymes from metabolizing the other drugs, which results in higher blood concentrations of drug with lower dosing, reducing adverse reactions. Cobicistat may be used with just one additional drug or multiple drugs such as the medication Stribild (also known as the Quad pill).

Uses

Antiretroviral drugs are used in the treatment of HBV, HIV infection, and AIDS. The combination drug emtricitabine and tenofovir disoproxil is the only antiretroviral approved to use for the prevention of HIV. The drug is used for pre-exposure prophylaxis (PrEP) when an adult is willing to engage in safer sex practices, is confirmed HIV-negative, and has a sexual high-risk relationship.

> **PRACTICE CONSIDERATIONS**
>
> PrEP is not a vaccine. PrEP uses antiretroviral drugs to keep the HIV from replicating. Vaccines, on the other hand, introduce the immune system to the virus in order to activate a response.

ADVERSE REACTIONS

Gastrointestinal System Reactions
- Nausea, vomiting
- Diarrhea
- Altered taste

Other Reactions
- Headache, fever, and chills
- Rash
- Numbness and tingling in the **circumoral** area (around the mouth) or peripherally, or both

CONTRAINDICATIONS

Do not administer antiretrovirals if the client has a history of allergies to the drug or other antiretrovirals. Women who are lactating should not use antiretroviral drugs. Antiretrovirals should not be prescribed to the client who is using cisapride, pimozide, triazolam, midazolam, or an ergot derivative. Ritonavir is contraindicated if the client is taking bupropion (Wellbutrin), zolpidem (Ambien), or an antiarrhythmic drug.

PRECAUTIONS

Antiretrovirals should be used cautiously in clients with diabetes mellitus, impaired hepatic function, pregnancy (pregnancy categories B and C), or hemophilia. Caution should be used for the client taking indinavir who has a history of kidney or bladder stone formation. Clients, especially older adults, taking didanosine are at higher risk for pancreatitis. If a client has a sulfonamide allergy, the drugs fosamprenavir and amprenavir should be used cautiously. Ergot derivatives (used in the treatment of migraine headaches) should not be prescribed if a client is taking a protease inhibitor because of the increased risk of peripheral ischemia. When taking protease inhibitors, grapefruit juice may increase drug concentration in the blood while garlic will reduce the effectiveness and both should not be consumed during treatment.

LASA ALERT

The following drugs may sound alike; be sure to clarify when they are ordered:

Drug Name	Sounds Like
Delavirdine	dalfampridine
Indinavir	Denavir
Kaletra	Keppra
Lexiva	Levitra, Pexeva
Nelfinavir	nevirapine
Norvir	Norvasc
Prezista	Prezcobix
Ritonavir	Retrovir
Saquinavir	SINEquan
Videx	Bidex, Lidex
Viracept	Viramune

Drugs that look like a similar drug are noted in the Summary Drug Tables of each chapter.

INTERACTIONS

The following interactions may occur when an antiretroviral is administered with another agent:

Interacting Drug	Common Use	Effect of Interaction
antifungals	Eliminate or manage fungal infections	Increased serum level of the antiretroviral
clarithromycin	Treat bacterial infection	Increased serum level of both drugs
sildenafil	Treat erectile dysfunction	Increased adverse reactions of sildenafil
opioid analgesics	Pain relief	Risk of toxicity with ritonavir
anticoagulant, anticonvulsant, antiparasitic agents	Prevent blood clots, seizures, parasitic infections, respectively	Decreased effectiveness when taking ritonavir
interleukins	Prevent severely low platelet counts usually related to chemotherapy	Risk of antiretroviral toxicity
fentanyl	Analgesia, used typically with procedures requiring anesthesia	Increased serum level of fentanyl
oral contraceptives	Birth control	Decreased effectiveness of the birth control agent
rifampin	Pulmonary tuberculosis	With efavirenz, nevirapine only; decreased serum levels of antivirals

Herbal Considerations

Individuals use St. John's wort (Fig. 11.3) for antibacterial, antidepressive, and antiviral effects of the supplement. This herbal supplement is one of the most commonly purchased herbal products in the United States. Studies show that the herb is effective in treating mild depression and has fewer adverse reactions than prescription antidepressants. Yet, researchers have found that in clients taking antiretroviral medications, the effectiveness of drug therapy is reduced if the client also takes St. John's wort. Clients need to be instructed to disclose the use of all over-the-counter medications and supplements to their primary health care provider to prevent potentially harmful interactions.

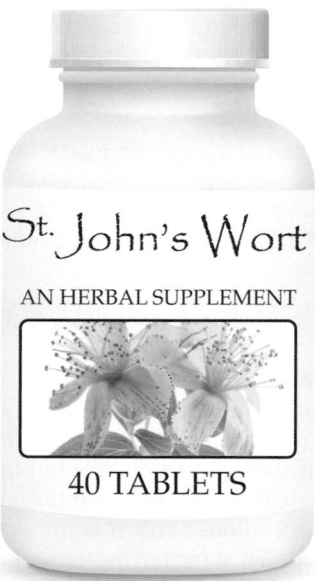

FIGURE 11.3 St. John's wort, used for antidepressive and antiviral properties.

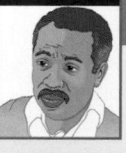

PHARMACOLOGY IN PRACTICE

PATHOPHYSIOLOGY

Why are viruses so difficult to treat even with the use of antiviral medications? Select all that apply.

1. Viruses are tiny
2. Viruses can develop resistance to antiviral drugs
3. Viruses have a hard-to-penetrate outer layer
4. Viruses are large
5. Viruses replicate inside human cells

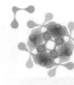

NURSING PROCESS STEPS TO BUILDING CLINICAL JUDGMENT
Client Receiving an Antiviral/Antiretroviral Drug

ASSESSMENT

Preadministration Assessment
Data gathering suggestions before the initial administration of the drug include:
Objective data

- Description of general appearance, resistance to infection (complete blood count)
- Vital signs (temperature, pulse, respirations, and blood pressure)
- Female clients—testing for pregnancy or inquiry regarding lactation if postnatal
- Inspect the body for signs of lesions (e.g., HSV-1 or HSV-2 infected clients—inspect the mouth, face, eyes, or genitalia) as a baseline for comparison during therapy

Many facilities have the capacity to take photographs of the area and include in the electronic health care record. This is helpful for comparison later in the treatment phase.
Subjective data

- Type and duration of symptoms (genitourinary and other systems)
- Remedies attempted before seeking care
- Exposure to ill individuals if immunocompromised

Lifespan Considerations

Childbearing/Menopausal Women
Ethinyl estradiol is known to cause an increase in liver function blood results when taken with Viekira Pak (combination HCV medication). Women of childbearing age treated for HCV should not take birth control pills or use hormonal vaginal rings. It is important to assess older women with HCV for hormone replacement or estrogen cream use as well.

Ongoing Assessment
The ongoing assessment depends on the reason for giving the antiviral drug. It is important to make a frequent assessment for improvement of the signs and symptoms identified in the initial assessment. Monitor for and report any adverse reactions from the antiviral drug. When appropriate, teach the client or caregivers to feel confident in inspecting the intravenous (IV) infusion site several times a day for redness, inflammation, or pain and report any signs of phlebitis.

NURSING DIAGNOSES

Drug-specific nursing diagnoses include the following:

- **Risk for malnutrition:** related to adverse reaction of antiviral drugs
- **Altered skin integrity** related to initial infection, adverse drug reactions, and administration of the antiviral drug

- **Injury risk** related to the client's mental status, peripheral neuropathy, and generalized weakness
- **Body image disturbance** related to body fat redistribution
- **Acute pain** related to kidney or bladder stones or inflammation caused by antiviral drugs

Nursing diagnoses that are related to drug administration are discussed in Chapter 4.

PLANNING

The expected outcomes for the client depend on the reason for administration of the antiviral drug but may include an optimal response to therapy, meeting of client needs related to the management of adverse reactions, and confidence in an understanding of the medication regimen.

IMPLEMENTATION

Promoting an Optimal Response to Therapy
Because these drugs may be used in the treatment of certain types of severe and sometimes life-threatening viral infections, the client may be concerned about the diagnosis and prognosis. Allow the client and family members time to talk and ask questions about treatment methods, especially when the drug is given IV and the client or family may be responsible for care in the home. It is important to prepare the antiviral drugs according to the manufacturer's directions. The administration rate is ordered by the primary health care provider.

Ribavirin
Ribavirin when used in HARRT is given orally. When it is used to treat RSV, it is given by inhalation using a small particle aerosol generator (called a *SPAG-2 aerosol generator*). It is important to discard and replace the solution every 24 hr. This drug can worsen respiratory status. Sudden deterioration of respiratory status can occur in infants receiving ribavirin, and it is important to monitor respiratory function closely throughout therapy. Report immediately any worsening of respiratory function to the primary health care provider. Female caregivers should know that the drug is a pregnancy category X drug, and women of childbearing age should take care not to inhale the drug as they prepare or give the drug to the client. In clients requiring mechanical ventilation, treatment should be provided only by health care providers familiar with the specific ventilator.

Administration
Rapid infusion or bolus administration of the antivirals has created toxicity in clients caused by excessive plasma levels of the drug. You should always check the recommended infusion rate of the drug and not exceed the rate.

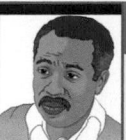

PHARMACOLOGY IN PRACTICE

DOSE CALCULATION

A primary health care provider has prescribed 5400 mg of foscavir per day to be administered intravenously. The strength of the drug in the available solution is 24 mg/mL. How many milliliters of solution in the syringe pump will the pharmacist have prepared for the nurse to administer one 5400-mg dose?

1. 250 mL
2. 225 mL
3. 275 mL
4. 200 mL

Monitoring and Managing Client Needs

Risk for Malnutrition

The metabolic needs of clients with HIV infection are demanding. Because the antiviral drugs may cause anorexia, nausea, or vomiting, providing adequate nutrition becomes a real challenge (see Chapter 38 for appetite stimulants). The gastrointestinal (GI) effects range from mild to severe. Many of the drugs can be given without regard to food. An exception is didanosine (Videx) when given in oral solution. Because it causes GI distress, the clinical pharmacist mixes the buffered powder with a liquid antacid and the mixture is dispensed this way to the client. This solution should be kept refrigerated and thoroughly shaken before being administered, which would be 30 minutes before or 2 hr after a meal.

The client may be able to tolerate small, frequent meals with soft, nonirritating foods if nausea is mild. Frequent sips of carbonated beverages or hot tea may be helpful for others. It is important to keep the atmosphere clean and free of odors. Provide good oral care before and after meals. Sometimes daily-dose drugs can be given at bedtime to reduce nausea. If nausea is severe or the client is vomiting, notify the primary health care provider.

Risk for Altered Skin Integrity

Monitor any skin lesions carefully for worsening or improvement. Should the lesions not improve, inform the primary health care provider. Accurate observation and documentation are essential. If an antiviral drug is administered topically, use gloves when applying to avoid spreading the infection. These drugs may also cause a rash as an adverse reaction. Note and report any rash to the primary health care provider.

When administering the drug by the IV route, closely observe the injection site for signs of phlebitis. Take care to prevent trauma because even slight trauma can result in bruising if the platelet count is low. If injections are given, pressure is applied at the injection site to prevent bleeding. Occasionally, headache or a slight fever may occur in clients taking antiviral drugs. An analgesic may be prescribed to manage these effects. Depending on the client's symptoms, monitor vital signs every 4 hr or as ordered by the primary health care provider.

Chronic Care Considerations

In the treatment of genital herpes, acyclovir treats the symptomatic lesions; it does not cure the virus. Clients should avoid intercourse when lesions/symptoms are present to reduce viral transmission.

Injury Risk

Some clients with a viral infection are acutely ill. Others may experience fatigue, lethargy, dizziness, or weakness as an adverse reaction to the antiviral/antiretroviral agent. Monitor these clients carefully. Call lights are placed in a convenient place for the hospitalized client and are answered promptly. If fatigue, dizziness, confusion, or weakness is present, the client may require assistance with ambulation or activities of daily living. Plan activities to provide adequate rest periods. Other drugs can damage the peripheral nerves, especially when used with other neurotoxic agents. Watch for signs of peripheral neuropathy (numbness, tingling, or pain in the feet or hands). It is important to report these signs immediately to the primary health care provider.

Disturbed Body Image

Clients taking the protease inhibitors (saquinavir, ritonavir, indinavir, nelfinavir, fosamprenavir, amprenavir, and atazanavir) have experienced redistribution of body fat. Adipose tissue moves to the center of the body, so clients appear to have thinner arms and legs with a rounder abdomen or enlarged breasts. Sometimes body fat relocates to the area behind the neck (frequently called a *buffalo hump*). Plan to spend time with these clients, encouraging them to verbalize their feelings regarding this change in appearance. It is also important to acknowledge these feelings as being both valid and important to the client.

Acute Pain

The drug indinavir (Crixivan) has been known to cause kidney or bladder stones in clients. Antiretroviral drugs have been known to cause acute pancreatitis. Clients should be assessed for pain. Any pain should be explored for location and intensity. When assessing the client for GI problems such as nausea, vomiting, abdominal pain, and jaundice, be alert because these are symptoms of pancreatitis, and particular care should be taken in assessment of pain. Acute, sudden-onset pain should be reported to the primary health care provider for both treatment and further assessment for more involved disease.

! NURSING ALERT

Clients receiving antiretroviral drugs for HIV infection may continue to contract opportunistic infections and other complications of HIV disease. Monitor all clients closely for signs of infection such as fever (even low-grade fever), malaise, sore throat, or lethargy. All caregivers are reminded to use good hand hygiene technique.

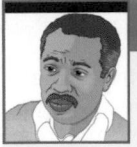

PHARMACOLOGY IN PRACTICE

CLIENT-CENTERED CARE

A nurse is caring for a client who is on antiretroviral therapy for HIV. The client has developed anorexia and nausea owing to the different drugs. Which of the following interventions should the nurse perform in the given situation? Select all that apply.

1. Reduce frequency of meals but increase quantity of meals.
2. Ensure that client's diet includes soft, nonirritating foods.
3. Keep the atmosphere clean and free of odors.
4. Eliminate carbonated beverages or hot tea from diet.
5. Provide good oral care before and after meals.

Educating the Client and Family

When an antiviral drug is given orally, explain the dosage schedule to the client and family, instructing the client to take the drug exactly as directed for the full course of therapy. If a dose is missed, the client should take it as soon as remembered but should not double the dose at the next dosage time. Any adverse reactions should be reported to the primary health care provider or the nurse. Help the client to understand that many of these drugs do not cure viral infections but they can decrease symptoms and increase feelings of well-being.

Instruct clients to report any symptoms of infection, such as an elevated temperature (even a slight elevation), sore throat, difficulty breathing, weakness, or lethargy. Again, review possible signs of pancreatitis (nausea, vomiting, abdominal pain, jaundice) and peripheral neuropathy (tingling, burning, numbness, or pain in the hands or feet). Any indication of pancreatitis or peripheral neuropathy must be reported at once.

Include the following information in the teaching plan for antiviral drugs:

- Many antiviral drugs do not cure viral infections, but they will shorten the course of disease outbreaks and promote healing of the lesions. The drugs will not prevent the spread of the disease to others. Topical drugs should not be applied more frequently than prescribed but should be applied with a finger cot or gloves. All lesions should be covered to prevent additional irritation. There should be no sexual contact while lesions are present on genitalia. Notify the primary health care provider if burning, stinging, itching, or rash worsens or becomes pronounced.
- Some drugs cause photosensitivity, so precautions should be taken when going outdoors, such as wearing sunscreen, head coverings, and protective clothing. Clients should also refrain from using tanning beds.
- Some clients have experienced an acute exacerbation of the disease when medications used to treat hepatitis B are stopped. Hepatic function should be closely monitored in these clients.

- Those taking antiretrovirals should be cautioned that there is an increased risk of adverse reactions (hypotension, visual disturbances, prolonged penile erection) when the erectile dysfunction drug sildenafil (Viagra) is used. Symptoms should be reported promptly to the primary health care provider.
- Some drugs affect mental status. Activities requiring mental alertness, such as driving a car, should be delayed until the effect of the drug is apparent because vision and coordination can be affected. Clients should rise slowly from a prone to a sitting position to decrease the possibility of lightheadedness caused by orthostatic hypotension. Changes such as nervousness, tremors, slurred speech, or depression should be reported.
- Some clients are on an alternate-dosage schedule. In this case, it is important to designate the days the drug is to be taken; calendars and cell phone apps are helpful aids to track schedules.
- Zanamivir (Relenza) may be taken daily or every 12 hr for up to a month using a "Diskhaler" delivery system. If a bronchodilator is also prescribed for use at the same time, the bronchodilator is used before the zanamivir. The drug may cause dizziness. The client should use caution when driving an automobile or operating dangerous machinery. Treatment with this drug does not decrease the risk of transmission of influenza to others.

EVALUATION

- Therapeutic response is achieved, and there is management of the infection and viral load.
- Adverse reactions are identified, reported to the primary health care provider, and managed successfully with appropriate nursing interventions:
  - Client maintains an adequate nutritional status.
  - Skin is intact and free of inflammation, irritation, infection, or ulcerations.
  - No evidence of injury is seen.
  - Perceptions of body changes are managed successfully.
  - Client is free of pain.
- Client and family express confidence and demonstrate an understanding of the drug regimen.

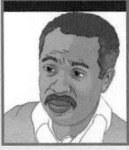

PHARMACOLOGY IN PRACTICE

USING CLINICAL REASONING

Mr. Park is staying in a long-term care facility following his hip replacement surgery. The primary health care provider prescribes acyclovir 200 mg every 4 hr during Mr. Park's waking hours for his outbreak of herpes zoster (shingles). Discuss what information you would give the skilled nursing facility staff concerning herpes zoster, the drug regimen, and the possible adverse reactions.

KEY POINTS

■ A virus is smaller than a bacterium. To reproduce, the virus needs cellular material of another living cell. Viral infections can range from the common cold to chronic systemic infections of the liver or immune system.

■ Antiviral drugs work by interfering with the virus's ability to reproduce in a cell. These drugs are used to reduce the effects of viral infections such as HSV-1 and HSV-2, CMV, and RSV. Diseases such as HBV and HCV have become chronic conditions when treated with antivirals. The effectiveness of antivirals is limited based on how well the virus can mutate, which results in viral resistance to the drug.

■ In most situations, antivirals have minor adverse reactions such as GI disturbances or flu-like symptoms.

■ Retroviruses attack cells and hamper the work of RNA in the cell. HIV is a retroviral disease.

■ RNA of the virus makes mutation of a retrovirus greater and harder to treat.

■ Antiretroviral drugs are used primarily to reduce viral load in clients with HIV and HBV. Multiple drugs are used to attack the virus at different parts of the life cycle; this is termed highly active antiretroviral therapy.

■ Adverse reactions range from minor GI issues to peripheral neuropathy or anaphylaxis. Shifts in body fat can be disturbing to clients taking these drugs.

SUMMARY DRUG TABLE
Antiviral Drugs

Generic Name	Trade Name	Uses	Adverse Reactions	Dosage Ranges
Antivirals				
Agents Used to Treat CMV-Related Infections				
cidofovir si-DOF-o-veer		CMV retinitis, acyclovir-resistant HSV	Headache, nausea, vomiting, diarrhea, anorexia, dyspnea, alopecia, rash, neutropenia, fever, chills	5 mg/kg IV once a week for 2 week, then once every 2 week for maintenance
foscarnet fos-KAR-net	Foscavir	CMV retinitis; acyclovir-resistant HSV-1 and -2	Headache, seizures, nausea, vomiting, diarrhea, anemia, abnormal renal function test results	CMV retinitis: 90–120 mg/kg/day IV; HSV: 40 mg/kg IV q8–12h
ganciclovir gan-SYE-kloe-veer	Cytovene	CMV retinitis; CMV prevention in transplant recipients	Anorexia, vomiting, diarrhea, fever, sweats, anemia, leukopenia	5 mg/kg IV q12h for 14–21 days, then daily
letermovir le-term-oh-vir	Prevymis	CMV prevention in transplant recipients	Headache, fatigue, diarrhea, nausea, vomiting, cough, peripheral edema	480 mg IV/orally daily in first month after transplant
valGANciclovir val-gan-SYE-kloe-veer	Valcyte	CMV retinitis, CMV prevention in transplant recipients	Headache, insomnia, diarrhea, nausea, vomiting, pancytopenia, fever	900 mg orally BID; transplant recipients: start 10 days before transplantation and continue 100 days after transplantation
Antiherpes Virus Agents				
acyclovir ay-SYE-kloe-veer	Sitavig, Zovirax	HSV, herpes zoster, varicella zoster	Nausea, vomiting, diarrhea, fever, headache, dizziness, confusion, rashes, myalgia	Oral: 200–800 mg q4h for 5 doses per day, treat for 5–10 days; IV: 5–10 mg/kg q8h; topical: apply to lesions q3h
famciclovir fam-SYE-kloe-veer		Acute herpes zoster, HSV-2	Fatigue, fever, nausea, vomiting, diarrhea, sinusitis, constipation, headache	Herpes zoster: 500 mg orally q8h for 7 days; HSV-2: 125 mg orally BID for 5 days
valACYclovir val-ay-SYE-kloe-veer	Valtrex	Herpes zoster; HSV-1 and -2	Nausea, headache	HSV-1: 2 g q12h for 1 day HSV-2 initial: 1 g BID for 10 days Recurrent infection: 500 mg orally BID for 5 days Herpes zoster: 1 g orally TID for 7 days

Continued

SUMMARY DRUG TABLE (continued)
Antibacterial Drugs That Disrupt Bacterial Cell Wall Synthesis

Generic Name	Trade Name	Uses	Adverse Reactions	Dosage Ranges
Agents Used to Treat Hepatitis B and C Infections				
adefovir dipivoxil a-DEF-o-veer	Hepsera	Chronic hepatitis B (HBV)	Asthenia, headache, abdominal pain	10 mg/day orally
⊘ **entecavir** en-TE-ka-veer	Baraclude	HBV	Dizziness, fatigue, headache	0.5–1 mg/day orally
sofosbuvir soe-FOS-bue-veer	Sovaldi	Chronic HCV, in combination with interferon or ribavirin	Headache, insomnia, nausea, decreased appetite, fatigue, itching	400 mg orally daily
elbasvir/grazoprevir ELB-as-veer graz-OH-pre-veer	Zepatier	Chronic HCV, in combination with ribavirin	Headache, nausea, fatigue	One tablet orally daily, 12–18 weeks
glecaprevir/pibrentasvir glek-A-pre-veer pi-BRENT-as-veer	Mavyret	Chronic HCV	Headache, nausea, fatigue	3 tablets orally, once daily 8 weeks
ledipasvir/sofosbuvir le-DIP-as-veer	Harvoni	Chronic HCV	Headache, fatigue	One tablet orally daily
ombitasvir/ paritaprevir/ ritonavir/dasabuvir	Viekira Pak	Chronic HCV	Nausea, fatigue, insomnia	Two tablets orally daily in morning
sofosbuvir/velpatasvir	Epclusa	Chronic HCV	Headache, fatigue	One tablet orally daily, 12 weeks
sofosbuvir/velpatasvir/ voxilaprevir	Vosevi	Chronic HCV	Headache, diarrhea, nausea, fatigue	One tablet orally daily, 12 weeks
ribavirin (inhalation) rye-ba-VYE-rin	Virazole	RSV	Worsening of pulmonary status, bacterial pneumonia, hypotension	Administered by aerosol with special aerosol generator
ribavirin/interferon combination		In combination with interferon for hepatitis C	Fatigue, headache, myalgia, anorexia, nausea, vomiting, insomnia, nervousness	800–1200 mg orally BID
Antivirals Agents and Neuraminidase Inhibitors to Treat Influenza				
baloxavir marboxil va-LOX-A-veer mar-BOX-el	Xofluza	Treatment of influenza A and B	Diarrhea, pharyngitis	40–80 mg orally within 48 hr of symptom onset
oseltamivir oh-sel-TAM-i-veer	Tamiflu	Prevention and treatment of influenza A and B	Nausea, vomiting, diarrhea	75 mg orally BID for 5 days
peramivir pe-RA-mi-veer	Rapivab	Same as oseltamivir	Diarrhea	600 mg IV
zanamivir za-NA-mi-veer	Relenza	Same as oseltamivir	Nausea, headache, rhinitis	5-mg inhalation q12hr
Antiretrovirals				
Protease Inhibitors				
atazanavir at-a-za-NA-veer	Reyataz	HIV infection	Nausea, rash	300–400 mg/day
darunavir dar-OO-na-veer	Prezista	HIV infection	Headache, diarrhea, constipation, and pain	600 mg orally BID
fosamprenavir FOS-am-pren-a-veer	Lexiva	HIV infection	Headache, nausea, vomiting, diarrhea, rash	1400 mg/day orally
indinavir in-DIN-a-veer	Crixivan	HIV infection	Headache, nausea, vomiting, diarrhea, kidney/bladder stones	800 mg orally q8h
nelfinavir nel-FIN-a-veer	Viracept	HIV infection	Diarrhea	750 mg orally TID or 1250 mg orally BID
ritonavir ri-TOE-na-veer	Norvir	HIV infection	Peripheral and circumoral paresthesias, nausea, vomiting, diarrhea, anorexia	600 mg orally BID

Generic Name	Trade Name	Uses	Adverse Reactions	Dosage Ranges
Antiretrovirals (continued)				
saquinavir *sa-KWIN-a-veer*	Invirase	HIV infection	Headache, nausea, diarrhea, heartburn, flatulence	Fortovase: six 200-mg capsules orally TID Invirase: three 200-mg capsules orally TID
tipranavir *tip-RA-na-veer*	Aptivus	HIV infection	Nausea, diarrhea, liver dysfunction, intracranial bleeding	500 mg orally BID
Nucleoside/Nucleotide Reverse Transcriptase Inhibitors (NRTIs)				
abacavir *a-BAK-a-veer*	Ziagen	HIV infection	Nausea, vomiting, diarrhea, anorexia, liver dysfunction	300 mg orally BID or 600 mg once daily
didanosine (ddI) *dye-DAN-oh-seen*	Videx	HIV infection	Headache, nausea, rash, vomiting, peripheral neuropathy, abdominal pain, diarrhea	Oral: 400 mg/day or 200 mg BID; for clients weighing less than 60 kg, 250 mg/day or 125 mg BID
emtricitabine *em-trye-SYE-ta-been*	Emtriva	HIV infection	Headache, nausea, vomiting, diarrhea, rash	200 mg/day orally
lamiVUDine (3TC) *la-MI-vyoo-deen*	Epivir, Epivir-HBV	HIV infection, chronic hepatitis B infection	Headache, nausea, diarrhea, nasal congestion, cough, fatigue	HIV: 150 mg orally BID HBV: 100 mg/day orally daily
remdesivir *rem-DE-si-vir*	Veklury	COVID-19	Nausea, rash, prolonged bleeding	200 mg IV, initially, then 100 mg daily
tenofovir disoproxil *ten-OF-oh-veer*	Viread	HIV infection, chronic hepatitis B	Nausea, vomiting, diarrhea, flatulence	300 mg/day orally
zidovudine (AZT) *zye-DOE-vyoo-deen*	Retrovir	HIV infection, prevention of maternal–fetal HIV transmission	Asthenia, malaise, weakness, headache, anorexia, diarrhea, nausea, abdominal pain, dizziness, insomnia, anemia, agranulocytosis	600 mg/day orally in divided doses; 1 mg/kg IV q4h
Nonnucleoside Reverse Transcriptase Inhibitors (NNRTIs)				
delavirdine *del-la-VEER-deen*	Rescriptor	HIV infection	Headache, nausea, diarrhea	400 mg orally TID
doravirine *DOR-a-VIR-een*	Pifeltro	HIV infection	Rash, nausea, diarrhea, dizziness, insomnia, fatigue	100 mg orally daily
efavirenz *e-FAV-e-renz*	Sustiva	HIV infection	Rash, pruritus, dizziness, insomnia, fatigue, nausea, vomiting	600 mg/day orally
etravirine *et-ra-VEER-een*	Intelence	HIV infection	Rash, nausea, diarrhea	200 mg orally BID
nevirapine *ne-VYE-ra-peen*	Viramune	HIV infection	Rash, fever, headache, nausea, stomatitis, liver dysfunction	200 mg orally BID
rilpivirine *ril-pi-VEER-een*	Edurant	HIV infection	Headache, insomnia, depression, rash	25 mg orally daily
Entry Inhibitors				
maraviroc *mah-RAV-er-rock*	Selzentry	HIV infection	Dizziness, cough, rash, abdominal and muscle pains	150–600 mg/day depending on other antiviral medications
enfuvirtide *en-FYOO-veer-tide*	Fuzeon	HIV infection	Injection site discomfort, induration, erythema	90 mg subcutaneous injection BID
Integrase Inhibitors				
raltegravir *ral-TEG-ra-veer*	Isentress	HIV infection	Headache, nausea, diarrhea, fever	400 mg orally BID
dolutegravir *doe-loo-TEG-ra-veer*	Tivicay	HIV infection	Insomnia	50 mg orally once daily

 This drug should be administered at least 1 hr before or 2 hr after a meal.

CHAPTER REVIEW

Know Your Drugs

Clients sometimes know a medication by the brand (or trade) name and not the generic name. To help you recognize both names, match the brand name with the generic name of the same medication.

Generic Name	Brand Name
1. acyclovir	A. Prezista
2. darunavir	B. Tamiflu
3. oseltamivir	C. Valtrex
4. valacyclovir	D. Zovirax

Calculate Medication Dosages

1. The client is prescribed acyclovir 200 mg. The drug is available in 100-mg tablets. The nurse administers _____.

2. The nurse is to administer 100 mg of zidovudine orally. The drug is available as syrup 50 mg/5 mL. The nurse administers _____.

Prepare for the NCLEX

RECALL THE FACTS

1. Which of the following statements about a virus is true?
   1. They are about the same size as a bacterium.
   2. Reproduction occurs by invading a host cell.
   3. Travel is exclusively by blood-borne routes.
   4. There are only a limited number of viruses.
2. How do a virus and a retrovirus differ?
   1. Require cellular material of another (host) cell to reproduce.
   2. Viral content reprograms the cell to reproduce virus.
   3. They attack the host cell RNA instead of DNA.
   4. The infected cell goes back to the original function.
3. Which of the following adverse reactions would the nurse expect in a client receiving acyclovir by the oral route?
   1. Nausea and vomiting
   2. Constipation and urinary frequency
   3. Conjunctivitis and blurred vision
   4. Nephrotoxicity

4. Which of the following would the nurse report immediately in a 3-month-old client receiving ribavirin?
   1. Any worsening of the respiratory status
   2. Refusal to take foods or fluids
   3. Drowsiness
   4. Constipation
5. The nurse is administering didanosine properly when _____.
   1. the antacid is not separated in the liquid
   2. the drug is prepared for subcutaneous injection
   3. the drug is given with meals
   4. the drug is given mixed with orange juice or apple juice
6. Administration of antiretrovirals can result in _____.
   1. abnormal hair growth
   2. body fat redistribution
   3. cardiac arrest
   4. discoloration of the skin

ANALYZE THE FACTS

7. *As a nurse on a pediatric unit, you are making the assignment to care for an infant receiving aerosol ribavirin for RSV. Which of the following nurses should be assigned to care for this client?
   1. Doris, a 22-year-old registered nurse
   2. Ariel, a female respiratory therapist
   3. Brad, a 26-year-old licensed practical nurse
   4. Vanessa, a 45-year-old pediatric certified nurse
8. *Mr. Park is to begin acyclovir treatment for his outbreak of shingles. As the nurse initiating care for him, you will check the medication administration record to see which drug he is taking for potential interactions?
   1. Cimetidine
   2. Ibuprofen
   3. Sildenafil
   4. Theophylline

ALTERNATE-FORMAT QUESTIONS

9. A client is prescribed one inhalation of zanamivir every 12 hr. The drug is available as one 5-mg blister per inhalation and is to be given with a Diskhaler device. How many milligrams will the nurse administer in a 24-hr period?

10. Match the viral infection with its site of infection.

1. Hepatitis C virus

2. Human immunodeficiency virus

3. Herpes zoster virus

4. Human papilloma virus

5. Respiratory syncytial virus

A. lies dormant in the nervous system

B. most common sexually transmitted infection (STI)

C. inflammation of the liver

D. respiratory infection primarily in children

E. destroys the immune system

To check your answers, see Appendix F.

―――――――――

*Indicates the question is directly linked to the NCLEX-PN test plan in Appendix G.

WANT TO KNOW MORE? A wide variety of resources are available to enhance your learning and understanding of this chapter.

▪ Visit the**Point** for resources such as:
  • NCLEX-Style Student Review Questions
  • Journal Articles
  • Dosage Calculations
  • Drug Monographs
  • Watch and Learn Videos
  • Concepts in Action Animations

▪ The *Study Guide to Accompany Introductory Clinical Pharmacology,* 12th edition, sold separately, will help you review and apply essential content.

▪ ✓*PrepU* is available to help students prepare for the NCLEX-PN examination.

Antifungal and Antiparasitic Drugs

Key Terms

candidiasis infection of the skin or mucous membrane with the yeast *Candida albicans*

cinchonism quinidine toxicity or poisoning

fungicidal deadly to fungi

fungistatic pertaining to agents that retard growth of fungi

fungus single-cell, colorless plant that lacks chlorophyll, such as yeast or mold

helminthiasis invasion by helminths (worms)

mycotic infections infection caused by fungi

over the counter (OTC) pertaining to drugs or other substances sold without a prescription; also known as *nonprescription*

parasite organism living in or on another organism (host) without contributing to the survival or well-being of the host

thrush candidiasis (candidal infection) of the mouth

Learning Objectives

On completion of this chapter, the student will:

1. Differentiate between superficial and systemic fungal infections.
2. Compare and contrast helminthic infections, protozoal infections, and amebiasis.
3. Explain the uses, general drug actions, adverse reactions, contraindications, precautions, and interactions of antifungal and antiparasitic drugs.
4. Distinguish important preadministration and ongoing assessment activities the nurse should perform on the client receiving an antifungal and antiparasitic drug.
5. Identify nursing diagnoses particular to a client taking an antifungal and antiparasitic drug.
6. List possible goals for a client taking an antifungal and antiparasitic drug.
7. Examine ways to promote an optimal response to therapy, how to manage adverse reactions, and important points to keep in mind when educating the client and family about antifungal and antiparasitic drugs.

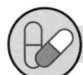 **Drug Classes**

| Antifungals | Anthelmintics | Antiprotozoals |

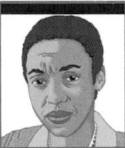 **PHARMACOLOGY IN PRACTICE**

Lillian Chase, age 36 years, is caring for her two grandchildren. She calls the clinic because she thinks they are unusually fussy during this visit. In asking about the children, there does not seem to be any indication they are ill. You discover that they typically play in a large sand lot at home. Think about questions to ask about the children as you read this chapter.

The drugs in this chapter fight infections caused by plants and insects. That is to say the drug classifications deal with infections caused by microscopic plants (the fungi and molds) and microscopic organisms (parasites and protozoa). Typically treated on an outpatient basis, these infections are seeing greater prominence in health care facilities owing to the vulnerability of clients who are immune compromised by disease or treatment for disease.

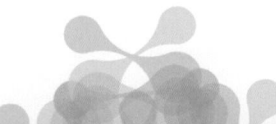

FUNGAL INFECTIONS

A **fungus** is a single-celled, colorless plant that lacks chlorophyll (Fig. 12.1). Fungi that cause disease in humans may be yeast-like or mold-like; the resulting infections are called fungal or **mycotic infections**.

Fungal infections range from superficial skin infections to life-threatening systemic infections. The superficial mycotic infections occur on the surface of, or just below, the skin or nails (see Chapter 52). *Systemic fungal infections* are serious infections that occur when fungi gain entrance into the interior of the body. These deep mycotic infections grow inside the body in sites such as in the lungs, brain, or gastrointestinal (GI) tract. Treatment of these deep mycotic infections is often difficult and prolonged.

Yeast infections caused by *Candida albicans* are known as **candidiasis**. Infection of the mouth by the microorganism *C. albicans* is commonly called **thrush**. Candidiasis also affects women in the vulvovaginal area and immunocompromised clients with chronic conditions in the perineum, the oral cavity, or systemically. Clients who are at an increased risk for candidal infections are those who have diabetes, are pregnant, or are taking oral contraceptives, antibiotics, or corticosteroids such as surgical clients.

Fungal infections are of great concern in those who receive organ transplants because of the ongoing use of antirejection drugs in this group of clients. The most common fungal infections seen in this population include candidiasis, aspergillosis (common mold), and *Cryptococcus neoformans* (cryptococcosis). The Summary Drug Table: Antifungal and Antiparasitic Drugs identifies drugs that are used to combat fungal infections.

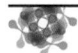 ## ANTIFUNGAL DRUGS

ACTIONS

Antifungal drugs may be **fungicidal** (destroy fungi) or **fungistatic** (slow or retard the multiplication of fungi). Amphotericin B, isavuconazonium (Cresemba), miconazole (Monistat), nystatin, voriconazole (Vfend), micafungin (Mycamine), and ketoconazole are thought to have an effect on the cell membrane of the fungus. The fungicidal or fungistatic effect of these drugs appears to be related to their concentration in body tissues. Fluconazole (Diflucan) has fungistatic activity that appears to result from the depletion of sterols (a group of substances related to fats) in the fungus cells.

Griseofulvin exerts its effect by being deposited in keratin precursor cells, which are then gradually lost (because of the constant shedding of top skin cells) and replaced by new, uninfected cells. The mode of action of flucytosine (Ancobon) is to inhibit DNA and RNA synthesis in the fungus. Clotrimazole (Lotrimin, Mycelex) binds with phospholipids in the fungal cell membrane, increasing permeability of the cell and resulting in loss of intracellular components.

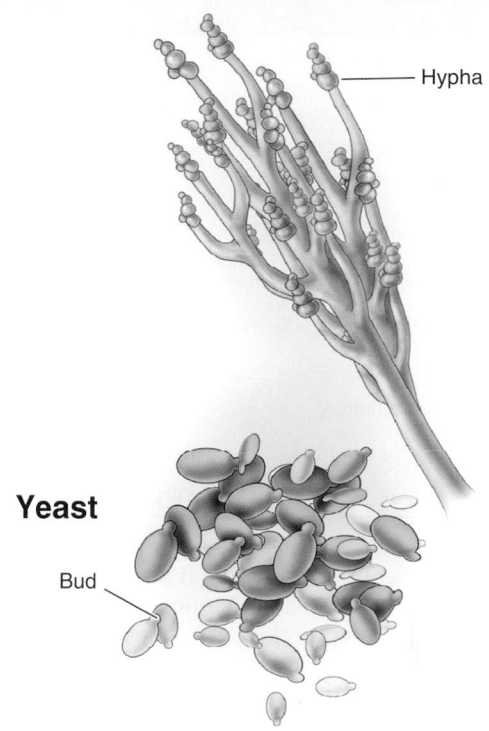

FIGURE 12.1 Examples of infection-causing fungi.

USES

Antifungal drugs are used prophylactically to prevent or to treat fungal infection in immunocompromised clients. They are also used to treat the following:

- Superficial and deep fungal infections
- Systemic infections such as aspergillosis, candidiasis, and cryptococcal meningitis
- Superficial infections of nail beds and oral, anal, and vaginal areas

The specific uses of antifungal drugs appear in the Summary Drug Table: Antifungal and Antiparasitic Drugs. Miconazole is an antifungal drug used to treat vulvovaginal "yeast" infections and is representative of all the vaginal antifungal agents. Fungal infections of the skin or mucous membranes may be treated with topical or vaginal preparations. A listing of the topical antifungal drugs appears in Table 12.1, and the vulvovaginal antifungal agents are listed in Table 12.2; these are also discussed in Chapter 52.

 H e r b a l   C o n s i d e r a t i o n s

Researchers have identified several antifungal herbs that are effective against skin infections, such as **tea tree oil** (*Melaleuca alternifolia*) and **garlic** (*Allium sativum*). Tea tree oil comes from an evergreen tree native to Australia. The herb has been used as a nonirritating antimicrobial

TABLE 12.1 Topical Antifungal Drugs

GENERIC NAME (FORM)	TRADE NAME(S)
butenafine HCl (cream)	Lotrimin, Mentax
ciclopirox (cream, lotion)	Ciclodan, Loprox, Penlac
clotrimazole (cream, solution, lotion)	Lotrimin
econazole (cream)	Ecoza
efinaconazole (solution)	Jublia
luliconazole (cream)	Luzu
miconazole (cream, solution, spray)	Monistat, Vusion
naftifine (cream, gel)	Naftin
oxiconazole (cream, lotion)	Oxistat
sulconazole (cream, solution)	Exelderm
tavaborole (solution)	Kerydin

for cuts, stings, wounds, burns, and acne. It can be found in shampoos, soaps, and lotions. Tea tree oil should not be ingested orally but is effective when used topically for minor cuts and stings. Topical application is most effective when used in a cream with at least 10% tea tree oil. Several commercially prepared ointments are available. The cream is applied to affected areas twice daily for several weeks.

Garlic is also used as an antifungal. A cream of 0.4% ajoene (the antifungal component of garlic) was found to relieve symptoms of athlete's foot and, like tea tree oil, is applied twice daily (DerMarderosian, 2003).

ADVERSE REACTIONS

Systemic Administration
- Headache
- Rash
- Anorexia and malaise
- Abdominal, joint, or muscle pain
- Nausea, vomiting, diarrhea

Topical Administration
- Site irritation
- Burning
- Crusting or drainage

CONTRAINDICATIONS

Antifungal drugs are contraindicated in clients with a history of allergy to the drug. Most of the systemic antifungal medications are contraindicated during pregnancy and lactation and are used only when the situation is life-threatening and outweighs the risk to the fetus.

Griseofulvin is not recommended for those with severe liver disease. Voriconazole is contraindicated when clients are taking the following medications: terfenadine, astemizole, sirolimus, rifampin, rifabutin, carbamazepine, ritonavir, ergot alkaloids, or long-acting barbiturates.

Both voriconazole and itraconazole are contraindicated in clients taking cisapride, pimozide, or quinidine. The

TABLE 12.2 Vaginal Antifungal Drugs

GENERIC NAME	SELECT TRADE NAME(S)
butoconazole nitrate	Gynazole-1
clotrimazole	Gyne-Lotrimin
miconazole	Monistat
nystatin	
terconazole	
tioconazole	Monistat-1

systemic agent itraconazole should not be used to treat fungal nail infections in clients with a history of heart failure.

PRECAUTIONS

Antifungals should be used cautiously in clients with renal dysfunction or hepatic impairment. Specific precautions include:

- Use amphotericin B cautiously in clients who have electrolyte imbalances or who currently use antineoplastic drugs (because severe bone marrow suppression can result).
- Administer griseofulvin cautiously with penicillin because of possible cross-sensitivity.
- Itraconazole should be used with caution in clients with human immunodeficiency virus (HIV) infection or hypochlorhydria (low levels of stomach acid).

INTERACTIONS

Possible interactions are dependent on each individual drug, and a number of interactions can occur. See Table 12.3 where drugs are listed in table format for better visualization.

LASA ALERT

The following drugs may sound alike; be sure to clarify when they are ordered:

Drug Name	*Sounds Like*
AmBisome	Ambisolm, Ambisom
Diflucan	diclofenac, Diprivan, disulfiram
fluconazole	flecainide, FLUoxetine, furosemide, itraconazole, voriconazole
itraconazole	fluconazole, posaconazole, voriconazole
miconazole	metroNIDAZOLE, Micronase, Micronor
Noxafil	minoxidil
Nystatin	atorvaSTATin, fluvastatin, lovastatin, pitavastatin, pravastatin, rosuvastatin, simvastatin, Nitrostat
Sporanox	Suprax, Topamax
terbinafine	terbutaline
Vfend	Venofer, Vimpat

Drugs that look alike are noted in the Summary Drug Tables of each chapter.

TABLE 12.3 Possible Interactions Between Antifungal and Other Drugs

INTERACTING DRUG	COMMON USE	EFFECT OF INTERACTION
Amphotericin B		
corticosteroids	Reduce inflammation	Risk for severe hypokalemia
digoxin	Management of cardiac problems	Increased risk of digitalis toxicity
aminoglycosides	Anti-infective agent	Increased risk of nephrotoxicity
cyclosporine	Immunosuppressant (particularly for transplant recipients)	Increased risk of nephrotoxicity
flucytosine	Antifungal	Drug toxicity
miconazole	Antifungal for vaginal infections	Decreased effectiveness of amphotericin B
Fluconazole		
oral hypoglycemics	Diabetes control	Increased effect of oral hypoglycemic
phenytoin	Seizure control	Decreased effectiveness of phenytoin
Griseofulvin		
barbiturates	Sedation	Decreased effectiveness of sedative
oral contraceptives	Birth control	Decreased effectiveness of birth control (breakthrough bleeding, pregnancy, or amenorrhea)
salicylates	Analgesia, pain relief	Decreased serum level of pain reliever
Itraconazole		
digoxin and cyclosporine	See above	Elevated blood levels of itraconazole
phenytoin, histamine antagonists	Antiseizure drug and GI acid suppressant, respectively	Decreased blood levels of itraconazole
isoniazid and rifampin	Antitubercular drugs	Decreased blood levels of itraconazole
Ketoconazole		
histamine antagonists and antacids	Control of GI upset	Decreased absorption of ketoconazole
rifampin or isoniazid	Antitubercular drugs	May decrease the blood levels of ketoconazole
Posaconazole		
cimetidine	GI acid suppressant	May decrease the blood levels of posaconazole
phenytoin	Seizure control	Increased effectiveness of phenytoin
rifabutin	Antitubercular drugs	May decrease the blood levels of posaconazole
statins	Reduce cholesterol	Increased effectiveness of statins
Voriconazole		
methadone, tacrolimus, the statins, benzodiazepines, calcium channel blockers	Addiction control and pain relief, immunosuppressant, lipid-lowering agents, sedative hypnotics, and blood pressure or angina control, respectively	Increased effectiveness of voriconazole
sulfonylureas	Diabetes control	Hypoglycemia
vinca alkaloids	Antineoplastic (chemotherapy) agents	Increased risk of neurotoxicity
Micafungin		
sirolimus	Immunosuppression	Risk of greater immunosuppression

TABLE 12.3 Possible Interactions Between Antifungal and Other Drugs (Continued)

INTERACTING DRUG	COMMON USE	EFFECT OF INTERACTION
nifedipine	Management of angina (chest pain)	Risk of nifedipine toxicity
Terbinafine		
Beta blockers and antidepressants	Cardiac problems and depression, respectively	Increased effectiveness of the beta blocker and antidepressant
Fluconazole, ketoconazole, itraconazole, voriconazole, or griseofulvin		
warfarin	Blood thinner	Increased risk of bleeding

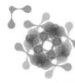

NURSING PROCESS STEPS TO BUILDING CLINICAL JUDGMENT
Client Receiving an Antifungal Drug

ASSESSMENT

Preadministration Assessment
Data gathering suggestions before giving the first dose of an antifungal drug include:
Objective data

- Vital signs (temperature, pulse, respirations, and blood pressure)
- Description of the infection—describe white plaques or sore areas on mucous membranes of the oral or perineal areas, as well as any vaginal discharge
- If the client is scheduled to receive amphotericin or flucytosine for a systemic fungal infection, be sure to weigh the client because the dosage of the drug is determined according to the client's weight

Subjective data

- Current symptoms of the infection (especially pain)
- Allergy history, particularly a drug allergy
- Drug history, particularly other antifungals, medicated creams, or home remedies used for this infection

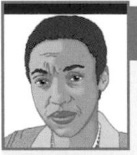

PHARMACOLOGY IN PRACTICE

ASSESSMENT
A nurse is required to assess a client for symptoms of a systemic mycotic infection. In which body part is a systemic mycotic infection most likely to be found?
1. Spleen
2. Lungs
3. Toe
4. Heart

Ongoing Assessment
When these drugs are used to treat systemic fungal infections, ongoing assessment involves careful observation of the client every 2–4 hr for adverse drug reactions. When these drugs are administered topically or on an outpatient basis, instruct the client in what to look for when gathering ongoing assessment data. This should include signs of improvement and adverse reactions, both minor and severe (requiring immediate notification of the primary health care provider).

NURSING DIAGNOSES
Drug-specific nursing diagnoses are the following:

- **Impaired comfort** related to intravenous (IV) administration of amphotericin B
- **Altered tissue perfusion: renal** related to adverse reactions of the antifungal drug

Nursing diagnoses related to drug administration are discussed in Chapter 4.

PLANNING
The expected outcomes for the client depend on the reason for administering the antifungal drug but may include a therapeutic response to the antifungal drug, client needs related to the management of adverse reactions, and confidence in an understanding of the medication regimen.

IMPLEMENTATION

Promoting an Optimal Response to Therapy: Administering Specific Antifungal Drugs

Amphotericin B
Amphotericin B is given only under close supervision typically in the hospital or clinic setting. Its use is reserved for serious and potentially life-threatening fungal infections. This drug is administered daily or every other day over several days or months.

The IV solution of amphotericin B is light sensitive and should be protected from exposure to light. If the solution is used within 8 hr, there is negligible loss of drug activity. Therefore, once the drug is reconstituted, administer the medication immediately, because the typical IV infusion is for a period of 6 hr or more. Consult the clinical pharmacist regarding whether to use a protective covering for the infusion container.

NURSING ALERT
Renal damage is the most serious adverse reaction to the use of amphotericin B. Renal impairment usually improves with a modification of the dosage regimen (reduced dosage or increased time between doses). Serum creatinine levels and blood urea nitrogen (BUN) levels are checked frequently during the course of therapy to monitor

kidney function. If the BUN exceeds 40 mg/dL or the serum creatinine level exceeds 3 mg/dL, the primary health care provider may discontinue the drug or reduce the dosage until renal function improves.

Nonsystemic Antifungal Infection Preparations

When a vaginal fungal infection is treated with miconazole during pregnancy, a vaginal applicator may be contraindicated. Manual insertion of the vaginal tablets may be preferred. Because small amounts of these drugs may be absorbed from the vagina, they are used only when essential during the first trimester.

Oral thrush infections (candidiasis) may be treated with oral solutions. Instruct the client to swish and hold the solution in the mouth for several seconds (or as long as possible), gargle, and swallow the solution. Oral infections also may be treated with medication lozenges. Sometimes the vaginal troche preparation of an antifungal medication is prescribed for oral use. The client needs specific instructions on how to use the medication to prevent confusion and improper use.

Monitoring and Managing Client Needs

Impaired Comfort: Medication Administration

When administering amphotericin B by IV infusion, be aware that immediate adverse reactions can occur. Nausea, vomiting, hypotension, tachypnea, fever, and chills (sometimes called *rigors*) may occur within 15–20 min of beginning the IV infusion. To prevent these adverse reactions, clients may be premedicated with antipyretics, antihistamines, or antiemetics. It is important to monitor the client's temperature, pulse, respirations, and blood pressure carefully during the first 30 min–1 hr of treatment. Monitor vital signs every 2–4 hr during therapy, depending on the client's condition. Also check the IV infusion rate and the infusion site frequently during administration of the drug. This is especially important if the client is restless or confused.

Clients should be taught before the drug is given that the side effects can be uncomfortable. Warm blankets should be provided for client comfort. Reassure the client that the medications administered before the antifungal will help to ease the adverse reactions. Instruction should include that the reactions decrease with ongoing therapy.

Altered Tissue Perfusion: Renal

When the client is taking a drug that is potentially toxic to the kidneys, carefully monitor fluid intake and output. If the client is known to have renal compromise, perform hourly measurements of urine output. Periodic laboratory tests are usually ordered to monitor the client's response to therapy and detect toxic reactions. Serum creatinine and BUN levels are checked frequently during the course of therapy to monitor kidney function. If the BUN exceeds 40 mg/dL or if the serum creatinine level exceeds 3 mg/dL, the primary health care provider may discontinue the drug therapy or reduce the dosage until renal function improves.

 Lifespan Considerations

Gerontology

Before administering fluconazole to an older adult or a client with renal impairment, the primary health care provider may order a creatinine clearance test. Watch for and report the laboratory results to the primary health care provider because the dosage may be adjusted based on the test results.

Educating the Client and Family

If the client is being treated in the ambulatory care setting, include the following points in the teaching plan:

- Clean the involved area and apply the ointment or cream to the skin as directed by the primary health care provider.
- Do not increase or decrease the amount used or the number of times the ointment or cream should be applied unless directed to do so by the primary health care provider.

Drug-specific teaching points include:

- Flucytosine—Nausea and vomiting may occur with this drug. Reduce or eliminate these effects by taking a few capsules at a time during a 15-min period. If nausea, vomiting, or diarrhea persists, notify the primary health care provider as soon as possible.
- Griseofulvin—Beneficial effects may not be noticed for some time; therefore, take the drug for the full course of therapy. Avoid exposure to sunlight and sunlamps because an exaggerated skin reaction (which is similar to severe sunburn) may occur even after a brief exposure to ultraviolet light. Notify the primary health care provider if fever, sore throat, or skin rash occurs.
- Ketoconazole—Complete the full course of therapy as prescribed by the primary health care provider. Do not take this drug with an antacid. In addition, avoid the use of nonprescription drugs unless use of a specific drug is approved by the primary health care provider. This drug may produce headache, dizziness, and drowsiness. If drowsiness or dizziness occurs, use caution while driving or performing other hazardous tasks. Notify the primary health care provider if pronounced abdominal pain, fever, or diarrhea occurs.
- Itraconazole—The drug is taken with food. Therapy continues for at least 3 months until infection is controlled. Report unusual fatigue, yellow skin, darkened urine, anorexia, nausea, and vomiting.
- Miconazole—If the drug (cream or tablet) is administered vaginally, insert the drug high in the vagina using the applicator provided with the product. Wear a panty liner after insertion of the drug to prevent staining of the clothing and bed linen. Continue taking the drug during the menstrual period if the vaginal route is being used. Do not have intercourse while taking this drug, or advise the partner to use a condom to avoid reinfection. To prevent recurrent infections, avoid nylon, thong underwear, and tight-fitting garments. If there is no improvement in 5–7 days, stop using the drug and consult the primary care provider, because a more serious infection may be present. If abdominal pain,

pelvic pain, rash, fever, or offensive-smelling vaginal discharge is present, do not use the drug, but notify the primary health care provider.

EVALUATION

• Therapeutic response is achieved and there is no evidence of infection.

• Adverse reactions are identified, reported to the primary health care provider, and managed successfully with appropriate nursing interventions:
  • Client reports comfort, without fever or chills.
  • Kidney perfusion is maintained.
• Client and family express confidence and demonstrate understanding of the drug regimen.

PARASITIC INFECTIONS

A **parasite** is an organism that lives in or on another organism (the host) without contributing to the survival or well-being of the host. These infections are infrequent in most populations in the United States except the immunocompromised. **Helminthiasis** (invasion of the body by parasitic worms) and protozoal infections (invasion of the body by single-celled parasites or malaria) are worldwide health problems. What makes these diseases especially worthy of concern is the frequency of global air travel in modern society. Conditions once confined to specific parts of the world can now be spread in hours or days by air travel.

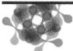 ## ANTHELMINTIC DRUGS

Roundworms, pinworms, whipworms, hookworms, and tapeworms are examples of helminths. The most common parasitic worm across the world is the roundworm. In the United States, the most common worm seen is the pinworm. *Anthelmintic* (against helminths) drugs are used to treat helminthiasis.

ACTIONS AND USES

Although the actions of anthelmintic drugs vary, their primary purpose is to kill parasites.

Albendazole (Albenza) interferes with the synthesis of the parasite's microtubules, resulting in death of susceptible larvae. This drug is used to treat larval forms of pork tapeworm and to treat liver, lung, and peritoneal disease caused by the dog tapeworm.

Mebendazole blocks the uptake of glucose by the helminth, resulting in depletion of the helminth's own glycogen. This drug is used to treat whipworm, pinworm, roundworm, American hookworm, and the common hookworm.

The activity of pyrantel is probably because of its ability to paralyze the helminth. Paralysis causes the helminth to release its grip on the intestinal wall, after which it can be excreted in the feces. Pyrantel is used to treat roundworm and pinworm.

ADVERSE REACTIONS

Generalized adverse reactions include the following:

• Drowsiness, dizziness
• Nausea, vomiting
• Abdominal pain and cramps, diarrhea

Adverse reactions associated with the anthelmintic drugs, if they do occur, are usually mild when the drug is used in the recommended dosage. Rash is a serious adverse reaction to pyrantel, which is sold **over the counter** (OTC), without a prescription. As such, clients may begin self-treatment before notifying their primary health provider. Therefore, it is important to ask the client about skin reactions when use of this medication is disclosed to the provider. For more information, see the Summary Drug Table: Antifungal and Antiparasitic Drugs.

CONTRAINDICATIONS AND PRECAUTIONS

The anthelmintic drugs are contraindicated in clients with known hypersensitivity to the drugs and during pregnancy (pregnancy category C). They should be used cautiously in lactating clients, clients with hepatic or renal impairment, and clients with malnutrition or anemia.

INTERACTIONS

The following interactions may occur when a specific anthelmintic drug is administered with another agent:

Interacting Drug	Common Use	Effect of Interaction
albendazole (Albenza)		
dexamethasone	Inflammation or immunosuppression	Increased effectiveness of albendazole
cimetidine	Relief of GI problems, such as heartburn	Increased effectiveness of albendazole
mebendazole		
hydantoins and carbamazepine	Seizure control	Lower levels of mebendazole

LASA ALERT

The following drugs may sound alike; be sure to clarify when they are ordered:

Drug Name	Sounds Like
Albenza	Aplenzin, Relenza

Drugs that look alike are noted in the Summary Drug Tables of each chapter.

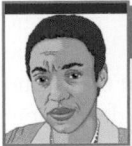

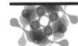 ANTIPROTOZOAL DRUGS

One of the greatest protozoal problems worldwide is the treatment and prevention of malaria. Although malaria is rare in the United States, on a worldwide scale, almost 200 million new cases of malaria occur yearly, with a yearly death rate of more than half million people (WHO, 2020). As global travel increases, more people may be at risk depending on where they go. The protozoal infections seen in the United States include giardiasis (contracted from contaminated food or water), trichomoniasis, toxoplasmosis, and opportunistic infections (such as pneumonia seen in immunocompromised clients). Examples of antiprotozoal drugs in use today are listed in the Summary Drug Table: Antifungal and Antiparasitic Drugs.

ACTIONS

Protozoa are single-celled animals. The protozoan that causes malaria is *Plasmodium falciparum*. Malaria is used as an example of how protozoa infect people. It is transmitted from person to person by certain species of the *Anopheles* mosquito. Figure 12.2 illustrates the life cycle

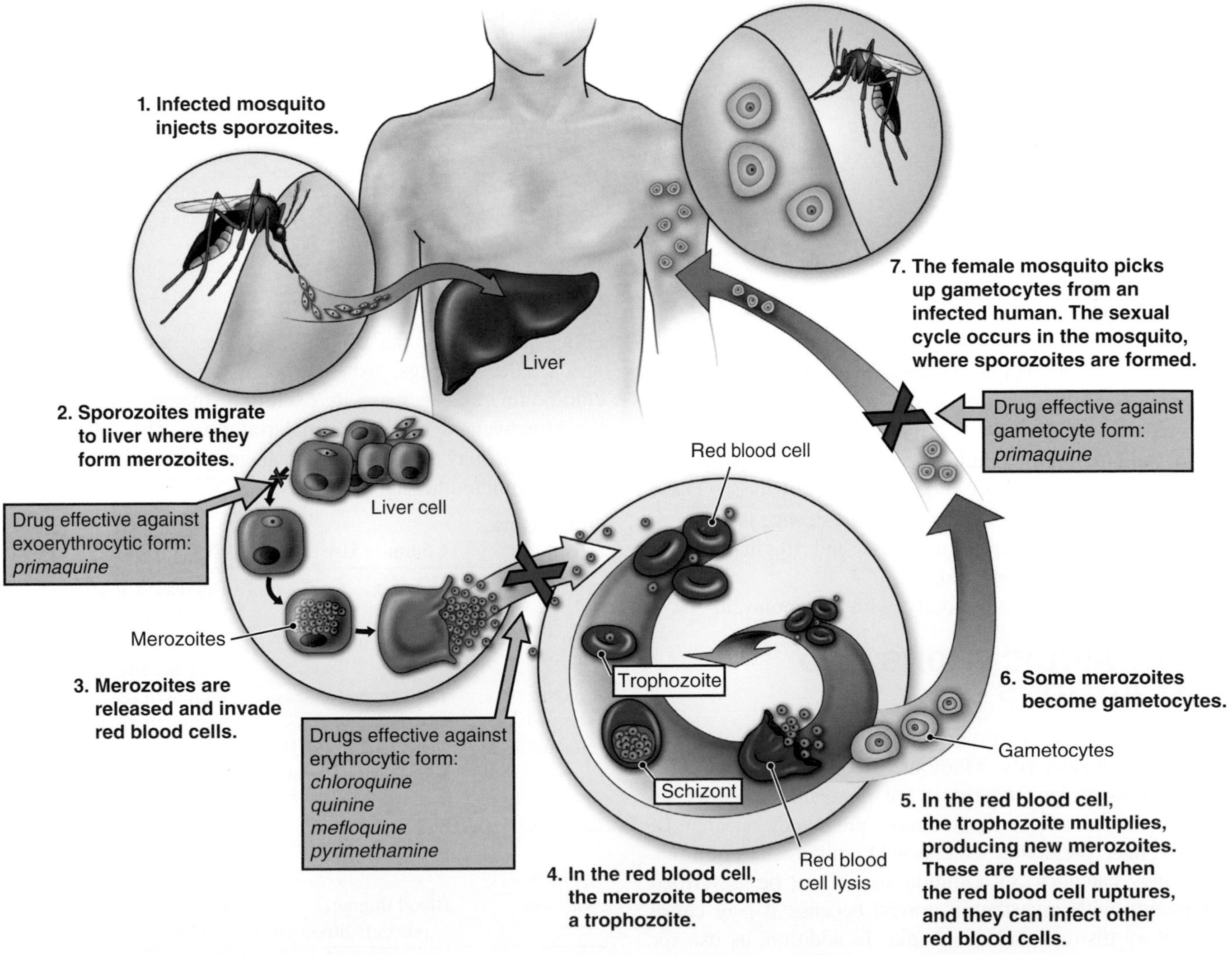

1. Infected mosquito injects sporozoites.

2. Sporozoites migrate to liver where they form merozoites.

Drug effective against exoerythrocytic form: *primaquine*

Liver cell

Liver

Merozoites

3. Merozoites are released and invade red blood cells.

Drugs effective against erythrocytic form:
chloroquine
quinine
mefloquine
pyrimethamine

Red blood cell

Trophozoite

Schizont

4. In the red blood cell, the merozoite becomes a trophozoite.

Red blood cell lysis

5. In the red blood cell, the trophozoite multiplies, producing new merozoites. These are released when the red blood cell ruptures, and they can infect other red blood cells.

6. Some merozoites become gametocytes.

Gametocytes

7. The female mosquito picks up gametocytes from an infected human. The sexual cycle occurs in the mosquito, where sporozoites are formed.

Drug effective against gametocyte form: *primaquine*

FIGURE 12.2 Life cycle of the malarial parasite and the sites of action of antimalarial drugs.

of malaria transmission and the drugs used in treatment. On the other hand, transmission of the more common protozoans (*Giardia, Trichomonas,* and *Toxoplasma* spp.) occurs through contaminated food or water, by fecal matter, or through sexual intercourse. In immunocompromised clients, the organism *Pneumocystis jirovecii* causes pneumonia. Antiprotozoal drugs interfere with, or are active against, the life cycle of the protozoan.

USES

Infectious Disease

Antiprotozoal drugs may be used to treat infections such as:

- Malaria
- Giardiasis
- Toxoplasmosis
- Intestinal amebiasis
- Sexually transmitted infections (trichomoniasis)
- *Pneumocystis* pneumonia (PCP)

Prophylaxis

Antimalarial drugs are used for suppressing (i.e., preventing) malaria.

ADVERSE REACTIONS

GI reactions include the following:

- Anorexia
- Nausea, vomiting
- Abdominal cramping and diarrhea

Other Reactions
- Headache and dizziness
- Visual disturbances or tinnitus
- Hypotension or changes detected on an electrocardiogram (associated with chloroquine)
- **Cinchonism**—a group of symptoms associated with quinine administration, including tinnitus, dizziness, headache, GI disturbances, and visual disturbances. These symptoms usually disappear when the dosage is reduced
- Peripheral neuropathy (numbness and tingling of the extremities), with metronidazole
- Nephrotoxicity and ototoxicity, with paromomycin

CONTRAINDICATIONS AND PRECAUTIONS

Antiprotozoal drugs are contraindicated in clients with known hypersensitivity. Many of the drugs are contraindicated during pregnancy (most are pregnancy category C; except metronidazole, nitazoxanide, pregnancy category B; doxycycline, pregnancy category D; miltefosine, quinine, pregnancy category X). Quinine should not be prescribed for clients with myasthenia gravis, because it may cause respiratory distress and dysphagia. In addition, its use for

leg cramps is discouraged because of the hematologic reactions that may occur. Antiprotozoal drugs should be used cautiously in children, lactating clients, and those who have hepatic or renal disease or bone marrow depression. Pregnancy category B antiprotozoals should be used cautiously in clients during pregnancy and lactation (can be given during the second and third trimesters) and in clients with blood dyscrasias, seizure disorders, severe hepatic impairment (metronidazole), bowel disease (paromomycin use interferes with absorption causing ototoxicity and renal impairment), or history of alcohol dependency. Clients with a history of mental health issues should not be prescribed mefloquine.

LASA ALERT

The following drugs may sound alike; be sure to clarify when they are ordered:

Drug Name	Sounds Like
hydroxychloroquine	hydrocortisone, hydroxyurea
malarone	mefloquine
metroNIDAZOLE	mebendazole, meropenem, metFORMIN, methotrexate, metoclopramide, miconazole
Plaquenil	Platinol
primaquine	primidone

Drugs that look alike are noted in the Summary Drug Tables of each chapter.

INTERACTIONS

Foods that acidify the urine (cranberries, plums, prunes, meats, cheeses, eggs, fish, and grains) may interact with chloroquine and increase its excretion, thereby decreasing the effectiveness of the antimalarial drug. The following interactions may also occur when an antiprotozoal is administered with another agent:

Interacting Drug	Common Use	Effect of Interaction
antacids	GI upset	Decreased absorption of the antimalarial
iron	Treat anemia	Decreased absorption of the antimalarial
digoxin	Treat cardiac disease	Increased risk of digoxin toxicity
cimetidine	Management of GI upset or heartburn	Decreased metabolism of metronidazole
phenobarbital	Sedative	Increased metabolism of metronidazole
Quinine		
warfarin	Blood thinner, prevents blood clots	Increased risk of bleeding

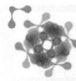

NURSING PROCESS STEPS TO BUILDING CLINICAL JUDGMENT
Client Receiving an Antiparasitic Drug

ASSESSMENT

Preadministration Assessment

Clients with parasitic infections may or may not be acutely ill. The acutely ill client requires hospitalization, but many individuals with parasitic infections can be treated on an outpatient basis.

Data gathering suggestions before administering an antiparasitic drug include:

Objective data

- General client appearance and vital signs
- Collection of stool specimens, typically serial collection needs to be made to see and identify the parasite

Subjective data

- Description of bowel movements—number, consistency, color, and frequency of stools if parasitic infection is suspected to be transmitted by the GI route
- History of travel or routine if no symptoms are identified

A relatively common infection, especially in pediatric populations, is the pinworm (helminth) infection. When a pinworm infection is suspected, instruct the parent on how to take a specimen from the anal area, preferably early in the morning before the client gets out of bed. Specimens are taken by swabbing the perianal area with a cellophane tape-covered swab.

Ongoing Assessment

Unless ordered otherwise, instruct the parent to observe all stools that are passed after the drug is given. It is important to inspect each stool visually for passage of the helminth. If stool specimens are to be saved for laboratory examination, follow facility procedure for saving the stool and transporting it to the laboratory. If the client is acutely ill or has a massive infection, it is important to monitor vital signs every 4 hr and measure and record fluid intake and output. Observe the client for adverse drug reactions, as well as severe episodes of diarrhea. It is important to notify the primary health care provider if these occur.

NURSING DIAGNOSES

The nursing diagnoses depend on the client and the type of parasitic infection. Drug-specific nursing diagnoses are the following:

- **Diarrhea** related to parasitic invasion of body
- **Hypovolemia/dehydration** related to parasitic invasion of body
- **Malnutrition** related to adverse effects of drug therapy
- **Ineffective airway clearance** related to adverse effects of drug therapy

Nursing diagnoses related to drug administration are discussed in Chapter 4.

PLANNING

The expected outcomes for the client depend on the reason for administering the antiparasitic but may include an optimal response to drug therapy, meeting client needs related to management of common adverse reactions, and confidence in an understanding of the therapeutic regimen.

IMPLEMENTATION

Promoting an Optimal Response to Therapy: Proper Administration

When treating a client for a parasitic infection, instruct the family on methods to prevent reinfection or passing the infection on to other persons. Instruct the family in frequent changing and washing of bed linens and undergarments. Caregivers need to also take care in obtaining or handling stool specimens. Instruct the client to wash their hands thoroughly after personal care and before meals.

When taking the drug pentamidine, clients should be placed in a reclining or supine position to prevent adverse effects should a sudden decrease in blood pressure occur. The client should be monitored for hypotension over a number of doses to be sure the client remains stable during treatments.

When administering an antimalarial drug, such as chloroquine, for prophylaxis (prevention), therapy should begin 2 weeks before exposure and continue for 6–8 weeks after the client leaves the area where malaria is prevalent.

Monitoring and Managing Client Needs

Diarrhea and Hypovolemia/Dehydration

Daily stool specimens may be ordered to be sent to the laboratory for examination. Keep a record of the number, consistency, color, and frequency of stools. Immediately deliver all stool specimens saved for examination to the laboratory because the organisms may die (and therefore cannot be seen microscopically). Inform laboratory personnel that the client has a parasite, because the specimen must be kept at or near body temperature until examined under a microscope.

Also monitor fluid intake and output and symptoms of a fluid volume deficit, and make sure the client is clean and the room free of odor. If dehydration is apparent, notify the primary health care provider. If the client is or becomes dehydrated, oral or IV fluid and electrolyte replacement may be necessary.

Malnutrition

GI upset may occur, causing nausea, vomiting, abdominal pain, and diarrhea. Taking the drug with food often helps to alleviate the nausea. The client may require frequent, small meals of easily digested food. A discussion of eating habits, food preferences, and food aversions assists in meal planning. Monitor body weight daily to identify any changes (increase or decrease). Make sure that meals are well balanced nutritionally, appetizing, and attractively served. Consult the registered dietitian if necessary.

Ineffective Airway Clearance

Bronchospasm or cough is more likely to occur when inhaled treatments of pentamidine are given. The primary health care provider may prescribe a bronchodilator to be given before the pentamidine treatment. Instruct the client and caregivers in the proper methods of administration and care of the respiratory equipment used at home with pentamidine (see Client Teaching for Improved Outcomes: Administering Pentamidine at Home).

Educating the Client and Family

When an antiparasitic is prescribed on an outpatient basis, give the client or family member complete instructions about taking the drug, as well as household precautions that should be followed until the parasite is eliminated from the intestine. Should the family have limited English proficiency, be sure to include language-appropriate written materials. When developing a client education plan, be sure to include the following:

- Follow the dosage schedule exactly as printed on the prescription container. It is absolutely necessary to follow the directions for taking the drug to eradicate the parasite.
- Follow-up stool specimens will be necessary because this is the only way to determine the success of drug therapy.
- When an infection is diagnosed, multiple members of the family may be infected, and all household members may need to be treated. Playmates of the infected child may also need to be treated.
- It is important to wash all bedding and bed clothes once treatment has started.
- Daily bathing (showering is best) is recommended. Disinfect toilet facilities daily, and disinfect the bathtub or shower stall immediately after bathing. Use the disinfectant recommended by the primary health care provider or use chlorine bleach. Scrub the surfaces thoroughly and allow the disinfectant to remain in contact with the surfaces for several minutes.
- During treatment for a ringworm infection, keep towels and facecloths for bathing separate from those of other family members to avoid the spread of the infection. It is important to keep the affected area clean and dry.
- Wash the hands thoroughly after urinating or defecating and before preparing and eating food. Clean under the fingernails daily and avoid putting fingers in the mouth or biting the nails.
- Food handlers should not resume work until a full course of treatment is completed and stools do not contain the parasite.
- Child care workers should be especially careful of diaper disposal and proper hand washing to prevent the spread of infections.
- Report any symptoms of infection (low-grade fever or sore throat) or thrombocytopenia (easy bruising or bleeding).
- Albendazole can cause serious harm to a developing fetus. Inform women of childbearing age of this. Explain that a barrier contraceptive is recommended during the course of therapy and for 1 month after discontinuing the therapy.
- When an antimalarial drug is used for preventing malaria and taken once a week, the client also must take the drug on the same day each week. The prevention program is usually started 1 week before the individual departs to an area where malaria is prevalent.

Client Teaching for Improved Outcomes

Administering Pentamidine at Home

The client may be required to receive aerosol pentamidine at home. Before discharge, the nurse checks to make sure arrangements have been made to deliver the specialized equipment and supplies, such as nebulizer and diluent, to the home.

When you teach, make sure your client and the caregiver understand the following:

✔ Prepare the solution immediately before use.
✔ Dissolve the contents in the proper amount of sterile water and protect the solution from light.
✔ Place the entire solution in the nebulizer's reservoir. Do not put any other drugs into the reservoir.
✔ Attach the tubing to the nebulizer and reservoir.
✔ Place the mouthpiece in your mouth and turn on the nebulizer.
✔ Breathe in and out deeply and slowly. The entire treatment should last 30–45 min.
✔ Tap the reservoir periodically to ensure that the entire drug is aerosolized.
✔ When the treatment is finished, turn off the nebulizer.
✔ Clean the equipment according to the manufacturer's instructions.
✔ Allow tubing, reservoir, and mouthpiece to air dry.
✔ Store the equipment in a clean plastic bag and put it away for the next dose.
✔ Use a calendar to mark the days you are to receive the drug and check off each time you have done the treatment.

EVALUATION

- Therapeutic response is achieved, and there is no evidence of infection.
- Adverse reactions are identified, reported to the primary health care provider, and managed successfully with appropriate nursing interventions:
  - Client reports adequate bowel movements.
  - Adequate fluid volume is maintained.
  - Client maintains an adequate nutritional status.
  - Lungs function effectively.
- Client and family express confidence and demonstrate understanding of the drug regimen.

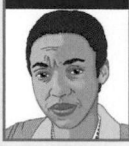

PHARMACOLOGY IN PRACTICE

USING CLINICAL REASONING

While listening to Lillian Chase talk about her grandchildren, the primary health care provider suspects the children may have pinworms. Determine what you would include in teaching Lillian how to collect a specimen for examination and a teaching plan to prevent the spread of pinworms to other family members.

KEY POINTS

■ A fungus is a single-celled plant that can cause yeast-like infections. These are called fungal or mycotic infections. Antifungal drugs slow the growth of or destroy fungi.

■ Superficial fungal infections to the skin, nails, and genital area are bothersome and are treated topically or by oral preparations. Systemic infections happen when the fungi gain entry into the body; these are serious infections, especially for those who are immunocompromised.

■ Most antifungals used for superficial infections cause minimal adverse reactions such as headache, rash, or minor GI disturbances. Antifungals used for systemic infections can cause greater adverse reactions. Clients are premedicated with antipyretics, antihistamines, and antiemetics because of the adverse reactions (chills, fever, rigors, etc.) caused by amphotericin B. Renal function should be moni-

tored when older adults and renal clients take these medications.

■ Helminthiasis and protozoal infections are caused when a parasite invades a host organism. Although these infections are found infrequently in the United States, they of concern because travelers can bring them back home. Because many more people travel worldwide, many travelers are treated prophylactically to prevent infection.

■ Many of these infections are treated on an outpatient basis, so client and caregiver confidence in managing the treatment and adverse reactions is important. Clients and caregivers need teaching to separate items of the infected person from those of other family members to prevent infection or reinfection.

SUMMARY DRUG TABLE
Antifungal Drugs and Antiparasitic Drugs

Generic Name	Trade Name	Uses	Adverse Reactions	Dosage Ranges
Antifungal Drugs				
amphotericin B *am-foe-TER-i-sin bee*	Abelcet, AmBisome, Amphotec	Systemic life-threatening fungal infections, cryptococcal meningitis in clients with HIV infection	Headache, hypotension, fever, shaking, chills, malaise, nausea, vomiting, diarrhea, abnormal renal function, joint and muscle pain	Desoxycholate: 1–1.5 mg/kg/day IV Lipid-based: 3–6 mg/kg/day IV
anidulafungin *ay-nid-yoo-la-FUN-jin*	Eraxis	Abdominal and esophageal candidiasis	Headache, rash, nausea, vomiting	100- to 200-mg loading dose IV, followed by 50–100 mg/day IV for at least 14 days
caspofungin *kas-poe-FUN-jin*	Cancidas	Invasive aspergillosis, esophageal candidiasis	Headache, rash, nausea, vomiting, abdominal pain, hematologic changes, fever	70-mg loading dose IV, followed by 50 mg/day IV for at least 14 days
fluconazole *floo-KOE-na-zole*	Diflucan	Oropharyngeal and esophageal candidiasis, vaginal candidiasis, cryptococcal meningitis	Headache, nausea, vomiting, diarrhea, skin rash	50–400 mg/day orally, IV
flucytosine (5-FC) *floo-SYE-toe-seen*	Ancobon	Systemic fungal infections	Nausea, diarrhea, rash, anemia, leukopenia, thrombocytopenia, renal insufficiency	50–150 mg/kg/day orally q6h
griseofulvin *gri-see-oh-FUL-vin*		Ringworm infections of the skin, hair, nails	Nausea, vomiting, diarrhea, oral thrush, headache, rash, urticaria	For ringworm and jock itch: 330–375 mg orally in a single or divided dose For athlete's foot: 660–750 mg/day orally in divided doses; take for 2–6 week until the infection is completely gone
isavuconazonium *eye-sa-vue-koe-na-ZOE-nee-um*	Cresemba	Systemic *Aspergillus* infections	Nausea, vomiting, abdominal pain, headache	372 mg IV/orally every 8 hr for 6 doses, 372 mg daily

Continued

SUMMARY DRUG TABLE (continued)
Antifungal Drugs and Antiparasitic Drugs

Generic Name	Trade Name	Uses	Adverse Reactions	Dosage Ranges
itraconazole *i-tra-KOE-na-zole*	Sporanox, Tolsura	Systemic fungal infections, may be used for nail infections	Nausea, vomiting, diarrhea, rash, abdominal pain, edema, hypokalemia in dosages over 600 mg/day	200–400 mg/day orally; IV as a single or divided dose Nail infections: 200 mg BID for 1 week, then repeat in 3 week
ketoconazole *kee-toe-KOE-na-zole*		Treatment of resistant systemic fungal infections	Nausea, vomiting, abdominal pain, headache, pruritus	200 mg/day orally; may increase to 400 mg/day orally
micafungin *my-ka-FUN-jin*	Mycamine	Esophageal candidiasis, candidal infection prevention in stem cell transplantation	Rash, pruritus, facial swelling, vasodilation, flushing, headache, dizziness, anorexia, nausea, vomiting	150 mg/day IV
miconazole *my-KON-a-zole*	Oravig	Oropharyngeal candidiasis	Headache, nausea	50 mg oral cavity daily
nystatin, oral *nye-STAT-in*	Bio-Statin	Nonesophageal GI membrane candidiasis	Rash, diarrhea, nausea, vomiting	500,000–1 million units TID
posaconazole *poe-sa-KON-a-zole*	Noxafil	Oral/pharyngeal candidiasis, prophylaxis of fungal infections	Headache; fever; abdominal pain; diarrhea; low potassium, red and white cells, and platelets	100–200 mg orally, 1–3 times daily
terbinafine *TER-bin-a-feen*		Nail fungal infections	Headache, nausea, flatulence, diarrhea, rash	250 mg/day for 6–12 week
voriconazole *vor-i-KOE-na-zole*	Vfend	*Aspergillus* systemic fungal infections	Visual disturbances, fever, rash, headache, anorexia, nausea, vomiting, diarrhea, peripheral edema, photosensitivity	Loading dose: 6 mg/kg q12h for the first day Maintenance: If tolerated orally: 200 mg q12h; if unable to take orally: 4 mg/kg q12h IV until able to switch to oral drug

Antiparasitic Drugs
Anthelmintic Drugs

albendazole *al-BEN-da-zole*	Albenza	Parenchymal neurocysticercosis caused by pork tapeworms, hydatid disease (caused by the larval form of the dog tapeworm)	Abnormal liver function test results, abdominal pain, nausea, vomiting, headache, dizziness	Weight greater than or equal to 60 kg: 400 mg Weight less than 60 kg: 15 mg/kg/day
ivermectin *eye-ver-MEK-tin*	Stromectol	Treatment of threadworm	Pruritus, rash, lymph node tenderness	Single dose of 200 µg/kg
mebendazole *me-BEN-da-zole*	Emverm	Treatment of whipworm, pinworm, roundworm, common and American hookworm	Transient abdominal pain, diarrhea	100 mg orally morning and evening for 3 consecutive days Pinworm: 100 mg orally as a single dose
praziquantel *Pray-zi-KWON-tel*	Biltricide	Treatment of liver flukes	Malaise, headache, dizziness, abdominal pain	25 mg/kg TID for 1 day
pyrantel *pi-RAN-tel*	Reese's pinworm	Treatment of pinworm and roundworm	Anorexia, nausea, vomiting, abdominal cramps, diarrhea, rash (serious)	11 mg/kg orally as a single dose; maximum dose, 1000 mg
triclabendazole *try-KLUH-bend-uh-zole*	Egaten	Treatment of flatworm	Headache, nausea, abdominal cramps, diarrhea	10 mg/kg/dose orally every 12 hr for 1 day

Generic Name	Trade Name	Uses	Adverse Reactions	Dosage Ranges
Antiprotozoal Drugs				
Primary Antimalarial Drugs				
chloroquine *KLOR-oh-kwin*		Treatment and prevention of malaria, extraintestinal amebiasis	Hypotension, electrocardiographic changes, headache, nausea, vomiting, anorexia, diarrhea, abdominal cramps, visual disturbances	Treatment: 160–200 mg IM and repeat in 6 hr if necessary Prevention: 300 mg orally weekly; begin 1–2 week before travel and continue for 4 week after return from endemic area
doxycycline *doks-i-SYE-kleen*	Vibramycin	Short-term prevention of malaria	Photosensitivity, anorexia, nausea, vomiting, diarrhea, superinfection, rash	100 mg orally daily, 1–2 days before travel and for 4 week after return from endemic area
quiNINE *KWYE-nine*	Qualaquin	Treatment of malaria	Nausea, vomiting, cinchonism, skin rash, visual disturbances	260–650 mg TID for 6–12 days
Other Antiprotozoal Drugs				
artemether and lumefantrine *ar-TEM-e-ther* and *loo-me-FAN-treen*	Coartem	Treatment of malaria	Headache, nausea, anorexia, muscle aches	3-day treatment of 4 tablets twice daily
atovaquone *a-TOE-va-kwone*	Mepron	Prevention and treatment of PCP	Nausea, vomiting, diarrhea, headache, rash	750 mg orally BID for 21 days
atovaquone and proguanil *a-TOE-va-kwone* and *pro-GWA-nil*	Malarone	Prevention and treatment of malaria	Headache, fever, myalgia, abdominal pain, diarrhea	Prevention: 1–2 days before travel, 1 tablet orally per day during period of exposure and for 7 days after exposure Treatment: 4 tablets orally daily for 3 days
benznidazole *benz-NID-a-zole*		Chagas disease	Abdominal pain, weight loss, rash	5–8 mg/kg/day in 2 doses for 60 days
hydroxychloroquine *hye-droks-ee-KLOR-oh-kwin*	Plaquenil	Prevention and treatment of malaria, systemic lupus erythematosus, and rheumatoid arthritis	Nausea, vomiting, diarrhea, headache	Prevention: begin 1–2 week before travel, 310 mg/week orally, continue for 4 week after return from endemic area Treatment: 620 mg orally in 2 doses
mefloquine *ME-floe-kwin*		Prevention and treatment of malaria	Vomiting, dizziness, disturbed sense of balance, nausea, fever, headache, visual disturbances	Prevention: begin 1 week before travel, 250 mg/week orally, continue for 4 week after return from endemic area Treatment: 5 tablets orally as a single dose
metroNIDAZOLE *metroe-NYE-da-zole*	Flagyl	Treatment of intestinal amebiasis, trichomoniasis, anaerobic microorganisms	Headache, nausea, peripheral neuropathy, disulfiram-like interaction with alcohol	750 mg orally TID for 5–10 days
miltefosine *mil-TEF-oh-seen*	Impavido	Treatment of leishmaniasis—tropical parasitic disease	Nausea, vomiting	50 mg orally TID
nitazoxanide *nye-ta-ZOX-a-nide*	Alinia	Diarrhea caused by *Giardia lamblia*	Abdominal pain, nausea, vomiting, diarrhea, headache	500 mg orally q12h with food

Continued

SUMMARY DRUG TABLE (continued)
Antifungal Drugs and Antiparasitic Drugs

Generic Name	Trade Name	Uses	Adverse Reactions	Dosage Ranges
paromomycin *par-oh-moe-MYE-sin*		Treatment of intestinal amebiasis	Nausea, vomiting, diarrhea	25–35 mg/kg/day in 3 divided doses with meals for 5–10 days
pentamidine *pen-TAM-i-deen*	Pentam, Nebupent	Prevention and treatment of PCP	IM: pain at injection site; fatigue, metallic taste, anorexia, shortness of breath, dizziness, rash, cough	Injection: 4 mg/kg IM or IV daily, for 14 days Aerosol (preventative): 300 mg/week for 4 week by nebulizer
primaquine *PRIM-ah-kwin*		Treatment of malaria	Nausea, vomiting, epigastric distress, abdominal cramps	26.3. mg/day orally for 14 days
pyrimethamine *peer-i-METH-a-meen*	Daraprim	Prevention and treatment of malaria, toxoplasmosis	Nausea, vomiting, hematologic changes, anorexia	Prevention: 25 mg orally once weekly Treatment: 50 mg/day for 2 days
secnidazole *sek-NID-a-zole*	Solosec	Bacterial vaginosis	Secondary vaginal fungal infection	2-g single dose vaginally
tafenoquine *ta-FEN-oh-kwin*	Arakaoda, Krintafel	Prevention of malaria	Headache, diarrhea, back pain, keratopathy	200 mg orally day for 3 days

CHAPTER REVIEW

Know Your Drugs

Clients sometimes know a medication by the brand (or trade) name and not the generic name. To help you recognize both names, match the brand name with the generic name of the same medication.

Generic Name	Brand Name
1. secnidazole	A. Reese's
2. pyrantel	B. Abelcet
3. doxycycline	C. Solosec
4. amphotericin B	D. Vibramycin

Calculate Medication Dosages

1. The primary care provider has prescribed fluconazole 200 mg orally initially, followed by 100 mg orally daily. On hand are fluconazole 100-mg tablets. What should the nurse administer as the initial dose?
2. Pyrantel 360 mg is prescribed. The drug is available in 180-mg capsules. The nurse teaches the caregiver to administer.

Prepare for the NCLEX

RECALL THE FACTS

1. Mycotic infections are caused by:
   1. bacteria.
   2. fungi.
   3. parasites.
   4. viruses.

2. A client asks how antimalarial drugs prevent or treat malaria. The nurse correctly responds that this group of drugs:
   1. kills the mosquito that carries the protozoa.
   2. interferes with the life cycle of the protozoa causing the malaria.
   3. ruptures the red blood cells that contain merozoites.
   4. increases the body's natural immune response to the protozoa.

3. Which of the following laboratory tests would the nurse monitor in clients receiving flucytosine?
   1. Liver function tests
   2. Complete blood count
   3. Renal functions tests
   4. Prothrombin levels

4. When discussing the adverse reactions of an anthelmintic, the nurse correctly states that:
   1. clients must be closely observed for 2 hr after the drug is given.
   2. adverse reactions are usually mild when recommended doses are used.
   3. most clients experience severe adverse reactions and must be monitored closely.
   4. no adverse reactions are associated with these drugs.

5. When preparing a client for pentamidine administration, the correct position is:
   1. lying on left side.
   2. reverse Trendelenburg.
   3. prone.
   4. reclining position.

ANALYZE THE FACTS

6. When giving one of the topical antifungals, the nurse assesses the client for the most common adverse reactions, which are _____.
   1. related to the GI tract
   2. urinary retention
   3. hypotension
   4. related to the nervous system

7. *A client is receiving amphotericin B for a systemic fungal infection. Which of the following would most likely indicate to the nurse that the client is experiencing an adverse reaction to amphotericin B?
   1. Fever and chills
   2. Abdominal pain
   3. Drowsiness
   4. Flushing of the skin

8. The nurse is teaching preschool mothers about pyrantel treatment for pinworm infection. Which adverse reaction should the mothers report immediately to the primary health care provider?
   1. Nausea
   2. Rash
   3. Diarrhea
   4. Headache

ALTERNATE-FORMAT QUESTIONS

9. Identify the household precautions to prevent spread of parasitic infections. **Select all that apply.**
   1. Wash all bedding in the home.
   2. Provide separate towels for bathing.
   3. Wash hands after using the bathroom or changing diapers.
   4. Sterilize toys with boiling water.

10. A client weighs 140 lb. If amphotericin B 1.5 mg/kg/day is prescribed, what is the total daily dosage of amphotericin B for this client?

To check your answers, see Appendix F.

---

*Indicates the question is directly linked to the NCLEX-PN test plan in Appendix G.

WANT TO KNOW MORE? A wide variety of resources are available to enhance your learning and understanding of this chapter.
- Visit thePoint for resources such as:
  - NCLEX-Style Student Review Questions
  - Journal Articles
  - Dosage Calculations
  - Drug Monographs
  - Watch and Learn Videos
  - Concepts in Action Animations
- The *Study Guide to Accompany Introductory Clinical Pharmacology*, 12th edition, sold separately, will help you review and apply essential content.
- ✓PrepU is available to help students prepare for the NCLEX-PN examination.

UNIT 3
Drugs Used to Manage Pain

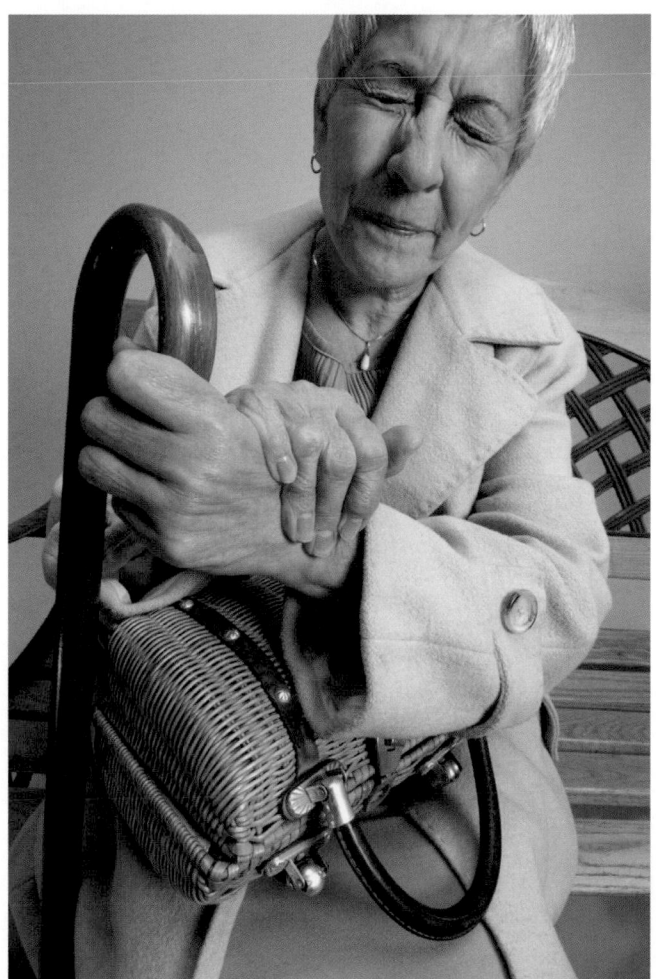

This unit examines how pain affects the entire body. The basic concepts in understanding pain are introduced, and many of the drugs used to reduce or alleviate pain are discussed. No one wants to be in pain, yet, it serves a very useful purpose. The body uses pain to warn about potential or actual danger to tissues. Typically, when a danger is present the tissues send a signal to the brain to pull away from the harmful object or situation. The danger can be something outside the body, such as heat, or inside the body, such as a blood clot. Pain is a protective sensation; it lets our body know there is an injury or the potential for an injury.

Yet, when pain lingers it affects client outcomes. For example, when clients recover more slowly than expected from injury and illness, pain may be the key factor. In this unit, you will learn about assessing pain, which drugs target the cause of pain, and, when pain cannot be prevented, which drugs are used to reduce the discomfort and help improve quality of life for clients. Because pain management is a complex skill to master, different concepts related to pain are highlighted in the four chapters of this unit. In this way, you can better learn how certain drug categories work best depending upon the pain presenting.

The nonopioid analgesics used to relieve mild to moderate pain are discussed in Chapters 13 and 14. They can be divided into three categories: salicylates, nonsalicylates (acetaminophen), and nonsteroidal anti-inflammatory drugs (NSAIDs). In Chapter 13, pain basics are discussed as well as the salicylates and acetaminophen. Because these drugs are typically purchased over the counter and taken without health care supervision, client teaching and outpatient interactions are highlighted. NSAIDs are covered in Chapter 14, along with discussion of pain assessment. This is as vital as knowing the temperature, pulse, and respiration and is often termed the fifth vital sign. Drugs used to treat migraine headaches are also covered in Chapter 14.

Chapter 15 discusses the major uses of the opioid analgesics in the relief or management of moderate to severe

acute and chronic pain. The ability of an opioid analgesic to relieve pain depends on several factors, such as the drug, the dose, the route of administration, the type of pain, the client, and the length of time the drug has been administered. Treatment of moderate to severe pain may include both an opioid and a nonopioid analgesic. You will gain knowledge to better understand client pain management strategies in this chapter. A number of people with chronic pain are turning to illicit drug use for relief. Although used for medical purposes, marijuana is one such option. Chapter 15 gives you objective information to better understand this client pain management alternative. When too much opioid is taken, an opioid antagonist may be used, these drugs are also discussed in Chapter 15.

To complete this unit's discussion of pain management, Chapter 16 reviews the use of drugs for anesthesia—the elimination of sensation and the perception of pain.

By understanding the basics of pain, its assessment, and the drugs used to treat pain, you can help clients deal with pain and promote quality of life.

13

Nonopioid Analgesics: Salicylates and Nonsalicylates

Key Terms

aggregation   clumping of blood elements

analgesic   drug that relieves pain

antipyretic   fever-reducing agent

jaundice   yellow discoloration of the skin because of liver disease

pain   unpleasant sensory or emotional perception

pancytopenia   reduction in all cellular elements of the blood

prostaglandins   fatty acid derivative found in almost every tissue and fluid of the body that affects the uterus and other smooth muscles; also thought to increase the sensitivity of peripheral pain receptors to painful stimuli

Reye syndrome   acute and potentially fatal disease of childhood; associated with a previous viral infection

salicylism   adverse reaction to a salicylate characterized by dizziness; impaired hearing; nausea; vomiting; flushing; sweating; rapid, deep breathing; tachycardia; diarrhea; mental confusion; lassitude; drowsiness; respiratory depression; and possibly coma

tinnitus   ringing in the ears

Learning Objectives

On completion of this chapter, the student will:

1. Discuss in general terms how pain is defined and the challenges of understanding the client's pain experience.
2. Distinguish the types, uses, general drug actions, common adverse reactions, contraindications, precautions, and interactions of the salicylates and acetaminophen.
3. Explain important preadministration and ongoing assessment activities the nurse should perform for the client taking salicylates or acetaminophen.
4. Identify nursing diagnoses particular to a client taking salicylates or acetaminophen.
5. Discuss the ways to promote an optimal response to therapy, how to manage common adverse reactions, and important points to keep in mind when educating clients about the use of salicylates or acetaminophen.

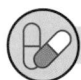 **Drug Classes**

Salicylates   Acetaminophen

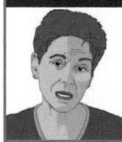 **PHARMACOLOGY IN PRACTICE**

Betty Peterson is at the outpatient clinic with complaints of a cold, muscular aches, and pain. She is currently taking a nonprescription aspirin product. She states she is experiencing some gastric upset and tells you that she plans to begin taking Tylenol because she has heard that it does not cause upset stomach. As you read this chapter consider whether this is a good change for Betty.

Pain can be described as "the unpleasant sensory and emotional perception associated with actual or potential tissue damage" (International Association for the Study of Pain, 1979). To treat pain, both opioid and nonopioid analgesics are used. This chapter discusses a simplistic understanding of pain as well as treating pain with the nonopioid analgesics: the salicylates and acetaminophen.

UNDERSTANDING PAIN

The nervous system is the mechanism involved in the recognition and perception of pain. The pain perception pathway in Figure 13.1 illustrates how pain signals that a noxious stimulus has or may cause injury to the body tissues. Nerve fibers in the tissue are stimulated by a noxious substance, such as heat from a hot pan, flame, or by stretching (an example would be the swelling by a blood clot that would force the nerve to stretch). In the illustration, heat activates the nerve endings (or receptors) and sends a message to the spinal cord. Then, in the spinal cord, the nerve impulses are transferred across different nerve pathways in the central nervous system and sent to the brainstem. From this area, the message goes to the brain cortex, where the perception of pain occurs, and in turn a message is sent back and the person removes the hand from the heat source, thus eliminating the heat sensation, reducing the perception of pain, and subsequently preventing further injury to the nerve endings in the hand.

Defining Pain

There are several factors to help in defining pain. No matter how pain is defined by the client, the best way for providers to understand the pain is by duration and location. Here we discuss duration, location, and the client's sensation.

Acute pain and chronic pain are used when discussing duration. *Acute pain* is brief and lasts less than 3–6 months. Causes range from a sunburn to postoperative, procedural, or traumatic pain. Acute pain usually subsides when the injury heals. A finger burned by the flame of a hot burner (as illustrated in Fig. 13.1) is an example of acute pain.

Chronic pain lasts more than 6 months and is often associated with specific diseases, such as cancer, sickle cell anemia, and end-stage organ or system failure. Various neuropathic and musculoskeletal disorders, such as headaches, fibromyalgia, rheumatoid arthritis, and osteoarthritis, are also causes of chronic pain.

Another important factor is location. It is important to have the client show or tell you where the pain is located on their body. With the ability of clients to attempt self-diagnosis using the Internet, naming what is the perceived origin or cause of pain may happen. This can lead to treating the pain incorrectly. An example being mid-sternal pain. The client may tell you they are experiencing heartburn, owing to where the pain they feel is located. The location of pain in the chest could also be symptoms of a heart attack. Therefore, it is important to have the client describe for you where the pain is located, not tell you what type of origin they think it is making the pain.

The Pain Experience

The *sensation* of pain is what the client feels. It can be modified at the site (peripherally) when the cause is treated or by modifying the signal in the brain (centrally). Pain, such as a burned finger, can be reduced when treated at the site of injury.

To treat pain effectively, you need a good understanding of the client's pain experience. This is challenging, because sometimes clients feel the provider is too busy to worry about the pain, or a previous bad pain management situation will make the client think you do not know how to treat the pain. In addition, clients sometimes offer only a vague or poor description of their pain experience. The sensation of pain is a complex phenomenon that is uniquely experienced by each individual. Therefore, the client's report of pain should always be taken seriously.

Medications to treat pain deal with the sensation experienced—drugs correct or help to heal the site of tissue damage or nerve stimulation (peripherally) or change or modulate the brain's perception of the pain signal (centrally). Peripheral pain (such as a burned finger) can be treated using nonopioid analgesics. The nonopioid analgesics such as the salicylates and nonsalicylates are used to treat mild to moderate peripheral pain. Many of these products can be obtained without a prescription. This fact sometimes makes clients think they are harmless drugs. This chapter discusses both routine use and harmful adverse reactions of salicylates and nonsalicylate analgesics.

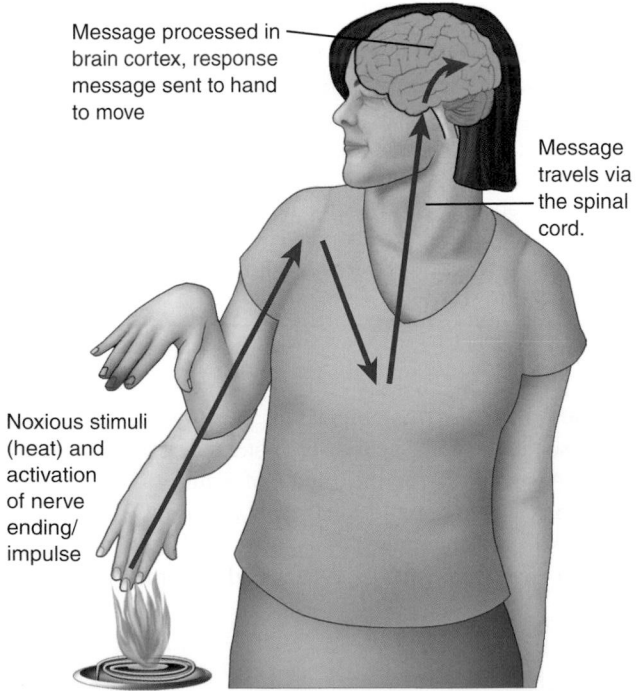

FIGURE 13.1 Example of pain perception pathway in response to heat. (Adapted from Taylor, C., Lillis, C., Lynn, P., & LeMone, P. (2015). *Fundamentals of nursing* (8th ed.). Wolters Kluwer.)

Message processed in brain cortex, response message sent to hand to move

Message travels via the spinal cord.

Noxious stimuli (heat) and activation of nerve ending/impulse

SALICYLATES

The salicylates are drugs derived from salicylic acid. Salicylates are useful in pain management because of their

analgesic (pain-relieving), **antipyretic** (fever-reducing), and anti-inflammatory effects. Examples include aspirin (acetylsalicylic acid) and magnesium salicylate. Specific salicylates are listed in the Summary Drug Table: Nonopioid Analgesics: Salicylates and Nonsalicylates.

ACTIONS

The antipyretic effect of salicylates is caused by the lowering of body temperature by the dilation of peripheral blood vessels. The blood flows out to the extremities, resulting in the dissipation of the heat of fever, which in turn cools the body.

The analgesic action of the salicylates is caused by the inhibition of prostaglandins. **Prostaglandins** are found in almost every tissue of the body and body fluid. When prostaglandins are released, the sensitivity of pain receptors in the tissue increases, making the client more likely to feel pain. Salicylates inhibit the production of prostaglandins, making pain receptors less likely to send the pain message to the brain. The reduction in prostaglandins is also thought to account for the anti-inflammatory activity of salicylates.

Aspirin more potently inhibits prostaglandin synthesis and has greater anti-inflammatory effects than other salicylates. In addition, aspirin prolongs the bleeding time by inhibiting the **aggregation** (clumping) of platelets. When bleeding time is prolonged, it takes a longer time for the blood to clot after a cut, surgery, or other injury to the skin or mucous membranes. This is why clients are asked to stop aspirin products a week or so before surgical procedures. Other salicylates do not have as great an effect on platelets as aspirin. This effect of aspirin on platelets is irreversible and lasts for the life of the platelet (7–10 days).

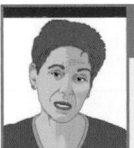

PHARMACOLOGY IN PRACTICE

PATHOPHYSIOLOGY
Which body system is involved in the recognition and perception of pain?

1. Nervous system
2. Cardiovascular system
3. Integumentary system
4. Endocrine system

Herbal Considerations

Willow bark has a long history of use as an analgesic from early Egyptians to members of various Native American tribes. Willow trees or shrubs grow in moist places, often along river banks in temperate or cold climates. When used as a medicinal herb, willow bark is collected in early spring from young branches. In addition to the use of the bark as a pain reliever, the bark and leaves of various willow species have been used to lower fever and reduce inflammation. The salicylates were isolated from willow bark and

identified as the most likely source of the bark's anti-inflammatory effects. The chemical structure was replicated in the laboratory and mass produced as synthetic salicylic acid. Years later, a modified version (acetylsalicylic acid) was first sold as aspirin. Aspirin became the most widely used pain reliever, fever reducer, and anti-inflammatory agent, leaving willow bark to be cast aside. The synthetic anti-inflammatory drugs work quickly and have a higher potency than willow bark. Willow bark takes longer to work, and fairly high doses may be needed to achieve a noticeable effect. However, fewer adverse reactions are associated with willow bark than with the salicylates. Although adverse reactions are rare with willow bark, it should be used with caution in clients with peptic ulcers and medical conditions in which aspirin is contraindicated (DerMarderosian, 2003).

USES

Salicylate nonopioid analgesics are used for:

- Relieving mild to moderate pain
- Reducing elevated body temperature
- Treating inflammatory conditions, such as rheumatoid arthritis, osteoarthritis, and rheumatic fever
- Decreasing the risk of myocardial infarction in those with unstable angina or previous myocardial infarction (aspirin only)
- Reducing the risk of transient ischemic attacks or strokes in men who have had transient ischemia of the brain because of fibrin platelet emboli (aspirin only). This use has been found to be effective in men (and women older than 65 years only).
- Helping maintain pregnancy in special at-risk populations (low-dose aspirin therapy). For example, it may be used to prevent or treat inadequate uterine–placental blood flow.

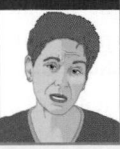

PHARMACOLOGY IN PRACTICE

SAFE DRUG ADMINISTRATION
In which of the following clients is acetaminophen preferred over aspirin?
1. Clients with severe pain
2. Clients with high fever
3. Clients with bleeding tendencies
4. Clients with inflammatory disorders

ADVERSE REACTIONS

Gastrointestinal (GI) system reactions include:

- Gastric upset, heartburn, nausea, vomiting
- Anorexia
- GI bleeding

Although salicylates are relatively safe when taken as recommended on the label or by the primary health care provider, their use can occasionally result in more serious reactions. Loss of blood through the GI tract may occur with salicylate use. The amount of blood lost is insignificant when a single dose is taken. However, use of these drugs over a long period, even in normal doses, can result in significant blood loss. Some individuals are allergic to aspirin and other salicylates. Allergy to salicylates may be manifested by hives, rash, angioedema, bronchospasm with asthma-like symptoms, and anaphylactoid (allergic) reactions.

CONTRAINDICATIONS

Salicylates are contraindicated in clients with known hypersensitivity to salicylates or nonsteroidal anti-inflammatory drugs (NSAIDs). Because salicylates prolong bleeding time, they are contraindicated in those with bleeding disorders or tendencies. These include clients with GI bleeding (from any cause), clients with blood dyscrasias (abnormalities), and clients receiving anticoagulant or antineoplastic drugs. Salicylates are classified as pregnancy category D (aspirin) and C drugs and should be used cautiously during pregnancy and lactation.

 Lifespan Considerations

Pediatric
Children or teenagers with influenza or chickenpox should not take salicylates, particularly aspirin, because their use appears to be associated with **Reye syndrome** (a life-threatening condition characterized by vomiting and lethargy progressing to coma). Acetaminophen is recommended for managing symptoms associated with these disorders.

PRECAUTIONS

Salicylates should be used cautiously in clients during lactation and in those with hepatic or renal disease, preexisting hypoprothrombinemia (low levels of prothrombin, which hampers clotting ability), and vitamin K deficiency. The drugs are also used with caution in clients with GI irritation, such as peptic ulcers, and in clients with mild diabetes or gout.

 Chronic Care Considerations

Aspirin is an over-the-counter (OTC) medication that clients may use to self-treat for pain. Some may take more aspirin than the recommended dosage, and toxicity can then result in a condition called **salicylism**. Signs and symptoms of salicylism include dizziness; **tinnitus** (a ringing sound in the ear); impaired hearing; nausea; vomiting; flushing; sweating; rapid, deep breathing; tachycardia; diarrhea; mental confusion; lassitude; drowsiness; respiratory depression; and

coma (from large doses). Mild salicylism usually occurs with repeated administration of large doses of a salicylate. This condition is reversible with reduction of the drug dosage.

LASA ALERT
The following drugs may sound alike; be sure to clarify when they are ordered:

Drug Name	*Sounds Like*
Aspirin	Afrin

Drugs that look like a similar drug are noted in the Summary Drug Tables of each chapter.

INTERACTIONS

Foods containing salicylates (e.g., curry powder, paprika, licorice, prunes, raisins, and tea) may increase the risk of adverse reactions. The following interactions may occur when a salicylate is administered with another agent:

Interacting Drug	Common Use	Effect of Interaction
Anticoagulant	Blood thinner	Increased risk for bleeding
NSAIDs	Pain relief	Increased serum levels of the NSAID
Activated charcoal	Antidote (usually to poisons)	Decreased absorption of the salicylates
Antacids	Relief of gastric upset, heartburn	Decreased effects of the salicylates
Carbonic anhydrase inhibitors	Reduction of intraocular pressure; also used as diuretic	Increased risk for salicylism

 # NONSALICYLATES

The major drug classified as a nonsalicylate analgesic is acetaminophen. It is the most widely used aspirin substitute for clients who are allergic to aspirin or who experience extreme gastric upset when taking aspirin. Acetaminophen is also the drug of choice for treating children with fever and flu-like symptoms.

ACTIONS

Acetaminophen is a nonsalicylate, nonopioid analgesic whose mechanism of action is unknown. The analgesic and antipyretic activity of acetaminophen is the same as salicylates. However, acetaminophen does not possess anti-inflammatory action and is of no value in the treatment

TABLE 13.1 Comparison of Drug Properties

TYPE OF ANALGESIC	ASPIRIN	ACETAMINOPHEN
Analgesic (pain reliever)	Yes	Yes
Antipyretic (fever reducer)	Yes	Yes
Anti-inflammatory (reduce swelling)	Yes	No
Anticoagulant (blood thinner)	Yes	No

of inflammation or inflammatory disorders (Table 13.1). Acetaminophen does not inhibit platelet aggregation; therefore, it is the analgesic of choice when bleeding tendencies are an issue.

USES

Acetaminophen is used for:

- Treating mild to moderate pain
- Reducing elevated body temperature (fever)
- Managing pain and discomfort associated with arthritic disorders

The drug is particularly useful for those with aspirin allergy and bleeding disorders, such as bleeding ulcer or hemophilia; those receiving anticoagulant therapy; and those who have recently had minor surgical procedures.

ADVERSE REACTIONS

Adverse reactions to acetaminophen are rare when the drug is used as directed. Adverse reactions associated with acetaminophen usually occur with chronic use or when the recommended dosage is exceeded. They include the following:

- Skin eruptions, urticaria (hives)
- Hemolytic anemia
- **Pancytopenia** (a reduction in all cellular components of the blood)
- Hypoglycemia
- **Jaundice** (yellow discoloration of the skin), hepatotoxicity (damage to the liver), and hepatic failure

Acute acetaminophen poisoning or toxicity can occur after a single 10- to 15-g dose of acetaminophen. Doses of 20–25 g may be fatal. With excessive doses, the liver cells undergo necrosis (die), and death can result from liver failure. The risk of liver failure increases in clients who drink alcohol habitually. Signs of acute acetaminophen toxicity include nausea, vomiting, confusion, liver tenderness, hypotension, cardiac arrhythmias, jaundice, and acute hepatic and renal failure.

 Chronic Care Considerations

Because renal function diminishes with age, those over 65 years should limit acetaminophen to 3000 mg daily, and if liver impairment is present the client should not exceed 2000 mg daily.

CONTRAINDICATIONS AND PRECAUTIONS

Hypersensitivity to acetaminophen is a contraindication to its use. Hepatotoxicity has occurred in habitual alcohol users after therapeutic dosages. The individual taking acetaminophen should avoid alcohol if taking more than an occasional dose of acetaminophen and avoid taking acetaminophen concurrently with the salicylates or the NSAIDs. Acetaminophen is classified as a pregnancy category B drug and is used cautiously during pregnancy and lactation. If an analgesic is necessary, it appears safe for short-term use. The drug is used cautiously in clients with severe or recurrent pain or high or continued fever because this may indicate a serious untreated illness. If pain persists for more than 5 days or if redness or swelling is present, the primary health care provider should be consulted.

 Lifespan Considerations

Adolescents
Many people use acetaminophen for pain relief because it does not cause GI distress. Because acetaminophen is contained in many cold preparations, it is recommended that the maximum daily level should be 3250 mg instead of 4 g. This 3-g daily maximum can be quickly and unintentionally surpassed when combining cold and pain relievers. You should instruct parents to be aware of the different drug preparations being used especially when teens and adolescents may self-administer these drugs for cold or flu symptoms. Examples of non-pain relievers containing acetaminophen are Actifed, Benadryl, Cepacol, Dayquil, Formula 44, Nyquil, Robitussin, Sudafed, and Theraflu.

LASA ALERT

The following drugs may sound alike; be sure to clarify when they are ordered:

Drug Name	Sounds Like
Tylenol	atenolol, timolol, Tylenol PM, Tylox

Drugs that look like a similar drug are noted in the Summary Drug Tables of each chapter.

INTERACTIONS

The following interactions may occur when acetaminophen is administered with another agent:

Interacting Drug	Common Use	Effect of Interaction
Barbiturates	Sedation, central nervous system depressants	Increased possibility of toxicity and decreased effect of acetaminophen
Hydantoins	Anticonvulsants	Increased possibility of toxicity and decreased effect of acetaminophen
Isoniazid and rifampin	Tuberculosis medications	Increased possibility of toxicity and decreased effect of acetaminophen
Loop diuretics	Control of fluid imbalance	Decreased effectiveness of the diuretic

Chronic Care Considerations

You should be aware of polypharmacy interactions when administering acetaminophen to clients with diabetes; care needs to be taken when blood glucose testing is done. Acetaminophen may alter blood glucose test results, resulting in falsely lower blood glucose values. As a result, inaccurate and lower doses of antidiabetic medications may be given to the client taking acetaminophen.

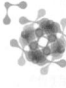

NURSING PROCESS —STEPS TO BUILDING CLINICAL JUDGMENT
Client Receiving a Salicylate or a Nonsalicylate

ASSESSMENT

Preadministration Assessment

Typically, a client taking a nonopioid analgesic is not hospitalized. Because of this reason, it is important to ask how long the client has taken the medication before seeing you or the primary health care provider.

Data gathering suggestions before the initial administration of the drug include:
Objective data

- Location of pain
- Description of site that is the cause of the pain (e.g., drainage, redness, swelling)
- Palpate for tenderness in the location of pain, examine joints if involved
- Vital signs (temperature, pulse, respirations, and blood pressure)

Subjective data

- Pain experience—onset, type (e.g., sharp, dull, squeezing), radiation, location, intensity, and duration
- Type and duration of symptoms (has it impacted ability to work or concentrate)
- If fever is present, client's description of type and duration of symptoms (general malaise, chills, and sweating)
- Allergy history, especially a history of drug allergies
- Alcohol use, especially if using acetaminophen
- Remedies attempted before seeking care

⚠ NURSING ALERT

Clients who are malnourished or who consume alcohol habitually (more than 3 drinks/day on a regular basis) are at greater risk for developing hepatotoxicity (damage to the liver) with the use of acetaminophen. It is recommended that use of acetaminophen should be limited to 1000–2000 mg daily for those who drink alcohol on a consistent daily basis.

Ongoing Assessment

As part of the ongoing assessment, monitor the client for relief of pain and ask the client to check the pain 30–60 min after administration of the drug. If pain persists, it is important to assess and document its severity, location, and intensity. (Examples of questions to ask the client appear in Chapter 14.) When nonopioid analgesics are given for fever, ask the family to monitor the temperature every 4 hr or more frequently, if necessary. Hot, dry, flushed skin and a decrease in urinary output may develop. If temperature elevation is prolonged, dehydration can occur. When given for any length of time, instruct the client and family to report adverse reactions, such as unusual or prolonged bleeding or dark stools, to the primary care provider.

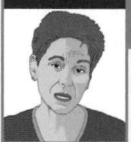

PHARMACOLOGY IN PRACTICE

ASSESSMENT

A client has been administered acetaminophen. Which of the following tasks should the nurse perform as part of the ongoing assessment?
1. Reassess client's pain rating 3 hr after administration
2. Monitor the client's vital signs every 8 hr
3. If stools are dark, send a sample for testing immediately
4. Assess for decrease in inflammation and greater mobility

NURSING DIAGNOSES

Drug-specific nursing diagnoses are the following:

- **Impaired comfort** related to fever or the disease process (e.g., infection or surgery)
- **Chronic** or **acute pain** related to peripheral nerve damage and/or tissue inflammation because of the disease process
- **Impaired physical mobility** related to muscle and joint stiffness
- **Risk for poisoning** related to increased salicylate or acetaminophen use

Nursing diagnoses related to drug administration are discussed in Chapter 4.

PLANNING

The expected outcomes of the client depend on the reason for administering a nonopioid analgesic but may include an optimal response to drug therapy, which includes relief of pain and fever; supporting client needs related to the management of adverse drug reactions; and confidence in an understanding of the medication regimen.

IMPLEMENTATION

Promoting an Optimal Response to Therapy

Salicylates

The client should be instructed to avoid salicylates for at least 1 week before any type of major or minor surgery, including dental surgery, because of the possibility of postoperative bleeding. In addition, the client should not use salicylates after any type of surgery until complete healing has occurred because of the effects of salicylates on platelets. The client may use acetaminophen or an NSAID after surgery or a dental procedure, when relief of mild pain is necessary.

You should observe the client for adverse drug reactions. When high doses of salicylates are administered (e.g., to those with severe arthritic disorders), instruct how to observe for signs of salicylism. Should signs of salicylism occur, instruct the client to notify the primary health care provider before the next dose is taken because a reduction in dose or determination of the plasma salicylate level may be necessary. Therapeutic salicylate levels are between 100 and 300 µg/mL. See Table 13.2 for symptoms associated with salicylate poisoning.

> **(!) NURSING ALERT**
> Serious GI toxicity can cause bleeding, ulceration, and perforation and can occur at any time during therapy, with or without symptoms. Although minor GI distress

TABLE 13.2 Symptoms of Salicylism

PLASMA LEVEL OF SALICYLATE	SYMPTOMS
Levels greater than 150 µg/mL (mild salicylism)	Tinnitus (ringing sound in the ear), difficulty hearing, dizziness, nausea, vomiting, diarrhea, mental confusion, central nervous system depression, headache, sweating, and hyperventilation (rapid, deep breathing)
Levels greater than 250 µg/mL	Symptoms of mild salicylism plus headache, diarrhea, thirst, and flushing
Levels greater than 400 µg/mL	Respiratory alkalosis, hemorrhage, excitement, confusion, asterixis (involuntary jerking movements especially of the hands), pulmonary edema, convulsions, tetany (muscle spasms), fever, coma, shock, and renal and respiratory failure

may be common, remain alert for symptoms indicating ulceration and bleeding in clients receiving long-term therapy, even if no previous gastric symptoms have been experienced.

Acetaminophen

Acetaminophen should be taken with a full glass of water. The client may take this drug with meals or on an empty stomach. Symptoms of overdosage include nausea, vomiting, diaphoresis, and generalized malaise.

Monitoring and Managing Client Needs

Impaired Comfort

If the client is receiving the analgesic for reduction of elevated body temperature, teach caregivers to check the temperature immediately before and 45–60 min after administration of the drug. If a suppository form of the drug is used, it is important to check the client after 30 min for retention of the suppository. If the drug fails to lower an elevated temperature, notify the primary health care provider because other means of temperature control, such as a cooling blanket, may be necessary. Clients can be made more comfortable by changing the clothing and bedding when it becomes damp because of the fluid loss during fever.

However, some health care providers may not prescribe an antipyretic for the client with an elevated temperature because evidence suggests that fever is the result of the immune system's production of disease-fighting antibodies. When a fever is below 102 °F (38.9 °C), the decision to treat an elevated temperature with an antipyretic is an individual one, based on the cause of the fever, the amount of discomfort to the client, and the client's physical condition.

Pain

Teach the client or caregiver to notify the primary health care provider if the salicylate or acetaminophen fails to relieve the client's pain or discomfort. Give the salicylate with food, milk, or a full glass of water to prevent gastric upset. If gastric distress does not resolve with food or drink, you should notify the primary health care provider because other drug therapies may be necessary. An antacid may be prescribed to minimize GI distress. Ask the client to check the color of the client's stools. Black or dark stools or bright red blood in the stool may indicate GI bleeding. The client should report any change in the color of stools to the primary health care provider.

 Lifespan Considerations

Gerontology
Salicylates are prescribed for the pain and inflammation associated with arthritis. Because older adults have a higher incidence of both rheumatoid arthritis and osteoarthritis and may use the nonopioid analgesics on a long-term basis, they are particularly vulnerable to GI bleeding. Encourage the client to take the drug

with a full glass of water or with food because this may decrease the GI effects.

Impaired Physical Mobility

The client may have an acute or chronic disorder with varying degrees of mobility. The client may be in acute pain or have long-standing mild to moderate pain. Along with the pain there may be skeletal deformities, such as the joint deformities seen with advanced rheumatoid arthritis. Considering the nature of the client's condition, you may suggest physical therapy or occupational therapy consultation to recommend assistive devices to aid with ambulation or other activities of daily living.

Risk for Poisoning

When clients contact you regarding fever, pain, or cold or flu symptoms, always ask what the client has been using to treat the condition and for how long. Clients are not always aware of the medications that contain salicylates or acetaminophen that are or are not pain-relieving medications (Table 13.3). By combining pain relievers and cold medications, a client can inadvertently take more than the 3250 mg maximum of acetaminophen for a couple of days before contacting the primary health care provider. Acute overdosage may be treated with administration of the drug acetylcysteine (Mucomyst) to prevent liver damage.

NURSING ALERT

Early diagnosis of acute acetaminophen toxicity is important because liver failure can be reversible. Toxicity is treated with gastric lavage, preferably within 4 hr of ingestion of the acetaminophen. Liver function studies are performed frequently. Acetylcysteine (Mucomyst) is an antidote to acetaminophen toxicity and acts by protecting liver cells and destroying acetaminophen metabolites. It is administered by nebulizer within 24 hr after ingestion of the drug and after the gastric lavage.

Teach the client about the signs and symptoms of acute salicylate toxicity or salicylism when using aspirin. Initial treatment for an overdose of salicylates includes induction of emesis or gastric lavage to remove any unabsorbed drug from the stomach. Activated charcoal diminishes salicylate absorption if given within 2 hr of ingestion. Further therapy is supportive (reduce hyperthermia and treat severe convulsions with diazepam). Hemodialysis is effective in removing the salicylate but is used only in clients with severe salicylism.

Educating the Client and Family

In some instances, a nonopioid analgesic may be prescribed for a prolonged period, such as when the client has arthritis. Some clients may discontinue use of the drug, fail to take the drug at the prescribed or recommended intervals, increase the dose, or decrease the time interval between doses, especially if there is an increase or decrease in their symptoms. The client and family should feel confident in their understanding of how the drug is to be taken. Instruct clients and family members on how to read and understand OTC medication labels (see Client Teaching for Improved Outcomes: Using Over-the-Counter Nonopioid Analgesic Drugs). Because clients frequently will begin use of OTC pain relievers before discussing with health care providers, develop teaching plans to include the following general points about these medications at any teaching session:

- Keep a record of when you take OTC pain relievers, and notify the primary health care provider or dentist of use at your next office visit.
- Take the drug with food or a full glass of water unless indicated otherwise by the primary health care provider. If gastric upset occurs, take the drug with food or milk. If the problem persists, contact the primary health care provider.
- If the drug is used to reduce fever, contact the primary health care provider if the temperature continues to remain elevated for more than 24 hr.
- Do not self-treat chronic pain using an OTC nonopioid analgesic without first consulting the primary health care provider.
- All drugs deteriorate with age. Salicylates often deteriorate more rapidly than many other drugs. If there is a vinegar odor to the salicylate, discard the entire contents of the container.
- The ingredients of some OTC drugs include aspirin or acetaminophen. The name of the salicylate may not appear in the name of the drug, but it is listed on the label. Ask your health care provider before use of these products. Consult the clinical pharmacist about the product's ingredients if in doubt.
- If surgery or a dental procedure, such as tooth extraction or gum surgery, is anticipated, notify the primary health care provider or dentist. Salicylates may be discontinued 1 week before the procedure because of the possibility of postoperative bleeding.
- If taking medication for arthritis, do not change from aspirin to acetaminophen without consulting the primary health care provider. Acetaminophen lacks the anti-inflammatory properties of aspirin.
- Avoid the use of alcoholic beverages.

TABLE 13.3 Common Combination Drugs Containing Acetaminophen

PAIN RELIEVERS	AMOUNT OF ACETAMINOPHEN
Saleto tablets	115 mg/tab
Excedrin migraine tablets	250 mg/tab
Excedrin aspirin-free caplets	500 mg/caplet
Axocet tablets	600 mg/tab
Non-Pain Relievers	Amount of Acetaminophen
NyQuil/DayQuil	650 mg/2 tablespoons (30 mL)
Zicam	650 mg/2 tablespoons (30 mL)
Benadryl allergy and sinus	500 mg/tab

Client Teaching for Improved Outcomes

Using Over-the-Counter Nonopioid Analgesic Drugs
Most nonopioid analgesics can be purchased without a prescription. A wide array of pain and fever reducers is readily available OTC; therefore, a client may be taking these medications for a period of time before consulting with a health care provider.

The potential for interaction with prescribed medications is high, especially when people view OTC preparations as harmless since they are readily available. This is why it is important for you to take any client interaction as an opportunity to educate about these products.
When you teach, make sure your client understands the following:

✔ Always read the label before you buy a product.
✔ What is the active ingredient? Are you taking that in any other drug?
✔ What is this drug supposed to do?
✔ Who should or should not take this drug?
✔ When should you consult your primary health care provider?
✔ Product tampering: Does the container still have a safety seal intact?
✔ How should this product be stored? Is it packaged in a safety container to prevent opening by children?

EVALUATION

• Therapeutic response is achieved, and pain is relieved.
• Adverse reactions are identified, reported to the primary health care provider, and managed successfully with appropriate nursing interventions:
  • Client reports comfort without fever.
  • Discomfort is reduced or eliminated.
  • Client maintains adequate mobility.
  • Toxic levels of medications are recognized before harm.
  • Client and family express confidence and demonstrate an understanding of the drug regimen.

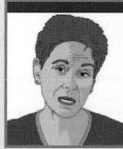

PHARMACOLOGY IN PRACTICE

USING CLINICAL JUDGMENT

What assessments would be important for you to make regarding the aspirin product she is taking and her gastric complaints? What other medications should you ask Betty about that may contain either aspirin or acetaminophen? What questions would you ask, and what information would you give Betty concerning Tylenol?

KEY POINTS

■ Pain is the unpleasant sensory and emotional perception associated with actual or potential tissue damage.

■ The sensation of pain is sent from the peripheral tissue to the brain where it is interpreted. Pain medications change the sensation in the tissues or modulate the signal in the brain.

■ Acute pain has a short duration of less than 3–6 months, whereas chronic pain lasts more than 6 months.

■ Salicylates and acetaminophen are used to treat mild to moderate pain and fever. Inflammation and blood thinning are additional properties of salicylates.

■ Gastric distress is the primary adverse reaction of salicylates. Long-term users should be monitored for potential bleeding from the GI tract. Ringing in the ears (tinnitus) can be an early sign of salicylism (toxic reaction). Children should refrain from aspirin use because of Reye syndrome.

■ Acetaminophen is used because it has less gastric adverse reactions. The daily maximum amount is 3250 mg and even less for those with liver function issues.

■ Multiple OTC products contain salicylates or acetaminophen. Clients need confidence in understanding how to purchase and take these products since the majority of users do so without health care provider supervision.

SUMMARY DRUG TABLE
Nonopioid Analgesics: Salicylates and Nonsalicylates

Generic Name	Trade Name	Uses	Adverse Reactions	Dosage Ranges
Salicylates				
aspirin (acetylsalicylic acid) *AS-pir-in*	Bayer, Ecotrin, Ecotrin (enteric coated), Empirin Buffered: Ascriptin, Asprimox, Bufferin, (multiple trade names)	Analgesic, antipyretic, anti-inflammatory, stroke prevention in men (and women older than 65 years only)	Nausea, vomiting, epigastric distress, gastrointestinal bleeding, tinnitus, allergic and anaphylactic reactions; salicylism with overuse	325–650 mg orally or rectally q4h, up to 8 g/day
diflunisal *dye-FLOO-ni-sal*		Same as aspirin, osteo/ rheumatoid arthritis	Same as aspirin	250–500 mg q8–12h (maximum dose, 1.5 g/day)
magnesium salicylate *mag-NEE-zhum* *sa-LIS-i-late*	Bufferin, Trilsate, Mobidin	Same as aspirin	Same as aspirin	650 mg orally q3h or 1090 mg TID
Nonsalicylate				
acetaminophen *a-seet-a-MIN-oh-fen*	APAP, Tempra, Tylenol (multiple trade names)	Analgesic, antipyretic	Rare when used as directed; skin eruptions, urticaria, hemolytic anemia, pancytopenia, jaundice, hepatotoxicity	325–650 mg/day orally q 4–6 hr; maximum dose, 3 g/day

CHAPTER REVIEW

Know Your Drugs

Clients sometimes know a medication by the brand (or trade) name and not the generic name. To help you recognize both names, match the brand name with the generic nonopioid pain reliever (either aspirin or acetaminophen) contained in the brand-name medication.

Generic Name	Brand Name
1. aspirin	A. Aspergum
2. acetaminophen	B. Cepacol
	C. Dayquil
	D. Pepto-Bismol
	E. Theraflu

Calculate Medication Dosages

1. The primary health provider orders acetaminophen elixir 180 mg orally. Acetaminophen elixir is available in a 120-mg/mL solution. The nurse administers _____.

2. Aspirin 650 mg orally is prescribed. On hand is aspirin in 325-mg tablets. The nurse administers _____.

Prepare for the NCLEX

RECALL THE FACTS

1. The best measurement of pain is:
   1. blood pressure.
   2. medication plasma levels.
   3. family observations.
   4. client self-report.

2. At a team conference, the nurse explains that the anti-inflammatory actions of the salicylates are most likely because of:
   1. a decrease in the prothrombin time.
   2. a decrease in the production of endorphins.
   3. the inhibition of prostaglandins.
   4. vasodilation of the blood vessels.

3. Which of the following symptoms would the nurse expect in a client experiencing salicylism?
   1. Dizziness, tinnitus, mental confusion
   2. Diarrhea, nausea, weight loss
   3. Constipation, anorexia, rash
   4. Weight gain, hyperglycemia, urinary frequency

4. When taking a salicylate, the drug is correctly administered:
   1. between meals.
   2. with a carbonated beverage.
   3. with food or milk.
   4. dissolved in juice.

5. While taking acetaminophen, clients who consume alcohol habitually are monitored by the nurse for symptoms of toxicity, which include:
   1. hypertension.
   2. visual disturbances.
   3. liver tenderness.
   4. skin lesions.

6. When hospitalized, which of the following drugs would the nurse most likely administer to a child with an elevated temperature?
   1. Baby aspirin
   2. Acetaminophen
   3. Fenoprofen
   4. Diflunisal

ANALYZE THE FACTS

7. A nurse instructs the client taking aspirin to avoid foods containing salicylates because this increases the risk of adverse reactions. Which foods should the client avoid?
   1. Salt, soft drinks
   2. Broccoli, milk
   3. Prunes, tea
   4. Liver, pepper

8. A client calls the clinic and tells the nurse a medication for aches smells like vinegar. The nurse's best response is:
   1. "Bring the medicine into the clinic"
   2. "Throw it away down your toilet"
   3. "Take it and let us know how your stomach feels in an hour"
   4. "Dispose of the drug where children and animals cannot get it"

ALTERNATE-FORMAT QUESTIONS

9. *Teens seek cold remedies when visiting the school nurse's office. To assess for the amount of acetaminophen taken, the nurse asks about which of the following products? **Select all that apply.**
   1. Actifed
   2. Alka-Seltzer Cold Tablets
   3. Bufferin
   4. Formula 44
   5. Sudafed

10. *Look at the drug label provided; the maximum amount of drug would be met by how many tablets?

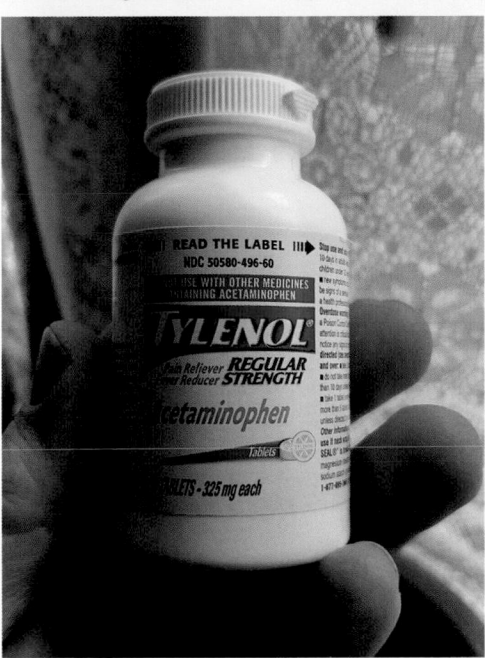

To check your answers, see Appendix F.

_____

*Indicates the question is directly linked to the NCLEX-PN test plan in Appendix G.

_____

WANT TO KNOW MORE? A wide variety of resources are available to enhance your learning and understanding of this chapter.
- Visit thePoint for resources such as:
  - NCLEX-Style Student Review Questions
  - Journal Articles
  - Dosage Calculations
  - Drug Monographs
  - Watch and Learn Videos
  - Concepts in Action Animations
- The *Study Guide to Accompany Introductory Clinical Pharmacology*, 12th edition, sold separately, will help you review and apply essential content.
- ✓*PrepU* is available to help students prepare for the NCLEX-PN examination.

Nonopioid Analgesics: Nonsteroidal Anti-inflammatory Drugs and Migraine Headache Medications

Key Terms

cyclooxygenase enzyme responsible for prostaglandin synthesis; contributes to integrity of stomach lining, pain, and inflammation

dysmenorrhea painful cramping during menstruation

dysuria painful or difficult urination

ecchymosis bruise-like subcutaneous hemorrhage

fifth vital sign inclusion of pain inquiry when temperature, pulse, respirations, and blood pressure readings are taken

jaundice yellow discoloration of the skin caused by liver disease

nociception chemical and mechanical process of sensation and perception

referred pain pain felt in an area remote from the site of origin, possibly along the same dermatome

oliguria reduced urine output

phenylketonuria (PKU) a genetic birth defect causing the amino acid phenylalanine to build up to toxic levels in the body

polyuria increased urination

purpura excessive skin hemorrhage causing red-purple patches under the skin

somnolence excessive drowsiness or sleepiness

stomatitis inflammation of a cavity opening, such as the oral cavity

transient ischemic attack (TIA) temporary interference with blood supply to the brain causing symptoms related to the portion of the brain affected (i.e., temporary blindness, aphasia, dizziness, numbness, difficulty swallowing, or paresthesias); may last a few moments to several hours, after which no residual neurologic damage is evident

Learning Objectives

On completion of this chapter, the student will:

1. Discuss the importance of good pain assessment.
2. Compare and contrast standardized methods to assess pain in different client populations.
3. Explain the types, uses, general drug actions, common adverse reactions, contraindications, precautions, and interactions of the nonsteroidal anti-inflammatory drugs (NSAIDs).
4. Describe the types, general drug actions, common adverse reactions, contraindications, precautions, and interactions of drugs used to treat migraine headaches.
5. Distinguish important preadministration and ongoing assessment activities the nurse should perform on the client taking an NSAID.
6. List nursing diagnoses particular to a client taking an NSAID.
7. Examine the ways to promote an optimal response to therapy, how to manage common adverse reactions, and important points to keep in mind when educating clients about the use of NSAIDs.

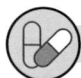 **Drug Classes**

Nonsteroidal anti-inflammatory
Migraine agents
- Calcitonin gene-related peptide (CGRP) receptor antagonist
- Selective serotonin agonists
- Ergotamine Derivatives
- Biologic agents

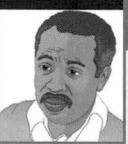 **PHARMACOLOGY IN PRACTICE**

Mr. Park has osteoarthritis and has been taking buffered aspirin for almost a year. He is confused at times and has difficulty hearing; his hearing loss concerns his daughter, who is visiting. As you read about pain assessment and the NSAID drugs, consider whether changing to celecoxib for the osteoarthritis pain would be a consideration.

When discussing the mode of action of NSAIDs, some texts include the salicylates in the NSAID group. Although the chemical and physiologic effects are similar, this text discusses the salicylates in a separate chapter (see Chapter 13). This is because salicylates and acetaminophen are used by many people independent of health care consultation. NSAIDs are nonopioid analgesics like the salicylates; the NSAIDs have anti-inflammatory, antipyretic, and analgesic effects. Although the NSAIDs can be purchased without a prescription, they are often recommended as important drugs as the first step in the treatment of the chronic pain and inflammation associated with disorders such as rheumatoid arthritis and osteoarthritis. As part of this first step, clients experiencing either acute or chronic pain need to be assessed thoroughly. In this chapter, pain assessment as well as general information on the NSAIDs is covered. NSAIDs are used for mild to moderate pain and are primarily taken on an outpatient basis; these drugs are listed in the Summary Drug Table: Nonsteroidal Anti-inflammatory Drugs and Migraine Medications.

PAIN ASSESSMENT

A key nursing role in administering pain relievers is a careful assessment of pain and the monitoring of the client's response to the pain medications. Pain assessment has a prominent place in any basic client encounter. You will find it is often considered the "**fifth vital sign**" in nursing assessment. When performing this component of your vital sign routine, two basic measures are needed in any pain assessment: *location* and *intensity*. Assessment of location helps the primary health care provider prescribe drugs that target the pain peripherally or centrally. The strength of the analgesic is determined by the client's report of the pain intensity.

The intensity of pain is subjective and individualized. Because of this subjectivity, it is sometimes difficult to measure objectively the signs of pain that match the level of distress reported by the client. The client's description of pain should always be taken seriously. Because failure to assess pain adequately is a major factor in the undertreatment of pain, guidelines to help you form questions to ask the client about pain are listed in Box 14.1.

Assessment Technique

As noted earlier, to prescribe effective analgesics for pain, the primary health care provider needs two key assessments about pain: location and intensity. To assess location, ask the client to describe or point to where the pain is at; be cautious of labeling the pain, since pain on the jaw could be from either a toothache or **referred pain**. Help teach your clients to describe their pain (see Client Teaching for Improved Outcomes: Talking to Providers About Pain).

Standardized pain measurement tools are used to provide consistency in assessing intensity (see examples in Fig. 14.1). The most common method used is to have a client rate the pain on a scale of 0–10, with 0 being "no pain" and 10 being the "most severe pain imagined" by the client.

Some population groups are known to have difficulty in assigning a number value to pain. For these clients it is hard to think about their pain experience in a quantitative

---

| **BOX 14.1** | **Guidelines and Questions for a Pain Assessment** |

Known as the *fifth vital sign*, the assessment of pain is just as important as the assessment of temperature, pulse, respirations, and blood pressure. The following points help to guide your ability to assess pain.

Assessment Guidelines
- Client's subjective description of the pain (What does the pain feel like?)
- Location(s) of the pain
- Intensity, severity, and duration
- Any factors that influence the pain
- Quality of the pain
- Patterns of coping
- Effects of previous therapy (if applicable)
- Nurses' observations of client's behavior

Sample Assessment Questions
Questions to include in the assessment of pain are as follows:
- Does the pain keep you awake at night? Prevent you from falling asleep or staying asleep?
- What makes your pain worse? What makes it better?
- Can you describe what your pain feels like? Sharp, stabbing, burning, or throbbing?
- Does the pain affect your mood? Are you depressed? Irritable? Anxious?
- What over-the-counter (OTC) or herbal remedies have you used for the pain?
- Does the pain affect your activity level? Are you able to walk? Perform self-care activities?

---

manner, like assigning a number to it. Box 14.2 gives examples of populations you should note may need alternate pain assessment tools. As with any group or individual suspected of limited health literacy, alternate ways to describe pain intensity are offered. All these tools help to assess the pain of clients no matter whether they are being treated with strong opioids or nonopioid analgesics such as the NSAIDs.

Barriers to Assessment and Treatment

Pain management in acute and chronic illness is an important responsibility in nursing. As pain managers, you need to be aware of and overcome the three main barriers to proper pain management having to do with assessment, intervention, and evaluation:

- Primary health care providers do not prescribe proper pain medicine doses.
- Nurses do not administer adequate medication for relief of pain.
- Clients do not report accurate levels of pain.

You can lessen these barriers to good pain management by showing sensitivity to client needs and learning techniques to conduct a good assessment.

Pain intensity scales

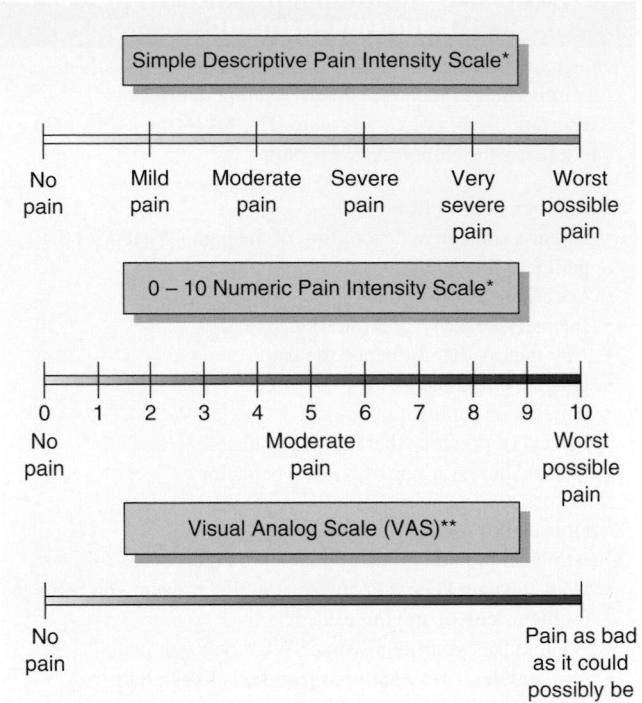

* If used as a graphic rating scale, a 10-cm baseline is recommended.
** A 10-cm baseline is recommended for VAS scales.

FIGURE 14.1 Examples of standardized pain assessment tools. (From Smeltzer, S. C., & Bare, B. G. (2000). *Brunnar & Suddarth's textbook of medical-surgical nursing* (9th ed.). Lippincott Williams & Wilkins.)

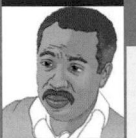

PHARMACOLOGY IN PRACTICE

ASSESSMENT
Which of the following assessments would be considered the fifth vital sign?
1. Blood pressure
2. Pain level
3. Respiration rate
4. Temperature

BOX 14.2 Populations at Higher Risk for Poor Pain Assessment

Clients at risk for inadequate pain management are frequently those who are not assessed well. Consider using standardized visual analog tools to assess pain in these high-risk client populations:
• Infants and children
• Older adults, especially those cognitively impaired
• Developmentally disabled children and adults
• Those with communication problems such as limited English proficiency or limited health literacy
• Those unable to communicate because of the illness or treatment process

NONSTEROIDAL ANTI-INFLAMMATORY DRUGS

ACTIONS

The NSAIDs are so named because they have anti-inflammatory effects, but they do not belong to the steroidal group of substances and thus do not possess the adverse reactions associated with the steroids (see Chapter 41). In addition, NSAIDs have analgesic and antipyretic properties. Although their exact mechanisms of action are not known, the NSAIDs are thought to inhibit prostaglandin synthesis by blocking the action of the enzyme **cyclooxygenase**. This enzyme is responsible for prostaglandin synthesis, which controls the process of inflammation. The NSAIDs inhibit the activity of two cyclooxygenase enzymes:

• *cyclooxygenase-1* (COX-1), an enzyme that helps to maintain the stomach lining
• *cyclooxygenase-2* (COX-2), an enzyme that triggers pain and inflammation

Traditional NSAIDs, such as ibuprofen and naproxen, are thought to regulate pain and inflammation by blocking COX-2. However, these drugs also inhibit COX-1, the enzyme that helps maintain the lining of the stomach. When NSAIDs are taken they block the effects of COX-2, producing pain relief, but they also block the effects of COX-1, which in turn produces adverse reactions. This inhibition of COX-1 causes unwanted gastrointestinal (GI) reactions such as stomach irritation and ulcers. Combination drugs (that include a proton pump inhibitor) are being used to reduce the risk of gastric and duodenal ulcers; examples are listed in Table 14.1.

The NSAID celecoxib (Celebrex) appears to work by specifically inhibiting the COX-2 enzyme without inhibiting the COX-1 enzyme. Celecoxib relieves pain and inflammation with less potential for GI adverse reactions.

TABLE 14.1 NSAID Combinations Offering Gastric/Intestinal Protection

GENERIC DRUGS	COMBINATION DRUG TRADE NAME
diclofenac/misoprostol	Arthrotec
ibuprofen/famotidine	Duexis
naproxen/esomeprazole	Vimovo
naproxen/lansoprazole	generic only offered

These drug combinations consist of an NSAID and a protein pump inhibitor. They are taken 30 min before meals twice daily. Arthrotec should not be taken by pregnant women.

Concept Mastery Alert

History of cardiac disease is an important factor to assess in a client initiating celecoxib therapy.

NURSING ALERT

Celecoxib is associated with an increased risk of serious cardiovascular thrombosis, myocardial infarction, and stroke, all of which can be fatal. All NSAIDs may carry a similar risk. Always question the client regarding a history of risk for actual cardiovascular disease before administering NSAIDs. Because of this risk, celecoxib as well as many of the other NSAIDs should not be used to relieve postoperative pain from a coronary artery bypass graft (CABG).

USES

The NSAIDs are used for the treatment of the following:

- Mild to moderate pain
- Primary **dysmenorrhea** (menstrual cramps)
- Fever (reduction)
- Pain associated with musculoskeletal disorders such as osteoarthritis and rheumatoid arthritis

Disease-modifying antirheumatic drugs are also used in the treatment of osteoarthritis and rheumatoid arthritis. These drugs are covered in Chapter 29.

 Lifespan Considerations

Pediatric
Ibuprofen is available to individuals as an over-the-counter (OTC) drug that may be purchased without a prescription. When assessing clients with pain, you should ask what medications the client is currently taking or has tried for pain relief already. Because of the risk of Reye syndrome from aspirin, ibuprofen is used in treatment of children with juvenile arthritis and for fever reduction in children 6 months–12 years of age.

ADVERSE REACTIONS

Gastrointestinal System Reactions
- Nausea, vomiting, dyspepsia
- Anorexia, dry mouth
- Diarrhea, constipation
- Epigastric pain, indigestion, abdominal distress or discomfort, bloating
- Intestinal ulceration, **stomatitis**
- **Jaundice**

Central Nervous System Reactions
- Dizziness, anxiety, lightheadedness, vertigo
- Headache
- Drowsiness, **somnolence** (sleepiness), insomnia
- Confusion, depression
- Stroke, psychic disturbances

Cardiovascular System Reactions
- Decrease or increase in blood pressure
- Congestive heart failure, cardiac arrhythmias
- Myocardial infarction

Renal System Reactions
- **Polyuria** (excessive urination), **dysuria** (painful urination), **oliguria** (reduced urine output)
- Hematuria (blood in the urine), cystitis
- Elevated blood urea nitrogen
- Acute renal failure in those with impaired renal function

Hematologic System Reactions
- Pancytopenia (reduction in blood cell components), thrombocytopenia (reduced platelet count)
- Neutropenia (abnormally few neutrophils), eosinophilia (low eosinophil count), leukopenia (reduced white blood cell count), agranulocytosis (reduced granulocyte count)
- Aplastic anemia

Integumentary System Reactions
- Rash, erythema (redness), irritation, skin eruptions
- **Ecchymosis** (subcutaneous hemorrhage), **purpura** (excessive skin hemorrhage causing red-purple patches under the skin)
- Exfoliative dermatitis, Stevens–Johnson syndrome

Metabolic/Endocrine System Reactions
- Decreased appetite, weight increase or decrease
- Flushing, sweating
- Menstrual disorders, vaginal bleeding
- Hyperglycemia or hypoglycemia (high or low blood sugar)

Sensory and Other Reactions
- Taste change
- Rhinitis (runny nose)
- Tinnitus (ringing in the ears)
- Visual disturbances, blurred or diminished vision, diplopia (double vision), swollen or irritated eyes, photophobia (sensitivity to light), reversible loss of color vision
- Thirst, fever, chills
- Vaginitis

CONTRAINDICATIONS

The NSAIDs are contraindicated in clients with known hypersensitivity. There is a cross-sensitivity to other NSAIDs, meaning if a client is allergic to one NSAID, there is an increased risk of an allergic reaction with any other NSAID. Hypersensitivity to aspirin is a contraindication for all NSAIDs. In general, NSAIDs are contraindicated during the third trimester of pregnancy and during lactation. Also, they are not to be used for postoperative pain following CABG surgery. Some NSAIDs are not used to treat rheumatoid arthritis or osteoarthritis; these include ketorolac, mefenamic, and meloxicam. Celecoxib is contraindicated in clients who are allergic to sulfonamides or have a history of cardiac disease or stroke. Ibuprofen is contraindicated in those who have hypertension, peptic ulceration, or GI bleeding. Arthrotec combines diclofenac and misoprostol (abortifacient), and should not be taken by pregnant women.

PRECAUTIONS

The NSAIDs should be used cautiously during pregnancy (pregnancy category B), by older adults (increased risk of ulcer formation in clients older than 65 years), and by clients with bleeding disorders, renal disease, cardiovascular disease, or hepatic impairment.

LASA ALERT

The following drugs may sound alike; be sure to clarify when they are ordered:

Drug Name	Sounds Like
CeleBREX	CeleXA, Cerebyx, Cervarix, Clarinex
Feldene	FLUoxetine
Indocin	Imodium, Lincocin, Minocin, Vicodin
Motrin	Neurontin
Naproxen	Natacyn, Nebcin, Naprosyn
Oxaprozin	oxazepam, OXcarbazepine
Piroxicam	PARoxetine
Tolmetin	tolcapone

Drugs that look like a similar drug are noted in the Summary Drug Tables of each chapter.

INTERACTIONS

The following interactions may occur when an NSAID is administered with another agent:

Interacting Drug	Common Use	Effect of Interaction
Anticoagulants	Blood thinner	Increased risk of bleeding
Lithium	Antipsychotic drug used for bipolar disorder	Increased effectiveness and possible toxicity of lithium
Cyclosporine	Antirejection agent (immunosuppressant)	Increased effectiveness of cyclosporine
Hydantoins	Anticonvulsant	Increased effectiveness of anticonvulsant
Diuretics	Excretion of extra body fluid	Decreased effectiveness of diuretic

Interacting Drug	Common Use	Effect of Interaction
Antihypertensive drugs	Blood pressure control	Decreased effectiveness of antihypertensive drug
Acetaminophen in long-term use	Pain relief	Increased risk of renal impairment

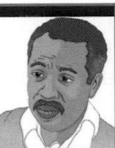

PHARMACOLOGY IN PRACTICE

SAFE DRUG ADMINISTRATION
Why is celecoxib not used to relieve postoperative pain for a client who has undergone coronary artery bypass graft (CABG) surgery?
1. Increased risk of duodenal ulcer
2. Increased risk of gastric bleeding
3. Increased risk of myocardial infarction
4. Increased risk of diarrhea

Herbal Considerations

Capsicum (hot pepper) has been cultivated in almost every society. Peppers are valued as a spice and flavoring for food. Capsaicin is the substance in peppers that, when applied topically, produces sensations varying from warmth to burning. For years, herbalists assumed that capsaicin worked by simply dilating blood vessels and increasing the supply of nutrients to injured joints. That may be a factor, but capsaicin actually works in a very different way.

People suffering from osteoarthritis have elevated levels of decapeptide substance P (DSP) in their blood and in the synovial fluid that bathes their joints. DSP has two undesirable functions. First, it breaks down the cartilage cushions in joints, contributing to osteoarthritis. Second, it serves as a pain neurotransmitter in both osteoarthritis and rheumatoid arthritis.

Researchers have discovered that capsaicin inhibits the activity of DSP. A cream containing capsaicin, when rubbed on the skin, penetrates arthritic joints, where it stops the destruction of cartilage, relieves pain, and increases flexibility. Side effects include a localized burning sensation during the first few weeks of use, which diminishes with continued application.

People suffering from ulcers are usually warned to avoid spicy foods. But new research suggests that capsaicin produces the opposite effect—that capsaicin might actually protect against peptic ulcers. A number of experiments over the years have found that capsaicin protects the gastric mucosal membrane against damage from alcohol and aspirin (DerMarderosian, 2003).

DRUGS USED IN THE TREATMENT OF MIGRAINE HEADACHES

About 12% of the population suffers from migraine headaches (Parikh, 2019). Although the cause is still relatively unknown, migraines are thought to start with chemical changes deep within the brain. Changes in sensory neurons cause pain and sensitivity to light/sound and may be accompanied by nausea and vomiting. Pain associated with migraine headaches is a complex process as illustrated in Figure 14.2.

Drugs used to treat migraine headaches are given prophylactically (preventative) to reduce brain chemical changes, thus reducing the process that causes the migraine or to treat the acute pain when a migraine occurs (abortive treatment). The mechanism of action and classification of the drugs to prevent migraine headaches are different from those used to treat the acute pain of the migraine attack.

Prophylactic treatment may include drugs from the following categories: beta blockers (see Chapter 24), calcium channel blockers (see Chapter 34), antidepressant medications (see Chapter 21), or antiepileptic drugs (see Chapter 28). CGRP monoclonal antibodies have been added to the list of drugs that help prevent migraines and are covered in Chapter 49.

The selective serotonin (5-HT) agonists used to relieve the acute pain are covered in this chapter and are listed in the Summary Drug Table: Nonsteroidal Anti-inflammatory Drugs and Migraine Medications.

ACTIONS AND USES

Preventative medications work by blocking the process of various chemicals in the brain to reduce the stimulation of nerve fibers, causing acute pain, vasodilation, and other cellular events. Most agents work to block serotonin, GABA, or calcium. Newer prophylactic drugs (CGRP antagonists) block the calcitonin gene-related peptide (CGRP) from attaching to other proteins or neurons thus preventing the steps involved in a migraine. CGRP, a peptide, is a portion of a protein. This protein portion is produced in neuro tissues and is involved in **nociception** (process of sensation and perception). By blocking this process of neurotransmission, the nerves are not stimulated and pain and vasodilation does not occur.

Acute medications work by activation of the 5-HT receptors, which causes vasoconstriction and reduces the neurotransmission, which in turn produces pain relief. Selective serotonin drugs are used for the relief of moderate to severe pain and inflammation related to migraine headaches. Because reduced GI motility can happen during a migraine event, delayed absorption of oral drugs may occur and alternative routes of administration are needed: rectal, internasal, or subcutaneous injection. Serotonin (5-HT) agonists are not used to prevent migraine headaches. Some clients find that a combination of medications or the addition of caffeine is helpful; therefore, a number of combination drugs are available to consumers; see Table 14.2.

TABLE 14.2 Acute Migraine Combination Medications

GENERIC DRUGS	COMBINATION DRUG TRADE NAME
Ergotamine Tartrate/Caffeine	Cafergot, Migergot
Isometheptene/Dichloralphenazone/ Acetaminophen	Nodolor
Isometheptene Mucate/Caffeine/ Acetaminophen	MigraLam, Prodrin, Treximet

ADVERSE REACTIONS

These agents are generally well tolerated, with most adverse reactions mild and transient. The most common are dizziness, nausea, fatigue, pain, dry mouth, and flushing.

Cardiovascular System Reactions
- Coronary artery vasospasm
- Cardiac arrhythmias and tachycardia
- Myocardial infarction

CONTRAINDICATIONS AND PRECAUTIONS

These drugs are contraindicated in clients with a known hypersensitivity to selective serotonin agonists and should only be used when a clear diagnosis of migraine headache has been established. 5-HT agonists should not be used in clients with ischemic heart disease (such as angina or myocardial infarction), **transient ischemic attacks** (TIAs), or uncontrolled hypertension or those clients taking monoamine oxidase inhibitor antidepressants. These drugs should be used cautiously in clients with hepatic or renal function impairment, such as the elderly or clients requiring dialysis. Because these are pregnancy category C drugs, they should be used during pregnancy only when the benefit outweighs the risk to the fetus. Caution should be exercised when administering them to lactating mothers.

The ergot derivatives (see Summary Drug Table: Nonsteroidal Anti-inflammatory Drugs and Migraine Medications) should not be used by HIV clients using protease inhibitors or clients taking macrolide antibiotics because of the risk of peripheral ischemia.

LASA ALERT

The following drugs may sound alike; be sure to clarify when they are ordered:

Drug Name	Sounds Like
Amerge	Altace, Amaryl
Reyvow	Revatio
SUMAtriptan	SAXagliptin, SITagliptin, somatropin, ZOLMitriptan

Drugs that look like a similar drug are noted in the Summary Drug Tables of each chapter.

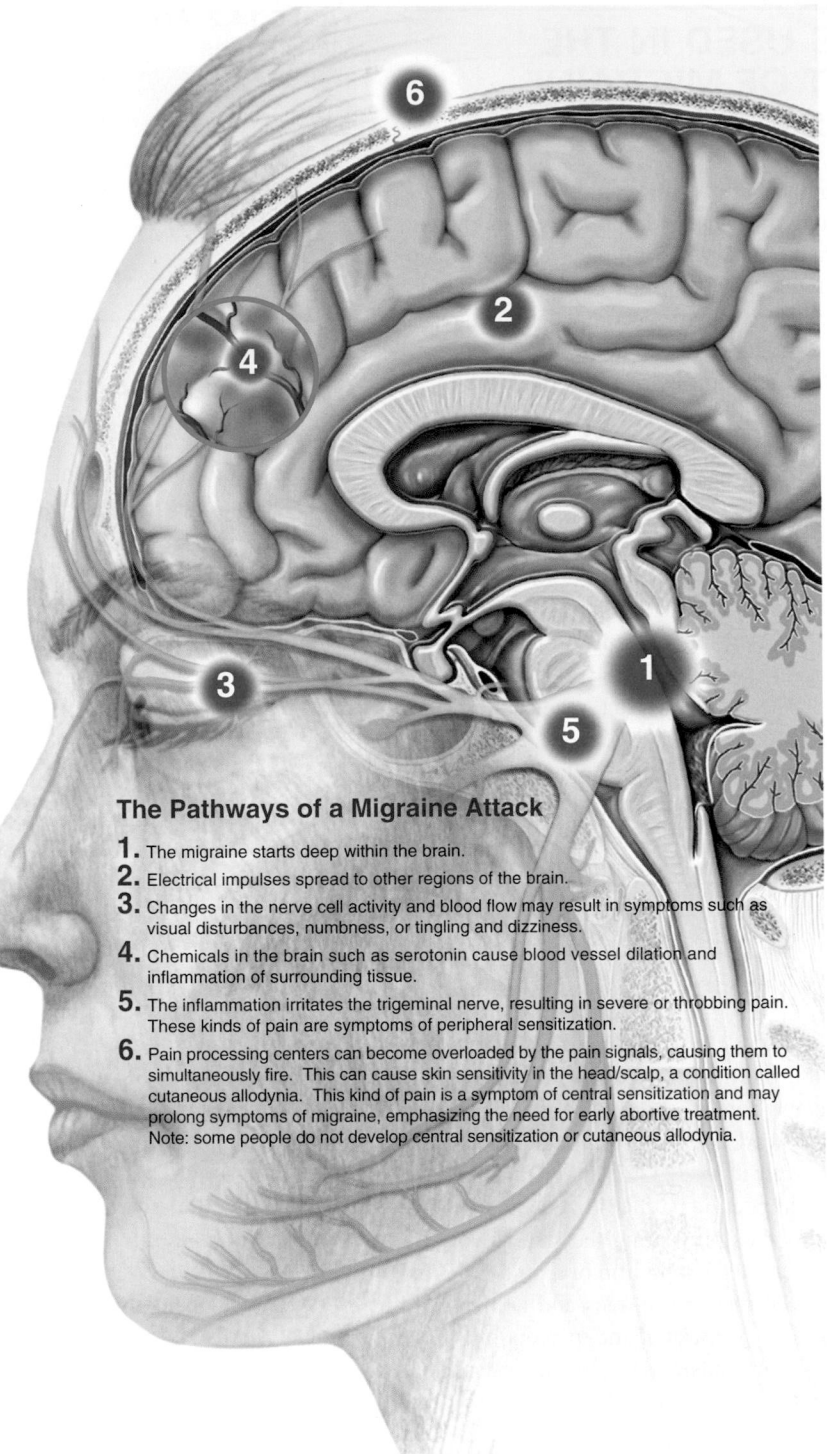

The Pathways of a Migraine Attack

1. The migraine starts deep within the brain.

2. Electrical impulses spread to other regions of the brain.

3. Changes in the nerve cell activity and blood flow may result in symptoms such as visual disturbances, numbness, or tingling and dizziness.

4. Chemicals in the brain such as serotonin cause blood vessel dilation and inflammation of surrounding tissue.

5. The inflammation irritates the trigeminal nerve, resulting in severe or throbbing pain. These kinds of pain are symptoms of peripheral sensitization.

6. Pain processing centers can become overloaded by the pain signals, causing them to simultaneously fire. This can cause skin sensitivity in the head/scalp, a condition called cutaneous allodynia. This kind of pain is a symptom of central sensitization and may prolong symptoms of migraine, emphasizing the need for early abortive treatment. Note: some people do not develop central sensitization or cutaneous allodynia.

FIGURE 14.2 Pathways of a migraine attack. (Courtesy of Anatomical Chart Co.)

INTERACTIONS

The following interactions may occur when a selective serotonin drug is administered with another agent:

Interacting Drug	Common Use	Effect of Interaction
Cimetidine	Decrease gastric secretions	Increased effectiveness of the 5-HT agonist
Oral contraceptives	Birth control	Increased effectiveness of the 5-HT agonist

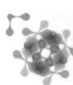

NURSING PROCESS STEPS TO BUILDING CLINICAL JUDGMENT
Client Receiving a Nonsteroidal Anti-inflammatory Drug or Migraine Medication

ASSESSMENT

Preadministration Assessment

Data gathering suggestions before the initial administration of the drug include:

Objective data

- Location of pain
- Description of site that is the cause of the pain (such as drainage, redness, swelling)
- Palpate for tenderness in the location of pain, examine joints if involved
- Vital signs (temperature, pulse, respirations, and blood pressure)

Subjective data

- Pain experience—onset, type (e.g., sharp, dull, squeezing), radiation, location, intensity, and duration
- Type and duration of symptoms (has it impacted ability to work or concentrate)
- If fever is present, client's description of type and duration of symptoms (general malaise, chills, and sweating)
- Allergy history, especially a history of aspirin or other NSAID allergies
- History of GI bleeding, cardiovascular disease, stroke, hypertension, peptic ulceration, or impaired hepatic or renal function
- Remedies attempted before seeking care

It is advantageous to teach the client how to rate their pain using one of the standardized pain scales. A visual analog tool known as the Wong–Baker FACES Pain Rating Scale (shown in Fig. 14.3) can be used for those who find it difficult to quantify pain numerically. There are many of these visual tools that can be useful with scales made of colors or facial expressions. Reassure clients that health care providers want to know about the pain episode and consistent measurement makes it easier to treat (see Client Teaching for Improved Outcomes: Talking to Providers About Pain).

Client Teaching for Improved Outcomes

Talking to Providers About Pain

Frequently clients are asked about pain, yet teaching the client the essentials of measuring pain infrequently does not happen until the person is in a painful situation. Here are some principles to cover with a client at any encounter so they are prepared to discuss pain when it happens.

When you teach, make sure your client understands the following:

- Tell your provider where the pain is at. Not all pain originates from the area that hurts. Pain can be referred to a different area; for example, gallbladder inflammation might present as pain in the shoulder.
- Tell your provider how much it hurts. Intensity is measured using standardized scales so everyone treats your pain the same. Learn to rate your pain on a scale of 0–10, with 0 being no pain and 10 being the most severe pain imagined by the client.
- Tell your provider what the most severe pain you can imagine is; this will help your health care provider gauge how well you handle pain.
- If you cannot measure pain with a number, there are other ways you can show how much it hurts. There are many scales, called visual analog scales, that you can use when you just do not think about pain as a number. You can use *mild, moderate,* or *severe pain* if those terms help you describe your pain. If you use a pain tool, bring it with you so your pain is measured consistently.
- How do you express that you are in pain? Some people are very stoic and may not show pain with moans or facial grimacing until the pain is hard to tolerate. How do you react when you hurt—do you withdraw or become irritable? Tell us what to look for when you have pain.
- What is your pain pattern? Are there times it hurts less or more? How does pain affect your activities?
- What helps? What do you do to make the pain tolerable? What have you tried that makes it worse? We do not want to do something to hurt you more.

Wong-Baker FACES® Pain Rating Scale

  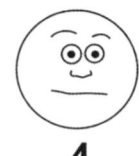   

0	2	4	6	8	10
No Hurt	Hurts Little Bit	Hurts Little More	Hurts Even More	Hurts Whole Lot	Hurts Worst

FIGURE 14.3 Wong–Baker FACES Pain Rating Scale, (c) 2020. (Wong-Baker FACES Foundation (2020). *Wong-Baker FACES® Pain Rating Scale*. With permission from http://www.WongBakerFACES.org)

Ongoing Assessment

Drugs used for mild to moderate pain are primarily administered at home or in long-term care settings. The responsibility of monitoring the relief of pain falls upon the client or caregiver in these settings with follow-up made by a nurse. You should instruct the client or caregiver to reassess the client's pain 30–60 min after administration of the drug and emphasize using the same pain rating tool the client chooses to use. If pain persists, it is important to note its severity, location, and intensity and relay this information to the nurse or primary health care provider. Hot, dry, flushed skin and a decrease in urinary output may develop if temperature elevation is prolonged; consequently, dehydration can occur. Ask the client or caregiver to make note if these problems arise and the client is at risk for dehydration. Also instruct how to monitor joints for a decrease in inflammation and greater mobility. Provide instruction, using written materials in the preferred language to explain adverse reactions, such as unusual or prolonged bleeding or dark-colored stools, and when to report these observations to the primary health care provider.

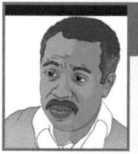

PHARMACOLOGY IN PRACTICE

ASSESSMENT

A client is prescribed an NSAID for osteoarthritis. What assessments should the nurse perform before administration of the NSAID?

1. Document limitations in mobility
2. Examine the level of consciousness in the client
3. Check the level of mental stability of the client
4. Determine the client's body temperature

NURSING DIAGNOSES

Drug-specific nursing diagnoses are the following:

- **Acute or chronic pain** related to peripheral tissue damage caused by the disease process or GI bleeding or inflammation from NSAID therapy
- **Impaired physical mobility** related to muscle and joint stiffness
- **Injury risk** related to adverse reaction of NSAID causing damage to optical field
- **Altered skin integrity** related to photosensitivity when using 5-HT agonists for migraine

Nursing diagnoses related to drug administration are discussed in Chapter 4.

PLANNING

The expected outcomes for the client depend on the reason for administration of the NSAID but may include an optimal response to drug therapy, which includes relief of pain and fever; supporting the client's needs related to the management of adverse reactions; and confidence in an understanding of the medication regimen.

IMPLEMENTATION

Promoting an Optimal Response to Therapy

A majority of the NSAID medications are taken in the outpatient setting; therefore, client teaching is an important nursing task. Teach the client to take the NSAID with food, milk, or antacids. Clients who do not experience adequate pain relief using one NSAID may have success using another NSAID. However, several weeks of treatment may be necessary to achieve full therapeutic response.

 Chronic Care Considerations

Migraine headache sufferers with **phenylketonuria (PKU)** should be informed that rizatriptan (Maxalt) and zolmitriptan (Zomig) contain phenylalanine and should be avoided.

Subcutaneous Injection for Migraine Headache Pain
The drug is dispensed in prefilled syringes. Each manufacturer makes a slightly different type of dispenser; therefore, be sure the client understands the device before they are is expected to self-administer the medication. Each dispenser should be used for only one injection and disposed of properly, even if the entire amount in the syringe is not used. Instruct the client to never use the drug if it is yellow or cloudy in the dispenser. Administration of sumatriptan should be just below the skin in the subcutaneous tissue. This drug should be given at the onset of the headache but can be administered anytime during the attack. A second injection can be delivered after 1 hr if pain has not been relieved. No more than two injections should be given in any 24-hr period. You should observe the client administering their first dose of sumatriptan by subcutaneous injection to be sure proper technique is used.

Monitoring and Managing Client Needs

Pain

NSAIDs are prescribed for the pain and inflammation associated with arthritis. Because older adults have a higher incidence of both rheumatoid arthritis and osteoarthritis and may use the NSAID on a long-term basis, they are particularly vulnerable to GI bleeding. Encourage the client to take the drug with a full (8-ounce) glass of water or with food, because this may decrease adverse GI effects.

Lifespan Considerations

Gerontology

Age appears to increase the possibility of adverse reactions to the NSAIDs. The risk of serious ulcer disease in adults older than 65 years is increased with higher doses of the NSAIDs. Use greater care and begin with reduced dosages in older clients, increasing the dosage slowly.

Impaired Physical Mobility

Teach caregivers to provide comfort measures to the client with pain in the limbs or joints affected by the various musculoskeletal disorders. Support limbs with proper positioning; applications of heat or cold, joint rest, and avoidance of joint overuse are additional comfort measures. Various orthopedic devices, such as splints and braces, may be used to support inflamed joints. The use of assistive mobility devices, such as canes, crutches, and walkers, eases pain by limiting movement or stress from weight bearing on painful joints. Walking with a physically impaired client gives you the opportunity to encourage ambulation as well as assess the increase in function provided by the NSAIDs (Fig. 14.4). Clients with osteoarthritis using NSAIDs should exhibit an increased range of motion and a reduction in tenderness, pain, stiffness, and swelling.

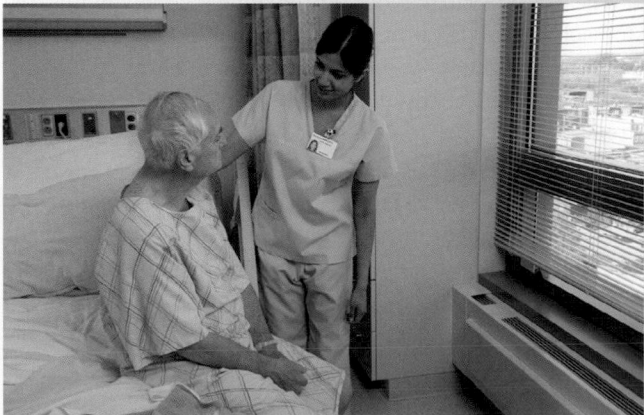

FIGURE 14.4 The nurse assesses the effects of pain medication while assisting the elderly client with ambulation.

It is important to teach the client receiving an NSAID about adverse drug reactions throughout therapy. GI reactions are the most common and can be severe, especially in those prone to upper GI tract disease. Cardiovascular reactions can be severe and even lead to death. Because of the severity of some of these adverse drug reactions, instruct the client to notify the primary health care provider of any complaints.

! NURSING ALERT

Instruct the client and caregivers that sudden or extremely painful gastric or cardiac symptoms may indicate an emergent problem. In these situations, clients should contact emergency services immediately and withhold the next dose.

Injury Risk

NSAIDs may cause visual disturbances, which can lead to an injury. Report any complaints of blurred or diminished vision or changes in color vision to the primary health care provider. Corneal deposits and retinal disturbances may also occur. The primary health care provider may discontinue therapy if ocular changes are noted. Blurred vision may be significant and warrants thorough examination. Because visual changes may be asymptomatic, clients on long-term therapy require periodic eye examinations.

Altered Skin Integrity: Photosensitivity

The skin can become more sensitive to sunlight when a client takes 5-HT agonists for migraine headache pain relief. Clients should be cautioned to wear protective clothing and sunscreen when outside. Teach clients that exposure to ultraviolet light in tanning salons can also cause a reaction; therefore, tanning should be discouraged when using these drugs until tolerance is determined.

! NURSING ALERT

Clients taking medications for migraine headache and using antidepressants (SSRI or SNRI—see Chapter 21 for full names) should be monitored for serotonin syndrome. Symptoms of serotonin syndrome include mental changes, tachycardia, blood pressure or temperature elevation, tightness in muscles, and difficulty walking (see Chapter 21).

Educating the Client and Family

In many instances, an NSAID may be prescribed for a prolonged period, such as when the client has arthritis. Some clients may discontinue their drug use, fail to take the drug at the prescribed or recommended intervals, increase the dose, or decrease the time interval between doses, especially if there is an increase or decrease in their symptoms. The client and family should feel confident in understanding that the drug is to be taken, even though symptoms have been relieved and the client may be pain free. As you develop a teaching plan include the following information:

- Take the drug exactly as prescribed by the primary health care provider. Do not increase or decrease the dosage, and do not take aspirin, other salicylates, or any OTC drugs without first consulting the primary health care provider. Notify the primary health care provider or dentist if pain is not relieved.

- Take the drug with food or a full glass of water unless indicated otherwise by the primary health care provider. If gastric upset occurs, take the drug with food or milk. If the problem persists, contact the primary health care provider.
- Whether taking an NSAID on a regular or occasional basis, inform all health care providers, including dentists, that you are taking it.
- If the drug is used to reduce fever, contact the primary health care provider if the temperature remains elevated for more than 24 hr after beginning therapy. Severe or recurrent pain or high or continued fever may indicate serious illness. If pain persists more than 10 days in adults, or if fever persists more than 3 days, consult the primary health care provider.
- Do not self-treat chronic pain with an OTC nonopioid analgesic; consult your primary health care provider.
- The drug may take several days to produce an effect (relief of pain and tenderness). If some or all of the symptoms are not relieved after 2 weeks of therapy, continue taking the drug, but notify the primary health care provider.
- These drugs may cause drowsiness, dizziness, or blurred vision. Use caution while driving or performing tasks that require alertness.
- Notify the primary health care provider if any of the following adverse reactions occur: skin rash, itching, visual disturbances, weight gain, edema, diarrhea, black stools, nausea, vomiting, chest/leg pain, numbness, or persistent headache.

Instructions for using selective serotonin agonists for migraine headache pain include the following:

- These drugs are used to treat actual migraine headache pain; they will not prevent or reduce the number of migraine headaches.
- Administer the drug at the onset of migraine symptoms. Doses can be repeated one time after 1 hr (2 hr for nasal spray).
- Never take more than two doses in a 24-hr period. Notify the primary health care provider when the headache is not relieved.

EVALUATION

- Therapeutic response is achieved and discomfort is reduced.
- Adverse reactions are identified, reported to the primary health care provider, and managed successfully with appropriate nursing interventions:
  - Client reports reduced or eliminated pain.
  - Client reports improved mobility.
  - Client is free of injury or uses adaptive devices for visual deficits.
  - Skin is intact and free of inflammation, irritation, or ulcerations.
- Client and family express confidence and demonstrate an understanding of the drug regimen.

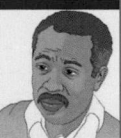 **PHARMACOLOGY IN PRACTICE**

USING CLINICAL REASONING

With the information learned about the client's pain experience and assessment of pain, discuss how you would perform a pain assessment with Mr. Park. What history of pain treatment is important for you to gather to help the primary health care provider determine the best pain management strategies for Mr. Park?

KEY POINTS

■ A key component to good pain management is the pain assessment. Location and intensity are the basic components of an assessment.

■ The sensation of pain is subjective—effort is taken with standardized pain measurement tools to help the client relay information needed to provide pain relief.

■ NSAIDs reduce inflammation differently than steroids by inhibiting prostaglandins. NSAIDs are used to treat mild to moderate pain, fever, and inflammation. They are used to treat a variety of chronic musculoskeletal disorders.

■ These drugs also block an enzyme that maintains the stomach lining; therefore, GI adverse reactions are common. Clients also need to be monitored for serious cardiovascular problems such as thrombosis, myocardial infarction, and stroke.

■ Migraine headaches are believed to be caused by vascular constriction and nerve stimulation. Selective serotonin agonists work to relieve the acute pain associated with the headache; they do not prevent the migraine attack.

SUMMARY DRUG TABLE
Nonopioid Analgesics: Nonsteroidal Anti-inflammatory Drugs and Migraine Headache Medications

Generic Name	Trade Name	Uses	Adverse Reactions	Dosage Ranges
Nonsteroidal Anti-inflammatory Drugs (NSAIDs)				
diclofenac *dye-KLOE-fen-ak*	Cambia, Flector (transdermal), Voltaren (gtts/gel), Zipsor, Zorvolex	Acute or chronic pain of rheumatoid arthritis, osteoarthritis, ankylosing spondylitis, and dysmenorrhea	Nausea, gastric or duodenal ulcer formation, GI bleeding	50–200 mg orally divided into 2 or 3 doses
etodolac *ee-toe-DOE-lak*		Osteoarthritis, rheumatoid arthritis, and acute pain	Dizziness, nausea, dyspepsia, rash, constipation, bleeding, diarrhea, tinnitus	300–500 mg BID; maximum daily dose 1200 mg
fenoprofen *fen-oh-PROE-fen*	Nalfon	Same as etodolac	Same as etodolac	300–600 mg orally 3 or 4 times daily; maximum daily dose 3.2 g
flurbiprofen *flure-BI-proe-fen*		Same as etodolac	Same as etodolac	Up to 300 mg/day orally in divided doses
ibuprofen *eye-byoo-PROE-fen*	Advil, Motrin, Caldolor (injectable)	Mild to moderate pain, rheumatoid disorders, dysmenorrhea, fever	Nausea, dizziness, dyspepsia, gastric or duodenal ulcer, GI bleeding, headache	400 mg orally q 4–6 hr; maximum daily dose 3.2 g
indomethacin *in-doe-METH-a-sin*	Indocin, Tivorbex	Rheumatoid disorders	Nausea, constipation, gastric or duodenal ulcer, GI bleeding, hematologic changes	25–50 mg orally, 3–4 times daily
ketoprofen *kee-toe-PROE-fen*		Mild to moderate pain, rheumatoid disorders, dysmenorrhea, aches, and fever	Dizziness, visual disturbances, nausea, constipation, vomiting, diarrhea, gastric or duodenal ulcer formation, GI bleeding	12.5–75.0 mg orally TID
ketorolac *KEE-toe-role-ak*	Sprix (nasal spray)	Episodic acute moderate to severe pain (less than 1-week duration)	Dyspepsia, nausea, GI pain and bleeding	Single dose: 60 mg IM or 30 mg IV Multiple dosing: 10 mg q 4–6 hr; maximum daily dose 40 mg
meclofenamate *me-kloe-fen-AM-ate*		Rheumatoid arthritis, mild to moderate pain, dysmenorrhea with heavy menstrual flow	Headache, dizziness, tiredness, insomnia, nausea, dyspepsia, constipation, rash, bleeding	50–400 mg orally q 4–6 hr; maximum dose 400 mg/day
mefenamic *me-fe-NAM-ik*	Ponstel	Episodic acute mild to moderate pain (less than 1-week duration)	Dizziness, tiredness, nausea, dyspepsia, rash, constipation, bleeding, diarrhea	250–500 mg q 6 hr
meloxicam *mel-OKS-i-kam*	Mobic, Vivlodex	Osteoarthritis	Nausea, dyspepsia, GI pain, headache, dizziness, somnolence, insomnia, rash	7.5–15.0 mg/day orally
nabumetone *na-BYOO-me-tone*		Rheumatoid arthritis and osteoarthritis	Dizziness, tiredness, nausea, dyspepsia, rash, constipation, bleeding, diarrhea	1000–2000 mg/day orally
naproxen *na-PROKS-en*	Aleve, Naprosyn, Naprelan	Rheumatoid arthritis, juvenile arthritis, osteoarthritis, mild to moderate pain, dysmenorrhea, general aches, and fever	Dizziness, headache, nausea, vomiting, gastric or duodenal ulcer, GI bleeding	250–500 mg q 6–8 hr orally; maximum daily dose 1.25 g
oxaprozin *oks-a-PROE-zin*	Daypro	Rheumatoid arthritis and osteoarthritis	Dizziness, nausea, dyspepsia, rash, constipation, GI bleeding, diarrhea	1200 mg/day orally

Continued

SUMMARY DRUG TABLE (continued)
Nonopioid Analgesics: Nonsteroidal Anti-inflammatory Drugs and Migraine Headache Medications

Generic Name	Trade Name	Uses	Adverse Reactions	Dosage Ranges
Nonsteroidal Anti-inflammatory Drugs (NSAIDs)				
piroxicam *peer-OKS-i-kam*	Feldene	Mild to moderate pain, rheumatoid arthritis, and osteoarthritis	Nausea, vomiting, diarrhea, gastric or duodenal ulcer, GI bleeding	20 mg/day orally as a single dose or 10 mg orally BID
sulindac *SUL-in-dak*		Mild to moderate pain, rheumatoid arthritis, ankylosing spondylitis, osteoarthritis, gouty arthritis	Nausea, vomiting, diarrhea, constipation, gastric or duodenal ulcer, GI bleeding	150–200 mg orally BID
tolmetin *TOLE-met-in*		Rheumatoid arthritis, juvenile arthritis, and osteoarthritis	Nausea, vomiting, diarrhea, constipation, gastric or duodenal ulcer, GI bleeding	400 mg orally TID or BID; maximum daily dose 1800 mg
Primarily COX-2 Inhibitor				
celecoxib *se-le-KOKS-ib*	Celebrex	Acute pain, rheumatoid arthritis, ankylosing spondylitis, primary dysmenorrhea, and osteoarthritis; reduction of colorectal polyps in familial adenomatous polyposis	Headache, dyspepsia, rash, increased risk of cardiovascular events	100–200 mg orally BID
Agents for Migraines				
Serotonin 5-HT Receptor Agonists				
almotriptan *al-moh-TRIP-tan*		Acute migraine headache pain	Headache, dizziness, fatigue, somnolence, nausea, dry mouth, flushing, hot/cold sensations, pain in chest or neck, paresthesias	6.25–12.5 mg orally; may be repeated in 2 hr
eletriptan *el-e-TRIP-tan*	Relpax	Acute migraine headache pain	Same as almotriptan	20–40 mg orally at onset of symptoms; may be repeated in 2 hr, not to exceed 80 mg/day
frovatriptan *froe-va-TRIP-tan*	Frova	Acute migraine headache pain	Same as almotriptan	2.5 mg orally at onset of symptoms; may be repeated in 2 hr, not to exceed 7.5 mg/day
lasmiditan *las-MID-i-tan*	Reyvow	Acute migraine headache pain	Dizziness	50–200 mg orally, in single dose, do not repeat for 24 hr
naratriptan *NAR-a-trip-tan*	Amerge	Acute migraine headache pain	Same as almotriptan	1.0–2.5 mg orally at onset of symptoms; may be repeated in 4 hr, not to exceed 5 mg/day
rizatriptan *rye-za-TRIP-tan*	Maxalt	Acute migraine headache pain	Same as almotriptan	5–10 mg orally at onset of symptoms; may be repeated in 4 hr, not to exceed 30 mg/day
SUMAtriptan *soo-ma-TRIP-tan*	Imitrex, Zembrace	Acute migraine and cluster headache pain	Same as almotriptan	25–100 mg orally; 20 mg nasally; 6 mg subcutaneously; 25 mg rectally; may be repeated in 2 hr, not to exceed 100 mg/day
ZOLMitriptan *zohl-mi-TRIP-tan*	Zomig	Acute migraine headache pain	Same as almotriptan	2.5–5.0 mg orally; 5 mg nasally; may be repeated in 2 hr, not to exceed 10 mg/day
Ergotamine Derivatives				
dihydroergotamine *dye-hye-droe-er-GOT-a-meen*	DHE 45, Migranal	Acute migraine and cluster headache pain	Nausea, rhinitis, altered taste	Nasally: total dose of 2 mg; parenterally: no more than 3 mg injected in 24 hr
ergotamine *er-GOT-a-meen*	Ergomar	Vascular headaches	Nausea, rhinitis, altered taste	2 mg sublingually; may be repeated in 30 min, not to exceed 6 mg/day

SUMMARY DRUG TABLE (continued)
Nonopioid Analgesics: Nonsteroidal Anti-inflammatory Drugs and Migraine Headache Medications

Generic Name	Trade Name	Uses	Adverse Reactions	Dosage Ranges
Calcitonin Gene-Related Peptide (CGRP) receptor antagonist				
rimegepant ri-ME-je-pant	Nurtec ODT	Acute migraine headache pain		75 mg daily sublingually
ubrogepant ue-BROE-je-pant	Ubrelvy	Acute migraine headache pain	Drowsiness	50–100 mg per dose orally
CGRP Biologics				
eptinezumab EP-ti-NEZ-ue-mab	Vyepti	Migraine prophylaxis	Nasopharyngitis	100 mg IV infusion, given 4 times yearly
erenumab e-REN-ue-mab	Aimovig	Migraine prophylaxis	Constipation, injection site reaction, antibody development	70 or 140 mg subcut monthly
fremanezumab free-ma-NEZ-ue-mab	Ajovy	Migraine prophylaxis	Injection site reaction, antibody development	225 mg subcut monthly, or 675 mg every 3 months
galcanezumab GAL-ka-NEZ-ue-mab	Emgality	Cluster and migraine prophylaxis	Injection site reaction, antibody development	Cluster: 300 mg subcut at onset; migraine: 120 mg subcut monthly

CHAPTER REVIEW

Know Your Drugs

Clients sometimes know a medication by the brand (or trade) name and not the generic name. To help you recognize both names, match the brand name with the generic name of the same medication.

Generic Name	Brand Name
1. celecoxib	A. Advil
2. ibuprofen	B. Aleve
3. naproxen	C. Celebrex
4. zolmitriptan	D. Zomig

Calculate Medication Dosages

1. Naproxen (Naprosyn) oral suspension 250 mg is prescribed. The dosage on hand is oral suspension 125 mg/5 mL. The nurse administers _____.

2. The physician orders celecoxib (Celebrex) 200 mg orally. The nurse has celecoxib 100-mg tablets on hand. The nurse administers _____.

Prepare for the NCLEX

RECALL THE FACTS

1. NSAIDs inhibit the action of _____.
   1. DNA synthesis
   2. prostaglandins
   3. cardiac muscles
   4. nerve fibers
2. The two basic measures of pain assessment are:
   1. time and intensity.
   2. site and time.
   3. duration and location.
   4. location and intensity.

3. The nurse monitors for which of the common adverse reactions when administering naproxen to a client?
   1. Headache, dyspepsia
   2. Blurred vision, constipation
   3. Anorexia, tinnitus
   4. Stomatitis, confusion
4. An older client is receiving sulindac. The nurse is aware that older adults taking NSAIDs are at increased risk for _____.
   1. ulcer disease
   2. stroke
   3. myocardial infarction
   4. gout
5. When a client is receiving an NSAID, the nurse must monitor the client for _____.
   1. agitation, which indicates nervous system involvement
   2. urinary retention, which indicates renal insufficiency
   3. decrease in white blood cell count, which increases the risk for infection
   4. GI symptoms, which can be serious and sometimes fatal
6. Which of the following statements would the nurse be certain to include in a teaching plan for the client taking an NSAID?
   1. "If GI upset occurs, take this drug on an empty stomach."
   2. "Avoid the use of aspirin or other salicylates when taking these drugs."
   3. "These drugs can cause extreme confusion and should be used with caution."
   4. "Relief from pain and inflammation should occur within 30 min after the first dose."

ANALYZE THE FACTS

7. *The nurse teaches a client to self-administer sumatriptan; when is this injection contraindicated?
1. At the onset of a migraine headache
2. When a visual aura is seen
3. Two hours following a previous dose
4. For weekly prophylactic use

8. Which of the following statements if made by the client taking an NSAID would indicate that he needs to see the primary health care provider immediately?
1. "I'm able to walk around without my cane at the grocery store."
2. "My wife has a fever so I gave her one of my pills."
3. "That leg still hurts and now it is red, warm, and swollen."
4. "I only have three pills left and the weekend is soon."

ALTERNATE-FORMAT QUESTIONS

9. *Because of the nausea experienced during a migraine headache and reduced GI motility, migraine medications are available in forms other than oral pills and tablets for administration. In which forms are they available? **Select all that apply.**
1. Sublingual
2. Internasal
3. Subcutaneous
4. Rectal

10. *Which pain assessment tool would be easiest to understand for a person with limited English reading ability? **Select all that apply.**
1. Wong–Baker FACES Pain Rating Scale
2. Simple Descriptive Pain Intensity Scale
3. 0–10 Numeric Pain Intensity Scale
4. Visual Analog Scale

To check your answers, see Appendix F.

---

*Indicates the question is directly linked to the NCLEX-PN test plan in Appendix G.

WANT TO KNOW MORE? A wide variety of resources are available to enhance your learning and understanding of this chapter.
- Visit the**Point** for resources such as:
  - NCLEX-Style Student Review Questions
  - Journal Articles
  - Dosage Calculations
  - Drug Monographs
  - Watch and Learn Videos
  - Concepts in Action Animations
- The *Study Guide to Accompany Introductory Clinical Pharmacology*, 12th edition, sold separately, will help you review and apply essential content.
- ✓**PrepU** is available to help students prepare for the NCLEX-PN examination.

15

Opioid Analgesics and Antagonists

Key Terms

adjuvant therapy used in addition to the primary treatment

agonist a drug that binds with a receptor and stimulates the receptor to produce a therapeutic response

agonist–antagonist drug with both agonist and antagonist properties

antagonist substance that counteracts the action of something else

cachectic malnourished, in poor health, physically wasted

cell surface receptor area built into cell membrane, which binds with chemical signs and causes a response by the cell

compounding medications made under the supervision of a licensed pharmacist, combining, mixing, or altering the ingredients of a drug to create a medication tailored to the needs of an individual client

miosis constriction of the pupil of the eye

opioid drug having opiate properties but not necessarily derived from opium; used to relieve moderate to severe pain

opioid naive no previous use or infrequent use of opioid medications

partial agonist agent that binds to a receptor but produces a limited response

patient-controlled analgesia drug pump and delivery system that allows clients to administer their own analgesic medication intravenously within a preset protocol

tolerance the body's physical adaptation to a drug

Learning Objectives

On completion of this chapter, the student will:

1. Explain how pain intensity is used to determine treatment using opioids and nonopioid analgesics.
2. Discuss the uses, general drug actions, general adverse reactions, contraindications, precautions, and interactions of the opioid analgesics and antagonists.
3. Distinguish important preadministration and ongoing assessment activities the nurse should perform on the client taking an opioid analgesic or antagonist.
4. List nursing diagnoses particular to a client taking an opioid analgesic or antagonist.
5. Examine ways to promote optimal response to therapy, how to manage adverse reactions, and important points to keep in mind when educating clients about the use of opioid analgesics and antagonists.

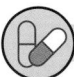 **Drug Classes**

Opioid agonists
Opioid agonist–antagonists

Opioid antagonists

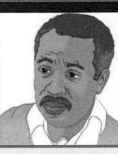 **PHARMACOLOGY IN PRACTICE**

When Mr. Park came to the preoperative unit, he complained that the pain on his back (where the shingles rash was erupting) was greater than the pain in his broken hip and leg. On rounds before the surgical procedure to repair his femur, the primary health care provider assured him that the acyclovir would begin to alleviate some of the pain from the rash. Following the surgical procedure, the surgeon ordered meperidine (Demerol) for postoperative pain management. In assessing Mr. Park, he reported his pain is "8 out of 10" on a 0–10 pain scale. The nurse promptly gives the drug, and approximately 20 min after receiving an injection of meperidine, the nurse discovers Mr. Park's vital signs are as follows: blood pressure 80/50 mm Hg, pulse rate 130 bpm, and respiratory rate 8 breaths/min.

Now that you have read almost all the chapters in this unit, determine whether you could have anticipated Mr. Park's risks for opioid toxicity and discuss what actions should be taken for a proper pain assessment and medication administration.

The discussion in this unit has focused on pain and its treatment as universal issues. In this chapter, the opioid drugs used for severe pain are discussed as well as how the intensity of pain determines the use of these drugs. Issues related to opiate use and subsequent resuscitation are a big concern in the United States; therefore, the antagonist drugs used to reverse opiates are also featured. Understanding their use and purpose is significant in pain management.

The World Health Organization (WHO) developed a three-step analgesic protocol based on intensity as a guideline for treating pain. These steps are envisioned as a ladder, and this "pain ladder" directs the use of both opioid and nonopioids in the treatment of pain using three steps. For mild pain, a health care provider uses Step 1, which stipulates prescribing a nonopioid analgesic, such as a nonsteroidal anti-inflammatory drug (NSAID) or acetaminophen. If necessary, an **adjuvant** (extra helping) agent may be used to promote the pain-relieving effect. These agents include drugs that affect the neurologic or musculoskeletal systems and are covered in Units 4–6. If pain persists or worsens even with appropriate dosage increases, a provider moves to Step 2 or Step 3, changing or adding to an analgesic as indicated. Step 2 and Step 3 analgesics typically contain opioid substances. Most clients with severe pain require treatment at a Step 2 or Step 3 level. Using the pain ladder from Steps 1–3 works well when describing acute pain, yet what about chronic or severe pain that comes from long-term treatment? Vargas-Shaffer proposed that a new step should be integrated into the ladder (2010). A fourth step would include the drugs and techniques used to treat chronic pain when a severe, crisis situation arises. During these episodes nerve stimulators, blocks using anesthetic drugs (Chapter 16), or continuous pump infusions are employed. Figure 15.1 illustrates this updated model of pain management using the WHO ladder.

OPIOID ANALGESICS

Opioid is the general term used for the opium-derived or synthetic analgesics used to treat moderate to severe pain. The opioid analgesics are controlled substances (see Chapter 1). The analgesic properties of opium have been known for hundreds of years. These drugs do not change the tissues where the pain sensation originates; instead, they change how the client perceives the pain in the brain.

The opiates are natural substances and include morphine sulfate,[1] codeine, opium alkaloids, and tincture of opium. Synthetic opioids are those manufactured analgesics with properties and actions similar to the natural opioids. Examples of synthetic opioid analgesics are methadone, levorphanol, remifentanil, and meperidine. Morphine sulfate, when extracted from raw opium and treated chemically, yields the semisynthetic opioids hydromorphone, oxymorphone, oxycodone, and heroin. Hydrocodone is a semisynthetic drug made from codeine.

Heroin is an illegal narcotic substance in the United States and is not used in medicine. *Narcotic* is a term that refers to the properties of a drug to produce numbness or a stupor-like state. Although the terms *opioid* and *narcotic* were once interchangeable, law enforcement agencies have generalized the term *narcotic* to mean a drug that is addictive and abused or used illegally. Health care providers use the term *opioid* to describe drugs used in pain relief. Additional analgesics are listed in the Summary Drug Table: Opioid Analgesics.

ACTIONS

Cells in the central nervous system (CNS) have receptor sites called *opiate receptors*. Although opiates are attracted to many different receptor sites, the mu (μ) and kappa (κ) receptors produce the analgesic, sedative, and euphoric effects associated with analgesic drugs.

---

[1] Numerous drug errors are attributed to using drug name suffixes (e.g., sulfate or HCl at the end of the drug name), according to the Institute for Safe Medicine Practices. Therefore, they have been removed from this book. Because morphine sulfate is considered a drug at greater risk for error when abbreviated, you will see it listed as such in this chapter (ISMP, 2012).

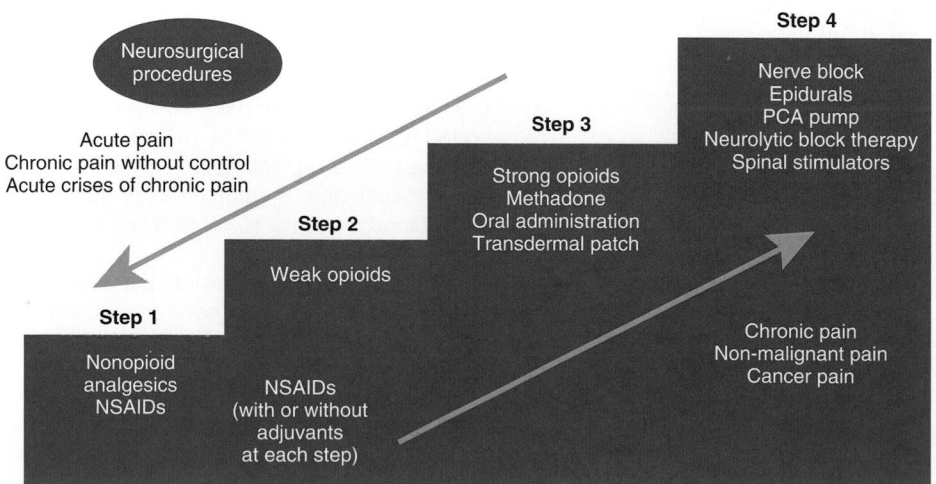

FIGURE 15.1 World Health Organization pain relief ladder with chronic pain fourth step adaption. (Adapted with permission from the Canadian Family Physician, 2020.)

Drugs that bind well to a receptor are called **agonist** agents. An opioid analgesic may be classified as an agonist, partial agonist, or mixed agonist–antagonist. The agonist binds to a receptor and causes a response. A **partial agonist** binds to a receptor, but the response is limited (i.e., is not as great as with the agonist). An **agonist–antagonist** has properties of both the agonist and antagonist. These drugs have some agonist activity and some antagonist activity at the receptor sites. Antagonists bind to a receptor and cause no response. An **antagonist** can reverse the effects of the agonist. This reversal is possible because the antagonist competes with the agonist for a receptor site.

In addition to the pain-relieving effects, other nonintended responses occur when the opiate receptor sites are stimulated. These include respiratory depression, decreased gastrointestinal (GI) motility, and **miosis** (pinpoint pupils). Table 15.1 identifies the responses in the body associated with three of the opiate receptors. The actions of the opioid analgesics on the various organs and structures of the body (also called *secondary pharmacologic effects*) are shown in Box 15.1. With long-term use, the client's body adapts to these secondary effects. The only bodily system that does not adapt and compensate is the GI system. Slow GI motility and the resulting constipation are always a problem in opioid therapy.

The most widely used opioid, morphine sulfate, is an effective drug for moderately severe to severe pain. Morphine sulfate is considered the prototype (model), or gold standard in pain management—morphine sulfate's actions, uses, and ability to relieve pain are the standards against which other opioid analgesics are often compared. Charts called *equal-analgesic conversions* compare other opioid doses with the doses of morphine sulfate that would be used for the same level of pain control. This conversion process is helpful when drugs are changed because of lessening or increasing pain and if adverse effects worsen to the point that they are unmanageable for the client. These conversions are particularly helpful when drugs change form, such as intravenous (IV) infusion to oral doses. More information on equal-analgesic conversion is explained in Chapter 54. Examples of

BOX 15.1 Secondary Pharmacologic Effects of the Opioid Analgesics

- **Cardiovascular**—peripheral vasodilation, decreased peripheral resistance, inhibition of baroreceptors (pressure receptors located in the aortic arch and carotid sinus that regulate blood pressure), orthostatic hypotension, and fainting
- **Central nervous system**—euphoria, drowsiness, apathy, mental confusion, alterations in mood, reduction in body temperature, feelings of relaxation, dysphoria (depression accompanied by anxiety); nausea and vomiting are caused by direct stimulation of the emetic chemoreceptors located in the medulla. The degree to which these occur usually depends on the drug and the dose
- **Dermatologic**—histamine release, pruritus, flushing, and red eyes
- **Gastrointestinal**—decrease in gastric motility (prolonged emptying time); decrease in biliary, pancreatic, and intestinal secretions; delay in digestion of food in the small intestine; increase in resting tone, with the potential for spasms, epigastric distress, or biliary colic (caused by constriction of the sphincter of Oddi). These drugs can cause constipation and anorexia.
- **Genitourinary**—urinary urgency and difficulty with urination, caused by spasms of the ureter. Urinary urgency also may occur because of the action of the drugs on the detrusor muscle of the bladder. Some clients may experience difficulty voiding because of contraction of the bladder sphincter.
- **Respiratory**—depressant effects on respiratory rate (caused by a reduced sensitivity of the respiratory center to carbon dioxide).
- **Cough**—suppression of the cough reflex (antitussive effect) by exerting a direct effect on the cough center in the medulla. Codeine has the most noticeable effect on the cough reflex.
- **Medulla**—nausea and vomiting can occur when the chemoreceptor trigger zone located in the medulla is stimulated. To a varying degree, opioid analgesics also depress the chemoreceptor trigger zone. Therefore, nausea and vomiting may or may not occur when these drugs are given.

websites that include equal-analgesic calculators are included in the bibliography.

Other opioids, such as meperidine and levorphanol, are effective for the treatment of moderate to severe pain. For moderate pain, the primary health care provider may order an opioid such as hydrocodone, codeine, or pentazocine.

USES

The opioid analgesics are used primarily for the treatment of moderate to severe acute and chronic pain and in the treatment and management of opiate dependence. In

TABLE 15.1 Bodily Responses Associated With Opioid Receptor Sites

RECEPTOR	BODILY RESPONSE
Mu (μ)	Morphine-like supraspinal analgesia, respiratory and physical depression, miosis, reduced GI motility
Delta (δ)	Dysphoria, psychotomimetic effects (e.g., hallucinations), respiratory and vasomotor stimulations caused by drugs with antagonist activity
Kappa (κ)	Sedation and miosis (pinpoint pupils)

addition, the opioid analgesics may be used for the following reasons:

- To decrease anxiety and sedate the client before surgery. Clients who are relaxed and sedated when an anesthetic agent is given are easier to anesthetize (requiring a smaller dose of an induction anesthetic), as well as easier to maintain under anesthesia
- To support anesthesia (i.e., as an adjunct during anesthesia)
- To promote obstetric analgesia
- To relieve anxiety in clients with dyspnea (breathing difficulty) associated with pulmonary edema
- Administered intrathecally (a single injection into spinal cord space) or epidurally (catheter placed into spinal cord space for multiple injections), to control pain for extended periods without apparent loss of motor, sensory, or sympathetic nerve function
- To relieve pain associated with a myocardial infarction (morphine sulfate is the agent of choice)
- To manage opiate dependence
- To induce conscious sedation before a diagnostic or therapeutic procedure in the hospital setting
- To treat severe diarrhea and intestinal cramping (camphorated tincture of opium may be used)
- To relieve severe, persistent cough (codeine may be helpful, although the drug's use has declined)

ADVERSE REACTIONS

Central Nervous System Reactions
- Euphoria, weakness, headache
- Lightheadedness, dizziness, sedation
- Miosis, insomnia, agitation, tremor
- Increased intracranial pressure, impairment of mental and physical tasks

Respiratory System Reactions
- Depression of rate and depth of breathing

Gastrointestinal System Reactions
- Nausea, vomiting
- Dry mouth, biliary tract spasms
- Constipation, anorexia

Cardiovascular System Reactions
- Facial flushing
- Tachycardia, bradycardia, palpitations
- Peripheral circulatory collapse

Genitourinary System Reactions
- Urinary retention or hesitancy
- Spasms of the ureters and bladder sphincter

Allergic and Other Reactions
- Pruritus, rash, and urticaria
- Sweating, pain at injection site, and local tissue irritation

Concept Mastery Alert

Although the respiratory system will adapt to secondary effects of opioids, the GI system does not. Adverse effects such as constipation and slow GI motility do not dissipate.

CONTRAINDICATIONS

All opioid analgesics are contraindicated in clients with known hypersensitivity to the drugs. These drugs are contraindicated in clients with acute bronchial asthma, emphysema, or upper airway obstruction and in clients with head injury or increased intracranial pressure. The drugs are also contraindicated in clients with convulsive disorders, severe renal or hepatic dysfunction, and acute ulcerative colitis. The opioid analgesics are pregnancy category C drugs (oxycodone is in pregnancy category B) and are not recommended for use during pregnancy or labor because they may prolong labor or cause respiratory depression in the neonate. The use of opioid analgesics is recommended during pregnancy only if the benefit to the mother outweighs the potential harm to the fetus.

PRECAUTIONS

Opioid analgesics should be used cautiously in older adults and in clients considered **opioid naive**, that is, who have not been medicated with opioid drugs before and who are consequently at greatest risk for respiratory depression. Example of this is a client undergoing their first surgical procedure as shown in Figure 15.2. The drugs should be administered

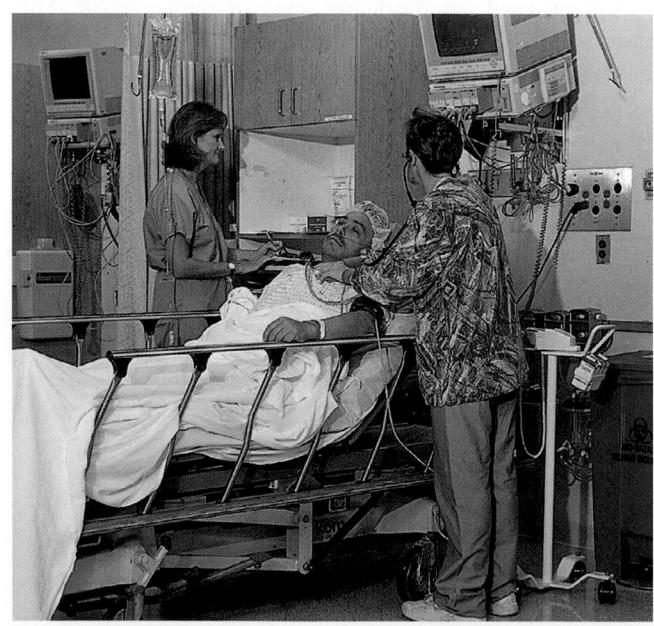

FIGURE 15.2 Clients who are in acute pain following a surgical procedure and do not use opioids routinely are at highest risk for respiratory depression. (Photo by B. Proud.)

cautiously in clients undergoing biliary surgery (because of the risk for spasm of the sphincter of Oddi, between the bile duct and small intestine; in these clients, meperidine is the drug of choice). Clients who are lactating should wait at least 4–6 hr after taking the drug to breastfeed the infant. Additional precautions apply to clients with undiagnosed abdominal pain, hypoxia, supraventricular tachycardia, prostatic hypertrophy, and renal or hepatic impairment.

LASA ALERT

The following drugs may sound alike; be sure to clarify when they are ordered:

Drug Name	Sounds Like
Alfenta	Sufenta
Alfentanil	Anafranil, fentaNYL, remifentanil, sufentanil
Buprenex	Brevibloc, Bumex
Codeine	Cardene, Cordran, iodine, Lodine
Demerol	Demulen, Desyrel, Dilaudid, Pamelor
Dilaudid	Demerol, Dilantin
HYDROcodone	HYDROmorphone, OxyCODONE, OxyMORphone
HYDROmorphone	morphine, buprenorphine
Meperidine	meprobamate
Methadone	dexmethylphenidate, ketorolac, memantine, Mephyton, methylphenidate, Metadate CD, Metadate ER, metOLazone, morphine
Morphine	magnesium sulfate, HYDROmorphone, methadone
MS Contin	OxyCONTIN
Roxanol	OxyFast, Roxicet, Roxicodone
Tapentadol	Tramadol

Drugs that look like a similar drug are noted in the Summary Drug Tables of each chapter.

INTERACTIONS

The following interactions may occur when an opioid analgesic is administered with another agent:

Interacting Drug	Common Use	Effect of Interaction
Alcohol	Social occasions	Increased risk for CNS depression
Antihistamines	Prevent or relieve allergic reactions	Increased risk for CNS depression
Antidepressants	Alleviate depression	Increased risk for CNS depression
Sedatives	Sedation	Increased risk for CNS depression
Phenothiazines	Relief of agitation, anxiety, vomiting	Increased risk for CNS depression

Interacting Drug	Common Use	Effect of Interaction
Opioid agonist–antagonist	Gynecologic or obstetric pain relief	Opioid withdrawal symptoms (if long-term opioid use)
Barbiturates	Used in general anesthesia	Respiratory depression, hypotension, or sedation

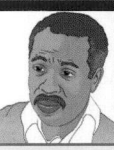

PHARMACOLOGY IN PRACTICE

ASSESSMENT
A nurse is caring for a client who is prescribed opioid analgesics. Which of the following is an allergic reaction to opioid analgesics?
1. Constipation
2. Urticaria
3. Palpitations
4. Facial flushing

THE OPIATE CRISIS

Diminishing pain and creating a sense of euphoria is one of the many reasons opiates have been an addicting agent ever since these substances were discovered (Ostling et al., 2018). This is also the reason their use has been feared by health care providers, knowing that the effect of these drugs on the nervous system can lead to reducing vital body functions and ultimately causing death.

In efforts to overcome these perceptions of fear, Pain Initiatives were launched in individual states in the United States to recognize and treat pain. Learning that strong opiates could make treatment for diseases like cancer more tolerable, pain became acknowledged as the fifth vital sign. At the same time, drug manufacturers were producing opiates more powerful than morphine sulfate and drugs like oxycodone and fentanyl in easier to use forms. As a result, we have to ask ourselves, has the pendulum of pain relief swung too far on the opposite side, resulting in a multitude of overdoses from opioids?

Opiate addiction is a complex topic, too broad to be covered adequately in a pharmacology textbook, yet here are some of the facts we know:

• More than 750,000 people have died since 1999 from a drug overdose (Wonder, 2020).
• Two of three drug overdose deaths in 2018 involved an opioid (Wilson et al., 2020).
• Cost and accessibility entice younger users to switch to heroin, still fentanyl is often cut with the drug making the chance of overdose greater (Painter, 2017).

The highest rates, nationally, of opioid prescriptions occurred in 2012, with a prescribing rate of 81 prescriptions per 100 people (CDC, 2020). By 2018, that rate declined to 51 prescriptions per 100 people. Despite the decrease in prescribing, overdoses involving opioids resulted in almost 47,000 deaths in 2018, with over one-third of those deaths involving a prescription opioid (Wilson et al., 2020).

In addition to being good pain managers, nurses need to be able to assess and respond to issues of opiate overuse and methods for both immediate rescue and long-term treatment of opiate addiction. The administration of opiate antagonist drugs is an important link in the cycle of pain management.

OPIATE ANTAGONISTS

An antagonist is a substance that counteracts the action of something else. Administration of an opiate antagonist prevents or reverses the effects of opioid drugs. For example, one of the most severe adverse reactions to opioid treatment is respiratory depression. In the brain, the antagonist drug "bumps" or replaces the opioid drug off of the receptor and the signal to breathe is reestablished.

ACTIONS

A drug that is an opioid antagonist has a greater affinity for a **cell surface receptor** than an opioid drug (agonist), and by binding to the cell it prevents the cell from responding to the opioid. Thus, an opioid antagonist reverses the actions of an opioid. An antagonist drug is not selective for specific adverse reactions. What this means is that when an antagonist is given to reverse a specific adverse reaction, such as respiratory depression, it is important to remember the antagonist drug reverses *all* effects. Therefore, a client who receives an antagonist to reverse respiratory effects will also experience a reversal of pain relief; that is, the pain will return. If the individual has not taken or received an opioid, an antagonist has no drug effect.

USES

The opioid antagonist you will typically see (naloxone) is used for the treatment of the following:

- Postoperative acute respiratory depression
- Opioid adverse effects (reversal)
- Suspected acute opioid overdosage

TABLE 15.2 Opioid/Antagonist Combinations

BRAND NAME	OPIOID	ANTAGONIST
Acurox	oxycodone	Niacin
Embeda	morphine	naltrexone
Suboxone	buprenorphine	Naloxone
Targniq	oxycodone	Naloxone

Other opioid antagonists are used for the treatment of opioid addiction. These antagonist drugs help those addicted to opiates (heroin or prescription medications such as oxycodone) by removing the pleasurable, euphoric effect of the drugs. This is accomplished by making a combined opiate/antagonist drug. Table 15.2 lists the agents used in some of these combination drugs.

ADVERSE REACTIONS

Generalized reactions include:

- Nausea and vomiting
- Sweating
- Tachycardia
- Increased blood pressure
- Tremors

CONTRAINDICATIONS, PRECAUTIONS, AND INTERACTIONS

Antagonists are contraindicated in those with a hypersensitivity to the opioid antagonists. Antagonists are used cautiously in those who are pregnant (pregnancy category B), in infants of opioid-dependent mothers, and in clients with an opioid dependency or cardiovascular disease. These drugs also are used cautiously during lactation.

These drugs may produce withdrawal symptoms in individuals who are physically dependent on the opioid. Antagonists may prevent the action or intended use of opioid antidiarrheals, antitussives, and analgesics.

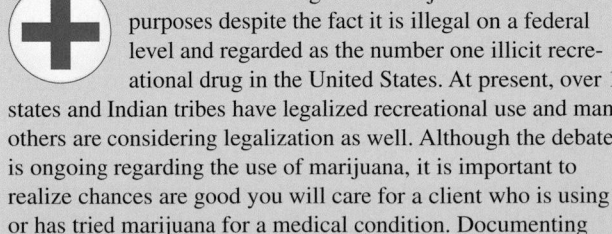

BOX 15.2	**Use of Medical Marijuana**

Most states have legalized marijuana for medical purposes despite the fact it is illegal on a federal level and regarded as the number one illicit recreational drug in the United States. At present, over 15 states and Indian tribes have legalized recreational use and many others are considering legalization as well. Although the debate is ongoing regarding the use of marijuana, it is important to realize chances are good you will care for a client who is using or has tried marijuana for a medical condition. Documenting use in the medical record is important so that all members of the health care team are aware of its use and possible interactions with other drugs.

Historically, medical use of marijuana (*cannabis*) dates back 4000 years. It was initially introduced into Western medicine as early as the 1850s. Legitimized by inclusion in the US Pharmacopeia (USP), it was prescribed by physicians for many reasons such as an analgesic to its use on a sore as a wart remover. In 1942, cannabis was removed from the USP and by 1970s was classified as a C-I controlled substance by the Drug Enforcement Agency and the Food and Drug Administration. Because of

BOX 15.2 Use of Medical Marijuana (Continued)

this classification, our understanding of medical use is based on antidotal evidence without formalized research (Kapur, 2015).

California was the first state to legalize medical marijuana in 1996. Client registries set up in each state help provide a better idea of why clients are consuming marijuana for medical purposes. To date, 90% of the clients use marijuana for pain management, with the second reason to reduce muscle spasm. Providers (MD, DO, Naturopath, or Nurse Practitioner) may *recommend* use for a qualified condition, which is unrelieved by standard treatments or medications. Medical marijuana is not *prescribed* to date because this would be a violation of federal laws.

Therapeutic Uses of Medical Marijuana

Cancer	Human immunodeficiency virus
Chronic renal failure	Intractable pain
Crohn disease with debilitating symptoms	Multiple sclerosis
Epilepsy or other seizure disorder	Muscle spasms, or spasticity
Glaucoma, acute or chronic	Posttraumatic stress disorder
Hepatitis C with debilitating nausea or intractable pain	Traumatic brain injury

Cannabis is a flowering herbal plant grown for hemp (rope fiber) as well as its drug properties. Cannabinoids are the chemical compounds in the plant that produce the effects sought by users. Tetrahydrocannabinol (THC) is the primary psychoactive component. Another compound, Cannabidiol (CBD), appears to relieve inflammation, anxiety, and nausea. Dronabinol (Marinol C-III class) and nabilone (Cesamet, C-II) are synthetic THC drugs used for chemotherapy-induced nausea and HIV-associated anorexia. A client using these drugs will experience the psychoactive effects of the drug, whereas products derived from CBD alone are being researched to produce the GI effects without the psychoactive effects, too.

Medical marijuana is available to smoke, vaporize, apply topically, or as an edible option such as infusions of oil, butters, tinctures made into candy-like products, lollipops, mints, drinks, and baked goods. As with other herbal products, consistent quality and purity is not regulated. For example, a typical cigarette may contain 0.5 g of marijuana, yet the THC content may be anywhere from 12% to 23%. Rate of onset

is also variable. Smoking may produce an effect in 10 min, whereas ingestion requires at least 30–60 min. Because of this lag time for edible products, people may feel they have not taken enough for effect and may ingest more resulting in a dangerous overdose. In addition to the intended effects, clients should be taught to recognize potential adverse effects of the drug.

Acute Adverse Effects

CNS	Cardiac
Anxiety	Increase heart rate
Panic reaction	Fluctuation in blood pressure
Psychotic symptoms	

Chronic Adverse Effects

CNS	Respiratory (When Inhaled)
Memory cognitive impairment	Chronic bronchitis
Psychotic symptoms	Decreased pulmonary function Pulmonary infection

The following interactions may occur when medical marijuana is taken with another agent:

Interacting Drug	Common Use	Effect of Interaction
Anticoagulants, antiplatelet, NSAIDs	Blood thinner	Increased risk of bleeding
Oral antidiabetic, insulin	To control blood sugar	Reduces blood sugar
Antihypertensive drugs	Blood pressure control	Reduces blood pressure
Sedatives and hypnotics	To relax and produce sleep	Increased effectiveness
Antihistamines	Prevent or relieve allergic reactions, induce sleep	Increased drowsiness
Opioids and muscle relaxants	Pain relief	Increased depressive effect
Phenytoin	Anti-seizures	Increases anti-seizure effect
Alcohol	Social occasions	Increased depressive effect

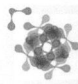

NURSING PROCESS: STEPS TO BUILDING CLINICAL JUDGMENT
Client Receiving an Opioid Analgesic for Pain/Rescue From Respiratory Depression

ASSESSMENT

Preadministration Assessment

Assessment for severe pain can be difficult because it is hard for the pain distracted client to discuss the situation. Be sure that you address each different pain like it is a new pain by doing a thorough assessment. Here are data gathering suggestions before the initial administration of the drug:
Objective data

- Location of pain
- Description of site that is the cause of the pain (such as drainage, redness, swelling)
- Palpate for tenderness in the location of pain, examine joints if involved
- Vital signs (temperature, pulse, respirations, and blood pressure)
- Medications on electronic health record if in clinical setting

If promethazine is used with an opioid to enhance the effects and reduce the dosage of the opioid, be mindful of the vital signs, especially respirations. Promethazine can increase the sedation effect and respiratory depression when used with an opiate.

Subjective data

- Pain experience—onset, type (e.g., sharp, dull, stabbing, throbbing), radiation, location, intensity, and duration
- Type and duration of symptoms (has it impacted ability to work or concentrate)
- When did it start and history of this pain, is it different, is the quality different, is the location different
- Remedies attempted before seeking care, both drug therapies and nonpharmaceutical
- Response to previous medications given for pain relief, such as nausea and hives

Risk Considerations for Respiratory Depression

Clients involved in long-term opioid therapy for pain relief build **tolerance** to the physical adverse effects of the drugs. Individuals at greater risk for respiratory depression when undergoing a surgical procedure with analgesic drugs include:

- long-term opioid users, who have a chronic or an acute respiratory issue.
- opioid-naive clients, those who do not use opioids routinely and who are being given an opioid drug for acute pain relief.

Ongoing Assessment

You can measure the effect of the opioid by taking the blood pressure, pulse, respiratory rate, and pain rating in 5–10 min if the drug is given intravenously (IV), 20–30 min if the drug is administered intramuscularly (IM) or subcutaneously (subcut), and 30 or more minutes if the drug is given orally. It is important to notify the primary health care provider if the analgesic is ineffective, because a higher dose or a different opioid analgesic may be required.

During the ongoing assessment, it is important for you to ask about the pain regularly and to accept the client and family's reports of pain. Nursing judgment must be exercised, because not all instances of a change in pain type, location, or intensity require notifying the primary health care provider. For example, if a client recovering from recent abdominal surgery experiences pain in the calf of the leg (suggesting venous thrombosis), you should immediately notify the primary health care provider. However, it is not necessary to contact the primary health care provider for pain that is slightly worse because the client has been moving in bed.

Fears of Respiratory Depression

The opioid-naive client who does not use opioids routinely and is being given an opioid drug for acute pain relief or a surgical procedure is at greatest risk for respiratory depression after opioid administration (see Fig. 15.2). Respiratory depression may occur in clients receiving a normal dose if the client is vulnerable (e.g., in a weakened or debilitated state). Older, **cachectic** (malnourished/in general poor health), or debilitated clients should receive a reduced initial dose until their response to the drug is known.

Sometimes the somnolence and pain relief produced by the opioid drug will slow the client's breathing pattern. This can be alarming if the respiratory rate you have been monitoring has been rapid because of anxiety and pain. The first step is to make efforts to arouse the client and coach their breathing pattern, if possible. If the client's respiratory rate is 10 breaths/min or less, monitor the client at more frequent intervals and notify the primary health care provider immediately. Before administration of the antagonist drug, note the blood pressure, pulse, and respiratory rate, and review the record for the drug suspected of causing the symptoms of respiratory depression. After the client has shown a response to the antagonist, monitor vital signs every 5–15 min. Notify the anesthesiologist or primary health care provider if any adverse drug reactions occur because additional medical treatment may be needed. Continue to monitor the respiratory rate, rhythm, and depth; pulse; blood pressure; and level of consciousness until the effects of the opioid wear off.

! NURSING ALERT

The effects of some opioids may last longer than the effects of naloxone. A repeat dose of naloxone may be ordered if results obtained from the initial dose are unsatisfactory. The duration of close client observation depends on the client's response to the administration of the opioid antagonist.

When an opiate is used as an antidiarrheal drug, document each bowel movement, as well as its appearance, color, and consistency. Notify the primary health care provider immediately if diarrhea is not relieved or becomes worse, if the client has severe abdominal pain, or if blood in the stool is noted.

NURSING DIAGNOSES

Drug-specific nursing diagnoses are the following:

- **Altered breathing pattern** related to pain and effects on breathing center by opioids
- **Injury risk** related to dizziness or lightheadedness from opioid administration
- **Constipation** related to the decreased GI motility caused by opioids
- **Malnutrition: less than body requirements** related to anorexia caused by opioids

When an antagonist is administered:

- **Impaired self-ventilation** related to brain response to slow breathing induced by the opioid drug
- **Acute pain** related to the antagonist drug displacing the opioid drug at cell receptor sites

Nursing diagnoses related to drug administration are discussed in Chapter 4.

PLANNING

The expected outcomes of the client may include relief of pain, supporting the client needs related to the management of adverse reactions, an understanding of **patient-controlled analgesia** (PCA; when applicable), absence of injury, adequate nutrition intake, and when using an antagonist providing adequate ventilation until a return to normal respiratory rate, rhythm, and depth, confidence in an understanding of the medication regimen.

IMPLEMENTATION

Promoting an Optimal Response to Therapy

Relieving Acute Pain

Acute pain can be severe following a surgical procedure. For acute pain, the goal is to control the pain, then reduce the dosage as the tissues heal. Many postoperative clients require less opioid when they can self-administer the medicine for pain. PCA allows postsurgical clients to administer their own analgesic by means of an IV pump system (Fig. 15.3). Pumps are preset to dispense small amounts of the opioid medication that the client can administer by pushing a button on the pump. The medication can be delivered, for example, when the client begins to feel pain or when the client wishes to ambulate but wants some medication to prevent pain on getting out of bed. The client does not have to wait for the nurse to administer the medicine. As a result, clients medicate before they cannot tolerate the pain, use less medication, and resume activity faster. When clients take less opioid, they also experience fewer unpleasant adverse reactions, such as nausea and constipation. Because the self-administration system is under the control of the nurse, who adds the drug to the infusion pump and sets the time interval (or lockout interval) between doses, the client cannot receive an overdose of the drug.

Not all acute pain requires IV medication. Clients may complain of moderate to severe pain with many dental and outpatient procedures. In addition, dealing with pain management in the home environment makes oral pain relief a necessity. That is why the number one prescription drug in the United States is a combination pain reliever: hydrocodone + acetaminophen. Using the concept of the modified WHO pain ladder for chronic pain management, medications that work to relieve pain both peripherally and centrally are ordered. For ease of administration and to provide good pain relief based on the pain ladder, drugs that combine a nonopioid and an opioid analgesic are available. These drugs work well at

dealing with the inflammation at the peripheral site, as well as modifying the pain perception centrally in the brain. Table 15.3 lists many of these drugs and their combination ingredients.

Until recent years, hydrocodone has only been available in a combination drug formula. In this combination form, it was easier to purchase because it was deemed a C-III controlled substance, leading to what many believe as an easy-to-abuse opioid (most opiates are designated C-II, requiring tighter prescriptive procedures). The drug is chemically similar to oxycodone, yet it works in the body like hydromorphone and has potency similar to morphine sulfate. Orally it is used for severe pain that is either acute or chronic. Hydrocodone (Zohydro ER and Hysingla ER) is now available as a C-II controlled substance in a solitary (hydrocodone only) drug form.

Sufentanil used for severe, acute pain is now available in a sublingual form to be used for treatment in an inpatient setting only. Gloves need to be worn during preparation and administration to prevent provider absorption. In addition, the client should not eat or drink for at least 10 min after administration.

Relieving Chronic Severe Pain

Morphine sulfate is the most widely used drug in the management of chronic severe pain. The fact that this drug can be given orally, nasally, subcutaneously, IM, IV, and rectally in the form of a suppository makes it tremendously versatile. Medication for chronic pain should be scheduled around the clock and not given on a PRN (as-needed) basis. With any chronic pain medication, the oral route is preferred as long as the client can swallow or can tolerate sublingual administration.

Controlled-release forms of opioids are indicated for the management of moderate to severe pain when a continuous, around-the-clock analgesic is needed for an extended time. Examples of these drugs include oxycodone (OxyContin) and morphine sulfate (MS Contin). The medication is given once every 8–12 hr; the actual drug is slowly released over time so the client does not get all the medication at once. Controlled-release drugs are not intended for use as a PRN analgesic. The client may experience fewer adverse reactions with oxycodone products than with morphine sulfate, and the drug is effective and safe for older adults. Controlled-release

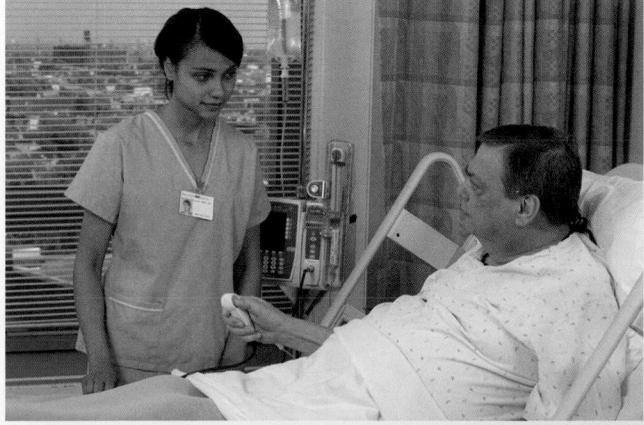

FIGURE 15.3 Patient-controlled analgesia (PCA) allows the client to self-administer medication as necessary to control pain.

TABLE 15.3 Opioid/Nonopioid Combination Oral Analgesics

BRAND NAME	OPIOID	NONOPIOID
Tylenol #3	codeine 30 mg	acetaminophen 300 mg
Vicoprofen	hydrocodone 7.5 mg	ibuprofen 200 mg
Vicodin	hydrocodone 5 mg	acetaminophen 300 mg
Vicodin ES	hydrocodone 7.5 mg	acetaminophen 750 mg
Percodan	oxycodone 5 mg	aspirin 325 mg
Percocet	oxycodone 5 mg	acetaminophen 325 mg
Roxicet	oxycodone 5 mg	acetaminophen 325 mg

tablets should be swallowed whole and are not to be broken, chewed, or crushed.

When long-acting forms of the opioids are used, a fast-acting form may be given for breakthrough pain. These are typically ordered on a PRN basis to be used between the long-acting doses for acute pain episodes. Morphine sulfate in oral or sublingual tablets is commonly used. Oral transmucosal fentanyl (Actiq) is also used to treat breakthrough cancer pain for clients who cannot swallow a pill.

Fentanyl transdermal is a transdermal system that is effective in the management of severe pain associated with diseases like cancer. This drug should be used only when other opioids or routes are proven unsuccessful; it should never be used on an opiate-naive client. The transdermal system allows for a timed-release patch containing the drug fentanyl to be activated over a 72-hr period. A small number of clients may require systems applied every 48 hr. When used, you should monitor for adverse reactions in the same manner as for other opioid analgesics.

Lifespan Considerations

Gerontology
The transdermal route should be used with caution in older adults, because the amount of subcutaneous tissue is reduced in the aging process. The transdermal route of drug administration for pain is used because it treats severe pain when other methods are not successful; it should not be used simply for the convenience of administration.

Compounded Medications
Sometimes pain is accompanied by symptoms such as anxiety or restlessness and is best relieved by a combination of drugs and not just the opioid analgesics alone. For better administration, especially if the client is at home, a mixture of an oral opioid and other drugs may be used to obtain relief; this is referred to as **compounding medications**. Brompton mixture is one of the most commonly used compounded pain relief solutions. In addition to the opioid, such as morphine sulfate or methadone, other drugs may be used in the compounded preparation, including antidepressants, stimulants, aspirin, acetaminophen, and sedatives. The clinical pharmacist prepares the medication as a solution, salve, or suppository depending on the best method to administer the preparation to the specific client. As the nurse, you are frequently required to teach the client or caregivers how to store and self-administer these preparations. It is necessary to monitor for the adverse reactions of each drug contained in the preparation. The time interval for administration varies. Some primary health care providers may order the mixture on a PRN basis; others may order it given at regular intervals.

Tolerance Versus Dependence
Over time, the client taking an opioid analgesic develops a tolerance to the drug. This is different from *physical dependence,* where the body experiences adverse effects if the medicine is stopped. With tolerance, the body physically adapts to the drug, and greater amounts are

needed to achieve the same effects. The rate at which tolerance develops varies according to the dosage, the route of administration, and the individual. Clients taking oral medications develop tolerance more slowly than those taking the drugs parenterally. Some clients develop tolerance quickly and need larger doses every few weeks, whereas others are maintained on the same dosage schedule throughout the course of the illness.

The fear of respiratory depression is a concern for many nurses when they administer an opioid, and some nurses may even hesitate to administer the drug. However, respiratory depression rarely occurs in clients using an opioid for chronic pain. In fact, these clients usually develop tolerance to the respiratory depressant effects of the drug very quickly. You should be more concerned about adverse effects on the GI system. The decrease in GI motility causes constipation, nausea, acute abdominal pain, and anorexia. It is important to provide a thorough, aggressive bowel program to clients when they are taking opioid medications.

Using Transdermal System Pain Management
When using a transdermal system, it is important to ensure that only one patch is on at a time to prevent additive effects of the drug. Find and remove the old patch before replacing it with a new one. To discard, fold the patch so the sticky side adheres to itself, and discard in the toilet or a "sharps" container. Never dispose in a waste container accessible to children or pets. Before the new transdermal patch is applied, date and initial the patch with a water-resistant pen. Use only water to cleanse the site before application, because soaps, oils, and other substances may irritate the skin. Rotate the site of application and do not apply over hair. To ensure complete contact with the skin surface, press for 10–20 seconds (Fig. 15.4). After 72 hr, remove the system and, if continuous therapy is prescribed, apply a new patch.

! NURSING ALERT
Heat can increase the absorption of the drug in a transdermal system, causing overdose of the drug. Caution clients and families never to place a heating blanket or pad over the patch. Also, teach clients to be aware of other heat sources as well such as tanning lamps, hot tubs, saunas, or hot baths.

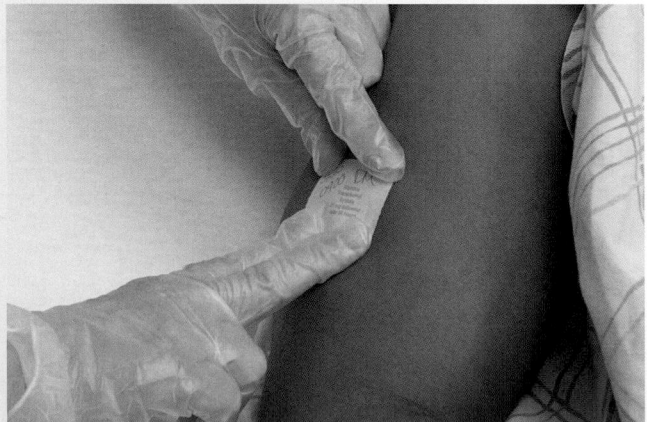

FIGURE 15.4 The nurse applies the transdermal patch securely.

Using Epidural Pain Management
Administration of morphine sulfate and fentanyl by the epidural route has provided an alternative to the IM or oral route. This approach was introduced with the idea that very small doses of opioid would provide long-lasting pain relief with significantly fewer systemic adverse reactions; hence it is thought of as Step 4 in the modified WHO pain ladder (see Fig. 15.1).

Epidural administration offers several advantages over other routes, including lower total dosages of the drug used, fewer adverse reactions, and greater client comfort. This type of pain management is used for postoperative pain, labor pain, and intractable chronic pain. The administration of the opioid is either by bolus or by continuous infusion pump.

Clients experience pain relief with fewer adverse reactions; the adverse reactions experienced are those related to processes under direct CNS control. The most serious adverse reaction associated with the epidurally administered opioids is respiratory depression. Clients using epidural analgesics for chronic pain are monitored for respiratory problems with an apnea monitor. The client may also experience sedation, confusion, nausea, pruritus, or urinary retention. Fentanyl is increasingly used as an alternative to morphine sulfate because clients experience fewer adverse reactions.

NURSING ALERT

Epidural analgesia should be administered only by those specifically trained in the use of IV and epidural anesthetics. Oxygen, resuscitative, and intubation equipment should be readily available.

Nursing care includes close monitoring of the client for respiratory depression immediately after insertion of the epidural catheter and throughout therapy. Vital signs are taken every 30 min, apnea monitors are used, and an opioid antagonist, such as naloxone, is readily available.

Policies and procedures for administering, monitoring, and documenting drugs given through the epidural route must be specific to the nurse practice act in each state and in accordance with federal and state regulations. This type of analgesia is most often managed by registered nurses with special training in the care and management of epidural catheters.

Monitoring and Managing Client Needs
You should contact the primary health care provider immediately if any of the following are present:

- Significant decrease in the respiratory rate or a respiratory rate of 10 breaths/min or less
- Significant increase or decrease in the pulse rate or a change in the pulse quality
- Significant decrease in blood pressure (systolic or diastolic) or a systolic pressure below 100 mm Hg

Altered Breathing Pattern
Opioids may depress the cough reflex. Encourage clients receiving an opioid, even for a few days, to cough and breathe deeply every 2 hr. This task prevents the pooling of secretions in the lungs, which can lead to hypostatic pneumonia and other lung problems. The client may be fearful that exercise will cause even greater pain. Teach the client that these activities are designed to help the body recover better. Performing tasks (such as getting out of bed) and therapeutic activities (such as deep breathing, coughing, and leg exercises) when the drug is producing its greatest analgesic effect, usually 1–2 hr after administering the opioid, aids in recovery. If the client experiences nausea and vomiting, notify the primary health care provider. A different analgesic or an antiemetic may be necessary.

Injury Risk
Opioids may produce orthostatic hypotension, which in turn results in dizziness. Report any significant change in the client's vital signs to the primary health care provider. Particularly vulnerable are postoperative clients and individuals whose ability to maintain blood pressure has been compromised. You should assist the client with ambulatory activities and with rising slowly from a sitting or lying position to assess for hypotensive problems. Miosis (pinpoint pupils) may occur with the administration of some opioids and is most pronounced with morphine sulfate, hydromorphone, and opium alkaloids. Miosis decreases the ability to see in dim light. If miosis occurs, teach the client and family to keep the room well lit during daytime hours and advise the client to seek assistance when getting out of bed at night.

Constipation
Most clients should begin taking a stool softener or laxative with the initial dose of an opioid analgesic. Decreased GI motility because of the opioids, in addition to lower food and water intake and decreased mobility, causes the constipation. Teach the client to keep a record of bowel movements and inform the primary health care provider if constipation appears to be a problem. Many clients need to continue taking a laxative for as long as they take an opioid analgesic. If the client is constipated despite the use of a stool softener or laxative, the primary health care provider may prescribe an enema or other means of relieving constipation.

Malnutrition
When an opioid is prescribed for a prolonged time, anorexia (loss of appetite) may occur. Those receiving an opioid for pain relief caused by a terminal illness often have severe anorexia from the disease and the opioid. Note food intake after each meal. When anorexia is prolonged, weigh the client as ordered by the primary health care provider. It is important to encourage caregivers to discuss with the primary health care provider treatment plans for continued weight loss and anorexia. Supplements may be ordered and administered orally, enterally, or parenterally.

A decision may be made to support the terminal client as they become anorexic and provide comfort measures without attempting to increase the weight or encourage eating.

Impaired Self-Ventilation
Depending on the client's condition, you may need to use cardiac monitoring, oxygen therapy, artificial ventilation (respirator), and other drugs during and after the administration of naloxone. It is important to keep suction equipment readily available because abrupt reversal of opioid-induced respiratory depression may cause vomiting. The goal is to maintain a patent airway, so you may need to turn and suction the client to achieve this.

If naloxone is given by IV infusion, the anesthesiologist or primary health care provider orders the IV fluid and amount, the drug dosage, and the infusion rate. Giving the drug by IV infusion requires use of a secondary line, an IV piggyback, or an IV push (see Chapter 54).

NURSING ALERT
When naloxone is used to reverse respiratory depression and the resulting somnolence, the drug is given by slow IV push until the respiratory rate begins to increase and somnolence abates. Keep in mind that giving a rapid bolus will cause withdrawal and return of intense pain.

Acute Pain
When the antagonist drug is given to clients, the pain experience returns abruptly; this is because the opioid no longer works in the body. Assess the pain level and begin to treat the pain again. As the client's breathing returns, review the circumstances that led to the use of the antagonist as an opioid reversal drug. Steps can then be taken to resume pain relief without the adverse reaction.

Monitor fluid intake and output and notify the primary health care provider of any change in the fluid intake–output ratio. Again, notify the primary health care provider if there is any sudden change in the client's condition.

PHARMACOLOGY IN PRACTICE

MANAGING NEEDS
A client in a postsurgical recovery unit is prescribed a dose of naloxone. Which of the following interventions should the nurse perform during and after naloxone administration when caring for this client? Select all that apply.
1. Monitor the client for symptoms of hypotension.
2. Make the suction equipment available.
3. Turn and suction the client when needed.
4. Provide oxygen or artificial ventilation if necessary.
5. Monitor hematologic changes.

Opioid Physical Dependence in Acute Pain Management
Clients receiving the opioid analgesics for short-term, acute pain do not develop physical dependence. Delays in medication administration cause clients to ask repeatedly for pain medication. This behavior is sometimes interpreted as drug-seeking behavior, or it may be associated with the fear (of the nurse) of making a client drug dependent. Nurses are also fearful that clients with a history of psychologic dependence might become dependent again when given pain medication. These individuals experience pain, too. They need to be provided adequate pain relief to *prevent* returning to dependency behaviors. Typically, it is the behavior of the nurses and primary health care providers in delaying administration of opioids for good pain control that causes the problems associated with appearances of dependence.

Drug dependence can, however, occur in a newborn whose mother was dependent on opiates during pregnancy. Withdrawal symptoms in the newborn usually appear during the first few days of life. Symptoms include irritability, excessive crying, yawning, sneezing, increased respiratory rate, tremors, fever, vomiting, and diarrhea.

Drug enforcement efforts to curb abuse are a way to reduce drug dependence. Sustained-release, extended-release, or controlled-release opioids are drugs formulated to release a set amount of drug over time making it a long-acting drug and to reduce the administration intervals for those who have difficulty taking a medication. These are also one of the biggest items in the drug abuse markets, because they can be crushed allowing for large amounts of the drug to be taken at one time. Pharmaceutical manufacturers have produced tamper deterrent products of long-acting opiate drugs, which when smashed up cannot provide an immediate release sensation to the user. Their effectiveness is questionable since there are no prescribing requirements in place to monitor their use (Ostling et al., 2018).

Management of Opioid Dependence
Two opioids are used in the treatment and management of opiate dependence: levomethadyl and methadone. Levomethadyl is given in an opiate dependency clinic to maintain control over the delivery of the drug. Because of its potential for serious and life-threatening prearrhythmic effects, levomethadyl is reserved for treating addicted clients who have had no response to other treatments. Levomethadyl is not taken daily; the drug is administered three times a week (Monday/Wednesday/Friday or Tuesday/Thursday/Saturday). Daily use of the usual dose will cause serious overdose.

NURSING ALERT
If a client is transferring from levomethadyl to methadone, the nurse should wait 48 hr after the last dose of levomethadyl before administering the first dose of methadone or other opioid.

Methadone, a synthetic opioid, may be used for the relief of pain, but it is also used in the detoxification and maintenance treatment of those dependent on opioids. Detoxification involves withdrawing the client from the opioid while minimizing withdrawal symptoms. Maintenance therapy is designed to reduce the client's desire to return to the drug that caused dependence, as well as to prevent withdrawal symptoms. Dosages vary with the client, the length of time the individual has been dependent, and the average amount of drug used

---

BOX 15.3 Symptoms of the Abstinence Syndrome

Early Symptoms
Yawning, tearing, runny nose, sweating

Intermediate Symptoms
Pupil dilation, tachycardia, twitching, tremor, restlessness, irritability, anxiety, anorexia

Late Symptoms
Muscle spasm, fever, nausea, vomiting, kicking movements, weakness, depression, body aches, weight loss, severe backache, abdominal and leg pains, hot and cold flashes, insomnia, repetitive sneezing; increased blood pressure, respiratory rate, and heart rate

---

each day. Clients enrolled in an outpatient methadone program for detoxification or maintenance therapy on methadone must continue to receive methadone when hospitalized. In adults, withdrawal symptoms are known as the *abstinence syndrome* (see Box 15.3 for more information).

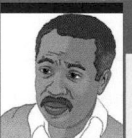

PHARMACOLOGY IN PRACTICE

INTERVENTIONS
A nurse is caring for a client who has delivered a baby. The client was opioid dependent during her pregnancy. Which of the following withdrawal symptoms should the newborn be monitored for due to the client's dependency? Select all that apply.
1. Excessive crying
2. Vomiting
3. Yawning
4. Coughing
5. Sneezing

Educating the Client and Family
Teach the client about the drug they are receiving for pain. Provide written materials in the preferred language about how often the drug can be given, adverse reactions to monitor for, and what to do if the client runs short of the drug.

If a client is to receive drugs through a PCA infusion pump, the client is taught how to use the machine during the preoperative visit rather than waiting until the client is in pain in the postoperative unit (see Client Teaching for Improved Outcomes: Using Client-Controlled Analgesia for Postoperative Pain). Notify the anesthesiologist or surgeon if the client does not understand the PCA procedure so that an alternative method of pain relief can be ordered.

Opioids for outpatient use may be prescribed in the oral form or as a timed-release transdermal patch. In certain cases, such as when terminally ill clients are being cared for at home, the nurse may give the family instruction in the parenteral administration of the drug or use of an IV pump.

Because opioid-related deaths are becoming more prevalent in our society, a *new form of drug delivery* of antagonist drug has been developed. In a medical setting, suspected opioid overdose can be dealt with by professionals. Evzio (naloxone) is a single-dose autoinjector made for administration by emergency responders, a family member, or caregiver to a person experiencing respiratory depression because of overdose. It works as an audio device (similar to an automated defibrillator) providing verbal instructions on how to deliver the injection, including staying with the client until emergency help arrives and to give the provider the used drug cartridge. The intent of the drug device is to begin treatment earlier with the intent to save lives. Family members requesting this device need to be taught how to use the device as well as be aware that opioid withdrawal symptoms may occur (see Box 15.3) and what to do if these occur.

When an opioid has been prescribed, include the following points in the teaching plan:

- This drug may cause drowsiness, dizziness, and blurring of vision. Use caution when driving or performing tasks requiring alertness.
  🍷 Avoid the use of alcoholic beverages unless use has been approved by the primary health care provider. Alcohol may intensify the action of the drug and cause extreme drowsiness or dizziness. In some instances, the use of alcohol and an opioid can have extremely serious and even life-threatening consequences that may require emergency medical treatment.
- Take the drug as directed on the container label and do not exceed the prescribed dose. Contact the primary health care provider if the drug is not effective.
- If GI upset occurs, take the drug with food.
- Notify the primary health care provider if nausea, vomiting, and constipation become severe.

EVALUATION

- Therapeutic response is achieved and discomfort is reduced. If PCA is ordered, the client demonstrates the ability to use PCA effectively.

Client Teaching for Improved Outcomes

Using Patient-Controlled Analgesia for Postoperative Pain

In some situations, IV opioid analgesics may be ordered for pain relief following a surgical procedure. If the client is able to participate, the anesthesiologist may offer PCA. The purpose of this is to allow the client to manage pain to recuperate faster and return to daily activities of life sooner.

When you teach, make sure your client understands the following:

✔ How the pump works; the machine regulates the dose of the drug as well as the time interval between doses.

✔ The location of the control button that activates the administration of the drug; the difference between the control button and the button to call the nurse (especially when both are similar in appearance and feel).

✔ Use the machine to prevent pain, such as when the client feels the need for pain relief or is about to engage in an activity that might cause pain (e.g., coughing, exercises, or getting out of bed).

✔ Push the button once; the button does not need to be depressed to keep the drug flowing in the IV.

✔ The dose of drug is ordered by the primary health care provider and set by the nurse. If the control button is used too soon after the last dose, the machine will not deliver the drug until the correct time; therefore, the client and family members do not need to worry about taking too much drug.

- Adverse reactions are identified, reported to the primary health care provider, and managed successfully with appropriate nursing interventions:
  - An adequate breathing pattern is maintained.
  - No evidence of injury is seen.
  - Client reports adequate bowel movements.
  - Client maintains an adequate nutritional status.
  If an opiate antagonist is used:
  - Client's respiratory rate, rhythm, and depth are normal.
  - Pain relief is resumed.
- Client and family express confidence and demonstrate an understanding of the drug regimen.

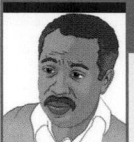

PHARMACOLOGY IN PRACTICE

USING CLINICAL REASONING

From your assessment, determine whether you think Mr. Park could be considered *opioid naive* and more likely to experience respiratory depression. What factors were neglected during the pain assessment that resulted in his respiratory depression?

KEY POINTS

■ A four-step analgesic protocol based on intensity can be used as a guideline for treating pain. The pain ladder directs the use of both opioids and nonopioids in the treatment of moderate to severe pain.

■ *Opioid* is a term used for drugs that change the pain sensation by attaching to receptor sites in the brain producing an analgesic, sedative, and euphoric effect. Most of these are derived from opium or a synthetic substance like opium.

■ These drugs are used to treat moderate to severe pain.

■ *Narcotic* is a term referring to the properties of a drug to produce numbness or a stupor-like state. Although the terms *opioid* and *narcotic* were once interchangeable, law enforcement agencies have generalized the term *narcotic* to mean a drug that is addictive and abused or used illegally. Health care providers use the term *opioid* to describe drugs used in pain relief.

■ Morphine sulfate is a drug used through multiple routes for relief of chronic and acute pain. Other opioids are com-

pared with this drug (the gold standard) when attempting to determine dosing or conversion between drug types.

■ Patient-controlled analgesia is a self-administered IV pump that clients use following painful procedures. By allowing clients to control administration, they tend to use less of the drug and recuperate faster.

■ The more common non–pain relief effects (known as secondary effects) of these drugs include respiratory depression, decreased GI motility, and miosis. Constipation is the one side effect to which the body does not build a tolerance.

■ An opioid antagonist reverses the effects of an opioid drug. This is used when clients experience extreme adverse reactions such as respiratory depression.

■ These drugs reverse all effects of the opioids and the client will experience pain.

■ Clients who seldom use opioid pain relievers are termed opioid naive; they are at the greatest risk of experiencing respiratory depression when administered opioids.

SUMMARY DRUG TABLE
Opioid Analgesics

Generic Name	Trade Name	Uses	Adverse Reactions[a]	Dosage Ranges
Agonists (Activate Receptors and Cause Action)				
Alfentanil *al-FEN-ta-nil*	Alfenta	Anesthetic adjunct	Respiratory depression, skeletal muscle rigidity, constipation, nausea, vomiting	Individualize dosage and titrate to obtain desired effect
codeine[b] *KOE-deen*		Moderate to severe pain, antitussive, anesthetic adjunct	Sedation, sweating, headache, dizziness, lethargy, confusion, lightheadedness	Analgesic: 15–60 mg every 4–6 hr orally, subcut, IM
fentaNYL[b] *FEN-ta-nil*	Abstral, Actiq, Fentora, Lazanda (nasal spray), Onsolis, Subsys	Severe pain, anesthetic adjunct, management of breakthrough cancer pain	Sweating, headache, vertigo, lethargy, confusion, nausea, vomiting, respiratory depression	Same as alfentanil 200–1600 µg/dose, depending on pain severity
fentanyl transdermal system[b]	Duragesic	Chronic pain unmanaged by other opioids	Sedation, sweating, headache, vertigo, lethargy, confusion, lightheadedness, nausea, vomiting	Individualized dosage: 25- to 175-µg transdermal patch (dose is amount absorbed per hour)
HYDROcodone[b] *hye-droe-KOE-done*	Hysingla ER, Zohydro ER	Severe pain	Sedation, sweating, headache, vertigo, lethargy, confusion, lightheadedness, nausea, vomiting	20–50 mg orally daily, greater than 80 mg daily only if opioid tolerant
HYDROmorphone[b] *hye-droe-MOR-fone*	Dilaudid,	Moderate to severe pain	Sedation, vertigo, lethargy, confusion, lightheadedness, nausea, vomiting	2–4 mg orally q4–6hr; 3 mg rectally every 6–8 hr; 1–2 mg IM or subcut every 4–6 hr
levorphanol[b] *lee-VOR-fa-nole*		Moderate to severe pain, preoperative sedation	Dizziness, nausea, vomiting, dry mouth, sweating, respiratory depression	2 mg orally every 3–6 hr; 1 mg IV every 3–8 hr
meperidine[b] *me-PER-i-deen*	Demerol	Acute moderate to severe pain, preoperative sedation, anesthetic adjunct	Lightheadedness, constipation, dizziness, nausea, vomiting, respiratory depression	50–150 mg orally, IM, subcut every 3–4 hr
methadone[b] *METH-a-done*	Dolophine	Severe pain; treatment of opioid dependence	Lightheadedness, dizziness, sedation, nausea, vomiting, constipation	Analgesic: 2.5–10 mg orally, IM, subcut every 4 hr; detoxification: 10–40 mg orally, IV
morphine[b] *MOR-feen*	Astramorph, Kadian, Duramorph; timed release: MS Contin	Acute/chronic pain, preoperative sedation, anesthetic adjunct, dyspnea	Sedation, hypotension, increased sweating, constipation, dizziness, drowsiness, nausea, vomiting, dry mouth, somnolence, respiratory depression	Acute pain relief: 10–30 mg every 4 hr; chronic pain relief: individualized
oxyCODONE[b] *oks-i-KOE-done*	Roxicodone, Oxaydo; timed release: OxyContin, Xtampza ER	Moderate to severe pain	Lightheadedness, sedation, constipation, dizziness, nausea, vomiting, sweating, respiratory depression	10–30 mg orally every 4 hr
oxyMORphone[b] *oks-i-MOR-fone*		Moderate to severe pain, preoperative sedation, obstetric analgesia	Lightheadedness, sedation, constipation, dizziness, nausea, vomiting, respiratory depression	1–1.5 mg subcut or IM every 4–6 hr
remifentanil *rem-i-FEN-ta-nil*	Ultiva	Anesthetic adjunct	Lightheadedness, skeletal muscle rigidity, nausea, vomiting, respiratory depression, sweating	Same as alfentanil
SUFentanil[b] *soo-FEN-ta-nil*	Dsuvia, Sufenta	Anesthetic adjunct, severe pain management	Same as alfentanil	Same as alfentanil

Continued

SUMMARY DRUG TABLE (continued)
Opioid Analgesics

Generic Name	Trade Name	Uses	Adverse Reactions[a]	Dosage Ranges
tapentadol[b] *ta-PEN-ta-dol*	Nucynta	Moderate to severe pain, neuropathic pain	Lightheadedness, nausea, vomiting, respiratory depression, sweating, serotonin syndrome	50–100 mg orally every 4–6 hr; max dose 700 mg on day 1; after 600 mg daily
traMADol[b] *TRA-ma-dole*	ConZip, Ultram	Moderate to severe chronic pain	Same as morphine	Titrate individual dose starting at 25 mg up to 100 mg/day
Agonists–Antagonists (Activate/Blocks Receptors, Causing Effect to a Lesser Extent)				
buprenorphine[b] *byoo-pre-NOR-feen*	Buprenex, Suboxone, Belbuca, Probuphine	Moderate to severe chronic pain, treatment of opioid dependence	Lightheadedness, sedation, dizziness, nausea, vomiting, respiratory depression	Sublingual, buccal, injectable, tablet, implant doses depending on route
butorphanol *byoo-TOR-fa-nole*		Acute pain, anesthetic adjunct	Lightheadedness, sedation, constipation, dizziness, nausea, vomiting, respiratory depression	1–4 mg IM, 0.5–2 mg IV Nasal spray (NS): 1 mg (spray), repeat in 60–90 min; may repeat every 3–4 hr
nalbuphine *NAL-byoo-feen*		Moderate to severe chronic pain, anesthetic adjunct	Lightheadedness, sedation, constipation, dizziness, nausea, vomiting, respiratory depression	10 mg/70 kg subcut, IM, or IV every 3–6 hr
pentazocine *pen-TAZ-oh-seen*		Same as nalbuphine	Same as nalbuphine	30–60 mg IM, subcut, IV every 3–4 hr; maximum daily dose 360 mg
Antagonists (Blocks Receptors, Reverses the Effect of the Opiate)				
naloxone *nal-OKS-one*	Narcan, Evzio	Complete or partial reversal of opioid effects after surgery or overdose	Nausea, vomiting, tachycardia, hypertension, return of postoperative pain, fever, dizziness	Postoperative opioid reversal: 0.1–0.2 mg IV at 2- to 3-min intervals Suspected opioid overdose: 0.4–2.0 mg IV at 2- to 3-min intervals
naltrexone *nal-TREKS-one*		Alcohol detox, opioid overdose	Nausea, vomiting, dizziness, fainting, headache, injection site reaction	50–100 mg/day

[a]Adverse reactions of opioid analgesics are discussed extensively in the chapter. Some of the reactions may be less severe or intense than others.
[b]REMS program (see Chapter 1).

CHAPTER REVIEW

Know Your Drugs

Clients sometimes know a medication by the brand (or trade) name and not the generic name. To help you recognize both names, match the brand name with the generic name of the same medication.

Generic Name	Brand Name
1. fentanyl	A. Demerol
2. hydromorphone	B. Dilaudid
3. meperidine	C. Duragesic
4. oxycodone	D. OxyContin

Calculate Medication Dosages

1. A client is prescribed oral morphine sulfate 12 mg. The dosage available is 10 mg/mL. The nurse administers _____.

2. A client is prescribed 0.8 mg naloxone IV for postoperative respiratory depression caused by morphine. Available is a vial with 1 mg/mL. The nurse administers _____.

Prepare for the NCLEX

RECALL THE FACTS

1. The nurse explains to the client that some opioids may be used as part of the preoperative medication regimen to _____.
    1. increase intestinal motility
    2. facilitate passage of an endotracheal tube
    3. enhance the effects of the skeletal muscle relaxant
    4. lessen anxiety and sedate the client

2. Each time the client requests an opioid analgesic, the nurse must _____.
    1. check the client's diagnosis
    2. talk to the client to see if he is awake
    3. determine the exact location and intensity of the pain
    4. administer the drug with food to prevent gastric upset

3. *When administering opioid analgesics to an older client, the nurse monitors the client closely for

    _____.
    1. an increased heart rate
    2. euphoria
    3. confusion
    4. a synergistic reaction

4. What is the action when an opioid antagonist is administered?
    1. increases renal clearance of the opioid drug
    2. speeds up the cardiovascular system
    3. displaces the opioid drug from the receptor site
    4. causes the respiratory center to stop functioning

ANALYZE THE FACTS

5. The client on opioid therapy complains of abdominal pain. What is the nurse's best response?
    1. "Let's see when you had your last pain medicine."
    2. "Can you rate your pain for me?"
    3. "Show me where on your tummy it hurts."
    4. "When was your last bowel movement?"

6. *Which of the following drug combinations would follow Step 1 of the WHO modified pain ladder?
    1. morphine sulfate orally 10 mg every 4 hr and morphine sulfate sublingual 1 mg PRN
    2. hydrocodone orally 5 mg and acetaminophen 500 mg
    3. naproxen orally 200 mg twice daily and acetaminophen 325 mg at bedtime
    4. meperidine 20 mg with Phenergan IM

7. Which of the following findings requires the nurse to immediately contact the primary health care provider?
    1. pulse rate of 80 beats/min
    2. complaint of breakthrough pain
    3. respiratory rate of 20 breaths/min
    4. systolic blood pressure of 140 mm Hg

ALTERNATE-FORMAT QUESTIONS

8. Which opiate receptors in the brain produce the analgesic, euphoric effects? **Select all that apply.**
    1. alpha
    2. delta
    3. kappa
    4. mu

9. *A client is prescribed Vicodin for pain relief following a surgical procedure. If the client takes 1 tablet every 4 hr, how much acetaminophen will the client take in 24 hr?

10. *In the recovery room, the physician prescribes naloxone 0.4 mg by injection as the initial dose for opioid-induced respiratory depression; it may be followed in 5 min with 0.2 mg. Orders read that the nurse should contact the primary health care provider when a total of 1 mg is given. How many times can the nurse give the drug before contacting the primary health care provider?

To check your answers, see Appendix F.

_____

*Indicates the question is directly linked to the NCLEX-PN test plan in Appendix G.

WANT TO KNOW MORE? A wide variety of resources are available to enhance your learning and understanding of this chapter.
- Visit the**Point** for resources such as:
    - NCLEX-Style Student Review Questions
    - Journal Articles
    - Dosage Calculations
    - Drug Monographs
    - Watch and Learn Videos
    - Concepts in Action Animations
- The *Study Guide to Accompany Introductory Clinical Pharmacology*, 12th edition, sold separately, will help you review and apply essential content.
- √**PrepU** is available to help students prepare for the NCLEX-PN examination.

16

Anesthetic Drugs

Key Terms

anesthesia loss of feeling or sensation

anesthesiologist physician with special training in administering anesthesia

anesthetist nurse with special training who administers anesthesia; also called *nurse anesthetist*

conscious sedation induced reduction in consciousness where client is able to maintain function while in a relaxed state

conduction block type of regional anesthesia produced by injection of a local anesthetic drug into or near a nerve trunk; examples include epidural, transsacral (caudal), and brachial

general anesthesia sensation-free state of entire body

local anesthesia provision of a pain-free state in a specific body area

neuroleptanalgesia altered state of consciousness or sensation

preanesthetic drug pertaining to status before administration of an anesthetic agent

regional anesthesia injection of a local anesthetic around nerves to block sensation

spinal anesthesia type of regional anesthesia produced by injection of a local anesthetic drug into the subarachnoid space of the spinal cord

Learning Objectives

On completion of this chapter, the student will:

1. State the uses of local anesthesia, methods of administration, and nursing responsibilities when administering a local anesthetic.
2. Describe the purpose of a preanesthetic drug and the nursing responsibilities associated with the administration of a preanesthetic drug.
3. Identify several drugs used for local, regional, conscious sedation, and general anesthesia.
4. List and briefly describe the four stages of general anesthesia.
5. Discuss important nursing responsibilities associated with caring for a client receiving a preanesthetic drug and during the postanesthesia care (recovery room) period.

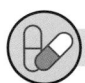 **Drug Classes**

Local anesthetics   General anesthetic agents
Preanesthetics

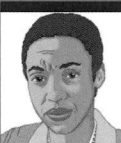 **PHARMACOLOGY IN PRACTICE**

Lillian Chase has asked her primary health care provider to remove a mole on her arm. You are asked to draw up into a syringe the medication to numb the area. After reading this chapter, see if you can make the appropriate selection.

A nesthesia is a loss of feeling or sensation. Anesthesia may be induced by various drugs that can bring about partial or complete loss of sensation. For the purposes of this book our discussion divides anesthesia into four types: local anesthesia, regional anesthesia, conscious sedation, and general anesthesia. **Local anesthesia**, as the term implies, is the provision of a sensation-free state in a specific area. With a local anesthetic, the client is often awake enough to follow directions but does not feel pain in the area that has been anesthetized. However, some procedures performed under local anesthesia may require the client to be sedated. Although not fully awake, sedated clients may still hear what is going on around them. **Regional anesthesia**, as implied by the name, offers a numbing sensation to a larger area or region of the body, such as the lower limbs or the pelvic area. **Conscious sedation** involves reducing the client's level of consciousness, producing a relaxed state while the client can still follow directions but does not remember the procedure. **General anesthesia** is the provision of a sensation-free state for the entire body. When a general

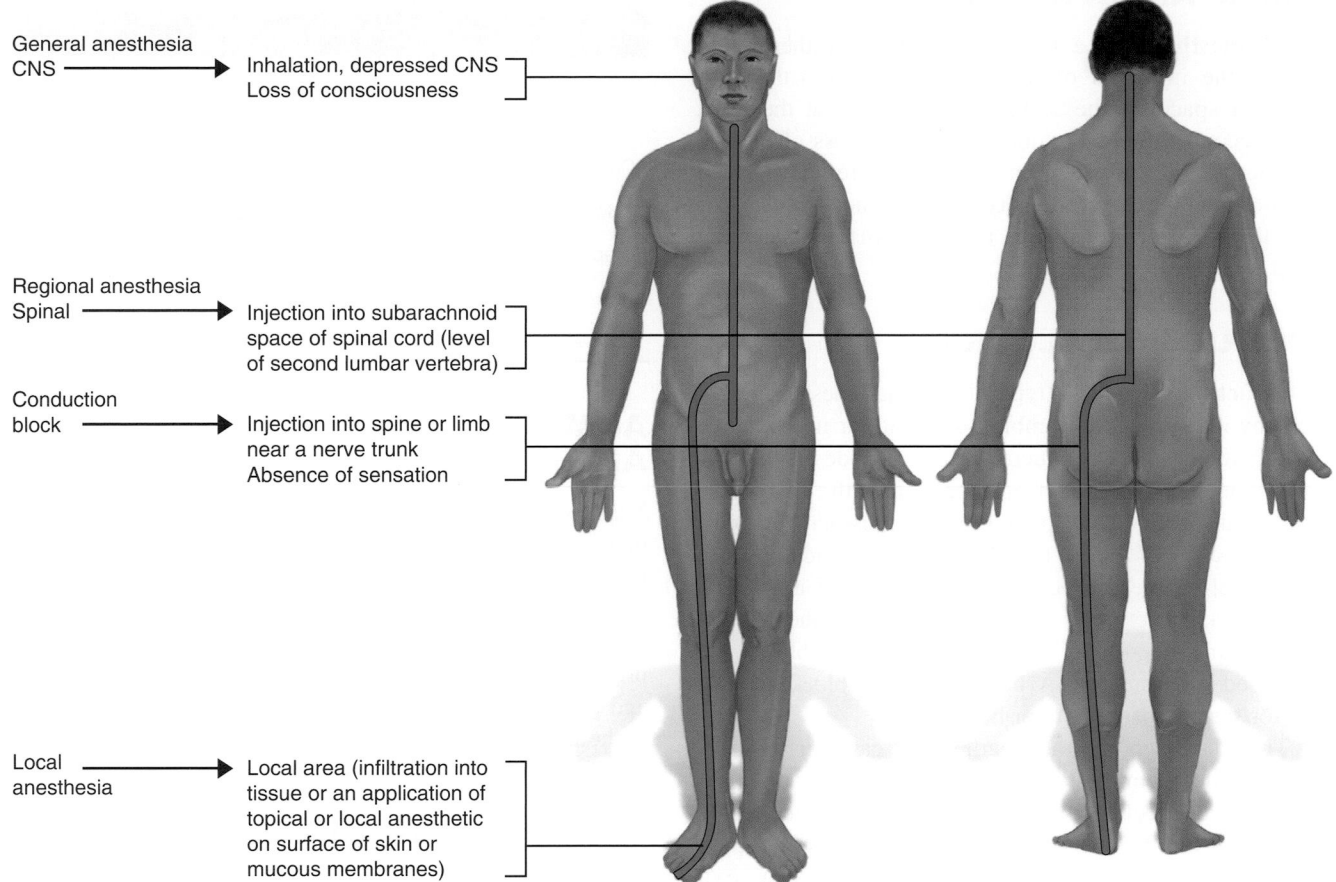

General anesthesia
CNS ──────→ Inhalation, depressed CNS
Loss of consciousness

Regional anesthesia
Spinal ──────→ Injection into subarachnoid
space of spinal cord (level
of second lumbar vertebra)

Conduction
block ──────→ Injection into spine or limb
near a nerve trunk
Absence of sensation

Local
anesthesia ──────→ Local area (infiltration into
tissue or an application of
topical or local anesthetic
on surface of skin or
mucous membranes)

FIGURE 16.1 Sites and mechanisms of action of drugs used for anesthesia. (Adapted from Timby, B. K. (2017). *Fundamental nursing skills and concepts* (11th ed.). Wolters Kluwer, Lippincott Williams & Wilkins.)

anesthetic is given, the client loses consciousness, has no control, and feels no pain. Reflexes, such as the swallowing and gag reflexes, are lost during deep general anesthesia (Fig. 16.1). Anesthetic drugs are included here in Unit 3 because they eliminate the sensation of pain, which completes the spectrum of pain management.

An **anesthesiologist** is a physician with special training in administering anesthesia. A nurse **anesthetist** is a registered nurse with at least a master's degree and special training who is qualified to administer anesthetics. Both physicians and nurses administer anesthesia. These providers are also responsible for monitoring the vital functions in the body as the surgical procedure is carried out.

LOCAL ANESTHESIA

The various methods of administering a local anesthetic include topical application and local infiltration.

TOPICAL ANESTHESIA

Topical anesthesia involves the application of the anesthetic to the surface of the skin, open area, or mucous membrane. The anesthetic may be applied with a cotton swab or

sprayed on the area. This type of anesthesia may be used to desensitize the skin or mucous membrane to the injection of a deeper local anesthetic. In some instances, topical anesthetics are dispensed in a transdermal form for chronic pain relief.

LOCAL INFILTRATION ANESTHESIA

Local infiltration anesthesia is the injection of a local anesthetic drug into tissues. This type of anesthesia may be used for dental procedures, the suturing of small wounds, or making an incision into a small area, such as that required for removing a superficial piece of tissue for biopsy. In palliative care, pain medication may be delivered into the subcutaneous tissue using a pump.

REGIONAL ANESTHESIA

Regional anesthesia is the injection of a numbing drug around nerves so that the area supplied by these nerves will not send pain signals to the brain. The anesthetized area is usually larger than the area affected by local infiltration anesthesia. Spinal anesthesia and conduction blocks are two types of regional anesthesia.

SPINAL ANESTHESIA

Spinal anesthesia is a type of regional anesthesia that involves the injection of a numbing drug into the subarachnoid space of the spinal cord, usually at the level of the second lumbar vertebra. There is a loss of feeling (anesthesia) and movement in the lower extremities, lower abdomen, and perineum. This type of anesthesia is used for surgeries of lower limbs, such as a total knee replacement or hip surgery.

CONDUCTION BLOCKS

A **conduction block** is a type of regional anesthesia produced by injection of a numbing drug into or near a nerve trunk. Examples of a conduction block include an epidural block (injection of a local anesthetic into the space surrounding the dura of the spinal cord), a transsacral (caudal) block (injection of a local anesthetic into the epidural space at the level of the sacrococcygeal notch), and a brachial plexus block (injection of a local anesthetic into the brachial plexus). Epidural—especially—and transsacral blocks are often used in obstetrics. A brachial plexus block may be used for surgery of the arm or hand.

The placement of the needle or a catheter requires strict aseptic technique by a skilled physician or anesthetist. Drug injected through the catheter spreads freely throughout the tissues in the space, interrupting pain conduction at the points where sensory nerve fibers exit from the spinal cord.

A catheter may be placed to give intermittent injections to maintain anesthesia over time such as the immediate postoperative period. This method is also used in palliative care for pain unrelieved by other methods.

PREPARING THE CLIENT FOR LOCAL ANESTHESIA

Depending on the procedure performed, preparing the client for local anesthesia may or may not be similar to preparing the client for general anesthesia. For example, administering a local anesthetic for dental surgery or for suturing a small wound may require that you explain to the client how the anesthetic will be administered, take the client's allergy history, and, when applicable, prepare the area to be anesthetized, which may involve cleaning the area with an antiseptic or shaving the area. Other local anesthetic procedures may require the client to be fasting (taking in nothing by mouth), because a sedative may also be administered. This conscious sedation would include starting an intravenous (IV) line and administering an IV sedative, such as the central nervous system (CNS) depressant drug midazolam, during some local anesthetic procedures, such as cataract surgery or a colonoscopy.

TABLE 16.1 Example of Local Anesthetics

GENERIC NAME	TRADE NAME
Articaine	Septocaine
Bupivacaine	Marcaine
Chloroprocaine	Nesacaine
Lidocaine	Xylocaine
Mepivacaine	Carbocaine, Isocaine
Prilocaine	
Ropivacaine	Naropin

ADMINISTERING LOCAL ANESTHESIA

The physician or dentist administers a local injectable anesthetic. These drugs may be mixed with epinephrine to cause local vasoconstriction. The drug stays in the tissue longer when epinephrine is used. This is contraindicated, however, when the local anesthetic is used on an extremity. When preparing these medications, you should proceed cautiously and be aware of when epinephrine is to be used and when it should not be used. Table 16.1 lists the more commonly used local anesthetics.

NURSING RESPONSIBILITIES

When caring for a client receiving local anesthesia, you may be responsible for applying a dressing to the surgical area if appropriate. Typically, when using local anesthesia, you will instruct the family or caregiver how to observe the area for bleeding, oozing, or other problems after the administration of the anesthetic and when to contact the primary health care provider.

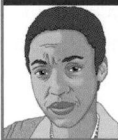

PHARMACOLOGY IN PRACTICE

INTERVENTION
Which of the following can be mixed in certain situations with an injectable local anesthetic to cause local vasoconstriction?
1. Epinephrine
2. Phenylephrine
3. Oxymetazoline
4. Diphenhydramine

 PREANESTHETIC DRUGS

A **preanesthetic drug** is one given before the administration of anesthesia. These drugs are to relax or sedate the client for the surgical procedure. They may be taken at home by the client, given by a nurse in the preanesthesia unit, or administered right before general anesthesia. The preanesthetic agent may consist of one drug or a combination of drugs.

USES OF PREANESTHETIC DRUGS

The general purpose, or use, of the preanesthetic drug is to prepare the client for anesthesia. Common preoperative medications include one or more of the following:

- *Antianxiety* drugs, such as lorazepam, reduce preoperative anxiety, cause slight sedation, slow motor activity, and promote the induction of anesthesia.
- *Histamine-2 receptor antagonists*, such as cimetidine, decrease gastric acidity and volume.
- *Anticholinergics*, such as glycopyrrolate, decrease respiratory secretions, dry mucous membranes, and prevent vagus nerve stimulation during endotracheal intubation.
- *Neuromuscular blocking agents,* such as succinylcholine, promote skeletal muscle relaxation during procedure, allow for rapid intubation.
- *Opioids*, such as fentanyl, sedate and decrease the amount of anesthesia.
- *Sedatives*, such as midazolam, promote sleep or amnesia and decrease anxiety.
- *Antibiotics*, such as kanamycin, destroy enteric microorganisms.

Lifespan Considerations

Gerontology

Preanesthetic drugs may be omitted in clients who are 60 years or older because many of the medical disorders for which these drugs are contraindicated are seen in older individuals. For example, atropine and glycopyrrolate, drugs that can be used to decrease secretions of the upper respiratory tract, are contraindicated in certain medical disorders, such as prostatic hypertrophy, glaucoma, and myocardial ischemia. Other preanesthetic drugs that depress the CNS, such as opioids, barbiturates, and antianxiety drugs, with or without antiemetic properties, may be contraindicated in the older individual.

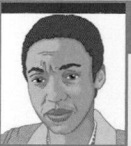

PHARMACOLOGY IN PRACTICE

SAFE MEDICATION ADMINISTRATION
A client is prescribed the drug midazolam by the anesthesiologist. The nurse knows that which of the following are the effects of midazolam?
1. Produces mild stimulation of respiratory and bronchial secretions
2. Brings about a reduction in anxiety levels
3. Depresses CNS to produce hypnosis and anesthesia
4. Decreases secretions in the upper respiratory tract

NURSING RESPONSIBILITIES

When caring for a client receiving a preanesthetic drug, assess the client's physical status and give an explanation of the anesthesia. In some hospitals, the anesthesiologist examines the client at an outpatient visit, a few days or a week before surgery, although this may not be possible in emergency situations. Some hospitals use operating room or postanesthesia care unit (PACU) staff members to visit the client before surgery to explain certain facts, such as the time of surgery, the effects of the preanesthetic drug, preparations for surgery, and the PACU. Proper explanation of anesthesia, the surgery itself, and the events that may occur in preparation for surgery, as well as care after surgery, requires a team approach. As the nurse on the team, your responsibilities include the following:

- Describe or explain the preparations for surgery ordered by the physician. Examples of preoperative preparations include fasting from midnight (or the time specified by the physician), enema, shaving of the operative site, use of a hypnotic for sleep the night before, and the preoperative injection about 30 minutes before surgery.
- Describe or explain immediate postoperative care, such as that given in the PACU (also called the *recovery room*) or a special postoperative surgical unit, and the activities of the health care team during this period. Explain that the client's vital signs will be monitored frequently and that other equipment, such as IV lines and fluids and hemodynamic (cardiac) monitors, may be used.
- Demonstrate, describe, and explain postoperative client activities, such as deep breathing, coughing, and leg exercises.
- Emphasize the importance of pain control, and make sure the client understands that relieving pain early on is better than trying to hold out, not take the medicine, and later attempt to relieve the pain. Teach the client how to use the patient-controlled analgesia pump.
- Tailor the preoperative explanations to fit the type of surgery scheduled. Not all of these teaching points may require inclusion in every explanation.
- Provide written instructions in the language of preference for the client to take home and read to reinforce the teachings.

CONSCIOUS SEDATION

When a procedure requires a client to be somewhat awake and relaxed, but still be able to follow directions, conscious sedation is employed. Conscious sedation involves keeping a client awake with medications to minimize anxiety and produce a calm, relaxed state, while at the same time reducing the sensation of pain to an area as well. This form of anesthesia is used in outpatient centers, ambulatory surgery, and procedural clinics as well as in dental offices and pediatric settings.

The use of nitrous oxide, or laughing gas, has been used for many years in dental practice and pediatrics (Karakashian & Caple, 2019). Conscious sedation includes not only the inhalation of gas but the administration of sedatives, intravenously (Chapter 20). For the client, it may be referred to as "twilight sleep," because clients report they feel like they have just taken a nap. Rivera (2015) in a literature review found that in 2007 about 25% of all endoscopy procedures used a form of conscious sedation. Today, many more outpatient procedures use this form of anesthesia.

Basically, conscious sedation differs from general anesthesia in that a complete loss of consciousness during the procedure does not happen. This anesthetic is defined using three different stages as outlined in Box 16.1. These stages are different from general anesthesia where the client loses consciousness and is not arousable and is unable to respond to repeated or painful stimuli. When a general anesthetic is used, client typically requires interventions to maintain airway patency and adequate ventilation (Rivera, 2015).

An important concept is that during the procedure the client may hear and remember what is happening. The nurse should provide verbal reassurance to the client even when they do not appear awake. This minimizes both discomfort and adverse responses to stress. Reassurance and preprocedural teaching will additionally promote cooperation and potentially lessen the amount of sedation and analgesia required.

GENERAL ANESTHESIA

The administration of general anesthesia requires the use of one or more drugs. The choice of anesthetic drug depends on many factors, including:

- General physical condition of the client
- Area, organ, or system being operated on
- Anticipated length of the surgical procedure

The anesthesiologist selects the anesthetic drugs that will produce safe anesthesia, analgesia (absence of pain), and, in some surgeries, effective skeletal muscle relaxation. A regional anesthesia with sedation may be used for procedures in both outpatient and inpatient surgical centers. General anesthesia is most commonly achieved with anesthetic vapors of volatile liquids, which are inhaled as vapors or by nitrous oxide.

STAGES OF GENERAL ANESTHESIA

General surgical anesthesia is divided into the following stages:

- Stage I—analgesia (induction)
- Stage II—delirium
- Stage III—surgical analgesia
- Stage IV—respiratory paralysis

Box 16.2 describes the stages of general anesthesia more completely. With newer drugs and techniques, the stages of anesthesia may not be as prominent as those described in Box 16.1. In addition, movement through the first two stages is usually very rapid.

Anesthesia begins with a loss of consciousness. This is part of the induction phase (stage I). The client is now relaxed and can no longer comprehend what is happening. After consciousness is lost, additional anesthetic drugs are administered. Some of these drugs are also used as part of the induction phase, as well as for deepening anesthesia. Depending on the type of surgery, an endotracheal tube also may be inserted to provide an adequate airway and to assist in administering oxygen and other anesthetic drugs. The endotracheal tube is removed during the postanesthesia period once the gag and swallowing reflexes have resumed. If an IV line was not inserted before the client's arrival in surgery, it is inserted by the anesthesiologist before the administration of an induction drug.

DRUGS USED FOR GENERAL ANESTHESIA

Barbiturate and Similar Agents

Methohexital (Brevital), which is an ultrashort-acting barbiturate, is used for the following:

- Induction of anesthesia
- Short surgical procedures with minimal painful stimuli
- In conjunction with or as a supplement to other anesthetics

These types of drugs have a rapid onset and a short duration of action. They depress the CNS to produce hypnosis and anesthesia but do not produce analgesia. Recovery after a small dose is rapid.

Etomidate, a nonbarbiturate, is used for induction of anesthesia. Etomidate also may be used to supplement other anesthetics, such as nitrous oxide, for short surgical procedures. It is a hypnotic without analgesic activity.

Propofol (Diprivan) is used for induction and maintenance of anesthesia. It also may be used for sedation during diagnostic procedures and procedures that use a local anesthetic. This drug also is used for continuous sedation of intubated or respiratory-controlled clients in intensive care units.

Benzodiazepines

Midazolam, a short-acting benzodiazepine CNS depressant, is used as a preanesthetic drug to relieve anxiety; for induction of anesthesia; for conscious sedation before minor procedures, such as endoscopy; and to supplement nitrous oxide and oxygen for short surgical procedures. When the drug is used for induction anesthesia, the client gradually loses consciousness over a period of 1–2 minutes.

Ketamine

Ketamine (Ketalar) is a rapid-acting general anesthetic. It produces an anesthetic state characterized by profound analgesia, cardiovascular and respiratory stimulation, normal or enhanced skeletal muscle tone, and occasionally mild respiratory depression. Ketamine is used for diagnostic and surgical procedures that do not require relaxation of skeletal muscles, for induction of anesthesia before the administration of other anesthetic drugs, and as a supplement to other anesthetic drugs.

Gases and Volatile Liquids

Nitrous oxide is the most commonly used anesthetic gas. It is a weak anesthetic and is usually used in combination with other anesthetic drugs. It does not cause skeletal muscle relaxation. The chief danger in the use of nitrous oxide is hypoxemia. Nitrous oxide is nonexplosive and is supplied in blue cylinders (oxygen tanks are green).

Sevoflurane (Ultane) is a volatile liquid anesthetic that is delivered by inhalation. Induction and recovery from anesthesia are rapid. It is used for induction and maintenance of general anesthesia in adult and pediatric clients for both inpatient and outpatient surgical procedures.

Hypotension may occur when anesthesia deepens.

Isoflurane (Forane) is a volatile liquid given by inhalation. It is used for induction and maintenance of anesthesia.

Desflurane (Suprane), a volatile liquid, is used for induction and maintenance of anesthesia. A special vaporizer is used to deliver this anesthetic, because delivery by mask results in irritation of the respiratory tract.

Opioids

The opioid analgesic fentanyl (Sublimaze) and the neuroleptic drug (major sedative) droperidol (Inapsine) may be used together. The combination of these two drugs results in **neuroleptanalgesia**, which is characterized by general quietness, reduced motor activity, and profound analgesia. Complete loss of consciousness may not occur unless other anesthetic drugs are used. The use of droperidol as a sedative, as an antiemetic to reduce nausea and vomiting during the immediate postanesthesia period, as an induction drug, and as an adjunct to general anesthesia has decreased because of its association with fatal cardiac dysrhythmias. Fentanyl may be used alone as a supplement to general or regional anesthesia. It may also be administered alone or with other drugs as a preoperative drug and as an analgesic during the immediate postoperative period.

Remifentanil (Ultiva) is used for induction and maintenance of general anesthesia and for continued analgesia during the immediate postoperative period. This drug is used cautiously in clients with a history of hypersensitivity to fentanyl.

TABLE 16.2 Examples of Muscle Relaxants Used During General Anesthesia

GENERIC NAME	TRADE NAME
Cisatracurium	Nimbex
Pancuronium	
Succinylcholine	Anectine

Skeletal Muscle Relaxants

The various skeletal muscle relaxants that may be used during general anesthesia are listed in Table 16.2. These drugs are administered to produce relaxation of the skeletal muscles during certain types of surgeries, such as those involving the chest or abdomen. They may also be used to facilitate the insertion of an endotracheal tube. Their onset of action is usually rapid (45 seconds to a few minutes), and their duration of action is 30 minutes or more.

NURSING RESPONSIBILITIES

Preanesthesia

Before surgery, and during the administration of general anesthesia, as the nurse, you have the following responsibilities:

- Performing the required tasks and procedures as prescribed by the physician and hospital policy before surgery and documenting these tasks on the client's chart. Examples of these tasks include administering a hypnotic agent before surgery, shaving the operative area, taking vital signs, seeing that the operative consent form is signed, checking that all jewelry or metal objects are removed from the client, inserting a catheter, inserting a nasogastric tube, and teaching.
- Outpatient: Be sure a caregiver is available to take the person home and to monitor the client after the procedure.
- Checking the chart for any recent abnormal laboratory test results. If a recent abnormal laboratory test finding was included in the client's chart shortly before surgery, alert the surgeon and the anesthesiologist to the abnormality.
- Flagging the list of known or suspected drug allergies or idiosyncrasies
- Administering the preanesthetic (preoperative) drug
- Instructing the client to remain in bed and placing the bed's side rails up once the preanesthetic drug has been given

> ⚠️ **NURSING ALERT**
>
> Preanesthetic drugs must be administered on time to produce their intended effects. Failure to give the preanesthetic drug on time may result in such events as increased respiratory secretions caused by the irritating effect of anesthetic gases and the need for an increased dose of the induction drug because the preanesthetic drug has not had time to sedate the client.

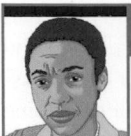

PHARMACOLOGY IN PRACTICE

INTERVENTION

A client in an acute care facility is about to have general anesthesia for an operation. Which of the following preanesthetic drugs will be administered to reduce the incidence of upper respiratory tract secretions in the client? Select all that apply.
1. Cholinergic blocking drug
2. Scopolamine and glycopyrrolate
3. Opioid or antianxiety drug
4. Diazepam or Valium

Postanesthesia: Postanesthesia Care Unit

After surgery, your responsibilities vary according to where you first come into contact with the postoperative client:

- Admitting the client to the unit according to hospital procedure or policy
- Checking the airway for patency, assessing the respiratory status, and giving oxygen as needed
- Positioning the client to prevent aspiration of vomitus and secretions
- With regional anesthesia, check limbs and body for proper position to prevent injury.
- Checking the patency of IV lines, catheters, drainage tubes, surgical dressings, and casts
- Reviewing the client's surgical and anesthesia records
- Monitoring the blood pressure, pulse, and respiratory rate every 5–15 minutes until the client is discharged from the area
- Checking the client every 5–15 minutes for emergence from anesthesia. Suctioning is provided as needed.
- Exercising caution in administering opioids. The nurse must check the client's respiratory rate, blood pressure, and pulse before these drugs are given and in 20–30 minutes assess pain level after administration (see Chapter 15). The physician is contacted if the respiratory rate is below 10 breaths/minute before the drug is given or if the respiratory rate falls below 10 breaths/minute after the drug is given.
- Discharging the client from the area to their room or other specified area. You should complete documentation of all drugs administered and nursing tasks performed before the client leaves the PACU.
- Outpatient: Ensure the client is able to ambulate (if appropriate) and has voided and vital signs are stable. Provide written instructions for care and follow-up.

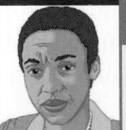

PHARMACOLOGY IN PRACTICE

USING CLINICAL REASONING

Lillian Chase requires a local anesthetic to remove a mole on her arm. There are two vials sitting on the counter: lidocaine 2% solution and lidocaine 2% with epinephrine 1:100,000 in solution. After reading this chapter, can you determine the appropriate choice for the injection?

KEY POINTS

■ Anesthesia is the loss of feeling or sensation. Local and general anesthesia are provided for pain relief and to perform otherwise painful procedures.

■ Local anesthesia includes topical, local infiltration and regional pain relief and is used when dealing with a specific area of the body and the client can remain conscious.

■ General anesthesia requires multiple drugs and stages to achieve a state where surgical procedures can be performed without pain, movement, or memory.

■ Conscious sedation and regional anesthesia allow pain-free surgical areas with clients who may be awake or able to follow commands.

■ A greater number of body systems are involved when a general anesthetic is administered; clients need assistance and coaching to resume respiratory, gastrointestinal, and musculoskeletal function following the procedure.

■ Nursing responsibility includes tasks to assist, maintain, and recover a client who has been given an anesthetic.

CHAPTER REVIEW

Know Your Drugs

Clients sometimes know a medication by the brand (or trade) name and not the generic name. To help you recognize both names, match the brand name with the generic name of the same medication.

Generic Name	Brand Name
1. lidocaine	A. Demerol
2. meperidine	B. Diprivan
3. propofol	C. Marcaine
4. bupivacaine	D. Xylocaine

Calculate Medication Dosages

1. As a preoperative medication for a client going to surgery, the anesthesiologist prescribes meperidine (Demerol) 50 mg IM. Meperidine is available in a solution of 50 mg/mL. The nurse prepares to administer _____.

Prepare for the NCLEX

RECALL THE FACTS

1. The type of anesthesia used when a small cut or wound is sutured is called _____.
   1. topical
   2. regional
   3. local
   4. conduction block

2. When planning preoperative care, the nurse expects that a preanesthetic medication is given before the client is transported to surgery.
   1. 10 minutes
   2. 30 minutes
   3. 40 minutes
   4. 60 minutes

3. Which of the following drugs is the most commonly used gas for general anesthesia?
   1. ethylene
   2. Forane
   3. nitrous oxide
   4. sevoflurane

4. Neuroleptanalgesia is used to promote general quietness, reduce motor activity, and induce profound analgesia. Which of the following two drugs are used in combination to accomplish neuroleptanalgesia?
   1. fentanyl and droperidol
   2. morphine and glycopyrrolate
   3. atropine and meperidine
   4. fentanyl and midazolam

5. One use of skeletal muscle relaxants as part of general anesthesia is to:
   1. prevent movement during surgery.
   2. facilitate insertion of the endotracheal tube.
   3. allow for deeper anesthesia.
   4. produce additional anesthesia.

ANALYZE THE FACTS

6. Which group of individuals is at a particularly higher risk for complications from preanesthetic drugs?
   1. infants
   2. adolescents and teens
   3. individuals who are obese
   4. older adults

7. Following general anesthesia, a client is rolled to the side during the recovery period to:
   1. assess respiratory status.
   2. prevent the endotracheal tube from being swallowed.
   3. assess vital signs better.
   4. prevent aspiration during recovery.

ALTERNATE-FORMAT QUESTIONS

8. *Match the medication with its intended action related to anesthetic procedures.

1. opioid	A. decrease chance of nausea
2. antiemetic	B. depress the central nervous system
3. cholinergic blocker	C. relieve pain and decrease anxiety
4. benzodiazepine	D. decrease secretions

9. Arrange the following actions as they happen during the stages of general anesthesia:
   1. respiratory paralysis
   2. moving about and mumbling may occur
   3. consciousness is lost
   4. muscles become ridged and sounds exaggerated
10. Glycopyrrolate (Robinul) is prescribed for a client as part of the preoperative preparation for surgery. The drug dose recommendation is 0.002 mg/lb. The client weighs 150 lb. The nurse expects the anesthesiologist to prescribe _____.

To check your answers, see Appendix F.

---

*Indicates the question is directly linked to the NCLEX-PN test plan in Appendix G.

WANT TO KNOW MORE? A wide variety of resources are available to enhance your learning and understanding of this chapter.
- Visit thePoint for resources such as:
  - NCLEX-Style Student Review Questions
  - Journal Articles
  - Dosage Calculations
  - Drug Monographs
  - Watch and Learn Videos
  - Concepts in Action Animations
- The *Study Guide to Accompany Introductory Clinical Pharmacology*, 12th edition, sold separately, will help you review and apply essential content.
- √*PrepU* is available to help students prepare for the NCLEX-PN examination.

UNIT 4
Drugs That Affect the Central Nervous System

The nervous system is a complex part of the human body sending messages to and from the brain. This brain-to-body connection helps with the regulation and coordination of activities such as movement, behavior, digestion, and sleep. There are two main divisions in the nervous system: the central nervous system (CNS) and the peripheral nervous system (PNS). The CNS consists of the brain and the spinal cord. The CNS receives, integrates, and interprets nerve impulses, whereas, the PNS is the messenger system, connecting all parts of the body with the CNS.

In this unit, drugs that affect the CNS are presented. Drugs that affect the CNS alter mood, sensation, and the interpretation of information in the brain. These drugs are used to enhance mental health well-being in both inpatient and outpatient settings. In this unit, you will learn about a range of drugs that stimulate and dampen signals in the CNS.

Drugs that stimulate the CNS are presented in Chapter 17. CNS stimulants are used to stimulate the body and reverse respiratory depression. You will also learn how drugs can strengthen one signal and dampen others, such as in the treatment of children and adults with attention-deficit hyperactivity disorder (ADHD) using stimulant drugs.

Chapter 18 discusses the drugs used to enhance neurotransmission to maintain and sometimes enhance the cognitive function of persons with dementia. Currently, Alzheimer disease (AD) is the ninth leading cause of death in adults older than 65 years. Close to $305 billion is spent annually to care for people with AD (including both direct and indirect costs) (AA, 2020). Although a cure is not known for this degenerative disease, the dementia experienced can be slowed by the use of drugs called *cholinesterase inhibitors*, which are covered in Chapter 18. Typically, an individual lives on average 8 years after diagnosis; yet, some people have been known to live up to 20 years after AD is discovered with the use of drugs to combat dementia symptoms.

Technology and the information age keep us going and tuned in to each other 24/7, which means there is no downtime. People feel stressed, fatigued, and anxious. Whereas

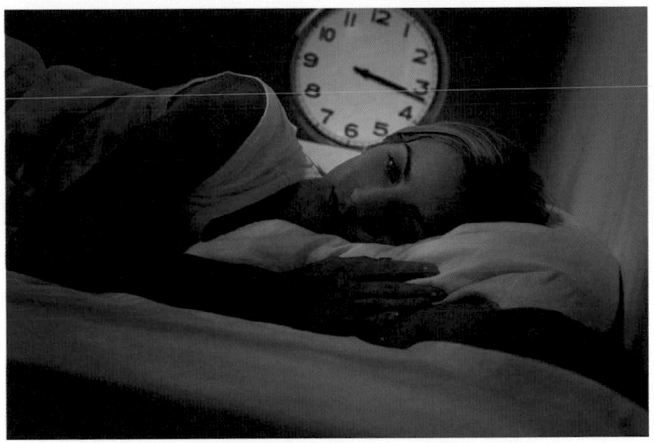

some individuals complain of frequently feeling anxious, others may have a diagnosis of an anxiety disorder. Drugs that have a depressing effect on neurotransmission in the CNS are used to treat anxiety (Chapter 19). Additionally, the sedative/hypnotic drugs (Chapter 20) are used to treat insomnia or to produce a calming effect when clients are about to undergo a surgical or diagnostic procedure.

Drugs that act on the CNS are also used to change mood or behavior. These drugs may take many days or even weeks to produce a therapeutic response. Chapter 21 discusses drugs used to treat depression, which is one of the most common mental health disorders in our country today. Depression is characterized by impaired functioning and feelings of intense sadness, helplessness, and worthlessness. People experiencing major depressive episodes exhibit physical and psychological symptoms, such as appetite disturbances, sleep disturbances, and loss of interest in job, family, and other activities usually enjoyed.

A psychotic disorder, on the other hand, is characterized by extreme personality disorganization and the loss of contact with reality. Drugs given to clients with a psychotic disorder, such as schizophrenia, are called *antipsychotic drugs* or *neuroleptics*. The antipsychotic drugs are discussed in Chapter 22.

Central Nervous System Stimulants

Learning Objectives

On completion of this chapter, the student will:

1. List the three classes of CNS stimulants.
2. Explain the uses, general drug actions, general adverse reactions, contraindications, precautions, and interactions of CNS stimulants.
3. Distinguish important preadministration and ongoing assessment activities the nurse should perform on the client taking a CNS stimulant.
4. List nursing diagnoses particular to a client taking a CNS stimulant.
5. Examine ways to promote an optimal response to drug therapy, how to manage common adverse drug reactions, and important points to keep in mind when educating clients about the use of CNS stimulants.

 Drug Classes

Amphetamines
Analeptics
Anorexiants

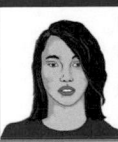

PHARMACOLOGY IN PRACTICE

Janna Wong is a 16-year-old high-school gymnast. Mrs. Wong has brought her to the clinic after reading on the Internet about attention-deficit hyperactivity disorder (ADHD). She is worried that Janna's lack of focus on training may be because of this disorder. She is here to have medications prescribed for her daughter.

This chapter discusses the drugs that stimulate the CNS and the nursing implications related to their administration. The three basic classes of stimulants are amphetamines, analeptics, and anorexiants. The definitions of these classes are presented in Box 17.1. These drugs are used with caution because the CNS stimulants have a high abuse potential owing to their ability to produce euphoria and wakefulness.

BOX 17.1 | **Central Nervous System Stimulants and Definitions**

Amphetamines. Drugs used to treat children with ADHD.
Analeptics. Drugs that stimulate the respiratory center of the brain and cardiovascular system, used with narcolepsy and as an adjuvant treatment for obstructive sleep apnea.
Anorexiants. Drugs used to suppress the appetite.

CENTRAL NERVOUS SYSTEM STIMULANTS

ACTIONS

Amphetamines stimulate the release of norepinephrine in the sympathetic nerve pathway of the brain and are called **sympathomimetic** (i.e., adrenergic) drugs. Basically, this means they stimulate the CNS to speed up (Rothman et al., 2001). You will learn more about these nerve pathways and how they work in Unit 5 (see Chapter 23). The amphetamine drug action results in an elevation of blood pressure, wakefulness, and an increase or decrease in pulse rate. Amphetamines also stimulate the dopamine and serotonin pathways of the brain producing a **euphoric** state; this pleasurable feeling is what increases their dependency potential.

! NURSING ALERT

Stimulants enhance dopamine transmission to areas of the brain that interpret well-being. To maintain pleasurable feelings, people continue the use of stimulants, which leads to their abuse and the potential for addiction.

One condition successfully treated by amphetamines is **attention-deficit hyperactivity disorder** (ADHD) in children. Amphetamines work by blocking the reuptake of norepinephrine and dopamine. This lessens the action of other neurotransmitters; enhancement of neurotransmission on a selected pathway is what helps clients with ADHD to focus concentration and attention.

One of the most widely used CNS stimulants is caffeine. It is a mild to potent analeptic CNS stimulant. Analeptics increase the depth of respirations by stimulating special receptors located in the carotid arteries and upper aorta. These special receptors (called *chemoreceptors*) are sensitive to the amount of oxygen in arterial blood. Stimulation of these receptors results in an increase in the depth of respirations. Caffeine is an analeptic that stimulates the CNS at all levels, including the cerebral cortex, the medulla, and the spinal cord. Individuals consume caffeine typically to reduce fatigue and increase wakefulness in **sleep–wake disturbances** (issues of lack of rest) (Pirschel, 2018). Caffeine also has mild diuretic activity. People take caffeine on their own in the form of coffee, tea, or even chocolate, yet caffeine's use as a therapeutic drug for stimulation in the neonatal setting is growing. Other actions of analeptics include cardiac stimulation (which may produce tachycardia), dilation of coronary and peripheral blood vessels, constriction of cerebral blood vessels, and skeletal muscle stimulation.

Analeptics used to treat **narcolepsy** (a disorder that causes an uncontrollable desire to sleep during normal waking hours, even though the individual has a normal nighttime sleeping pattern) include modafinil, armodafinil, pitolisant, and solriamfetol. The exact mechanism of action is not known, but the drugs are thought to bind to dopamine keeping it at the neural synapse and not being reabsorbed, thereby reducing the number of sleep episodes. They do not cause cardiac and other systemic stimulatory effects like other CNS stimulants. These drugs are sometimes used in the treatment of obstructive sleep apnea to promote daytime wakefulness (not to replace continuous positive airway pressure during sleep). Clients should be cautioned that it may take up to 8 weeks to have a satisfactory response to the drugs used to treat narcolepsy.

The anorexiants are drugs pharmacologically similar to the amphetamines. Their ability to suppress the appetite is thought to be caused by their action on the appetite center in the hypothalamus. Studies show that drugs when used with diet modification and exercise result in typically no more than 10% weight loss overall (Cummings, 2020). Use of CNS stimulants for weight control is being replaced with drugs used for type 2 diabetes, see Chapter 40.

USES

The CNS stimulants are used in the treatment of the following:

- ADHD
- Drug-induced respiratory depression
- Postanesthesia respiratory depression, without reduction of analgesia
- Narcolepsy
- Obstructive sleep apnea
- Exogenous obesity
- Sleep–wake disturbances (caffeine)
- Alzheimer's apathy

! NURSING ALERT

ADHD is a condition of both children and adults and is characterized by inattention, hyperactivity, and impulsivity. Because these behaviors, when independently present, can be normal in any individual, it is important that the child receive a thorough examination and appropriate diagnosis by a well-qualified professional before drug therapy is initiated (Fig. 17.1).

ADVERSE REACTIONS

Neuromuscular System Reactions
- Excessive CNS stimulation, headache, dizziness
- Apprehension, disorientation, hyperactivity

Other Reactions
- Nausea, vomiting, cough, dyspnea
- Urinary retention, tachycardia, palpitations

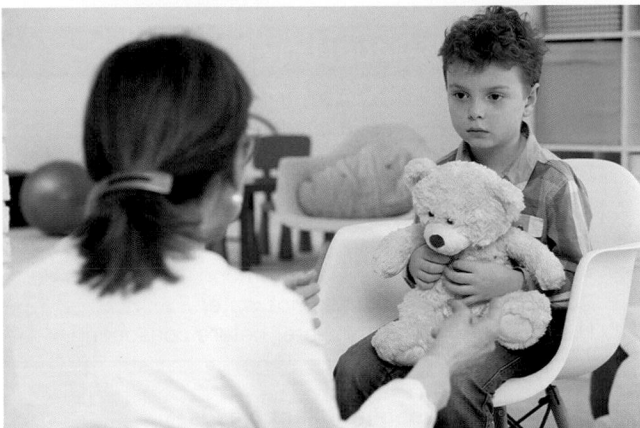

FIGURE 17.1 Children should always have a thorough examination before stimulants for attention-deficit hyperactivity disorder (ADHD) are prescribed.

For more information on adverse reactions, see the Summary Drug Table: Central Nervous System Stimulants.

CONTRAINDICATIONS

The CNS stimulants are contraindicated in clients with known hypersensitivity or convulsive disorders and in those with ventilation disorders (e.g., chronic obstructive pulmonary disease [COPD]). Do not administer CNS stimulants to clients with cardiac problems, severe hypertension, or hyperthyroidism. *CNS stimulants are not recommended as treatment for depression.* Amphetamines and anorexiants should not be taken concurrently or within 14 days of antidepressant medications. In addition, amphetamines are contraindicated in clients with glaucoma. Most anorexiants are classified as pregnancy category X and should not be used during pregnancy. All of the drugs used to treat narcolepsy cause hormonal changes in women and possibly congenital defects, therefore they should not be used during pregnancy.

PRECAUTIONS

The CNS stimulants should be used cautiously in clients with respiratory illness, renal or hepatic impairment, and history of substance abuse. The CNS stimulants do pass through breast milk and should be used cautiously in lactating women. Because of the hormonal changes in women on narcoleptic medications, they should use a barrier form of birth control.

LASA ALERT

The following drugs may sound alike; be sure to clarify when they are ordered:

Drug Name	Sounds Like
Dopram	DOPamine
Doxapram	doxazosin, doxepin, DOXOrubicin
Focalin	Focalgin-B, Folotyn
Methylphenidate	Methadone, Metadate
Pitolisant	Pitocin
Ritalin	Rifadin
Solriamfetol	solifFENacin
Vyvanse	Glucovance, Visanne, ViVAXIM, Vytorin, Vivactil

Drugs that look like a similar drug are noted in the Summary Drug Tables of each chapter.

INTERACTIONS

The following drugs may interact with a CNS stimulant when it is administered with them:

Interacting Drug	Common Use	Effect of Interaction
Anesthetics	Anesthesia during surgical procedures	Increased risk of cardiac arrhythmias
Theophylline	Respiratory problems, such as asthma	Increased risk of hyperactive behaviors
Oral contraceptives	Birth control	Decreased effectiveness of oral contraceptive when taken with modafinil

---

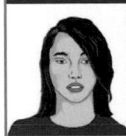

PHARMACOLOGY IN PRACTICE

SAFE DRUG ADMINISTRATION
Which of the following reactions could occur if theophylline is combined with CNS stimulants?
1. Decreased effectiveness of the CNS stimulant
2. Increased risk of cardiac arrhythmias
3. Increased risk of hyperactive behaviors
4. Decreased effectiveness of theophylline

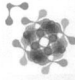

NURSING PROCESS—STEPS TO BUILDING CLINICAL JUDGMENT
Client Receiving a Central Nervous System Stimulant

ASSESSMENT
Assessment of the client receiving a CNS stimulant depends on the drug, the client, and the reason for administration.

Preadministration Assessment
Data gathering suggestions before the initial administration of the CNS stimulants include:

Objective data
- Description of general appearance, resistance to infection (complete blood count)
- Vital signs (temperature, pulse, respirations, and blood pressure)
- Weight and height especially for ADHD and obesity treatment, calculate body mass index (BMI)

- Female clients—testing for pregnancy or inquiry regarding lactation if postnatal
- Respiratory depression—note the depth of the respirations and any pattern to the respiratory rate, such as shallow respirations or alternating deep and shallow respirations
- Arterial blood gases readings for conditions of slowed breathing—depression/apnea

Subjective data

- Current history of symptoms, type, and duration
- Description of observed behavior patterns the child with ADHD demonstrates
- Review chart for drugs that may cause respiratory depression

Ongoing Assessment

Respiratory Depression

After administering an analeptic, carefully monitor the client's respiratory rate and pattern until the respirations return to normal. You should also monitor the level of consciousness, blood pressure, and pulse rate at 5- to 15-minute intervals or as ordered by the primary health care provider. Arterial blood gases may be drawn for analysis at intervals to determine the effectiveness of the analeptic, as well as the need for additional drug therapy. It is important to observe the client for adverse drug reactions and to report the occurrence immediately to the primary health care provider.

For those prescribed a stimulant for either weight loss or ADHD, clients will typically be seen on an outpatient basis. Behavior logs reviewed and weight measurements should be taken at each visit.

NURSING DIAGNOSES

Drug-specific nursing diagnoses are the following:

- **Sleep–wake disturbance** related to CNS stimulation and hyperactivity, nervousness, insomnia, other (specify)
- **Altered breathing pattern** related to respiratory depression
- **Malnutrition: less than body requirements** related to diminished appetite

Nursing diagnoses related to drug administration are discussed in Chapter 4.

PLANNING

The expected outcomes for the client depend on the reason for administration of a CNS stimulant but may include an optimal response to therapy, support of client needs related to management of adverse drug reactions, and confidence in an understanding of the medication regimen.

IMPLEMENTATION

Promoting an Optimal Response to Therapy
Stimulants are used long term for ADHD and may be used in the short-term treatment of exogenous obesity (obesity caused by a persistent calorie intake that is greater than needed by the body). However, their use in treating exogenous obesity has declined. This is because the long-term use of the amphetamines for obesity carries the potential for dependence and abuse.

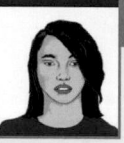

SAFE DRUG ADMINISTRATION
Which of the following points should the nurse include in the teaching plan for clients who are being administered CNS stimulants for attention deficit hyperactivity disorder (ADHD)?
1. Administer drug half an hour before breakfast.
2. Administer drug in the late afternoon.
3. Administer drug with milk, not water.
4. Dissolve drug in milk or water before consuming.

Monitoring and Managing Client Needs

Sleep–Wake Disturbance
When CNS stimulant therapy causes insomnia, teach the caregiver to administer the drug early in the day (when possible) to diminish sleep disturbances. The primary health care provider may choose a long-acting form of the drug to be given daily in the morning to help reduce sleep pattern issues. Provide the client with activities to distract them from napping during the day.

Other stimulants, such as coffee, tea, or cola drinks, are avoided. Be aware that energy drinks such as Red Bull, Rockstar, and Monster all contain caffeine in addition to the herbal products and vitamins marketed. In some clients, nervousness, restlessness, and palpitations may occur. Check vital signs every 6–8 hours or more often if tachycardia, hypertension, or palpitations occur. The adverse drug reactions that may occur with amphetamine use may be serious enough to require discontinuation of the drug. In some instances, the adverse drug effects are mild and may even disappear during therapy as physical tolerance builds. Teach the client to inform the primary care provider of any adverse reactions or behavior differences. An example would be if a client tells you they can sleep without problem while on a stimulant. This would indicate the client has built a tolerance to the drug, and in this case the dosage is not increased.

 Lifespan Considerations

Gerontology
Older adults are especially sensitive to the effects of the CNS stimulants and may exhibit excessive anxiety, nervousness, insomnia, and mental confusion. Cardiovascular disorders, common in the older adult, may be worsened by the CNS stimulants. Careful monitoring is important because these reactions may result in the need to discontinue use of the drug.

These drugs may also be helpful in managing narcolepsy, a disorder manifested by an uncontrollable desire to sleep during normal waking hours, even though the individual has a normal nighttime sleeping pattern. The individual with narcolepsy may fall asleep for a few minutes to a few hours many times in one day. The disorder begins in adolescence or young adulthood and persists throughout life.

Altered Breathing Pattern
Respiratory depression can be a serious event requiring administration of a respiratory stimulant. When an analeptic

drug is administered, document the rate, depth, and character of the respirations before the drug is given. This provides a baseline for evaluating the effectiveness of drug therapy. Before administering the drug, be sure that the client has a patent airway. Oxygen is usually administered before, during, and after drug administration. After administration, monitor respirations closely and document the effects of therapy.

When respiratory depression occurs in the postsurgical setting, carefully assess the client's level of pain. Respiratory depression can occur after a surgical procedure from the combination of drugs used to produce anesthesia. Opioid reversal drugs, such as naloxone (Narcan), that reverse the effects of opioid agents replace the pain relief drug at the receptor site of the cell. This means that the client can experience a sudden and severe return of pain because the pain relief effect of the drug is eliminated along with the reversal of respiratory depression. Use of analeptic drugs for respiratory stimulation can enhance the breathing pattern without changing the pain relief effect of the opioid drug. Therefore, breathing improves and pain relief continues for the client.

Nausea and vomiting may occur with the administration of an analeptic; therefore, you should keep a suction machine nearby in case the client vomits. Urinary retention may result from doxapram administration; be sure to measure intake and output, and notify the primary health care provider if the client cannot void or the bladder appears to be distended on palpation.

Malnutrition: Less Than Body Requirements
One of the adverse reactions of CNS stimulant use in the child with ADHD is decreased appetite. Although decreased appetite is a desired effect when treating a client with weight problems, it is not desirable when treating ADHD. Manos et al. (2007) suggest that the lack of appetite possibly minimizes growth in children because they do not eat due to the drug stimulation. Therefore, it is important to monitor weight and growth patterns of children on long-term treatment with the CNS stimulant drugs.

Teach the parents to monitor the eating patterns of the child while they are taking CNS stimulants and to feel confident in preparing nutritious meals and snacks. A good breakfast is important to provide, because the drug will cause the child to possibly not feel hungry at lunchtime in school where the parent cannot monitor nutritional intake. The child should be checked frequently for growth issues with height and weight measurements. During ADHD treatment, the drug regimen may be interrupted periodically under direction of the primary health provider to evaluate the effectiveness of drug management or to rest the body from the drug effects. Sometimes these breaks in medication administration are termed a *drug holiday.*

 Lifespan Considerations

Pediatric
An increased risk of suicidal ideation in children and adolescents has been found when using the drug atomoxetine (Strattera). Clients with ADHD started on atomoxetine should be monitored carefully for suicidal

thoughts or behaviors. Teach the family about specific behaviors to observe for and build confidence in how to ask their children about suicidal thinking that would indicate a need to contact the primary health care provider.

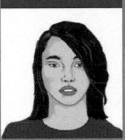 **PHARMACOLOGY IN PRACTICE**

MANAGING NEEDS
Children taking CNS stimulants for the long-term treatment of ADHD should be monitored closely for which of the following? Select all that apply.
1. Hyperglycemia
2. Growth
3. Hypotension
4. Weight loss
5. Respiratory depression

Educating the Client and Family
The type of information included in the teaching plan depends on the drug and the reason for its use. The client and family should feel confident in understanding what the purpose of the drug is and what possible adverse reactions may occur. It is important to emphasize the need to follow the recommended dosage schedule. As you develop the teaching plan, include the following additional teaching points:

- ADHD: Give the drug in the morning 30–45 minutes before breakfast and before lunch. Do not give the drug in the late afternoon. Keep a journal of the child's behavior, including the general patterns, socialization with others, and attention span. Bring this record to each primary health care provider or clinic visit, because this record may help the primary health care provider determine future drug dose adjustments or additional treatment modalities. The primary health care provider may prescribe drug therapy only on school days, when high levels of attention and performance are necessary.
- Narcolepsy: Keep a record of the number of times per day that periods of sleepiness occur, and bring this record to each visit to the primary health care provider or clinic.
- Amphetamines and anorexiants: These drugs are taken early in the day to avoid insomnia. These drugs are used in conjunction with a physical activity and food-reduction program. Do not increase the dose or take the drug more frequently, except on the advice of the primary health care provider. These drugs may impair the ability to drive or perform hazardous tasks and may mask extreme fatigue. If dizziness, lightheadedness, anxiety, nervousness, or tremors occur, contact the primary care provider. Avoid or decrease the use of coffee, tea, and energy drink/carbonated beverages containing caffeine (see Client Teaching for Improved Outcomes: Using Anorexiants for Weight Loss).
- Caffeine (oral, nonprescription): Over-the-counter caffeine preparations should be avoided if the individual has a history of heart disease, high blood pressure, or stomach ulcers. These products are intended for occasional use and should not be used if heart palpitations, dizziness, or light-headedness occurs.

Client Teaching for Improved Outcomes

Using Anorexiants for Weight Loss

When you teach, make sure your client understands the following:

✔ These drugs are intended for clients with chronic weight management issues when used with an approved diet and physical activity program.

✔ These drugs should only be used for obesity (BMI of 30 or greater) or overweight (BMI of 27) when comorbid conditions exist, such as hypertension, type 2 diabetes, or dyslipidemia.

✔ Never take over-the-counter weight loss preparations with these drugs.

✔ If you have not achieved 5% weight loss in 12 weeks, contact your primary health care provider; never increase the dose to speed up or increase weight loss.

✔ Call your primary health care provider immediately if you experience mental changes (agitation or hallucinations), rapid heartbeat, dizziness, lack of coordination, or feelings of warmth. This may be a condition called neuroleptic malignant syndrome, which needs emergent treatment.

✔ Be aware of possible impairment in the ability to drive or perform hazardous tasks.

✔ Avoid other stimulants, including those containing caffeine such as coffee, tea, and energy/cola drinks

✔ Read labels of foods and nonprescription drugs for possible stimulant content.

✔ Be aware of mental changes, especially if serotonin-based antidepressants have been taken. Notify your primary health care provider immediately to prevent serotonin syndrome (see Chapter 21).

✔ Women: Use pregnancy protection and do not breastfeed when using these drugs.

EVALUATION

• Therapeutic response is achieved and respiratory depression is reversed; the child's behavior and school performance are improved; or the desired weight loss is achieved.

• Adverse reactions are identified, reported to the primary health care provider, and managed successfully with appropriate nursing interventions:
  • Client reports fewer episodes of inappropriate sleep patterns.
  • Breathing pattern is maintained.
  • Client maintains an adequate nutritional status.

• Client and family express confidence and demonstrate an understanding of the drug regimen.

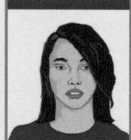

PHARMACOLOGY IN PRACTICE

USING CLINICAL REASONING

What are some assessment questions you will ask Janna about her daily routine to determine if she has the behavior patterns described as ADHD? Are there other reasons that Janna's mother may want her to take stimulants?

KEY POINTS

■ CNS stimulants enhance neurotransmission and stimulate receptors in different parts of the brain. These drugs are used for ADHD, narcolepsy, respiratory depression, and weight loss. They should not be used to treat clinical depression.

■ There is a high degree of addiction potential with these drugs because of stimulation of the brain's pleasure centers with enhanced neurotransmission of dopamine.

■ When used routinely, stimulants are offered in long-acting form or in the morning and at lunchtime to reduce the incidence of insomnia.

■ Stimulants can affect other organs; adverse reactions include tachycardia, palpitations, headache, dizziness, apprehension, nausea, vomiting, and urinary retention.

SUMMARY DRUG TABLE
Central Nervous System Stimulants

Generic Name	Trade Name	Uses	Adverse Reactions	Dosage Ranges
Amphetamines				
amphetamine *am-FET-a-meen*	Evekeo	Narcolepsy, ADHD, exogenous obesity	Insomnia, nervousness, headache, tachycardia, anorexia, dizziness, excitement	Narcolepsy: 5–60 mg/day orally in divided doses ADHD: 5 mg BID, increase by 10 mg/week until desired effect
amphetamine/ dextroamphetamine	Adderall XR	Narcolepsy, ADHD	Same as amphetamine	10–30 mg orally once daily
dexmethylphenidate *dex-meth-il-FEN-i-date*	Focalin	ADHD	Nervousness, insomnia, loss of appetite, abdominal pain, weight loss, tachycardia, skin rash	2.5 mg orally BID; maximum dosage, 20 mg/day
dextroamphetamine *deks-troe-am-FET-a-meen*	Dexedrine, Zenzedi	Narcolepsy, ADHD	Same as amphetamine	Narcolepsy: 5–60 mg/day orally in divided doses ADHD: up to 40 mg/day orally
lisdexamfetamine *lis-dex-am-FET-a-meen*	Vyvanse	ADHD	Same as amphetamine	30–70 mg/day orally in one morning dose
methamphetamine *meth-am-FET-a-meen*	Desoxyn	ADHD, exogenous obesity	Same as amphetamine	ADHD: up to 25 mg/day orally Obesity: 5 mg orally 30 minutes before meals
methylphenidate *meth-il-FEN-i-date*	Aptensio XR, Concerta, Metadate, Ritalin, Methylin, Quillivant, Daytrana (transdermal patch)	ADHD, narcolepsy	Insomnia, anorexia, dizziness, headache, abdominal pain	5–60 mg/day orally
Analeptics				
armodafinil *ar-moe-DAF-i-nil*	Nuvigil	Narcolepsy, obstructive sleep apnea, sleepiness caused by shift work	Headache, nausea, insomnia	150–250 mg/day orally in a single morning dose
caffeine *KAF-een*	Cafcit, 5-hour Energy, Vivarin	Fatigue, drowsiness, as adjunct in analgesic formulation, premature apnea, respiratory depression	Palpitations, nausea, vomiting, insomnia, tachycardia, restlessness	Respiratory depression: 500 mg/1 g IM, IV
doxapram *DOKS-a-pram*	Dopram	Respiratory depression: postanesthesia, drug-induced, acute respiratory insufficiency superimposed on COPD	Dizziness, headache, apprehension, disorientation, nausea, cough, dyspnea, urinary retention	0.5–1 mg/kg IV
modafinil *moe-DAF-i-nil*	Provigil	Narcolepsy, obstructive sleep apnea	Headache, nausea	200–400 mg/day orally
pitolisant *Pi-TOL-i-sant*	Wakix	Narcolepsy—promote wakefulness	Headache	17–36 mg orally in morning
solriamfetol *SOL-ri-AM-fe-tol*	Sunosi	Narcolepsy, obstructive sleep apnea	Headache	150 mg/day orally

Continued

SUMMARY DRUG TABLE (continued)
Central Nervous System Stimulants

Generic Name	Trade Name	Uses	Adverse Reactions	Dosage Ranges
Anorexiants				
phentermine FEN-ter-meen	Adipex-P	Obesity	Same as benzphetamine	8 mg orally TID or 15.0–37.5 mg orally as a single daily dose
phentermine/ topiramate FEN-ter-meen & toe-PYRE-a-mate	Qsymia	Obesity	Same as benzphetamine	One tablet daily
naltrexone/bupropion nal-TREKS-one & byoo-PROE-pee-on	Contrave	Obesity	Same as benzphetamine	2 tablets twice daily
Miscellaneous Drugs				
atoMOXetine AT-oh-mox-a-teen	Strattera	ADHD (acts like antidepressant rather than stimulant)	Headache, decreased appetite, abdominal pain, vomiting, cough	Initial dose: 40 mg/day orally, may increase up to 100 mg/day orally
cloNIDine KLON-i-deen	Kapvay	ADHD, opiate withdrawal (supervised only)	Drowsiness, dizziness, sedation, dry mouth, constipation, syncope, dreams, rash	0.4 mg/day (extended release only)
guanFACINE GWAHN-fa-seen	Intuniv	ADHD	Dry mouth, somnolence, asthenia, dizziness, headache, constipation, fatigue	1–3 mg/day orally at bedtime
sodium oxybate SOW-dee-um ox-i-BATE	Xyrem	Narcolepsy, excessive daytime sleepiness	Headache, dizziness, somnolence	4.5–9.0 g/night taken in 2 doses at least 2½ hours apart

CHAPTER REVIEW

Know Your Drugs

Clients sometimes know a medication by the brand (or trade) name and not the generic name. To help you recognize both names, match the brand name with the generic name of the same medication.

Generic Name	Brand Name
1. methylphenidate	A. Adderall XR
2. lisdexamfetamine	B. Concerta
3. amphetamine/dextroamphetamine	C. Strattera
4. atomoxetine	D. Vyvanse

Calculate Medication Dosages

1. Adderall XR 30 mg daily in the morning is prescribed. The drug comes in 15-mg capsules. The parent will administer _____.
2. Modafinil 400 mg is prescribed. The drug is available in 200-mg tablets. The nurse administers _____.

Prepare for the NCLEX

RECALL THE FACTS

1. Which of the listed drug categories is not included as a class of CNS stimulants?
   1. amphetamines
   2. analeptics
   3. analgesics
   4. anorexiants

2. Initial assessment of the child with ADHD includes _____.
   1. assessing which stimuli the child responds to the most
   2. determining the child's intelligence
   3. obtaining a record of the child's behavior pattern
   4. obtaining vital signs

3. When assessing the client receiving doxapram for chronic pulmonary disease, the nurse observes the client for adverse drug reactions, which may include _____.
   1. headache, dizziness, variations in heart rate
   2. diarrhea, drowsiness, hypotension
   3. decreased respiratory rate, weight gain, bradycardia
   4. fever, dysuria, constipation

4. When teaching a client who is receiving an amphetamine for a diagnosis of narcolepsy, the nurse instructs the client to _____.
   1. record the times of the day the medication is taken
   2. take the medication at bedtime as well as in the morning
   3. take the drug with meals
   4. keep a record of how often periods of sleepiness occur

5. When administering an amphetamine, the nurse first checks to see if the client is taking or has taken a monoamine oxidase inhibitor (MAOI) because _____.
   1. a lower dosage of the amphetamine may be needed
   2. a higher dosage of the amphetamine may be needed
   3. the amphetamine can be substituted as the antidepressant drug
   4. the amphetamine is not given within 14 days of the MAOI

ANALYZE THE FACTS

6. A child with ADHD is admitted to the pediatric unit for a fractured tibia. Dexmethylphenidate is prescribed 7.5 mg BID; when should these doses be given?
   1. 7 and 11 a.m..
   2. 7 a.m. and 5 p.m.
   3. 9 a.m. and 5 p.m.
   4. 9 a.m. and 9 p.m.

7. The parent of a child with ADHD asks why a stimulant is used on a child who is too stimulated already. The best answer is:
   1. The stimulation to the pleasure center relaxes the child.
   2. The drug strengthens the nerve pathway to focus concentration.
   3. The drug stimulates the child to wear themselves down enough to focus.
   4. The drug is additive with the behavior to cancel out the bad behaviors.

8. *An obese client is weighed at the clinic. The starting weight was 370 lb; after 12 weeks the client now weighs 348 lb. The best action at this time is to:
   1. continue the anorexiant.
   2. increase the anorexiant.
   3. reduce the anorexiant.
   4. stop the anorexiant.

ALTERNATE-FORMAT QUESTIONS

9. An obese female client is starting an anorexiant for weight loss. Select all the points the nurse should emphasize in teaching this client about the drug. Select all that apply.
   1. You should modify your diet and exercise when taking these drugs.
   2. Never take over-the-counter diet pills when taking these drugs.
   3. You may take these drugs if your BMI is 22.
   4. Stop the anorexiant if you plan to get pregnant.

10. *Phentermine 8 mg three times a day orally is prescribed as an adjunct for weight loss. The total amount of drug the client will receive daily is _____. Is this an appropriate dose for this drug?

To check your answers, see Appendix F.

_____

*Indicates the question is directly linked to the NCLEX-PN test plan in Appendix G.

WANT TO KNOW MORE? A wide variety of resources are available to enhance your learning and understanding of this chapter.
- Visit thePoint for resources such as:
  - NCLEX-Style Student Review Questions
  - Journal Articles
  - Dosage Calculations
  - Drug Monographs
  - Watch and Learn Videos
  - Concepts in Action Animations
- The *Study Guide to Accompany Introductory Clinical Pharmacology*, 12th edition, sold separately, will help you review and apply essential content.
- ✓*PrepU* is available to help students prepare for the NCLEX-PN examination.

18

Antidementia Drugs

Key Terms

acetylcholine neurotransmitter that sends impulses across the parasympathetic branch of the autonomic nervous system

Alzheimer disease (AD) progressive neurologic disorder that affects cognition, emotion, and movement

amyloid plaque tangles of protein in nerve tissue

delirium an acute, temporary state of mental confusion

dementia decrease in cognitive function

parasympathetic pertaining to the part of the autonomic nervous system concerned with conserving body energy

Learning Objectives

On completion of this chapter, the student will:

1. Compare and contrast the clinical manifestations of Alzheimer disease (AD).
2. Explain the uses, general drug actions, general adverse reactions, contraindications, precautions, and interactions associated with the administration of antidementia drugs.
3. Distinguish important preadministration and ongoing assessment activities the nurse should perform with the client taking an antidementia drug.
4. List nursing diagnoses particular to a client taking an antidementia drug.
5. Examine ways to promote an optimal response to therapy, how to manage common adverse reactions, and important points to keep in mind when educating clients about the use of antidementia drugs.

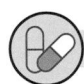 **Drug Classes**

Cholinesterase inhibitors
N-methyl-d-aspartate (NMDA) receptor antagonists

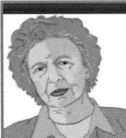 **PHARMACOLOGY IN PRACTICE**

Mrs. Moore, 85 years of age, has been experiencing progressive forgetfulness for about a year. Her daughter was in town last week and accompanied her to the clinic. After an initial examination, the primary health care provider decided to try a cholinesterase inhibitor. Mrs. Moore has called the clinic today complaining of gastrointestinal (GI) distress symptoms. She tells you to order an x-ray and find the ulcer in her tummy. You ask her to come to the clinic and she agrees. What assessment questions do you need to ask to determine if this is an appropriate request?

One of the greatest fears of aging is **dementia**. Used as an overall term for a variety of diseases and conditions, dementia involves the decrease in cognitive functioning, such as memory, attention, language or communication ability, and problem-solving skills. **Alzheimer disease** (AD) is the cause of about 60%–80% of all cases of dementia. The specific pathologic changes of AD occur in the cortex of the brain. These changes involve the degeneration of

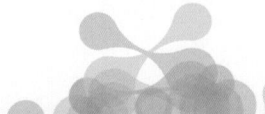

nerves by **amyloid plaques** and tangled nerve bundles, which slows or blocks transmission within the brain. When neurotransmission is impaired, the clinical symptoms of dementia result. Cholinesterase inhibitors and the newer NMDA receptor antagonists are drugs used to strengthen neurotransmission and improve or maintain memory in those with dementia.

Approximately 5.8 million people in the United States who are over the age of 65 years are diagnosed with AD (AA, 2020). AD progresses in a five-stage sequence as illustrated in Figure 18.1. This is a representation of the pathologic processes and not the "traditional" AD stages; these expanded stages help you understand the role of drug therapy in the treatment of the disease (Reisberg et al., 2012). Early on is a period of time called the preclinical stage when measurable changes are happening in the brain. The individual does not experience changes in cognitive or functional ability, yet these changes can be seen on magnetic resonance imaging and the biomarkers are present in blood and cerebrospinal fluid. Currently, drugs are not suitable for this time, which can occur up to 20 years before symptoms begin to appear.

The second stage is when cognitive changes appear and is termed mild cognitive impairment. Clients are often identified because of mild to moderate anxiety as changes in thinking ability become noticeable to the client or, as frequently occurs, to family members. This is when other acute or chronic causes should be ruled out as causing the thinking or memory changes.

PRACTICE CONSIDERATIONS

Hypothyroidism can present with cognitive impairment. Researchers have found that some clients are treated for dementia when thyroid dysfunction is the true medical problem. A study looking at those prescribed antidementia medications found only 32% had thyroid function testing done before prescription of the medication to rule out other medical conditions first (Sakata & Okumura, 2018).

During the second stage, a client's functional ability is intact, and this is when medications can help to limit the cognitive progression into later stages of the disease (Reisberg et al., 2012). Antianxiety and antidepressant drugs (Chapters 19 and 21) may be prescribed before antidementia medications. If mental ability does not improve then cholinesterase inhibitors or NMDA receptor antagonists are added to the treatment regime. Extensive mental function testing is indicated and can help delineate a course of treatment. Unfortunately, many individuals are not identified during this stage and best outcomes from the antidementia medications are not seen because they are not started early.

During the third through fifth stages of the disease, behaviors typically associated with the dementia of AD present, memory, thinking, and behavior changes, limit the ability to function independently (Jack et al., 2011). Reasoning and judgment become impaired. Socialization lessens due to behavioral changes, and variable degrees of assistance are needed for activities of daily living. Changes and additions in medications help to support function and behaviors. Refer to other chapters in Unit 4 to learn about the drugs used to support the client who is anxious (Chapter 19), depressed (Chapter 21), or may have difficulty controlling negative behaviors (Chapters 20 and 23).

The drugs used to treat dementia slow the progression. They do not cure or stop the symptoms or the disease. Other diseases, such as Parkinson disease, may have a dementia component, but cholinesterase inhibitors are approved primarily to treat mild to moderate dementia caused by AD. Drugs used to treat AD do not cure the disease but slow the progression of dementia. Two classes of drugs that are used include the cholinesterase inhibitors such as donepezil (Aricept) and the NMDA receptor antagonist such as memantine (Namenda). Other drug classes are used for specific symptomatic relief. For example, wandering, irritability, and aggression in people with AD are treated with antipsychotics, such as risperidone and olanzapine. Other drugs, such as

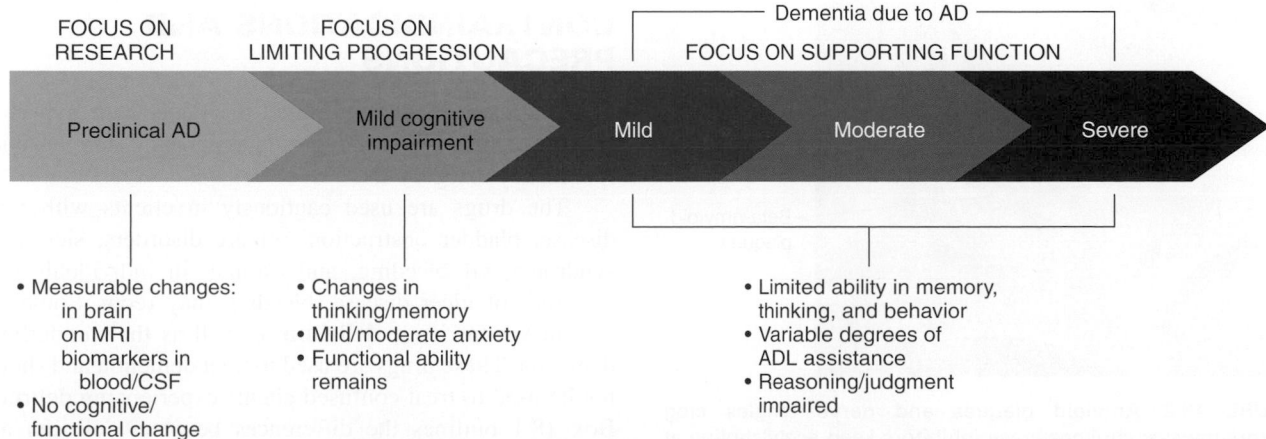

FIGURE 18.1 Continuum of Alzheimer disease progression.

antidepressants or antianxiety drugs may be helpful in AD for symptoms of depression and anxiety; these drugs are all discussed in individual chapters.

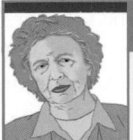

PHARMACOLOGY IN PRACTICE

PATHOLOGY
In the following stage of Alzheimer disease, there are brain changes detectable on an MRI but no cognitive changes. Which stage of the disease is being described?
1. Stage 1
2. Stage 3
3. Stage 5

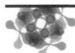 **ANTIDEMENTIA DRUGS**

ACTIONS

Acetylcholine is the transmitter substance in the **parasympathetic** (or cholinergic) neuropathway. Individuals with AD experience reduction in nerve impulse transmission because of plaques and tangles as illustrated in Figure 18.2. As a result, the client experiences problems with memory and thinking. The cholinesterase inhibitors act to increase the level of acetylcholine in the central nervous system (CNS) by inhibiting its breakdown and slowing neural destruction. However, the disease is progressive, and although these drugs alter the progress of the disease, they do not stop it. Cholinesterase inhibitors are not frequently used in late-stage AD.

A newer drug used to treat AD dementia is the NMDA receptor antagonist drug, memantine (Namenda). The NMDA receptor antagonist is thought to work by decreasing the excitability of neurotransmission caused by an excess of the amino acid glutamate in the CNS. Glutamate is also a transmitter to areas of learning and memory in the brain, yet too much of this substance can damage cells. The NMDA blocker attaches to nerve cell receptors and helps to prevent the cell damage.

USES

Cholinesterase inhibitors and the NMDA receptor antagonist are used to treat early and moderate stages of dementia associated with AD. Their use for severe cognitive decline as well as other dementias, such as vascular or Parkinson dementia, is being studied.

PRACTICE CONSIDERATIONS

Currently, methylphenidate (CNS stimulant) is being researched as a medication to diminish apathetic affect and improve cognition in clients with AD. Initial results demonstrate good short-term improvement (Kishi et al., 2020).

ADVERSE REACTIONS

Generalized adverse reactions include:

- Anorexia, nausea, vomiting, diarrhea
- Dizziness and headache

Additional adverse reactions are listed in the Summary Drug Table: Antidementia Drugs.

⚠ NURSING ALERT

Early diagnosis is the key to using drugs to slow AD symptoms. Brain imaging with positron emission tomography scans is enhanced with radioactive diagnostic drugs. Two drugs currently in use are flutemetamol (Vizamyl) and florbetapir (Amyvid). Adverse reactions of these drugs include flushing, headache, increased blood pressure, nausea, and dizziness.

CONTRAINDICATIONS AND PRECAUTIONS

These drugs are contraindicated in clients with hypersensitivity to the drugs and during pregnancy and lactation (pregnancy category B).

The drugs are used cautiously in clients with renal disease, bladder obstruction, seizure disorders, sick sinus syndrome, GI bleeding, and asthma. In individuals with a history of ulcer disease, bleeding may recur. Some clients may experience **delirium** as well as their underlying dementia. These drugs are used to treat dementia and should not be used to treat confused clients experiencing delirium. Box 18.1 outlines the differences between delirium and dementia.

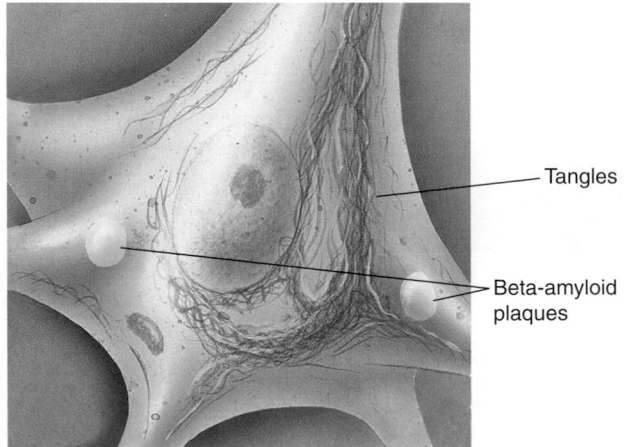

FIGURE 18.2 Amyloid plaques and nerve tangles clog neuropathways; cholinesterase inhibitors keep acetylcholine at the nerve junction longer to promote transmission.

BOX 18.1	**Differences Between Confusion of Delirium and Dementia**	
	Delirium	**Dementia**
Onset	Sudden change	Progressive change
Typical presentation	Affects senses (see, hear, feel)	Affects memory and judgment
Reversibility	Yes, when cause such as oxygen, chemical imbalances, or infection is found and treated	No, can slow progression with drugs, need to change environment for client to remain safe

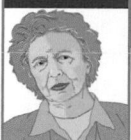

PHARMACOLOGY IN PRACTICE

ASSESSMENT
A client with dementia may also have delirium. Which of the following signs indicate a cognitive problem is due to delirium and not dementia? Select all that apply.
1. Sudden onset
2. Client feels itchy
3. Placing oxygen may resolve it
4. Progressive changes
5. Irreversible

LASA ALERT

The following drugs may sound alike; be sure to clarify when they are ordered:

Drug Name	*Sounds Like*
Aricept	Ascriptin, Azilect
Razadyne	Rozerem

Drugs that look like a similar drug are noted in the Summary Drug Tables of each chapter.

INTERACTIONS

The following interactions may occur when a cholinesterase inhibitor or NMDA receptor antagonist is administered with another agent:

Interacting Drug	Common Use	Effect of Interaction
Anticholinergics	Decrease of bodily secretions	Decreased effectiveness of anticholinergics
Nonsteroidal anti-inflammatory drugs	Pain relief	Increased risk of GI bleeding
Theophylline	Breathing problems	Increased risk of theophylline toxicity
Thiazide diuretics (with NMDA receptor antagonist)	Reduce fluid retention	Decreased effectiveness of the thiazide drug

SUPPLEMENTS FOR BRAIN HEALTH

Individuals are very fearful of memory loss leading to dementia. Here are two examples of supplements or herbal preparations clients may be taking to enhance memory and brain health—apoaequorin and ginko biloba.

Apoaequorin is a calcium-binding protein originally discovered in a species of jellyfish. The company marketing a popular product for memory enhancement, Quincy Bioscience, has published several studies speculating the neuroprotective effects of apoaequorin. In their studies, individuals received the supplement or a placebo with results showing marked memory improvement in the group taking the supplement (Martin, 2012). The use of the supplement is based on the idea that brain cell death and subsequent dementia has to do with the amount of calcium in the cells of the brain (Martin, 2012). When calcium is not bound to proteins, it fluctuates in the circulation of the brain. Over time, this fluctuation in and out of the brain cells can cause cell death leading to the advancement of the dementia of Alzheimer disease (Martin, 2012).

In an independent study, Bedlack (2013) was unable to replicate the calcium-binding capability of apoaequorin and found that it did not survive the process of digestion (destroyed by acid) and was not able to pass the blood–brain barrier. Any supplement should be discussed with a primary health care provider before starting self-treatment.

 Herbal Considerations

Ginkgo, one of the oldest herbs in the world, has many beneficial effects. It is thought to improve memory and brain function and enhance circulation to the brain, heart, limbs, and eyes. Conflicting research both supports and disputes ginkgo's ability to enhance memory. Medical studies in the United States and England (Snitz et al., 2009; UM, 2011) have not demonstrated increases in mental function. Despite this research, the "brain herb" is still taken by healthy adults hoping to retain their current memory and cognitive function. The recommended dose is 40 mg standardized extract ginkgo three times daily. The effects of ginkgo may not be evident until after 4–24 weeks of treatment. The most common adverse reactions include mild GI discomfort, headache, and rash. Excessively large doses have been reported to cause diarrhea, nausea, vomiting, and restlessness. Ginkgo is contraindicated in clients taking selective serotonin reuptake inhibitor or monoamine oxidase inhibitor antidepressants because of the risk of a toxic reaction. Moreover, individuals taking anticoagulants should take ginkgo only on the advice of a primary care provider.

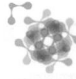

NURSING PROCESS—STEPS TO BUILDING CLINICAL JUDGMENT
Client Receiving an Antidementia Drug

ASSESSMENT

A client receiving an antidementia drug may be treated in the hospital, long-term care facility, or outpatient setting.

Preadministration Assessment

Data gathering suggestions before the initial administration of antidementia drugs include:

Objective data

- Description of general appearance, orientation to person, place, and time
- Vital signs (temperature, pulse, respirations, and blood pressure) and weight
- Observation of behavior during interview: poor eye contact, failure to answer questions completely, inappropriate answers to questions, monotone speech pattern, and inappropriate laughter, sadness, or crying, signifying varying stages of decline
- Cognitive screen with tools such as Mini-Mental Status Examination (MMSE)
- Battery of cognitive and functional ability testing, including orientation, calculation, recall, and language

Subjective data

- Current history of symptoms that bother the client
- Self-report compared with family members for ability to perform activities of daily living and self-care
- Unusual activity such as wandering or outbursts of anger or frustration
- Medical and mental health history
- Review chart for drugs that may cause changes in mental health

When the disease is advancing, clients with AD are not always able to give a reliable history of their illness. A family member or primary caregiver may be helpful in verifying or providing information needed for an accurate assessment.

Ongoing Assessment

Ongoing assessment of clients taking antidementia drugs includes both mental and physical assessments. Cognitive and functional abilities are assessed routinely for changes. Initial assessments will be compared with the ongoing assessments to monitor the client's improvement (if any) after taking the antidementia drugs.

Using standardized tools to obtain an accurate description of the client's behavior and cognitive ability aids the primary health care provider in planning therapy and thus becomes an important part of client management. Clients with poor response to drug therapy may require dosage changes, discontinuation of the drug therapy, or the addition of other therapies to the treatment regimen. However, response to these drugs may take several weeks. The symptoms that the client is experiencing may improve or remain the same, or the client may experience only a small response to therapy. It is important to remember that a treatment that slows the progression of symptoms in AD is a successful treatment.

NURSING DIAGNOSES

Drug-specific nursing diagnoses include the following:

- **Malnutrition: less than body requirements** related to anorexia, nausea, or vomiting
- **Injury risk** related to dizziness, syncope, clumsiness, or the disease process

Nursing diagnoses related to drug administration are discussed in Chapter 4.

PLANNING

The expected outcomes for the client may include an optimal response to drug therapy, meeting client needs related to the management of adverse reactions, an absence of injury, and confidence in an understanding of the medication regimen.

IMPLEMENTATION

Promoting an Optimal Response to Therapy

As you develop a care plan to meet the client's individual needs, keep in mind this is a progressive disease. When the drugs no longer provide memory enhancement, environmental factors may need to change rather than modifying the client's behavior.

If the client is hospitalized, it is important to monitor vital signs and other assessments to determine if changes may be from the dementia or if the client is experiencing delirium (acute confusion) caused by reversible causes (see Box 18.1).

ⓘ NURSING ALERT

Should cholinesterase inhibitor therapy be discontinued, individuals lose any benefit they have received from the drugs within 6 weeks.

Rivastigmine (Exelon) is available in a transdermal form of the drug. The patches are changed on a daily basis and rotated to a clean, dry, and hairless area. Because the client is experiencing dementia, the site for application should be where the client is not able to pick at or remove the patch. The upper or lower portions of the back are recommended for the patch administration. Because the same site should not be used more than once every 2 weeks, document or teach the caregiver to make a chart of the back and indicate where patches have been applied during the last 14 days.

Monitoring and Managing Client Needs

Malnutrition: Less Than Body Requirements
When taking an antidementia drug, clients may experience nausea and vomiting. Although this can occur with all of the cholinesterase inhibitors, clients taking rivastigmine (Exelon) appear to have more problems with nausea and severe vomiting. Attention to the dosing of medications can decrease adverse GI reactions and promote nutrition. The primary health care provider may discontinue use of the drug and then restart the drug therapy at the lowest

dose possible. Restarting therapy at the lower dose helps to reduce nausea and vomiting.

The antidementia drug can be taken with or without food. Although donepezil (Aricept) is administered orally once daily at bedtime, it can also be given with a snack. When administering rivastigmine as an oral solution, remove the oral dosing syringe provided in the protective container. The syringe provided is used to withdraw the prescribed amount. The dose may be swallowed directly from the syringe or first mixed with a small glass of water, cold fruit juice, or soda.

 Chronic Care Considerations

Namzaric is the first combined cholinesterase inhibitor and NMDA receptor antagonist drug on the market. By combining these medications, drug administration is reduced to one daily pill in the evening instead of up to six pills throughout the day. This may ease distress on clients with AD who have difficulty taking medications.

Weight loss and eating problems related to the inability to swallow are two major problems in the late stage of AD. These problems, coupled with anorexia and nausea associated with administration of cholinesterase inhibitors, present a challenge for caregivers. Typically, these drugs are not administered during the late stage of dementia, but there may be a period of worsening symptoms before the drugs are stopped entirely.

Mealtime should be simple and calm. Offer the client a well-balanced diet with foods that are easy to chew and digest. Frequent, small meals may be tolerated better than three regular meals. Offering foods of different consistency and flavor is important in case the client can handle one form better than another. Fluid intake of six to eight glasses of water daily is encouraged to prevent dehydration.

Injury Risk
Physical decline and the adverse reactions of dizziness and syncope place the client at risk for injury. The client may require assistance when ambulating. Assistive devices such as walkers or canes may reduce falls. To minimize the risk of injury, the client's environment should be controlled and safe. Encouraging the use of bed alarms, keeping the bed in low position, and using night lights, as well as frequent monitoring, will reduce the risk of injury. The client should wear medical identification, such as a MedicAlert bracelet, at all times.

Educating the Client and Family
Early in the disease, the client may be able to understand changes, yet suspicion and denial are classic symptoms of the disease; therefore, the client may not be amenable to treatment. As cognitive abilities decrease, focus on educating the family and primary caregiver of the client's needs. Depending on the degree of cognitive decline, discuss the drug regimen with the client, family member, or caregiver. It is important to evaluate accurately the client's ability to assume responsibility for taking drugs at home. The client and family should feel confident in understanding that the drugs used do not cure but rather control symptoms of the disease. It is your task to help

family members assume responsibility for medication administration when the client appears to be unable to manage their own drug therapy in the home.

Teach and provide written handouts in the preferred language about the drugs and adverse reactions that may occur with a specific drug, and encourage the caregiver or family members to contact the primary health care provider immediately when a serious drug reaction occurs.

As you develop a teaching plan for the client or family member, include the following points:

- Keep all appointments with the primary care provider or clinic, because close monitoring of therapy is essential. Dose changes may be needed to achieve the best results.
- Report any unusual changes or physical effects to the primary health care provider.
- Take the drug exactly as directed. Do not increase, decrease, or omit a dose or discontinue use of this drug unless directed to do so by the primary health care provider.
- Do not drive or perform other hazardous tasks if drowsiness occurs. Discuss with your primary health care provider when clients should be evaluated for their continued ability to drive.
- Do not take any nonprescription drug before talking to your primary health care provider.
- Keep track of when the drug is taken. Marking the calendar, cell phone alarms, or a pill counter that holds the medicine for each day of the week may be helpful tools to remind the client to take the medication or determine whether the medication has been taken for the day.
- Notify the primary care provider if the following adverse reactions are experienced for more than a few days: nausea, diarrhea, difficulty sleeping, vomiting, or loss of appetite.
- Immediately report the occurrence of the following adverse reactions: severe vomiting, dehydration, or changes in neurologic functioning.
- Notify the primary health care provider if the client has a history of ulcers, feels faint, experiences severe stomach pains, vomits blood or material that resembles coffee grounds, or has bloody or black stools.
- Remember that these drugs do not cure AD but slow the mental and physical degeneration associated with the disease. The drug must be taken routinely to slow the progression.

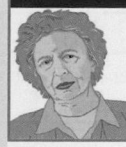 **PHARMACOLOGY IN PRACTICE**

MANAGING NEEDS
A client with moderate dementia of the Alzheimer type repeatedly spits out pills.
They are being changed to a transdermal patch. Where should the nurse place a cholinesterase inhibitor transdermal patch so that the client cannot easily remove it?
1. Upper arm
2. Side of thigh
3. Chest
4. Lower back

EVALUATION

- Therapeutic effect is achieved and cognitive function is maintained.
- Adverse reactions are identified, reported to the primary health care provider, and managed successfully through appropriate nursing interventions:
  - Client maintains an adequate nutritional status.
  - No injury is evident.
- Client (if able) and family express confidence and demonstrate an understanding of the drug regimen.

PHARMACOLOGY IN PRACTICE

USING CLINICAL REASONING

While Mrs. Moore is putting on a patient gown at the clinic, you notice she appears to have multiple "bandages" all over her body. Upon closer examination, the bandage reads EXELON PATCH. Does this explain her GI distress?

KEY POINTS

■ AD is one of the conditions in which dementia is a major issue. This occurs because of the buildup of plaques and tangles in the neurons of the brain. Acetylcholine is reduced, resulting in symptoms of dementia.

■ The progression of memory loss associated with dementia is treated with cholinesterase inhibitors/NMDA receptor antagonist agents. These drugs slow progression but do not cure dementia.

■ Clients with dementia may at times experience acute confusion, known as delirium. These drugs do not treat delirium.

■ Some of the most common adverse reactions of these drugs include dry mouth, nausea, and vomiting. Nutrition becomes a primary issue in treatment because clients with AD also may have reduced appetite and difficulty eating.

■ Involvement of family members or caregivers is essential for the treatment and management of the client with AD because of the cognitive and functional changes involved.

SUMMARY DRUG TABLE
Antidementia Drugs

Generic Name	Trade Name	Uses	Adverse Reactions	Dosage Ranges
Cholinesterase Inhibitors				
donepezil *doh-NEP-e-zil*	Aricept	Mild to severe dementia caused by AD, memory improvement in dementia caused by stroke, vascular disease, multiple sclerosis	Headache, nausea, diarrhea, insomnia, muscle cramps	5–10 mg/day orally
galantamine *ga-LAN-ta-meen*	Razadyne	Mild to moderate (AD) dementia	Nausea, vomiting, diarrhea, anorexia, dizziness	16–24 mg BID orally
rivastigmine *ri-va-STIG-meen*	Exelon (transdermal)	Mild to moderate dementia of AD and Parkinson disease	Nausea, vomiting, diarrhea, dyspepsia, anorexia, insomnia, fatigue, dizziness, headache	1.5–12 mg/day BID orally; 4.6, 9.5, 13.3 mg daily transdermal patch
NMDA Receptor Antagonist				
memantine *me-MAN-teen*	Namenda	Moderate to severe (AD) dementia	Dizziness, headache, confusion	5–10 mg BID orally
Combination Drugs				
memantine/donepezil	Namzaric	Moderate to severe (AD) dementia	See individual drugs above	14–28/10 mg orally every evening

CHAPTER REVIEW

Know Your Drugs

Clients sometimes know a medication by the brand (or trade) name and not the generic name. To help you recognize both names, match the brand name with the generic name of the same medication.

Generic Name	Brand Name
1. donepezil	A. Aricept
2. galantamine	B. Exelon
3. memantine	C. Namenda
4. rivastigmine	D. Razadyne

Calculate Medication Dosages

1. Rivastigmine oral solution 6 mg is prescribed. The drug is available as an oral solution of 2 mg/mL. The nurse administers _____.
2. Oral memantine (Namenda) 10 mg is prescribed for a client with AD. On hand are 5-mg tablets. The nurse administers _____.

Prepare for the NCLEX

RECALL THE FACTS

1. AD involves protein plaques and nerve tangles that limit which neurotransmitter?
   1. acetylcholine
   2. dopamine
   3. norepinephrine
   4. serotonin
2. Adverse reactions that the nurse would assess for in a client taking rivastigmine (Exelon) include _____.
   1. occipital headache
   2. vomiting
   3. hyperactivity
   4. hypoactivity
3. When administering donepezil (Aricept) to a client with AD, the nurse would most likely expect which diagnostic test to have been prescribed?
   1. complete blood count
   2. cholesterol levels
   3. brain scan
   4. electrolyte analysis
4. Which of the following nursing diagnoses would the nurse most likely place on the care plan of a client with AD that is related to adverse reactions of the cholinesterase inhibitors?
   1. Malnutrition
   2. Confusion
   3. Self-harm risk
   4. Bowel incontinence
5. The nurse correctly administers donepezil (Aricept) _____.
   1. three times daily around the clock
   2. twice daily 1 hour before meals or 2 hours after meals
   3. once daily in the morning
   4. once daily at bedtime

ANALYZE THE FACTS

6. When a client's dementia causes them to pick at items, the rivastigmine transdermal patch should be placed:
   1. on the abdomen.
   2. on the upper arms.
   3. between the shoulder blades.
   4. on the thigh.

7. *The nurse correctly disposes the rivastigmine transdermal patch by first:
   1. placing it in a tissue and discarding in trash can.
   2. flushing the patch in the client's toilet.
   3. folding it over so the adhesive side sticks together.
   4. disposing in a sharps contaminated box in the client's room.
8. Which of the following is an indicator of delirium?
   1. progressive, insidious onset
   2. caused by bladder infection
   3. ongoing confusion
   4. problems with memory

ALTERNATE-FORMAT QUESTIONS

9. Which of the following are used to monitor progression of AD? **Select all that apply.**
   1. MMSE
   2. brain scan
   3. blood studies
   4. urinalysis
   5. memory testing
10. For drug development purposes, AD is now defined in five stages. Cholinesterase inhibitors are used during which stage(s)? **Select all that apply.**
    1. stage 1
    2. stage 2
    3. stage 3

To check your answers, see Appendix F.

*Indicates the question is directly linked to the NCLEX-PN test plan in Appendix G.

> **WANT TO KNOW MORE?** A wide variety of resources are available to enhance your learning and understanding of this chapter.
> - Visit thePoint for resources such as:
>   - NCLEX-Style Student Review Questions
>   - Journal Articles
>   - Dosage Calculations
>   - Drug Monographs
>   - Watch and Learn Videos
>   - Concepts in Action Animations
> - The *Study Guide to Accompany Introductory Clinical Pharmacology*, 12th edition, sold separately, will help you review and apply essential content.
> - ✔**PrepU** is available to help students prepare for the NCLEX-PN examination.

19

Antianxiety Drugs

Key Terms

anxiety feelings of apprehension, worry, or uneasiness

anxiolytics drugs used to treat anxiety

ataxia unsteady gait; muscular incoordination

gamma (γ)-aminobutyric acid (GABA) a neurotransmitter inhibitor that is involved in the regulation of sleep and anxiety

generalized anxiety disorder (GAD) disorder of chronic anxiety, exaggerated worry, and tension

physical dependence habitual use of a drug, where negative physical withdrawal symptoms result from abrupt discontinuation

posttraumatic stress disorder (PTSD) a mental health condition triggered by a terrifying event

psychological dependence compulsion or craving to use a substance to obtain a pleasurable experience

tolerance increasingly larger dosages of a drug are required to obtain the desired effect

Learning Objectives

On completion of this chapter, the student will:

1. Explain the uses, general drug actions, general adverse reactions, contraindications, precautions, and interactions associated with the administration of antianxiety drugs.
2. Distinguish important preadministration and ongoing assessment activities the nurse should perform on the client taking an antianxiety drug.
3. List nursing diagnoses particular to a client taking an antianxiety drug.
4. Examine ways to promote an optimal response to therapy, how to manage common adverse reactions, and important points to keep in mind when educating clients about the use of antianxiety drugs.

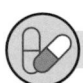 **Drug Classes**

Benzodiazepines   Antidote
Nonbenzodiazepines

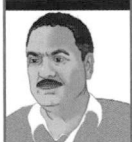 **PHARMACOLOGY IN PRACTICE**

Mr. Garcia, 55 years of age, is being seen in the clinic for an upper respiratory infection. Using an interpreter, he tells you that his shortness of breath makes him anxious. His respirations are 32 breaths/minute, heart rate is 98 beats/minute, and blood pressure is 161/92 mm Hg. The primary health care provider prescribes alprazolam (Xanax) 0.25 mg orally three times a day. As you read this chapter, determine if this is appropriate.

Anxiety is a feeling of apprehension, worry, or uneasiness that may or may not be based on reality. Anxiety may be seen in many types of situations, ranging from the "jitters" and excitement of a new job to the acute panic that may be seen during withdrawal from alcohol. Although a certain amount of anxiety is normal, excess anxiety interferes with day-to-day functioning and can cause undue stress in the lives of some individuals. Drugs used to treat anxiety are called *antianxiety drugs*. **Anxiolytics** is another term you may see when referring to the antianxiety drugs.

Antianxiety drug classes include the benzodiazepines and the nonbenzodiazepines. Examples of the benzodiazepines include alprazolam

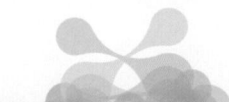

(Xanax), chlordiazepoxide (Librium), diazepam (Valium), and lorazepam (Ativan). **Physical dependence** and **psychological dependence** result from long-term use of the benzodiazepines. Owing to the risk of dependence, benzodiazepines are intended for short-term anxiety relief. In addition, these drugs are classified as schedule IV controlled substances (see Chapter 1) because of the ability to cause dependency. Typically, long-term psychiatric anxiety conditions such as **generalized anxiety disorder** or **posttraumatic stress disorder** are treated with antidepressant medications (Chapter 21), and anxiolytics are not the first-line choice of drug treatment for these disorders. The nonbenzodiazepines useful in reducing anxiety include buspirone, doxepin, and hydroxyzine.

ACTIONS

Anxiolytic drugs exert their tranquilizing effect by blocking certain neurotransmitter receptor sites. In turn, this prevents the neurotransmission of the anxious perception and the body's physical reaction to the anxiety. Benzodiazepines exert their tranquilizing effect by potentiating the effects of **gamma (γ)-aminobutyric acid** (GABA), an inhibitory transmitter (Fig. 19.1). Nonbenzodiazepines exert their action in various ways. For example, buspirone is thought to act on the brain's serotonin receptors. Hydroxyzine (Vistaril) produces its antianxiety effect by acting on the hypothalamus and brainstem reticular formation.

USES

Antianxiety drugs are used in the management of the following:

- Isolated episodes of intense anxiety
- Temporary use for those with severe functional impairment

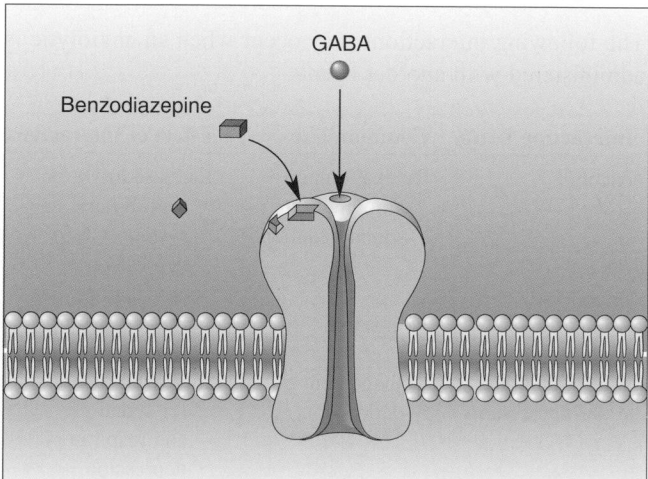

FIGURE 19.1 Benzodiazepine drugs bind to a site on the cell receptor, potentiating the effect of GABA (an inhibitory neurotransmitter) on the receptor. (Adapted from Bear, M. F., Connors, B. W., & Parasido, M. A. (2001). *Neuroscience—exploring the brain* (2nd ed.). Lippincott Williams & Wilkins.)

- Preanesthetic sedation and muscle relaxation
- Convulsions or seizures
- Alcohol withdrawal

ADVERSE REACTIONS

Frequent, early reactions include:

- Mild drowsiness or sedation
- Light-headedness or dizziness
- Headache

Other adverse body system reactions include:

- Lethargy, apathy, fatigue
- Disorientation
- Anger
- Restlessness
- Nausea, constipation or diarrhea, dry mouth
- Visual disturbances

See the Summary Drug Table: Antianxiety Drugs for more information.

Dependence

Some individuals have been prescribed benzodiazepines for decades in order to deal with anxiety issues. Long-term use of benzodiazepines results in physical dependence and **tolerance** (increasingly larger dosages required to obtain the desired effect). If these drugs should not be used for long-term therapy, then why not stop them? Because when used by a client on a daily basis (as a sedative) withdrawal symptoms can occur even if the drug is stopped after only 4–6 months of use. Should large doses be used, these withdrawal symptoms can appear after only 2–3 months of use. If abruptly withdrawn, acute withdrawal reactions may last from 5 to 28 days with the peak of symptoms in the second week (Box 19.1). Therefore, a gradually decreasing dosage schedule (known as *tapering*) should be used when stopping a benzodiazepine.

BOX 19.1 Symptoms of Benzodiazepine Withdrawal

- Increased anxiety and panic
- Fatigue
- Hypersomnia and nightmares
- Metallic taste
- Concentration difficulties
- Headache and tinnitus
- Tremors
- Numbness in the extremities
- Tachycardia, hypertension
- Nausea, vomiting, diarrhea
- Fever and sweating
- Muscle tension, aching, and cramps
- Psychoses and hallucination
- Agitation
- Memory impairment
- Convulsions (possible)

In addition, the client needs support and encouragement from the provider to enhance a successful discontinuation of the drug. Be aware that long-term users face increased anxiety when discontinuing the drug. This anxiety is generated from the fear of not knowing how they will respond when the medication is stopped. Subsequently, the client will display anxious behaviors and request to be put back on or increase the dose of the benzodiazepine. This behavior is frequently viewed by others as addiction to the benzodiazepine drugs rather than a fear reaction.

! NURSING ALERT

Withdrawal symptoms are more likely to occur when the benzodiazepine is taken for 3 months or more and is suddenly discontinued. Therefore, antianxiety drugs must never be discontinued abruptly.

The nonbenzodiazepine antianxiety drug buspirone is associated with less physical dependence potential and less effect on motor ability and cognition.

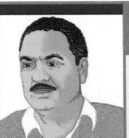

PHARMACOLOGY IN PRACTICE

ASSESSMENT

A client on benzodiazepine therapy for 4 weeks comes to an adult day health facility. The electronic health record indicates the drug was stopped abruptly. The nurse should monitor for which of the following?
1. Increased RBC count
2. Decreased pulse rate
3. Increased anxiety
4. Increased appetite

CONTRAINDICATIONS

Do not administer antianxiety drugs to clients with known hypersensitivity, psychoses, and acute narrow-angle glaucoma. The benzodiazepines are contraindicated during pregnancy (pregnancy category D drugs) and labor. Reports of floppy infant syndrome manifested by sucking difficulties, lethargy, and hypotonia have been seen in the newborn of a mother using benzodiazepines. Lactating women should also avoid the benzodiazepines because of the effect on the infant (lethargy and weight loss). Owing to a specific enzyme reaction, grapefruit or its juice should not be taken if the client is on buspirone and diazepam.

Buspirone is a pregnancy category B drug, and hydroxyzine is a pregnancy category C drug. Their safety is still questionable because adequate studies have not been performed in pregnant women. All of these drugs are contraindicated when clients are in a coma or shock and if the vital signs of the client in acute alcoholic intoxication are low.

PRECAUTIONS

Antianxiety drugs are used cautiously in elderly clients and in clients with impaired liver function, impaired kidney function, or debilitation.

Lifespan Considerations

Gerontology

Recent studies link the chronic use of benzodiazepines by those older than 65 years to a greater chance of developing dementia (Billioti, 2012).

LASA ALERT

The following drugs may sound alike; be sure to clarify when they are ordered:

Drug Name	Sounds Like
Ativan	Ambien, Atarax, Atgam, Avitene
busPIRone	buPROPion
chlordiazePOXIDE	chlorproMAZINE
clonazePAM	ALPRAZolam, cloBAZam, cloNIDine, clorazepate, cloZAPine, LORazepam
hydrOXYzine	hydrALAZINE, hydroCHLOROthiazide, hydroxyurea
KlonoPIN	cloNIDine, clorazepate, cloZAPine, LORazepam
LORazepam	ALPRAZolam, clonazePAM, diazePAM, KlonoPIN, Lovaza, temazepam, zolpidem
meprobamate	meperidine
oxazepam	oxcarbazepine, oxaprozin, quazepam
Vistaril	Restoril, Versed, Zestril

Drugs that look like a similar drug are noted in the Summary Drug Tables of each chapter.

INTERACTIONS

The following interactions may occur when an anxiolytic is administered with another agent:

Interacting Drug	Common Use	Effect of Interaction
Alcohol	Relaxation and enjoyment in social situations	Increased risk for central nervous system (CNS) depression or convulsions
Analgesics	Pain relief	Increased risk for CNS depression
Tricyclic antidepressants	Management of depression	Increased risk for sedation and respiratory depression
Antipsychotics	Control of psychotic symptoms	Increased risk for sedation and respiratory depression
Digoxin	Management of cardiac problems	Increased risk for digitalis toxicity

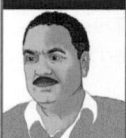

PHARMACOLOGY IN PRACTICE

SAFE DRUG ADMINISTRATION

A client visits a neighborhood clinic with symptoms of anxiety. The primary health care provider has prescribed hydroxyzine. Which of the following conditions should the nurse flag for possible contraindication or complications when administering hydroxyzine? Select all that apply.
1. Impaired liver function
2. Impaired pancreas function
3. Impaired kidney function
4. Bone marrow depression
5. Clients with debilitation

Herbal Considerations

Kava is a popular herbal remedy thought to relieve stress, anxiety, and tension; promote sleep; and provide relief from menstrual discomfort. Kava's benefits are not supported by science, and the US Food and Drug Administration (FDA) has issued an alert indicating that the use of kava may cause liver damage. Because kava-containing products have been associated with liver-related injuries (e.g., hepatitis, cirrhosis, and liver failure), the safest way to use kava is to take the herb occasionally for episodes of anxiety, rather than on a daily basis. It is important that individuals who use a kava-containing dietary supplement and experience signs of liver disease immediately consult their primary health care provider. Identifying kava-containing products can be difficult. Careful reading of the "Supplement Facts" information on the label may identify kava by any of the following names: kava, ava, ava pepper, awa, kava root, kava-kava, kew, *Piper methysticum* G. Forst, *Piper methysticum*, Sakau, tonga, or yanggona (FDA Consumer Advisory, 2009).

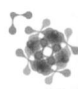

NURSING PROCESS—STEPS TO BUILDING CLINICAL JUDGMENT
Client Receiving an Antianxiety Drug

ASSESSMENT

Preadministration Assessment

Individuals with mild anxiety or depression do not necessarily require inpatient care. These clients are usually seen at periodic intervals in the primary health care provider's office or in a mental health outpatient setting. Treatment for anyone in the hospital or in an outpatient setting may be anxiety provoking, especially if the individual has reduced health literacy (Fig. 19.2). Assessment of both client groups is similar.

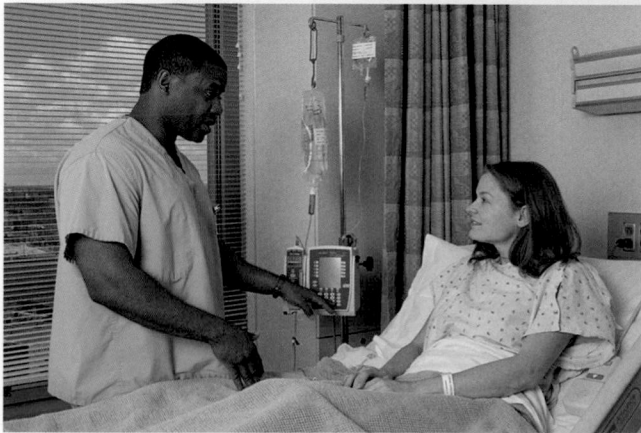

FIGURE 19.2 Hospitalization can be an anxious experience for clients. Anxiolytic medications can help the client focus on client teaching and activities of daily living to improve client outcomes.

Data gathering suggestions before the initial administration of antianxiety drugs include:
Objective data

- Description of general appearance; watch for cool or pale skin
- Vital signs and weight; watch for increases in pulse, respirations, and blood pressure
- Observation of behavior during interview: inability to focus, extreme restlessness, facial grimaces, muscle tension, or tense posture

Subjective data

- Rating of anxiety level (see below)
- Current history of symptoms, description of how the client reacts to stress
- Self-report compared with family members for episodes of behavioral change or escalation of symptoms
- Coping mechanisms used to deal with anxiety, especially self-medicating with alcohol or drugs
- Medical, social, and mental health history
- Review chart for drugs that may cause changes in mental health

Because anxiety is a subjective feeling, you may ask the client to rate their anxiety on a 0–10 scale, just as you would when asking about pain.

When asking about alcohol or drug intake, ask direct, nonjudgmental questions. More accurate intake information is obtained when using questions such as "How much alcohol do you drink daily?" or "Do you drink more or less than three alcohol beverages daily?"

Ongoing Assessment

An ongoing assessment is important for the client taking an antianxiety drug. Ask the client to rate the anxiety and compare this with the baseline rating. Check the client's blood pressure before drug administration. If systolic pressure has dropped 20 mm Hg, withhold the drug because the client is at greater risk to fall, and notify the primary health care provider. Periodically monitor the client's mental status and anxiety level during therapy and assess for improvement or decline of behavioral and functional ability.

During follow-up in the ambulatory setting, ask the client or a family member about adverse drug reactions or any other problems occurring during therapy. Flag these reactions or problems to be sure they come to the attention of the primary health care provider. Describe and document outward behavior and any complaints or problems in the client's record. Compare your new information with previous notations and observations.

NURSING DIAGNOSES

Drug-specific nursing diagnoses are the following:

- **Injury risk** related to dizziness or hypotension and gait problems
- **Impaired comfort** related to dryness in the gastrointestinal (GI) tract from medications
- **Coping impairment** related to situation causing anxiety

Nursing diagnoses related to drug administration are discussed in Chapter 4.

PLANNING

The expected client outcomes may include an optimal response to drug therapy, support of client needs related to the management of adverse drug reactions, and confidence in an understanding of the medication regimen.

IMPLEMENTATION

Promoting an Optimal Response to Therapy

During initial therapy, observe the client closely for adverse drug reactions. Some adverse reactions, such as episodes of postural hypotension and drowsiness or dry mouth, may need to be tolerated because drug therapy must continue. The antianxiety drugs are not recommended for long-term use. These drugs are meant to reduce anxiety in a short period, allowing the client to develop other coping skills to deal with anxious situations.

When the antianxiety drugs are used for short periods (1–2 weeks), tolerance, dependence, or withdrawal symptoms usually do not develop. Should any signs of tolerance or dependence develop (see Box 19.1), such as the client needing larger doses of drug or complaints of increased anxiety and agitation, contact the primary health care provider.

Monitoring and Managing Client Needs

Injury Risk

When these drugs are given in the outpatient setting, instruct both the client and family about adverse reactions (dizziness, light-headedness, or **ataxia**) that can cause a client to fall and become injured. This is very important when the drugs are administered to older adults.

Lifespan Considerations

Gerontology

Benzodiazepines are excreted more slowly in older adults, causing a prolonged drug effect. The drugs may accumulate in the blood, resulting in an increase in adverse reactions or toxicity.

Antianxiety drugs stay in the body of older adults longer, so the initial dose should be small and the dose increased gradually until a therapeutic response is obtained. However, if lorazepam and oxazepam are used, these are relatively safe for older adults when given in normal dosages. Buspirone also is a safer choice for older adults with anxiety, because it does not cause excessive sedation and the risk of falling is not as great.

When the client is hospitalized, develop a nursing care plan to meet the client's individual needs regarding the anxious behavior. Vital signs should be monitored at frequent intervals, usually three or four times daily, when antianxiety medication doses are adjusted. Clients should be monitored for symptoms such as dizziness or light-headedness. When antianxiety drugs are started or increased, instruct the client to stay in bed and call for assistance to get up out of the bed or chair, and consider the need for supervision for any ambulatory activities. Provide assistance with activities of daily living to the client experiencing any sedation effects. This includes help with eating, dressing, and ambulating. In some instances, such as when a hypotensive episode occurs, the vital signs are taken more often. Report any significant change in the vital signs to the primary health care provider. The sedation and drowsiness that sometimes occur with the use of an antianxiety drug may decrease as therapy continues.

Parenteral administration is indicated primarily in acute states when the client's behavior makes it difficult to take the medication by mouth. Choose a large muscle mass, such as the gluteus muscle, when administering the drug by the intramuscular (IM) route. Then observe the client closely for at least 3 hours after parenteral administration. The client is kept lying down (when possible) for 30 minutes to 3 hours after the drug is given.

Lifespan Considerations

Gerontology

Parenteral (intravenous [IV] or IM) administration to older adults, the debilitated, and those with limited pulmonary reserve requires extreme care because the client may experience apnea and cardiac arrest. Resuscitative equipment should be readily available during parenteral (particularly IV) administration. For specific information regarding administration of parenteral diazepam, see Chapter 28.

Impaired Comfort

Antianxiety drugs can cause both dryness of the mucous membranes and slower transit in the intestines, leading to constipation. Assess swallowing (because of a dry mouth) and give with lots of fluid, especially in the older, institutionalized adult. Nursing interventions to relieve some of these reactions may include offering frequent sips of water to relieve dry mouth and provide adequate hydration. The client may also chew sugarless gum or suck on hard candy to reduce discomfort from dry mouth. Administer oral antianxiety drugs with food or meals to decrease the possibility of GI upset. Meals should include fiber, fruits, and vegetables to aid in preventing constipation.

Coping Impairment

When the client is an outpatient, compare response to therapy at the time of each clinic visit. In some instances, question the client or a family member about the response to therapy. The type of questions asked depend on the client and the diagnosis and should include open-ended questions. The following are examples of questions that are not open ended: "Do you feel less nervous?" or "Would you like to tell me how everything is going?" Both questions could be answered, "yes" or "no." Instead ask the same question in an open-ended format such as, "How are you feeling?" This gives the client the ability to describe the feelings yet they may remain silent. At that point you can wait for a response or rephrase questions or direct the conversation toward other subjects until the client feels comfortable enough to discuss feelings.

Once the client has reduced the anxious behavior, you may be able to help them identify what is precipitating the panic attacks or causing anxiety. It is important for you to help the client understand that there are health care providers who can help them gain skills to cope with situations before the anxious behavior returns.

Although benzodiazepine toxicity is rare when the drug is used correctly, it may occur from an overdose of the drug. Benzodiazepine toxicity causes sedation, respiratory depression, and coma. Flumazenil is an antidote (antagonist) for benzodiazepine toxicity and acts to reverse the sedation, respiratory depression, and coma within 6–10 minutes after IV administration. Adverse reactions to flumazenil include agitation, confusion, seizures, and, in some cases, symptoms of benzodiazepine withdrawal. Adverse reactions to flumazenil, related to the symptoms of benzodiazepine withdrawal, are relieved by the administration of the benzodiazepine.

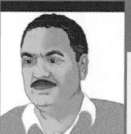

PHARMACOLOGY IN PRACTICE

MANAGING NEEDS

An adult family home client is prescribed chlordiazepoxide for anxiety. Which of the following dietary changes should the nurse instruct the caregivers to perform to prevent the occurrence of constipation in this client?
1. Provide vitamin supplements.
2. Restrict client's diet to fluids only.
3. Provide client with a fiber-rich diet and plenty of fluids.
4. Restrict client to a strict vegetarian diet.

Educating the Client and Family

Evaluate the client's ability to assume responsibility for taking drugs at home. You should explain and provide written materials in the preferred language of any adverse reactions that may occur with a specific antianxiety drug and encourage the client or family members to contact the primary health care provider immediately if a serious adverse reaction occurs. The client and family should feel confident in understanding that the drugs prescribed will help to reduce anxiety on a short-term basis. If anxiety persists, notify the primary health care provider so that other therapy options can be explored. As you develop a teaching plan for the client or family member, include the following:

- Take the drug exactly as directed. Do not increase, decrease, or omit a dose or discontinue use of this drug unless directed to do so by the primary health care provider.
- Do not discontinue use of the drug abruptly because withdrawal symptoms may occur.
- Avoid driving or performing other hazardous tasks if drowsiness occurs.
- Do not take any nonprescription drugs until discussing the specific drug with the primary health care provider.
- Inform physicians, dentists, and other health care providers of therapy with this drug.
  - Do not drink alcoholic beverages while taking this medication.
- If dizziness occurs when changing position, rise slowly when getting out of bed or a chair. If dizziness is severe, always have help when changing positions.
- If dryness of the mouth occurs, relieve it by taking frequent sips of water, sucking on hard candy, or chewing gum (preferably sugarless).
- Prevent constipation by eating high-fiber foods, increasing fluid intake, and exercising if the condition permits.
- Keep all appointments with the primary health care provider because close monitoring of therapy is essential.
- Report any unusual changes or physical effects to the primary health care provider.

EVALUATION

- Therapeutic response is achieved and client reports decrease in feelings of anxiety.
- Adverse reactions are identified, reported to the primary health care provider, and managed successfully with appropriate nursing interventions:
  - No evidence of injury is seen.
  - Client reports comfort without increased GI distress.
  - Client manages coping effectively.
- Client and family express confidence and demonstrate an understanding of the drug regimen.

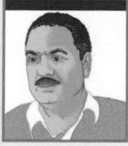

PHARMACOLOGY IN PRACTICE

USING CLINICAL REASONING

Discuss what assessment findings in the beginning of the chapter would indicate increased anxiety. As part of the client teaching, what precautions would you relay to Mr. Garcia about this medication? How will you determine if he understands the information correctly?

KEY POINTS

■ Anxiety involves a feeling of apprehension, worry, or uneasiness that may or may not be based on reality. Anxiety is a normal feeling, yet as anxiety increases it can interfere with day-to-day functioning.

■ Because it is a subjective feeling, clients can be asked to rate anxiety similar to rating pain.

■ Benzodiazepines and nonbenzodiazepine anxiolytics are used to treat anxiety on a short-term basis. Physical and psychological dependence can occur with use of these drugs; typically psychiatric anxiety disorders (which need long-term treatment) use antidepressants for treatment instead of benzodiazepines.

■ The anxiolytics work by blocking certain neurotransmitters, which in turn reduce anxiety; they additionally can reduce blood pressure, which can cause adverse reactions such as hypotension, dizziness, and drowsiness.

■ Benzodiazepine doses should always be tapered and never stopped abruptly; withdrawal can occur with symptoms such as a return of anxiety, concentration problems, tremor, and sensory disturbances.

■ Older adults do not eliminate these drugs as well as younger people and can experience adverse reactions with smaller doses than what younger people can tolerate.

SUMMARY DRUG TABLE
Antianxiety Drugs

Generic Name	Trade Name	Uses	Adverse Reactions	Dosage Ranges
Benzodiazepines				
alprazolam *al-PRAY-zoe-lam*	Xanax	Anxiety disorders, short-term relief of anxiety, panic attacks	Transient mild drowsiness, light-headedness, headache, depression, constipation, diarrhea, dry mouth	0.25–0.5 mg orally TID, may be increased to 4 mg/day in divided doses
chlordiazePOXIDE *klor-dye-az-a-POKS-ide*		Anxiety disorders, short-term relief of anxiety, acute alcohol withdrawal	Same as alprazolam	Anxiety: 5–25 mg orally 3 or 4 times daily Acute alcohol withdrawal: 50–100 mg IM, then 25–50 mg IM
clonazePAM *kloe-NA-ze-pam*	KlonoPIN	Panic disorder, anticonvulsant	Same as alprazolam	0.25 mg orally BID
clorazepate *klor-AZ-eh-pate*	Tranxene	Anxiety disorders, short-term relief of anxiety, acute alcohol withdrawal, anticonvulsant	Same as alprazolam	Anxiety: 15–60 mg/day orally in divided doses Acute alcohol withdrawal: up to 90 mg/day with taper-off schedule
diazePAM *dye-AZ-e-pam*	Valium	Anxiety disorders, short-term relief of anxiety, acute alcohol withdrawal, anticonvulsant, procedural relief of anxiety and tension	Same as alprazolam	Individualize dosage: 2–10 mg IM, IV, or orally 2–4 times daily
LORazepam *lor-A-ze-pam*	Ativan	Anxiety disorders, short-term relief of anxiety, preanesthetic	Same as alprazolam	1–10 mg/day orally in divided doses; when used as preanesthetic: up to 4 mg IM, IV
oxazepam *oks-A-ze-pam*		Anxiety disorders, short-term relief of anxiety, alcohol withdrawal syndrome	Same as alprazolam	10–30 mg orally 3–4 times daily

Generic Name	Trade Name	Uses	Adverse Reactions	Dosage Ranges
Nonbenzodiazepines				
busPIRone *byoo-SPYE-rone*		Anxiety disorders, short-term relief of anxiety	Dizziness, drowsiness	15–60 mg/day orally in divided doses
doxepin *DOKS-e-pin*	Silenor	Anxiety and depression, insomnia	Same as buspirone	75–150 mg/day, up to 300 mg/day for those severely ill
hydroxyzine *hye-drox'-ih-zeen*	Vistaril	Anxiety and tension associated with psychoneurosis, pruritus, preanesthetic sedative	Dry mouth, transitory drowsiness, involuntary motor activity	25–100 mg orally QID Preanesthetic: 50–100 mg orally or 25–100 mg IM
meprobamate *me-proe-BA-mate*		Anxiety disorders, short-term relief of anxiety	Drowsiness, ataxia, nausea, dizziness, slurred speech, headache, weakness, vomiting, diarrhea	1.2–1.6 g/day orally in 3–4 doses, not to exceed 2.4 g/day
Benzodiazepine Antidote				
flumazenil *FLOO-may-ze-nil*		Reverse sedation or drowsiness of benzodiazepines and some sleep aids, lessen benzodiazepine withdrawal symptoms	Tachycardia, panic	0.2 mg IV, may be repeated up to 4 doses

CHAPTER REVIEW

Know Your Drugs

Clients sometimes know a medication by the brand (or trade) name and not the generic name. To help you recognize both names, match the brand name with the generic name of the same medication.

Generic Name	Brand Name
1. alprazolam	A. Ativan
2. clonazepam	B. Klonopin
3. diazepam	C. Valium
4. lorazepam	D. Xanax

Calculate Medication Dosages

1. Hydroxyzine (Vistaril) 100 mg IM is prescribed. Available is a vial with 100 mg hydroxyzine per milliliter. The nurse administers _____.
2. The client is prescribed 30 mg oxazepam three times a day orally. The drug is available in 15-mg tablets. The nurse administers _____.

Prepare for the NCLEX

RECALL THE FACTS

1. Benzodiazepines potentiate which neurotransmitter?
   1. acetylcholine
   2. GABA
   3. norepinephrine
   4. serotonin

2. Alprazolam (Xanax) is contraindicated in clients with _____.
   1. glaucoma
   2. congestive heart failure
   3. diabetes
   4. hypertension

3. Which of the following drugs is a schedule IV controlled substance?
   1. hydroxyzine
   2. doxepin
   3. buspirone
   4. chlordiazepoxide

4. Which of the following is a sign of drug withdrawal and not an adverse reaction?
   1. dizziness
   2. metallic taste
   3. constipation
   4. sedation

5. The benzodiazepines are pregnancy category D drugs that should not be taken while lactating because the newborn may become _____.
   1. depressed
   2. excited and irritable
   3. lethargic and lose weight
   4. hypoglycemic

ANALYZE THE FACTS

6. Which condition is best treated with benzodiazepines?
   1. obsessive-compulsive anxiety disorder
   2. presurgical apprehension
   3. posttraumatic stress disorder
   4. grief reactions

7. *A family member calls the nurse to report that the client taking an antianxiety medication is hypotensive. The nurse instructs the family member to:
   1. give oral fluids to increase the blood pressure.
   2. have the client rise more slowly from a lying or sitting position.
   3. take the client to a local fire station three times a week to check blood pressure.
   4. stop the medication until the nurse checks with the primary health care provider.

8. Antianxiety medications are used cautiously in older adults because of the:
   1. inability to absorb the drugs because of decreased acid production.
   2. drug not being distributed as well because of poor circulation.
   3. liver metabolizing the drug faster, making it ineffective.
   4. reduced elimination, making it build up in the circulation.

ALTERNATE-FORMAT QUESTIONS

9. Describe the feelings of anxiety. Select all that apply.
   1. apprehension
   2. panic
   3. uneasiness
   4. worry
   5. jitters

10. A client is restless as they are prepared for a gastric procedure in the outpatient clinic. The primary health care provider asks you to draw up 4 mg of lorazepam (Ativan). Looking at the photo, how many milliliters will you draw up in the syringe?

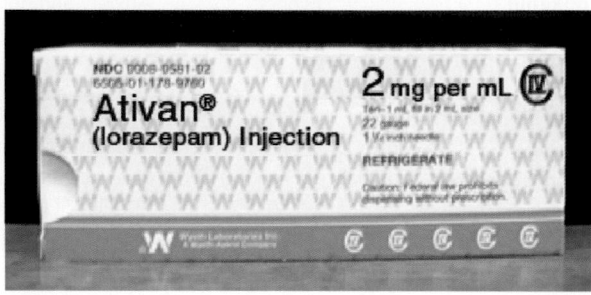

To check your answers, see Appendix F.

---

*Indicates the question is directly linked to the NCLEX-PN test plan in Appendix G.

Want to Know More? A wide variety of resources are available to enhance your learning and understanding of this chapter.
- Visit thePoint for resources such as:
  - NCLEX-Style Student Review Questions
  - Journal Articles
  - Dosage Calculations
  - Drug Monographs
  - Watch and Learn Videos
  - Concepts in Action Animations
- The *Study Guide to Accompany Introductory Clinical Pharmacology*, 12th edition, sold separately, will help you review and apply essential content.
- √*PrepU* is available to help students prepare for the NCLEX-PN examination.

Sedatives and Hypnotics

Key Terms

ataxia unsteady gait; muscular incoordination

hypnotic drug that induces sleep

paradoxical reaction when a drug or treatment has the opposite effect of the usual intent

sedative drug producing a relaxing, calming effect

somnolence sleepy or drowsy state

Learning Objectives

On completion of this chapter, the student will:

1. Differentiate between a sedative and a hypnotic.
2. Explain the uses, general drug actions, adverse reactions, contraindications, precautions, and interactions of sedatives and hypnotics.
3. Distinguish important preadministration and ongoing assessment activities the nurse should perform with the client taking a sedative or hypnotic.
4. List nursing diagnoses particular to a client taking a sedative or hypnotic.
5. Examine ways to promote an optimal response to therapy, how to manage common adverse reactions, and important points to keep in mind when educating clients about the use of sedatives or hypnotics.

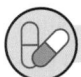 **Drug Classes**

Barbiturates

Nonbarbiturates
- Benzodiazepines
- Nonbenzodiazepines

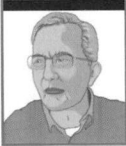 **PHARMACOLOGY IN PRACTICE**

Mr. Phillip's wife died in an automobile accident, and he has had trouble coping with the loss of his spouse. He complains about sleeping difficulties; he wakes frequently through the night. The primary health care provider prescribes a hypnotic, one capsule per night for use during the next 3 weeks. Read about the sedative and hypnotic drugs in this chapter, and see if you think this recommendation would be helpful for Mr. Phillip.

According to the National Sleep Foundation, insomnia affects approximately 30%–50% of the population in the United States—this means about 40 million people suffer routinely with sleeping problems (National Sleep Foundation, 2020). Sedatives and hypnotics, the drugs in this chapter, are used primarily to treat insomnia. Box 20.1 lists the criteria used to define insomnia. It may be caused by a number of factors, one of which is lifestyle changes such as a new job, moving to a new town, or returning to school as well as additional factors that may include jet lag, chronic pain, headaches, stress, or anxiety.

BOX 20.1 National Sleep Foundation Criteria for the Diagnosis of Insomnia

One or more of the following symptoms must occur:
- Difficulty falling asleep
- Waking often and trouble going back to sleep at night
- Waking too early in the morning
- Feeling tired upon waking

In many cases insomnia is treated in the outpatient setting. Yet, one of the most frequent client problems during hospitalization is insomnia. Clients are in an unfamiliar surrounding that is unlike the home setting. Noises and lights at night often interfere with or interrupt sleep, especially with multiple interruptions (Fig. 20.1). An important part of meeting client needs during illness is to help the client gain rest and sleep. Sleep deprivation may interfere with the healing process; therefore, a **hypnotic** may be given. A hypnotic is a drug that induces drowsiness or sleep, meaning it allows the client to fall asleep and stay asleep. Hypnotics are given at night or bedtime. These drugs may also be prescribed for short-term use to promote sleep after discharge as a client transitions back to the home environment.

A **sedative** is a drug that produces a relaxing, calming effect. Sedatives are usually given during daytime hours, and although they may make the client drowsy, they usually do not produce sleep.

Sedatives and hypnotics are divided into two classes: barbiturates and nonbarbiturates. The nonbarbiturates are classified into two groups: benzodiazepines and nonbenzodiazepines. Barbiturates were once the drugs of choice to treat insomnia and anxiety; however, the side effects proved to be too harsh. Currently, barbiturates may be used in cases where a deep, nonwaking sleep is desired, such as the few states where assisted suicide is legal. The nonbarbiturates are now used as sedatives in place of barbiturates, because they are more effective in treating insomnia and the adverse reactions are less than those of the barbiturates. Some of the benzodiazepines are also used as antianxiety drugs (see

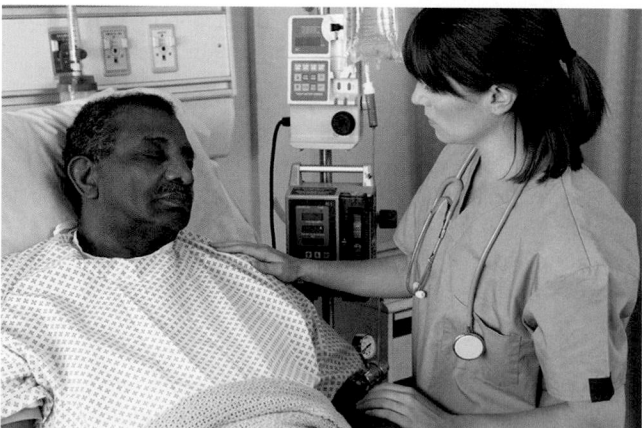

FIGURE 20.1 Noises and lights in the environment may cause insomnia for the hospitalized client.

Chapter 19). The benzodiazepines used primarily for sedation rather than anxiety are discussed in this chapter and include temazepam (Restoril) and triazolam (Halcion).

The nonbenzodiazepines are a group of unrelated drugs. Examples include eszopiclone (Lunesta) and zolpidem (Ambien). Barbiturates, benzodiazepines, and nonbenzodiazepines are listed in the Summary Drug Table: Sedatives and Hypnotics.

ACTIONS

Barbiturates

All barbiturates have essentially the same mode of action. These drugs are capable of producing central nervous system (CNS) depression and mood alterations ranging from mild excitation to mild sedation, hypnosis (sleep), and deep coma. These drugs also are respiratory depressants; the degree of depression usually depends on the dose taken. Barbiturates have a long half-life, which prolongs a sleepy or drowsy feeling. This is the reason they are used infrequently, if at all.

Benzodiazepines and Nonbenzodiazepines (the Nonbarbiturates)

Nonbarbiturate sedatives and hypnotics have essentially the same mode of action as the barbiturates—that is, they depress the CNS. The benzodiazepine effect on gamma-aminobutyric acid (γ-aminobutyric acid) (GABA) to potentiate neural inhibition is discussed in Chapter 19. However, these drugs have a lesser effect on the respiratory rate—another reason they are chosen over barbiturates for insomnia.

The nonbenzodiazepine effects diminish after approximately 2 weeks. Persons taking these drugs for longer than 2 weeks may have a tendency to increase the dose to produce the desired effects (e.g., sleep sedation). Physical tolerance and psychological dependence may occur, especially after prolonged use of high doses. However, their addictive potential appears to be less than that of the barbiturates. Discontinuing use of a sedative or hypnotic after prolonged use may result in mild to severe withdrawal symptoms.

USES

The sedative and hypnotic drugs are used in the treatment of:

- Insomnia
- Convulsions or seizures

They are also used as adjuncts for anesthesia and for:

- Preoperative sedation
- Conscious sedation

 Concept Mastery Alert

Sedatives and hypnotics are used primarily to treat insomnia. They may also be used to treat seizures or for preoperative sedation.

Lifespan Considerations

Gerontology

Older adult clients may require a smaller hypnotic dose, and in some instances, a sedative drug may act like a hypnotic and produce sleep.

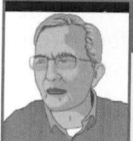

PHARMACOLOGY IN PRACTICE

PATHOPHYSIOLOGY

Which of the following drugs purposely induces drowsiness?

1. Anxiolytic
2. Sedative
3. Hypnotic
4. Opioid

ADVERSE REACTIONS

- Nervous system reactions include dizziness, drowsiness, and headache.
- A common gastrointestinal reaction is nausea.

CONTRAINDICATIONS

These drugs are contraindicated in clients with known hypersensitivity to sedatives or hypnotics. Do not administer these drugs to comatose clients, those with severe respiratory problems, those with a history of drug and alcohol habitual use, or pregnant or lactating women. Because of a specific enzyme reaction, grapefruit or its juice should not be taken if the client is on triazolam or zaleplon. The barbiturates are classified as pregnancy category D drugs.

Benzodiazepines (e.g., estazolam, temazepam, triazolam) used for sedation are classified as pregnancy category X drugs. Most nonbenzodiazepines are pregnancy category B or C drugs.

Lifespan Considerations

Childbearing Women

Women taking benzodiazepines should be warned of the potential risk to the fetus so that contraceptive methods may be instituted, if necessary. A child born to a mother taking benzodiazepines may experience withdrawal symptoms during the postnatal period.

PRECAUTIONS

Sedatives and hypnotics should be used cautiously in lactating clients and in clients with hepatic or renal impairment, habitual alcohol use, and mental health problems.

LASA ALERT

The following drugs may sound alike; be sure to clarify when they are ordered:

Drug Name	Sounds Like
Ambien	Abilify, Ativan, Ambi 10
Dayvigo	Daypro, Daysee, Daytrana
dexMEDEtomidine	dexAMETHasone
flurazepam	temazepam
Halcion	halcinonide, Haldol
Lunesta	Neulasta
quazepam	oxazepam
Precedex	Peridex
ramelteon	Razadyne, Remeron
Restoril	Resotran, RisperDAL, Vistaril, Zestril
triazolam	alPRAZolam
zaleplon	Zelapar, Zemplar, zolpidem, ZyPREXA, Zydis
zolpidem	lorazepam, zaleplon, Zyloprim

Drugs that look like a similar drug are noted in the Summary Drug Tables of each chapter.

INTERACTIONS

The following interactions may occur when a sedative or hypnotic is administered with another agent:

Interacting Drug	Common Use	Effect of Interaction
Antidepressants	Management of depression	Increased sedative effect
Opioid analgesic antihistamines	Pain relief, relief of allergy symptoms (runny nose and itching)	Increased sedative effect
Phenothiazines (e.g., Thorazine)	Management of agitation and psychotic symptoms	Increased sedative effect
Cimetidine	Management of gastric upset	Increased sedative effect
Alcohol	Relaxation and enjoyment in social situations	Increased sedative effect

Antihistamines have a sedating effect and may be used independently by clients at home because their purchase does not require a prescription. Other over-the-counter (OTC) sleep aids are also abundant; clients may not volunteer information regarding their use of these alternative or complementary remedies. Always inquire about use of herbal or OTC products. Although laboratory testing is not conclusive, medical reports indicate a possible interaction with eucalyptus products causing increased sedation.

Herbal Considerations

Melatonin is a hormone produced by the pineal gland in the brain. Melatonin has been used in treating insomnia, overcoming jet lag, improving the effectiveness of the immune system, and as an antioxidant. The most significant use—at low doses—is the short-term treatment of insomnia. Melatonin obtained from animal pineal tissue is not recommended for use because of the risk of contamination. The synthetic form of melatonin does not carry this risk. Supplements should be purchased from a reliable source to minimize the risk of contamination. Drowsiness may occur within 30 minutes after taking the supplement. The drowsiness may persist for an hour or more, affecting any activity that requires mental alertness, such as driving. Possible adverse reactions include headache and depression. Although uncommon, allergic reactions (difficulty breathing, hives, or swelling of the lips, tongue, or face) to melatonin have been reported (DerMarderosian, 2003).

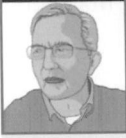

PHARMACOLOGY IN PRACTICE

SAFE DRUG ADMINISTRATION

A client undergoing treatment for an allergy is prescribed sedatives for anxiety. Which of the following may be a possible effect of the interaction between antihistamines and sedatives?
1. Restlessness
2. Increased sedation
3. Headache
4. Chronic pain

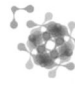

NURSING PROCESS: STEPS TO BUILDING CLINICAL JUDGMENT
Client Receiving a Sedative or Hypnotic

ASSESSMENT

Preadministration Assessment

Data gathering suggestions before the initial administration of sedative or hypnotic drugs include:

Objective data

- Vital signs—watch for changes in blood pressure, lowering after administration
- Level of consciousness—alert, confused, or lethargic
- Observation of behavior during interview: is pain preventing rest?
- Observations of the environment that may cause insomnia

Subjective data

- Current history of symptoms, description of typical sleep patterns, when does the client go to bed, awaken
- Methods used to deal with insomnia, especially self-medicating with alcohol or drugs
- Medical, social, and mental health history
- Review chart for drugs that may cause changes in sleep patterns (has consent been signed if preprocedural sedation)

⚠ NURSING ALERT

Clients taking hypnotics need enough time for the drug to wear off to be awake. This means 6–8 hours of uninterrupted sleep. If a client needs to awaken between 5 and 6 a.m., then the drug should be taken between 10 and 11 p.m. If the drug is given sooner or later, the person will either be awake earlier or sleepy and hard to arouse in the morning.

If the client is receiving one of these drugs for daytime sedation, assess the client's general mental state and level of consciousness. If the client appears sedated and difficult to awaken, you should withhold the drug and contact the primary health care provider as soon as possible.

Ongoing Assessment

Before administering the drug, focus assessment on reasons why the person cannot get rest or sleep. **Somnolence** (sleepy or drowsy state) is likely; therefore, after administration you will be assessing for results of the drug now rather than causes of insomnia. Ask the client about the circumstances causing insomnia and whether other factors such as pain, lights, or disruptive activity are bothersome. After assessing the client, make a decision regarding administration of the drug or if other interventions are more appropriate to try first.

Ask if the drug helped the client sleep on previous nights. If not, a different drug or dose may be needed; consult the primary health care provider regarding the drug's ineffectiveness.

If the client has a given-as-needed (PRN) order for an opioid analgesic or other CNS depressant and a hypnotic, discuss with the primary health care provider regarding the time interval between administrations of these drugs. Usually, at least 2 hours should elapse between administration of a hypnotic and any other CNS depressant, but this interval may vary, depending on factors such as the client's age and diagnosis.

⚠ NURSING ALERT

When giving a sedative or hypnotic, notify the primary health care provider if one or more vital signs significantly vary from the baseline, if the respiratory rate is less than 10 breaths/minute, or if the client appears lethargic.

NURSING DIAGNOSES

Drug-specific nursing diagnoses are the following:

- **Injury risk** related to drowsiness or impaired memory
- **Altered breathing pattern** related to respiratory depression
- **Coping impairment** related to excessive use of medication

Nursing diagnoses related to drug administration are discussed in Chapter 4.

PLANNING

The expected outcomes for the client depend on the reason for administration of a sedative or hypnotic but may include an optimal response to drug therapy (e.g., sedation or sleep), support of client needs related to management of adverse drug reactions, and confidence in an understanding of the medication regimen.

IMPLEMENTATION

Promoting an Optimal Response to Therapy

You should provide supportive care to promote the effects of the sedative or hypnotic drug. This includes interventions such as back rubs, night lights or a darkened room, and a quiet atmosphere. The client is discouraged from drinking beverages containing caffeine, such as coffee, cola, or energy drinks, which can contribute to wakefulness.

Never leave hypnotics and sedatives at the client's bedside to be taken at a later hour; hypnotics and sedatives are controlled substances (see Chapter 1). In addition, never leave these drugs unattended in the nurses' station, hallway, or other areas to which clients, visitors, or hospital personnel have direct access.

! NURSING ALERT

Some sleep medicines (zolpidem) may cause memory loss or amnesia. A person may not remember getting up out of bed, driving, or eating. These drugs should be taken only when a person plans for 7–8 hours of sleep.

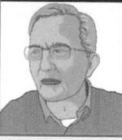

PHARMACOLOGY IN PRACTICE

MANAGING NEEDS

A nurse is caring for a client who is prescribed a sedative. Which of the following measures can ensure an optimal response to hypnotic therapy? Select all that apply.
1. Back rubs
2. Alcohol intake
3. Night lights
4. Darkened room
5. Bedtime coffee

Monitoring and Managing Client Needs

Injury Risk

It is important to observe the client for adverse drug reactions. During periods when the client is excited or confused, protect the client from harm and provide supportive care and a safe environment. Assess the client receiving a sedative dose and determine what safety measures must be taken.

After administration of a hypnotic, such as before a surgical or diagnostic procedure, raise the side rails of the bed and advise the client to remain in bed and to call for assistance if it is necessary to get out of bed. Observe the client receiving a hypnotic 1–2 hours after the drug is given to evaluate the effect of the drug. When used for insomnia, notify the primary health care provider if the client fails to sleep, awakens one or more times during the night, or experiences an adverse drug reaction. In some instances, supplemental doses of a hypnotic may be ordered if the client awakens during the night.

Excessive drowsiness and headache the morning after a hypnotic has been given (drug hangover) may occur in some clients. Report this problem to the primary health care provider because a smaller dose or a different drug may be necessary. When getting out of bed, the client is encouraged to rise to a sitting position first, wait a few minutes, and then rise to a standing position. When necessary, assist the ambulatory client if groggy.

Clients using these drugs in an outpatient setting are taught about the hazards of operating machinery or involvement in other potentially hazardous tasks until they are sure that concentration and focus are not affected.

Lifespan Considerations

Gerontology

The older adult is at greater risk for oversedation, dizziness, confusion, or **ataxia** (unsteady gait) when taking a sedative or hypnotic. Also be aware of and check elderly and debilitated clients for a **paradoxical reaction**, such as marked excitement, or confusion. If excitement or confusion occurs, observe the client at more frequent intervals (as often as every 5–10 minutes may be necessary) for the duration of this occurrence and institute safety measures to prevent injury. If oversedation, extreme dizziness, or ataxia occurs, notify the primary health care provider.

Altered Breathing Pattern

Sedatives and hypnotics depress the CNS and can cause respiratory depression. Carefully assess respiratory function (rate, depth, and quality) before administering a sedative, 30 minutes to 1 hour after administering the drug, and frequently thereafter.

Instruct the client not to drink alcohol when taking sedatives or hypnotics. Alcohol is a CNS depressant, as are the sedatives and hypnotics. When alcohol and a sedative or hypnotic are taken together, there is an additive effect and an increase in CNS depression, which has, on occasion, resulted in death. Emphasize the importance of abstaining from alcohol use while taking this drug and stress that the use of alcohol and any one of these drugs can result in serious effects.

Coping Impairment

Sedatives and hypnotics are best given for no more than 2 weeks and preferably for a shorter time. Sedatives and hypnotics can become less effective after they are taken for a prolonged period. Thus, there may be a tendency for a client to increase the dose without consulting the primary health care provider. To ensure compliance with the treatment regimen, emphasize the importance of not increasing or decreasing the dose unless a change in dosage is recommended by the primary health care provider. In addition, stress the importance of not repeating the dose during the night if sleep is interrupted or sleep lasts only a few hours, unless the primary health care provider has approved taking the drug more than once per night. There are time-release medications that may be appropriate if insomnia remains; encourage the client to talk to the primary health care provider about this option instead of changing dosing on their own.

Although the practice is not recommended, a client with sleep disturbances may be taking one of these drugs for an extended period of time. A sedative or hypnotic can cause drug dependency. Teach the client not to suddenly discontinue use of these drugs when there is a question of possible dependency. Clients who have been taking a sedative or hypnotic for several weeks should gradually withdraw from taking the drug to prevent withdrawal symptoms (see Chapter 19). Symptoms of withdrawal include restlessness, excitement, euphoria, and confusion. Withdrawal can result in serious consequences, especially in those with existing diseases or disorders.

Educating the Client and Family

When educating the client and family about sedatives and hypnotics, several general points must be considered. The client and family should feel confident in understanding that the drug is to help promote sleep and is a time-limited solution. As you develop a teaching plan, be sure to include one or more of the following items of information:

- The primary health care provider usually prescribes these drugs for short-term use only.
- If the drug appears to be ineffective, contact the primary health care provider. Do not increase the dose unless advised to do so by the primary health care provider.
- Notify the primary health care provider if any adverse drug reactions occur.
  - Do not drink any alcoholic beverage 2 hours before, with, or 8 hours after taking the drug.
- When taking the drug as a sedative, be aware that the drug can impair the mental and physical abilities required for performing potentially dangerous tasks, such as driving a car or operating machinery.

- After taking a drug to sleep, observe caution when getting out of bed at night. Keep the room dimly lit and remove any obstacles that may result in injury when getting out of bed. Never attempt to drive or perform any hazardous task after taking a drug intended to produce sleep.
- Do not use these drugs if you are pregnant, considering becoming pregnant, or breastfeeding.
- Do not use OTC cold, cough, or allergy drugs while taking this drug unless their use has been approved by the primary health care provider. Some of these products contain antihistamines or other drugs that also may cause mild to extreme drowsiness. Others may contain an adrenergic drug, which is a mild stimulant, and therefore will defeat the purpose of the sedative or hypnotic.
- Do not take zolpidem or tasimelteon with food. Eszopiclone, ramelteon, and zaleplon may be taken with food, yet meals or snacks high in fat can interfere with the absorption of these drugs.

EVALUATION

- Therapeutic response is achieved and sleep pattern is improved or the client is calm and relaxed for a procedure.
- Adverse reactions are identified, reported to the primary health care provider, and managed successfully with appropriate nursing interventions:
  - No evidence of injury is seen.
  - An adequate breathing pattern is maintained.
  - Client manages coping effectively.
- Client and family express confidence and demonstrate an understanding of the drug regimen.

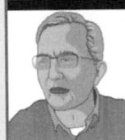

PHARMACOLOGY IN PRACTICE

USING CLINICAL REASONING

Two weeks following his initial prescription, Mr. Phillip calls the primary health care provider's office and asks for a refill of his sleep medication prescription. Determine what questions you would ask Mr. Phillip. Explain why you would ask them.

KEY POINTS

■ Sedatives produce a relaxing and calming effect. Hypnotic drugs produce sleep. These drugs work by depressing the CNS. Barbiturate use is rare because of a long half-life, dependency, and harsh adverse reactions. The nonbarbiturates include both benzodiazepines and nonbenzodiazepines.

■ Insomnia affects nearly 30%–50% of the population in the United States. Although it is often treated in the outpatient setting, many hospitalized clients suffer from insomnia, too. These drugs are meant to treat insomnia for only a short period of time, such as 2 weeks. If continued, longer dependency can occur.

■ Clients should always be asked about sleep aids they have tried before, because both herbal and OTC products are abundant.

■ Clients should be cautioned about activities requiring concentration and focus, such as driving, and be aware that blood pressure can drop, leading to dizziness and potential for injury. Doses should not be increased without consulting the primary health care provider.

■ Sedatives and hypnotics can also cause respiratory depression. Other CNS depressants, such as alcohol, should not be used with these drugs.

SUMMARY DRUG TABLE
Sedatives and Hypnotics

Generic Name	Trade Name	Uses	Adverse Reactions	Dosage Ranges
Benzodiazepines				
estazolam es-TA-zoe-lam		Hypnotic	Headache, heartburn, nausea, palpitations, rash, somnolence, vomiting, weakness, body and joint pain	1–2 mg orally
flurazepam flure-AZ-e-pam		Hypnotic	Same as estazolam	15–30 mg orally
quazepam KWAZ-e-pam	Doral	Sedative	Daytime drowsiness	7.5 mg orally
temazepam te-MAZ-e-pam	Restoril	Hypnotic	Same as estazolam	15–30 mg orally
triazolam trye-AY-zoe-lam	Halcion	Sedative, hypnotic	Same as estazolam	0.125–0.5 mg orally at bedtime
Nonbenzodiazepines				
dexMEDEtomidine deks-MED-e-toe-mi-deen	Precedex	Sedation during intubation/ ventilation, procedural sedation	Hypotension, nausea, bradycardia	1 mcg/kg over 10 minutes IV
eszopiclone es-zoe-PIK-lone	Lunesta	Insomnia	Headache, somnolence, taste changes, chest pain, migraine, edema	1–3 mg orally at bedtime
lemborexant lem-boe-REX-ant	Dayvigo	Insomnia	Headache, fatigue, drowsiness	10 mg/day orally at bedtime
ramelteon ra-MEL-tee-on	Rozerem	Insomnia	Dizziness, headache	8 mg orally at bedtime
suvorexant soo-voe-REX-ant	Belsomra	Insomnia	Drowsiness, headache	10–20 mg orally at bedtime
tasimelteon tas-i-MEL-tee-on	Hetlioz	Non–24 sleep disorder	Headache, nightmares, rhinitis, pharyngitis	20 mg orally at bedtime
zaleplon ZAL-e-plon		Transient insomnia	Dizziness, headache, rebound insomnia, nausea, myalgia	10 mg orally at bedtime
zolpidem zole-PI-dem	Ambien, Edluar, Intermezzo, Zolpimist	Transient insomnia	Drowsiness, headache, myalgia, nausea	10 mg orally at bedtime
Barbiturates				
pentobarbital pen-toe-BAR-bi-tal	Nembutal	Sedative, hypnotic, preoperative sedation	Respiratory and CNS depression, nausea, vomiting, constipation, diarrhea, bradycardia, hypotension, syncope, hypersensitivity reactions, headache	Available only in parenteral form: 100 mg deep IM or IV, may titrate up to 200–500 mg
secobarbital see-koe-BAR-bi-tal	Seconal	Hypnotic, preoperative sedation	Same as pentobarbital sodium	Hypnotic: 100 mg orally at bedtime Sedation: 200–300 mg orally 1–2 hours before procedure

 This drug should not be administered with food (especially high-fat meals).

CHAPTER REVIEW

Know Your Drugs

Clients sometimes know a medication by the brand (or trade) name and not the generic name. To help you recognize both names, match the brand name with the generic name of the same medication.

Generic Name	Brand Name
1. eszopiclone	A. Ambien
2. zaleplon	B. Intermezzo
3. zolpidem	C. Lunesta
	D. Sonata

Calculate Medication Dosages

1. Halcion 0.125 mg is prescribed. The drug is available in 0.125-mg tablets. The nurse administers _____.
2. Eszopiclone (Lunesta) 2 mg is prescribed for insomnia. The drug is available in 1-mg tablets. The nurse administers _____.

Prepare for the NCLEX

RECALL THE FACTS

1. Sedative and hypnotic drugs exert action to depress the _____.
   1. peripheral nervous system
   2. cardiovascular and respiratory systems
   3. musculoskeletal system
   4. CNS
2. Nonbarbiturates are used instead of barbiturates because they _____.
   1. produce better sleep patterns
   2. have fewer adverse reactions
   3. are newer formulas
   4. cause less amnesia
3. Which of these assessments should the nurse report immediately to the primary health provider?
   1. dizziness when arising from the chair
   2. heart rate of 80 beats/minute
   3. respiration rate of 8 breaths/minute
   4. joint pain
4. When giving a hypnotic to an older client, the nurse is aware that _____.
   1. smaller doses of the drug are usually given to older clients
   2. older clients usually require larger doses of a hypnotic
   3. older adults excrete the drug faster than younger adults
   4. dosages of the hypnotic may be increased each night until the desired effect is achieved
5. Which of the following points should be included in a teaching plan for a client taking a sedative or hypnotic?
   1. An alcoholic beverage may be served 1–2 hours before a sedative is taken without any ill effects.
   2. Dosage of the sedative may be increased if sleep is not restful.
   3. These drugs may safely be used for 6 months to 1 year when given for insomnia.
   4. Do not use any OTC cold, cough, or allergy medications while taking a sedative or hypnotic.
6. Which of the following sedatives/hypnotics is a pregnancy category X drug?
   1. zolpidem (Ambien)
   2. ramelteon (Rozerem)
   3. temazepam (Restoril)
   4. eszopiclone (Lunesta)

ANALYZE THE FACTS

7. *An elderly client has arthritis in the lower back, and the pain keeps them awake at night. The client asks if they can have a "sleeping pill." In considering this request, the nurse must take into account that hypnotic medications might _____.
   1. not be the drug of choice when pain causes insomnia
   2. be given instead of an analgesic to relieve pain
   3. increase the pain threshold
   4. be added to an analgesic to improve this situation
8. *The clinic nurse prepares teaching materials to give a client about use of a hypnotic. Which statement would prompt the nurse to contact the primary health care provider?
   1. "I plan to listen to some relaxing music tonight."
   2. "Stopping off at the tavern should help calm me before bedtime."
   3. "I will have a coworker pick me up tomorrow morning."
   4. "A nutritious meal may help me sleep better."

ALTERNATE-FORMAT QUESTIONS

9. Criteria for diagnosing insomnia include which of the items below? Select all that apply.
   1. waking too early
   2. sleeping in the middle of the day
   3. difficulty falling asleep
   4. trouble returning to sleep at night
10. When teaching about the nonbenzodiazepine hypnotics, certain foods should not be taken because they interfere with absorption. **Select all of the foods that should not** be taken with these drugs.
    1. peanut butter and crackers
    2. ice cream
    3. apple pie with ice cream
    4. chocolate pudding

To check your answers, see Appendix F.

_____

*Indicates the question is directly linked to the NCLEX-PN test plan in Appendix G.

WANT TO KNOW MORE? A wide variety of resources are available to enhance your learning and understanding of this chapter.
- Visit the**Point** for resources such as:
  - NCLEX-Style Student Review Questions
  - Journal Articles
  - Dosage Calculations
  - Drug Monographs
  - Watch and Learn Videos
  - Concepts in Action Animations
- The *Study Guide to Accompany Introductory Clinical Pharmacology*, 12th edition, sold separately, will help you review and apply essential content.
- ✓**PrepU** is available to help students prepare for the NCLEX-PN examination.

Antidepressant Drugs

Key Terms

bipolar disorder a mood disorder characterized by severe swings from extreme hyperactivity to depression

dysphoric characterized by extreme or exaggerated sadness, anxiety, or unhappiness

endogenous pertaining to something that normally occurs or is produced within the organism

mood disorders a spectrum of conditions that range from severe debilitation to an exhaustive elation

neurohormones secreted rather than transmitted neurosubstances

orthostatic hypotension decrease in blood pressure occurring after standing in one place for an extended period

priapism painful, persistent penile erection

serotonin syndrome potentially life-threatening drug reaction that causes the body to produce too much serotonin

tardive dyskinesia rhythmic, involuntary movements of the tongue, face, mouth, or jaw and sometimes the extremities

tyramine amino acid, commonly found in fermented foods such as cheese and red wine

unipolar depression mental disorder of low mood, low self-esteem, and loss of interest/pleasure; also known as major mood disorder

Learning Objectives

On completion of this chapter, the student will:

1. Define depression and identify symptoms of a major depressive disorder (MDD).
2. Compare and contrast the different types of antidepressant drugs.
3. Explain the uses, general drug actions, general adverse reactions, contraindications, precautions, and interactions of the antidepressant drugs.
4. Distinguish important preadministration and ongoing assessment activities that the nurse should perform on the client taking an antidepressant drug.
5. List nursing diagnoses particular to a client taking an antidepressant drug.
6. Examine ways to promote an optimal response to therapy, how to manage common adverse reactions, and important points to keep in mind when educating clients about the use of antidepressant drugs.

 Drug Classes

Selective serotonin reuptake inhibitors (SSRIs)

Serotonin/norepinephrine or dopamine/norepinephrine reuptake inhibitors (SNRIs or DNRIs)

Tricyclic antidepressants (TCAs)

Monoamine oxidase inhibitors (MAOIs)

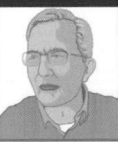 **PHARMACOLOGY IN PRACTICE**

Following the death of his wife in a car accident, Mr. Phillip has been severely depressed for about 2 months. A week ago, the primary care provider prescribed Zoloft 100 mg orally daily. His family is frustrated because he is still depressed. Mr. Phillip's daughter is concerned because he feels drowsy and cannot seem to get up until 11 a.m. or noon on most days. They are requesting that the dosage be increased. Read about the antidepressants and determine what should happen next.

Depression may be described as feeling sad, unhappy, or "down in the dumps." Most of us feel this way at one time or another for short periods of time, which is perfectly normal. On the other hand, major depressive disorder (MDD) is the medical diagnosis for one of the mental health conditions called **mood disorders** (a spectrum of conditions

BOX 21.1 Symptoms of Depression

- Feelings of hopelessness or helplessness
- Diminished interest in activities of life
- Significant weight loss or gain (without dieting)
- Insomnia (inability to sleep) or hypersomnia (excessive sleeping)
- Agitation, restlessness, or irritability
- Fatigue or loss of energy
- Feelings of worthlessness
- Excessive or inappropriate guilt
- Diminished ability to think or concentrate, or indecisiveness
- Recurrent thoughts of death or suicide (or suicide attempt)

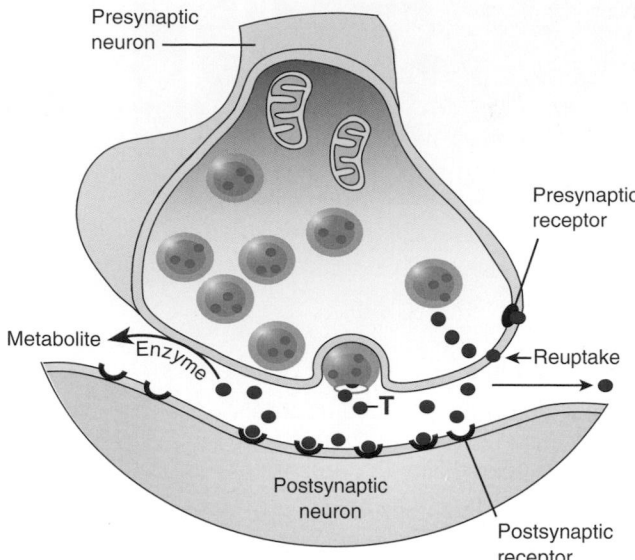

FIGURE 21.1 Antidepressant drugs inhibit the reuptake of the neurotransmitter (T) by presynaptic receptors, thus making it available to the more sensitive postsynaptic neuron.

that range from severe debilitation to an exhaustive elation), which is also called clinical depression by a number of people. Symptoms are not the result of normal bereavement such as the loss of a loved one, or caused by another disease, such as hypothyroidism. In fact, it is speculated that up to 33% of hospitalized clients suffer from depressive symptoms in addition to their medical disease and almost half of all long-term care residents suffer from depression (Wang et al., 2017).

Many of the drugs used to treat a major depressive episode (MDD), are meant to treat a condition called **unipolar depression**. Individuals with this diagnosis present with a **dysphoric** (extreme or exaggerated sadness, anxiety, or unhappiness) mood, which interferes with daily functioning. To diagnose this condition, five or more of the symptoms listed in Box 21.1 need to occur daily, or nearly every day, for a period of 2 weeks or more.

The depressive symptoms of mood disorders are treated with antidepressant drugs and psychotherapy. The four major classes of antidepressants are presented according to current use:

- Selective serotonin reuptake inhibitors (SSRIs)
- Serotonin/norepinephrine or dopamine/norepinephrine reuptake inhibitors (SNRIs or DNRIs)
- Tricyclic antidepressants (TCAs)
- Monoamine oxidase inhibitors (MAOIs)

The older antidepressants (TCAs and MAOIs) blocked the reuptake of the **endogenous** (produced by the body) neurotransmitters, norepinephrine and serotonin. This action resulted in stimulation of the central nervous system (CNS) by these neurotransmitters and alleviation of the depressed mood. As this theory was questioned, research turned to looking at the effects of antidepressants related to slowing adaptive changes in norepinephrine and serotonin receptor systems (Fuller & Wong, 1985). Treatment with antidepressants is thought to produce complex changes in the sensitivities of both presynaptic and postsynaptic receptor sites. Antidepressants increase the sensitivity of postsynaptic alpha-adrenergic (α-adrenergic) and serotonin receptors and decrease the sensitivity of the presynaptic receptor sites. This enhances recovery from the depressive episode by making neurotransmission activity more effective, as visualized in Figure 21.1.

SELECTIVE SEROTONIN REUPTAKE INHIBITORS

ACTIONS

The SSRIs inhibit CNS uptake of serotonin (a CNS neurotransmitter). The increase in serotonin levels is thought to act as a stimulant to reverse depression.

USES

The SSRIs are used in the treatment of the following:

- Depressive episodes
- Anxiety disorders (panic, posttraumatic stress disorder [PTSD], generalized anxiety disorder [GAD], and social phobias)
- Premenstrual dysphoric disorder
- Obsessive-compulsive disorder (OCD)
- Bulimia nervosa

Unlabeled uses include Raynaud disease, migraine headaches, diabetic neuropathy, and hot flashes. These drugs may be used with psychotherapy in severe cases.

ADVERSE REACTIONS

Neuromuscular System Reactions

- Somnolence, dizziness
- Headache, insomnia
- Tremor, weakness

Gastrointestinal and Genitourinary System Reactions

- Constipation, dry mouth, nausea
- Pharyngitis and runny nose
- Urinary retention and abnormal ejaculation

CONTRAINDICATIONS

The SSRIs are contraindicated in clients with hypersensitivity to the drugs and during pregnancy (pregnancy category C). Clients taking cisapride (Propulsid), pimozide (Orap), or carbamazepine (Tegretol) should not take fluoxetine (Prozac). Because of a specific enzyme reaction, grapefruit or its juice should not be consumed if the client is on sertraline (Zoloft).

PRACTICE CONSIDERATIONS

Pregnant Women

Researchers doing a systematic review of the literature found an increased risk of persistent pulmonary hypertension in newborns of women taking SSRI antidepressants during pregnancy (Grigoriadis et al., 2014). Ongoing research is attempting to see if there is a correlation between SSRI intake during the second and third trimesters of pregnancy and later autism spectrum disorder diagnosed in children (Boukhris et al., 2015).

PRECAUTIONS

The SSRI antidepressants should be used cautiously in clients with type 2 diabetes, cardiac disease, or impaired liver or kidney function and in those at risk for suicidal ideation or behavior. Clients should not be switched to an SSRI antidepressant drug within 2 weeks of stopping an MAOI antidepressant. Clients should be instructed regarding the potential for **serotonin syndrome** (Box 21.2).

 Herbal Considerations

Clients should be assessed for use of herbal preparations containing St. John's wort because of the potential for adverse reactions when taken with antidepressants and the increased risk of serotonin syndrome (DerMarderosian & Beutler, 2003).

BOX 21.2 Serotonin Syndrome

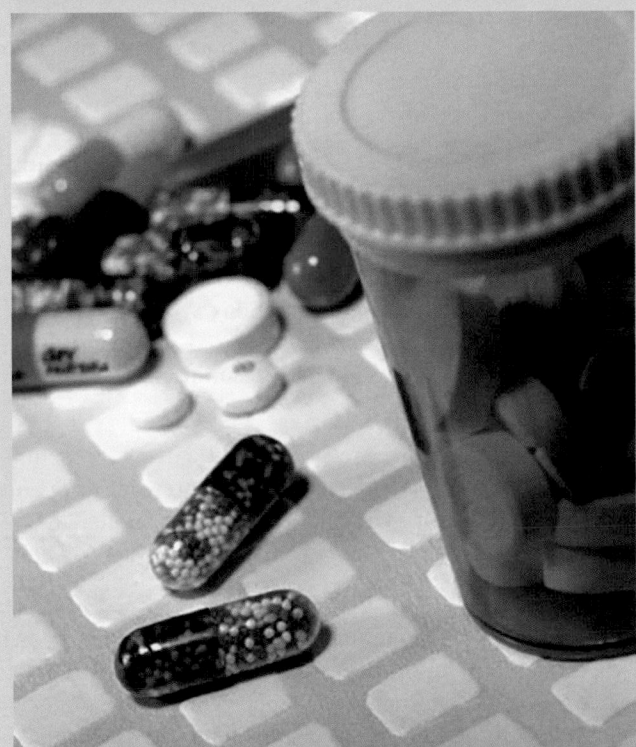

A client recently prescribed an SSRI antidepressant awakens feeling nauseated and restless. As they rush to the bathroom with diarrhea, they stumble. Are the heart palpitations a result from sudden GI distress and stumbling, or is this one more symptom indicating serotonin syndrome?

Serotonin syndrome is a potentially life-threatening adverse drug reaction in which the brain has too much serotonin. It most often occurs when two drugs affecting the body's level of serotonin are taken together. Clients are at greatest risk when an SSRI or SNRI antidepressant is prescribed. Other prescription and over-the-counter drugs that raise serotonin levels alone or in combination with the serotonin-based antidepressants include:
- mood-altering drugs such as the MAOIs, drugs used to treat anxiety such as buspirone and trazodone
- migraine relievers such as almotriptan, naratriptan, sumatriptan, rizatriptan, and zolmitriptan
- the pain relievers meperidine, fentanyl, tramadol, or pentazocine
- drugs prescribed for nausea such as granisetron, metoclopramide, and ondansetron
- cough and cold remedies containing dextromethorphan
- the herbal supplements St. John's wort and ginseng

To diagnose serotonin syndrome, your client must present with at least three of the following signs or symptoms:
- Agitation or confusion
- Nausea or diarrhea
- Dilated pupils (eyes)
- Rapid or irregular heart beat
- Increased temperature, shivering, and goose bumps
- Increased sweating not caused by activity
- Muscle spasms (myoclonus) or overactive reflexes (hyperreflexia)
- Tremor or restlessness
- Uncoordinated movements (ataxia)

Blood tests, scans, and toxicology screens are used to rule out other conditions such as infections, intoxication, metabolic and hormone problems, or drug withdrawal and overdose. Clients diagnosed with serotonin syndrome should be hospitalized at least 24 hours for close observation with treatment that includes:
- Benzodiazepines such as diazepam or lorazepam to decrease agitation, seizure-like movements, and muscle stiffness
- Cyproheptadine, a drug that blocks serotonin production
- Intravenous (through the vein) fluids
- Withdrawal of medicines that caused the syndrome

The FDA asks manufacturers to include warning labels on their products giving the potential risk of serotonin syndrome. Be sure you teach your clients to look at each medication, especially over-the-counter products like cold remedies, before purchasing.

INTERACTIONS

The following interactions may occur when an SSRI is administered with another agent:

Interacting Drugs	Common Use	Effect of Interaction
Other antidepressants	Treatment of depression	Increased risk of toxic effects
Cimetidine	Relief of gastric upset	Increased anticholinergic symptoms (dry mouth, urinary retention, blurred vision)
Nonsteroidal anti-inflammatory drugs (NSAIDs)	Relief of inflammation and pain	Increased risk for GI bleeding; decreased effectiveness of SSRI
Lithium (interaction with fluoxetine)	Treatment of bipolar disorder	Increased risk of lithium toxicity

Note that the effectiveness of fluoxetine is decreased in clients who smoke cigarettes during administration of the drug.

SEROTONIN/ NOREPINEPHRINE OR DOPAMINE/NOREPINEPHRINE REUPTAKE INHIBITORS

ACTIONS

It is thought that the mechanism of action of most of the SNRIs/DNRIs is to affect neurotransmission of serotonin, norepinephrine, and dopamine. Examples in this group of drugs include venlafaxine (Effexor XR) and bupropion (Wellbutrin).

USES

SNRIs/DNRIs may be used in conjunction with psychotherapy in severe cases or alone in the treatment of the following:

- Depressive episodes
- Depression accompanied by anxiety disorders (GAD, panic, social phobias, PTSD)
- Diabetic peripheral neuropathic pain, fibromyalgia, and chronic muscle pain

Unlabeled uses include enhancing weight loss and treating aggressive behaviors, menstrual disorders, cocaine withdrawal and alcohol cravings, migraine headache prevention, and stress incontinence.

ADVERSE REACTIONS

Neuromuscular System Reactions
- Somnolence, migraine headache
- Hypotension, dizziness, lightheadedness, and vertigo
- Blurred vision, photosensitivity, insomnia, nervousness or agitation, and tremor

Gastrointestinal System Reactions
- Nausea, dry mouth, anorexia, thirst
- Diarrhea, constipation, bitter taste

Other System Reactions
- Fatigue, tachycardia, and palpitations
- Change in libido, impotence
- Skin rash, itching, vasodilation resulting in flushing and excessive sweating

Additional adverse reactions and adverse reactions associated with the use of all the antidepressant drugs are listed in the Summary Drug Table: Antidepressants.

CONTRAINDICATIONS

SNRIs/DNRIs are contraindicated in clients with known hypersensitivity to the drugs. Among the SNRIs/DNRIs antidepressants, bupropion and maprotiline are pregnancy category B drugs. Other antidepressants discussed in this section are in pregnancy category C. Safe use of the antidepressants during pregnancy has not been established. They should be used during pregnancy only when the potential benefits outweigh the potential hazards to the developing fetus. Maprotiline should not be used with clients who have a seizure disorder or during the acute phase of a myocardial infarction. Clients taking cisapride, pimozide, or carbamazepine should not take nefazodone because of risk for hepatic failure. Because of a specific enzyme reaction, grapefruit or its juice should not be taken if the client is on vilazodone or trazodone.

A smoking cessation product which is a form of the antidepressant drug bupropion is marketed under the name Zyban as well as other names. Smokers should not use Zyban if they are currently taking bupropion for management of depression because of the possibility of bupropion overdose.

PRECAUTIONS

SNRIs/DNRIs should be used cautiously in clients with cardiac disease, renal or hepatic impairment, or hyperthyroid disease or those who are at risk of suicidal ideation or behavior. Clients should be instructed regarding the potential for serotonin syndrome (see Box 21.2).

LASA ALERT

The following drugs may sound alike; be sure to clarify when they are ordered:

Drug Name	Sounds Like
Aplenzin	Albenza, Relenza
buPROPion	busPIRone
Cymbalta	Symbyax
DULoxetine	Dexilant, FLUoxetine, PARoxetine, vortioxetine
Effexor	Enablex
Fetzima	Farxiga
Levomilnacipran	Milnacipran
Pristiq	PriLOSEC
Savella	cevimeline, sevelamer
Venlafaxine	Venclexta, venetoclax

Drugs that look like a similar drug are noted in the Summary Drug Tables of each chapter.

INTERACTIONS

The following interactions may occur when an SNRI/DNRI is administered with another agent:

Interacting Drug	Common Use	Effect of Interaction
Sedatives and hypnotics, analgesics	Sedation and pain relief, respectively	Increased risk of respiratory and nervous system depression
Warfarin	Anticoagulation (blood thinner)	Increased risk for bleeding
Cimetidine	Gastrointestinal (GI) upset	Increased anticholinergic symptoms (dry mouth, urinary retention, blurred vision)
Antihypertensive agents	Treatment of high blood pressure	Increased risk for hypotension
MAOIs	Antidepressant	Increased risk for hypertensive episodes, severe convulsions, and hyperpyretic episodes

POSSIBLE NEW ANTIDEPRESSANTS

Esketamine is a drug related to the general anesthetic ketamine. It has been found to be effective in clients with treatment-resistant depression and is administered nasally. One issue is the cost—it can be well over $5000/month, and the client must be observed for at least 2 hours post administration owing to the severe sedation reaction.

Brexanolone is another drug being used for postpartum depression. It acts like a steroid in the brain on the GABA receptors. Drawbacks to this drug again are the cost ($34,000) and the IV administration required—given over 60 hours.

TRICYCLIC ANTIDEPRESSANTS

Discovery of the role of dopamine in depression and the ability to be more selective in reuptake make the following classes of drugs less frequently prescribed than those already discussed.

ACTIONS

The TCAs, such as amitriptyline and doxepin, inhibit the reuptake of norepinephrine or serotonin in the brain.

USES

TCA drugs are used in the treatment of the following:

- Depressive episodes
- Bipolar disorder
- OCD
- Chronic neuropathic pain
- Depression accompanied by anxiety disorders
- Enuresis

Unlabeled uses include peptic ulcer disease, sleep apnea, panic disorder, bulimia nervosa, premenstrual symptoms, and some dermatologic problems. These drugs may be used with psychotherapy in severe cases.

ADVERSE REACTIONS

Generalized reactions include:

- Anticholinergic effects (e.g., sedation, dry mouth, visual disturbances, urinary retention)
- Constipation and photosensitivity

! NURSING ALERT

Although the TCAs are not considered antipsychotic agents, the drug amoxapine has been associated with **tardive dyskinesia** and neuroleptic malignant syndrome (NMS). Tardive dyskinesia is a syndrome of involuntary movement that may be irreversible. Symptoms of NMS are similar and include muscle rigidity, altered mental status, and autonomic system problems, such as tachycardia or sweating. These syndromes tend to occur more readily in elderly women; the drug should be discontinued, the primary health care provider notified immediately, and treatment of adverse effects begun quickly.

CONTRAINDICATIONS

The TCAs are contraindicated in clients with known hypersensitivity to the drugs. The TCAs are not given within 14 days of the MAOI antidepressants, to clients with a recent myocardial infarction, or to children or lactating mothers. These drugs are in pregnancy categories C and D, and the safety of their use during pregnancy has not been established. Doxepin is contraindicated in clients with glaucoma or in those with a tendency for urinary retention.

PRECAUTIONS

The TCAs should be used cautiously in clients with cardiac disease, hepatic or renal impairment, hyperthyroid disease, history of seizure activity, narrow-angle glaucoma or increased intraocular pressure, or urinary retention and in those at risk of suicidal ideation or behavior.

> **NURSING ALERT**
>
> The TCAs can cause cardiac-related adverse reactions, such as tachycardia and heart block. Give these drugs with caution to older adults or the person with preexisting cardiac disease.

LASA ALERT

The following drugs may sound alike; be sure to clarify when they are ordered:

Drug Name	Sounds Like
amitriptyline	aminophylline, imipramine, nortriptyline
amoxapine	amoxicillin, Amoxil
clomiPRAMINE	chlorproMAZINE, clevidipine, clomiPHENE, desipramine, Norpramin
desipramine	clomiPRAMINE, dalfampridine, diphenhydrAMINE, disopyramide, imipramine, nortriptyline
norpramin	clomiPRAMINE, imipramine, Normodyne, Norpace, nortriptyline, Tenormin
pamelor	Demerol

Drugs that look like a similar drug are noted in the Summary Drug Tables of each chapter.

INTERACTIONS

The following interactions may occur when a TCA is administered with another agent:

Interacting Drugs	Effect of Common Use	Interaction
Sedatives and hypnotics, analgesics	Sedation and pain relief, respectively	Increased risk of respiratory and nervous system depression
Cimetidine	Treatment of GI upset	Increased anticholinergic symptoms (dry mouth, urinary retention, blurred vision)
MAOIs	Antidepressant agents	Increased risk for hypertensive episodes, severe convulsions, and hyperpyretic episodes
Adrenergic agents	Neuromuscular agents	Increased risk for arrhythmias and hypertension

MONOAMINE OXIDASE INHIBITORS

ACTIONS

Drugs classified as MAOIs inhibit the activity of monoamine oxidase, a complex enzyme system responsible for inactivating certain neurotransmitters. Blocking monoamine oxidase results in an increase in *endogenous* epinephrine, norepinephrine, dopamine, and serotonin in the nervous system. An increase in these **neurohormones** (secreted rather than transmitted neurosubstances) stimulates the CNS.

USES

The MAOI antidepressants are less frequently used in the treatment of depressive episodes owing to the possible reaction of hypertensive crisis and other unwanted adverse reactions. Unlabeled uses include bulimia, night terrors, migraine headaches, seasonal affective disorder, and multiple sclerosis.

ADVERSE REACTIONS

- Neuromuscular reactions include **orthostatic hypotension**, dizziness, vertigo, headache, and blurred vision.
- GI and genitourinary system reactions include constipation, dry mouth, nausea, diarrhea, and impotence.
- A serious adverse reaction associated with MAOIs is hypertensive crisis (extremely high blood pressure), which may occur when foods containing **tyramine** (an amino acid) are eaten (Box 21.3 provides a list of foods containing tyramine).

> **NURSING ALERT**
>
> One of the earliest symptoms of hypertensive crisis is headache (usually occipital), followed by a stiff or sore neck, nausea, vomiting, sweating, fever, chest pain, dilated pupils, and bradycardia or tachycardia. If a hypertensive crisis occurs, immediate medical intervention is necessary to reduce the blood pressure. Strokes (cerebrovascular accidents) and death have been reported.

BOX 21.3	Foods Containing Tyramine to be Avoided if Taking MAOI Antidepressant

- Aged cheese (e.g., blue, Camembert, cheddar, Emmentaler, mozzarella, parmesan, Romano, Stilton, Swiss)
- Sour cream
- Yogurt
- Beef or chicken livers
- Pickled herring
- Fermented meats (e.g., bologna, pepperoni, salami, dried fish)
- Undistilled alcoholic beverages (e.g., imported beer; ale; red wine, especially Chianti and sherry)
- Caffeinated beverages (e.g., coffee, tea, colas)
- Chocolate
- Certain fruits and vegetables (e.g., avocado, bananas, fava beans, figs, raisins, sauerkraut)
- Yeast extracts
- Soy sauce

CONTRAINDICATIONS AND PRECAUTIONS

The MAOI antidepressants are contraindicated in the elderly and in clients with known hypersensitivity to the drugs, pheochromocytoma, liver and kidney disease, cerebrovascular disease, hypertension, history of headaches, or congestive heart failure. Safety has not been established for use in clients younger than 16 years or during pregnancy (pregnancy category C) or lactation.

The MAOIs should be used cautiously in clients with impaired liver function, history of seizures, parkinsonian symptoms, diabetes, or hyperthyroidism and in those at risk of suicidal ideation or behavior. Individuals on MAOIs should not take decongestants without the permission of their primary health care provider.

When stopping MAOI therapy, the drug must be tapered over a period of 2–4 weeks. Should the drug be stopped abruptly, withdrawal symptoms can occur effecting the GI system (e.g., nausea, vomiting, diarrhea) and neuro system (e.g., headaches, dizziness, tremors, paresthesia, somnolence, and sleep disturbances).

LASA ALERT

The following drugs may sound alike; be sure to clarify when they are ordered:

Drug Name	*Sounds Like*
Nardil	Norinyl
Phenelzine	Phenytoin

Drugs that look like a similar drug are noted in the Summary Drug Tables of each chapter.

❗ NURSING ALERT

Be sure to review the medical history for MAOI use when the anti-infective, linezolid, or the procedural dye, methylene blue, is prescribed. Both these drugs when used with an MAOI can result in serotonin syndrome (see Box 21.2)

INTERACTIONS

The following interactions may occur when an MAOI antidepressant is administered with another agent:

Interacting Drugs or Agent	Common Use	Effect of Interaction
Sedatives and hypnotics, analgesics	Sedation and pain relief, respectively	Increased risk for adverse reactions during surgery
Thiazide diuretic	Relief of fluid retention	Increased hypotensive effects of the MAOI
Meperidine	Pain relief	Increased risk for hypertensive episodes, severe convulsions, and hyperpyretic episodes
Adrenergic agents	Neuromuscular agent	Increased risk for cardiac arrhythmias and hypertension
Tyramine or tryptophan	Amino acids found in some foods	Hypertensive crisis, which may occur up to 2 weeks after the MAOI is discontinued
Antitussives	Relieve cough	Hypotension, fever, nausea, jerking motions to the leg, and coma

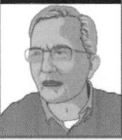

PHARMACOLOGY IN PRACTICE

DRUG RECOGNITION

Which of the following classes of antidepressants exert their effects by exclusively inhibiting the reuptake of serotonin?

1. SSRIs
2. Tricyclic antidepressants
3. MAOIs
4. Dopamine norepinephrine reuptake inhibitors

🦠 LITHIUM

Although lithium is not a true antidepressant drug, it is grouped with the antidepressants because of its use in regulating the severe fluctuations of the manic phase of **bipolar disorder** (a mood disorder characterized by severe swings from extreme hyperactivity to depression). During the manic phase, the person experiences altered thought processes, which can lead to bizarre delusions. The drug diminishes the frequency and intensity of hyperactive (manic) episodes.

Lithium is rapidly absorbed after oral administration. The most common adverse reactions include tremors, nausea, vomiting, thirst, and polyuria. Toxic reactions may occur when serum lithium levels are greater than 1.5 mEq/L (Table 21.1). Because some of these toxic reactions are serious, lithium blood level measurements are usually obtained during therapy, and the dosage of lithium is adjusted accordingly.

Lithium is contraindicated in clients with hypersensitivity to tartrazine (commonly used yellow food dye), renal or cardiovascular disease, sodium depletion, and dehydration and in clients receiving diuretics. Lithium is a pregnancy category D drug and is contraindicated during pregnancy and lactation. For women of childbearing age, contraceptives may be prescribed while they are taking lithium.

Antacids will decrease the effectiveness of lithium. Lithium is monitored carefully in clients who sweat profusely, experience diarrhea or vomiting, or have an infection or fever causing fluid loss. Clients taking diuretics or antipsychotic drugs should be monitored for lithium toxicity.

TABLE 21.1 Lithium Toxicity

SERUM LITHIUM	SIGNS OF TOXICITY
Level	
1.5–2.0 mEq/L	Diarrhea, vomiting, nausea, drowsiness, muscular weakness, lack of coordination (early signs of toxicity)
2–3 mEq/L	Giddiness, ataxia, blurred vision, tinnitus, vertigo, increasing confusion, slurred speech, blackouts, myoclonic twitching or movement of entire limbs, choreoathetoid (involuntary) movements, urinary or fecal incontinence, agitation or manic-like behavior, hyperreflexia, hypertonia, dysarthria
More than 3 mEq/L	May produce a complex clinical picture involving multiple organs and organ systems, including seizures (generalized and focal), arrhythmias, hypotension, peripheral vascular collapse, stupor, muscle group twitching, spasticity, coma

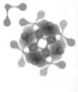

NURSING PROCESS: STEPS TO BUILDING CLINICAL JUDGMENT
Client Receiving an Antidepressant Drug

ASSESSMENT

A client receiving an antidepressant drug may be treated in the hospital or in an outpatient setting.

Preadministration Assessment
Data gathering suggestions before the initial administration of an antidepressant include:
Objective data

- Description of general appearance
- Vital signs
- Observation of behavior during interview: slowness to answer questions, a monotone speech pattern, or crying
- Laboratory testing—thyroid stimulating hormone, thyroid panel (rule out hypothyroidism)

Subjective data

- Mental status—Standardized tools typically include questions about *desire* to participate in activities, *withdrawal* from social interactions, and whether *dependency* on others has increased
- Has the client felt helpless or hopeless in the last 2 weeks?
- Comments about feelings of anxiety, sadness, guilt, or increased attachment to others
- Coping mechanisms used to deal with depression, especially self-medicating with alcohol or drugs
- Medical, social, and mental health history
- *Assess the potential for self-harm or suicide*

It is important to document the presence of suicidal thoughts. Providers sometimes think asking about suicidal thoughts is what causes clients to take their own lives; it does not. It is important to ask the questions in a straightforward manner using simple questions. Box 21.4 provides indications for those at risk for suicidal behavior. Accurately document and immediately report any statements to the primary health care provider concerning suicide or the ability of the client to carry out any suicidal intentions.

Ongoing Assessment
The therapeutic effects of the antidepressants may take 2–4 weeks to be seen. Therefore, many clients who are hospitalized when antidepressants are prescribed may be discharged before follow-up assessments are made. These clients are usually seen at periodic intervals in the primary health care provider's office or in a mental health outpatient setting.

Before the drug lifts the depressive mood, clients are monitored for the adverse reactions of the drugs, which can cause clients to stop taking them prematurely.

BOX 21.4 **Indications of Suicidal Behavior**

- Verbal cueing: statements of worthlessness or that a "situation" will be over soon
- *Coming out* of depressive mood: when a person is at the greatest risk for self-harm
- A "command" hallucination: when "voices" are telling a client they are worthless and should die
- Lack of alternatives: when a person who has relatively few coping skills/support networks has the false belief that they have ruled out all resources available and death is now the only solution

At the time of each visit to the primary health care provider or clinic, observe the client for a response to therapy. Question the client or family members about what they see or how they feel about the response to therapy. The type of questions asked depends on the client and the diagnosis and may include questions such as:

- How are you feeling?
- How would you describe your depressed feelings?
- How would you rate your depression?
- Would you like to tell me how everything is going?

You may need to rephrase questions or direct conversation toward other subjects until the client feels comfortable and can discuss therapy. Also, reinforce that it takes time for the client to see results and praise the client for continuing to take the medication even if they do not see a response yet.

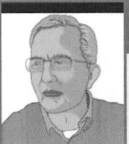

PHARMACOLOGY IN PRACTICE

ASSESSMENT
A quick assessment of depression includes asking questions about which of the following? Select all that apply.
1. Appetite increases
2. Desire to participate in activity
3. Unusual dependence on others
4. Withdrawal from social interaction

NURSING DIAGNOSES

Drug-specific nursing diagnoses are the following:

- **ADL deficit** related to inability to participate in activities of daily living secondary to somnolence, drowsiness, and depressive state
- **Sleep wake disturbance** related to depression and excessive drowsiness
- **Malnutrition risk** related to anorexia, constipation, and depression
- **Suicide attempt risk** related to suicidal ideation and adverse reaction to antidepressive drug
- **Acute pain** related to **priapism** (painful erection)
- **Dehydration** related to disregard for fluids causing lithium toxicity

Nursing diagnoses related to drug administration are discussed in Chapter 4.

PLANNING

The expected outcomes of the client depend on the reason for administration of an antidepressant but may include an optimal response to drug therapy, support of client needs related to the management of adverse drug reactions, and confidence in an understanding of the medication regimen.

IMPLEMENTATION

Promoting an Optimal Response to Therapy
Response to antidepressant medications is not rapid. It can take a number of weeks for the drugs to take effect. Fluoxetine is an example of a drug that may take as long as 4 weeks to attain a full therapeutic effect. Some adverse reactions, such as dry mouth, episodes of orthostatic hypotension, and drowsiness, appear long before the intended effect of the antidepressant. The inability to deal with the unpleasantness of these adverse reactions is one of the primary reasons clients stop taking antidepressants. The two adverse reactions that clients have the most trouble tolerating are somnolence and dry mouth. During initial therapy or whenever the dosage is increased or decreased, instruct the client what to expect in terms of the adverse reactions or behavioral changes. Teach the client when to report change in behavior or the appearance of adverse reactions to the primary health care provider, because a further increase or decrease in dosage may be necessary or use of the drug may need to be discontinued.

When caring for hospitalized clients with depression, develop a nursing care plan to meet the client's individual needs. Should client behavior require the antidepressants to be given parenterally, give these drugs intramuscularly (IM) in a large muscle mass, such as the gluteus muscle. Keep the client lying down (when possible) for about 30 minutes after administering the drug.

Monitoring and Managing Client Needs

Activities of Daily Living Deficit
Initially, the client may need assistance with self-care, because clients with depression often do not have the physical or emotional energy to perform self-care activities. This is complicated by the fact that many antidepressants cause excessive drowsiness during the initial stages of treatment, and clients may need assistance with ambulation and self-care activities. These problems usually subside as the depression lifts and tolerance to the adverse reactions builds with continued use of the antidepressant. To minimize the risk for injury, assist the client when necessary and make the environment as safe as possible. When orthostatic hypotension is an effect of drug therapy, instruct the client how to rise from a lying position to a sitting position. The client remains in a sitting position for a few minutes before rising to a standing position. Position changes are made slowly, with assistance offered if necessary.

If the client has a difficult time with self-care because of the depression or sedative effects of the antidepressants, arrange for assistance with activities of daily living, including help with eating, dressing, and ambulating. However, encourage self-care whenever possible, allowing sufficient time for the client to accomplish tasks to the fullest extent of their ability. It is important to provide positive feedback when appropriate. As a therapeutic effect of the drug is attained, the client will be able to resume self-care (if no other physical conditions interfere).

Document behavioral observations at periodic intervals, the frequency of which depends on hospital or unit guidelines. An accurate assessment of the client's behavior aids the primary health care provider in planning therapy and thus becomes an important part of nursing management. Clients with a poor response to drug therapy may require dosage changes, a change to another antidepressant drug, or the addition of other therapies to the treatment regimen.

Sleep Wake Disturbance

Many of the antidepressant drugs cause somnolence. This adverse reaction is one of the greatest reasons clients stop taking the medication. Teach the client or care providers to administer the drug at night—the sedative effects promote sleep, and the adverse reactions appear less troublesome. An exception to this is the SSRIs; it is best to administer those medications in the morning.

Assess the environment to help promote sleep at night and wakefulness during the day. Drapes should be shut at night and opened in the day to let in light, and clocks should be available for the client to see the time of day. These activities will help the client to reorient to daytime and nighttime, thereby promoting an effective sleep pattern.

Malnutrition Risk: Less Than Body Requirements

Depressed clients may not feel like eating; therefore, they lose weight. This can be potentiated by the adverse reactions of anorexia and constipation. Monitor dietary intake and help the registered dietician in providing nutritious meals, taking into consideration foods that the client likes and dislikes. Fluid intake and foods high in fiber are important for the client to prevent constipation. Weighing the client weekly is important for monitoring weight loss or gain. To minimize the dry mouth that frequently accompanies administration of antidepressants, teach good oral hygiene and provide frequent sips of fluids and sugarless gum or hard candy.

 Lifespan Considerations

Pediatric

Studies show that children and adolescents with MDDs have an increased risk of suicidal ideation when prescribed antidepressant medications.

Suicide Attempt Risk

Clients with a high suicide potential require a well-supervised environment and protection from suicidal acts. For clients with severe depression, suicide precautions are important until a therapeutic effect is achieved. When the client is hospitalized, policies of observation must be strictly followed for the client's protection.

Of greatest concern is the depressed client who has suicidal ideation but has not been identified as such (see Box 21.4 for indications of suicidal risk). Clients in a depressive state may lack the energy to carry out plans for ending their own life. Because the full therapeutic effect of the antidepressant may not be attained for 10 days–4 weeks, clients have time to gain enough energy to carry out an injurious act upon themselves. Clients with suicidal ideation must be monitored closely. Report any expressions of guilt, hopelessness, or helplessness; insomnia; weight loss; and direct or indirect threats of suicide.

When suicidal ideation is suspected, oral administration of medications requires greater consideration. After administration of an oral drug, inspect the client's oral cavity to be sure the drug has been swallowed. If the client resists having their oral cavity checked, report this refusal to the primary health care provider. Clients planning suicide may try to keep the drug on the side of the mouth or under the tongue and not swallow in an effort to hoard or save enough of the drug to attempt suicide at a later time. Other clients may refuse to take the drug. If the client refuses to take the drug, contact the primary health care provider regarding this problem because parenteral administration of the drug may be necessary.

 Lifespan Considerations

Gerontology

Older men with prostatic enlargement are at increased risk for urinary retention when they take antidepressants.

Acute Pain

An uncommon but potentially serious adverse reaction of trazodone is priapism (a persistent erection of the penis). This can be very painful, and if not treated within a few hours, priapism can result in impotence. Because this can be an embarrassing adverse reaction, instruct the client regarding self-treatment strategies using pseudoephedrine (see Chapter 47) and when to report any prolonged or inappropriate penile erection. The antidepressant drug is discontinued immediately by the client and the primary care provider notified. If self-treatment is not effective, injection of alpha-adrenergic stimulants (α-adrenergic stimulants) (e.g., norepinephrine) may be needed in treating priapism. In some cases, surgical intervention may be required.

Dehydration—Toxicity Potential When Taking Lithium

Fluid volume determines the concentration of lithium in the blood. The dosage of lithium is individualized according to serum levels and clinical response to the drug. The desirable serum lithium level is between 0.6 and 1.2 mEq/L. Blood samples are drawn immediately before the next dose of lithium (8–12 hours after the last dose) when lithium levels are relatively stable.

Lithium toxicity is closely related to serum lithium levels and can occur even when the drug is administered at therapeutic doses. This can happen because during the acute manic phase, clients may be so active that they do not realize they need to eat or drink and are at greater risk of dehydration, resulting in a higher serum lithium level. Hospitalized clients may be required to take "fluid" breaks, where they are taught to stop and drink fluid at specified times. Clients should maintain an oral intake of approximately 3000 mL/day. Adverse reactions are seldom observed at serum lithium levels of less than l.5 mEq/L, except in the client who is especially sensitive to lithium. See Table 21.1 for toxic symptoms that may occur. When clients are discharged, instruct them to notify the primary health care provider any time they experience fever, diarrhea, vomiting, or nausea to prevent dehydration and a possible increase in the serum lithium level.

Lifespan Considerations

Gerontology

Older adults are at increased risk for lithium toxicity because of a decreased rate of excretion. Lower dosages may be necessary to decrease the risk of toxicity.

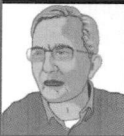

PHARMACOLOGY IN PRACTICE

MANAGING NEEDS

A nurse is caring for a male client under treatment with trazodone. Which of the following is an adverse reaction that the nurse should teach the client to report immediately?
1. Priapism
2. Orthostatic hypotension
3. Insomnia
4. Diarrhea

Educating the Client and Family

When some clients are discharged to the home setting, lack of adherence to drug therapy is a problem because of unpleasant adverse drug effects. It is very important to educate the client or family members thoroughly about the importance of managing the reactions so that the client will continue the proper drug regimen. Evaluate the client's ability to assume responsibility for taking drugs at home (see Client Teaching for Improved Outcomes: Empowering Client Responsibility for Antidepressant Drug Therapy). The administration of antidepressant drugs becomes a family responsibility if the outpatient appears to be unable to manage their own drug therapy.

The client and family should feel confident in understanding any adverse reactions that may occur with a specific antidepressant drug. Encourage the client or family member to contact the primary health care provider immediately if a serious drug reaction occurs. As you develop a teaching plan, include the following points for the client or family member:

- Inform the primary health care provider, dentist, and other medical personnel of therapy with this drug.
- If dizziness occurs when changing position, rise slowly when getting out of bed or a chair. If dizziness is severe, always have help when changing positions.
- Relieve dry mouth by taking frequent sips of water, sucking on hard candy, or chewing gum (preferably sugarless gum).
- Keep all clinic appointments or appointments with the primary health care provider because close monitoring of therapy is essential.
- Do not take the antidepressants during pregnancy. Notify the primary health care provider if you are pregnant or wish to become pregnant.
- Report any unusual changes or physical effects to the primary health care provider.
- Avoid prolonged exposure to sunlight or sunlamps because an exaggerated reaction to the ultraviolet light may occur (photosensitivity), resulting in a burn.

- For male clients who take trazodone and who experience prolonged, inappropriate, and painful erections, stop taking the drug and notify the primary care provider.
- Remember to take lithium with food or immediately after meals to avoid stomach upset. Drink at least 10 large glasses of fluid each day and add extra salt to food if permissible. Prolonged exposure to the sun may lead to dehydration. If any of the following occurs, do not take the next dose and immediately notify the primary health care provider: diarrhea, vomiting, fever, tremors, drowsiness, lack of muscle coordination, or muscle weakness.

Client Teaching for Improved Outcomes

Empowering Client Responsibility for Antidepressant Drug Therapy

Antidepressants are taken for long periods of time, requiring self-management on the part of the client. When people feel empowered in decision making, they are more likely to remain adherent to a plan of care.

When you teach, make sure your client understands the following:

✔ Explain the reason for drug therapy, including the type of antidepressant prescribed, drug name, dosage, and frequency of administration.
✔ Enlist the aid of family members to support adherence with therapy.
✔ Urge the client to take the drug exactly as prescribed and not to increase or decrease dosage, omit doses, or discontinue use of the drug unless directed to do so by the health care provider.
✔ Advise that full therapeutic effect may not occur for several weeks.
✔ Instruct in the signs and symptoms of behavioral changes indicative of therapeutic effectiveness or increasing depression and suicidal tendencies.
✔ Review measures to reduce the risk for suicidal ideation.
✔ Instruct about possible adverse reactions with instructions to notify the health care provider should any occur.
✔ Reinforce safety measures such as changing positions slowly and avoiding driving or hazardous tasks.
✔ Advise avoidance of alcohol and use of nonprescription drugs unless discussed with the primary health care provider.
✔ Encourage the client to inform other health care providers and medical personnel about drug therapy regimen.
✔ Instruct in measures to minimize dry mouth.
✔ Reassure results of therapy will be monitored by periodic laboratory tests and follow-up visits with the health care provider.
✔ Assist with arrangements for follow-up visits.

EVALUATION

- Therapeutic response is achieved and the depressive mood is improved.
- Adverse reactions are identified, reported to the primary health care provider, and managed successfully through appropriate nursing interventions:
  - Client resumes ability to care for self.
  - Client reports fewer episodes of disturbed sleep patterns.
  - Client maintains an adequate nutritional status.
  - Client does not attempt suicide.
  - Client is free of pain.
  - Adequate hydration is maintained.

- Client and family express confidence and demonstrate an understanding of the drug regimen.

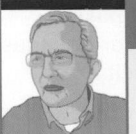

PHARMACOLOGY IN PRACTICE

USING CLINICAL REASONING

What information do you need to give Mr. Phillip and his family regarding the action and adverse reactions of these drugs? How might this drug be interacting with other drugs prescribed in earlier chapters of this unit?

KEY POINTS

■ Mood disorders are a spectrum of feelings that range from severe debilitation to an exhaustive elation.

■ MDD is also termed unipolar or clinical depression. This condition is characterized by a dysphoric mood lasting at least 2 weeks. Bipolar depression may or may not have the depressed component, yet it has the manic or energized portion.

■ Drugs used to treat unipolar depression include those that modify the neurotransmission of one or more of the following: serotonin, norepinephrine, or dopamine. Currently the most frequently used drugs are from the SSRIs or the SNRIs/DNRIs.

■ Antidepressants may take from 2–4 weeks for the intended response to occur. Unfortunately, adverse reactions can occur sooner, and clients may stop taking the drug before maximum benefit is obtained. These adverse reactions include drowsiness, dizziness and lightheadedness, dry mouth, thirst, and constipation.

■ These drugs increase the risk of suicidal ideation, and clients must be both questioned and observed for any suicidal behaviors.

■ Clients taking drugs for mania have behaviors (energized) that put them at risk for dehydration—a condition that can increase serum levels of lithium, a drug used for bipolar depression, resulting in toxicity.

SUMMARY DRUG TABLE
Antidepressants

Generic Name	Trade Name	Uses	Adverse Reactions	Dosage Ranges
Selective Serotonin Reuptake Inhibitors (SSRIs)				
citalopram *sye-TAL-oh-pram*	CeleXA	Major depressive disorder (MDD), panic disorder, posttraumatic stress disorder (PTSD), premenstrual disorder, dementia-associated agitation	Nausea, dry mouth, sweating, somnolence, insomnia, anorexia, diarrhea	20–90 mg/day orally
escitalopram *es-sye-TAL-oh-pram*	Lexapro	MDD, generalized anxiety disorder, panic disorder, OCD	Headache, insomnia, somnolence, nausea	10–20 mg/day orally
FLUoxetine *floo-OKS-e-teen*	PROzac, Sarafem	Depression (MDD and bipolar), bulimia, OCD, panic disorder, premenstrual dysphoric disorder (Sarafem only)	Anxiety, nervousness, somnolence, insomnia, drowsiness, asthenia, tremor, headache, nausea, diarrhea, constipation, dry mouth, anorexia	20 mg/day orally in the morning or up to 80 mg/day (dose split between morning and at noon)

Generic Name	Trade Name	Uses	Adverse Reactions	Dosage Ranges
fluvoxaMINE *floo-VOKS-a-meen*		OCD, depression (MDD), bulimia, PTSD	Headache, nervousness, somnolence, insomnia, nausea, diarrhea, dry mouth, constipation, dyspepsia, ejaculatory disturbances	50–300 mg/day orally in divided doses
PARoxetine *pa-ROKS-e-teen*	Paxil, Brisdelle, Pexeva	Depression (MDD), OCD, panic disorder, general anxiety disorder, social anxiety disorder, PTSD, premenstrual dysphoric disorder, menopausal flushing	Headache, tremors, somnolence, nervousness, dizziness, insomnia, nausea, diarrhea, constipation, dry mouth, sweating, weakness, sexual dysfunction	20–50 mg/day orally
sertraline *SER-tra-leen*	Zoloft	Depression (MDD), OCD, panic disorders, PTSD, social anxiety disorder	Headache, drowsiness, anxiety, dizziness, insomnia, fatigue, nausea, diarrhea, dry mouth, ejaculatory disturbances, sweating	50–200 mg/day orally
vilazodone *vil-AZ-oh-done*	Viibryd	Depression	Dry mouth, increased appetite, heartburn, dizziness, shakiness	40 mg daily orally
vortioxetine *vor-tye-OX-e-teen*	Trintellix	Depression (MDD)	Nausea, vomiting, constipation	5–20 mg daily orally
Serotonin/Norepinephrine and Dopamine/Norepinephrine Reuptake Inhibitors (SNRIs/DNRIs)				
buPROPion *byoo-PROE-pee-on*	Aplenzin, Wellbutrin	Depression, seasonal affective disorder (SAD), neuropathic pain, attention-deficit hyperactivity disorder (ADHD)	Agitation, dizziness, dry mouth, insomnia, sedation, headache, nausea, vomiting, tremor, constipation, weight loss, anorexia, excess sweating	100–300 mg/day orally in divided doses; sustained release, 1 tablet BID orally
desvenlafaxine *des-ven-la-FAX-een*	Pristiq	Depression (MDD)	Anxiety, constipation, decreased appetite, dizziness, insomnia, sexual dysfunction	50 mg daily orally
DULoxetine *doo-LOX-e-teen*	Cymbalta	Depression (MDD), generalized anxiety disorder, diabetic peripheral neuropathy, fibromyalgia, stress incontinence (men)	Insomnia, dry mouth, nausea, constipation	40–60 mg/day orally
levomilnacipran *lee-voe-mil-NA-ci-pran*	Fetzima	Depression (MDD)	Nausea, vomiting, constipation, sweating, increased heart rate, erectile dysfunction	120 mg once daily orally
milnacipran *mil-NAY-ci-pran*	Savella	Fibromyalgia	Constipation, dry mouth, tachycardia, hot flush, vomiting	12.5–50.0 mg twice daily orally
nefazodone *nef-AY-zoe-done*		Depression	Somnolence, insomnia, dizziness, nausea, dry mouth, constipation, headache, weakness	200–600 mg/day orally in divided doses
traZODone *TRAZ-oh-done*		Depression, alcohol craving	Drowsiness, dizziness, priapism, dry mouth, nausea, vomiting, constipation, fatigue, nervousness	150–400 mg/day orally in divided doses, not to exceed 600 mg/day
venlafaxine *ven-la-FAX-een*	Effexor XR	Depression (MDD), anxiety disorders, migraine, narcolepsy, neuropathic pain, premenstrual disorder	Headache, insomnia, dizziness, nervousness, weakness, anorexia, nausea, constipation, dry mouth, somnolence, sweating	75–215 mg/day orally in divided doses

Continued

SUMMARY DRUG TABLE (continued)
Antidepressants

Generic Name	Trade Name	Uses	Adverse Reactions	Dosage Ranges
Tricyclic Antidepressants				
amitriptyline *a-mee-TRIP-ti-leen*		Depression, neuropathic pain, eating disorders	Sedation, anticholinergic effects (dry mouth, dry eyes, urinary retention), constipation	Up to 150 mg/day orally in divided doses; 20–30 mg IM QID; severely depressed hospitalized client: up to 300 mg/day orally. Do not administer IV
amoxapine *a-MOKS-a-peen*		Depression accompanied by anxiety	Same as amitriptyline	50 mg orally 2–3 times daily up to 300 mg/day, if poor response may go up to 600 mg/day
clomiPRAMINE *kloe-MI-pra-meen*	Anafranil	OCD, MDD	Same as amitriptyline, sexual dysfunction	25–250 mg/day orally in divided doses
desipramine *des-IP-ra-meen*	Norpramin	Depression, eating disorders	Same as amitriptyline	100–200 mg/day orally, not to exceed 300 mg/day
doxepin DOKS-*e-pin*	Silenor	Anxiety or depression, emotional symptoms accompanying organic disease, insomnia	Same as amitriptyline	25–150 mg/day orally in divided doses
imipramine *im-IP-ra-meen*		Depression, enuresis, eating disorders	Same as amitriptyline	100–200 mg/day orally in divided doses Childhood enuresis (older than 6 years): 25 mg/day, 1 hour before bedtime, not to exceed 2.5 mg/kg/day
nortriptyline *nor-TRIP-ti-leen*	Pamelor	Depression, smoking cessation, neuralgia	Same as amitriptyline	25 mg orally 3–4 times/day; not to exceed 150 mg/day
protriptyline *proe-TRIP-ti-leen*		Depression	Same as amitriptyline	15–40 mg/day orally in 3–4 doses, not to exceed 60 mg/day
trimipramine *trye-MI-pra-meen*		Depression	Same as amitriptyline	75–150 mg/day orally in divided doses, not to exceed 300 mg/day
Monoamine Oxidase Inhibitors				
phenelzine *FEN-el-zeen*	Nardil	Atypical depression	Orthostatic hypotension, vertigo, dizziness, nausea, constipation, dry mouth, diarrhea, headache, restlessness, blurred vision, hypertensive crisis	45–90 mg/day orally in divided doses
tranylcypromine *tran-il-SIP-roe-meen*	Parnate	Major depressive disorder (unipolar depression)	Same as phenelzine	30–60 mg/day orally in divided doses
isocarboxazid *eye-soe-kar-BOKS-a-zid*	Marplan	Depression	Same as phenelzine	10–40 mg/day orally
Misc. Antidepressants				
ARIPiprazole *ay-ri-PIP-ray-zole*	Abilify	Adjunct for major depressive disorders, bipolar disorder, schizophrenia	Agitation, akathisia, anxiety, drowsiness, headache, constipation, dry mouth, nausea	10–30 mg/day orally
asenapine *a-SEN-a-peen*	Saphris	Adjunct for major depressive disorders, bipolar disorder, schizophrenia	Agitation, akathisia, anxiety, drowsiness, headache, constipation, dry mouth, nausea	5–10 mg orally twice daily

Generic Name	Trade Name	Uses	Adverse Reactions	Dosage Ranges
ªbrexanolone *brex-AN-oh-lone*	Zulresso	Postpartum depression	Excessive sedation, drowsiness, dizziness, dry mouth, skin flush	Titrated continuous IV infusion over 60 hours
brexpiprazole *breks-PIP-ray-zole*	Rexulti	Adjunct for major depressive disorders, schizophrenia	Restlessness, weight gain	0.5–4.0 mg orally daily
cariprazine *kar-IP-ra-zeen*	Vraylar	Adjunct for major depressive disorders, bipolar disorder, schizophrenia	Agitation, akathisia, anxiety, drowsiness, headache, constipation, dry mouth, nausea	1.5–6.0 mg orally daily
esketamine *es-KET-a-meen*	Spravato	Adjunct for treatment resistant depression	Sedation, dizziness, headache, nausea, taste changes	Intranasal, 56–84 mg twice weekly
maprotiline *ma-PROE-ti-leen*		Depression, anxiety, neuropathic pain	Sedation, dry mouth, constipation, orthostatic hypotension	75–150 mg/day orally; for severe depression, dosage may increase to 215 mg/day orally
mirtazapine *mer-TAH-za-peen*	Remeron	Depression, GAD, PTSD, insomnia, headaches, nausea and vomiting	Sedation, dry mouth, constipation, orthostatic hypotension	15–45 mg/day orally
Mood Stabilizer				
lithium *LITH-ee-um*	Lithobid	Manic episodes of bipolar disorder	Headache, drowsiness, tremors, nausea, polyuria (see Table 21.1)	Based on lithium serum levels; average dose range is 900–1800 mg/day orally in divided doses

ªREMS Alert.

CHAPTER REVIEW

Know Your Drugs

Clients sometimes know a medication by the brand (or trade) name and not the generic name. To help you recognize both names, match the brand name with the generic name of the same medication.

Generic Name	Brand Name
1. bupropion	A. Celexa
2. citalopram	B. Paxil
3. paroxetine	C. Wellbutrin
	D. Zyban

Calculate Medication Dosages

1. The primary care provider prescribes trazodone 150 mg orally. Available are 50-mg tablets. The nurse administers _____.

2. The primary care provider prescribes oral paroxetine (Paxil) 50 mg/day. The drug is available as oral suspension with strength of 10 mg/5 mL. The nurse administers _____.

Prepare for the NCLEX

RECALL THE FACTS

1. A client exhibits high energy and disorganized behavior on the mental health unit. This is best termed _____.
    1. clinical depression
    2. unipolar disorder
    3. major depressive disorder
    4. bipolar disorder

2. Which of the following adverse reactions would the nurse expect to find in a client taking amitriptyline?
    1. constipation and abdominal cramps
    2. bradycardia and double vision
    3. sedation and dry mouth
    4. polyuria and hypotension

3. Major depressive disorder is suspected in which of the following clients?
    1. woman who is crying about her mastectomy performed yesterday
    2. line worker who lost his job in a manufacturing plant 3 months ago
    3. person diagnosed with hypothyroidism
    4. child who had a parent die from suicide

4. Which of the following antidepressants would be most likely to cause the client to have a seizure?
    1. amitriptyline
    2. bupropion
    3. sertraline
    4. venlafaxine

5. Which of the following symptoms would indicate to the nurse that a client taking lithium is experiencing toxicity?
    1. constipation, abdominal cramps, rash
    2. stupor, oliguria, hypertension
    3. nausea, vomiting, diarrhea
    4. dry mouth, blurred vision, difficulty swallowing

ANALYZE THE FACTS

6. The nurse instructs the client taking an MAOI not to eat foods containing _____.
   1. glutamine
   2. sugar
   3. tyramine
   4. large amounts of iron

7. In giving discharge instructions to a client taking lithium, the nurse stresses that the client should:
   1. eat a diet high in carbohydrates and low in proteins
   2. increase oral fluid intake to approximately 3000 mL/day
   3. have blood drawn before each dose of lithium is administered
   4. avoid eating foods high in amines

8. When administering an antidepressant to a client with suicidal ideation, it is most important for the nurse to _____.
   1. have the client remain upright for at least 30 minutes after taking the antidepressant
   2. assess the client in 30 minutes for a therapeutic response to the drug
   3. monitor the client for an occipital headache
   4. inspect the client's oral cavity to be sure the drug was swallowed

ALTERNATE-FORMAT QUESTIONS

9. *A client with limited health literacy is prescribed controlled release fluoxetine for a depression. It will be prescribed to take one 90-mg capsule weekly. What methods should you use to help this client remember when to take the medication? **Select all that apply.**
   1. use a calendar on the wall
   2. ask a family member to call the client weekly
   3. set a cell phone to alarm weekly
   4. have the clinic receptionist call weekly

10. Antidepressant drugs prevent the reuptake of which neurotransmitter(s)? **Select all that apply.**
    1. acetylcholine
    2. dopamine
    3. norepinephrine
    4. serotonin

To check your answers, see Appendix F.

_____

*Indicates the question is directly linked to the NCLEX-PN test plan in Appendix G.

WANT TO KNOW MORE? A wide variety of resources are available to enhance your learning and understanding of this chapter.
- Visit the Point for resources such as:
  - NCLEX-Style Student Review Questions
  - Journal Articles
  - Dosage Calculations
  - Drug Monographs
  - Watch and Learn Videos
  - Concepts in Action Animations
- The *Study Guide to Accompany Introductory Clinical Pharmacology*, 12th edition, sold separately, will help you review and apply essential content.
- ✓PrepU is available to help students prepare for the NCLEX-PN examination.

Antipsychotic Drugs

Key Terms

agranulocytosis decrease or lack of granulocytes (a type of white blood cell [WBC])

akathisia extreme restlessness and increased motor activity

alogia inability to finish a sentence when communicating

anhedonia lack of joy or pleasurable feelings

avolition inability to determine and initiate goals and activities

blood dyscrasias abnormal condition of the blood cells

delusions false belief that cannot be changed with reason

dopamine primary neurotransmitter in the sympathetic nervous system that deals with pleasure and reward in the brain

dystonia prolonged muscle contractions that may cause twisting and repetitive movements of abnormal posture

extrapyramidal syndrome group of adverse reactions involving the extrapyramidal portion of the nervous system causing abnormal muscle movements, especially akathisia and dystonia

hallucinations false sensation or perception of reality

photophobia intolerance to light

photosensitivity abnormal sensitivity when exposed to light

psychosis spectrum of disorders that affect mood and behavior

recidivism act of repeating a behavior

tardive dyskinesia rhythmic, involuntary movements of the tongue, face, mouth, or jaw and sometimes the extremities

Learning Objectives

On completion of this chapter, the student will:

1. Explain the uses, general drug actions, general adverse reactions, contraindications, precautions, and interactions associated with the administration of antipsychotic drugs.
2. Distinguish important preadministration and ongoing assessment activities the nurse should perform on the client taking an antipsychotic drug.
3. List nursing diagnoses for a client taking an antipsychotic drug.
4. Examine ways to promote an optimal response to therapy, how to manage common adverse reactions, and important points to keep in mind when educating clients about the use of antipsychotic drugs.

 Drug Classes

- First-generation (conventional) antipsychotics
- Second-generation (atypical) antipsychotics

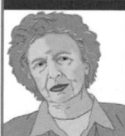 **PHARMACOLOGY IN PRACTICE**

Mrs. Moore's daughter calls the clinic. She tells you that her mother has been up at night, wandering the house, listening and speaking to people who are not there. If she tries to stop her, Mrs. Moore gets agitated and has tried to hit the daughter. The daughter tells you that she volunteers at a long-term care facility back where she lives and there are a number of people like her mother taking Seroquel. She asks if she can get this drug for her mother. After reading this chapter, determine if this is an appropriate medication for Mrs. Moore.

Antipsychotic drugs are administered to clients experiencing a psychotic disorder. The term **psychosis** refers to a spectrum of disorders that affect mood and behavior, with schizophrenia being the most recognized disorder. Schizophrenia is characterized by disordered thinking, perceptual disturbance, behavioral abnormality, affective problems, and impaired socialization. Symptoms of the disease are known as positive or negative symptoms (Box 22.1). Antipsychotic medications are designed to diminish these behaviors so people can function in society.

ACTIONS

Antipsychotic drugs act on the **dopamine** receptors of the brain. Neurobiologic theory suggests that it is higher levels of the neurotransmitter dopamine that cause problems. Positive symptoms result from misfiring at the nerve synapse. Anatomic changes coupled with misfiring cause the negative symptoms. Drugs work by inhibiting or blocking the release of the neurotransmitter dopamine in the brain and possibly regulate the firing of nerve cells in certain areas of the brain. These effects may be responsible for the ability of these drugs to suppress the symptoms of certain psychotic disorders (Fig. 22.1). The conventional or first-generation antipsychotics work to diminish the positive symptoms. Because these drugs block dopamine transmission, they unfortunately produce unpleasant **extrapyramidal** effects (see Adverse Reactions). Examples of antipsychotic drugs include chlorpromazine, haloperidol (Haldol), and fluphenazine.

A newer group of antipsychotic drugs classified as atypical antipsychotics or second-generation antipsychotics (SGAs) is believed to act on serotonin receptors as well as on the dopamine receptors in the brain. They are termed *atypical* because the typical extrapyramidal side effects are lessened, which in turn helps to both diminish the positive symptoms and enhance behaviors to reduce the negative symptoms. Examples of the atypical antipsychotic drugs include clozapine (Clozaril) and aripiprazole (Abilify). The Summary Drug Table: Antipsychotic Drugs gives a more complete listing of the antipsychotic drugs.

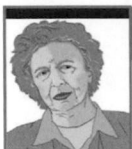

PHARMACOLOGY IN PRACTICE

PATHOPHYSIOLOGY
Which of the following are positive symptoms of schizophrenia? Select all that apply.
1. Concrete thinking
2. Delusions
3. Agitation
4. Alogia
5. No joy

USES

The antipsychotic drugs are used in the treatment of the following:

• Acute and chronic psychoses, such as schizophrenia
• Bipolar (manic phase) illness
• Agitation and behavioral disorders

Selected drugs may be used for their adverse effects to treat minor conditions; for example, chlorpromazine may be

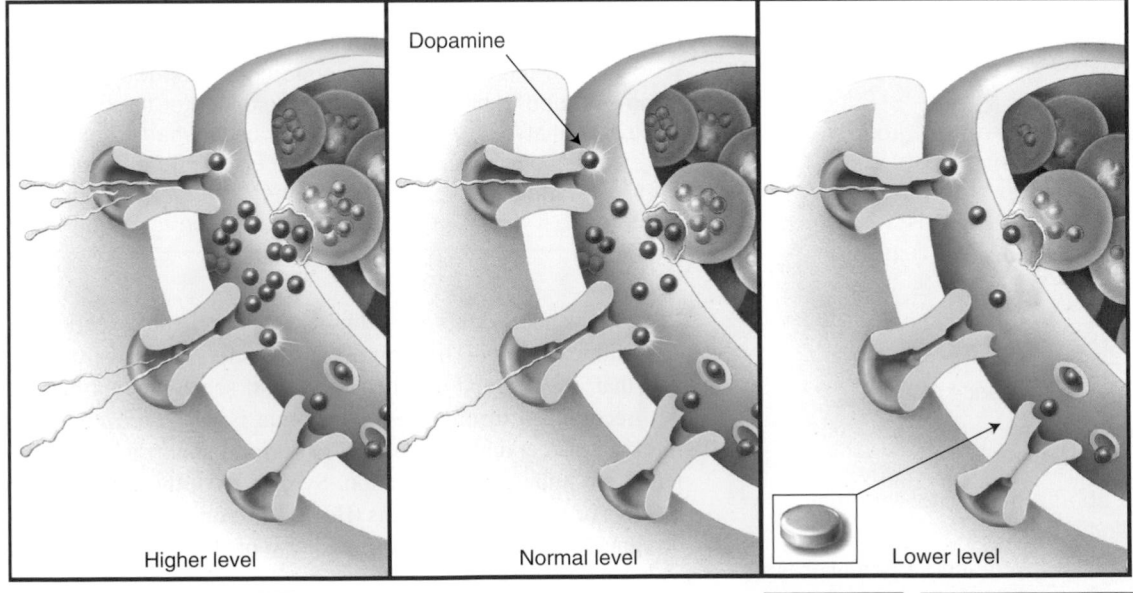

Too much transmission results in positive symptoms

Antipsychotic drug blocks dopamine transmission

Too little transmission results in extrapyramidal symptoms

FIGURE 22.1 Psychotic disorders involve too much dopamine transmission. The antipsychotic drugs block dopamine.

used to treat uncontrollable hiccoughs, and chlorpromazine and prochlorperazine are used as antiemetics.

ADVERSE REACTIONS

Generalized System Reactions

- Sedation, headache, hypotension
- Dry mouth, nasal congestion
- Urticaria, **photophobia** (intolerance to light), **photosensitivity** (abnormal sensitivity when exposed to light). Photosensitivity can result in severe sunburn when clients taking antipsychotic drugs are exposed to the sun or ultraviolet light, such as that used in a tanning bed.

Behavioral Changes

- Possible increase in the intensity of the psychotic symptoms
- Lethargy, hyperactivity, paranoid reactions, agitation, and confusion

Endocrine Changes (SGA)

- Weight gain
- Increased cholesterol, triglyceride, and blood sugar levels

NURSING ALERT

Studies indicate there is a higher incidence of diabetes in clients with schizophrenia than in the general population (Llorente & Urrutia, 2006). This is very likely due to adverse reactions of the (SGA) medications (Rojo et al., 2015) or lifestyle behaviors of this client population.

Neuroleptic malignant syndrome (NMS) is a rare reaction characterized by a combination of extrapyramidal effects, hyperthermia, and autonomic disturbance. It typically occurs within 1 month after the antipsychotic drugs are begun. NMS is potentially fatal and requires intensive symptomatic treatment and immediate discontinuation of the drug causing the syndrome. Once the antipsychotic drug is discontinued, recovery occurs within 7–10 days.

Recidivism

A major concern in the treatment of psychosis is adherence to a consistent medication regimen. Behaviors associated with the disease often cause people to be hospitalized. When medications are started the behavioral symptoms diminish (see Box 22.1), yet, in turn, adverse reactions occur. Some of the adverse reactions can be as uncomfortable to the client as the disorder itself. In addition, these medications take time to produce the optimal affect (sometimes 6–10 weeks). Clients may independently stop using the drug because of the unpleasantness of the reactions, thus causing the psychotic symptoms to return. Once psychotic symptoms return, the client typically engages in the behaviors that caused them to be hospitalized. This becomes a "revolving door" of hospitalizations and discharges and is known as

| **BOX 22.2** | **Extrapyramidal Syndrome** |

- Parkinson-like symptoms—fine tremors, muscle rigidity, mask-like appearance of the face, slowness of movement, slurred speech, and unsteady gait
- Akathisia—extreme restlessness and increased motor activity
- Dystonia—facial grimacing and twisting of the neck into unnatural positions

recidivism. The following sections describe the adverse reactions that are typically unacceptable to clients.

Extrapyramidal Syndrome

Among the most significant adverse reactions associated with the antipsychotic drugs are the extrapyramidal effects. The term **extrapyramidal syndrome** (EPS) refers to a group of adverse reactions affecting the extrapyramidal portion of the nervous system as a result of antipsychotic drugs. This part of the nervous system affects body posture and promotes smooth and uninterrupted movement of various muscle groups. Antipsychotics disturb the function of the extrapyramidal portion of the nervous system, causing abnormal muscle movement. Extrapyramidal effects include Parkinson-like symptoms, **akathisia**, and **dystonia** (Box 22.2). Extrapyramidal effects usually diminish with a reduction in the dosage of the antipsychotic drug. Switching to an SGA antipsychotic medication is helpful in reducing symptoms.

Tardive Dyskinesia

Tardive dyskinesia (TD) is a syndrome consisting of potentially irreversible, involuntary movements. TD is characterized by rhythmic, involuntary movements of the tongue, face, mouth, or jaw and sometimes the extremities. The tongue may protrude, and there may be chewing movements, puckering of the mouth, and facial grimacing. TD is a late-appearing reaction and may be observed in clients receiving an antipsychotic drug or after discontinuation of antipsychotic drug therapy. Because TD is nonreversible, drug therapy must be discontinued when symptoms initially occur during the course of therapy. Because of the risk of TD, it is best to use the smallest dose and the shortest duration of treatment that produces a satisfactory clinical response. The use of atypical (SGA) antipsychotic drugs has increased because they are less likely to cause TD effects.

CONTRAINDICATIONS

Antipsychotics are contraindicated in clients with known hypersensitivity to the drugs, in comatose clients, in those who are severely depressed, and in those who have bone marrow depression, **blood dyscrasias**, Parkinson disease (specifically, haloperidol), liver impairment, coronary artery disease, or severe hypotension or hypertension. Because of a specific enzyme reaction, grapefruit or its juice should not be taken if the client is on the drug quetiapine or pimozide.

Antipsychotic drugs are classified as pregnancy category C drugs (except for clozapine, which is pregnancy category B). Safe use of these drugs during pregnancy and lactation has not been clearly established. Antipsychotics should be used only when clearly needed and when the potential benefit outweighs any potential harm to the fetus.

PRECAUTIONS

Antipsychotic drugs are used cautiously in clients with respiratory disorders, glaucoma, prostatic hypertrophy, epilepsy, decreased renal function, and peptic ulcer disease.

Lifespan Considerations

Gerontology

Clients with dementia may exhibit agitated behaviors, which have resulted in treatment using antipsychotic drugs. There is an association between increased cerebrovascular problems and mortality with the use of antipsychotic medications (especially SGAs) in this population.

LASA ALERT

The following drugs may sound alike; be sure to clarify when they are ordered:

Drug Name	Sounds Like
Abilify	Ambien
ARIPiprazole	proton pump inhibitors (dexlansoprazole, esomeprazole, lansoprazole, omeprazole, pantoprazole, RABEprazole)
chlorproMAZINE	chlordiazePOXIDE, chlorproPAMIDE, clomiPRAMINE, prochlorperazine, promethazine

Drug Name	Sounds Like
Fanapt	Xanax
fluPHENAZine	fluvoxaMINE
Haldol	Halcion, Halog, Stadol
Iloperidone	domperidone
Invega	Intuniv
Latuda	Lantus
OLANZapine	olsalazine, QUEtiapine
Prochlorperazine	chlorproMAZINE
RisperDAL	lisinopril, reserpine, Restoril, rOPINIRole
RisperiDONE	reserpine, rOPINIRole
SEROquel	Desyrel, SEROquel XR, Serzone, SINEquan
Symbyax	Cymbalta
Thioridazine	thiothixene, Thorazine
Thiothixene	FLUoxetine, thioridazine
Ziprasidone	TraZODone
ZyPREXA	CeleXA, Reprexain, Zestril, ZyrTEC, Zelapar, zolpidem, zapelon

Drugs that look like a similar drug are noted in the Summary Drug Tables of each chapter.

INTERACTIONS

The following interactions may occur when an antipsychotic is administered with another agent:

Interacting Drug	Common Use	Effect of Interaction
Anticholinergic drugs	Management of gastrointestinal (GI) problems such as peptic ulcer disease	Increased risk for TD and psychotic symptoms
Immunologic drugs	Treatment of chronic illness such as cancer, arthritis, human immunodeficiency virus (HIV) infection	Increased severity of bone marrow suppression
Alcohol	Relaxation and enjoyment in social situations	Increased risk for central nervous system depression

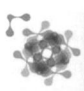

NURSING PROCESS—STEPS TO BUILDING CLINICAL JUDGMENT
Client Receiving an Antipsychotic Drug

ASSESSMENT

Preadministration Assessment

A client receiving an antipsychotic drug may be treated in the hospital or in an outpatient setting.

Objective data

• Description of dress, hygiene, and general appearance

• Observation of behavior during interview: poor eye contact, failure to answer questions completely, inappropriate answers to questions, a monotone speech pattern, and inappropriate laughter, sadness, or crying.

• Hands on assessment (e.g., vital signs) only if client allows

Frequently, clients in a psychotic episode do not perceive reality in the same manner as other clients and touch may be thought of as a threatening act against themselves instead of a therapeutic gesture as with other client populations. The client may strike out because of fear caused by the psychosis; therefore, touching can be perceived by the client as an aggressive gesture and should be avoided.

Subjective data

- Current history of symptoms, description of how the client reacts to environment (reaching out to or attending to stimuli not in the setting)
- Mental status: note the presence of both positive (**hallucinations** or **delusions**) and negative symptoms
- Self-report compared with family members for psychotic episodes, behavioral change or escalation of symptoms
- Coping mechanisms used to deal with psychosis, especially self-medicating with alcohol or drugs
- Medical, social, and mental health history
- *Assess the potential for self-harm or harm to others*

Some clients, such as those with controlled schizophrenia, do not require inpatient care. You may see these clients at periodic intervals in the mental health outpatient setting. The initial assessments of the outpatient are basically the same as those for the hospitalized client.

Ongoing Assessment

Many antipsychotic drugs are administered for a long time, which makes the ongoing assessment an important part of determining therapeutic drug effects and monitoring for adverse reactions, particularly EPS (see Box 22.2) and TD. Your role is important in the administration of these drugs in both the inpatient and clinic settings for the following reasons:

- The client's response to drug therapy on an inpatient basis requires around-the-clock assessments, because frequent dosage adjustments may be necessary during therapy.
- Accurate assessments for the appearance of adverse drug effects assume a greater importance when the client may be unable to verbalize physical changes to the primary health care provider or nursing staff.

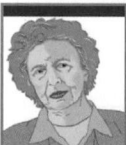

PHARMACOLOGY IN PRACTICE

ASSESSMENT

Before beginning antipsychotic drug therapy, a nurse is required to assess a client. Which of the following should the nurse record as deviations from normal behavior?
1. Shy or timid behavior
2. Brief replies to questions
3. Frequent laughter
4. Poor eye contact

NURSING DIAGNOSES

Drug-specific nursing diagnoses are the following:

- **Injury risk** related to hypotension or sedation

- **Impaired physical mobility** related to impaired motor ability
- **Infection risk** related to agranulocytosis
- **Hyperglycemia** related to medication and lifestyle

Nursing diagnoses related to drug administration are discussed in Chapter 4.

PLANNING

The expected outcomes for the client depend on the reason for drug administration but may include an optimal response to drug therapy, meeting of client needs related to management of adverse drug reactions, an absence of injury, and confidence in an understanding of the medication regimen.

IMPLEMENTATION

Promoting an Optimal Response to Therapy

You should develop a nursing care plan that helps to empower the client in dealing with the illness as well as meeting the client's individual needs.

Managing Care of the Inpatient

Notations of client behavioral patterns are written at periodic intervals (frequency depends on hospital or unit guidelines). An accurate description of the client's behavior aids the primary health care provider in planning therapy and thus becomes an important part of nursing management. Clients with a poor response to drug therapy may require dosage changes, a change to another psychotherapeutic drug, or the addition of other therapies to the treatment regimen. However, it is important to know that full response to antipsychotic drugs takes several weeks.

If the client's behavior is violent or aggressive, antipsychotic drugs may have to be given parenterally. You will require assistance in securing the client and should give the drugs intramuscularly (IM) in a large muscle mass, such as the gluteus muscle. Keep the client lying down (when possible) for about 30 min after administering the drug.

! NURSING ALERT

In combative clients or those who have serious manifestations of acute psychosis (e.g., hallucinations or loss of contact with reality), parenteral administration may be repeated every 1–4 hr until the desired effects are obtained. Monitor the client closely for cardiac arrhythmias or rhythm changes, or hypotension.

The practice of restrain and sedate is under review because it needs more personnel and may cause harm or injury to either or both the client and staff members (Zeller & Citrome, 2016). Instead, de-escalation approaches and the use of newer modes of drug delivery are being explored. Providing drugs in inhaled, sublingual, and intranasal formulations may be seen more frequently than injectables in situations of aggressive behaviors in the future (Zeller & Citrome, 2016).

Antipsychotic drugs are typically given as a single oral daily dose. Oral administration, especially in the long-term care setting, requires special attention, because some clients have difficulty swallowing (because of dry mouth or other causes). After administration of an oral drug, inspect the client's oral cavity to be sure the drug has been swallowed. If the client resists having their oral cavity checked, report this refusal to the primary health care provider.

Other clients may refuse to take the drug altogether. Never force a client to take an oral drug. If the client refuses the drug, and you cannot reason with the client to take the drug, contact the primary health care provider regarding this problem because parenteral administration of the medication may be necessary.

Oral liquid concentrates are available for clients who can more easily swallow a liquid. To aid in administration to debilitated or elderly clients, oral drugs can be mixed in liquids such as fruit juices, tomato juice, milk, or carbonated beverages. Semisolid foods, such as soups or puddings, may also be used.

Managing Care of the Outpatient

Great strides have been made in formulating drugs for extended time frames to better monitor and maintain medication compliance. Some clinics will offer clients the drug in an infrequent injection. Many clients are receptive to an injectable form when it is framed as reducing the need for hospitalization (because of compliance).

At the time of each visit of the client to the primary health care provider's office or the clinic, observe and document the client's behavior indicating a response to therapy. In some instances, you may question the client or a family member about the response to therapy. The questions asked depend on the client and the diagnosis, and may include:

- Are you feeling nervous or restless?
- Do you hear voices that others cannot hear?
- How is everything going?

You may need to rephrase questions or direct conversation toward other subjects until the client feels comfortable and is able to discuss therapy.

Ask the client or a family member about adverse drug reactions or any other problems occurring during therapy. Document in the client's record your observations of their outward behavior and any complaints or problems. Compare these notations with previous documentation of behavior. Any reactions or problems should be brought to the attention of the primary health care provider.

Monitoring and Managing Client Needs

The client may need to tolerate some adverse reactions, such as dry mouth, episodes of orthostatic hypotension, and drowsiness during drug therapy. Nursing interventions to relieve some of these reactions may include offering frequent sips of water, reminders or offering assistance to the client as they get out of the bed or chair, and supervising ambulatory activities.

Injury Risk

Antipsychotic drugs may cause extreme drowsiness and sedation, especially during the first or second week of therapy. This reaction may impair mental or physical abilities. The client may need assistance with activities of daily living because of the experience of extreme sedation.

This includes cueing or help with eating, dressing, and ambulating. If hypotension or sedation occurs with these drugs, administration at bedtime helps to minimize the risk of injury. During hypotensive episodes, if possible, it is important to monitor vital signs at least daily. Report any significant change in vital signs to the primary health care provider.

Drowsiness usually diminishes after 2 or 3 weeks of therapy. However, if the client continues to be troubled by drowsiness and sedation, the primary health care provider may decide to prescribe a lower dosage or different drug.

Impaired Physical Mobility

Clients can experience mobility problems if EPS occurs while taking the antipsychotic drugs. Extrapyramidal effects include muscular spasms of the face and neck, the inability to sleep or sit still, tremors, rigidity, or involuntary rhythmic movements. During initial therapy or whenever the dosage is increased or decreased, observe the client closely for adverse drug reactions to prevent the development of EPS and TD. You will want to use a standardized tool, such as the Abnormal Involuntary Movement Scale, to screen the client for symptoms (Box 22.3) and any behavioral changes. Because these adverse effects are considered "late stage," be alert to their presence. Report immediately to the primary health care provider any change in behavior or the appearance of adverse reactions. An immediate decrease in dosage will not change the condition but may prevent further deterioration of the client.

! NURSING ALERT

Because there is no known treatment for TD and it is irreversible in clients, immediately report symptoms. These include rhythmic, involuntary movements of the tongue, face, mouth, jaw, or extremities.

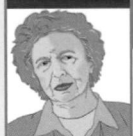

PHARMACOLOGY IN PRACTICE

MANAGING NEEDS
Which of the following are symptoms of tardive dyskinesia (TD) that the nurse should report immediately?
1. Dry feeling in mouth
2. Rhythmic facial movements
3. Orthostatic hypotension
4. Lethargy or drowsiness

Infection Risk

The use of the drug clozapine has been associated with severe **agranulocytosis**, or decreased white blood cell (WBC) count. This bone marrow suppression can make the client more susceptible to illness and infection. To ensure close monitoring for this adverse reaction, clozapine is available only through a client management system (a program that combines WBC testing, client monitoring, and pharmacy and drug distribution services). Only a 1-week supply of this drug is dispensed at a time. A weekly WBC count is done throughout therapy and for 4 weeks after therapy is discontinued. In addition, teach

BOX 22.3 Abnormal Involuntary Movement Scale Screening Tool

Client identification: _____ Date: _____
Rated by: _____

1. Either before or after completing the examination procedure, observe the client unobtrusively at rest (e.g., in waiting room).
2. The chair to be used in this examination should be a hard, firm one without arms.
3. After observing the client, they may be rated on a scale of 0 (none), 1 (minimal), 2 (mild), 3 (moderate), and 4 (severe) according to the severity of symptoms.
4. Ask the client whether there is anything in their teeth (i.e., gum, candy) and, if there is, to remove it.
5. Ask client about the current condition of their teeth. Ask client if they wear dentures. Do teeth or dentures bother client now?
6. Ask client whether they notice any movement in mouth, face, hands, or feet. If yes, ask to describe and to what extent the movements currently bother client or interfere with their activities.

0	1	2	3	4	Ask Client to tap thumb with each finger as rapidly as possible for 10–15 seconds, separately with right hand, then with left hand. (Observe facial and leg movements.)
0	1	2	3	4	Flex and extend client's left and right arms (one at a time).
0	1	2	3	4	ᵃAsk client to stand up. (Observe in profile. Observe all body areas again, hips included.)
0	1	2	3	4	Have client sit in chair with hands on knees, legs slightly apart, and feet flat on floor (look at entire body for movements while in this position).
0	1	2	3	4	Ask client to sit with hands hanging unsupported: if male, hands between legs; if female and wearing a dress, hands hanging over knees. (Observe hands and other body areas.)
0	1	2	3	4	Ask client to open mouth. (Observe tongue at rest within mouth.) Do this twice.
0	1	2	3	4	Ask client to protrude tongue. (Observe abnormalities of tongue movement.) Do this twice.
0	1	2	3	4	Ask client to extend both arms outstretched in front with palms down. (Observe trunk, legs, and mouth.)
0	1	2	3	4	ᵃHave client walk a few paces, turn, and walk back to chair. (Observe hands and gait.) Do this twice.

ᵃActivated movements.

the client to monitor for signs or symptoms indicating bone marrow suppression: lethargy, weakness, fever, sore throat, malaise, mucous membrane ulceration, or "flu-like" complaints.

Another issue with the medication clozapine is extreme constipation. As the dosage is increased so is the severity of adverse reactions to where serious bowel complications (e.g., necrotizing colitis) can occur. This is especially true when medications slowing GI motility (opioids, anticholinergics) are also being taken. Assessment and routine monitoring of bowel function should occur and possible prophylactic laxative treatment may be required.

Hyperglycemia

The tendency for diabetes and its risk factors (see Chapter 40) is greater for those clients with serious mental illness. These risk factors can include sedentary lifestyle, diet, or other factors such as obesity. The administration of atypical antipsychotic (SGA) drugs with the adverse reaction of weight gain can put the client at higher risk of acquiring type 2 diabetes (clozapine and olanzapine users gain the most weight). Before starting treatment with an SGA, the client should be weighed and a family history documented to indicate type 2 diabetes risk. Laboratory work for fasting blood sugar, total and low-density lipoprotein (LDL) cholesterol, and triglycerides should be taken and compared at periodic intervals.

Educating the Client and Family

Adherence to routine medication use is a problem with some clients once they are discharged. It is important to evaluate accurately the client's ability to assume responsibility for continuing to take the drugs. Some clients will have the benefit of family for assistance; others do not. The client should feel confident in understanding that the drug has the benefit of reducing positive and negative symptoms. Also, reporting adverse reactions allows the primary health care provider to modify the doses to reduce problems while the client still benefits from the drug.

As you develop a teaching plan for the client or family member, include the following points:

- Keep all primary care provider and clinic appointments, because close monitoring of therapy is essential.
- Report any unusual changes or physical effects to the primary health care provider.
- Take the drug exactly as directed. Do not increase, decrease, or omit a dose or discontinue use of this drug unless directed to do so by the primary health care provider.
- Do not drive or perform other hazardous tasks if drowsiness occurs.
- Do not take any nonprescription drug unless use of a specific drug has been approved by the primary health care provider.
- Inform physicians, dentists, and other medical personnel of therapy with this drug.
  - 🍷 Do not drink alcoholic beverages unless approval is obtained from the primary health care provider.
- If dizziness occurs when changing position, rise slowly when getting out of bed or a chair. If dizziness is severe, always have help when changing positions.

- To relieve dry mouth, take frequent sips of water, suck on hard candy, or chew gum (preferably sugarless).
- Notify your primary health care provider if you become pregnant or intend to become pregnant during therapy.
- Immediately report the occurrence of the following adverse reactions: restlessness, inability to sit still, muscle spasms, mask-like expression, rigidity, tremors, drooling, or involuntary rhythmic movements of the mouth, face, or extremities.
- Avoid exposure to the sun. If exposure is unavoidable, wear sunblock, keep arms and legs covered, and wear a sun hat.
- Report increased thirst, urination, and weight gain to the primary health care provider.
- Note that only a 1-week supply of clozapine is dispensed at a time. The drug is obtained through a special program designed to ensure the required blood monitoring. Weekly WBC laboratory tests are required. Immediately report any signs of weakness, fever, sore throat, malaise, or flu-like symptoms to the primary health care provider.
- Note that olanzapine is available as a disintegrating tablet. If using the orally disintegrating tablet, peel back the foil on the blister packaging. Using dry hands, remove the tablet, and place the entire tablet in the mouth. The tablet will disintegrate immediately with or without liquid.

EVALUATION

- Therapeutic effect is achieved and psychotic behavior is decreased.
- Adverse reactions are identified, reported to the primary health care provider, and managed successfully through appropriate nursing interventions:
  - No evidence of injury is seen.
  - Client maintains adequate mobility.
  - No evidence of infection is seen.
  - Blood glucose levels remain stable.
- Client and family express confidence and demonstrate an understanding of the drug regimen.

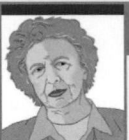

PHARMACOLOGY IN PRACTICE

USING CLINICAL REASONING

The behaviors described by Mrs. Moore's daughter could be considered positive symptoms of a psychotic disorder. Are there other reasons or conditions that might be causing her to exhibit these behaviors? Mrs. Moore has been diagnosed with dementia and heart failure. From the information you learned, what class of drug is Seroquel, are there indications here for its use, and are there contraindications based on her history? If this drug is prescribed, what assessments need to be done on an ongoing basis?

KEY POINTS

■ Psychosis is a spectrum of mood and behaviors, with schizophrenia being the most recognized. Symptoms of the disease are categorized as positive and negative. Antipsychotic medications are designed to diminish the behaviors so people can function in society.

■ First-generation (conventional) antipsychotics alleviate the positive symptoms such as agitation, delusions, and hallucinations. The newer second-generation (atypical) drugs reduce the negative symptoms—those that have an impact on affect, communication, initiative, thinking, and feeling.

■ These drugs reduce the amount of dopamine for neurotransmission. Sometimes the reduction is too much, which results in extrapyramidal symptoms. If the medications are not stopped TD (an irreversible disorder) can result. The atypical medications affect both dopamine and serotonin, and EPS reactions are fewer.

■ Although second-generation (atypical) antipsychotics have fewer extrapyramidal symptom reactions, caution needs to be exercised with clients with dementia because of the relationship between stroke and mortality. In addition, the weight gain and other factors may predispose an individual to type 2 diabetes.

■ Most medications need 6–10 weeks to demonstrate effect on the disorder. Unfortunately, adverse reactions begin much earlier; therefore, clients struggle with unpleasant symptoms of the disorder or reactions from the drugs. A revolving cycle of lack of adherence to therapy and rehospitalization occurs, called *recidivism*.

SUMMARY DRUG TABLE
Antipsychotic Drugs

Generic Name	Trade Name	Uses	Adverse Reactions	Dosage Ranges
First-Generation Antipsychotics (Conventional)				
chlorproMAZINE *klor-PROE-ma-zeen*		Psychotic disorders, nausea, vomiting, intractable hiccoughs	Hypotension, drowsiness, TD, nasal congestion, dry mouth, dystonia, EPS, behavioral changes, photosensitivity	Psychiatric disorders: up to 400 mg/day orally in divided doses Nausea and vomiting: 10–25 mg orally, 25–50 mg IM, 50–100 mg rectally
fluPHENAZine *floo-FEN-a-zeen*		Psychotic disorders	Drowsiness, tachycardia, EPS, dystonia, akathisia, hypotension	0.5–10.0 mg/day orally in divided doses, up to 20 mg/day; 1.25–10.0 mg/day IM in divided doses
haloperidol *ha-loe-PER-i-dole*	Haldol	Psychotic disorders, Tourette syndrome, hyperactivity, behavior problems in children	EPS, akathisia, dystonia, TD, drowsiness, headache, dry mouth, orthostatic hypotension	0.5–5.0 mg orally BID or TID with dosage up to 100 mg/day in divided doses; 2–5 mg IM Children: 0.05–0.075 mg/kg/day orally
loxapine *LOKS-a-peen*	Adasuve	Psychotic disorders	EPS, akathisia, dystonia, TD, drowsiness, headache, dry mouth, orthostatic hypotension	10–100 mg/day orally, not to exceed 250 mg/day
molindone *moe-LIN-done*		Psychotic disorders	EPS, akathisia, dystonia, TD, drowsiness, headache, dry mouth, orthostatic hypotension	50–75 mg/day orally, not to exceed 225 mg/day
perphenazine *per-FEN-a-zeen*		Psychotic disorders	Hypotension, postural hypotension, TD, photophobia, urticaria, nasal congestion, dry mouth, akathisia, dystonia, pseudoparkinsonism, behavioral changes, headache, photosensitivity	4–16 mg orally 2–4 times/day
pimozide *PI-moe-zide*		Tourette syndrome	Parkinson-like symptoms, motor restlessness, dystonia, oculogyric crisis, TD, dry mouth, diarrhea, headache, rash, drowsiness	Initial dose: 1–2 mg/day orally Maintenance dose: up to 10 mg/day orally
prochlorperazine *proe-klor-PER-a-zeen*		Psychotic disorders, nausea, vomiting, anxiety	EPS, sedation, TD, dry eyes, blurred vision, constipation, dry mouth, photosensitivity	Psychotic disorders: up to 150 mg orally, 10–20 mg IM Nausea, vomiting: 15–40 mg/day orally in divided doses Anxiety: 5 mg orally TID
thioridazine *thye-oh-RID-a-zeen*		Schizophrenia	Cardiac arrhythmias, drowsiness, TD, nausea, dry mouth, constipation, diarrhea	50–100 mg orally TID, not to exceed 800 mg/day
thiothixene *thye-oh-THIKS-een*		Schizophrenia	EPS, drowsiness, nausea, diarrhea, TD	6–30 mg/day orally, not to exceed 60 mg/day
trifluoperazine *trye-floo-oh-PER-a-zeen*		Psychotic disorders, anxiety	Drowsiness, pseudoparkinsonism, dystonia, akathisia, TD, photophobia, blurred vision, dry mouth, salivation, nasal congestion, nausea, discolored urine (pink to red-brown)	Psychosis: 4–20 mg/day orally in divided doses Anxiety: 1–2 mg orally BID

Continued

SUMMARY DRUG TABLE (continued)
Antipsychotic Drugs

Generic Name	Trade Name	Uses	Adverse Reactions	Dosage Ranges
Second Generation Antipsychotics (Atypical)				
ARIPiprazole *ay-ri-PIP-ray-zole*	Abilify	Schizophrenia, manic phase of bipolar disorders	Agitation, akathisia, anxiety, drowsiness, headache, constipation, dry mouth, nausea	10–30 mg/day orally
asenapine *a-SEN-a-peen*	Saphris, Secuado (TD)	Schizophrenia, manic phase of bipolar disorders	Agitation, akathisia, anxiety, drowsiness, headache, constipation, dry mouth, nausea	5–10 mg orally twice daily, TD 24-hr patch
brexpiprazole *breks-PIP-ray-zole*	Rexulti	Schizophrenia, agitation of dementia, major depressive disorder	Restlessness, weight gain	0.5–4.0 mg orally daily
cariprazine *kar-IP-ra-zeen*	Vraylar	Schizophrenia, major depressive disorder	Agitation, akathisia, anxiety, drowsiness, headache, constipation, dry mouth, nausea	1.5–6.0 mg orally daily
cloZAPine *KLOE-za-peen*	Clozaril, FazaClo	Severely ill schizophrenic clients with no response to other therapies	Drowsiness, sedation, akathisia, tachycardia, nausea, agranulocytosis, constipation	Initial dose: 25–50 mg/day, titrate up to 300–400 mg/day orally, not to exceed 900 mg/day
iloperidone *eye-loe-PER-i-done*	Fanapt	Schizophrenia	Agitation, dizziness, nervousness, akathisia, constipation, weight gain	12 mg twice daily orally
lumateperone *loo-ma-TE-per-one*	Caplyta	Schizophrenia	Drowsiness, sedation, dizziness, EPS, nausea	42 mg/day orally
lurasidone *loo-RAS-i-done*	Latuda	Schizophrenia	Somnolence, nervousness, akathisia, nausea, weight gain	40–80 mg/day orally
OLANZapine *oh-LAN-za-peen*	ZyPREXA	Schizophrenia, short-term treatment of manic episodes of bipolar disorder	Agitation, dizziness, nervousness, akathisia, constipation, fever, weight gain	5–20 mg/day orally
paliperidone *pal-ee-PER-i-done*	Invega	Psychotic disorders	Dizziness, weakness, headache, dry mouth, increased saliva, weight gain, stomach pain	6–12 mg/day orally
pimavanserin *pim-a-VAN-ser-in*	Nuplazid	Psychosis associated with Parkinson disease	Nausea, peripheral edema	34 mg/day orally
QUEtiapine *kwe-TYE-a-peen*	SEROquel	Psychotic disorders, manic episodes of bipolar disorder	Orthostatic hypotension, dizziness, vertigo, nausea, constipation, dry mouth, diarrhea, headache, restlessness, blurred vision	150–750 mg/day orally in divided doses
risperiDONE *ris-PER-i-done*	RisperDAL, Perseris	Psychotic disorders; adolescent schizophrenia and mania	Agitation, dizziness, nervousness, akathisia, constipation, fever, weight gain	1–3 mg orally BID; adolescents: 0.5–6.0 mg orally once daily
ziprasidone *zi-PRAS-i-done*	Geodon	Schizophrenia, bipolar mania, acute agitation	Somnolence, drowsiness, sedation, headache, arrhythmias, dyspepsia, fever, constipation, EPS	80 mg orally BID
aripiprazole lauroxil	Aristada	Schizophrenia	Same as aripiprazole	IM dosing to titrate to oral aripiprazole
olanzapine/fluoxetine	Symbyax	Bipolar depressive episodes	Same as olanzapine	6-mg/25-mg combination tablet taken in the evening orally

CHAPTER REVIEW

Know Your Drugs

Clients sometimes know a medication by the brand (or trade) name and not the generic name. To help you recognize both names, match the brand name with the generic name of the same medication.

Generic Name	Brand Name
1. clozapine	A. Clozaril
2. haloperidol	B. Geodon
3. risperidone	C. Haldol
4. zipraidone	D. Risperdal

Calculate Medication Dosages

1. A client is prescribed quetiapine (Seroquel) 100 mg BID. The drug is available in 50-mg tablets. The nurse would administer _____.

2. An agitated client is prescribed haloperidol 3 mg now. The drug is available in a 5 mg/1 mL preloaded syringe. How many milliliters will be administered?

Prepare for the NCLEX

RECALL THE FACTS

1. Schizophrenia involves an overabundance of which neurotransmitter?
   1. acetylcholine
   2. dopamine
   3. norepinephrine
   4. serotonin

2. Which of the following is a negative symptom associated with schizophrenia?
   1. hallucinations
   2. delusions
   3. flat affect
   4. agitation

3. History of which disease is significant when administering a second-generation antipsychotic?
   1. hypertension
   2. liver failure
   3. type 2 diabetes
   4. cardiac failure

4. Which of the following behaviors would the nurse expect to see in a client experiencing TD?
   1. muscle rigidity, dry mouth, insomnia
   2. rhythmic, involuntary movements of the tongue, face, mouth, or jaw
   3. muscle weakness, paralysis of the eyelids, diarrhea
   4. dyspnea, somnolence, muscle spasms

5. Which of the following drugs is least likely to produce extrapyramidal effects?
   1. chlorpromazine
   2. haloperidol
   3. fluphenazine
   4. risperidone

ANALYZE THE FACTS

6. *A client taking fluphenazine for schizophrenia is also prescribed an antiparkinson drug. What is the best explanation for adding an antiparkinson drug to the regimen?
   1. prevents severe allergic reaction from sun exposure
   2. promotes the effects of fluphenazine
   3. reduces fine tremors, muscle rigidity, and slow movement
   4. decreases hallucinations and delusions

7. *As a nurse on a mental health unit, you are ordering weekly lab draws for morning rounds. Three clients are taking the drug clozapine. Which of the following labs should be drawn on these clients?
   1. fasting blood glucose
   2. LDL
   3. complete blood count
   4. amylase

8. The nurse is leading a medication support group. Which is the best statement to make when a client says the drugs don't work?
   1. "They won't work if you don't take them."
   2. "I know it is hard to keep taking the medicine when you can't readily see the effects."
   3. "That's not appropriate to say in front of everyone else here."
   4. "Statements like that give me a headache."

ALTERNATE-FORMAT QUESTIONS

9. When administering a second-generation antipsychotic to a client, the nurse would most likely expect which diagnostic test(s) to be prescribed? **Select all that apply.**
   1. complete blood count
   2. fasting blood glucose levels
   3. cholesterol levels
   4. electrolyte analysis

10. Match the drug with its generation category:

1. Conventional (first generation)	A. aripiprazole
2. Atypical (second generation)	B. chlorpromazine
	C. Geodon
	D. quetiapine
	E. Zyprexa

To check your answers, see Appendix F.

---

*Indicates the question is directly linked to the NCLEX-PN test plan in Appendix G.

WANT TO KNOW MORE? A wide variety of resources are available to enhance your learning and understanding of this chapter.

- Visit thePoint for resources such as:
  - NCLEX-Style Student Review Questions
  - Journal Articles
  - Dosage Calculations
  - Drug Monographs
  - Watch and Learn Videos
  - Concepts in Action Animations
- The *Study Guide to Accompany Introductory Clinical Pharmacology*, 12th edition, sold separately, will help you review and apply essential content.
- √PrepU is available to help students prepare for the NCLEX-PN examination.

UNIT 5
Drugs That Affect the Peripheral Nervous System

Neurotransmission is a very complex concept and is key to how many drugs work in the body. In Unit 4, you learned how drugs almost exclusively affect the neurotransmitters working in the brain. In this unit you will come to better understand the nervous system as a whole and how drugs are used to enhance or block the nerve impulses as they travel through the rest of the body. To help you understand the complexity of the nervous system, think of it as a telephone system. Although many use a cell phone exclusively, think of our nerves like the landline telephone you may remember from your grandparents' or parents' homes. Our nerves are akin to long telephone wires that connect the brain to all parts of our body. When you make a call, a signal is sent over a series of wires to another person. When the person you are calling picks up the phone and answers, it begins a series of conversations back and forth across that telephone line. Our nervous system network is as complex as telephone lines. Someone can call and connect with many different houses. Some calls might be a friendly reminder of an event; others are an urgent call for help.

What is different in our bodies than the telephone system is that the pathway is not one long wire; rather it is like a series of wire segments that traverse your body. At the end of every nerve is a terminal end, and the message has to "jump" across the gap (or synapse) to a receptor on the beginning of the next nerve in the path. Substances called neurotransmitters are the elements that cross the synapse to keep the message conduction going. This synaptic area is where many of the drugs work.

Now that you can visualize the telephone network, think about this as we discuss the neural network. When one of our senses is stimulated (taste, see, smell, feel), a message is sent to the brain over a series of nerve pathways called the *afferent nerves* (the incoming pathway). The nerve message is processed by the brain and then a command message is sent via the *efferent nerves* from the brain to the various organs or tissues of the body where an action is carried out (outgoing pathway).

The peripheral nervous system (PNS) is a complex network of nerves from the spinal cord to the organs and other body structures. The PNS is divided into two branches: the somatic nervous system and the autonomic nervous system. The somatic branch of the PNS is concerned with sensation and voluntary movement. This sensory part of the somatic nervous system is covered in Unit 6. Briefly, in the somatic branch, messages are sent to the brain concerning the internal and external environment, such as sensations of heat, pain, cold, and pressure. The outgoing message in the somatic nervous system is concerned with the voluntary movement of skeletal muscles, such as those used in walking, talking, or chewing food.

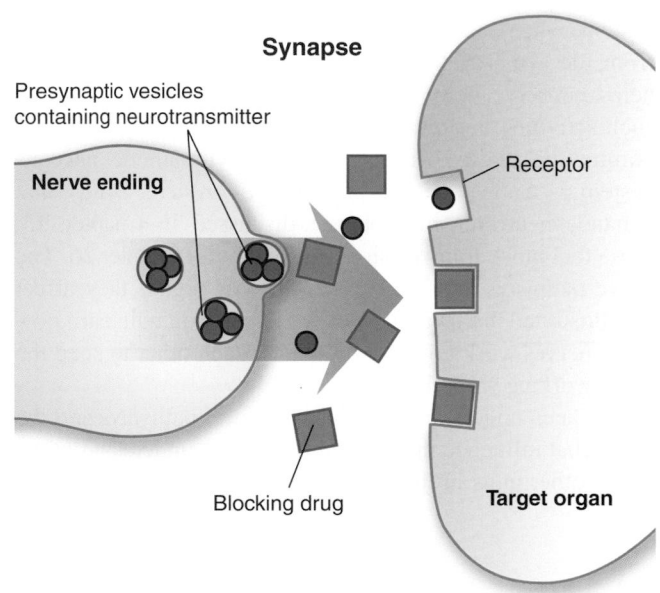

Chapters in this unit focus on drugs that affect the autonomic branch of the peripheral nerves. The autonomic branch of the PNS is concerned with functions essential to the survival of the organism. Functional activity of the autonomic nervous system is not controlled consciously (i.e., the activity is automatic). This system controls blood pressure, heart rate, gastrointestinal activity, and glandular secretions.

A clear understanding of the autonomic branch makes learning about these drugs much easier. The autonomic nervous system is divided into the sympathetic and the parasympathetic branches. The chapters of this unit follow the structure of the autonomic system, enhancing and blocking of the sympathetic branch, then enhancing and blocking the parasympathetic side. These two branches work as opposites to each other to make the body function properly. The sympathetic branch tends to regulate the expenditure of energy and activates when the organism is confronted with stressful situations. The language used to describe both systems and drugs can be confusing. The sympathetic system is also called the *adrenergic branch.* Repetition of terms will thread through all the chapters to help you understand these concepts. Chapter 23 discusses drugs that mimic the effects of the sympathetic system—the adrenergic drugs. Again, these drugs have an impact on many different body systems and organs; therefore, the focus of Chapter 23 is on the drugs used in the prevention (responding to allergic reactions) and the treatment of shock. Drugs that block or inhibit the system are called *antiadrenergic drugs, adrenergic blocking drugs,* or *sympatholytics.* One of the major body systems affected by adrenergic blocking drugs is the heart and vascular system. Some of the drugs used to treat hypertension are featured in Chapter 24.

The parasympathetic branch of the autonomic nervous system, when activated, attempts to do the opposite actions from the sympathetic branch. The parasympathetic branch helps conserve body energy and is partly responsible for such activities as slowing the heart rate, digesting food, and eliminating bodily wastes. The parasympathetic nervous system is known as the *cholinergic branch.* Drugs that enhance neurotransmission are discussed in Chapter 25; those that block transmission are covered in Chapter 26. The nerve pathways and the body tissues or organs they affect are illustrated in this unit. In each chapter you will learn how these nerves work together or against each other to keep the body working smoothly.

A keen understanding of these neural pathways and the drugs that influence them make it easier to understand many of the other units in this text.

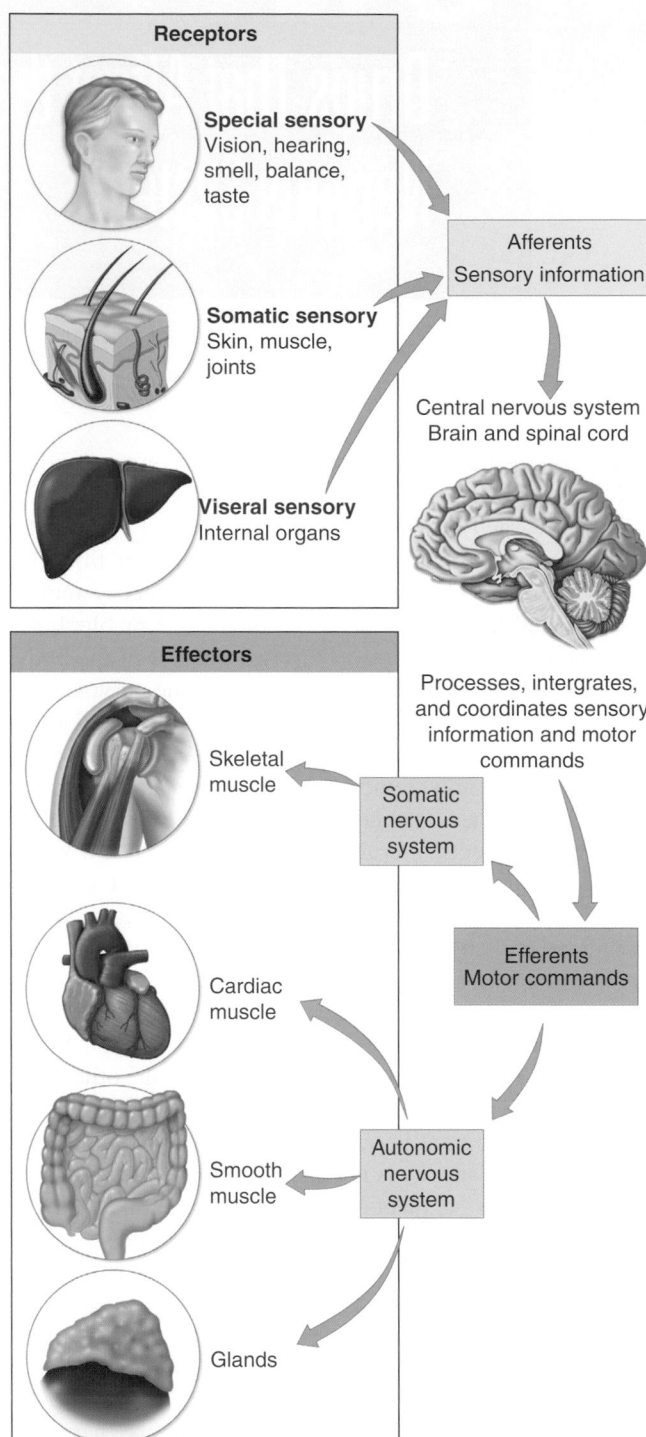

23

Adrenergic Drugs

Key Terms

adrenergic pertaining to the sympathetic branch of the nervous system, which controls heart rate, breathing rate, and the ability to divert blood to the skeletal muscles

autonomic nervous system (ANS) division of the peripheral nervous system concerned with functions essential to the life of the organism and not consciously controlled (e.g., blood pressure, heart rate, gastrointestinal activity)

catecholamine neurotransmitters that are released during the body's stress response and include norepinephrine, epinephrine, and dopamine

extravasation escape of fluid from a blood vessel into surrounding tissue

neurotransmitter chemical substances released at the nerve ending that facilitate the transmission of nerve impulses

norepinephrine neurotransmitter that transmits impulses across the sympathetic branch of the autonomic nervous system

parasympathetic pertaining to the part of the autonomic nervous system concerned with conserving body energy (i.e., slowing the heart rate, digesting food, and eliminating waste)

peripheral nervous system (PNS) all nerves outside of brain and spinal cord

shock inadequate blood flow to the bodily tissues

stroke volume the volume of blood ejected (leaving) from a ventricle at each heart beat

sympathetic pertaining to the sympathetic nervous system

sympathomimetic drugs that mimic the actions of the sympathetic nervous system; see *adrenergic*

vasopressors drugs that raise the blood pressure

Learning Objectives

On completion of this chapter, the student will:

1. Discuss the activity of the autonomic nervous system, specifically the sympathetic branch.
2. Compare and contrast the types of shock, physiologic responses of shock, and the use of adrenergic drugs in the treatment of shock.
3. Explain the uses, general drug actions, contraindications, precautions, interactions, and adverse reactions associated with the administration of adrenergic vasopressor drugs.
4. Distinguish important preadministration and ongoing assessment activities the nurse should perform on the client taking an adrenergic drug.
5. List nursing diagnoses particular to a client taking an adrenergic drug.
6. Examine ways to promote an optimal response to therapy, how to manage common adverse reactions, and important points to keep in mind when educating clients about the use of adrenergic drugs.

 Drug Classes

Adrenergic (sympathomimetics)
Short-acting beta$_2$ (β_2) agonists
Long-acting β_2 agonists
Optic agents (alpha$_2$ agonists/sympathomimetics)

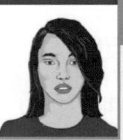 **PHARMACOLOGY IN PRACTICE**

Janna Wong is brought into the clinic by her mother. Yesterday she was in the yard and came into the house crying after being stung by a bee. Later in the evening she complained of itching around her throat and what Janna called a "fat tongue." As you read this chapter, think about what type of reaction this might have been.

The portion of the **peripheral nervous system (PNS)** studied in Unit 5 (Chapters 23–26) is a system of nerves that *automatically* regulates bodily functions; hence, it is called the **autonomic nervous system (ANS)**. Concepts such as this will be repeated many times in this unit to help solidify your understanding of how important the nervous system is to drug action. The ANS is divided into two branches: the **sympathetic** and the **parasympathetic**. This chapter focuses on the sympathetic branch, which is regulated by involuntary control. In other

281

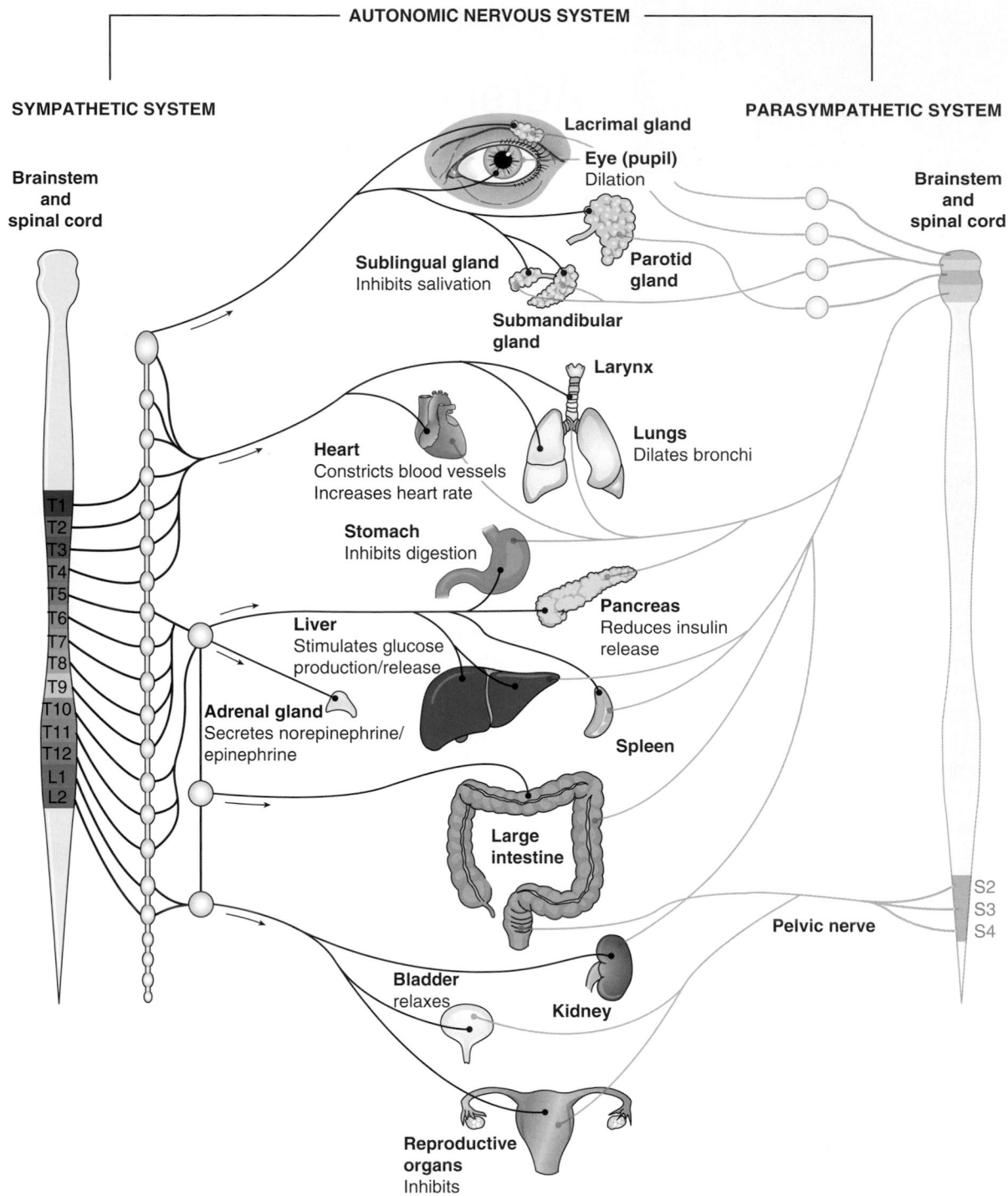

AUTONOMIC NERVOUS SYSTEM

SYMPATHETIC SYSTEM

PARASYMPATHETIC SYSTEM

Brainstem and spinal cord

Brainstem and spinal cord

Lacrimal gland

Eye (pupil)
Dilation

Sublingual gland
Inhibits salivation

Parotid gland

Submandibular gland

Larynx

Lungs
Dilates bronchi

Heart
Constricts blood vessels
Increases heart rate

Stomach
Inhibits digestion

Pancreas
Reduces insulin release

Liver
Stimulates glucose production/release

Adrenal gland
Secretes norepinephrine/epinephrine

Spleen

T1 T2 T3 T4 T5 T6 T7 T8 T9 T10 T11 T12 L1 L2

Large intestine

S2 S3 S4

Pelvic nerve

Bladder
relaxes

Kidney

Reproductive organs
Inhibits

FIGURE 23.1 Bodily responses to stimulation of the sympathetic nervous system cause organ responses shown here. (Adapted from Cohen, B. J. (2003). *Medical terminology* (4th ed.). Lippincott Williams & Wilkins.)

words, a person does not have willful control over what this system does. Activation of this branch is often called the *fight, flight,* or *freeze response.* These nerves are stimulated when the body is confronted with stressful situations, such as danger, intense emotion, or severe illness. The sympathetic branch controls a person's heart rate, breathing rate, and ability to divert blood to the skeletal muscles—for example, to enable a person to run (the flight response). Figure 23.1

illustrates autonomic pathways to specific organs of the body and highlights how the organs respond when the sympathetic branch stimulates those organs throughout the body.

AUTONOMIC TERMINOLOGY

Catecholamine is a term used for the natural neurohormone or **neurotransmitter** produced when the body is stressed.

BOX 23.1	Demystifying the Autonomic Nervous System—Sympathetic Branch	
Terminology		**Clue to Remembering**
Anatomic name	Sympathetic	*Sympathetic* to your plight
Functional name	Adrenergic	Like *adrenalin*, speeds it up
Primary neurotransmitter	Norepinephrine	Precursor to *epinephrine (adrenalin)*

Norepinephrine (produced in the medulla of the adrenal gland) is the primary naturally produced neurotransmitter. Other neurotransmitters include epinephrine and dopamine. To make it easier to remember and understand, Box 23.1 illustrates ways to remember the naming of various components of the sympathetic branch. Norepinephrine is the primary neurotransmitter in the sympathetic branch of the autonomic nervous system and the substance that keeps the nerve message (or impulse) going from the brain to the target organ. Because this system is activated by norepinephrine, which is the precursor of epinephrine (also called adrenalin), another term for the sympathetic pathway is the **adrenergic** branch. Therefore, the medicines used that work like the adrenergic branch are termed adrenergic drugs.

In the sympathetic branch of the autonomic nervous system, adrenergic drugs produce activity similar to the neurotransmitter norepinephrine. Another name for these drugs is **sympathomimetic** (i.e., mimicking the actions of the sympathetic nervous system) drugs. The adrenergic drugs produce pharmacologic effects similar to the effects that occur in the body when the sympathetic nerves (norepinephrine) and the adrenal gland medulla (epinephrine) are stimulated. Because these all have a similar structure, they are called catecholamine to reflect that likeness to each other. The primary effects of these drugs occur on the heart, the blood vessels, and the smooth muscles, such as the bronchi of the lungs. These terms may be very confusing; taking the time to understand the nervous system and the names associated will make learning about the drugs and their effects easier. Refer to Box 23.2 for a better understanding of the adrenergic class of drugs.

BOX 23.2	More Variation on Drug Classes

Drug terminology to help you understand the drug class differences:

Adrenergic system = sympathetic branch of the autonomic nervous system

Adrenergic drugs = sympatho*mimetic* drugs (to mimic transmission of the sympathetic nerve)

Adrenergic blocker drugs = sympatho*lytic* drugs (to stop the transmission of the sympathetic nerve)

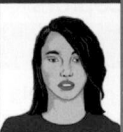

PHARMACOLOGY IN PRACTICE

DRUG RECOGNITION
Drugs that produce activity similar to the neurotransmitter norepinephrine are known as which of the following?
1. Sympatholytics
2. Antiadrenergic drugs
3. Sympathomimetics
4. Anticholinergic drugs

ACTIONS

The purpose of stimulating the sympathetic (adrenergic) nerves is to divert blood flow to the vital organs so that the body can deal with a stressful situation (the fight, flight, or freeze response). In general, adrenergic (sympathomimetic) drugs produce one or more of the following responses in varying degrees (see Fig. 23.1):

- Central nervous system—wakefulness, quick reaction to stimuli, quickened reflexes
- Autonomic nervous system—relaxation of the smooth muscles of the bronchi, constriction of blood vessels and sphincters of the stomach, dilation of coronary blood vessels, decrease in gastric motility
- Heart—increase in the heart rate
- Metabolism—increased use of glucose (sugar) and liberation of fatty acids from adipose tissue

Receptor Selectivity

The degree to which any organ is affected by the sympathetic nervous system depends on which postsynaptic nerve receptor sites are activated (Fig. 23.2). Adrenergic nerves have either alpha (α) or beta (β) receptors. Drugs that act on the receptors are called *selective* or *nonselective*. Adrenergic drugs may be selective (act on alpha receptors or beta receptors

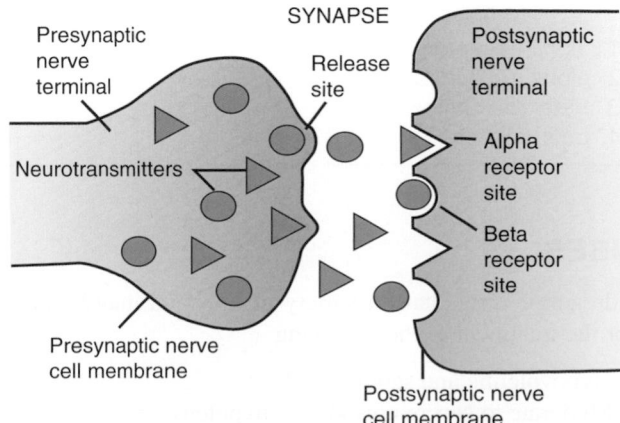

FIGURE 23.2 Neurotransmitter (e.g., norepinephrine) is released by the presynaptic nerve, crosses the synapse, and binds with alpha and beta receptors in the cell membrane of the postsynaptic nerve, continuing the transmission of the nerve impulse.

TABLE 23.1 Effects of the Adrenergic Receptors

RECEPTOR	SITE	EFFECT
Alpha$_1$	Peripheral blood vessels	Vasoconstriction of peripheral blood vessels
Alpha$_2$	Presynaptic neuron	Regulates release of neurotransmitters; decreases tone, motility, and secretions of gastrointestinal tract
Beta$_1$	Myocardium	Increased heart rate, increased force of myocardial contraction
Beta$_2$	Peripheral blood vessels	Vasodilation of peripheral vessels
	Bronchial smooth muscles	Bronchodilation

only) or nonselective (act on both alpha and beta receptors). For example, isoproterenol acts chiefly on beta receptors; therefore, it is considered a selective drug. Epinephrine is a nonselective drug because it does not act on (*select*) only one receptor; it acts on both alpha and beta receptors.

Whether an adrenergic drug acts on only alpha or beta, or alpha and beta receptors accounts for the variation of responses seen with this group of drugs. Table 23.1 lists the type of adrenergic nerve receptor that corresponds with each action of the autonomic nervous system on the body. The alpha and beta receptors can be further grouped as alpha$_1$ (α_1)- and alpha$_2$ (α_2)-adrenergic receptors and beta$_1$ (β_1)- and beta$_2$ (β_2)-adrenergic receptors. Compare this with the organ groups illustrated in Figure 23.1 to help you learn the connection between specific receptors and select drugs.

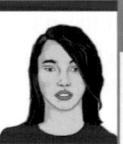

PHARMACOLOGY IN PRACTICE

PHYSIOLOGY

Which of the following adrenergic receptors is responsible for increased heart rate and increased force of myocardial contraction?
1. alpha$_1$ receptors
2. alpha$_2$ receptors
3. beta$_2$ receptors
4. beta$_1$ receptors

USES

Adrenergic drugs have a variety of uses and may be given for the treatment of the following:

- Hypovolemic and septic **shock**
- Moderate to severe episodes of hypotension
- Control of superficial bleeding during surgical and dental procedures of the mouth, nose, throat, and skin
- Cardiac decompensation and arrest
- Allergic reactions (anaphylactic shock, angioneurotic edema)

TABLE 23.2 Respiratory and Ophthalmic Sympathomimetics

GENERIC DRUG NAMES	BRAND DRUG NAMES
Short-Acting Beta$_2$ Agonists (SABAs—Used for Acute Respiratory Symptom Relief)^a	
albuterol	Proventil, Ventolin
epinephrine	Adrenalin
levalbuterol	Xopenex
metaproterenol	
terbutaline	
Long-Acting Beta$_2$ Agonists (LABAs—Used for Long-Term Respiratory Management)^a	
arformoterol	Brovana
formoterol	Foradil
indacaterol	Arcapta
salmeterol	Serevent Diskus
Alpha$_2$-Adrenergic Agonists (Optic Agents)^b	
brimonidine tartrate	Alphagan-P
Sympathomimetics^b	
apraclonidine	Iopidine
dipivefrin	Propine
epinephrine	

^{a}See Chapter 31 for detailed information.
^{b}See Chapter 53 for detailed information.

- Temporary treatment of heart block
- Ventricular arrhythmias (under certain conditions)
- Respiratory distress (as bronchodilators)
- Nasal congestion and glaucoma (topical formulation)

Clients at risk for life-threatening reactions to allergens, exercise, or unknown triggers may obtain and be instructed in the use of adrenergic drugs to lessen allergic reactions before emergency medical care is given.

Adrenergic drugs may also be used as a vasoconstricting adjunct to local anesthetics to prolong anesthetic action in the tissues. The adrenergic drugs used primarily as **vasopressors** (drugs that raise the blood pressure because of their ability to constrict blood vessels) are listed in the Summary Drug Table: Adrenergic Drugs. Sympathomimetics are also used as bronchodilators in the treatment of respiratory problems (see Chapter 31) or topically in the treatment of glaucoma (see Chapter 53). These drugs are listed in Table 23.2 by name only; more information is provided in the respective chapters.

Treating Shock

Adrenergic drugs are important in the care and treatment of clients in shock. Shock is a state of inadequate tissue perfusion. The three types of shock—hypovolemic shock,

TABLE 23.3 Types of Shock

TYPE[a]	DESCRIPTION
Hypovolemic	Occurs when the blood volume is significantly diminished. *Examples:* hemorrhage; fluid loss caused by burns, dehydration, or excess diuresis
Cardiogenic–obstructive shock	Occurs when cardiac output is insufficient and perfusion to the vital organs cannot be maintained. *Examples:* a result of acute myocardial infarction, ventricular arrhythmias, congestive heart failure, or severe cardiomyopathy Obstructive shock is categorized with cardiogenic shock. It occurs when obstruction of blood flow results in inadequate tissue perfusion. *Examples:* pericardial tamponade, restrictive pericarditis, and severe cardiac valve dysfunction
Distributive (vasogenic) shock	Occurs when there are changes to the blood vessels causing dilation, but no additional blood volume. The blood is redistributed within the body. This category is further differentiated: • Septic shock—circulatory insufficiency resulting from overwhelming infection (e.g., central line infection) • Anaphylactic shock—hypersensitivity resulting in massive systemic vasodilation (e.g., drug allergic reaction) • Neurogenic shock—interference with PNS control of blood vessels (e.g., spinal cord injury)

[a]Other causes of shock include hypoglycemia, hypothyroidism, and Addison disease.

cardiogenic shock, and distributive shock—are described in Table 23.3. During shock, the supply of arterial blood and oxygen is diverted and what does flow to the cells and tissues is inadequate for survival. A series of physiologic mechanisms are initiated by the body to counteract the symptoms of shock. The brain activates the hypothalamic–pituitary–adrenal (HPA) system. The HPA triggers the production of hormones and the release of epinephrine and norepinephrine. In some situations, the body is able to compensate and blood pressure is maintained. However, if shock is untreated and compensatory mechanisms of the body fail, irreversible shock occurs and death follows.

Various clinical manifestations may be present in a client who is in shock. For example, in the early stages of shock, the extremities may be warm because vasodilation is initiated and blood flow to the skin and extremities is maintained. If the condition is untreated, blood flow to the vital organs, skin, and extremities is compromised and the client becomes cool and clammy. Regardless of the type, shock results in a decrease in cardiac output, decrease in arterial blood pressure (hypotension), reabsorption of water by the kidneys (causing a decrease in urinary output), decrease in the exchange of oxygen and carbon dioxide in the lungs, increase in carbon dioxide and decrease in oxygen in the blood, hypoxia (decreased oxygen reaching the cells), and increased concentration of intravascular fluid. This scenario compromises the functioning of vital organs such as the heart, brain, and kidneys. The various physiologic responses caused by shock are listed in Table 23.4.

Management of shock is aimed at providing basic life support (airway, breathing, and circulation) while attempting to correct the underlying cause. Antibiotics, inotropes, hormones (e.g., insulin, thyroid), and other drugs may be used to treat the underlying disease. However, the initial pharmacologic intervention is aimed at supporting the circulation with vasopressors.

TABLE 23.4 Physiologic Manifestations of Shock

BODILY SYSTEM	POSSIBLE SIGNS AND SYMPTOMS
Integumentary (skin)	Pallor, cyanosis, cold and clammy, sweating
Central nervous system	Agitation, confusion, disorientation, coma
Cardiovascular	Hypotension, tachycardia, arrhythmias, wide pulse pressure, gallop rhythm
Respiratory	Tachypnea, pulmonary edema
Renal	Urinary output less than 20 mL/hr
Metabolic (endocrine)	Acidosis

Adrenergic (sympathomimetic) drugs improve hemodynamic status by improving myocardial contractility and increasing heart rate, which results in increased cardiac output. Peripheral resistance is increased by vasoconstriction. In cardiogenic shock or shock associated with low cardiac output, an adrenergic drug may be used with a vasodilating drug. A vasodilator, such as nitroprusside or nitroglycerin (see Chapter 35), improves myocardial performance because the adrenergic drug action on the cardiovascular system maintains blood pressure.

ADVERSE REACTIONS

Adverse reactions associated with the administration of adrenergic drugs depend on the drug used, the dose administered, and individualized client response. Some common adverse reactions include:

• Cardiac arrhythmias (bradycardia or tachycardia)
• Headache
• Nausea and vomiting
• Increased blood pressure (which may reach dangerously high levels)

Additional adverse reactions for specific adrenergic drugs are listed in the Summary Drug Table: Adrenergic Drugs.

 Lifespan Considerations

Gerontology

The older adult is especially vulnerable to adverse reactions of adrenergic drugs, particularly epinephrine. In addition, older adults are more likely to have preexisting cardiovascular disease that predisposes them to potentially serious cardiac arrhythmias. Closely monitor all older clients taking an adrenergic drug, and report any changes in the pulse rate or rhythm immediately. Also note, epinephrine may temporarily increase tremor and rigidity in older adults with Parkinson disease.

CONTRAINDICATIONS

Adrenergic drugs are contraindicated in clients with known hypersensitivity. Isoproterenol is contraindicated in clients with tachyarrhythmias or heart block caused by digitalis toxicity, ventricular arrhythmias, and angina pectoris. Dopamine is contraindicated in those with pheochromocytoma (adrenal gland tumor), unmanaged arrhythmias, and ventricular fibrillation. Epinephrine is contraindicated in clients with narrow-angle glaucoma and as a local anesthetic adjunct in fingers and toes. Norepinephrine is contraindicated in clients who are hypotensive from blood volume deficits.

NURSING ALERT

Supine hypertension is a potentially dangerous adverse reaction in the client taking midodrine. The drug should be given only to clients whose lives are impaired despite standard treatment offered. This reaction is minimized by administering midodrine during the day while the client is in an upright position. The suggested dosing schedule for the administration of midodrine is shortly before arising in the morning, midday, and late afternoon (not after 6:00 p.m.). Drug therapy should continue only in the client whose orthostatic hypotension improves during the initial treatment.

PRECAUTIONS

These drugs are used cautiously in clients with coronary insufficiency, cardiac arrhythmias, angina pectoris, diabetes, hyperthyroidism, occlusive vascular disease, or prostatic hypertrophy. Clients with diabetes may require an increased dosage of insulin. Adrenergic drugs are classified as pregnancy category C and are used with extreme caution during pregnancy.

INTERACTIONS

The following interactions may occur when an adrenergic drug is administered with another agent:

Interacting Drug	Common Use	Effect of Interaction
Antidepressants	Treatment of depression	Increased sympathomimetic effect
Oxytocin	Induction of uterine contractions	Increased risk of hypertension

There is an increased risk of seizures, hypotension, and bradycardia when dopamine is administered with phenytoin (Dilantin). There is an increased risk of hypertension when dobutamine is administered with the beta-adrenergic (β-adrenergic) blocking drugs.

 Herbal Considerations

Ephedra (Ma Huang) and the many substances of the *Ephedra* genus have been used medicinally (e.g., *Ephedra sinica* and *Ephedra intermedia*). Ephedra (ephedrine) preparations have traditionally been used to relieve cold symptoms and improve respiratory function and as an adjunct in weight loss. Large doses may cause a variety of adverse reactions, such as hypertension and irregular heart rate. The use of ephedra has shifted from relief of respiratory problems to an aid to weight loss and enhanced athletic performance, despite the US Food and Drug Administration warning to the public not to take ephedrine-containing dietary supplements. Before taking this herb, the client should consult a primary health care provider. Ephedra should not be used with the cardiac glycosides, halothane, guanethidine, monoamine oxidase inhibitor antidepressants, or oxytocin or by clients taking St. John's wort. Stroke and heart attack have resulted from taking these products. Many producers of weight loss supplements are removing the ephedra component because of potential legal liability (DerMarderosian, 2003).

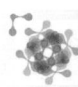

NURSING PROCESS—STEPS TO BUILDING CLINICAL JUDGMENT
Client Receiving an Adrenergic Drug

ASSESSMENT

Assessment of the client receiving an adrenergic drug differs depending on the drug, the client, and the reason for administration. For example, assessment of the client in shock who is to be treated with norepinephrine is different from that for the client receiving epinephrine with a local anesthetic while having a tooth cavity repaired. Both are receiving adrenergic drugs, but the circumstances are much different.

Preadministration Assessment

Data gathering suggestions before the initial administration of the drug include:
Objective data

- Description of signs of shock or allergen, such as cool skin, cyanosis, diaphoresis, and a change in the level of consciousness
- Vital signs (temperature, pulse, respirations, and blood pressure), continual monitoring if the situation is urgent/emergent
- Descriptions of trauma, infection, or blood loss if these are the causes of the hypotensive episode
- Intravenous (IV) access—is it patent for use of medications and increased fluid volume

Subjective data

- Type and duration of symptoms, if unresponsive may be from a witness of episode
- Allergy history, especially if severe reaction occurred in the past
- Remedies attempted before seeking care

Ongoing Assessment

During the ongoing assessment, observe the client for the effect of the drug, such as improved breathing of the client with asthma or response of blood pressure to the administration of the vasopressor. During therapy, evaluate and document the drug effect and vital signs. Comparison of assessments made before and after administration may help the primary health care provider determine future use of the drug for this client. It is important to report adverse drug reactions to the primary health care provider as soon as possible.

When a client has self-administered a drug for a life-threatening allergic reaction, try to get as much information as possible from the client about the incident leading up to using the drug. If the client was with family or friends, gain subjective data from these people regarding the events leading up to the need for drug injection.

NURSING DIAGNOSES

Drug-specific nursing diagnoses are the following:

- **Ineffective tissue perfusion** related to hypovolemia, blood loss, impaired distribution of fluid, impaired circulation, impaired transport of oxygen across alveolar and capillary bed, other (specify)

- **Decreased cardiac output** related to altered heart rate and/or rhythm
- **Sleep deprivation/insomnia** related to adverse reactions (nervousness) to the drug and the environment

Nursing diagnoses related to drug administration are discussed in Chapter 4.

PLANNING

The expected outcomes of the client depend on the reason for administering an adrenergic agent but may include an optimal response to drug therapy, meeting client needs related to management of adverse drug reactions, and confidence in an understanding of the medication regimen.

IMPLEMENTATION

Promoting an Optimal Response to Therapy

Management of the client receiving an adrenergic agent varies and depends on the drug used, the reason for administration, and the client's response to the drug. In most instances, adrenergic drugs are potent and potentially dangerous. Minimize distractions and exercise great care in the calculation and preparation of these drugs for administration. Although adrenergic drugs are potentially dangerous, proper supervision and management before, during, and after administration will minimize the occurrence of any serious problems. Report and document any complaint the client may have while taking an adrenergic drug. However, nursing judgment is necessary when reporting adverse reactions. Report adverse effects immediately, such as the development of cardiac arrhythmias, regardless of the time of day or night. Yet, for other adverse effects, such as a nervous feeling, reassure the client these feelings are expected; reporting of this event need not be dealt with immediately.

Monitoring and Managing Client Needs

Ineffective Tissue Perfusion
If the client is being given an adrenergic drug for hypotension, there is already a problem with tissue perfusion. Administration of the adrenergic drug may correct the problem or, if the blood pressure becomes too high, tissue perfusion may again be a problem. By maintaining the blood pressure at the systolic rate prescribed by the primary health care provider, tissue perfusion will be maintained.

When a client is in shock and experiencing ineffective tissue perfusion, there is a decrease in oxygen, resulting in an inability of the body to nourish its cells at the capillary level. If the client has marked hypotension, the administration of a vasopressor is required. The primary health care provider determines the cause of the hypotension and then selects the best method of treatment. Some hypotensive episodes require the use of a less potent vasopressor; at other times, a more potent vasopressor, such as dobutamine, dopamine, or norepinephrine, is necessary.

Consider the following points when administering the potent vasopressors such as dopamine and norepinephrine:

- Use an electronic infusion device to administer these drugs.
- Do not mix dopamine with other drugs, especially sodium bicarbonate or other alkaline IV solutions. Check with the clinical pharmacist before adding a second drug to an IV solution containing this drug.
- Do not dilute norepinephrine or dopamine IV solutions before administration. The primary health care provider orders the drug dosage based on the drug concentration; any change in the amount of drug added to the solution would change the amount of drug infused.
- Blood pressure is monitored continuously from the beginning of therapy until the desired blood pressure is achieved and until the client is transferred to a less supervised unit.
- Adjust the rate of drug administration according to the client's blood pressure. The rate of administration of the IV solution is increased or decreased to maintain the client's blood pressure at the systolic pressure ordered by the primary health care provider.
- Readjustment of the rate of flow of the IV solution is often necessary. The frequency of adjustment depends on the client's response to the vasopressor.
- Inspect the needle site and surrounding tissues at frequent intervals for leakage (**extravasation**, infiltration) of the solution into the subcutaneous tissues surrounding the needle site. If leakage occurs, establish another IV line immediately, then discontinue the IV containing the vasopressor, and notify the primary health care provider. These drugs are particularly damaging when they leak into surrounding tissues. You should know the extravasation protocol and have orders signed by the primary health provider to implement the protocol whenever these drugs are used.
- Never leave the client receiving these drugs unattended.

 Concept Mastery Alert

Nurses who are caring for clients who have been prescribed dopamine should inspect the needle site and surrounding tissues for leakage.

Infiltration into the surrounding tissues can cause tissue death, and blood pressure should be measured continuously because dopamine is vasoactive and may work very quickly.

Monitoring the client in shock requires your vigilance. The client's heart rate, blood pressure, and electrocardiogram are monitored continuously. Urine output is measured often (usually hourly), and accurate intake and output measurements are taken. Monitoring of central venous pressure by a central venous catheter provides an estimate of the client's fluid status. Sometimes additional hemodynamic monitoring is necessary with a pulmonary artery catheter. The use of a pulmonary artery catheter allows nurses to monitor a number of parameters, such as cardiac output and peripheral vascular resistance. Therapy is adjusted according to the primary health care provider's instructions.

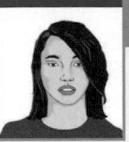 **PHARMACOLOGY IN PRACTICE**

SAFE DRUG ADMINISTRATION
A nurse is required to administer dopamine to a client. Which of the following nursing interventions should the nurse perform when caring for the client? Select all that apply.
1. Administer dopamine only via IV route.
2. Mix dopamine with alkaline solutions before administering.
3. Use an electronic infusion device to administer these drugs.
4. Monitor blood pressure every 30 min.
5. Inspect needle site and surrounding tissues at frequent intervals.

Decreased Cardiac Output

The heart rate and **stroke volume** (volume of blood leaving the heart) determine cardiac output. The stroke volume is determined in part by the contractile state of the heart and the amount of blood in the ventricle available to be pumped out. The interventions listed to support tissue perfusion also help to support cardiac output of the client in shock.

When the client is in shock, it is important to continually monitor vital signs (heart rate and rhythm, respiratory rate, and blood pressure) carefully to determine the severity of shock. For example, as cardiac output decreases, compensatory tachycardia (rapid heartbeat) develops to increase cardiac output. As shock deepens, the pulse volume becomes progressively weaker and assumes a "thready" feel. The heart rate increases and the heart rhythm may become irregular. Initially, the respiratory rate is rapid, as the client experiences air hunger, but in profound shock, the respiratory rate decreases. Blood pressure decreases as shock progresses.

! NURSING ALERT

Regardless of the actual numeric reading of the blood pressure, a progressive decrease in blood pressure is serious. Report any progressive decrease in blood pressure, a decrease in systolic blood pressure below 100 mm Hg, or any decrease of 20 mm Hg or more of the client's normal blood pressure.

Sleep Deprivation/Insomnia

Often adrenergic drugs are used in the critical care setting. These units can be as busy in the middle of the

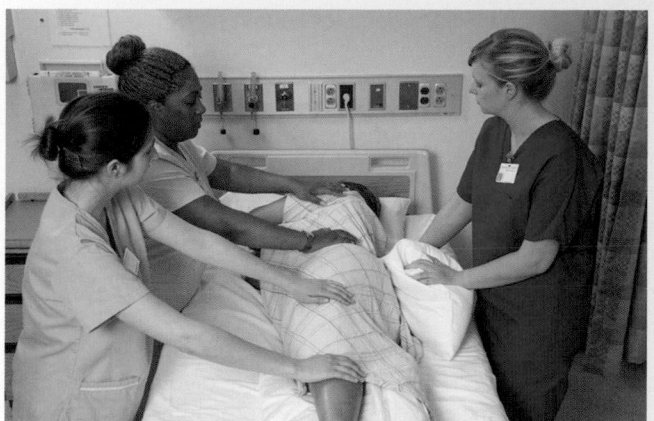

FIGURE 23.3 Nursing activities are clustered together to minimize the disruption in sleep patterns.

night as they are in the middle of the day. Clients can easily get confused regarding the time of day, which can cause a great deal of stress in the client. It is helpful to identify circumstances that disturb sleep, such as when the nursing staff enter the room during the night or turn the overhead light on during the night (Fig. 23.3). Plan care with as few interruptions as possible or make modifications. For example, to filter light, curtains

can be drawn over windows and between clients in critical care units. Weigh the importance of monitoring client status and combine with comfort interventions when administering the adrenergic drugs. A thorough explanation of the reason for close monitoring of the vital signs is necessary, especially to family members who are present. In addition, caffeinated beverages are avoided, especially after 5:00 p.m. Other sleep aids may be used (e.g., warm milk, back rub, progressive relaxation, or bedtime snack).

Potential Medical Complication: Responding to Allergens

Once a client has experienced an allergic reaction, they are at risk for having another reaction. Triggers can include foods, stinging insects, latex, chemical or environmental items, and even exercise. Clients who have experienced an allergic reaction may be instructed in the use of epinephrine via an autoinjection device such as the EpiPen (Fig. 23.4) so they may carry out normal daily activities without fear of an incident occurring when help is unavailable. Sometimes clients are fearful and wonder if the situation calls for use of the drug or if they should seek out care instead. During an allergic reaction, the drug should be administered first, then medical care obtained.

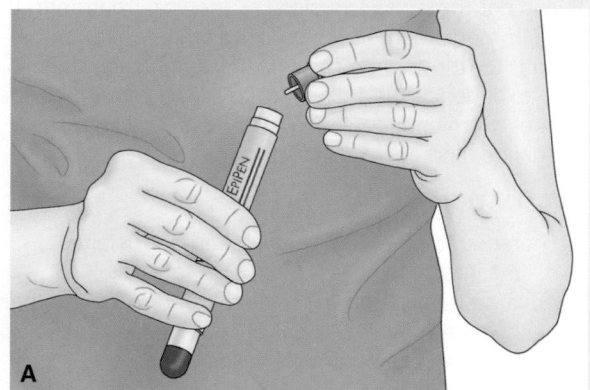
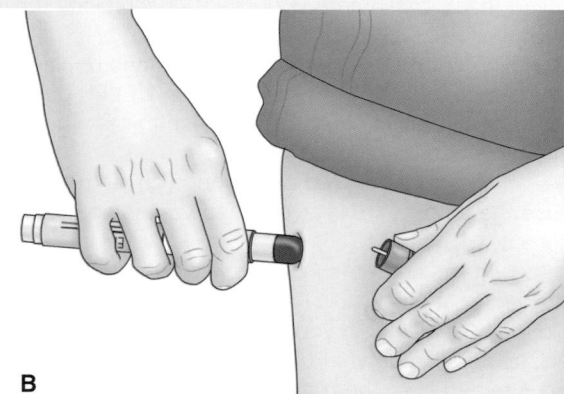
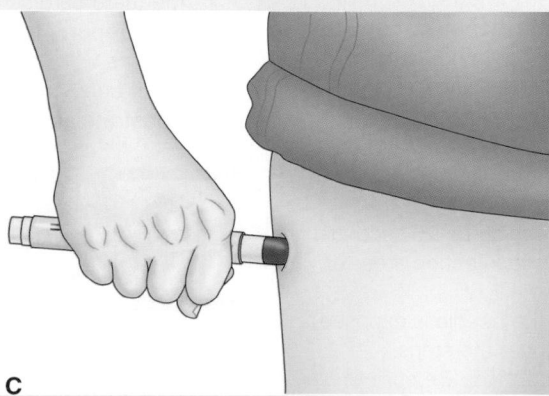

FIGURE 23.4 Example of preloaded autoinjection device for use in treating allergic reactions. (From Timby, B. K., & Smith, N. E. (2009). *Introductory medical-surgical nursing* (10th ed.). Lippincott Williams & Wilkins.)

Chronic Care Considerations

Research conducted by Chaudhry, Portnoy, and Purser (2012) found that almost all lay persons taught to use an autoinjector had forgotten the skill within 3 months of instruction. Be sure to discuss and review procedures at every client visit when a client is given one of these devices to use.

Client Teaching for Improved Outcomes

Using an Autoinjector for Allergic Reactions

If an individual has experienced an allergic reaction or is at risk of having a reaction, they may be prescribed a self-administering antidote. It is important to carry this device at all times. It should not be exposed to extreme temperatures (e.g., do not store in refrigerator or put in glove box of car). The device is an autoinjector, meaning it is designed to inject the medication with minimal training, therefore minimizing fear of use. When the device is used it is still important to seek medical treatment as soon as possible. If alone, the client should call the emergency number first, then administer the dose. Use of these devices should not be considered in place of medical care and advice; the client should be taken to an emergency department as soon as possible. *When you teach, make sure your client understands the following:*

✔ Depending on the device, there is an orange or black tip on the small end of the autoinjector. NEVER put your fingers or hand over this, because this is where the needle comes out.

✔ Take off the activation cap only when you are ready to use the autoinjector, never when you do not plan to use it.

✔ Use only if the contents in the "window" of the autoinjector are clear.

✔ Hold the autoinjector in your fist with the orange or black tip pointing down. Pull off the activation cap (opposite end from the black tip) with your other hand.

✔ Hold the orange or black tip near the outer thigh of the person who is getting the injection. Most devices are designed to be used through clothing. Note: if the person is obese, be sure to teach the individual to ensure that the needle correctly penetrates.

✔ Gently, but FIRMLY, swing and jab the black tip into the outer thigh so that the autoinjector is perpendicular to the thigh.

✔ Hold the autoinjector firmly in the thigh for 10 seconds.

✔ Remove the unit and massage the injection area for 10 seconds.

✔ Check the orange or black tip. If the needle is exposed, the dose was received. If not, repeat the steps.

✔ DO NOT THROW AWAY THE DEVICE. Be sure to take the used device to the emergency department with you.

It is important that clients be taught how to recognize symptoms and use the device. Teach the client to recognize the symptoms of an allergic reaction, which include hives, itching, flushing, and swelling of the lips, tongue, or inside of the mouth. Clients may feel tightness of the throat or chest if the airway is affected. Other symptoms can include chest pain, dizziness, and headache as the blood pressure gets lower. Specific instructions for using autoinjecting epinephrine are provided in Client Teaching for Improved Outcomes: Using an Autoinjector for Allergic Reactions.

Educating the Client and Family
Specially trained health care providers give some adrenergic drugs, such as the vasopressors. Your responsibility focuses on monitoring for and teaching about the treatment and drug to the client or family. Depending on the situation, you may include facts such as how the drug will be given (e.g., the route of administration) and what results are expected. Use your judgment regarding some of the information given to the client or family regarding administration of an adrenergic drug in life-threatening situations, because certain facts, such as the seriousness of the client's condition, are usually best explained by the primary health care provider.

When teaching the client about self-administration of epinephrine, make sure the client and family understand this is not to be used in place of medical treatment. It is an immediate intervention used while treatment is sought for the allergic reaction. After injection the client may experience the following reactions: faster heartbeat, nausea, vomiting, sweating, dizziness, weakness, headache, and nervousness.

EVALUATION

- Therapeutic effect is achieved and perfusion is maintained.
- Adverse reactions are identified, reported to the primary health care provider, and managed successfully through appropriate nursing interventions:
  - Adequate tissue perfusion is maintained.
  - Adequate cardiac output is maintained.
  - Client reports fewer episodes of inappropriate sleep patterns.
- Client (if able) and family express confidence and demonstrate an understanding of the drug regimen.

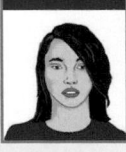 **PHARMACOLOGY IN PRACTICE**

USING CLINICAL REASONING

The primary health care provider has prescribed an autoinjector rescue drug for Janna to use. Her mother feels this is too much responsibility for a 16-year-old. How would you approach the mother to help her understand the significance of the reaction and ease of use of this device?

KEY POINTS

■ The sympathetic branch of the autonomic nervous system regulates involuntary body functions. The primary neurotransmitter of the sympathetic branch is norepinephrine; activation of this system is often called the fight, flight, or freeze response.

■ When the sympathetic nerves are stimulated, the purpose is to divert blood flow to the vital organs so the body can deal with the stressful situation. A person becomes wakeful with quicker reflexes and pupils dilate. The smooth muscles of the bronchi relax as do the coronary vessels, and the heart rate increases. Blood flow is constricted to areas such as the gastrointestinal (GI) and genitourinary systems.

■ Drugs that mimic the sympathetic response are called sympathomimetic or adrenergic (because the primary transmitter is adrenalin or epinephrine). Actions in the body are modified depending on how the drug acts on different cell receptors. Drugs can be selective for alpha or beta receptors. Drugs can also be nonselective.

■ These drugs are used to treat shock, hypotension, allergic reactions, heart conditions, and bronchoconstriction. Topical formulas are used for glaucoma and nasal congestion. Older individuals are very susceptible to adverse reactions, especially to epinephrine.

■ Adverse reactions include increased blood pressure, nausea, vomiting, headache, and cardiac arrhythmias.

SUMMARY DRUG TABLE
Adrenergic Drugs

Generic Name	Trade Name	Uses	Adverse Reactions	Dosage Ranges
Adrenergic (Sympathomimetic) Drugs Used Primarily for Vasopressor Effects				
DOBUTamine *doe-BYOO-ta-meen*		Cardiac decompensation because of depressed contractility caused by organic heart disease or cardiac surgical procedures	Headache, nausea, increased heart rate, increase in systolic blood pressure, palpitations, anginal and nonspecific chest pain	2.5–10.0 µg/kg/min IV (up to 40 µg/kg/min); titrate to client's hemodynamic and renal status
DOPamine *DOE-pa-meen*		Shock caused by myocardial infarction, trauma, open heart surgery, renal failure, and chronic cardiac decompensation in congestive heart failure	Nausea, vomiting, ectopic beats, tachycardia, anginal pain, palpitations, hypotension, dyspnea	2–50 µg/kg/min IV (infusion rate determined by client's response)
droxidopa *drox-i-DOE-pa*	Northera	Neurogenic orthostatic (supine) hypotension	Dizziness, syncope, headache, urinary retention	100–600 mg three times daily orally
EPINEPHrine *ep-i-NEF-rin*	EpiPen	Ventricular standstill; treatment and prophylaxis of cardiac arrest, heart block; mucosal congestion and acute sinusitis; prolong regional/local anesthetics; anaphylactic reactions	Anxiety, restlessness, headache, lightheadedness, dizziness, nausea, dysuria, pallor	Cardiac arrest: 0.5–1.0 mg IV Respiratory distress (e.g., anaphylaxis): 0.1–0.25 mg of hay fever, rhinitis
isoproterenol *eye-soe-proe-TER-e-nole*	Isuprel	Shock, bronchospasm during anesthesia, cardiac standstill and arrhythmias	Anxiety, sweating, flushing, headache, lightheadedness, dizziness, nausea, vomiting, tachycardia	Shock: 4 µg/mL diluted solution IV Cardiac arrhythmias, cardiac standstill: 0.02–0.06 mg of diluted solution IV, or 1:5000 solution intracardiac injection
midodrine *MI-doe-dreen*		Orthostatic hypotension, only when client is considerably impaired	Paresthesias, headache, pain, dizziness, supine hypertension, bradycardia, piloerection, pruritus, dysuria, chills	10 mg orally TID during daylight hours when client is upright
norepinephrine (levarterenol) *nor-ep-i-NEF-rin*	Levophed	Shock, hypotension, cardiac arrest	Restlessness, headache, dizziness, bradycardia, hypertension	2–4 µg/min, rate adjusted to maintain desired blood pressure
phenylephrine *fen-il-EF-rin*	Biorphen, Vazculep	Hypotension in cardiac shock	Restlessness, headache, dizziness, bradycardia, hypertension	0.5–0.6 µg/kg/min, rate adjusted to maintain desired blood pressure

CHAPTER REVIEW

Know Your Drugs

Clients sometimes know a medication by the brand (or trade) name and not the generic name. To help you recognize both names, match the brand name with the generic name of the same medication.

Generic Name	Brand Name
1. epinephrine	A. Levophed
2. isoproterenol	B. Isuprel
3. norepinephrine	C. EpiPen

Calculate Medication Dosages

1. The physician orders 2 mg of 1:1000 epinephrine solution IV. The drug is available in 1:1000 solution 1 mg/mL. The nurse administers _____.

2. The physician orders 0.5 mg of 1:1000 epinephrine in a subcutaneous injection. The drug is available in 1:1000 solution 1 mg/mL. The nurse administers _____.

Prepare for the NCLEX

RECALL THE FACTS

1. What is the primary transmitting substance in the sympathetic branch of the nervous system?
   1. Serotonin
   2. Norepinephrine
   3. Dopamine
   4. Acetylcholine

2. Shock is described as:
   1. result of blood loss.
   2. compensation for bodily assault.
   3. inadequate tissue perfusion.
   4. the fight, flight, or freeze response.

3. The physician prescribes norepinephrine, a potent vasopressor, to be administered to a client in shock. The rate of the administration of the IV fluid containing the norepinephrine is:
   1. maintained at a set rate of infusion.
   2. adjusted per protocol to maintain the client's blood pressure.
   3. given at a rate not to exceed 5 mg/min.
   4. discontinued when the blood pressure is 100 mm Hg systolic.

4. At what intervals would the nurse monitor the blood pressure of a client administered norepinephrine?
   1. Continuously
   2. Every 30 min
   3. Every hr
   4. Every 4 hr

5. Which of the following are the common adverse reactions the nurse would expect with the administration of the adrenergic drugs?
   1. Bradycardia, lethargy, bronchial constriction
   2. Increase in appetite, nervousness, drowsiness
   3. Anorexia, vomiting, hypotension
   4. Headache, nervousness, nausea

6. When dobutamine is administered with the beta-adrenergic blocking drugs, the nurse is aware of an increased risk for _____.
   1. seizures
   2. arrhythmias
   3. hypotension
   4. hypertension

ANALYZE THE FACTS

7. *If a client uses an autoinject epinephrine device, the best disposal would be:
   1. container the injector is packaged in.
   2. after being seen by emergency personnel.
   3. hard plastic container.
   4. sharps box or needle container.

8. When norepinephrine is transmitted in the sympathetic nervous system, which of the following occurs?
   1. Heart rate slows
   2. Blood pressure lowers
   3. GI system speeds up
   4. Bronchi relax

ALTERNATE-FORMAT QUESTIONS

9. Select the terms that describe drugs that stimulate the sympathetic branch of the ANS. Select all that apply.
   1. Sympathomimetic
   2. Sympatholytic
   3. Adrenergic
   4. Cholinergic

10. *An adult with an allergy to honeybees is stung and calls the nurse at the clinic. The client has two EpiPens at home. The solution is 1 mg/mL and each EpiPen contains 0.3 mL. What drug dose has the client taken if two injections were given?

To check your answers, see Appendix F.

---

*Indicates the question is directly linked to the NCLEX-PN test plan in Appendix G.

> **WANT TO KNOW MORE?** A wide variety of resources are available to enhance your learning and understanding of this chapter.
> - Visit **thePoint** for resources such as:
>   - NCLEX-Style Student Review Questions
>   - Journal Articles
>   - Dosage Calculations
>   - Drug Monographs
>   - Watch and Learn Videos
>   - Concepts in Action Animations
> - The *Study Guide to Accompany Introductory Clinical Pharmacology*, 12th edition, sold separately, will help you review and apply essential content.
> - ✔**PrepU** is available to help students prepare for the NCLEX-PN examination.

Adrenergic Blocking Drugs

Key Terms

alpha (α)-adrenergic alpha receptors of the adrenergic nerves that control the vascular system

antiadrenergic blocks the neurotransmission of the sympathetic nervous system

beta (β)-adrenergic beta receptors of the adrenergic nerves that primarily control the heart

cardiac arrhythmia abnormal rhythm of the heart, also known as cardiac *dysrhythmias*

first-dose effect marked adverse reaction with the first dose

glaucoma group of diseases of the eye characterized by increased intraocular pressure; results in changes within the eye, visual field defects, and eventually blindness (if left untreated)

heart failure (HF) condition in which the heart cannot pump enough blood to meet the tissue needs of the body, may also be called *congestive heart failure* (*CHF*)

orthostatic hypotension decrease in blood pressure occurring after standing in one place for an extended period

pheochromocytoma tumor of the adrenal medulla characterized by hypersecretion of epinephrine and norepinephrine

postural hypotension decrease in blood pressure after a sudden change in body position

sympatholytic blocking the sympathetic nervous system

Learning Objectives

On completion of this chapter, the student will:

1. List the four types of adrenergic blocking drugs.
2. Explain the uses, general drug actions, general adverse reactions, contraindications, precautions, and interactions of the adrenergic blocking drugs.
3. Distinguish important preadministration and ongoing assessment activities the nurse should perform on the client taking an adrenergic blocking drug.
4. List nursing diagnoses particular to a client taking an adrenergic blocking drug.
5. Examine ways to promote an optimal response to therapy, how to manage common adverse reactions, nursing actions that may be taken to minimize orthostatic or postural hypotension, and important points to keep in mind when educating clients about the use of adrenergic blocking drugs.

 Drug Classes

Alpha (α)-adrenergic blocking	Alpha/beta-adrenergic blocking
Beta (β)-adrenergic blocking	Centrally and peripherally acting antiadrenergic

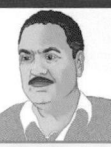 **PHARMACOLOGY IN PRACTICE**

Alfredo Garcia is accompanied by his wife to the clinic. He came in with complaints of an upper respiratory tract infection. While taking vital signs you discover a blood pressure of 210/120. He has never been diagnosed with hypertension. As you read, think about what antiadrenergic drugs do to blood vessels and blood pressure.

In this chapter, we continue our discussion of the sympathetic branch of the autonomic nervous system and what happens when the nerve impulses are blocked.

AUTONOMIC TERMINOLOGY

Norepinephrine is the primary substance that transmits nerve impulses across the sympathetic branch of the autonomic nervous system. Activation of these nerves is sometimes called our *fight, flight, or freeze response.* Drugs that facilitate the transmission of norepinephrine were featured in Chapter 23. In Chapter 23, you learned that the classes of drugs were called sympathomimetic or adrenergic. In this chapter, drugs that prevent the response are typically called *adrenergic blocking*. Two additional drug terms that are less frequently used are **antiadrenergic** or **sympatholytic**, because again these agents block the transmission of norepinephrine in the sympathetic portion of the autonomic nervous system (Box 24.1).

Figure 24.1 shows how the body organs respond when sympathetic nerve impulses are blocked by these medications.

BOX 24.1	**More Variation on Drug Class Names**
Sympatholytic Antiadrenergic Adrenergic blockers	All terms meaning—to stop the neurotransmission of norepinephrine along the sympathetic branch of the autonomic nervous system

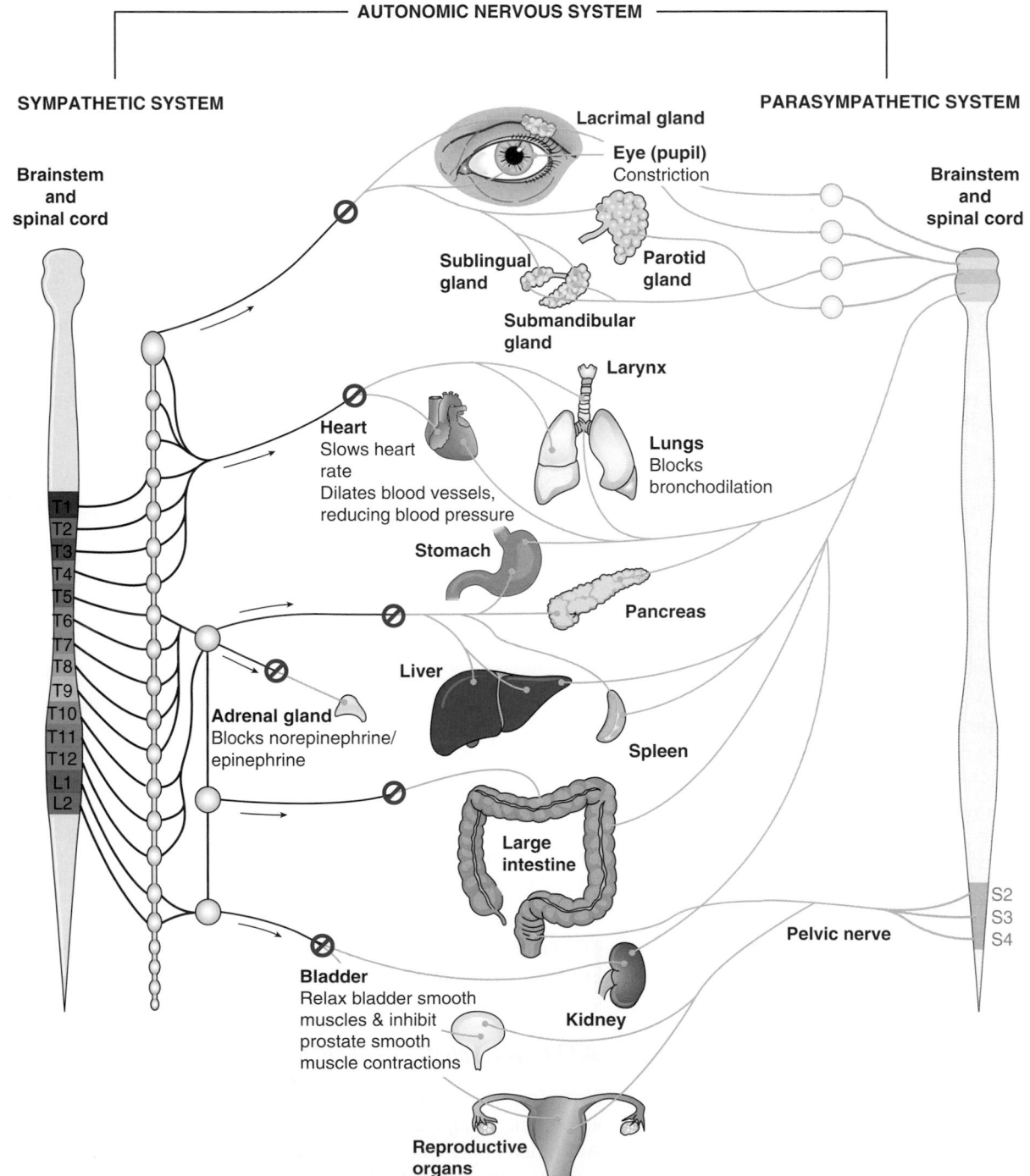

FIGURE 24.1 Bodily responses to blocking the stimulation of the sympathetic nervous system. (Adapted from Cohen, B. J. (2003). *Medical terminology* (4th ed.). Lippincott Williams & Wilkins.)

Drugs blocking neurotransmission in the sympathetic nervous system may work *directly* by blocking the receptor or *indirectly* by preventing release of norepinephrine. These drugs are clustered into four different groups:

- **Alpha (α)-adrenergic blocking** drugs—drugs that block alpha-adrenergic receptors. These drugs produce their greatest effect on the alpha receptors of the adrenergic nerves that control the vascular system.
- **Beta (β)-adrenergic blocking** drugs—drugs that block beta-adrenergic receptors. These drugs produce their greatest effect on the beta receptors of adrenergic nerves, primarily the beta receptors of the heart.
- α/β-Adrenergic blocking drugs—drugs that block both alpha- and beta-adrenergic receptors. These drugs act on both alpha and beta nerve fibers.
- Centrally and peripherally acting antiadrenergic drugs— drugs that prevent the release of the neurotransmitter (norepinephrine). These drugs block the adrenergic nerve impulse in both the central and peripheral nervous systems.

Each of these drug groups is discussed individually, followed by an example of the Nursing Process for the group as a whole. The focal group of drugs in this chapter is the beta-adrenergic blocking drugs. See the Summary Drug Table: Adrenergic Blocking Drugs for a more complete listing of these drugs.

ALPHA-ADRENERGIC BLOCKING DRUGS

ACTIONS

From the last chapter, we know stimulation of alpha-adrenergic nerves results in vasoconstriction. If stimulation of alpha-adrenergic nerves is interrupted or blocked, the result is the opposite—*vasodilation*. Alpha-adrenergic blocking drugs produce the direct opposite effect of an adrenergic drug with alpha activity. Drugs used in this category cause vasodilation by relaxing the smooth muscle of blood vessels. Alpha-adrenergic blockers are used primarily in ophthalmic preparations that constrict the pupil and are discussed in Chapter 53.

USES

Alpha-adrenergic blocking drugs are used in the treatment of the following:

- Hypertension caused by pheochromocytoma (a tumor of the adrenal gland that produces excessive amounts of epinephrine and norepinephrine)
- Hypertension during preoperative preparation
- Reduce ocular pressure during laser surgery
- Prevent or treat tissue damage caused by extravasation of the drug—dopamine

ADVERSE REACTIONS

Administration of an alpha-adrenergic blocking drug may result in weakness, orthostatic hypotension, cardiac arrhythmias, hypotension, and tachycardia. See the Summary Drug Table: Adrenergic Blocking Drugs for more information.

CONTRAINDICATIONS, PRECAUTIONS, AND INTERACTIONS

Alpha-adrenergic blocking drugs are contraindicated in clients who are hypersensitive to the drugs and in clients with coronary artery disease. These drugs are used cautiously during pregnancy (pregnancy category C) and lactation, after a recent myocardial infarction (MI), and in clients with renal failure or Raynaud disease. When phentolamine (Regitine) is administered with epinephrine (a sympathomimetic), there is decreased vasoconstrictor and hypertensive action.

BETA-ADRENERGIC BLOCKING DRUGS

Beta-adrenergic blocking drugs are commonly called *beta blockers* by both health care providers and clients alike.

ACTIONS

These drugs decrease or block the stimulation of the sympathetic nervous system on select tissues. Beta-adrenergic receptors are found mainly in the heart. *Stimulation* of beta receptors of the heart results in an increase in the heart rate. By blocking the nerve impulse of beta-adrenergic nerves it decreases the heart rate and dilates the blood vessels. These drugs work by blocking the nerve impulse from jumping the synapse area and continuing to the adjoining nerve ending (Fig. 24.2). These drugs decrease the heart's excitability, decrease cardiac workload and oxygen consumption, and provide membrane-stabilizing effects thus contributing to the antiarrhythmic activity of the beta-adrenergic blocking drugs. Examples of beta-adrenergic blocking drugs used for cardiac purposes are esmolol (Brevibloc) and propranolol (Inderal).

The same properties work when used to treat **glaucoma** of the eye. Glaucoma is a condition of the eye where narrowing or blockage of the drainage channels (canals of Schlemm) between the anterior and posterior chambers happens. This results in a buildup of pressure (increased intraocular pressure [IOP]) in the eye. Blindness may occur if glaucoma is left untreated. Beta-adrenergic blocking drugs such as betaxolol (Betoptic) and timolol (Timoptic) are used to treat glaucoma. When used topically as ophthalmic drops, they appear to reduce the production of aqueous humor in the anterior chamber of the eye, lessening the effects of glaucoma.

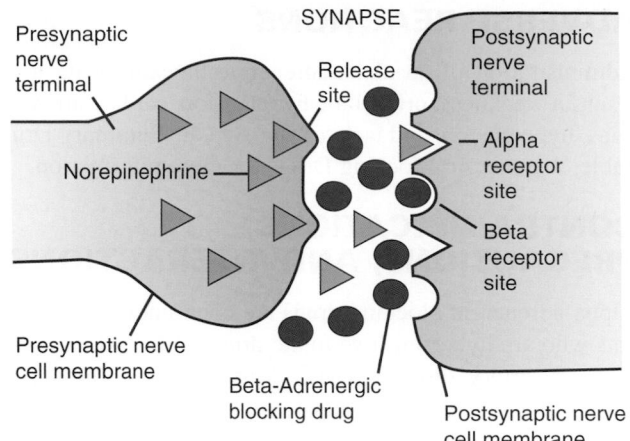

FIGURE 24.2 Beta-adrenergic blocking drugs prevent epinephrine and norepinephrine from occupying receptor sites on cell membranes.

USES

Beta-adrenergic blocking drugs are used in the treatment of the following:

- Hypertension (first-choice drug for clients with stable angina or CAD)
- Cardiac arrhythmia (abnormal rhythm of the heart), such as ventricular or supraventricular tachycardia
- Migraine headaches
- Heart failure (HF)
- Angina pectoris
- Glaucoma (topical ophthalmic eye drops)

Beta-adrenergic blockers are also used to prevent reinfarction in clients with a recent MI (1–4 weeks after the MI).

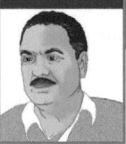

PHARMACOLOGY IN PRACTICE

ASSESSMENT
A nurse is caring for a client with glaucoma. The client is administered a beta-adrenergic blocking ophthalmic preparation, such as timolol. How will the effectiveness of the drug be determined?
1. Measure intraocular pressure of the client.
2. Monitor blood pressure of the client.
3. Monitor respiratory rate of the client.
4. Measure pulse rate of the client.

C h r o n i c C a r e C o n s i d e r a t i o n s

Hypertension research studies demonstrate better client outcomes for African Americans when beta blockers are used in combination with diuretics than other drugs alone to treat hypertension, such as angiotensin-converting enzyme inhibitors (Ferdinand, 2007).

ADVERSE REACTIONS

- Generalized reactions that affect the body include orthostatic hypotension, bradycardia, dizziness, vertigo, and headache.
- Gastrointestinal (GI) reactions include hyperglycemia, nausea, vomiting, and diarrhea.
- Bronchospasm (especially in those with a history of asthma).

Many of these reactions are mild and may disappear with therapy. More serious adverse reactions include symptoms associated with heart failure (i.e., dyspnea, weight gain, peripheral edema).

L i f e s p a n C o n s i d e r a t i o n s

Gerontology
Older adults are at increased risk for adverse reactions when taking beta-adrenergic blocking drugs. Monitor the older adult closely for confusion, worsening of angina, shortness of breath, and peripheral vascular insufficiency (e.g., cold extremities, paresthesia of the hands, weak peripheral pulses).

CONTRAINDICATIONS, PRECAUTIONS, AND INTERACTIONS

These drugs are contraindicated in clients with an allergy to beta blockers; in clients with sinus bradycardia, second- or third-degree heart block; and in those with asthma, emphysema, and hypotension. When discontinuing the drug, beta blockers should always be tapered slowly, not abruptly stopped. The drugs are used cautiously in clients with diabetes, thyrotoxicosis, or peptic ulcer.

LASA ALERT

The following drugs may sound alike; be sure to clarify when they are ordered:

Drug Name	Sounds Like
Betapace	Betapace AF
betaxolol	bethanechol, labetalol
Brevibloc	Brevital, Bumex, Buprenex
esmolol	Osmitrol
Inderal	Adderall, Enduron, Imdur, Imuran, Inderide, Isordil, Toradol
pindolol	Parlodel, Plendil
propranolol	prasugrel, Pravachol, Propulsid
Sotalol	Stadol, Sudafed
Timolol	atenolol, Tylenol

Drugs that look like a similar drug are noted in the Summary Drug Tables of each chapter.

The following interactions may occur when a beta-adrenergic blocker is administered with another agent:

Interacting Drug	Common Use	Effect of Interaction
Antidepressants (monoamine oxidase inhibitors [MAOIs], selective serotonin reuptake inhibitors [SSRIs])	Management of depression	Increased effect of the beta blocker, bradycardia
Nonsteroidal anti-inflammatory drugs (NSAIDs), salicylates	Pain relief	Decreased effect of the beta blocker
Loop diuretics	Management of cardiovascular problems	Increased risk of hypotension
Clonidine	Management of cardiovascular problems	Increased risk of paradoxical hypertensive effect
Cimetidine	Management of GI problems	Increased serum level of the beta blocker and higher risk of beta blocker toxicity
Lidocaine	Management of cardiac problems	Increased serum level of the beta blocker and higher risk of beta blocker toxicity

ALPHA/BETA-ADRENERGIC BLOCKING DRUGS

ACTIONS

Alpha/beta-adrenergic blocking drugs block the stimulation of both the alpha- and beta-adrenergic receptors, resulting in peripheral vasodilation. The two drugs in this category are carvedilol (Coreg) and labetalol.

USES

Carvedilol is used to treat essential hypertension and in HF to reduce progression of the disease. Labetalol is used in gestational hypertension, either alone or in combination with another drug, such as a diuretic.

ADVERSE REACTIONS

Most adverse effects of alpha/beta-adrenergic blocking drugs are mild and do not require discontinuation of therapy. General body system adverse reactions include fatigue,

dizziness, hypotension, drowsiness, insomnia, weakness, diarrhea, dyspnea, chest pain, bradycardia, and skin rash.

CONTRAINDICATIONS, PRECAUTIONS, AND INTERACTIONS

Alpha/beta-adrenergic blockers are contraindicated in clients with hypersensitivity to the drugs, bronchial asthma, decompensated HF, and severe bradycardia. The drugs are used cautiously in clients with drug-controlled HF, chronic bronchitis, or impaired hepatic or cardiac function; in those with diabetes; and during pregnancy (pregnancy category C) and lactation.

LASA ALERT

The following drugs may sound alike; be sure to clarify when they are ordered:

Drug Name	Sounds Like
carvedilol	atenolol, captopril, carbidopa, carteolol
Coreg	Corgard, Cortef, Cozaar
labetalol	betaxolol, LaMICtal, lamoTRIgine, Lipitor

Drugs that look like a similar drug are noted in the Summary Drug Tables of each chapter.

The following interactions may occur when an alpha/beta-adrenergic blocker is administered with another agent:

Interacting Drug	Common Use	Effect of Interaction
Antidepressants (tricyclics and SSRIs)	Management of depression	Increased risk of tremors
Cimetidine	Management of GI problems	Increased effect of the adrenergic blocker
Clonidine	Management of cardiovascular problems	Increased effect of the clonidine
Digoxin	Management of cardiac problems	Increased serum level of the digoxin and higher risk of digoxin toxicity

CENTRALLY AND PERIPHERALLY ACTING ANTIADRENERGIC DRUGS

ACTIONS

One group of antiadrenergic drugs inhibits the release of norepinephrine from certain adrenergic nerve endings in the peripheral nervous system. This group is composed of *peripherally acting* (i.e., acting on peripheral structures) antiadrenergic drugs. An example of a peripherally acting antiadrenergic drug for treating hypertension is prazosin (Minipress). These drugs are also used to treat benign prostatic hypertrophy (BPH).

Another group of antiadrenergic drugs is called the *centrally acting* antiadrenergic drug group because they act on the central nervous system (CNS) rather than on the peripheral nervous system. This group affects specific CNS centers, thereby decreasing some of the activity of the sympathetic nervous system. Although the action of both types of antiadrenergic drugs is somewhat different, the results are basically the same. An example of a centrally acting antiadrenergic drug is clonidine (Catapres).

USES

Antiadrenergic drugs are used mainly for the treatment of certain cardiac arrhythmias, hypertension, and BPH (see the Summary Drug Table: Adrenergic Blocking Drugs).

ADVERSE REACTIONS

- Peripherally acting antiadrenergic: hypotension, weakness, lightheadedness, and bradycardia
- Centrally acting antiadrenergic: dry mouth, drowsiness, sedation, anorexia, rash, malaise, and weakness

CONTRAINDICATIONS, PRECAUTIONS, AND INTERACTIONS

The peripherally acting antiadrenergic drugs are contraindicated in clients with a hypersensitivity to any of the drugs. Reserpine is contraindicated in clients who have an active peptic ulcer or ulcerative colitis and in clients who are mentally depressed. Reserpine is used cautiously in clients with a history of depression, in those with renal impairment or cardiovascular disease, and during pregnancy and lactation.

Centrally acting antiadrenergic drugs are contraindicated in active hepatic disease, in antidepressant therapy using MAOIs, and in clients with a history of hypersensitivity to these drugs. The centrally acting antiadrenergic drugs are used cautiously in clients with a history of liver disease or renal impairment and during pregnancy and lactation.

 Lifespan Considerations

Pregnancy

Methyldopa (centrally acting) or labetalol (alpha/beta adrenergic blocker) are recommended for pregnant women over other hypertensive drugs because the risk to the fetus is less with these drugs than with other antiadrenergics or hypertensive medications.

The following interactions may occur when an antiadrenergic drug is administered with another agent:

Interacting Drug	Common Use	Effect of Interaction
Adrenergic drugs	Management of cardiovascular problems	Increased risk of hypertension
Levodopa	Management of Parkinson disease	Decreased effect of the levodopa, hypotension
Anesthetic agents	Surgical anesthesia	Increased effect of the anesthetic
Beta blockers	Management of cardiovascular problems	Increased risk of hypertension
Lithium	Treatment of psychosis	Increased risk of lithium toxicity
Haloperidol	Treatment of psychosis	Increased risk of psychotic behavior

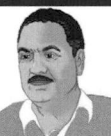 **PHARMACOLOGY IN PRACTICE**

SAFE DRUG ADMINISTRATION
A nurse is caring for a client taking both an antidepressant and an adrenergic blocking drug. Which of the following actions should the nurse perform when the client receiving adrenergic blocking drugs shows a dramatic decrease in blood pressure?
1. Monitor for excessive perspiration
2. Monitor for confusion
3. Adjust into a more comfortable position
4. Hold the drug dose

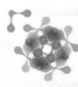

NURSING PROCESS: STEPS TO BUILDING CLINICAL JUDGMENT
Client Receiving an Adrenergic Blocking Drug

ASSESSMENT

Assessment depends on the drug, the client, and the reason for administration.

Preadministration Assessment

Data gathering suggestions before an adrenergic blocking drug is administered for the first time include:

Objective data

- General client appearance, look for cardiac-specific signs such as dyspnea (especially on exertion), peripheral edema, distended neck veins, and cough
- Vital signs (temperature and respirations)
- Blood pressure–specific measurements—both arms in sitting, standing, and supine positions
- Pulse—rate and rhythm
- Electrocardiogram may also be ordered

Subjective data

- Current symptoms (malaise, fatigue)
- Pain experience—onset, type (e.g., sharp, dull, squeezing), radiation, location, intensity, and duration
- Precipitating factors of anginal pain, such as exertion or emotional stress
- Allergy history, particularly a drug allergy
- History of other chronic health conditions

Ongoing Assessment

It is important to perform an ongoing assessment of the client receiving adrenergic blocking drug therapy. This assessment often depends on the reason the drug is administered. For all adrenergic blocking drugs, it is important to observe these clients continually for the appearance of adverse reactions. Some adverse reactions are mild, whereas others, such as diarrhea, may cause a problem, especially if the client is older or debilitated.

Typically, hypertensive clients will be asked to monitor their own blood pressures between clinic visits. This can be accomplished by obtaining equipment for the home or periodic visits to a local fire station or pharmacy. If a client gets a significantly different reading when using a public machine, be sure they learn to ask when the machine was last calibrated. An odd reading can be machine error and should be authenticated with another reading elsewhere. More in-depth information regarding care of the client with hypertension is provided in Chapter 34.

NURSING DIAGNOSES

Drug-specific nursing diagnoses are the following:

- **Impaired comfort** related to drying of secretions secondary to medication
- **Ineffective tissue perfusion: peripheral** related to hypotension
- **Injury risk** related to vertigo, dizziness, weakness, and syncope secondary to hypotension

Nursing diagnoses related to drug administration are discussed in Chapter 4.

PLANNING

The expected outcomes for the client depend on the reason for administration of an adrenergic blocking drug but may include an optimal response to drug therapy, meeting of client needs related to the management of adverse reactions, and confidence in an understanding of the medication regimen.

IMPLEMENTATION

Promoting an Optimal Response to Therapy

Most adrenergic blocking drugs may be given with food. Sotalol (Betapace) is given on an empty stomach because food may reduce absorption of the drug. Important to note is that the drugs preventing release of neurotransmitters (antiadrenergics) should be taken at the same time each day because the fluctuation in blood level can affect blood pressure.

When adrenergic blocking drugs are given to clients to control hypertension, angina, or cardiac arrhythmias, it is important to communicate with the primary health care provider about the client's response to therapy. When given for a cardiac arrhythmia, these drugs can provoke new or worsen existing ventricular arrhythmias. If angina worsens or does not appear to be controlled by the drug, the client needs to feel confident to contact the primary health care provider immediately.

When the drug is administered for hypertension, the client is monitored for a decrease in blood pressure. On the other hand, if there is a significant *increase* in blood pressure, administer the ordered dose and notify the primary health care provider immediately because additional drug therapy may be necessary.

When a beta-adrenergic blocking ophthalmic preparation, such as timolol, is used by clients with glaucoma, it is important they continue periodic follow-up examinations with an ophthalmologist. At these examinations, the intraocular pressure is measured to determine the effectiveness of drug therapy.

Monitoring and Managing Client Needs

Impaired Comfort

Some clients may experience one or more adverse drug reactions during treatment with adrenergic blocking drugs. Adverse reactions that pose no serious threat to the client's well-being, such as dry mouth or mild constipation, are reactions that impair comfort.

Even minor adverse drug reactions can be distressing to the client, especially when they persist for a long time. Therefore, when possible, you can relieve minor adverse reactions with simple nursing measures. For example, assist or teach the client with dry mouth to take frequent sips of water or suck on a piece of hard candy (provided that the client does not have diabetes or is not on a special diet that limits sugar intake) to relieve the dryness. Help relieve a client's constipation by encouraging increased intake of high-fiber foods and fluids, unless extra fluids are contraindicated. The primary health care provider also may order a laxative or stool softener. It is important for you to maintain a daily record of bowel elimination for the hospitalized client. Dryness, slower GI motility, and immobility all make constipation a greater risk for the hospitalized client. Other GI side effects, such as anorexia, diarrhea, and constipation, can be minimized by administering drugs at a specific time in relation to meals, with food, or with antacids.

Ineffective Tissue Perfusion: Peripheral

During initial therapy, or if in an institutional setting when an adrenergic blocking drug is given for hypertension, the client's blood pressure is taken before each dose is given. Some clients can have an unusual response to the drugs and an increase in blood pressure may occur. In addition, for some individuals, these drugs may decrease the blood pressure at a more rapid rate than other drugs. It is important to monitor the client's blood pressure on both arms and in the sitting, standing, and supine positions for the first week or more of therapy. Once the client's blood pressure has stabilized, take the blood pressure before each drug administration using the same arm and position for each reading until the client is ready to return home. To ensure safe administration, with most electronic medication administration records (MARs), you cannot access the entry for the medication without making a notation regarding results of a blood pressure reading. Measuring the blood pressure near the end of the dosing interval or near the end of the day after the last dose of the day helps to determine if the blood pressure is controlled throughout the day.

> **! NURSING ALERT**
>
> When administering a sympatholytic drug, such as propranolol (Inderal), take an apical pulse rate and blood pressure before giving the drug. If the pulse is below 60 beats/min, or if there is any irregularity in the client's heart rate or rhythm, or if systolic blood pressure is less than 90 mm Hg, withhold the drug and contact the primary health care provider.

The client with a life-threatening arrhythmia may receive an adrenergic blocking drug, such as propranolol, by the intravenous (IV) route. When these drugs are administered IV, cardiac monitoring is necessary. Clients not in a monitored unit are usually transferred to one as soon as possible. When administering these drugs for a life-threatening arrhythmia, it is important to monitor the client continually with cardiac, blood pressure, and respiratory rate frequently.

When propranolol is administered orally for a less serious cardiac arrhythmia, cardiac monitoring is usually not necessary. Typically, notation of the last reading is required in an electronic MAR. When at home, periodically monitor the client's blood pressure and pulse rate and rhythm at varying intervals, depending on the length of treatment and the client's response to the drug.

Injury Risk

Administration of the adrenergic blocking drugs may cause hypotension. If the drug is administered for hypertension, then a decrease in blood pressure is expected. If a significant decrease in blood pressure (a drop of 20 mm Hg systolic or a systolic pressure below 90 mm Hg) occurs after a dose of an adrenergic blocking drug, withhold the next drug dose and notify the primary health care provider immediately. A dosage reduction or discontinuation of the drug may be necessary.

> **! NURSING ALERT**
>
> Some adrenergic blocking drugs (e.g., prazosin or terazosin) may cause a first-dose effect. A first-dose effect occurs when the client experiences marked hypotension (or postural hypotension) and syncope with sudden loss of consciousness with the first few doses of the drug.

The **first-dose effect** may be minimized by decreasing the initial dose and administering the dose at bedtime. The dosage can then be slowly increased every 2 weeks until a full therapeutic effect is achieved. If the client experiences syncope (lightheadedness or fainting), place the client in a recumbent position and treat supportively. This effect is self-limiting and in most cases does not recur after the initial period of therapy. Lightheadedness and dizziness are more common than loss of consciousness. On occasion, clients receiving an adrenergic blocking drug may experience postural or orthostatic hypotension. **Postural hypotension** is characterized by a feeling of lightheadedness and dizziness when the client suddenly changes from a lying to a sitting or standing position, or from a sitting to a standing position. **Orthostatic hypotension** is characterized by similar symptoms and occurs when the client changes or shifts position after standing in one place for a long period. Box 24.2 provides tips on how to minimize these adverse reactions.

Symptoms of postural or orthostatic hypotension often lessen with time, and the client may be allowed to get out of bed or a chair slowly without assistance. You should exercise good judgment in this matter. Allowing the client to rise from a lying or sitting position without help is done only when the determination has been made that the symptoms have lessened and ambulation poses no danger of falling.

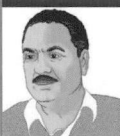

PHARMACOLOGY IN PRACTICE

MANAGING NEEDS

A nurse is caring for a client on beta-adrenergic blocker therapy. The client is going to be administered lidocaine at the dental clinic. Which of the following interactions may occur and the nurse should instruct the client to warn the dental clinic staff is possible?
1. Increased risk of hypotension
2. Increased serum level of the beta blocker
3. Increased risk of paradoxical hypertensive effect
4. Increased effect of the beta blocker

BOX 24.2 Minimizing the Effects of Adrenergic Blocking Drugs

Assisting clients to minimize the uncomfortable effects of adrenergic blocking drugs can be challenging. The following measures may be useful:

- Instruct clients to rise slowly from a sitting or lying position.
- Provide assistance for the client getting out of bed or a chair if symptoms of postural hypotension are severe. Place the call light nearby and instruct clients to ask for assistance when they get in and out of bed or a chair.
- Assist the client in bed to a sitting position and have the client sit on the edge of the bed for about 1 min before ambulating.
- Help seated clients to a standing position and instruct them to stand in one place for about 1 min before ambulating.
- Remain with the client while they are standing in one place, as well as during ambulation.
- Instruct the client to avoid standing in one place for prolonged periods. This is rarely a problem in the hospital but should be included in the client and family discharge teaching plan.
- Teach the client to avoid taking hot showers or baths, which tend to increase vasodilation.

Educating the Client and Family

Some clients do not adhere to the prescribed drug regimen for a variety of reasons, such as failure to comprehend the prescribed treatment, the cost of drug therapy, or failure to understand the importance of continued and uninterrupted therapy when they do not feel symptoms. If a stable client has a sudden blood pressure increase, investigate the possibility of one of these factors causing the problem. In some instances where the price of drugs is an issue, financial assistance may be necessary; in other instances, clients need to know why they are taking a drug and why therapy must be continuous to attain and maintain an optimal state of health and well-being.

Support your client's health literacy by describing the drug protocol and stress the importance of continued and uninterrupted therapy when teaching the client who is prescribed an adrenergic blocking drug. Client education will differ according to the reason the adrenergic blocking drug was prescribed. Hypertension and coronary artery disease (CAD) do not always present overtly. In other words, people may not feel like they have a heart-related condition and decide to stop taking a beta blocker because they do not see a benefit to taking or a risk if stopping the medication. Educate clients regarding the signs of cardiac conditions that can occur if a beta blocker is stopped suddenly. Clients can experience severe anginal pain, myocardial infarction, and even cardiac arrhythmias. These drugs need to be tapered (taking less of the drug over time) if there is a plan to discontinue the drug and clients should be monitored for the development of symptoms and the dose modified to reduce those symptoms.

In some instances, the primary health care provider may advise the hypertensive client to lose weight or eat a special diet, such as the DASH (Dietary Approaches to Stop Hypertension) diet. A special diet also may be recommended for the client with angina or a cardiac arrhythmia. When appropriate, enlist the help of a registered dietician to stress the importance of diet and weight loss in the therapy of hypertension.

It is important to include the following additional points in the teaching plan for the client with hypertension, angina, or a cardiac arrhythmia:

- Do not stop taking the drug abruptly. Most of these drugs require that the dosage be gradually decreased to prevent precipitation or worsening of adverse effects.
- Notify the primary health care provider promptly if adverse drug reactions occur.
- Observe caution while driving or performing other hazardous tasks because these drugs (beta-adrenergic blockers) may cause drowsiness, dizziness, or lightheadedness.
- Immediately report any signs of HF (weight gain, difficulty breathing, or edema of the extremities).
- Do not use any nonprescription drug (e.g., cold or flu preparations or nasal decongestants) unless you have discussed use of a specific drug with the primary health care provider.
- Inform dentists and other primary health care providers of therapy with this drug.
- Keep all primary health care provider appointments because close monitoring of therapy is essential.
- Check with a primary health care provider or clinical pharmacist to determine if the drug is to be taken with food or on an empty stomach.

In addition, when an adrenergic blocking drug is prescribed for hypertension, the primary health care provider may want the client to monitor their own blood pressure between office visits (see Client Teaching for Improved Outcomes: Monitoring Blood Pressure at Home).

Client Teaching for Improved Outcomes

Monitoring Blood Pressure at Home

Clients taking medications for high blood pressure typically require frequent monitoring. Although blood pressure readings need to be taken frequently, they do not need to be done at the office of a health care provider when the client has the proper equipment at home. *When you teach, make sure your client understands the following:*

✔ Assess the client and a family member's ability to see numbers on equipment and handle the apparatus as you help the client determine the best equipment to be used in the home. Be sure the proper size cuff is purchased for the client to minimize inaccurate readings. Remind the client to deflate the cuff completely before putting on or taking off the device.

✔ Teach the client and a family member how to inflate and deflate the device and have them demonstrate use before doing the procedure independently. Be sure the arm used is stretched out and at the level of the heart. Many devices have digital readings; if using a sphygmomanometer, teach what to look for on the dial.

✔ Teach the client and a family member to use the same extremity for taking the blood pressure and to be in a comfortable, relaxed place and to roll up the sleeve or remove tight-fitting clothing before placing the cuff.

✔ Explain that blood pressure can vary slightly with emotion, time of day, and position of the body. It is typically not necessary to take multiple readings during the day unless requested by the primary health care provider.

✔ Instruct the client to continue taking the medication regardless of the readings of the blood pressure. Give the parameters of when to call the primary health care provider or emergency services if needed.

✔ Instruct the client to keep an accurate list of medications being taken with the blood pressure equipment. This will provide easy reference for any changes you are asked to make.

✔ Explain how to document the blood pressure readings so both the client and primary health care provider can see the trends of the readings.

EVALUATION

• Therapeutic effect is achieved and hypertension or other disease is controlled.
• Adverse reactions are identified, reported to the primary health care provider, and managed successfully through appropriate nursing interventions.
  • Dryness is managed and comfort maintained.
  • Peripheral tissue perfusion is maintained.
  • No evidence of injury is seen.
• Client and family express confidence and demonstrate an understanding of the drug regimen.

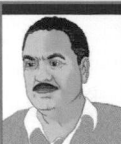

PHARMACOLOGY IN PRACTICE

USING CLINICAL REASONING

Mr. Garcia is prescribed metoprolol 100 mg after breakfast daily. His wife is concerned about him getting up early in the mornings to urinate. When is he most likely to have hypotensive reactions and when is he least likely? How will you teach him to deal with the possibility of orthostatic hypotension?

KEY POINTS

■ The sympathetic branch of the autonomic nervous system regulates involuntary body functions. The antiadrenergic drugs block the neurotransmitter norepinephrine in the sympathetic branch.

■ The purpose of adrenergic blocking drugs is to block or interrupt the signals that divert blood flow to the vital organs. Instead, the blood vessels dilate and relax smooth muscle. The heart rate decreases and the blood pressure is lowered.

■ Drugs that block the sympathetic system are called sympatholytic or antiadrenergic. Actions in the body are modified depending on how the drug acts on different cell receptors. Drugs can be selective for alpha or beta receptors. Drugs can also be nonselective.

■ These drugs are used to treat hypertension, cardiac arrhythmias, BPH, glaucoma, and a rare condition called pheochromocytoma. As with the adrenergic drugs, older individuals are very susceptible to adverse reactions with these drugs.

■ Adverse reactions include decreased blood pressure, weakness, increased heart rate, nausea, vomiting, headache, and bronchospasm in those with asthma.

■ When starting therapy with antiadrenergic drugs, clients should be monitored and taught about orthostatic hypotension—the sudden drop in blood pressure when going from a lying to a sitting or standing position. This information can help prevent falls and injury.

SUMMARY DRUG TABLE
Adrenergic Blocking Drugs

Generic Name	Trade Name	Uses	Adverse Reactions	Dosage Ranges
Alpha-Adrenergic Blocking Drugs				
phentolamine *fen-TOLE-a-meen*		Diagnosis of pheochromocytoma, hypertensive episodes before and during surgery, prevention/treatment of dermal necrosis after IV administration of norepinephrine or dopamine	Weakness, dizziness, flushing, nausea, vomiting, orthostatic hypotension	5 mg IV, IM Tissue necrosis: 5–10 mg in 10 mL saline solution infiltrated into affected area

Generic Name	Trade Name	Uses	Adverse Reactions	Dosage Ranges
Beta-Adrenergic Blocking Drugs (Beta Blockers)				
acebutolol *a-se-BYOO-toe-lole*		Hypertension, ventricular arrhythmias	Bradycardia, dizziness, weakness, hypotension, nausea, vomiting, diarrhea, nervousness	Hypertension: 400 mg orally in 1–2 doses Arrhythmias: 400–1200 mg/day orally in divided doses
atenolol *a-TEN-oh-lole*	Tenormin	Hypertension, angina, acute MI	Bradycardia, dizziness, fatigue, weakness, hypotension, nausea, vomiting, diarrhea, nervousness	Hypertension/angina: 50–200 mg/day orally Acute MI: 5 mg IV over 5 min, may be repeated
betaxolol *be-TAKS-oh-lol*		Hypertension	Same as acebutolol	10–40 mg orally daily
bisoprolol *bis-OH-proe-lol*		Hypertension	Same as acebutolol	2.5–10.0 mg orally daily; maximum dose: 20 mg orally daily
esmolol *ES-moe-lol*	Brevibloc	Supraventricular tachycardia, noncompensatory tachycardia	Hypotension, weakness, lightheadedness, urinary retention	50–200 µg/kg/min IV, loading dose may be as high as 500 µg/kg over 1 min
metoprolol *me-toe-PROE-lol*	Lopressor, Toprol-XL	Hypertension, angina, MI, HF	Dizziness, hypotension, HF, cardiac arrhythmia, nausea, vomiting, diarrhea	Hypertension/angina: 100–450 mg/day orally Extended release: 50–100 mg/day orally HF: 25–200 mg/day orally Acute MI: 3 bolus doses of 5 mg IV
nadolol *NAY-doe-lol*	Corgard	Hypertension, angina	Dizziness, hypotension, nausea, vomiting, diarrhea, HF, cardiac arrhythmia	Hypertension: 40–80 mg/day orally Angina: 40–80, may go to 240 mg/day orally
nebivolol *ne-BIV-oh-lol*	Bystolic	Hypertension	Dizziness, headache, nausea, diarrhea, tingling extremities	5–40 mg orally daily
pindolol *PIN-doe-lol*		Hypertension	Bradycardia, dizziness, hypotension, nausea, vomiting, diarrhea	5–60 mg/day orally BID
propranolol *proe-PRAN-oh-lol*	Inderal	Cardiac arrhythmias, MI, angina, hypertension, migraine prophylaxis, hypertrophic subaortic stenosis, pheochromocytoma, essential tremor	Bradycardia, dizziness, hypotension, nausea, vomiting, diarrhea, bronchospasm, hyperglycemia, pulmonary edema	Arrhythmias: 10–30 mg orally TID, QID Hypertension: 120–240 mg/day orally in divided doses Angina: 80–320 mg/day orally in divided doses Migraine: 160–240 mg/day orally in divided doses
⊘ **sotalol** *SOE-ta-lol*	Betapace, Betapace AF, Sorine	Ventricular arrhythmias (maintain normal sinus rhythm—Betapace AF only)	Dizziness, hypotension, nausea, vomiting, diarrhea, respiratory distress	160–320 mg/day orally in divided doses
timolol *TIM-oh-lol*		Hypertension, MI, migraine prophylaxis	Dizziness, hypotension, nausea, vomiting, diarrhea, pulmonary edema	Hypertension: 10–40 mg/day orally in divided doses MI: 10 mg orally BID Migraine: 20 mg/day orally
Topical Preparations				
betaxolol (ophthalmic) *be-TAKS-oh-lol*	Betoptic	Glaucoma	Brief ocular discomfort, tearing	1 gtt BID
carteolol *KAR-tee-oh-lol*	Ocupress	Glaucoma	Same as betaxolol	1 gtt in affected eye(s) TID

Continued

SUMMARY DRUG TABLE (continued)
Adrenergic Blocking Drugs

Generic Name	Trade Name	Uses	Adverse Reactions	Dosage Ranges
Topical Preparations (continued)				
levobetaxolol *lee'-voe-beh-tax'-oh-lahl*	Betaxon	Glaucoma	Same as betaxolol	1 gtt in affected eye(s) BID
levobunolol *lee-voe-BYOO-noe-lol*	AKBeta, Liquifilm	Glaucoma	Same as betaxolol	0.5% Solution: 1–2 gtt in affected eye(s) daily 0.25% Solution: 1–2 gtt in affected eye(s) BID
metipranolol *met-i-PRAN-oh-lol*		Treatment of elevated IOP in clients with ocular hypertension or open-angle glaucoma	Ocular irritation, tearing	1 gtt in affected eye(s) BID
timolol (ophthalmic) *TIM-oh-lole*	Betimol, Timoptic	Glaucoma	Ocular irritation, tearing	1 gtt BID
Alpha/Beta-Adrenergic Blocking Drugs				
carvedilol *KAR-ve-dil-ole*	Coreg	Hypertension, HF, left ventricular dysfunction	Bradycardia, hypotension, cardiac insufficiency, fatigue, dizziness, diarrhea	6.25–25.0 mg orally BID
labetalol *la-BET-a-lole*		Hypertension (severe, incl. preeclampsia)	Fatigue, drowsiness, insomnia, hypotension, impotence, diarrhea	200–400 mg/day orally in divided doses IV: 20 mg over 2 min with blood pressure monitoring, may repeat
Antiadrenergic Drugs: Centrally Acting				
cloNIDine *KLON-i-deen*	Catapres, Catapres-TTS (transdermal)	Hypertension, ADHD, severe pain in clients with cancer, opiate withdrawal (supervised only)	Drowsiness, dizziness, sedation, dry mouth, constipation, syncope, dreams, rash	100–600 µg/day orally Transdermal: release rate 0.1–0.3 mg/24 hr
guanFACINE *GWAHN-fa-seen*	Intuniv	Hypertension, ADHD	Dry mouth, somnolence, asthenia, dizziness, headache, constipation, fatigue	1–3 mg/day orally at bedtime
methyldopa *meth-il-DOE-pa*		Hypertension, hypertensive crisis, preeclampsia	Bradycardia, aggravation of angina pectoris, HF, sedation, headache, rash, nausea, vomiting, nasal congestion	250 mg orally BID or TID; maintenance dose: 2 g/day; 250–500 mg q6hr IV
Antiadrenergic Drugs: Peripherally Acting				
alfuzosin *al-FYOO-zoe-sin*	Uroxatral	BPH	Headache, dizziness	10 mg orally daily
doxazosin *doks-AY-zoe-sin*	Cardura	Hypertension, BPH	Headache, dizziness, fatigue	Hypertension: 1–8 mg orally daily BPH: 1–16 mg orally daily
phenoxybenzamine *fen-oks-ee-BEN-za-meen*	Dibenzyline	Phenocytocromia	Dizziness, postural hypotension, drowsiness, palpitation, nasal congestion	10–20 mg orally, 1–2 times daily
prazosin *PRAZ-oh-sin*	Minipress	Hypertension	Dizziness, postural hypotension, drowsiness, headache, loss of strength, palpitation, nausea	1–20 mg orally daily in divided doses
silodosin *SI-lo-doe-sin*	Rapaflo	BPH, dislodge ureteral stones	Dizziness, lightheadedness, headache, diarrhea, nasal congestion	8 mg orally daily
tamsulosin *tam-SOO-loe-sin*	Flomax	BPH, dislodge ureteral stones	Headache, ejaculatory dysfunction, dizziness, rhinitis	0.4 mg orally daily
terazosin *ter-AY-zoe-sin*		Hypertension, BPH, dislodge ureteral stones	Dizziness, postural hypotension, headache, dyspnea, nasal congestion	Hypertension: 1–20 mg orally daily BPH: 1–10 mg orally daily

This drug should be administered at least 1 hr before or 2 hr after a meal.

CHAPTER REVIEW

Know Your Drugs

Clients sometimes know a medication by the brand (or trade) name and not the generic name. To help you recognize both names, match the brand name with the generic name of the same medication.

Generic Name	Brand Name
1. carvedilol	A. Cardura
2. clonidine	B. Catapres
3. doxazosin	C. Coreg
4. nadolol	D. Corgard

Calculate Medication Dosages

1. A client in long-term care is ordered 50 mg of atenolol. The drug bubble pack card comes in 25-mg tablets per dose. How many tablets does the nurse remove from the bubble pack card?
2. The physician orders 0.4 mg of tamsulosin (Flomax) daily before breakfast. The drug is available in 0.4-mg capsules. The nurse instructs the client to take _____.

Prepare for the NCLEX

RECALL THE FACTS

1. Antiadrenergic drugs block which of the following transmitters?
   1. Serotonin
   2. Norepinephrine
   3. Dopamine
   4. Acetylcholine
2. A client is to receive a beta-adrenergic drug for hypertension. Before the drug is administered, the most important assessment the nurse performs is _____.
   1. weighing the client
   2. obtaining blood for laboratory tests
   3. taking a past medical history
   4. taking the blood pressure on both arms
3. When an adrenergic blocking drug is given for a life-threatening cardiac arrhythmia, which of the following activities would the nurse expect to be a part of client care?
   1. Daily electrocardiograms
   2. Fluid restriction to 1000 mL/day
   3. Daily weights
   4. Continual cardiac monitoring

4. To prevent complications when administering a beta-adrenergic blocking drug to an elderly client, the nurse would be particularly alert for _____.
   1. vascular insufficiency (e.g., weak peripheral pulses and cold extremities)
   2. complaints of an occipital headache
   3. insomnia
   4. hypoglycemia
5. The client with glaucoma will likely receive a(n) _____.
   1. alpha/beta-adrenergic blocking drug
   2. alpha-adrenergic blocking drug
   3. beta-adrenergic blocking drug
   4. antiadrenergic drug

ANALYZE THE FACTS

6. When norepinephrine is blocked in the sympathetic nervous system, which of the following occurs?
   1. Heart rate increases
   2. Blood pressure lowers
   3. GI system slows
   4. Bronchi constrict
7. Mr. Garcia was seen with a blood pressure of 210/120 and has taken one dose of metoprolol and returned for a blood pressure reading. Which of the following blood pressures should be reported to the primary health care provider immediately?
   1. 150/100
   2. 200/100
   3. 250/130
   4. 170/80

ALTERNATE-FORMAT QUESTIONS

8. *The primary health care provider prescribes 60 mg propranolol to be given via the GI tube. The drug is available in an oral solution of 5 mg/mL. The nurse uses a total of 30 mL of warm water to flush before and after administering the drug. The total volume of fluid for this procedure was:
   1. 35 mL of water and drug solution.
   2. 42 mL of water and drug solution.
   3. 65 mL of water and drug solution.
   4. 72 mL of water and drug solution.

9. Select the terms that describe drugs that block the sympathetic branch of the autonomic nervous system. **Select all that apply.**
   1. Sympathomimetic
   2. Sympatholytic
   3. Antiadrenergic
   4. Anticholinergic
10. A client has just had a dose increase to 12.5 mg of carvedilol. The client has a bottle with 3.125-mg tablets and insists on finishing the bottle before buying a different strength. The nurse tells the client to take

   _____.

To check your answers, see Appendix F.

---

*Indicates the question is directly linked to the NCLEX-PN test plan in Appendix G.

Cholinergic Drugs

Key Terms

acetylcholine neurotransmitter that transmits impulses across the parasympathetic branch of the autonomic nervous system

acetylcholinesterase enzyme that can inactivate the neurotransmitter acetylcholine

cholinergic crisis cholinergic drug toxicity

micturition voiding of urine

miosis constriction of the pupil of the eye

muscarinic receptors neurologic receptors that stimulate smooth muscle in the parasympathetic branch of the autonomic nervous system

myasthenia gravis neuromuscular condition characterized by weakness and fatigability of the muscles

nicotinic receptors neurologic receptors that stimulate skeletal muscles in the parasympathetic branch of the autonomic nervous system

parasympathomimetic mimic the activity of the parasympathetic nervous system; also called *cholinergic drugs*

synergistic the effect is greater than that of each of the two drugs separately

Learning Objectives

On completion of this chapter, the student will:

1. Discuss important aspects of the parasympathetic nervous system.
2. Explain the uses, drug actions, general adverse reactions, contraindications, precautions, and interactions of cholinergic drugs.
3. Distinguish important preadministration and ongoing assessment activities the nurse should perform on the client taking a cholinergic drug.
4. List nursing diagnoses particular to a client taking a cholinergic drug.
5. Examine ways to promote an optimal response to therapy, how to manage common adverse reactions, and important points to keep in mind when educating the client about the use of cholinergic drugs.

Drug Classes

Direct acting
Indirect acting (anticholinesterase)

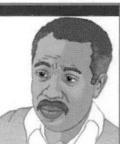

PHARMACOLOGY IN PRACTICE

Mr. Park is in the perioperative area, having just been given his preoperative medications for hip surgery. He is very concerned about the function of his bladder and bowels, because after falling in the garden he was unable to get up to urinate and needed to be straight-catheterized in the emergency room. Mr. Park is fearful that the surgery will lead to more retention issues and another infection, this time in his bladder.

Discussion now turns to another portion of the autonomic nervous system—the parasympathetic branch. To best understand how the parasympathetic nervous system and drugs associated with it work—*think opposites*! Stimulation of the parasympathetic pathway results in the body responding with opposite reactions to those triggered by the sympathetic system. The blood vessels dilate, sending blood to the gastrointestinal (GI) tract; secretions and peristalsis are activated and salivary glands increase production; the heart slows and pulmonary bronchioles constrict; the smooth muscle of the bladder contracts and the pupils of the eyes constrict (Fig. 25.1), all the opposite of what happens when the sympathetic system is stimulated.

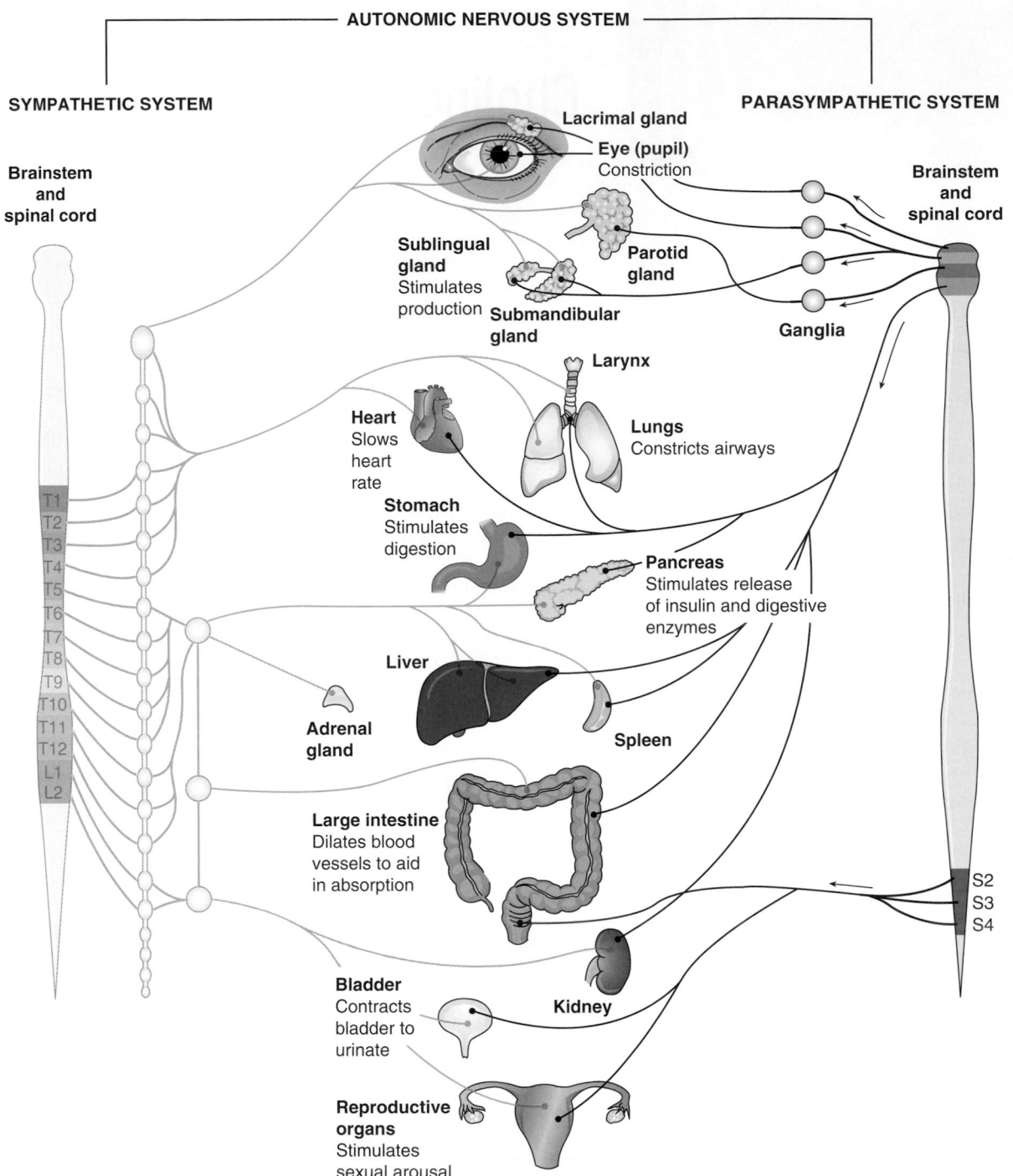

FIGURE 25.1 Responses of body organs and structures when the parasympathetic nervous system is stimulated. (Adapted from Cohen, B. J. (2003). *Medical terminology* (4th ed.). Lippincott Williams & Wilkins.)

AUTONOMIC TERMINOLOGY

We can say the response is the opposite of the flight, fight, or freeze concept. In fact, activation of these nerves is sometimes called the *rest-and-digest response*. To make it easier to remember and understand, Box 25.1 illustrates ways to remember the naming of various components of the parasympathetic branch.

Acetylcholine (ACh) is the neurotransmission substance that carries nerve impulses across the parasympathetic branch of the autonomic nervous system. There are two types of

receptors in the parasympathetic nervous branch: **muscarinic receptors** (which stimulate smooth muscle) and **nicotinic receptors** (which stimulate skeletal muscle).

Cholinergic drugs mimic the activity of the parasympathetic nervous system. They are also called **parasympathomimetic** drugs. What makes the parasympathetic system function differently is the enzyme **acetylcholinesterase** (AChE). AChE is an enzyme that can inactivate the neurotransmitter ACh, thereby preventing the nerve synapse

BOX 25.1 Demystifying the Autonomic Nervous System— Parasympathetic Branch

Terminology		Clue to Remembering
Anatomic Name	Parasympathetic	*Para*—beside, watches, not participate in the quick action
Functional Name	Cholinergic	Sounds like "colon"—digest connection
Primary Neurotransmitter	Acetylcholine (Ach)	
Enzymatic Blocker	Acetylcholinesterase (AChE)	

from continuing the nerve impulse. Again, this is very confusing terminology, and the information in Box 25.2 is meant to help you make these important distinctions. This interruption in neurotransmission can diminish cognitive function, which is seen in illnesses such as Alzheimer disease. Drugs that inhibit the enzyme AChE are called *anticholinesterases* or *acetylcholinesterase inhibitors*. These drugs are discussed specifically in Chapter 18.

ACTIONS

Drugs acting on the sympathetic nervous system more prominently impact the cardiac, circulatory, or respiratory systems. Cholinergic drugs that act on the parasympathetic nervous system more prominently impact vision, digestion, elimination, and the reproductive system. Drugs like the

BOX 25.2 More Variation on Drug Classes

Drug terminology to help you understand the drug class differences:

Cholinergic System = Parasympathetic branch of the autonomic nervous system

Cholinergic drugs = Parasympatho*mimetic* drugs (to mimic transmission of the parasympathetic nerve)

Anticholinergic = Cholinergic blocker drugs— Parasympatho*lytic* drugs (to stop the transmission of the parasympathetic nerve)

Opposite actions:

Adrenergic drugs *act like* Cholinergic blockers

Adrenergic blockers *act like* Cholinergic drugs

Enzymes make the difference in the Parasympathetic system:

Acetylcholinesterase (AChE)—inactivates neurotransmission in the parasympathetic nerve

The Double Negative:

Anticholinesterase or Acetylcholinesterase inhibitors—these **BLOCK** the activity of the enzyme (AChE) that **BLOCKS** parasympathetic transmission—in other words it makes it flow!

neurotransmitter ACh are called *direct-acting cholinergics.* An example of cholinergic influence is on the act of **micturition** (voiding of urine). Micturition is both a voluntary and an involuntary act. The parasympathetic branch of the autonomic nervous system partly controls the (involuntary) process of micturition by constricting the detrusor muscle and relaxing the bladder sphincter (Fig. 25.1). Urinary retention (not caused by a mechanical obstruction, such as a stone in the bladder) results when micturition is impaired. Treatment of urinary retention with direct-acting cholinergic drugs causes contraction of the bladder smooth muscles and passage of urine.

An example of indirect action is the use of cholinergic drugs to treat **myasthenia gravis**, a disease that involves rapid fatigue of skeletal muscles. This is because of the lack of ACh released at the nerve endings of parasympathetic nerves. Cholinergic drugs that prolong the activity of ACh by inhibiting the release of AChE are called *indirect-acting cholinergics* or *anticholinesterase muscle stimulants*. Primary treatment of this disease is accomplished with immunotherapy. Anticholinesterase drugs are additionally used to treat the symptoms of this disorder by acting indirectly to inhibit the activity of AChE and promote muscle contraction.

Treatment of glaucoma with an indirect-acting cholinergic drug produces **miosis** (constriction of the iris). Although used for many years, these drugs are rarely used today because of the frequency of dosing and side effects experienced. See the Summary Drug Table: Cholinergic Drugs for a more complete listing of these drugs.

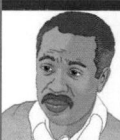

PHARMACOLOGY IN PRACTICE

PHYSIOLOGY
Which of the following is the substance responsible for transmission of nerve impulses across the parasympathetic nervous system?
1. Acetylcholine
2. Norepinephrine
3. Dopamine
4. Acetylcholinesterase

USES

Major uses of the cholinergic drugs are in the treatment of the following:

- Urinary retention (when drug therapy is indicated)
- Neurogenic bladder when retention is an issue
- Myasthenia gravis (for symptom management)

ADVERSE REACTIONS

General adverse reactions include the following:

- Nausea, diarrhea, abdominal cramping
- Salivation
- Flushing of the skin
- Cardiac arrhythmias and muscle weakness

CONTRAINDICATIONS

These drugs are contraindicated in clients with known hypersensitivity to the drugs, asthma, peptic ulcer disease, coronary artery disease, and hyperthyroidism. Bethanechol is contraindicated in those with mechanical obstruction of the GI or genitourinary tracts. Clients with secondary glaucoma, iritis, corneal abrasion, or any acute inflammatory disease of the eye should not use the ophthalmic cholinergic preparations.

PRECAUTIONS

These drugs are used cautiously in clients with hypertension, epilepsy, cardiac arrhythmias, bradycardia, recent coronary occlusion, and megacolon. The safety of these drugs has not been established for use during pregnancy (pregnancy category C) or lactation, or in children.

LASA ALERT

The following drugs may sound alike; be sure to clarify when they are ordered:

Drug Name	Sounds Like
bethanechol	betaxolol
guanidine	guanFACINE

Drugs that look like a similar drug are noted in the Summary Drug Tables of each chapter.

INTERACTIONS

The following interactions may occur when a cholinergic drug is administered with another agent:

Interacting Drug	Common Use	Effect of Interaction
Aminoglycoside antibiotics	Anti-infective agent	Increased neuromuscular blocking effect
Corticosteroids	Treatment of inflammation/ respiratory problems	Decreased effect of the cholinergic

When cholinergic drugs are administered with other cholinergics, there is a **synergistic** effect of the drugs and greater risk for toxicity. Concurrent use of more than one anticholinergic drug antagonizes the effects of cholinergic drugs. Because anticholinergic drugs can have this additive effect, atropine is the drug used as an antidote for overdosage of cholinergic drugs.

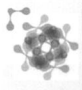

NURSING PROCESS—STEPS TO BUILDING CLINICAL JUDGMENT
Client Receiving a Cholinergic Drug

ASSESSMENT

Preadministration Assessment
Data gathering suggestions before the initial administration of the drug for urinary retention include:
Objective data

- General observation and palpation of abdomen, especially rounded swelling over the pelvis
- Bladder scanning and measurement of residual urine
- Vital signs (temperature, pulse, respirations, and blood pressure)
- Renal function tests, and urinalysis

Subjective data

- Client's description of retention, including pain, pressure, and incontinence
- Type and duration of symptoms, including bowel
- Drug and surgical history
- Remedies attempted before seeking care

Data gathering suggestions before the initial administration of the drug for management of symptoms associated with myasthenia gravis include:

- Complete neurologic assessment
- Interdisciplinary assessments—speech or occupational therapy (signs of muscle weakness, such as drooling

[i.e., the lack of ability to swallow], inability to chew and swallow, drooping of the eyelids, inability to perform repetitive movements [e.g., walking, combing hair, using eating utensils], difficulty breathing, and extreme fatigue.

Typically, the ocular symptoms, such as drooping eyelids or double vision, are less likely to improve than other symptoms.

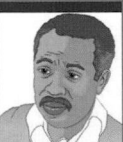

PHARMACOLOGY IN PRACTICE

ASSESSMENT
A primary health care provider has prescribed bethanechol to a client for acute urinary retention. What should the nurse check for in the client before the administration of bethanechol?
1. Tachyarrhythmias
2. Myocardial infarction
3. Coronary occlusion
4. Fecal contents in the large intestine

Ongoing Assessment
While the client is receiving a cholinergic drug, it is important to monitor for drug toxicity or cholinergic crisis.

NURSING ALERT

Cholinergic crisis (cholinergic drug toxicity) symptoms include severe abdominal cramping, diarrhea, excessive salivation, muscle weakness, rigidity and spasm, and clenching of the jaw. Clients exhibiting these symptoms require immediate medical treatment. In the case of drug overdose, an antidote such as atropine (0.4–0.6 mg intravenously) is administered.

Urinary Retention

Ongoing assessment for a client with urinary retention includes measuring and documenting fluid intake and output. If the amount of each voiding is insufficient or the client fails to void, palpate the bladder to determine its size, use the bladder scanner after the client attempts to void, and measure for urine residual. Notify the primary health care provider of the amount of urine the client is unable to eliminate or if the client fails to void after drug administration.

Myasthenia Gravis

Once therapy is under way, document any increase in symptoms of the disease or adverse drug reactions before giving each dose of the drug. Assess the client for the presence or absence of the symptoms of myasthenia gravis before each drug dose. In clients with severe myasthenia gravis, carry out these assessments between drug doses as well as immediately before drug administration. Document each symptom as well as the client's response or lack of response to drug therapy.

Assessment is important because the dosage frequently is increased or decreased early in therapy, depending on the client's response. Regulation of dosage is important in keeping the symptoms of myasthenia gravis from incapacitating the client. For many clients, the symptoms are fairly well controlled with drug therapy once the optimal drug dose is determined.

NURSING DIAGNOSIS

Drug-specific nursing diagnosis includes:

• **Diarrhea** related to adverse drug reaction

Nursing diagnoses related to drug administration are discussed in Chapter 4.

PLANNING

The expected outcomes of the client depend on the reason for administration of the cholinergic drug but may include an optimal response to therapy, meeting client needs related to the management of adverse reactions, and confidence in an understanding of the medication regimen.

IMPLEMENTATION

Promoting an Optimal Response to Therapy

The care of a client receiving a cholinergic drug depends on the drug used, the reason for administration, and the client's response to the drug.

Managing Urinary Retention

Voiding usually occurs in 5–15 min after subcutaneous drug administration and 30–90 min after oral administration. For institutionalized clients, place the call light and any other items the client might need, such as the urinal or the bedpan, within easy reach. However, should the client feel a sense of urinary urgency and not be able to handle these aids easily, promptly answer the client's call light.

Managing Myasthenia Gravis

Oral drug administration is typically the route used to manage symptoms. At the start of therapy, determining the dosage that will control symptoms may be difficult. In many cases, the dosage must be adjusted upward or downward until optimal drug effects are obtained. Clients with severe symptoms of the disease require the drug every 2–4 hr, even during the night. Sustained-release tablets are available that allow less frequent dosing and help the client to have longer undisturbed periods during the night.

NURSING ALERT

Because of the need to make frequent dosage adjustments, observe the client closely for symptoms of drug overdosage or underdosage. Signs of drug overdosage include muscle rigidity and spasm, salivation, and clenching of the jaw. Signs of drug underdosage are signs of the disease itself, namely, rapid fatigability of the muscles, drooping of the eyelids, and difficulty breathing. If symptoms of drug overdosage or underdosage develop, contact the primary health care provider immediately.

Monitoring and Managing Client Needs

When a cholinergic drug is given by the oral or parenteral route, adverse drug reactions may affect many systems of the body, such as the heart, respiratory and GI tracts, and central nervous system. Observe the client closely for the appearance of adverse drug reactions, such as a change in vital signs or an increase in symptoms. You should document any complaints the client may have and notify the primary health care provider.

Diarrhea

When these drugs are used orally, they occasionally result in excessive salivation, abdominal cramping, flatus, and sometimes diarrhea. Inform the client that these reactions will continue until tolerance develops, usually within a few weeks. Until tolerance develops, you need to ensure that proper facilities, such as a bedside commode, bedpan, or bathroom, are readily available. The client is encouraged to ambulate to assist the passing of flatus. If needed, a rectal tube may be used to assist in the passing of flatus. Document fluid intake and output and track the number, consistency, and frequency of stools if diarrhea is present. The primary health care provider is informed if diarrhea is excessive because this may be an indication of toxicity.

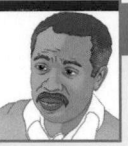

PHARMACOLOGY IN PRACTICE

MANAGING NEEDS
What drug is used to counteract a cholinergic crisis?
1. Zyban
2. Pyridostigmine
3. Corticosteroids
4. Atropine

Educating the Client and Family

Clients required to take a drug over a long period may incur lapses in their drug schedule. For some, it is a matter of occasionally forgetting to take a drug; for others, a lapse may be caused by other factors, such as failure to understand the importance of drug therapy, the cost of the drug, or unfamiliarity with the consequences associated with discontinuing the drug therapy.

When developing a teaching plan for the client and family, emphasize the importance of uninterrupted drug therapy. Allow the client and family time to ask questions, especially when dealing with clients who are older or for whom English is not their first language. Explore any problems that appear to be associated with the prescribed drug regimen and then report them to the primary health care provider. Be sure confidence in understanding the purpose of the drug therapy is evident from the client and family, as well as an understanding of the adverse reactions that may occur.

Myasthenia Gravis
Clients with myasthenia gravis learn to adjust their drug dosage according to their needs, because dosage needs may vary slightly from day to day. Teach the client and family members to feel confident in recognizing

symptoms of overdosage and underdosage, as well as what steps the primary health care provider wishes them to take if either occurs. The dosage regimen is explained and instruction is given in how to adjust the dosage upward or downward.

Be sure that written or printed descriptions of the signs and symptoms of drug overdosage or underdosage are in the preferred language if the client does not understand English. Demonstrate for the client how to keep a record of the response to drug therapy (e.g., time of day, increased or decreased muscle strength, fatigue) and to bring this to each primary health care provider or clinic visit until the symptoms are well controlled and the drug dosage is stabilized. Make sure these clients have identification (such as a Medic Alert tag) indicating that they have myasthenia gravis.

EVALUATION

- Therapeutic effect is achieved.
- Adverse reactions are identified, reported to the primary health care provider, and managed successfully through appropriate nursing interventions:
  - Client reports adequate bowel movements.
- Client and family express confidence and demonstrate an understanding of the drug regimen.

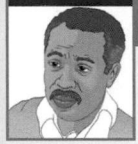

PHARMACOLOGY IN PRACTICE

USING CLINICAL REASONING
When urinary retention leads to placement of a urinary catheter, it results in putting the client at risk for infection. With the information learned about the cholinergic drugs, what can you tell Mr. Park that will help calm him before surgery?

KEY POINTS

■ The parasympathetic branch of the autonomic nervous system functions the opposite of the sympathetic branch. The neurotransmitter of the parasympathetic branch is acetylcholine; activation of this system is often called the rest-and-digest response. What makes this system different is the enzyme acetylcholinesterase. This enzyme inactivates acetylcholine in the nerve synapse.

■ The purpose of cholinergic drugs is to send blood flow to the digestive tract, stimulating secretions and peristalsis. The heart rate slows and lung bronchi constrict. Smooth muscle of the bladder contracts and voiding is made possible.

■ Drugs that mimic the response are called parasympathomimetic or cholinergic (because the primary transmitter is acetylcholine). Actions in the body are modified depending on how the drug acts on different cell receptors. Drugs can be selective for muscarinic or nicotinic receptors. Drugs can be direct acting or indirect acting.

■ These drugs are used to treat urinary retention, the disease myasthenia gravis, and infrequently glaucoma. Adverse reactions are typically GI in nature, ranging from nausea to diarrhea and abdominal cramping.

SUMMARY DRUG TABLE
Cholinergic Drugs

Generic Name	Trade Name	Uses	Adverse Reactions	Dosage Ranges
Direct-Acting Cholinergics				
bethanechol *be-THAN-e-kole*	Urecholine	Acute nonobstructive urinary retention, neurogenic atony of urinary bladder with urinary retention	Abdominal discomfort, headache, diarrhea, nausea, salivation, urgency	10–50 mg orally BID to QID; 2.5–5 mg subcutaneously TID to QID
Indirect-Acting (Anticholinesterase) Muscle Stimulants				
guanidine *GWAHN-i-deen*		Myasthenic syndrome (Eaton–Lambert disease)	Palpitations, numbness in lips/extremities, dry mouth, nausea, abdominal cramping	10–30 mg/kg/day, titrate until adverse reaction occurs
pyridostigmine *peer-id-oh-STIG-meen*	Mestinon, Regonol	Myasthenia gravis	Increased bronchial secretions, cardiac arrhythmias, muscle weakness	Average dose is 600 mg/day orally at spaced intervals

See Chapter 18 for Cholinesterase Inhibitors.

CHAPTER REVIEW

Know Your Drugs

Clients sometimes know a medication by the brand (or trade) name and not the generic name. To help you recognize both names, match the brand name with the generic name of the same medication.

Generic Name	Brand Name
1. bethanechol	A. Duvoid
2. pyridostigmine	B. Mestinon
	C. Urecholine

Calculate Medication Dosages

1. The primary care provider prescribes 2.5 mg of bethanechol subcutaneously. The drug is available in a solution of 5 mg/mL. The nurse administers _____.

Prepare for the NCLEX

RECALL THE FACTS

1. What is the transmitting substance in the parasympathetic branch of the nervous system?
   1. Serotonin
   2. Norepinephrine
   3. Dopamine
   4. Acetylcholine
2. In which condition are drugs used to stop the enzyme that prevents neurotransmission?
   1. Urinary retention
   2. Myasthenia gravis
   3. Glaucoma
   4. Alzheimer disease
3. A client has received a diagnosis of myasthenia gravis and begins a regimen of pyridostigmine. The nursing assessment is important because the dose of the drug _____.
   1. usually must be increased every 4 hr early in therapy
   2. frequently is increased or decreased early in therapy
   3. is titrated according to the client's blood pressure
   4. is gradually decreased as a therapeutic response is achieved

ANALYZE THE FACTS

4. *When acetylcholine is transmitted in the parasympathetic nervous system, which of the following occurs?
   1. Heart rate increases
   2. Pupils of the eye dilate
   3. Digestion is stimulated
   4. Bronchi relax

ALTERNATE-FORMAT QUESTIONS

5. Select the terms that describe drugs that affect the parasympathetic branch of the autonomic nervous system. **Select all that apply.**
   1. Parasympathomimetic
   2. Parasympatholytic
   3. Adrenergic
   4. Cholinergic
6. The dosage of pyridostigmine (Mestinon) is 600 mg/day. How many 60 mg tablets will the client take?

To check your answers, see Appendix F.

_____

*Indicates the question is directly linked to the NCLEX-PN test plan in Appendix G.

WANT TO KNOW MORE? A wide variety of resources are available to enhance your learning and understanding of this chapter.
- Visit the**Point** for resources such as:
  - NCLEX-Style Student Review Questions
  - Journal Articles
  - Dosage Calculations
  - Drug Monographs
  - Watch and Learn Videos
  - Concepts in Action Animations
- The *Study Guide to Accompany Introductory Clinical Pharmacology*, 12th edition, sold separately, will help you review and apply essential content.
- ✓**PrepU** is available to help students prepare for the NCLEX-PN examination.

Cholinergic Blocking Drugs

26

Key Terms

anticholinergic blocks the neurotransmission of the parasympathetic nervous system

cholinergic blocking blocks the effect of the parasympathetic branch of the autonomic nervous system; also called anticholinergics

cycloplegia paralysis of the ciliary muscle, resulting in an inability to focus the eye

drug idiosyncrasy any unusual or abnormal response that differs from the response normally expected to a specific drug and dosage

mydriasis dilation of the pupil

parasympatholytic blocking the parasympathetic nervous system

xerostomia drying of oral secretions

Learning Objectives

On completion of this chapter, the student will:

1. Explain the uses, general drug actions, general adverse reactions, contraindications, precautions, and interactions of the cholinergic blocking drugs (also called anticholinergic drugs and cholinergic blockers).
2. Distinguish important preadministration and ongoing assessment activities the nurse should perform on the client taking a cholinergic blocking drug.
3. List nursing diagnoses particular to the client taking a cholinergic blocking drug.
4. Examine ways to promote an optimal response to therapy, how to manage common adverse reactions, and important points to keep in mind when educating clients taking cholinergic blocking drugs.

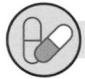 **Drug Classes**

Anticholinergics	Anti-Parkinson cholinergic
Cholinergic blocking urinary	blocking
antispasmodics	Respiratory cholinergic blocking

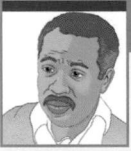 **PHARMACOLOGY IN PRACTICE**

Mr. Park is in the perioperative area having just been given his preoperative medications for hip surgery. He is very concerned about the function of his bladder and bowels. His stomach feels "rumbly" and he is very concerned that he will be incontinent of stool in the bed. After reading this chapter, decide whether his concerns are valid.

The **cholinergic blocking** drugs discussed in this chapter block the effects of cholinergic drugs on the parasympathetic system; this interaction is similar to how adrenergic and adrenergic blocking drugs interact with the sympathetic nervous system. The difference on the autonomic system is the opposite; blocking the parasympathetic system is like stimulating the sympathetic system.

AUTONOMIC TERMINOLOGY

Acetylcholine (ACh) is the primary neurotransmitter in the parasympathetic branch of the autonomic nervous system. Cholinergic blocking drugs block the action of the neurotransmitter ACh in

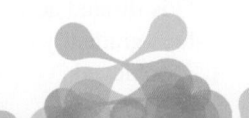

BOX 26.1	More Variation on Drug Class Names
Parasympatholytic Anticholinergic Cholinergic blockers	All terms meaning—to stop the neurotransmission of acetylcholine along the parasympathetic branch of the autonomic nervous system

the parasympathetic nervous system. Cholinergic blocking drugs are also called **anticholinergic** drugs, or **parasympatholytic**, and less frequently cholinergic blockers (Box 26.1). Parasympathetic nerves reach many areas of the body; therefore, the effects of the cholinergic blocking drugs are numerous.

ACTIONS

Cholinergic blocking drugs inhibit the activity of ACh at the parasympathetic nerve synapse. When the activity of ACh is inhibited, impulses traveling along the parasympathetic nerve cannot pass from the nerve ending to an organ or structure.

As mentioned in Chapter 25, two types of receptors are found in the parasympathetic nerve branch: muscarinic and nicotinic receptors. Cholinergic blocking drugs most often are selective and target just one of these two types of receptors. The receptor type targeted is dependent on the drug.

For example, antispasmodic drugs used to treat an overactive urinary bladder are selective and work by inhibiting the action of the muscarinic receptors in the parasympathetic nervous system. As a result, the detrusor muscle of the bladder does not contract, which prevents the sensations of urinary urgency. Because they are selective, a urinary antispasmodic drug has no effect on skeletal muscles, because it does not inhibit the nicotinic receptors in the parasympathetic nervous system that innervate the skeletal muscles.

Another example involves drugs selective for muscarinic receptors that are used as maintenance treatment of chronic respiratory conditions such as chronic obstructive pulmonary disease (COPD) and asthma. In obstructive lung disease (e.g., asthma) stimulation of the parasympathetic nerves seems to make disease symptoms worse. When drugs such as ipratropium are used to manage bronchodilation in nonacute conditions, these drugs block the release of ACh in airway smooth muscles, thus reducing bronchial constriction. Use of these drugs once or twice daily helps to reduce breathing distress and increase lung function. Because the drugs are selective for M₃ muscarinic receptors, they have less adverse reactions in other body systems (Buels & Fryer, 2012). Consequently, when a nonselective drug is used and because of the wide distribution of parasympathetic nerves, many organs and structures of the body, including the eyes, the respiratory and gastrointestinal (GI) tracts, the heart, and the bladder can be affected (Fig. 26.1). Looking back at Chapter 23, you will note that responses caused by blocking the

parasympathetic nervous system are similar to those that activate the sympathetic response.

As you gain an understanding of the complexity of the interaction of drug and nerve synapse, a word of caution, responses may not follow the patterns explained in this unit all the time. For example, scopolamine (an anticholinergic drug) may occasionally cause excitement, delirium, and restlessness, which are responses different than anticipated. This reaction is considered a **drug cidiosyncrasy** (an unexpected or unusual drug effect).

 Lifespan Considerations

Gerontology
Because older clients taking a cholinergic blocking drug have exhibited symptoms such as excitement, agitation, mental confusion, drowsiness, urinary retention, or other adverse effects, it is recommended that many of these drugs not be used for those older than 65 years. These effects may be seen even with small doses. The benefit of the medication reducing the intended symptoms should outweigh the risk of injury when prescribed.

USES

The primary uses of cholinergic blocking drugs are in the treatment of the following:

- Maintenance treatment of asthma and COPD
- Ureteral or biliary colic and bladder overactivity
- Pylorospasm and peptic ulcer
- Vagal nerve–induced bradycardia

In addition, the cholinergic blocking drugs are administered for the preoperative reduction of oral secretions. The Summary Drug Table: Cholinergic Blocking Drugs lists the uses of specific cholinergic blocking drugs.

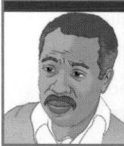 **PHARMACOLOGY IN PRACTICE**

PHYSIOLOGY
Oxybutynin, used for the treatment of overactive bladder, exerts its effect by inhibiting the action of which of the following receptors?
1. Nicotinic receptors
2. Alpha-adrenergic (α-adrenergic) receptors
3. Muscarinic receptors
4. Beta-adrenergic (β-adrenergic) receptors

ADVERSE REACTIONS

The severity of many adverse reactions is often dose dependent—that is, the larger the dose, the more intense the adverse reaction. Adverse reactions of selected body systems occurring with the administration of a cholinergic blocking drug are listed below.

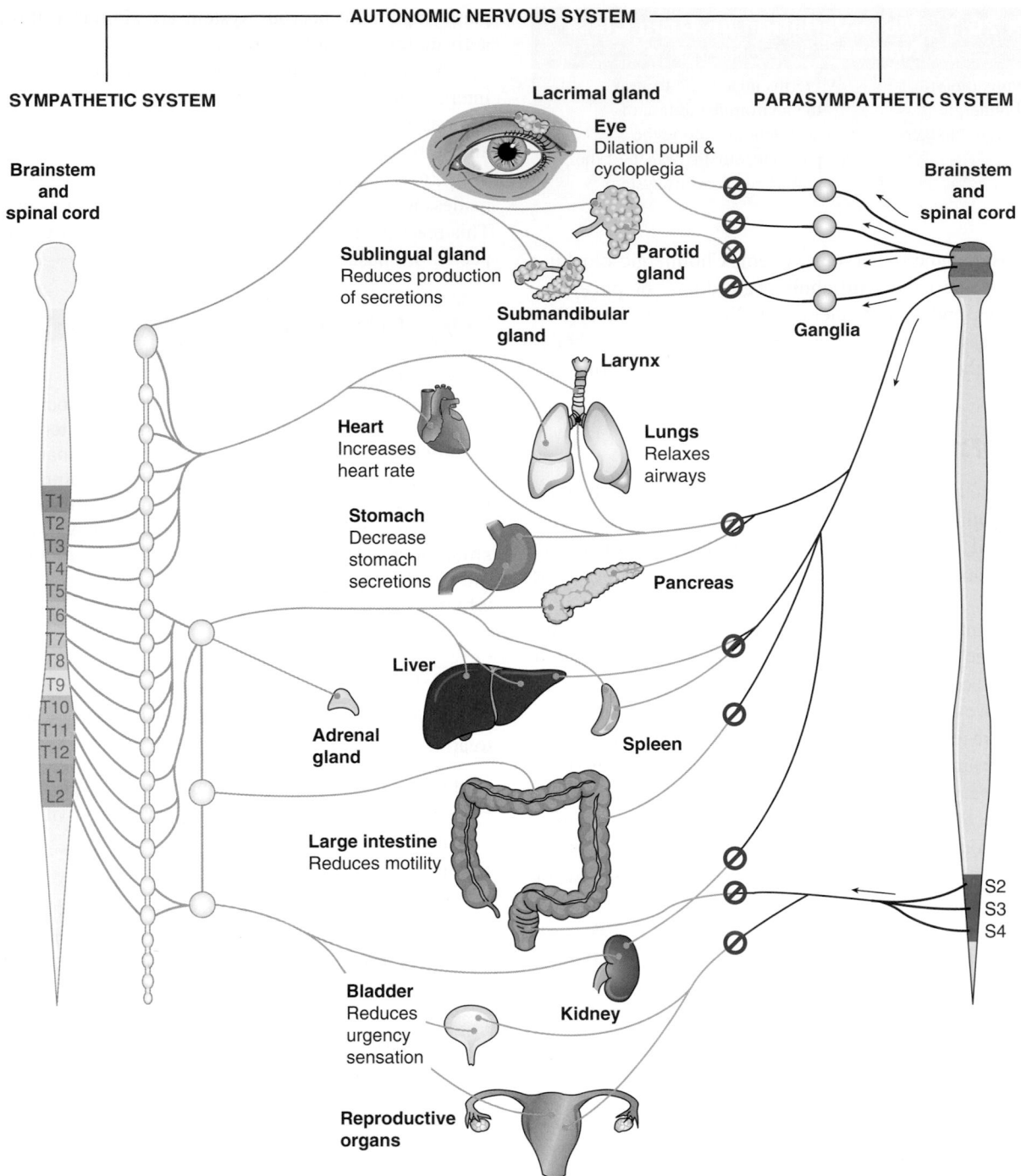

AUTONOMIC NERVOUS SYSTEM

SYMPATHETIC SYSTEM

PARASYMPATHETIC SYSTEM

Lacrimal gland

Eye
Dilation pupil &
cycloplegia

Brainstem
and
spinal cord

Brainstem
and
spinal cord

Sublingual gland
Reduces production
of secretions

**Parotid
gland**

**Submandibular
gland**

Ganglia

Larynx

Heart
Increases
heart rate

Lungs
Relaxes
airways

Stomach
Decrease
stomach
secretions

Pancreas

Liver

**Adrenal
gland**

Spleen

T1
T2
T3
T4
T5
T6
T7
T8
T9
T10
T11
T12
L1
L2

Large intestine
Reduces motility

S2
S3
S4

Bladder
Reduces
urgency
sensation

Kidney

**Reproductive
organs**

FIGURE 26.1 Bodily responses of blocking the stimulation of the parasympathetic nervous system. (Adapted from Cohen, B. J. (2003). *Medical terminology* (4th ed.). Lippincott Williams & Wilkins.)

Gastrointestinal System Reactions
- Dry mouth, nausea, vomiting
- Difficulty in swallowing, heartburn
- Constipation

Central Nervous System Reactions
- Headache, flushing, nervousness
- Drowsiness, weakness, insomnia
- Nasal congestion, fever

Visual Reactions
- Blurred vision
- Mydriasis (dilation of the pupil)
- Photophobia
- **Cycloplegia** (paralysis of accommodation or inability to focus the eye)
- Increased ocular tension

Genitourinary System Reactions

- Urinary hesitancy and retention
- Dysuria

Cardiovascular System Reactions

- Palpitations
- Bradycardia (after low doses of atropine)
- Tachycardia (after higher doses of atropine)

Other Reactions

- Urticaria
- Decreased sweat production
- Anaphylactic shock
- Rash

Sometimes a secondary adverse reaction is as desirable as the intended use. An example of this includes drowsiness when atropine is used before surgery to reduce respiratory secretions. Although drying up the respiratory system is the reason the drug is given, drowsiness is a benefit in addition to the desired response.

During hot summer months, clients receiving a cholinergic blocking drug should be instructed to watch for signs of heat prostration (e.g., fever; tachycardia; flushing; warm, dry skin; mental confusion) because these drugs decrease the person's ability to sweat.

CONTRAINDICATIONS

Cholinergic blocking drugs are contraindicated in clients with known hypersensitivity to the drugs or glaucoma. Other clients for whom cholinergic blocking drugs are contraindicated are those with myasthenia gravis, tachyarrhythmia, myocardial infarction, and heart failure (unless bradycardia is present).

PRECAUTIONS

These drugs are used with caution in clients with GI infections, benign prostatic hypertrophy, urinary retention, hyperthyroidism, hepatic or renal disease, and hypertension. Use atropine with caution in clients with asthma, because of generalized reactions. Caution is used in prescribing these drugs for clients over the age of 65 years, yet the indication for use may be due to aging of the body. The benefit of the drug should always outweigh the risk of the adverse reactions when prescribed. Cholinergic blocking drugs are classified as pregnancy category C drugs and are used only when the benefit to the woman outweighs the risk to the fetus. This caution also applies to over-the-counter preparations available for the relief of allergy and cold symptoms and as aids to induce sleep. Some of these products contain atropine, scopolamine, or other cholinergic blocking drugs. Although this warning is printed on the container or package, many users fail to read drug labels carefully.

LASA ALERT

The following drugs may sound alike; be sure to clarify when they are ordered:

Drug Name	*Sounds Like*
benztropine	Bromocriptine
dicyclomine	diphenhydrAMINE, doxycycline, dyclonine
Ditropan	Detrol, diazepam, Diprivan, dithranol
Enablex	Effexor XR
fesoterodine	fexofenadine, tolterodine
flavoxATE	fluvoxaMINE
oxybutynin	OxyCONTIN
revefenacin	darifenacin, Revlimid
Spiriva	Apidra, Inspra, Serevent
trihexyphenidyl	Trifluoperazine
tiotropium	ipratropium
Tudorza	Jolessa, Lodosyn, Taclonex, Tekturna HCT, Tekturna, Tikosyn, Tobrex, Toradol, Truvada, Tubersol, Zaditor

Drugs that look like a similar drug are noted in the Summary Drug Tables of each chapter.

INTERACTIONS

The following interactions may occur when a cholinergic blocking drug is administered with another agent:

Interacting Drug	Common Use	Effect of Interaction
Antibiotics/ antifungals	Fight infection	Decreased effectiveness of anti-infective drug
Meperidine, flurazepam, phenothiazines	Preoperative sedation	Increased effect of the cholinergic blocker
Tricyclic antidepressants	Management of depression	Increased effect of the cholinergic blocker
Haloperidol	Antianxiety/ antipsychotic agent	Decreased effectiveness of the antipsychotic drug
Digoxin	Management of cardiac problems	Increased serum levels of digoxin

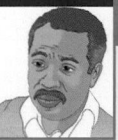

PHARMACOLOGY IN PRACTICE

SAFE DRUG ADMINISTRATION

A client who was prescribed a cholinergic blocking drug is concerned about drug interactions. The client informs the nurse that he is taking the antidepressant Wellbutrin. What antidepressant drug class interacts with cholinergic blockers?

1. Selective serotonin reuptake inhibitors
2. Serotonin–norepinephrine reuptake inhibitors
3. Tricyclics
4. Monoamine oxidase inhibitors

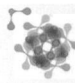

NURSING PROCESS: STEPS TO BUILDING CLINICAL JUDGMENT
Client Receiving a Cholinergic Blocking Drug

ASSESSMENT

Maintenance of chronic respiratory symptoms and urinary bladder spasm is the primary use of cholinergic blockers. Because separate chapters are devoted to these issues, the focus of nursing concerns in this chapter will be for surgical or ulcer management.

Preadministration Assessment

Data gathering suggestions before the initial administration of the drug include:
Objective data

- Vital signs (temperature, pulse, respirations, and blood pressure)
- Description of signs, such as occult blood in stool for peptic ulcer, visual acuity for glaucoma
- Measure for weight loss, or look for dehydration (e.g., poor skin turgor, dry lips/mouth)

Subjective data

- History of general health and well-being
- Pain experience—onset, type (e.g., sharp, dull, burning), radiation, location, intensity, and duration
- Client's description of symptoms of the current disorder and remedies attempted before seeking care

Ongoing Assessment

When administering a cholinergic blocking drug, check vital signs, observe for adverse drug reactions, and evaluate the symptoms and complaints related to the client's diagnosis. For example, question the client with a peptic ulcer regarding current symptoms, and then make a comparison of these symptoms with the symptoms present before the start of therapy. Document any increase in the severity of symptoms and notify the primary health care provider.

NURSING DIAGNOSES

Drug-specific nursing diagnoses include:

- **Impaired comfort** related to **xerostomia**
- **Constipation** related to slowing of peristalsis in the GI tract
- **Injury risk** related to dizziness, drowsiness, mental confusion, impaired vision, or heat prostration
- **Ineffective tissue perfusion** related to impaired heart pumping action

Nursing diagnoses related to drug administration are discussed in Chapter 4.

PLANNING

The expected outcomes for the client depend on the reason for administration of a cholinergic blocking drug but may include an optimal response to therapy, meeting client needs related to the management of adverse reactions, and confidence in an understanding of and adherence to the prescribed medication regimen.

IMPLEMENTATION

Promoting an Optimal Response to Therapy

If a cholinergic blocking drug is administered before surgery, be sure to give it at the exact time prescribed because the drug must be given time to produce the greatest effect (i.e., the drying of upper respiratory and oral secretions) before the administration of a general anesthetic. Before administration, instruct the client to void. Inform the client and family members that drowsiness and extreme dryness of the mouth and nose will occur about 20–30 min after the drug is given. This is normal, and fluid is not to be taken. The side rails of the bed are raised, and the client is instructed to remain in bed after administration of the preoperative drug.

Lifespan Considerations

Gerontology

Cholinergic blocking drugs are usually not included in the preoperative drugs of clients older than 60 years.

Monitoring and Managing Client Needs

Impaired Comfort: Xerostomia

When taking these drugs on a daily basis, mouth dryness may be severe and extremely uncomfortable. The client may complain of a "cottonmouth" sensation, in which oral dryness feels like a mouthful of cotton. The client may have moderate to extreme difficulty swallowing drugs and food. The client's speech may be impeded and hard to understand because of the dry mouth.

Encourage the client to take a few sips of water before and while taking an oral drug and to sip water at intervals during meals. If allowed, hard candy slowly dissolved in the mouth and frequent sips of water during the day may help relieve persistent oral dryness. Check the oral cavity frequently for soreness or ulcerations. Refer to the Client Teaching for Improved Client Outcomes: Combating Dry Mouth for suggestions on diminishing the discomfort.

Constipation

Constipation caused by decreased gastric motility can be a problem with cholinergic blocking drugs. Encourage the client to increase fluid intake up to 2000 mL daily (if health conditions permit), eat a diet high in fiber, and engage in adequate exercise. Clients being treated for an overactive bladder may be hesitant to increase fluids because of fear of an episode of urinary incontinence. Reassure the client that increasing fluids will help minimize the adverse reactions of constipation and dry mouth, whereas the cholinergic blocking drug helps to eliminate the sensations of urinary frequency and urgency (Fig. 26.2). The primary health care provider may prescribe a stool softener, if necessary, to prevent constipation.

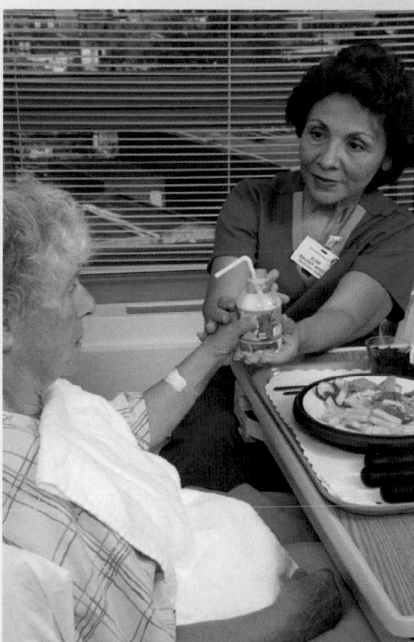

FIGURE 26.2 Because of the reduction in secretions caused by anticholinergic drugs, encourage fluids during all client interactions.

Injury Risk

These drugs may cause drowsiness, dizziness, and blurred vision. Clients (especially older adults) may require assistance with ambulation. Blurred vision and photophobia are commonly seen with the administration of a cholinergic blocking drug. The severity of this adverse reaction is commonly dose dependent; that is, the larger the dose, the more intense the adverse reaction.

Monitor the client for any disturbance in vision. If photophobia is a problem, the client may need to wear shaded glasses when going outside, even on cloudy days. Those with photophobia may be more comfortable in a semi-darkened room, especially on sunny days. Rooms are kept dimly lit and curtains or blinds closed to eliminate bright sunlight in the room. Unfortunately, this will increase the risk of fall injury. Clients should be taught to call for assistance to prevent injury when ambulation is required.

Mydriasis (prolonged pupillary dilation) and **cycloplegia** (paralysis of the ciliary muscle, resulting in difficulty focusing), if they occur, may interfere with reading, watching television, and similar activities. Screen time should be avoided to reduce strain on the eyes. If these drug effects upset the client, discuss the problem with the primary health care provider. At times, these visual impairments will have to be tolerated because drug therapy cannot be changed or discontinued. Encourage the client to engage in other forms of diversional therapy, such as interaction with others or listening to the radio.

Client Teaching for Improved Outcomes

Combating Dry Mouth

One of the most common and uncomfortable adverse effects occurring with the use of cholinergic blocking drugs is a dry mouth. There are strategies to help both reduce the discomfort and maintain a healthy oral cavity. *When you teach, make sure your client understands the following:*

✔ Perform frequent mouth care, including brushing, rinsing, and flossing.
✔ Keep a glass or sports bottle filled with fluid on hand at all times.
✔ Sip small amounts of cool water or fluids throughout the day and with meals.
✔ Try one of the flavor additives or a slice of lemon, lime, or cucumber in the water.
✔ Take a few sips of water before taking any oral drugs.
✔ Suck on ice chips or frozen ices, such as popsicles.
✔ Chew gum, preferably sugarless.
✔ Suck on sugar-free hard candies.
✔ Avoid alcohol-based mouthwashes.

 Lifespan Considerations

Gerontology

Discuss with the family of an older client possible visual and mental impairments (blurred vision, confusion, agitation) that may occur during therapy with these drugs. Objects or situations that may cause falls, such as throw rugs, footstools, and wet or newly waxed floors, are removed or avoided whenever possible. Show the family how to place items with the potential to obstruct walkways against the walls (e.g., footstools, chairs, stands).

The physiologic mechanism of sweating may decrease and can be followed by heat prostration. Make sure the client is observed at frequent intervals for signs of overheating, especially if the client is older or debilitated. Avoid going outside on hot, sunny days; use fans to cool the body if the day is extremely warm; sponge the skin with cool water if other cooling measures are not available; and wear loose-fitting clothes in warm weather. In cases of suspected heat prostration, the next dose of the drug is withheld and the primary health care provider contacted immediately. The older adult client receiving a cholinergic blocking drug is also observed at frequent intervals for excitement, agitation, mental confusion, drowsiness, urinary retention, or other adverse effects. If any of these should occur, the next dose of the drug should be withheld and the primary health care provider contacted. Client safety must be ensured until these adverse reactions subside.

Ineffective Tissue Perfusion

The client receiving atropine for third-degree heart block is placed on a cardiac monitor during and after administration of the drug. The monitor is watched for a change in pulse rate or rhythm. Tachycardia, other cardiac arrhythmias, or failure of the drug to increase the heart rate is reported to the primary health care provider immediately because other drugs or medical management may be necessary.

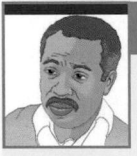

PHARMACOLOGY IN PRACTICE

MANAGING CLIENT NEEDS

Which of the following interventions should a nurse perform when caring for a client receiving a cholinergic blocking drug and who is experiencing constipation?

1. Place items against walls to ensure clear path to bathroom.
2. Engage in handwork activities.
3. Monitor food intake to be sure the client is eating fiber-rich foods.
4. Monitor for a change in pulse rate or rhythm.

Educating the Client and Family

A cholinergic blocking drug may be prescribed for a prolonged period. Some clients may discontinue drug use, especially if their original symptoms have been relieved. Make sure that the client and family understand that the prescribed drug is to be continued even though symptoms have been relieved.

When a cholinergic blocking drug is prescribed for outpatient use, teach the client about the more common adverse reactions associated with these drugs, such as dry mouth, drowsiness, dizziness, and visual impairments. Warn the client that if drowsiness, dizziness, or blurred

vision occurs, caution must be observed while driving or performing other tasks requiring alertness and clear vision.

Some of the adverse reactions associated with the cholinergic blocking drugs may be uncomfortable or distressing. Encourage the client to discuss these problems with the primary health care provider. You can offer suggestions to lessen the intensity of some of these adverse reactions.

EVALUATION

- Therapeutic effect is achieved.
- Adverse reactions are identified, reported to the primary health care provider, and managed successfully through appropriate nursing interventions:
  - Mucous membranes remain moist.
  - Client reports adequate bowel movements.
  - No evidence of injury is seen.
  - Tissue perfusion is maintained.
- Client and family express confidence and demonstrate an understanding of the drug regimen.

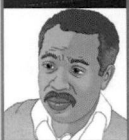

PHARMACOLOGY IN PRACTICE

USING CLINICAL REASONING

A nurse assistant comes to you because they are having difficulty with Mr. Park. The nursing assistant is frustrated with his continual struggles to get out of bed and asks you about the purpose of preoperative drugs and why clients cannot get out of bed after receiving a preoperative drug. Describe how you would explain this to the nurse assistant.

KEY POINTS

■ The parasympathetic branch of the autonomic nervous system regulates both involuntary body functions and skeletal muscles. The anticholinergic drugs block the neurotransmitter acetylcholine in the parasympathetic branch.

■ The purpose of cholinergic blocking drugs is to block or interrupt the signals that send blood flow to the digestive tract, including salivary secretions and colon peristalsis. These drugs also reduce spasms of the overactive bladder, reducing urinary urgency.

■ Drugs that block the parasympathetic system are called parasympatholytic or anticholinergic. Actions in the body

are modified depending on how the drug acts on different cell receptors. Drugs can be selective for muscarinic or nicotinic receptors. Drugs can also affect skeletal muscles.

■ These drugs are used to treat gastric sphincter spasm, ureteral and biliary colic, bladder overactivity, bradycardia, respiratory distress, and Parkinson disease.

■ Adverse reactions include decreased oral secretions, slower GI motility, constipation, nasal congestion, vision problems, and urinary retention. Mental reactions of excitement, agitation, confusion, and drowsiness may occur, especially in the older client.

SUMMARY DRUG TABLE
Cholinergic Blocking Drugs

Generic Name	Trade Name	Uses	Adverse Reactions	Dosage Ranges
atropine *A-troe-peen*	AtroPen	Pylorospasm, reduction of bronchial and oral secretions, excessive vagal-induced bradycardia, anticholinesterase poisoning	Drowsiness, blurred vision, tachycardia, dry mouth, urinary hesitancy	0.4–0.6 mg orally, IM, subcut, IV
dicyclomine *dye-SYE-kloe-meen*	Bentyl	Functional bowel/irritable bowel syndrome	Same as atropine	80–160 mg orally QID
glycopyrrolate *glye-koe-PYE-roe-late*		Oral: peptic ulcer Parenteral: in conjunction with anesthesia to reduce bronchial and oral secretions, to block cardiac vagal inhibitory reflexes during induction of anesthesia and intubation; protection against the peripheral muscarinic effects of cholinergic agents (e.g., neostigmine)	Blurred vision, dry mouth, altered taste perception, nausea, vomiting, dysphagia, urinary hesitancy and retention	Oral: 1–2 mg BID or TID Parenteral: peptic ulcer, 0.1–0.2 mg IM, IV, TID, QID Preanesthesia: 0.002 mg/lb IM Intraoperative: 0.1 mg IV
methscopolamine *meth-skoe-POL-a-meen*		Adjunctive therapy for peptic ulcer	Same as atropine	2.5 mg 30 min before meals and 2.5–5 mg orally at bedtime
propantheline *proe-PAN-the-leen*		Adjunctive therapy for peptic ulcer	Dry mouth, constipation, hesitancy, urinary retention, blurred vision	15 mg orally 30 min before meals and at bedtime
scopolamine *skoe-POL-a-meen*		Preanesthetic sedation, motion sickness	Confusion, dry mouth, constipation, urinary hesitancy, urinary retention, blurred vision	0.32–0.65 mg IM, subcut, IV, diluted with sterile water for injections Transdermal: apply 1 patch 4 hr before travel q3days
Cholinergic Blocking Urinary Antispasmodics				
darifenacin *dar-i-FEN-a-sin*	Enablex	Overactive bladder	Dry mouth, constipation	7.5 mg orally daily
fesoterodine *fes-oh-TER-oh-deen*	Toviaz	Overactive bladder	Dry mouth, constipation	4–8 mg orally daily
flavoxATE *fla-VOKS-ate*		Urinary symptoms caused by cystitis, prostatitis, and other urinary problems	Dry mouth, drowsiness, blurred vision, headache, urinary retention	100–200 mg orally 3–4 times/day
oxybutynin *oks-i-BYOO-ti-nin*	Ditropan XL	Overactive bladder, neurogenic bladder	Dry mouth, nausea, headache, drowsiness, constipation, urinary retention	5 mg orally, 2–3 times/day; 3.9 mg transdermal, use 3–4 days
solifenacin *sol-i-FEN-a-sin*	Vesicare	Overactive bladder	Dry mouth, constipation, blurred vision, dry eyes	5 mg orally daily
tolterodine *tole-TER-oh-deen*	Detrol, Detrol LA (long acting, extended release)	Overactive bladder	Dry mouth, constipation, headache, dizziness	2 mg orally, TID; extended release: 4 mg daily
trospium *TROSE-pee-um*		Overactive bladder	Dry mouth, constipation, headache	20 mg orally TID

Continued

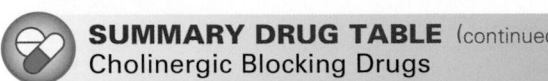

SUMMARY DRUG TABLE (continued)
Cholinergic Blocking Drugs

Generic Name	Trade Name	Uses	Adverse Reactions	Dosage Ranges
Cholinergic Blocking Drugs for Parkinson Disease				
benztropine mesylate *BENZ-troe-peen*	Cogentin	Parkinson disease, drug-induced extrapyramidal syndrome (EPS)	Dry mouth, blurred vision, dizziness, nausea, nervousness, skin rash, urinary retention, dysuria, tachycardia, muscle weakness, disorientation, confusion	0.5–6 mg/day orally Acute dystonia: 1–2 mL IM or IV
trihexyphenidyl *trye-heks-ee-FEN-i-dill*		Parkinsonism symptoms, drug-induced EPS	Same as benztropine mesylate	1–15 mg/day orally in divided doses
Cholinergic Blocking Drugs for Nonacute Respiratory Symptom Relief				
aclidinium *a-kli-DIN-ee-um*	Tudorza Pressair	Maintenance treatment of COPD	Headache, cough, sinus irritation, vomiting, diarrhea, toothache, urinary tract infection	400 mcg inhalation twice daily
ipratropium *ih-prah-troe'-pee-um*	Atrovent	Bronchospasm associated with chronic obstructive pulmonary disease, chronic bronchitis and emphysema, rhinorrhea	Dryness of the oropharynx, nervousness, irritation from aerosol, dry mouth, runny nose, upper respiratory symptoms (URI), dizziness, headache, GI distress, nausea, palpitations	Aerosol: 2 inhalations QID, not to exceed 12 inhalations; Solution: 500 mg (1 unit dose vial) TID, QID by oral nebulization Nasal spray: 2 sprays per nostril BID, TID of 0.03%, or 2 sprays per nostril TID, QID of 0.06%
revefenacin *REV-e-FEN-a-sin*	Yupelri	Maintenance treatment of COPD	Headache, dizziness, URI symptoms	Daily inhalation, 175 mcg/dose
tiotropium *ty-oh-TRO-pee-um*	Spiriva	Maintenance treatment of COPD	Same as revefenacin, increased stroke potential	1 capsule per day using inhalation device, not for oral use
umeclidinium *ue-me-kli-DIN-ee-um*	Incruse Ellipta	Prevention of bronchospasm associated with COPD, chronic bronchitis, and emphysema	Stuffy nose, cough, sore throat, muscle-joint–tooth pain, rapid heartbeat	62.5 mcg inhalation once daily

 This drug should be administered at least 1 hr before or 2 hr after a meal.

CHAPTER REVIEW

Know Your Drugs

Clients sometimes know a medication by the brand (or trade) name and not the generic name. To help you recognize both names, match the brand name with the generic name of the same medication.

Generic Name	Brand Name
1. benztropine mesylate	A. Cogentin
2. fesoterodine	B. Ditropan XL
3. oxybutynin	C. Spiriva
4. tiotropium	D. Toviaz

Calculate Medication Dosages

1. A client is prescribed glycopyrrolate 0.1 mg intramuscularly (IM). The drug is available in a solution of 0.2 mg/mL. The nurse administers _____.

2. Oral trihexyphenidyl 4 mg is ordered. The drug is available as an elixir with a strength of 2 mg/5 mL. The nurse administers _____.

Prepare for the NCLEX

RECALL THE FACTS

1. Anticholinergic drugs block which of the following transmitters?
   1. Acetylcholine
   2. Dopamine
   3. Norepinephrine
   4. Serotonin
2. A client taking solifenacin (Vesicare) for an overactive bladder complains of dry mouth. The nurse should _____.
   1. consider this to be unusual and contact the primary health care provider
   2. encourage the client to take frequent sips of water
   3. give the client salt-water mouth rinses
   4. ignore this reaction because it is only temporary
3. Which of the following adverse reactions would the nurse expect after the administration of atropine as part of a client's preoperative medication regimen?
   1. Enhanced action of anesthesia
   2. Reduced secretions of the upper respiratory tract
   3. Prolonged action of the preoperative opioid
   4. Increased gastric motility
4. Because of the effect of cholinergic blocking drugs on intestinal motility, the nurse must monitor the client taking these drugs for the development of _____.
   1. esophageal ulcers
   2. diarrhea
   3. heartburn
   4. constipation
5. Cholinergic blocking drugs are contraindicated in clients with _____.
   1. gout
   2. glaucoma
   3. diabetes
   4. bradycardia
6. A cholinergic blocking drug is administered and the client becomes acutely confused; this is an example of _____.
   1. synergism
   2. agonist–antagonist effect
   3. drug idiosyncrasy
   4. sympathetic nervous system response

ANALYZE THE FACTS

7. When acetylcholine is blocked in the parasympathetic nervous system, which of the following occurs?
   1. Pupils constrict.
   2. Heart rate decreases.
   3. GI system becomes active.
   4. Salivary glands secrete less.

8. *The nurse has administered a presurgical anticholinergic drug about 30 min ago. Which of the following responses would be of concern and should be reported immediately?
   1. "Nurse, my throat is dry."
   2. "I'm feeling a bit anxious. When will the surgeon be here?"
   3. "I need to leave. I have important business to do!"
   4. "My nose is suddenly stuffy. I wonder if I have a cold."

ALTERNATE-FORMAT QUESTIONS

9. Select the terms that describe drugs that block the parasympathetic branch of the ANS. **Select all that apply.**
   1. Parasympathomimetic
   2. Parasympatholytic
   3. Antiadrenergic
   4. Anticholinergic
10. A client says he is stopping the anticholinergic drug because of dry mouth and constipation. What are some teaching tips the nurse can offer to reduce these adverse reactions? **Select all that apply.**
    1. Add more fiber to diet.
    2. Limit fluid intake.
    3. Swish mouth with water periodically.
    4. Add a cucumber to drinking water.
    5. Brush and floss teeth regularly.

To check your answers, see Appendix F.

_____

*Indicates the question is directly linked to the NCLEX-PN test plan in Appendix G.

WANT TO KNOW MORE? A wide variety of resources are available to enhance your learning and understanding of this chapter.

- Visit thePoint for resources such as:
  • NCLEX-Style Student Review Questions
  • Journal Articles
  • Dosage Calculations
  • Drug Monographs
  • Watch and Learn Videos
  • Concepts in Action Animations
- The *Study Guide to Accompany Introductory Clinical Pharmacology*, 12th edition, sold separately, will help you review and apply essential content.
- ✓*PrepU* is available to help students prepare for the NCLEX-PN examination.

UNIT 6
Drugs That Affect the Neuromuscular System

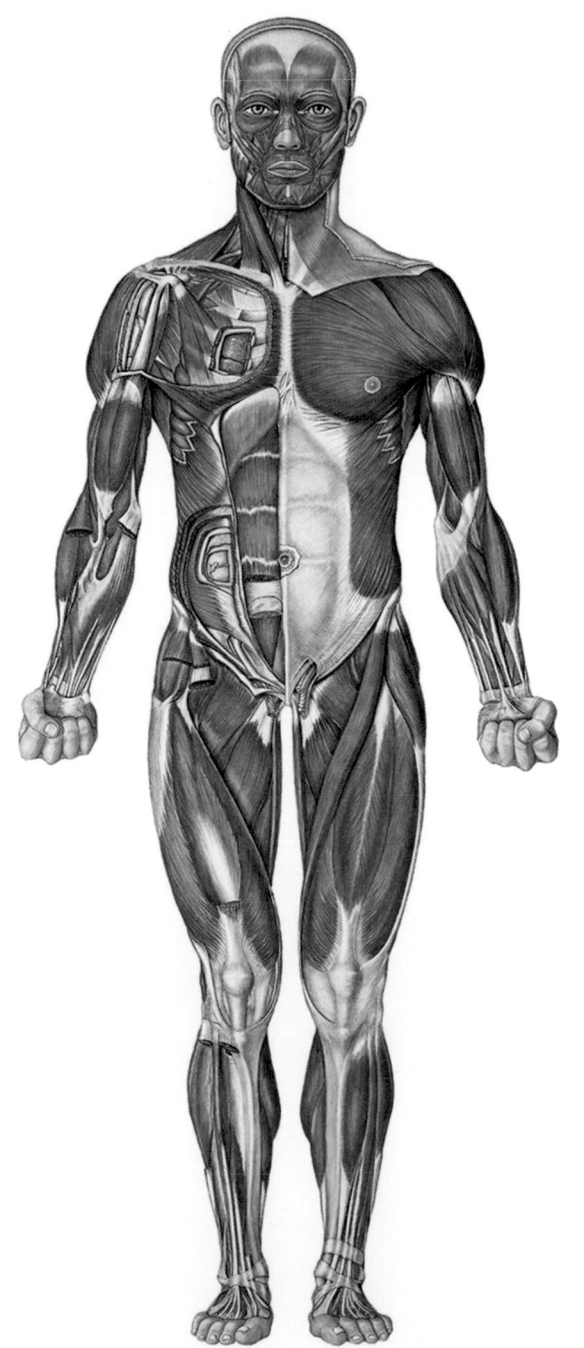

Previous units in this book have examined both the central and peripheral nervous systems of our bodies and how drugs affect function both in those systems and in other selected bodily systems. The focus of Unit 6 is on how drugs can help connect the nervous system with the muscles in our bodies to help produce movement.

In this unit, you will learn more about the somatic branch of the peripheral nervous system, which is concerned with sensation and voluntary movement. In the somatic branch, messages are sent to the brain concerning the internal and external environment, such as sensations of heat, pain, cold, and pressure. The outgoing message in the somatic nervous system is concerned with the voluntary movement of skeletal muscles, such as those used in walking, talking, or writing a letter.

The musculoskeletal system comprises the bones, joints, and muscles that provide the body with a means of movement. Although separate from the nervous system, they work together and are referred to as the neuromuscular system—providing our bodies with the ability to live, work, and play. A number of degenerative diseases (Parkinson disease, epilepsy, and fibromyalgia) affect both the musculoskeletal and neurologic systems.

Many drugs are designed to strengthen or diminish motor messages from the brain to the muscles and other tissues. Some of these drug categories, which are covered in this unit, include antiparkinson, antiepileptic (or antiseizure), and muscle relaxant drugs.

Parkinsonism is a general term that refers to a group of symptoms involving motor movement. The name comes from Parkinson disease, a progressive neurologic disease with symptoms that worsen over time. In earlier chapters, you learned about drugs that can have adverse reactions similar to the symptoms of Parkinson disease. Select drugs can reduce the symptoms that impact the neuromuscular system when caused by the disease or by other drugs. These drugs are covered in Chapter 27 and relieve the symptoms of both Parkinson disease and adverse reactions of other drugs that assist in maintaining the client's mobility and functioning capability for as long as possible.

Neurotransmission of the brain can be overexcited by injury or disease. When this happens, seizures occur. The newest guidelines for defining seizures as presented by the International League Against Epilepsy will help you understand the drugs used to treat epilepsy and other seizure disorders. Chapter 28 discusses the antiepileptic drugs used to depress abnormal brain activity and lessen or prevent seizure activity.

The promotion of mobility and function of bones and joints is the focus of Chapter 29. Drugs used for both acute and chronic conditions are included in this chapter. When muscles are injured and need to heal, drugs are provided to relax and allow for healing. The drugs used to prevent injury or fracture from osteoporosis or to treat conditions such as rheumatoid arthritis are discussed.

Antiparkinson Drugs

Key Terms

achalasia   failure to relax; usually referring to the smooth muscle fibers of the gastrointestinal (GI) tract, especially failure of the lower esophagus to relax, causing difficulty swallowing and a feeling of fullness in the sternal region

agonist   a drug that binds with a receptor and stimulates the receptor to produce a therapeutic response

akathisia   extreme restlessness and increased motor activity

blood–brain barrier   ability of the nervous system to prohibit large and potentially harmful molecules from crossing from the blood into the brain

bradykinesia   slow movement

choreiform movements   involuntary muscular twitching of the limbs or facial muscles

dystonic   muscular spasms most often affecting the tongue, jaw, eyes, and neck

extrapyramidal symptoms (EPS)   group of adverse reactions involving the extrapyramidal portion of the nervous system causing abnormal muscle movements, especially akathisia and dystonia

on–off phenomenon   fluctuation in levodopa therapy where inconsistent absorption causes alternating improved status and loss of therapeutic effect

parkinsonism   referring to a cluster of symptoms associated with Parkinson disease (i.e., fine tremors, slowing of voluntary movements, muscular weakness)

Parkinson disease   degenerative disorder caused by an imbalance of dopamine and acetylcholine in the CNS

restless leg syndrome   disorder with an irresistible urge to move the legs; urge lessens with movement but worsens with rest

Learning Objectives

On completion of this chapter, the student will:

1. Define the terms "Parkinson disease" and "parkinsonism".
2. Explain the uses, general drug actions, adverse drug reactions, contraindications, precautions, and interactions of antiparkinson drugs.
3. Distinguish important preadministration and ongoing assessment activities the nurse should perform on the client taking an antiparkinson drug.
4. List nursing diagnoses particular to a client taking an antiparkinson drug.
5. Examine ways to promote an optimal response to therapy, how to manage adverse reactions, and important points to keep in mind when educating clients about the use of antiparkinson drugs.

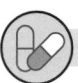 **Drug Classes**

Dopaminergic agents
Dopaminergic monoamine oxidase B inhibitors (MAOIs)
Dopamine receptor agonists
Catechol-O-methyltransferase (COMT) inhibitors
Cholinergic blocking agents (anticholinergic drugs)

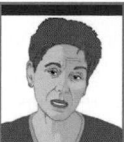 **PHARMACOLOGY IN PRACTICE**

A woman in the clinic waiting room comes to the front desk and says, "That lady over there is odd. She looks like she is keeping tune to a song with her hand and her head, but there is no music playing. I don't feel comfortable sitting here in the waiting area." The client is Betty Peterson, and she been taking amitriptyline for depression.

Parkinson disease (PD) is seen yearly in approximately 1 million US citizens (PD Foundation, 2020). This disease affects the messages sent from the central nervous system (CNS) to the skeletal muscles of the body via the somatic branch of the peripheral nervous system (PNS). The somatic branch of the PNS relies on dopamine as the primary neurotransmitter. An imbalance of dopamine and acetylcholine in the CNS occurs in Parkinson disease. This happens because the substantia nigra (an area of the brain) loses cells, which reduces the supply of the neurotransmitter dopamine. As a result, too much acetylcholine (ACh) affects this area of the brain.

An overabundance of ACh results in symptoms such as trembling, rigidity, difficulty walking, and problems with balance. Together with slow movement (**bradykinesia**), these symptoms make up what is referred to as the cardinal signs of Parkinson disease. Other symptoms of Parkinson disease include slurred speech, a mask-like and emotionless facial appearance, difficulty chewing, and swallowing. As the spine assumes a rigid, bent-forward posture, the gait becomes unsteady and shuffled. This group of symptoms is termed **extrapyramidal symptoms** (EPSs).

In addition to a diagnosis of Parkinson disease, this cluster of symptoms may be seen with the use of certain drugs (as in the chapter case study), head injuries, and encephalitis. The drugs featured in this chapter are used to treat both Parkinson disease and adverse reactions of other medications. Drugs used to treat **parkinsonism** (or more frequently called Parkinson-like symptoms) are called *antiparkinson drugs*. These drugs either supplement the dopamine in the brain or block excess acetylcholine (ACh) so that better transmission of nerve impulses occurs. The Summary Drug Table: Antiparkinson Drugs provides a listing of the drugs used to treat Parkinson disease and EPSs.

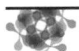 # DOPAMINERGIC DRUGS

Dopaminergics are drugs that affect the dopamine content of the brain. These drugs include levodopa, carbidopa (Lodosyn), amantadine, and carbidopa/levodopa combination (Sinemet). Other drugs that work to enhance dopamine include agonists such as bromocriptine or monoamine oxidase inhibitors (MAOIs) such as selegiline, which may be prescribed initially in early PD (see Summary Drug Table: Antiparkinson Drugs).

ACTIONS

As discussed earlier, the Parkinson-like symptoms are caused by a depletion of dopamine in the CNS. Unfortunately, supplementing dopamine is difficult because of a structure called the **blood–brain barrier**. The blood–brain barrier is a meshwork of tightly packed cells in the walls of the brain's capillaries that work to protect the brain by screening out certain substances. This unique meshwork of cells in the CNS prohibits large and potentially harmful molecules from leaving the blood and crossing into the brain. This ability to screen out certain substances has important implications for drug therapy, because different drugs can pass through the blood–brain barrier more easily than others. Dopamine is not easy to supplement because when taken as an oral medication it does not easily cross the blood–brain barrier.

Levodopa is a chemical formulation found in plants and animals and is converted into dopamine by the body. Dopamine, in the form of levodopa, crosses the

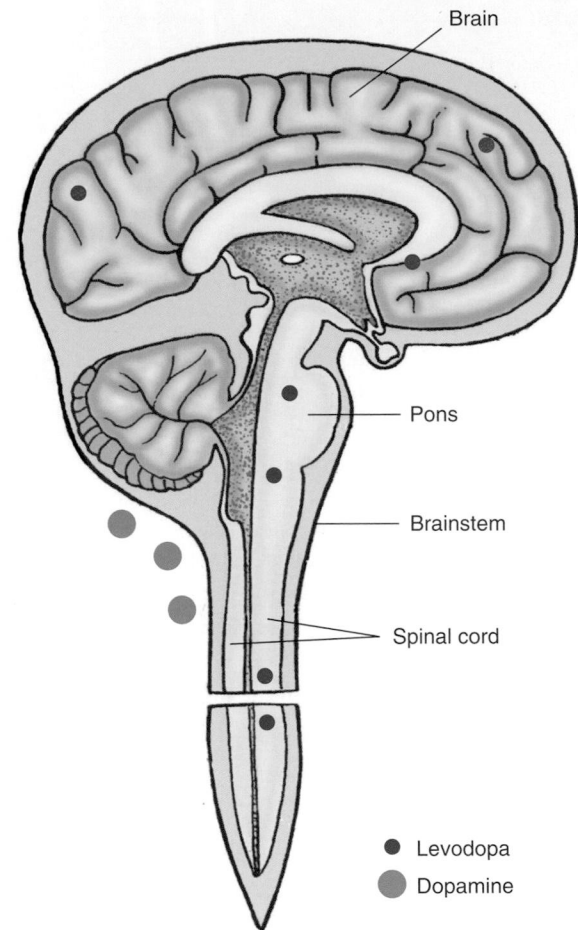

FIGURE 27.1 The blood–brain barrier selectively inhibits certain substances from entering the brain and spinal fluid. Cells in the brain form tight junctions that prevent or slow the passage of certain substances. Levodopa can pass the blood–brain barrier, whereas dopamine cannot.

blood–brain barrier but only in small quantities. At one time, levodopa, used alone, caused severe adverse reactions because too much dopamine stayed in the PNS. Combining levodopa with another drug (carbidopa) allows more levodopa to reach the brain, which in turn permits the drug to have a better pharmacologic effect in clients with Parkinson disease (Fig. 27.1). Carbidopa has no effect when given alone. Therefore, the combination makes more levodopa available to the brain and, as a result, the dosage of levodopa may be reduced, decreasing peripheral effects. Combination tablets of carbidopa and levodopa are available in several strengths of the two drugs and as a timed-release medication.

Drugs that work to stimulate the dopamine receptors are called **agonists**. An example of this drug category includes bromocriptine. Other drugs work to increase the availability of dopamine. The action of amantadine is to make more of the dopamine available at the receptor site. Rasagiline (Azilect) and selegiline inhibit monoamine oxidase type B, again making more dopamine available.

USES

Dopaminergic drugs are used to treat the Parkinson-like symptoms of the following:

- Parkinson disease
- Parkinson-like symptoms (extrapyramidal) as a result of injury, drug therapy, or encephalitis
- **Restless leg syndrome** (RLS)

ADVERSE REACTIONS

During early treatment with levodopa/carbidopa, adverse reactions are usually not a problem, because of the resolution of Parkinson-like symptoms. As the medication's effectiveness lessens, generalized adverse reactions include the following:

- Dry mouth and difficulty in swallowing
- Anorexia, nausea, and vomiting
- Abdominal pain and constipation
- Increased hand tremor
- Headache and dizziness

The most serious adverse reactions seen with levodopa include **choreiform movements** (involuntary muscular twitching of the limbs or facial muscles) and **dystonic** movements (muscular spasms most often affecting the tongue, jaw, eyes, and neck). Amantadine can reduce these symptoms when added to levodopa-based drugs. Less common but still serious reactions include mental changes such as dementia, depression, psychotic episodes, paranoia, and suicidal tendencies (covered in Unit 4—Drugs that Affect the Central Nervous System).

CONTRAINDICATIONS AND PRECAUTIONS

The dopaminergic drugs are contraindicated in clients with known hypersensitivity to the drugs. Levodopa is contraindicated in clients with narrow-angle glaucoma and those receiving MAOI antidepressants. The client should be screened for unusual skin lesions, because levodopa can activate malignant melanoma. Levodopa is used cautiously in clients with cardiovascular or pulmonary diseases, peptic ulcer disease, renal or hepatic disease, and psychosis. Levodopa and combination antiparkinson drugs (e.g., carbidopa/levodopa) are classified in pregnancy category C and are used with caution during pregnancy and lactation.

NURSING ALERT

When pain medications are prescribed for clients with PD, review the medication list for selegiline, safinamide, or rasagiline. The opioid meperidine (Demerol) combined with the dopamine agonists causes a dangerous antimetabolite conversion. Caution should be taken with any other opioid used with these antiparkinson drugs as well.

INTERACTIONS

The following interactions may occur when a dopaminergic drug is administered with another agent:

Interacting Drug	Common Use	Effect of Interaction
Tricyclic antidepressants	Management of depression	Increased risk of hypertension and dyskinesia
Antacids	Relief of GI upset and heartburn	Increased effect of levodopa
Antiepileptic	Seizure control	Decreased effect of levodopa

Foods high in pyridoxine (vitamin B_6) or vitamin B_6 preparations reduce the effect of levodopa. However, when carbidopa is used with levodopa, pyridoxine has no effect on the action of levodopa. In fact, when levodopa and carbidopa are given together, pyridoxine may be prescribed to decrease the adverse effects associated with levodopa.

DOPAMINE RECEPTOR AGONISTS

ACTIONS

It is thought that nonergot dopamine receptors act directly on postsynaptic dopamine receptors of nerve cells in the brain, mimicking the effects of dopamine in the brain.

USES

Dopamine receptor agonists are used for the treatment of the signs and symptoms of Parkinson disease. It is also used in the treatment of RLS, a disorder where the client has an irresistible urge to move the legs, which lessens with movement but worsens with rest. The symptoms of this disorder worsen in the evening, causing difficulty with sleep. Another drug approved for treatment of RLS is gabapentin (see Chapter 28). The drug apomorphine (Apokyn) is used for the rapid event of **on–off phenomena** in Parkinson disease. This injectable drug must be specially ordered and antiemetic therapy must be initiated with this drug.

ADVERSE REACTIONS

The most common adverse reactions include the following:

- Nausea, dizziness, vomiting
- Somnolence, hallucinations, confusion, visual disturbances
- Postural hypotension, abnormal involuntary movements
- Headache

PRACTICE CONSIDERATIONS

Rotigotine transdermal patches contain a small amount of metal. These should be removed prior to cardioversion or MRI scans.

CONTRAINDICATIONS AND PRECAUTIONS

Dopamine receptor agonists are contraindicated in clients with known hypersensitivity to the drugs. Dopamine receptor agonists are used with caution in clients with dyskinesia, orthostatic hypotension, hepatic or renal impairment, cardiovascular disease, and a history of hallucinations or psychosis. Both ropinirole and pramipexole are pregnancy category C drugs, and safety during pregnancy has not been established.

There is an increased risk of CNS depression when the dopamine receptor agonists are administered with other CNS depressants. When administered with levodopa, dopamine receptor agonists increase the effects of levodopa (a lower dosage of levodopa may be required). In addition, when dopamine receptor agonists are administered with levodopa, there is an increased risk of hallucinations. When administered with ciprofloxacin, there is an increased effect of the dopamine receptor agonist.

LASA ALERT

The following drugs may sound alike; be sure to clarify when they are ordered:

Drug Name	Sounds Like
Mirapex	Hiprex, Mifeprex, MiraLax
Neupro	Neupogen
Requip	Reglan
ROPINIRole	RisperDAL, risperiDONE, ropivacaine

Drugs that look like a similar drug are noted in the Summary Drug Tables of each chapter.

INTERACTIONS

The following interactions may occur when a dopamine receptor agonist is administered with another agent:

Interacting Drug	Common Use	Effect of Interaction
Cimetidine, ranitidine	Management of GI problems	Increased dopamine agonist effectiveness
Verapamil, quinidine	Management of cardiac problems	Increased dopamine agonist effectiveness
Estrogen	Female hormonal supplement	Increased dopamine agonist effectiveness
Phenothiazines	Antipsychotic agent	Decreased dopamine agonist effectiveness

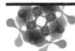 # COMT INHIBITORS

Another classification of antiparkinson drugs is the catechol-O-methyltransferase (COMT) inhibitors. Examples of the COMT inhibitors are entacapone (Comtan) and tolcapone (Tasmar).

ACTIONS

These drugs are thought to prolong the effect of levodopa by blocking an enzyme, COMT, which eliminates dopamine. When given with levodopa, the COMT inhibitors increase the plasma concentrations and duration of action of levodopa.

USES

The COMT inhibitors are used as adjuncts to levodopa/carbidopa in treating Parkinson disease. Entacapone is a mild COMT inhibitor and is used to help manage fluctuations in the response to levodopa in individuals with Parkinson disease. Tolcapone is a potent COMT inhibitor that easily crosses the blood–brain barrier. However, the drug is associated with liver damage and liver failure. Because of the danger to the liver, tolcapone is reserved for people who do not respond to other therapies.

ADVERSE REACTIONS

Adverse reactions most often associated with the administration of COMT inhibitors include the following:

- Dizziness
- Dyskinesias, hyperkinesias, **akathisia** (extreme restlessness and increased motor activity)
- Nausea, anorexia, and diarrhea
- Orthostatic hypotension, sleep disorders, excessive dreaming
- Somnolence and muscle cramps

CONTRAINDICATIONS AND PRECAUTIONS

These drugs are contraindicated in clients with hypersensitivity to the drugs and during pregnancy and lactation (pregnancy category C). Tolcapone is contraindicated in clients with liver dysfunction. The COMT inhibitors are used with caution in clients with hypertension, hypotension, and decreased hepatic or renal function.

LASA ALERT

The following drugs may sound alike; be sure to clarify when they are ordered:

Drug Name	Sounds Like
Azilect	Aricept
selegiline	Salagen, sertraline, Serzone, Stelazine
rasagiline	repaglinide
Zelapar	zaleplon, Zemplar, zolpidem, ZyPREXA, Zydis

Drugs that look like a similar drug are noted in the Summary Drug Tables of each chapter.

INTERACTIONS

The following interactions may occur when a COMT inhibitor is administered with another agent:

Interacting Drug	Common Use	Effect of Interaction
MAOI antidepressants	Management of depression	Increased risk of toxicity of both drugs
Adrenergic drugs	Treatment of cardiac and blood pressure problems	Increased risk of cardiac symptoms

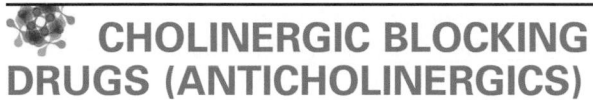

CHOLINERGIC BLOCKING DRUGS (ANTICHOLINERGICS)

ACTIONS

ACh, a neurotransmitter, is produced in excess in Parkinson disease. Drugs with cholinergic blocking activity block ACh in the CNS, enhancing dopamine transmission. Drugs with cholinergic blocking activity are generally less effective than levodopa in treating parkinsonism and are limited in dose by peripheral adverse reactions. Antihistamines, such as diphenhydramine (Benadryl), are used in older adult clients because they produce fewer adverse effects.

USES

Drugs with cholinergic blocking activity are used as adjunctive therapy in all forms of Parkinson-like symptoms and in the control of drug-induced extrapyramidal disorders (Box 27.1).

ADVERSE REACTIONS

Adverse reactions to drugs with cholinergic blocking activity include the following:

- Dry mouth
- Blurred vision
- Dizziness, mild nausea, and nervousness

These reactions may become less pronounced as therapy progresses. Other adverse reactions may include:

- Skin rash, urticaria (hives)
- Urinary retention, dysuria
- Tachycardia, muscle weakness
- Disorientation and confusion

If any of these reactions are severe, the drug may be discontinued for several days and restarted at a lower dosage, or a different antiparkinson drug may be prescribed.

CONTRAINDICATIONS AND PRECAUTIONS

These drugs are contraindicated in those with a hypersensitivity to the anticholinergic drugs, glaucoma (angle-closure glaucoma), pyloric or duodenal obstruction, peptic ulcers, prostatic hypertrophy, **achalasia** (failure of the muscles of the lower esophagus to relax, causing difficulty swallowing), myasthenia gravis, and megacolon.

These drugs are used with caution in clients with tachycardia, cardiac arrhythmias, hypertension, or hypotension; those with a tendency toward urinary retention; those with decreased liver or kidney function; and those with obstructive disease of the urinary system or GI tract. The cholinergic blocking drugs are given with caution to the older adult.

 Lifespan Considerations

Gerontology

Individuals older than 60 years frequently develop increased sensitivity to anticholinergic drugs and require careful monitoring. Confusion and disorientation may occur. Lower doses may be required.

INTERACTIONS

The following interactions may occur when a cholinergic blocking drug is administered with another agent:

Interacting Drug	Common Use	Effect of Interaction
Amantadine	Treatment of parkinsonism	Increased anticholinergic effects
Digoxin	Management of cardiac disease	Increased digoxin serum levels
Haloperidol	Antipsychotic agent	Increased psychotic behavior
Phenothiazines	Antipsychotic agent	Increased anticholinergic effects

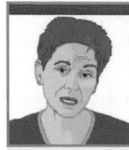

PHARMACOLOGY IN PRACTICE

SAFE DRUG ADMINISTRATION
Cholinergic blocking drugs are contraindicated in which category of client?
1. Clients with bone marrow depression
2. Clients with cardiac disorders
3. Clients with visual impairment
4. Clients with prostatic hypertrophy

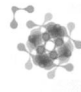

NURSING PROCESS: STEPS TO BUILDING CLINICAL JUDGMENT
Client Receiving an Antiparkinson Drug

ASSESSMENT

Preadministration Assessment
Data gathering suggestions before the initial administration of an antiparkinson drug include:
Objective data

- Description of signs (especially PD cardinal signs) and effects on change in activities of daily living
- Neuromuscular assessment (see Box 27.2)
- Mental condition (e.g., impairment in memory, signs of depression, or withdrawal)
- Vital signs (temperature, pulse, respirations, and blood pressure)
- Neurological studies and scans
- Liver function laboratory tests if COMT inhibitors are being prescribed

Subjective data

- Current history of symptoms, type, and duration
- Should memory impairment make this difficult for the client, solicit data from family or friends
- Drug history, particularly drugs with EPS reactions

Ongoing Assessment
Evaluate the client's response to drug therapy by observing the client or asking about various neuromuscular signs (Box 27.2). Compare these observations with the data obtained during the initial physical assessment. For example, the client is assessed for clinical improvement of the symptoms of the disease, such as improvement of tremor of head or hands at rest, muscular rigidity, mask-like facial expression, and ambulation stability. Although drug response may occur slowly in some clients, these observations aid the primary health care provider in adjusting the dosage to obtain the desired therapeutic results.

A serious and potentially fatal adverse reaction to tolcapone is liver dysfunction. Regular blood testing to monitor liver function is usually prescribed. Testing of

BOX 27.2 Neuromuscular Assessment

The neuromuscular assessment includes observation for the following:
- Tremors of the hands or head while the client is at rest
- Mask-like facial expression
- Changes (from normal) in walking
- Type of speech pattern (halting, monotone)
- Postural deformities
- Muscular rigidity
- Drooling, difficulty in chewing or swallowing
- Changes in thought processes
- Ability of the client to carry out any or all of the activities of daily living (e.g., bathing, ambulating, dressing)

serum aminotransferase levels is ordered at frequent intervals (e.g., every 2 weeks for the first year and every 8 weeks thereafter). Treatment is discontinued if the alanine aminotransferase (ALT; previously, serum glutamic pyruvic transaminase [SGPT]) exceeds the upper normal limit or signs or symptoms of liver failure develop. The client is observed for indicators of liver dysfunction such as persistent nausea, fatigue, lethargy, anorexia, jaundice, dark urine, pruritus, and right upper quadrant tenderness.

NURSING DIAGNOSES

Drug-specific nursing diagnoses include the following:

- **Malnutrition:** related to nausea, dry mouth
- **Constipation** related to neurologic changes in the bowel
- **Injury risk** related to dizziness, lightheadedness, orthostatic hypotension, loss of balance
- **Impaired physical mobility** related to alterations in balance, unsteady gait, dizziness
- **Impaired sleep** related to involuntary movement at rest

Nursing diagnoses related to drug administration are discussed in Chapter 4.

PLANNING

The expected outcomes for the client may include an optimal response to drug therapy, meeting client needs related to the management of adverse reactions, absence of injury, and confidence in an understanding of the medication regimen.

IMPLEMENTATION

Promoting an Optimal Response to Therapy

Effective management of the client with Parkinson disease requires careful monitoring of the drug therapy. Optimal response to these drugs often requires titration of doses based on client activities. To accomplish this requires psychological support, with emphasis on client and family teaching. Often clients and family members may be given a range of drug dosages to administer to find the best response with the fewest adverse reactions.

The antiparkinson drugs also may be used to treat the Parkinson-like symptoms that occur with the administration of some of the psychotherapeutic drugs. When used for this purpose, antiparkinson drugs may exacerbate mental symptoms and precipitate a psychotic event. Review Chapter 22 for intervention strategies and monitoring.

Clients who have difficulty taking drugs orally may be administered medications via enteral tube feeding. Those with advanced symptoms of Parkinson disease can be administered a combination of carbidopa/levodopa (Duopa) directly into the small intestine. This has diminished motor symptoms greatly (Vacca, 2019).

Drugs administered as transdermal patches (rotigotine or selegiline) are applied daily at approximately the same time to maintain blood level. Rotation of sites (front of the abdomen, thigh, hip, flank, shoulder, or upper arm) should be set up on a 2-week schedule of different areas, and the patch should be applied to clean, dry, hairless skin. Mark and note location, time, and date. Exposing transdermal patches to external heat sources (e.g., heating pad, electric blanket, hot tub/shower, direct sunlight) will cause an increase in medication distribution. If patch falls off, immediately apply a new one to a new site.

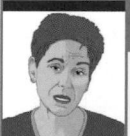

PHARMACOLOGY IN PRACTICE

DOSE CALCULATION

Ropinirole is titrated for restless leg syndrome. The pharmacy has provided the client with a 2-month supply of 0.25-mg tablets. The client is on week 4 and is to take 2 mg ropinirole 1–3 hr before bedtime. How many tablets will the client take for each evening dose during week 4?

Monitoring and Managing Client Needs

Teach the client or a family member how to journal daily for the development of adverse reactions. By using a chart or journal describing adverse reactions, these can be reported in an easier fashion to the primary health care provider, because a dosage adjustment or change to a different antiparkinson drug may be necessary with the occurrence of more serious adverse reactions. Teach the client or family how to describe movements and to be alert for those such as facial grimacing, protruding tongue, exaggerated chewing motions and head movements, and jerking movements of the arms and legs. If these occur, the client should not take the next dose of the drug and should notify the primary health care provider immediately.

Malnutrition

Clients may experience multiple adverse reactions that can affect their dietary intake and cause them to lose weight. Some adverse reactions, although not serious, may be uncomfortable. An example of a less serious but uncomfortable adverse reaction is dryness of the mouth. Teach the client to relieve dry mouth by taking frequent sips of water, ice chips, or hard candy (if allowed). If dry mouth is so severe that there is difficulty in swallowing or speaking, or if loss of appetite and weight loss occur, the dosage of the antiparkinson drug may be reduced.

Some clients taking the antiparkinson drugs experience GI disturbances such as nausea, vomiting, or constipation. This can affect the client's nutritional status. Help the family to learn to create a calm environment; serve small, frequent meals; and serve foods the client prefers to help improve nutrition. For those with eating issues, monitor the client's weight frequently. GI disturbances are sometimes helped by taking the drug with meals. Severe nausea or vomiting may necessitate discontinuing the drug and changing to a different antiparkinson drug. With continued use of the drug, nausea usually decreases or resolves.

Constipation

Neurologic changes cause changes in peristalsis and dilation of the bowel, leading to chronic constipation. Also, some clients with Parkinson disease may have difficulty communicating and are not able to tell the caregiver or nurse that bodily urges are occurring. Observe the client with Parkinson disease for outward changes that may indicate the need to eliminate. For example, a sudden change in the facial expression or changes in posture may indicate abdominal pain or discomfort, which may be caused by urinary retention, paralytic ileus, or constipation. If constipation is a problem, stress the need for a diet high in fiber and increasing fluids in the diet. A stool softener may be needed to help prevent constipation.

Injury Risk

Minimizing the risk for injury is an important aspect in the care of the client with Parkinson disease. The client with visual difficulties may need assistance with ambulation. Visual difficulties (e.g., adverse reactions of blurred vision and diplopia) may be evidenced only by the client's sudden refusal to read or watch television or by the client bumping into objects when ambulating. Lack of balance is an issue for those with Parkinson disease. Research indicates a reduction in injury when clients participate in activities to improve balance, such as Tai Chi (Li, 2012). You can refer clients to occupational or activity directors who may have listings of exercise programs that cater to individuals with balance issues.

Carefully evaluate any sudden changes in the client's behavior or activity and report them to the primary health care provider. Sudden changes in behavior may indicate hallucinations, depression, or other psychotic episodes.

 Lifespan Considerations

Gerontology
Hallucinations occur more often in the older adult than in the younger adult receiving antiparkinson drugs. This is especially likely when taking dopamine receptor agonists.

Adverse reactions such as dizziness, muscle weakness, and ataxia (lack of muscular coordination) may further increase difficulty with ambulatory activities. Clients with Parkinson disease are especially prone to falls and other accidents because of the disease process and possible adverse drug reactions. The client should learn to ask for assistance in getting out of the bed or a chair, walking, and other self-care activities. In addition, assistive devices such as a cane or walker may help with ambulation (Fig. 27.2). You may suggest that the client wear shoes with rubber soles to minimize the possibility of slipping. When hospitalized, slipper socks are typically color coded to indicate a fall risk for this client. The room should be kept well lighted, the use of scatter or throw rugs should be avoided, and any small pieces of furniture or objects that might increase the risk of falling should be removed. Carefully assess the environment and make necessary adjustments to ensure the client's safety.

Clients who are prone to orthostatic hypotension as a result of the drug regimen are instructed to arise slowly from a sitting or lying position, especially after sitting or lying for a prolonged time.

Impaired Physical Mobility
The on–off phenomenon may occur in clients taking levodopa. In this condition, the client may suddenly alternate between improved clinical status and loss of therapeutic effect. This effect is associated with long-term levodopa treatment. Low doses of the drug, reserving the drug for severe cases, or the use of a *drug holiday* may be prescribed. Should symptoms occur, the primary health care provider may order a drug holiday that includes complete withdrawal of levodopa for 5–14 days, followed by gradually restarting drug therapy at a lower dose. Clients on a drug holiday need to be monitored for complications.

Impaired Sleep
Clients with RLS have difficulty in sleeping because of leg movements that increase during periods of rest. To facilitate sleep, teach the client to engage in activities to promote rest as they prepare for sleep. Bedtime rituals such as a hot bath, engaging the mind in a pleasant activity (crossword puzzle or reading), and leg massage may help to improve the ability to sleep. Antidepressants (such as escitalopram) may be prescribed, too.

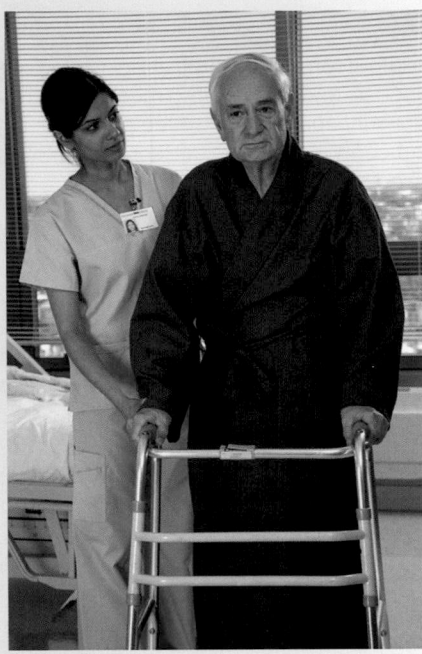
FIGURE 27.2 Nurses promote client safety by providing ambulatory assistance to the client with Parkinson-like (extrapyramidal) symptoms.

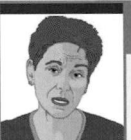 **PHARMACOLOGY IN PRACTICE**

MANAGING NEEDS
A nurse is caring for a client receiving an antiparkinson drug. The client is complaining of constipation. What instructions should the nurse offer the client to help relieve constipation? **Select all that apply**.
1. Decrease the intake of carbohydrates.
2. Use a stool softener.
3. Increase intake of fiber in the diet.
4. Increase intake of fluids in the diet.
5. Increase intake of vitamin C.

Educating the Client and Family
Provide a referral to the discharge planning coordinator or social worker if you find issues with the client's ability to understand the therapeutic drug regimen, ability to perform self-care in the home environment, or ability to adhere to the prescribed drug therapy.

If the client requires supervision or help with daily activities and the drug regimen, encourage the family to create a home environment that is least likely to result in accidents or falls. Changes such as removing throw rugs, installing a hand rail next to the toilet, and moving obstacles that can result in tripping or falling can be made at little or no expense to the family. As you develop a teaching plan for the client or family member, include the following points:

- If dizziness, drowsiness, or blurred vision occurs, avoid driving or performing other tasks that require alertness.

- Avoid the use of alcohol unless use has been approved by the primary health care provider.
- Relieve dry mouth by sucking on hard candy (unless the client has diabetes) or taking frequent sips of water. Consult a dentist if dryness of the mouth interferes with wearing, inserting, or removing dentures or causes other dental problems.
- Keep all appointments with the primary health care provider or clinic personnel because close monitoring of therapy is necessary.
- Ask your primary health care provider before buying vitamin supplements when taking levodopa. Vitamin B$_6$ (pyridoxine) may interfere with the action of levodopa.

EVALUATION

- Therapeutic effect is achieved and the Parkinson-like symptoms are controlled.
- Adverse reactions are identified, reported to the primary health care provider, and managed successfully through appropriate nursing interventions.

- Client maintains an adequate nutritional status.
- Client has adequate bowel movements.
- No evidence of injury is seen.
- Client maintains adequate mobility.
- Client reports restful sleep.
- Client and family express confidence and demonstrate an understanding of the drug regimen.

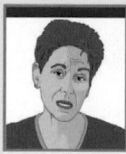

PHARMACOLOGY IN PRACTICE

USING CLINICAL REASONING

You ask Betty to follow you into an examination room. There you assess a repetitive hand tremor, and she appears to open her mouth frequently with a dry, sticky sound. What do you think she is experiencing, and how will you document these findings for the primary health care provider?

KEY POINTS

■ Parkinson disease is a progressive neurologic disease caused by reduction in dopamine in the brain. Cardinal signs include tremors, rigidity, and bradykinesia.

■ When drugs or other illnesses cause adverse reactions like the cardinal symptoms of Parkinson disease, this is termed Parkinson-like or extrapyramidal symptoms.

■ The drugs used to treat Parkinson disease and Parkinson-like symptoms either supplement dopamine or block excess acetylcholine to enhance neurotransmission. Blood–brain barrier issues make supplementing dopamine difficult.

■ Client and family participation is crucial since frequent titration of the drugs leads to better client outcomes.

■ The most common adverse reactions are dry mouth and GI distress such as nausea, vomiting, and constipation. When combined with other drugs less common reactions such as involuntary muscle twitching and spasm can occur.

SUMMARY DRUG TABLE
Antiparkinson Drugs

Generic Name	Trade Name	Uses	Adverse Reactions	Dosage Ranges
Dopaminergic Drugs				
amantadine *a-MAN-ta-deen*	Gocovri, Osmolex ER	Parkinson disease/drug-induced extrapyramidal symptoms	Lightheadedness, dizziness, insomnia, confusion, nausea, constipation, dry mouth, orthostatic hypotension, depression	200–400 mg/day orally in divided doses
bromocriptine *broe-moe-KRIP-teen*	Cycloset, Parlodel	Parkinson disease, female endocrine imbalances, acromegaly, fibrocystic breast disease, diabetes mellitus type2	Drowsiness, sedation, dizziness, faintness, epigastric distress, anorexia	10–40 mg/day orally
carbidopa *kar-bi-DOE-pa*	Lodosyn	Used with levodopa in the treatment of Parkinson disease	None by itself; adverse reactions are those of levodopa	70–100 mg/day orally

Continued

SUMMARY DRUG TABLE (continued)
Antiparkinson Drugs

Generic Name	Trade Name	Uses	Adverse Reactions	Dosage Ranges
carbidopa/levodopa *kar-bi-DOE-pa/lee-voe-DOE-pa*	Rytary, Sinemet, Sinemet CR, Duopa (enteral only)	Parkinson disease	Anorexia, nausea, vomiting, abdominal pain, dysphagia, dry mouth, mental changes, headache, dizziness, increased hand tremor, choreiform, or dystonic movements	Begin with 10 mg/100 mg tablet orally TID, titrated dose combination to minimize symptoms
levodopa *lee-voe-DOE-pa*		Parkinson disease	Same as carbidopa/levodopa	0.5–1 g/day orally initially, not to exceed 8 g/day
Dopaminergic Drugs—MAOB-Is				
rasagiline *ra-SA-ji-leen*	Azilect	Parkinson disease	Headache, arthralgia, depression, dyspepsia, flu syndrome	0.5–1 mg/day orally
safinamide *Sa-FIN-a-mide*	Xadago	Agonist for levodopa/carbidopa in Parkinson disease	Nausea, dyskinesia	50–100 mg orally daily
selegiline *se-LE-ji-leen*	Zelapar	Agonist for levodopa/carbidopa in Parkinson disease	Nausea, dizziness	5 mg orally at breakfast and lunch, transdermal
Dopamine Receptor Agonists, Nonergot				
apomorphine *a-poe-MOR-feen*	Apokyn	Parkinson disease "off" episode	Profound hypotension, nausea, vomiting	0.2 mL as needed for "off" episode
pramipexole *pra-mi-PEKS-ole*	Mirapex	Parkinson disease, restless leg syndrome (RLS)	Dizziness, somnolence, insomnia, hallucinations, confusion, nausea, dyspepsia, syncope	0.125–1.5 mg orally TID
ROPINIrole *roe-PIN-i-role*	Requip XL	Parkinson disease, RLS	Dizziness, somnolence, insomnia, hallucinations, confusion, nausea, dyspepsia, syncope	0.25–1 mg orally TID
rotigotine *Roe-TIG-oh-teen*	Neupro	Parkinson disease, RLS	Dizziness, drowsiness, fatigue, malaise, hypotension, peripheral edema	2–8 mg patch replaced daily
COMT Inhibitors				
entacapone *en-TA-ka-pone*	Comtan	As adjunct to levodopa/carbidopa in Parkinson disease	Dyskinesia, hyperkinesia, nausea, diarrhea, urine discoloration	200–1600 mg/day orally
tolcapone *TOLE-ka-pone*	Tasmar	Parkinson disease when refractory to levodopa/carbidopa	Orthostatic hypotension, dyskinesia, sleep disorders, dystonia, excessive dreaming, somnolence, dizziness, nausea, anorexia, muscle cramps, liver failure	100–200 mg orally TID
Cholinergic Blocking Drugs (Anticholinergics)				
benztropine mesylate *BENZ-troe-peen*	Cogentin	Parkinson disease, drug-induced EPS	Dry mouth, blurred vision, dizziness, nausea, nervousness, skin rash, urinary retention, dysuria, tachycardia, muscle weakness, disorientation, confusion	0.5–6 mg/day orally Acute dystonia: 1–2 mL IM or IV
trihexyphenidyl *trye-heks-ee-FEN-i-dill*		Parkinson disease, drug-induced EPS	Same as benztropine	1–15 mg/day orally in divided doses

Generic Name	Trade Name	Uses	Adverse Reactions	Dosage Ranges
Miscellaneous Drugs				
diphenhydrAMINE *dye-fen-HYE-dra-meen*	Benadryl	Drug-induced EPS, allergies	Same as benztropine	25–50 mg orally TID or QID
istradefylline *IS-tra-DEF-i-lin*	Nourianz	Treat PD off episodes, adjuvant to levodopa/carbidopa	Dizziness, insomnia, dyskinesia	40 mg orally daily
Combination Drugs				
carbidopa, **levodopa**, **entacapone**	Stalevo	Parkinson disease	See individual drugs	Titrated to individual need of assorted drugs

CHAPTER REVIEW

Know Your Drugs

Clients sometimes know a medication by the brand (or trade) name and not the generic name. To help you recognize both names, match the brand name with the generic name of the same medication.

Generic Name	Brand Name
1. bromocriptine	A. Zelapar
2. carbidopa	B. Lodosyn
3. pramipexole	C. Mirapex
4. selegiline	D. Parlodel

Calculate Medication Dosages

1. Oral levodopa 0.75 g is prescribed. The drug is available in 100-mg tablets, 250-mg tablets, and 500-mg tablets. The nurse administers _____.

2. Oral ropinirole 6 mg is prescribed. The drug is available in 2-mg tablets. The nurse administers _____.

Prepare for the NCLEX

RECALL THE FACTS

1. Parkinson disease or parkinsonism occurs because of the lack of which neurotransmitter?
   1. Acetylcholine
   2. Dopamine
   3. Serotonin
   4. GABA

2. The most serious adverse reactions seen with levodopa include _____.
   1. choreiform and dystonic movements
   2. depression
   3. suicidal tendencies
   4. paranoia

3. Older clients prescribed one of the dopamine receptor agonists are monitored closely for which of the following adverse reactions?
   1. Occipital headache
   2. Hallucinations
   3. Paralytic ileus
   4. Cardiac arrhythmias

4. Clients should be monitored closely for EPS when taking antiparkinson drugs with which class of drugs?
   1. Anticoagulants
   2. Vitamins
   3. Antidepressants
   4. Antihypertensives

5. The client taking tolcapone for Parkinson disease is monitored closely for _____.
   1. kidney dysfunction
   2. liver dysfunction
   3. agranulocytosis
   4. the development of an autoimmune disease

ANALYZE THE FACTS

6. The nurse reports which of the following as a diminished response to antiparkinson drug treatment rather than an adverse reaction?
   1. Dry mouth and difficulty in swallowing
   2. Anorexia, nausea, and vomiting
   3. Abdominal pain and constipation
   4. Increased hand tremor

7. *When taking a cholinergic blocking drug for Parkinson-like symptoms, the client most likely would experience which of the following adverse reactions?
   1. Constipation, urinary frequency
   2. Muscle spasm, convulsions
   3. Diarrhea, hypertension
   4. Dry mouth, dizziness

8. A family member asks the nurse which exercise is best to help a client with Parkinson disease maintain balance. Which is the best response?
   1. Swimming
   2. Tai Chi
   3. Jogging
   4. Mind puzzles

ALTERNATE-FORMAT QUESTIONS

9. Identify the interventions to use to help promote sleep for the client with RLS. **Select all that apply.**
   1. Take a hot bath.
   2. Watch a fast-paced show on television.
   3. Do a crossword puzzle.
   4. Take a brisk walk in the night air.
   5. Take vitamin B_6.
10. Arrange the following steps of dopamine distribution to a client with Parkinson disease:
    1. Levodopa targets the nerve to complete neurotransmission.
    2. The tablet(s) are swallowed.
    3. The carbidopa allows the levodopa to cross the blood–brain barrier.
    4. The levodopa and carbidopa combine together and are absorbed into the circulation.

To check your answers, see Appendix F.

---

*Indicates the question is directly linked to the NCLEX-PN test plan in Appendix G.

WANT TO KNOW MORE? A wide variety of resources are available to enhance your learning and understanding of this chapter.
- Visit thePoint for resources such as:
  - NCLEX-Style Student Review Questions
  - Journal Articles
  - Dosage Calculations
  - Drug Monographs
  - Watch and Learn Videos
  - Concepts in Action Animations
- The *Study Guide to Accompany Introductory Clinical Pharmacology*, 12th edition, sold separately, will help you review and apply essential content.
- ✓*PrepU* is available to help students prepare for the NCLEX-PN examination.

Antiepileptics

28

Key Terms

ataxia unsteady gait; muscular incoordination

atonic generalized seizure with loss of muscle tone; person suddenly drops

convulsion sudden, involuntary muscular contractions

epilepsy chronic, recurring seizure disorder

generalized seizures loss of consciousness during seizure

gingival hyperplasia overgrowth of gum tissue

focal seizures localized seizure in the brain, with/without impaired consciousness, sometimes called partial seizure

myoclonic sudden, forceful muscular contraction

nystagmus involuntary and constant movement of the eyeball

pancytopenia reduction in all cellular elements of the blood

precipitation condensation of a solid from a solution during a chemical reaction

seizure cluster of symptoms resulting from abnormal electrical activity in the brain

status epilepticus emergency situation characterized by continual seizure activity

Stevens–Johnson syndrome (SJS) fever, cough, muscular aches and pains, headache, and lesions of the skin, mucous membranes, and eyes; the lesions appear as red wheals or blisters, often starting on the face, in the mouth, or on the lips, neck, and extremities

tonic–clonic generalized seizure activity consisting of alternating contraction (tonic) and relaxation of muscles (clonic)

Learning Objectives

On completion of this chapter, the student will:

1. Compare and contrast the different types of drugs used as antiepileptics.
2. Explain the general drug actions, uses, adverse reactions, contraindications, precautions, and interactions of antiepileptics.
3. Distinguish important preadministration and ongoing assessment activities the nurse should perform with the client receiving an antiepileptic.
4. List nursing diagnoses particular to a client taking an antiepileptic.
5. Examine ways to promote an optimal response to therapy, how to manage common adverse reactions when administering the antiepileptics, and important points to keep in mind when educating a client about the use of antiepileptics.

 Drug Classes

Hydantoins
Carboxylic acid derivatives
Succinimides

Benzodiazepines
Nonspecified drugs

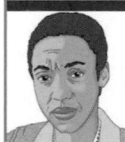 **PHARMACOLOGY IN PRACTICE**

Lillian Chase was in a car accident last year and had a seizure on the way to the hospital. As you review her medication list and ask about her drugs, she tells you that since she has been taking phenytoin she has had no seizures.

Drugs used for managing seizure disorders are called antiepileptics (AEDs). In some references, you will also see the terms antiseizure or anticonvulsant drugs—all of these terms describe the same group of drugs. Pharmacologically, they are classified as anticonvulsant, yet not all seizures have convulsions, hence the name change. This leads to discussing another set of terms that may appear confusing—*convulsion* and *seizure*. These terms are often used interchangeably yet have very different meanings. The term **convulsion** refers to a behavior— the sudden, involuntary contraction of the muscles of the body, often accompanied by loss of consciousness. A **seizure**, on the other hand, may be defined as an event; it is the periodic disturbances of the brain's electrical activity (Fisher, 2014). In other words, a person can experience a convulsion when they have a seizure. However, not all seizure activity will result in a convulsion.

SEIZURE DISORDERS

Seizure disorders are generally categorized as idiopathic, hereditary, or acquired.

- Idiopathic seizures—have no known cause
- Hereditary seizure disorder—passed from parent to child in their genetic makeup
- Acquired seizure disorders—have a known cause (such as, high fever, electrolyte imbalances, uremia, hypoglycemia, hypoxia, brain tumors or injury, and some drug withdrawal reactions)

The primary goal is to treat the underlying pathologic process to stop the seizures. Sometimes when the cause is not clear, and the seizures cannot be stopped, the activity needs to be controlled on a chronic basis. Medications play a significant role in this chronic management of seizure activity.

Seizures caused by disease, such as in **epilepsy**, may not be easy to eliminate. Epilepsy is characterized by recurrent unprovoked seizures (Fisher, 2014). Examples of the known causes of epilepsy include brain injury at birth, head injuries, and inborn errors of metabolism. In some clients, the cause of epilepsy is never determined. Epileptic seizures are classified according to the International League Against Epilepsy (ILAE) as illustrated in Figure 28.1. Each different type of seizure disorder is characterized by a specific pattern of events, as well as a different pattern of motor or sensory manifestation.

Drugs are the first-line treatment for most seizures. Lamotrigine is considered the drug of first choice for **focal seizures** and valproate for **generalized seizures**. Yet with newer medications on the market, any single or combination of drugs may be used with these goals in mind: (1) control of seizures and (2) minimal adverse reactions. Other factors considered are type of seizure, age, gender, other medical conditions, and cost. Most antiepileptics have specific uses; that is, they are of value in treating certain types of seizure disorders. The drug categories used as antiepileptics include the hydantoins, carboxylic acid derivatives, succinimides,

Generalized Seizures (40% of seizures)

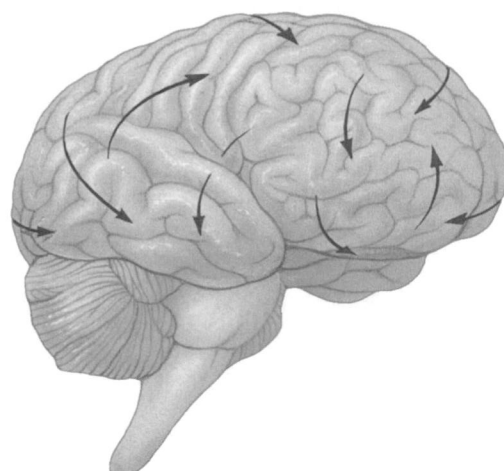

Focal Seizures (60% of seizures)

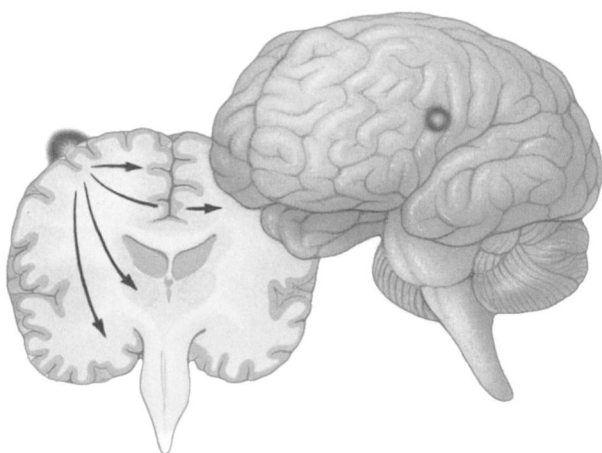

Absence
Involve a loss of consciousness with vacant stare or unresponsiveness.

Myoclonic
Involve sudden, forceful contractions of single or multiple groups of muscles.

Clonic
Longer jerking activity.

Tonic–clonic
Include alternate contraction (tonic phase) and relaxation (clonic phase) of muscles, a loss of consciousness, and abnormal behavior.

Atonic
Loss of muscle tone, person suddenly drops.

Simple
Consciousness is not impaired, can involve senses (flashing lights or a change in taste or speech) or motor ability (uncontrolled stiffening or jerking in one part of the body such as the finger, mouth, hand, or foot), nausea, déjà vu feeling.

Complex
Consciousness is impaired and variable (unconscious repetitive actions), staring gaze, hallucination/delusion.

Focal evolving to generalized
Begins as focal seizure and becomes generalized.

FIGURE 28.1 Classification of seizures by the International League Against Epilepsy (ILAE, 2020). (Adapted with ILAE criteria and Courtesy of Anatomical Chart Co.)

and benzodiazepines. In addition, several newer drugs are used as antiepileptics and do not fit in a specific category. They all possess the ability to depress abnormal neural discharges in the central nervous system (CNS), thereby inhibiting seizure activity. The Summary Drug Table: Antiepileptics provides a listing of the drugs used to treat seizure disorders.

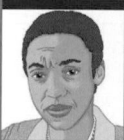

PHARMACOLOGY IN PRACTICE

PHYSIOLOGY
Which of the following are ways to categorize seizure disorders? Select all that apply.
1. Voluntary
2. Hereditary
3. Idiopathic
4. Acquired

ACTIONS

Antiepileptics depress abnormal nerve impulse discharges in the CNS. The six categories of antiepileptics achieve this effect through different modes of action:

- **Hydantoins** stabilize the hyperexcitability postsynaptically in the motor cortex of the brain.
- **Carboxylic acid derivatives** increase the levels of gamma (γ)-aminobutyric acid (GABA), which stabilizes cell membranes.
- **Succinimides** depress the motor cortex, creating a higher threshold before nerves react to the convulsive stimuli.
- **Benzodiazepines** elevate the seizure threshold by decreasing postsynaptic excitation.
- **Nonspecified drugs** have differing properties; for example, gabapentin is a GABA agonist and topiramate blocks the seizure activity rather than raising the threshold.

Seizures are theoretically reduced in intensity and frequency of occurrence or, in some instances, are virtually eliminated. For some clients, only partial control of the seizure disorder may be obtained with antiepileptic drug therapy.

USES

Antiepileptics are used prophylactically to prevent seizures after trauma or neurosurgery or in clients with a tumor and in the treatment of the following:

- Seizures of all types
- Neuropathic pain
- Bipolar disorders
- Anxiety disorders

Occasionally, **status epilepticus** (an emergency characterized by continual seizure activity with no interruptions) can occur. Lorazepam (Ativan) is the drug of choice for this condition. However, because the effects of lorazepam last less than 1 hr, longer-lasting antiepileptics, such as

phenytoin (Dilantin) are given to control the seizure activity on an ongoing basis. Another specific example is the drug clobazam, which is a benzodiazepine approved solely as an adjuvant to treatment of Lennox–Gastaut syndrome, a very rare form of epilepsy.

ADVERSE REACTIONS

At least 25% of those who experience adverse reactions will stop taking their medication (Kwan, 2000). Clients report side effects are intolerable. Adverse reactions that may occur with the administration of an antiepileptic drug include the following.

Central Nervous System Reactions
- Drowsiness, weakness, dizziness
- Headache, somnolence
- **Nystagmus** (constant, involuntary movement of the eyeball)
- **Ataxia** (loss of control of voluntary movements, especially gait)
- Slurred speech

Gastrointestinal System Reactions
- Nausea, vomiting
- Anorexia
- Constipation, diarrhea
- **Gingival hyperplasia** (overgrowth of gum tissue)
- Acute liver failure (with the drug felbamate)

OTHER REACTIONS

- Skin rashes, pruritus, urticaria
- Serious skin reactions, such as **Stevens–Johnson syndrome**, have been associated with the use of lamotrigine (Lamictal)
- Hematologic changes, such as **pancytopenia** (decrease in all the cellular components of the blood), leukopenia, aplastic anemia, and thrombocytopenia, have occurred with administration of selected drugs, including carbamazepine (Tegretol) and felbamate (Felbatol). See the Summary Drug Table: Antiepileptics for more information.

 Lifespan Considerations

Pregnant Women
Research suggests an association between the use of antiepileptics by pregnant women with epilepsy and an increased incidence of birth defects (ILAE, 2017). The Epilepsy Foundation has established the North American AED Pregnancy Registry for women to gain information about the safety of AEDs while pregnant and maintaining seizure control. This is sponsored by researchers from Massachusetts General Hospital and a number of pharmaceutical companies. Well over 10,000 women have enrolled to date.

CONTRAINDICATIONS

All categories of antiepileptics are contraindicated in clients with known hypersensitivity to the drugs. Phenytoin is contraindicated in clients with sinus bradycardia, sinoatrial block, Adams–Stokes syndrome, and second- and third-degree atrioventricular block; it also is contraindicated during pregnancy and lactation (ethotoin and phenytoin are pregnancy category D drugs). Ethotoin (Peganone) is contraindicated in clients with hepatic abnormalities. The succinimides are contraindicated in clients with bone marrow depression or hepatic or renal impairment. A higher incidence of systemic lupus erythematosus has been found in clients taking succinimides.

The drug category oxazolidinedione has been associated with serious adverse reactions and fetal malformations; therefore, the last drug in that category was taken off the market.

Carbamazepine should not be given within 14 days of monoamine oxidase inhibitor antidepressants. Carbamazepine is contraindicated in clients with bone marrow depression or hepatic or renal impairment and during pregnancy (pregnancy category D). Valproic acid (Depakote) is not administered to clients with renal impairment or during pregnancy (pregnancy category D). Oxcarbazepine (Trileptal), a nonspecified antiepileptic, may exacerbate dementia.

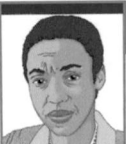

PHARMACOLOGY IN PRACTICE

SAFE DRUG ADMINISTRATION
A nurse is caring for a client who has a history of status epilepticus. Which drug should be available in parenteral form should this happen to the client again?
1. Phenytoin
2. Lorazepam
3. Barbiturate
4. Diazepam

PRECAUTIONS

Antiepileptics should be used cautiously in clients with liver or kidney disease and those with neurologic disorders. The newer medications, eslicarbazepine and oxcarbazepine, can cause hyponatremia. The benzodiazepines are used cautiously during pregnancy (pregnancy category D) and in clients with psychoses, clients with acute narrow-angle glaucoma, and older or debilitated clients. Phenytoin and lacosamide are used cautiously in clients with hypotension, severe myocardial insufficiency, and hepatic impairment.

Nonspecified antiepileptics are used cautiously in clients with glaucoma or increased intraocular pressure; a history of cardiac, renal, or liver dysfunction; and psychiatric disorders. Valproic acid is associated with, in addition to hepatic failure and birth defects, an increased risk for pancreatitis. Vigabatrin (Sabril) used to help treat refractory complex focal seizures may cause progressive and permanent vision loss.

LASA ALERT

The following drugs may sound alike; be sure to clarify when they are ordered:

Drug Name	Sounds Like
acetazolamide	acetaminophen
Ativan	Ambien, Atarax, Atgam, Avitene
Cerebyx	CeleBREX, CeleXA, Cerezyme, Cervarix
cloBAZam	clonazePAM
clonazePAM	ALPRAZolam, cloBAZam, cloNIDine, clorazepate, cloZAPine, LORazepam
Dilantin	Dilaudid, dilTIAZem, Dipentum
epitol	Epinal
ethosuximide	methsuximide
gabapentin enacarbil	gabapentin, gemfibrozi
Keppra	Kaletra
KlonoPIN	cloNIDine, clorazepate, cloZAPine, LORazepam
lacosamide	zonisamide
LaMICtal	labetalol, LamISIL, Lomotil
lamoTRIgine	labetalol, LamISIL, lamiVUDine, levETIRAcetam, levothyroxine, Lomotil
levETIRAcetam	lamoTRIgine, levOCARNitine, levoFLOXacin
LORazepam	ALPRAZolam, clonazePAM, diazePAM, KlonoPIN, Lovaza, temazepam, zolpidem
Lyrica	Hydrea, Lopressor
magnesium sulfate	manganese sulfate, morphine sulfate
OXcarbazepine	carBAMazepine, oxaprozin, oxazepam
phenytoin	phenelzine, phentermine, PHENobarbital
Primidone	predniSONE, primaquine, pyridoxine
TEGretol	Mebaral, Topamax, Toprol-XL, Toradol, TRENtal
tiaGABine	tiZANidine
Topamax	Sporanox, TEGretol, Toprol-XL
Trileptal	TriLipix
Vimpat	Venofer, Vfend, Vimovo
Zarontin	Neurontin, Xalatan, Zantac, Zaroxolyn
Zonegran	SINEquan

Drugs that look like a similar drug are noted in the Summary Drug Tables of each chapter.

INTERACTIONS

The following interactions may occur when an antiepileptic is administered with another agent:

Interacting Drug	Common Use	Effect of Interaction
Antibiotics/ antifungals	Fight infection	Increased effect of the antiepileptic
Tricyclic antidepressants	Manage depression	Increased effect of the antiepileptic
Salicylates	Pain relief	Increased effect of the antiepileptic
Cimetidine	Control gastrointestinal (GI) upset	Increased effect of the antiepileptic
Theophylline	Treatment of respiratory problems	Decreased serum levels of the antiepileptic
Antiepileptics medications	Reduce seizure activity	May increase seizure activity
Protease inhibitors	Treatment of human immunodeficiency virus (HIV) infection	Increased carbamazepine levels, resulting in toxicity
Oral contraceptives	Birth control	Decreased effectiveness of birth control, resulting in breakthrough bleeding or pregnancy (Box 28.1)

Interacting Drug	Common Use	Effect of Interaction
Analgesics or alcohol	CNS depressants	Increased depressant effect
Antidiabetic medications	Manage diabetes mellitus	Increased blood glucose levels

---

BOX 28.1 Pregnancy Prevention

Women taking birth control (i.e., pills, patch, ring) and one of the listed AEDs are at a greater risk of failure and becoming pregnant:

carbamazepine	phenobarbital
felbamate	phenytoin
oxcarbazepine	primidone
	topiramate

Other forms of birth control should be prescribed for women taking any of the above AEDs.

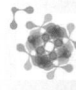

NURSING PROCESS
Client Receiving an Antiepileptic

ASSESSMENT

Preadministration Assessment

Seizures that occur in the outclient setting are almost always seen first by family members or friends, rather than by a member of the health care profession. The occurrence of abnormal behavior patterns or convulsive movements usually prompts the client to visit the primary health care provider's office or a neurologic clinic. A thorough client history is necessary to identify the type of seizure disorder.

Data gathering suggestions before the initial administration of the drug include:
Objective data

- Description of the seizures (the motor or psychic activity occurring during the seizure)
- Frequency of the seizures (approximate number per day)
- Average length of a seizure
- Vital signs (temperature, pulse, respirations, and blood pressure)
- Neurological diagnostic testing—electroencephalogram, computed axial tomography scan, and magnetic resonance imaging scan

- Laboratory tests—complete blood count, lumbar puncture, and hepatic and renal function tests (to rule out organic causes)

Subjective data

- Description of the aura (a subjective sensation preceding a seizure), if any has occurred
- Description of the degree of impairment of consciousness
- Description of what, if anything, appears to bring on the seizure
- Medical history, history of head or other injury
- Family history of seizure activity
- Drug therapy (list of all current drugs)

Ongoing Assessment

Antiepileptics control, but do not cure, epilepsy. Therefore, these medications will be taken indefinitely. An accurate ongoing assessment is important for obtaining the desired effect of the antiepileptic. The dosage of the antiepileptic may require frequent adjustments during the initial treatment period. Dosage adjustments are based on the client's

BOX 28.2 Quick Bedside Assessment

Ask the following questions or have client describe the behavior:
- What is your name?
- What are you feeling?
- What do you see? (*Hold up two fingers in front of client.*)
- Where are you and where do you live?
- Touch your left ear.
- What is this called? (*Hold up an item like your pen.*)

response to therapy (e.g., the control of the seizures) as well as the occurrence of adverse reactions. Depending on the client's response to therapy, a second antiepileptic may be added to the therapeutic regimen, or one antiepileptic may be changed to another. Regularly, serum plasma levels of the antiepileptic are measured to monitor for toxicity.

The client's seizures, along with response to drug therapy, should be documented when a hospitalized client is receiving an antiepileptic. Most seizures occur without warning, and others may not see the client until after the seizure has begun or after the seizure is over. Box 28.2 illustrates questions for a bedside assessment. Responses are documented in the client record. Any observations made during and after the seizure are important and may aid in the diagnosis of the type of seizure, as well as assist the primary health care provider in evaluating the effectiveness of drug therapy.

Part of the adherence issue in taking AEDs consistently has to do with unpleasant adverse reactions experienced in other body systems thought by the client to be completely unrelated to the seizure activity (Kwan, 2000). Clients may decide to reduce or stop taking medications because of how they feel. It is important to monitor for adverse reactions, especially those that may occur in a body system other than the neurological system. For example, a client may not connect the reduced ability to fight infections with an antiepileptic medication. Table 28.1 illustrates the blood levels that are monitored on a routine basis when clients are taking AEDs. When issues are identified early and treated, this will reduce noncompliance.

NURSING DIAGNOSES

Drug-specific nursing diagnoses include the following:

- **Injury risk** related to seizure disorder, drowsiness, ataxia, and vision disturbances
- **Altered skin integrity** related to adverse reactions (rash)
- **Infection risk** related to immunosuppression secondary to drug therapy
- **Impaired oral mucous membranes** related to gum overgrowth secondary to hydantoins

Nursing diagnoses related to drug administration are discussed in Chapter 4.

PLANNING

The expected outcomes for the client depend on the type and severity of the seizure but may include an optimal response to therapy (control of seizure), meeting client needs related to the management of adverse reactions, and confidence in an understanding of the medication regimen.

TABLE 28.1 Specific Routine Laboratory Monitoring While Taking Select Antiepileptic Medication

ANTIEPILEPTIC DRUG (AED)	LABORATORY TESTS
Carbamazepine	White blood cells
Eslicarbazepine	Serum sodium
Felbamate	Liver function study
Oxcarbazepine	Serum sodium
Phenytoin	Serum phenytoin levels
Valproic acid	Platelet count/serum ammonia

IMPLEMENTATION

Promoting an Optimal Response to Therapy

When administering an antiepileptic, do not omit or miss a dose (except by order of the primary health care provider).

> **NURSING ALERT**
>
> Recurrence of seizure activity may result from abrupt discontinuation of the drug, even when the antiepileptic is being administered in small daily doses.

Document and flag in the care plan antiepileptic administration. If the primary health care provider discontinues the antiepileptic therapy, the dosage is gradually withdrawn or another drug is gradually substituted.

Special Considerations for Hydantoins

Phenytoin remains a commonly prescribed antiepileptic because of its effectiveness, low toxicity, and relatively low cost. However, a genetically linked inability to metabolize phenytoin has been identified. For this reason, it is important to monitor serum concentrations of the drug on a regular basis to detect signs of toxicity (slurred speech, ataxia, lethargy, dizziness, nausea, and vomiting). Phenytoin plasma levels between 10 and 20 mcg/mL give optimal antiepileptic effect. However, many clients achieve seizure control at lower serum concentration levels. Levels greater than 20 mcg/mL are associated with toxicity. Clients with plasma levels greater than 20 mcg/mL may exhibit nystagmus, and at concentrations greater than 30 mcg/mL, ataxia and mental changes are common. Phenytoin can be administered orally and parenterally. When taken orally, the drug should be taken with meals to avoid GI upset. If the drug is administered parenterally, the intravenous (IV) route is preferred over the intramuscular (IM) route, because erratic absorption of phenytoin causes pain and muscle damage at the injection site.

> **NURSING ALERT**
>
> Lower-than-average plasma levels have been found in clients administered phenytoin by enteral feeding tubes. More frequent monitoring of blood levels is suggested for this client population.

Special Considerations for Benzodiazepines
The dosage of a benzodiazepine is highly individualized; increase the dose cautiously to avoid adverse reactions, particularly in older and debilitated clients. IV lorazepam may bring seizures under control quickly. However, for some clients, seizure activity may resume because of the short duration of the drug's effects. Drug **precipitation** can occur when diazepam (Valium) is administered IV. Never mix diazepam with other drugs. When used to control seizures, diazepam is administered by IV pushed slowly as close as possible to the IV site, allowing at least 1 min for each 5 mg of drug.

Lifespan Considerations

Gerontology
Apnea and cardiac arrest have occurred when diazepam is administered to older adults, very ill clients, and individuals with limited pulmonary reserve. Older or debilitated adults may require a decreased dosage of diazepam to reduce ataxia and oversedation.

Monitoring and Managing Client Needs

Injury Risk
Drowsiness is a common adverse reaction to antiepileptic drugs, especially early in therapy. Assist the client with all ambulatory activities until the client is stable. Remind the client to rise from the bed slowly and sit for a few minutes before standing. Drowsiness decreases with continued use.

Use caution when giving an oral preparation because aspiration of the tablet, capsule, or liquid may occur if the client experiences drowsiness. Test the client's swallowing ability by offering small sips of water before giving the drug. If the client has difficulty swallowing, withhold the drug and notify the primary health care provider as soon as possible. A different route of administration may be necessary. Because injury may occur when the client has a seizure, take precautions to prevent falls and other injuries until seizures are controlled by the drug.

Visual disturbances may occur with antiepileptic therapy. Permanent vision loss has been associated with vigabatrin, and clients on this medication and other drugs causing visual disturbances should be regularly evaluated by an ophthalmologist. The client with a visual disturbance is assisted with ambulation and oriented carefully to the environment. The client may be especially sensitive to bright lights and want the room light dimmed. Because photosensitivity can occur, the client should stay out of the sun if possible and wear sunscreens and protective clothing as needed until the individual effects of the drug are known.

Altered Skin Integrity
Carbamazepine, eslicarbazepine, lamotrigine, and phenytoin are most often the drugs that will produce a hypersensitivity rash. Should a rash occur, notify the primary health care provider immediately because the primary health care provider may discontinue the drug. If the rash is exfoliative (red rash with scaling of the skin),

purpuric (small hemorrhages or bruising on the skin), or bullous (skin vesicle filled with fluid, i.e., blister), use of the drug is not resumed. If the rash is milder (e.g., acne/sunburn-like), therapy may be resumed after the rash completely disappears. As the rash heals, keep the client's nails short, apply an antiseptic cream (if prescribed), and instruct the client to avoid using soap until the rash subsides.

Lifespan Considerations

Caucasian and Asian populations
Skin rashes are seen in Caucasian populations at a rate of 6 per 10,000 users of the drug carbamazepine. Risk for severe skin rashes (Stevens–Johnson and epidermal necrolysis) is estimated to be 10 times greater in some Asian populations when prescribed this drug. The increased risk is linked to a genetic variation. Genetic testing should be performed if this drug is prescribed for clients with Asian history, and if positive, the drug should be used only if the benefit outweighs the risk (Trivedi, 2016).

Infection Risk
You should be alert for the signs of pancytopenia, such as sore throat, fever, general malaise, bleeding of the mucous membranes, epistaxis (bleeding from the nose), and easy bruising. Antiepileptics such as carbamazepine, felbamate, and phenytoin may cause aplastic anemia and agranulocytosis. The succinimides are also particularly toxic. Routine laboratory tests, such as complete blood counts and differential counts, should be performed periodically. If bone marrow depression is evident (e.g., the client's platelet count and white blood cell count decrease significantly), the primary health care provider may discontinue or change antiepileptic drugs. When pancytopenia is present and blood cell counts are low, using a soft-bristled toothbrush may protect the mucous membranes from bleeding and easy bruising. The extremities also need to be protected from trauma or injury.

! NURSING ALERT
Hematologic changes (e.g., aplastic anemia, leukopenia, and thrombocytopenia) need to be reported immediately. Teach the client how to identify signs of thrombocytopenia (bleeding gums, easy bruising, increased menstrual bleeding, tarry stools) or leukopenia (sore throat, chills, swollen glands, excessive fatigue, or shortness of breath) and to contact the primary health care provider.

Impaired Oral Mucous Membrane
Long-term administration of hydantoins can cause gingivitis and gingival hyperplasia (overgrowth of gum tissue). It is important to inspect periodically the mouth, teeth, and gums of clients in a hospital or long-term clinical setting who are receiving one of these drugs. Any changes in the gums or teeth are reported to the primary health care provider. Teach the client to perform oral care after each meal.

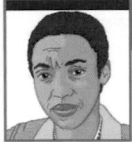

PHARMACOLOGY IN PRACTICE

MANAGING NEEDS

A client prescribed an antiepileptic complains of a chronic pain and requests an analgesic to be taken over time. Which possible interaction of analgesics with antiepileptics should the nurse monitor for in this client?

1. Increased carbamazepine levels
2. Increased seizure activity
3. Increased blood glucose levels
4. Increased depressant effect

Educating the Client and Family

When the client receives a diagnosis of epilepsy, you can assist the client and the family in adjustment to the diagnosis. Instruct family members in the care of the client before, during, and after a seizure. Explain the importance of restricting some activities until the seizures are controlled by drugs. Restriction of activities often depends on the age, sex, and occupation of the client. For some clients, the restriction of activities may create problems with such activities as employment, management of the home environment, or child care. For example, the client may be prohibited from driving while the primary health care provider attempts to control the seizure activity. You may assist the client to look for other modes of transportation to continue typical activities or employment. If a problem is recognized, a referral to a social worker, discharge planning coordinator, or public health nurse may be needed.

Review adverse drug reactions associated with the prescribed antiepileptic with the client and family members. The client and family members are instructed to contact the primary health care provider if any adverse reactions occur before the next dose of the drug is due. The client must not stop taking the drug until the problem is discussed with the primary health care provider.

Some clients, once their seizures are under control (e.g., stop occurring or occur less frequently), may have a tendency to stop the drug abruptly or begin to omit a dose occasionally. The drug must never be abruptly discontinued or doses omitted. If the client experiences drowsiness during initial therapy, a family member should be responsible for administering the drug. As you develop a teaching plan for the client or family member, include the following points:

- Do not omit, increase, or decrease the prescribed dose.
- Antiepileptic blood levels must be monitored at regular intervals, even if the seizures are well controlled.
- This drug should never be abruptly discontinued; AEDs must be tapered when stopped; consult the primary health care provider.
- Do not attempt to put anything in the mouth of a person having a seizure.

- If the primary health care provider finds it necessary to stop the drug, another drug usually is prescribed. Start taking this drug immediately (at the time the next dose of the previously used drug was due).
- Antiepileptic drugs may cause drowsiness or dizziness. Observe caution when performing hazardous tasks. Do not drive unless the adverse reactions of drowsiness, dizziness, or blurred vision are not significant. Driving privileges will be approved or reinstated by the primary health care provider based on seizure control.
- Avoid the use of alcohol unless use has been approved by the primary health care provider.
- Wear medical identification, such as a Medic Alert tag or bracelet, indicating drug use and the type of seizure disorder.
- Do not use any nonprescription drug unless the preparation has been approved by the primary health care provider.
- Keep a record of all seizures (date, time, length), as well as any minor problems (e.g., drowsiness, dizziness, lethargy), and take the record to each clinic or office visit.
- Contact the local branches of agencies, such as the Epilepsy Foundation of America, for information and assistance with problems, such as legal matters, insurance, driver's license, low-cost prescription services, and job training or retraining.

Hydantoins

- Inform the dentist and other primary health care providers of use of this drug.
- Brush and floss the teeth after each meal and make periodic dental appointments for oral examination and care.
- Take the medication with food to reduce GI upset.
- Thoroughly shake a phenytoin suspension immediately before use.
- Do not take capsules that are discolored.
- Notify the primary health care provider if any of the following occurs: skin rash, bleeding, swollen or tender gums, yellowish discoloration of the skin or eyes, unexplained fever, sore throat, unusual bleeding or bruising, persistent headache, malaise, or pregnancy.

Succinimides

- If GI upset occurs, take the drug with food or milk.
- Notify the primary health care provider if any of the following occurs: skin rash, joint pain, unexplained fever, sore throat, unusual bleeding or bruising, drowsiness, dizziness, blurred vision, or pregnancy.

Vigabatrin

- Periodic vision assessment and restricted administration through the SHARE program is required to recognize and reduce vision loss.

EVALUATION

- Therapeutic effect is achieved and convulsions are controlled.

- Adverse reactions are identified, reported to the primary health care provider, and managed successfully through appropriate nursing interventions:
  - No injury is evident.
  - Skin remains intact.
  - No evidence of infection is seen.
  - Mucous membranes are moist and intact.
- Client and family express confidence and demonstrate an understanding of the drug regimen.

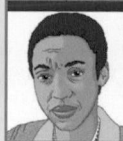

PHARMACOLOGY IN PRACTICE

USING CLINICAL REASONING
As you talk with Lillian she tells you that she has omitted one or two doses over the last month because she is "doing so well." How would you respond to Ms. Chase's statement?

KEY POINTS

■ *Convulsion* and *seizure* are terms often used interchangeably to describe a convulsion, which is the sudden, involuntary muscle contraction caused by changes in brain electrical activity. Seizures may be caused by disease, injury, or metabolic changes or be inherited at birth.

■ Antiepileptic drugs are used to depress the abnormal nerve impulses discharged in the brain. When discontinued, the drugs should be tapered down or seizure activity may return.

■ The most common adverse reactions are GI distress such as nausea, vomiting, constipation, or diarrhea, as well as drowsiness, dizziness, sleepiness, or headache. Prolonged use of the hydantoins can cause overgrowth of gum tissue. Twenty-five percent of clients will stop, reduce, or change their own AED because of the unpleasant adverse reactions.

■ Monitoring for the more serious adverse reactions such as life-threatening skin rashes and decreased blood counts should be done regularly.

SUMMARY DRUG TABLE
Antiepileptics

Generic Name	Trade Name	Uses	Adverse Reactions	Dosage Ranges
Hydantoins				
ethotoin *ETH-oh-toyn*	Peganone	Tonic–clonic seizures	Ataxia, CNS depression, headache, hypotension, nystagmus, mental confusion, slurred speech, dizziness, drowsiness, nausea, vomiting, gingival hyperplasia, rash	2–3 g/day orally in 4–6 divided doses
fosphenytoin *FOS-fen-i-toyn*	Cerebyx	Status epilepticus	Same as ethotoin	Loading dose: 15–20 mg/kg IV Maintenance dose: 4–6 mg/kg/day IV
phenytoin *FEN-i-toyn*	Dilantin	Tonic–clonic seizures, status epilepticus, prophylactic seizure prevention	Same as ethotoin	Oral: loading dose: 1 g divided into three doses prevention (400, 300, 300 mg) orally q2hr Maintenance dose: started 24 hr after loading dose, 300–400 mg/day Parenteral: 10–15 mg/kg IV
Carboxylic Acid Derivatives				
valproic acid *val-PROE-ik* **(divalproex)**	Depakote	Epilepsy, migraine headache, mania	Headache, somnolence, dizziness, tremor, nausea, vomiting, diplopia	10–60 mg/kg/day orally; if dosage is more than 250 mg/day, give in divided doses
Succinimides				
ethosuximide *eth-oh-SUKS-i-mide*	Zarontin	Focal seizures	Drowsiness, ataxia, dizziness, nausea, vomiting, urinary frequency, pruritus, urticaria, gingival hyperplasia	Up to 1.5 g/day orally in divided doses; children, 250 mg/day orally
methsuximide *meth-SUKS-i-mide*	Celontin	Focal seizures	Same as ethosuximide	300–1200 mg/day orally

Continued

SUMMARY DRUG TABLE (continued)
Antiepileptics

Generic Name	Trade Name	Uses	Adverse Reactions	Dosage Ranges
Benzodiazepines				
clonazePAM *kloe-NA-ze-pam*	KlonoPIN	Seizure disorders, panic disorders	Drowsiness, depression, ataxia, anorexia, diarrhea, constipation, dry mouth, palpitations, visual disturbances, rash	Initial dose: do not exceed 1.5 mg/day orally in three divided doses; increase in increments of 0.5–1 mg q3day; do not exceed 20 mg/day
clobazam *KLOE-ba-zam*	Onfi, Sympazan	Adjunct to other AED to treat Lennox–Gastaut syndrome	Lethargy, somnolence, ataxia, aggression, fatigue, insomnia	Initial dose: 5–10 mg orally, titrate to no more than 40 mg
clorazepate *klore-AZ-eh-pate*	Tranxene	Focal seizures, anxiety disorders, alcohol withdrawal	Same as clonazepam	Initial dose: 7.5 mg orally TID, maximum dose 90 mg/day
diazePAM *dye-AZ-e-pam*	Valium, Valtoco (nasal form)	Status epilepticus, seizure disorders (all forms), anxiety disorders, alcohol withdrawal	Same as clonazepam	Seizure control: 2–10 mg/day orally BID to QID Status epilepticus: 5–10 mg IV initially, maximum dose 30 mg Rectally: 0.2–0.5 mg/kg
LORazepam *lor-A-ze-pam*	Ativan	Status epilepticus, preanesthetic	Same as clonazepam	Status epilepticus: 4 mg IV over 2 min
Nonspecified Preparations				
acetaZOLAMIDE *a-set-a-ZOLE-a-midee*		Epilepsy, altitude sickness	Drowsiness, dizziness, nausea, diarrhea, constipation, visual disturbances	8–30 mg/kg/day in divided doses
brivaracetam *briv-a-RA-se-tam*	Briviact	Adjunct for focal seizures	Dizziness, lethargy, malaise, fatigue, nausea, vomiting	25–100 mg orally daily
cannabidiol *kan-a-bi-DYE-ol*	Epidiolex	Treat Lennox–Gastaut or Dravet syndromes	Drowsiness, lethargy, malaise, insomnia, decreased appetite, weight loss, anemia, fatigue	10 mg orally twice daily
carBAMazepine *kar-ba-MAZ-e-peen*	TEGretol, Carbatrol, Epitol, Equetro	Epilepsy, bipolar disorder, trigeminal/postherpetic neuralgia	Dizziness, nausea, drowsiness, unsteady gait, nausea, vomiting	Maintenance: 800–1200 mg/day orally in divided doses
cenobamate *SEN-oh-BAM-ate*	Xcopri	Complex focal seizures	Hypersomnia, dizziness, drowsiness, lethargy, malaise, fatigue, headache	12.5 mg orally daily
eslicarbaxepine *es-li-kar-BAZ-e-peen*	Aptiom	Focal seizures	Dizziness, drowsiness, headache, nausea, vomiting	400–1200 mg orally once daily
felbamate *FEL-ba-mate*	Felbatol	Focal seizures in clients who fail other drug therapy first	Insomnia, headache, anxiety, acne, rash, dyspepsia, vomiting, constipation, diarrhea, upper respiratory tract infection, fatigue, rhinitis, aplastic anemia, hepatic disorders	1200–3600 mg/day orally in divided doses
gabapentin *GA-ba-PEN-tin*	Fanatrex, Gralise, Neurontin	Focal seizures (adults), postherpetic neuralgia	Somnolence, dizziness, ataxia	900–1800 mg/day orally in 3–4 divided doses
gabapentin enacarbil *GA-ba-PEN-tin en-a-KAR-bil*	Horizant	Restless leg syndrome, postherpetic neuralgia	Same as gabapentin	600 mg orally twice daily
lacosamide *la-KOE-sa-mide*	Vimpat	Focal seizures (adults)	Dizziness, headache, nausea, double vision	100–400 mg orally in two divided doses
lamoTRIgine *la-MOE-tri-jeen*	Lamictal	Focal seizures (used with other antiepileptics), bipolar disorder	Dizziness, insomnia, somnolence, ataxia, nausea, vomiting, diplopia, headache, Stevens–Johnson syndrome rash	50–500 mg/day orally in two divided doses

Generic Name	Trade Name	Uses	Adverse Reactions	Dosage Ranges
levETIRAcetam *lee-va-tye-RA-se-tam*	Keppra, Elepsia XR	Focal seizures, tonic–clonic seizures, bipolar disorder, migraine headache	Headache, dizziness, asthenia, somnolence, infection	500 mg BID orally, increasing dose every 2 weeks until reach 3000 mg daily
magnesium sulfate *mag-NEE-zhum SUL-fate*		Hypomagnesemia, seizures associated with eclampsia and acute nephritis (children)	Flushing, sweating, hypothermia, depressed reflexes, hypotension, cardiac and CNS depression	Nephritis: 20–40 mg/kg IM in a dilute solution Eclampsia: 4 g IV in dilute solution, titrate continued infusion per serum level
OXcarbazepine *ox-car-BAZ-e-peen*	Oxtellar XR, Trileptal	Focal seizures, epilepsy	Headache, dizziness, fatigue, somnolence, ataxia, diplopia, nausea, vomiting, abdominal pain	600–1200 mg orally BID
perampanel *per-AM-pa-nel*	Fycompa	Focal seizures, tonic–clonic seizures (used with other antiepileptics)	Dizziness, somnolence, fatigue, irritability	2–12 mg orally at bedtime
pregabalin *pre-GAB-a-lin*	Lyrica	Focal seizures (adults), neuropathic pain, postherpetic neuralgia	Dizziness, somnolence	Seizure activity: 150 mg/day in 2–3 divided doses
primidone *PRI-mi-done*	Mysoline	Epilepsy	Dizziness, somnolence, nausea, vomiting	Up to 500 mg orally QID
rufinamide *roo-FIN-a-mide*	Banzel	Seizures (associated with Lennox–Gastaut syndrome)	Dizziness, fatigue, headache, somnolence, nausea	400–3200 mg orally BID
tiaGABine *tye-AG-a-been*	Gabitril	Focal seizures	Dizziness, somnolence, asthenia, nervousness, nausea	4–56 mg/day orally
topiramate *toe-PYRE-a-mate*	Topamax	Focal/tonic–clonic seizures, migraine headache	Fatigue, concentration problems, somnolence, anorexia	Seizure activity: 200–400 mg/day orally in divided doses
vigabatrin *vye-GA-ba-trin*	Sabril, Vigadrone	Focal seizures, infantile spasms	Somnolence, fatigue, dizziness, headache, weight gain, upper respiratory tract infection symptoms, visual loss	1.5 g orally twice daily, titrated for infants by body weight
zonisamide *zoe-NIS-a-mide*	Zonegran	Focal seizures of epilepsy	Somnolence, anorexia, dizziness, headache, rash, heat stroke	100–400 mg/day orally

CHAPTER REVIEW

Know Your Drugs

Clients sometimes know a medication by the brand (or trade) name and not the generic name. To help you recognize both names, match the brand name with the generic name of the same medication.

Generic Name	Brand Name
1. carbamazepine	A. Dilantin
2. diazepam	B. Lyrica
3. phenytoin	C. Tegretol
4. pregabalin	D. Valium

Calculate Medication Dosages

1. Zonisamide 200 mg is prescribed. The drug is available in 100 mg tablets. The nurse administers _____.
2. The primary health care provider prescribes ethosuximide syrup 500 mg for a client with absence seizures. The drug is available in a strength of 250 mg/5 mL. The nurse administers _____.

Prepare for the NCLEX

RECALL THE FACTS

1. A convulsion is best described as _____.
   1. loss of consciousness
   2. disturbances in brain electrical activity
   3. sudden, involuntary contractions
   4. disrupted CNS neurologic impulses
2. Focal seizures make up what percentage of total seizures?
   1. 20%
   2. 40%
   3. 60%
   4. 100%
3. A client is prescribed phenytoin for a recurrent epileptic disorder. The nurse teaches the client that the most common adverse reactions are _____.
   1. related to the gastrointestinal system
   2. associated with the reproductive system
   3. associated with kidney function
   4. related to the CNS

4. When administering diazepam to an older client, the nurse should monitor the client for unusual effects of the drug such as _____.
   1. marked excitement
   2. excessive sweating
   3. heart arrhythmias
   4. agitation
5. Some antiepileptics may cause birth defects. The nurse should instruct the female client regarding:
   1. birth control methods.
   2. prenatal vitamins and supplements.
   3. alternative therapy for seizure control.
   4. how to stop taking the drugs to get pregnant.

ANALYZE THE FACTS

6. When caring for a client taking a succinimide for seizure control, the nurse monitors the client for blood dyscrasias. Which of the following symptoms would indicate that the client may be developing a blood dyscrasia?
   1. Constipation, blood in the stool
   2. Diarrhea, lethargy
   3. Sore throat, general malaise
   4. Hyperthermia, excitement
7. Which statement would be included when educating the client taking carbamazepine for seizures?
   1. Take this drug with milk to enhance absorption.
   2. Wear a sunscreen and protective clothing when exposed to sunlight.
   3. To minimize adverse reactions, take this drug once daily at bedtime.
   4. Visit a dentist frequently because this drug increases the risk of gum disease.
8. Which of the following adverse reactions, if observed in a client prescribed phenytoin, would indicate that the client may be developing phenytoin toxicity?
   1. Severe occipital headache
   2. Ataxia
   3. Hyperactivity
   4. Somnolence

ALTERNATE-FORMAT QUESTIONS

9. *The nurse is preparing to administer an antiepileptic for status epilepticus. The primary health care provider prescribes lorazepam (Ativan) 4 mg IV. Look at the package provided. The nurse will administer _____.

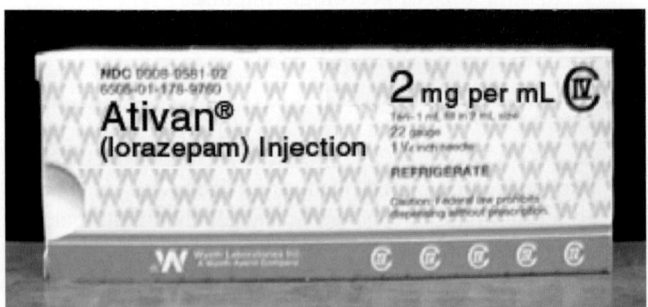

10. Look at the image provided. Which drug is most likely to cause gingival hyperplasia?

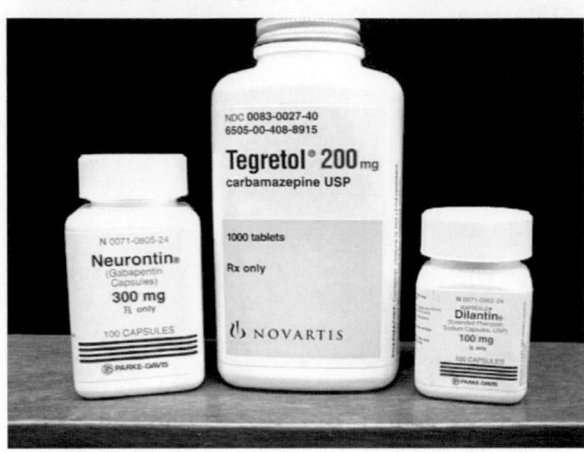

Neurontin   Tegretol   Dilantin

To check your answers, see Appendix F.

_____

*Indicates the question is directly linked to the NCLEX-PN test plan in Appendix G.

WANT TO KNOW MORE? A wide variety of resources are available to enhance your learning and understanding of this chapter.
- Visit the**Point** for resources such as:
  - NCLEX-Style Student Review Questions
  - Journal Articles
  - Dosage Calculations
  - Drug Monographs
  - Watch and Learn Videos
  - Concepts in Action Animations
- The *Study Guide to Accompany Introductory Clinical Pharmacology,* 12th edition, sold separately, will help you review and apply essential content.
- ✓*PrepU* is available to help students prepare for the NCLEX-PN examination.

Skeletal Muscle, Bone, and Joint Disorder Drugs

Key Terms

alopecia abnormal loss of hair; baldness

autoimmune a response where antibodies are formed against one's own body

dyspepsia fullness or epigastric discomfort

gout a metabolic disorder resulting in increased levels of uric acid and causing severe joint pain

hypercalcemia abnormally high level of serum calcium

musculoskeletal pertaining to the bones and muscles

osteoporosis skeletal disorder characterized by porous bone, making weaker bone strength and greater risk of fracture of a bone

Paget disease condition where bones grow too large and become weak

rheumatoid arthritis (RA) inflammatory changes in connective tissue

Stevens–Johnson syndrome (SJS) fever, cough, muscular aches and pains, headache, and lesions of the skin, mucous membranes, and eyes; the lesions appear as red wheals or blisters, often starting on the face, in the mouth, or on the lips, neck, and extremities

Learning Objectives

On completion of this chapter, the student will:

1. List the types of drugs used to treat musculoskeletal disorders.
2. Explain the uses, general drug actions, adverse reactions, contraindications, precautions, and interactions of the drugs used to treat musculoskeletal disorders.
3. Distinguish important preadministration and ongoing assessment activities the nurse should perform on the client taking a drug used to treat musculoskeletal disorders.
4. List nursing diagnoses particular to a client taking a drug for the treatment of musculoskeletal disorders.
5. Examine ways to promote an optimal response to therapy, how to manage adverse reactions, and important points to keep in mind when educating the client about drugs used to treat musculoskeletal disorders.

 Drug Classes

Skeletal muscle relaxants
Disease-modifying antirheumatic drugs (DMARDs)
Bone resorption inhibitors—bisphosphonates
Uric acid inhibitors

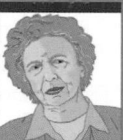

PHARMACOLOGY IN PRACTICE

A call was taken at the clinic from Mrs. Moore's daughter, who lives out of town. When you return her call, she expresses concern about her mother's balance and possible risk for falls. She asks if she (Mrs. Moore) should be taking a pill to strengthen her bones. Consider this request as you read this chapter.

A variety of drugs are used in treating **musculoskeletal** (bone and muscle) injuries and disorders. In this chapter, drugs used for both acute and chronic conditions are discussed. In an acute situation, such as when muscles are injured and if surgery is not warranted, then medications, exercise, and physical therapy are used to heal the injury. Skeletal muscle relaxants may be used to promote healing; our discussion in this chapter will start with these drugs.

Later in the chapter, you will learn about drugs used with chronic musculoskeletal conditions.

SKELETAL MUSCLE RELAXANTS

In addition to pain relievers (Unit 3), skeletal muscle relaxants are used to assist in relaxing certain muscle groups as strains and sprains repair themselves.

ACTIONS

The mode of action of many skeletal muscle relaxants, such as carisoprodol, baclofen, and chlorzoxazone, is not clearly understood. Many of these drugs do not directly relax skeletal muscles, but their ability to relieve acute painful musculoskeletal conditions may be because of their sedative action. Cyclobenzaprine appears to have an effect on muscle tone, thereby reducing muscle spasm.

The exact mode of action of diazepam (Valium), an antianxiety drug (see Chapter 19), in the relief of painful musculoskeletal conditions is unknown. The drug does have a sedative action, which may account for some of its ability to relieve muscle spasm and pain.

USES

Skeletal muscle relaxants are used in various acute painful musculoskeletal conditions, such as muscle strains and back pain.

ADVERSE REACTIONS

Drowsiness is the most common reaction seen with the use of skeletal muscle relaxants. Additional adverse reactions are given in the Summary Drug Table: Drugs Used to Treat Musculoskeletal, Bone, and Joint Disorders. Some of the adverse reactions that may occur with the administration of diazepam include drowsiness, sedation, sleepiness, lethargy, constipation or diarrhea, bradycardia or tachycardia, and rash.

CONTRAINDICATIONS

Skeletal muscle relaxants are contraindicated in clients with known hypersensitivity to the drugs. Baclofen is contraindicated in skeletal muscle spasms caused by rheumatic disorders. Carisoprodol is contraindicated in clients with a known hypersensitivity to meprobamate. Cyclobenzaprine is contraindicated in clients with a recent myocardial infarction, cardiac conduction disorders, and hyperthyroidism. In addition, cyclobenzaprine is contraindicated within 14 days of the administration of a monoamine oxidase inhibitor (MAOI). Oral dantrolene is contraindicated during lactation and in clients with active hepatic disease and muscle spasm caused by rheumatic disorders.

PRECAUTIONS

Skeletal muscle relaxants are used with caution in clients with a history of cerebrovascular accident, cerebral palsy, parkinsonism, or seizure disorders and during pregnancy

and lactation (pregnancy category C). Hepatitis is of concern when women and those older than 35 years are prescribed dantrolene. Carisoprodol is used with caution in clients with severe liver or kidney disease and during pregnancy (category unknown) and lactation. Cyclobenzaprine is used cautiously in clients with cardiovascular disease and during pregnancy and lactation (pregnancy category B). Dantrolene, a pregnancy category C drug, is used with caution during pregnancy.

LASA ALERT

The following drugs may sound alike; be sure to clarify when they are ordered:

Drug Name	Sounds Like
Baclofen	Bactroban
Cyclobenzaprine	cycloSERINE, cyproheptadine
Metaxalone	mesalamine, metOLazone
Skelaxin	Robaxin
tiZANidine	nizatidine, tiaGABine.
Zanaflex	Xiaflex

Drugs that look like a similar drug are noted in the Summary Drug Tables of each chapter.

INTERACTIONS

The following interactions may occur when a skeletal muscle relaxant is administered with another agent:

Interacting Drug	Common Use	Effect of Interaction
Central nervous system (CNS) depressants, such as alcohol, antihistamines, opiates, and sedatives	Promote a calming effect or provide pain relief	Increased CNS depressant effect
Cyclobenzaprine		
MAOIs	Manage depression	Risk for high fever and convulsions
Orphenadrine		
Haloperidol	Treat psychotic behavior	Increased psychosis
Tizanidine		
Antihypertensives	Reduce blood pressure	Increased risk of hypotension

When you review the medical record of a postsurgical client, look for use of muscle relaxants during the operative procedure. This category of drugs is used to relax muscle tone throughout the body or to relax specific muscles. During anesthesia induction (insertion of an endotracheal tube) these drugs relax the muscles in the neck and throat, which makes tube insertion easier and less likely to result in an injury to tissues. Muscle relaxants also reduce muscle tension in the abdomen or chest for surgery and allow for easier movement of joints and limbs when a client is positioned for surgery. Examples of muscle relaxants used during surgery are included in Table 29.1.

TABLE 29.1 Examples of Muscle Relaxants Used for Surgical Procedures

GENERIC NAME	TRADE NAME
Cisatracurium	Nimbex
Mivacurium	Mivacron
Pancuronium	
Rocuronium	
Succinylcholine	Anectine
Vecuronium	

When chronic disease affects skeletal muscles, it typically causes limitations in function. Drugs are frequently used to maintain function caused by the chronic illness. Examples of the drugs used for musculoskeletal disorders include disease-modifying antirheumatic drugs (DMARDs), bone resorption inhibitors (used to treat osteoporosis), and uric acid inhibitors (used to treat gout). A description of these and other musculoskeletal disorders is given in Table 29.2.

The following drug classes are used in the treatment of a variety of chronic diseases noted in each section.

DISEASE-MODIFYING ANTIRHEUMATIC DRUGS

Rheumatoid arthritis (RA) is an **autoimmune** disorder, in which antibodies are formed against one's own body. As a defense mechanism white blood cells are mobilized and lodge in the joints, causing swelling, pain, and inflammation (Fig. 29.1). This condition is typically treated using three classifications of drugs: nonsteroidal anti-inflammatory drugs (NSAIDs), corticosteroids, and DMARDs. Early stages of the disease process may respond well to the NSAIDs alone. As RA advances, pain medication and

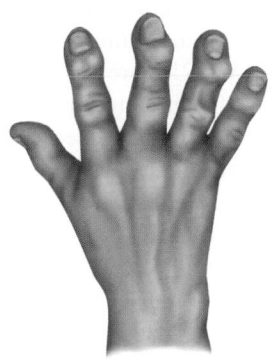

FIGURE 29.1 Example of acute rheumatoid arthritis in the joints of the fingers on the hand. (From Bickley, L. S., & Szilagyi, P. (2017). *Bates' guide to physical examination and history taking* (12th ed.). Wolters Kluwer.)

TABLE 29.2 Selected Musculoskeletal Disorders

DISORDER	DESCRIPTION
Synovitis	Inflammation of the synovial membrane of a joint resulting in pain, swelling, and inflammation. It occurs in disorders such as rheumatic fever, RA, and gout
Arthritis	Inflammation of a joint. The term is frequently used to refer to any disease involving pain or stiffness of the musculoskeletal system
Osteoarthritis or degenerative joint disease (DJD)	Noninflammatory DJD marked by degeneration of the articular cartilage, changes in the synovial membrane, and hypertrophy of the bone at the margins
Rheumatoid arthritis	Chronic systemic disease that produces inflammatory changes throughout the connective tissue in the body. It affects joints and other organ systems of the body. Destruction of articular cartilage occurs, affecting joint structure and mobility. RA primarily affects individuals between 20 and 40 years of age
Gout	Form of arthritis in which uric acid accumulates in increased amounts in the blood and often is deposited in the joints. The deposit or collection of urate crystals in the joints causes the symptoms (pain, redness, swelling, joint deformity)
Osteoporosis	Loss of bone density occurring when the loss of bone substance exceeds the rate of bone formation. Bones become porous, brittle, and fragile. Compression fractures of the vertebrae are common. This disorder occurs most often in postmenopausal women but can occur in men as well
Hypercalcemia of malignancy	Advanced-stage malignant disease. It can occur with 10%–50% of tumors. It is associated with parathyroid hormone production and can be difficult to manage. Symptoms include lethargy, anorexia, nausea, vomiting, thirst, polydipsia, constipation, and dehydration. If untreated, it may lead to cognitive difficulties, confusion, obtundation (extreme dullness, near-coma), and coma
Paget disease (osteitis deformans)	Chronic bone disorder characterized by abnormal bone remodeling. The disease disrupts the growth of new bone tissue, causing the bone to thicken and become soft. This weakens the bone, which increases susceptibility to fracture or collapse of the bone (e.g., the vertebrae) even with slight trauma

corticosteroids may be used for quick relief and the DMARDs to suppress the immune response.

This section describes the disease-modifying antirheumatic drugs, frequently called DMARDs. The NSAIDs and corticosteroids are discussed in Chapters 14 and 41, respectively.

ACTIONS AND USES

When the immobility and pain of RA can no longer be controlled by pain relief agents and anti-inflammatory drugs, DMARDs are used. The most commonly used DMARDs include methotrexate, sulfasalazine, hydroxychloroquine, and leflunomide. These drugs have properties to produce immunosuppression, which in turn decreases the body's autoimmune response. Therefore, in RA treatment, DMARDs are useful for their immunosuppressive ability. Other autoimmune diseases treated with DMARDs include Crohn disease and fibromyalgia. Methotrexate is used in cancer therapy, in which the immunosuppression is considered an adverse reaction rather than an intended effect.

Drugs called tumor necrosis factor (TNF) inhibitors are used in persons with RA and related inflammatory conditions. TNF-alpha is a small protein that regulates the body's immune cells and produces inflammation. These drugs are termed biologic DMARDs and work to suppress the body's natural immune response (see Chapter 49). Biologic DMARDs include etanercept (Enbrel), adalimumab (Humira), infliximab (Remicade), certolizumab pegol (Cimzia), and golimumab (Simponi).

Cytotoxic drugs, such as azathioprine (Imuran), cyclophosphamide (Cytoxan), cyclosporine, and gold salts are extremely toxic and reserved for life-threatening problems (such as systemic vasculitis) or when other drugs fail to achieve remission and are only mentioned in this chapter because you may hear of their use, such as in a history intake.

ADVERSE REACTIONS

Immunosuppressive drugs can cause the following adverse reactions:

- Nausea
- Stomatitis
- **Alopecia** (hair loss)

The adverse reactions to sulfa-based drugs, such as sulfasalazine, include ocular changes, gastrointestinal (GI) upset, and mild pancytopenia. Biologic DMARDs produce flu-like symptoms. Because they reduce the immune response, infectious diseases such as tuberculosis are a concern. The most common adverse reaction to the drugs given by injection is skin irritation. For more information, see the Summary Drug Table: Drugs Used to Treat Musculoskeletal, Bone, and Joint Disorders.

CONTRAINDICATIONS

All categories of DMARDs are contraindicated in clients with known hypersensitivity to the drugs. Clients with renal insufficiency, liver disease, alcohol abuse, pancytopenia, or folate deficiency should not take methotrexate. Women who are pregnant or attempting to become pregnant should not use leflunomide. Biologic DMARDs should not be used in clients with heart failure or neurologic demyelinating diseases. Anakinra (Kineret) should not be used in combination with etanercept, adalimumab, or infliximab.

PRECAUTIONS

These drugs should be used with caution in clients with obesity, diabetes, and hepatitis B or C. Hepatoxicity is of concern when taking leflunomide. Women should not become pregnant, and sexual partners should use barrier contraception to prevent transmission of the drug by semen.

Sulfasalazine is selected over methotrexate for clients with liver disease. Clients taking etanercept, adalimumab, or infliximab should be screened for preexisting tuberculosis because of the increase in opportunistic infections presenting after treatment.

LASA ALERT

The following drugs may sound alike; be sure to clarify when they are ordered:

Drug Name	Sounds Like
Hydroxychloroquine	hydrocortisone, hydroxyurea
Leflunomide	lenalidomide
Methotrexate	mercaptopurine, methylPREDNISolone sodium succinate, metOLazone, metroNIDAZOLE, mitoXANTRONE, MXT Patch, PRALAtrexate.
Plaquenil	Platinol
sulfasalazine	cefuroxime, salsalate, sulfADIAZINE
Orencia	Oracea
anakinra	amikacin, Ampyra
Humira	Humulin, Humalog
Cimzia	Cyramza
sarilumab	adalimumab, certolizumab, golimumab, tocilizumab
inFLIXimab	idaruCIZUmab, riTUXimab
Remicade	Renacidin, Rituxan

Drugs that look like a similar drug are noted in the Summary Drug Tables of each chapter.

INTERACTIONS

The following interactions may occur when a DMARD, such as methotrexate, is administered with another agent:

Interacting Drug	Common Use	Effect of Interaction
Sulfa antibiotics	Fight infection	Increased risk of methotrexate toxicity
Aspirin and NSAIDs	Pain relief	Increased risk of methotrexate toxicity

> **NURSING ALERT**
> Because DMARDs are designed to produce immunosuppression, clients need to be monitored routinely for infections. Instruct clients to report any problem, no matter how minor, such as a cold or open sore—even these can become life-threatening.

BONE RESORPTION INHIBITORS: BISPHOSPHONATES

Approximately 54 million Americans have **osteoporosis** (porous bone) or low bone mass (NOF, 2020). Osteoporosis involves the loss of bone mass, seen typically in postmenopausal women. It is estimated that 700,000 spinal fractures and 290,000 hip fractures occur yearly in the United States because of this disease (Black & Rosen, 2016). The bisphosphonates and newer biologic drugs are helping to reduce these fractures and those of **Paget disease** (bone growth and weakening).

ACTIONS

Bisphosphonates act primarily on the bone by inhibiting normal and abnormal bone resorption. This results in increased bone mineral density, reversing the progression of osteoporosis.

USES

Bisphosphonates are used in the treatment of the following:

- Osteoporosis in postmenopausal women and men (caused by glucocorticoid use)
- **Hypercalcemia** (increased serum calcium) of malignant diseases and bony metastasis of some solid tumors
- Paget disease of the bone

ADVERSE REACTIONS

Adverse reactions with bisphosphonates include:

- Nausea, diarrhea
- Increased or recurrent bone pain
- Headache
- **Dyspepsia** (GI discomfort), acid regurgitation, dysphagia
- Abdominal pain

Bisphosphonates are typically not an issue when the client is instructed in the proper administration of the drug (see Nursing Process section). Asking the client to teach-back understanding of the procedures will help clarify issues before they happen and reduce adverse reactions.

CONTRAINDICATIONS AND PRECAUTIONS

These drugs are contraindicated in clients who are hypersensitive to the bisphosphonates. Alendronate (Fosamax) and risedronate (Actonel) are contraindicated in clients with hypocalcemia. Alendronate is a pregnancy category C drug and is contraindicated during pregnancy. These drugs are also contraindicated in clients with delayed esophageal emptying or renal impairment. Concurrent use of these drugs with hormone replacement therapy is not recommended.

Administration of the biologic, denosumab (Prolia), is associated with hypokalemia, osteonecrosis of the jaw, infection, skin reactions, and atypical femoral fractures. Benefit of the drug versus harsh and unusual adverse reactions are monitored by the US Food and Drug Administration (FDA) in a program called Risk Evaluation and Mitigation Strategy (REMS). With this program, specific instruction and monitoring must occur and documentation sent to the FDA regarding administration of the drug and client knowledge of potential adverse reactions.

Although these drugs have not been studied, if a pregnant woman presents with malignancy, their use during the pregnancy may be justified if the potential benefit outweighs the potential risk to the fetus.

PRACTICE CONSIDERATIONS

Standard drug treatment of osteoporosis includes approximately 5 years of bisphosphonate administration. At that time a "drug holiday" is recommended. Current studies indicate that the best estimate regarding drug holiday is the client's baseline risk—if high, then longer treatment is recommended (McClung, 2013).

LASA ALERT

The following drugs may sound alike; be sure to clarify when they are ordered:

Drug Name	Sounds Like
alendronate	Risedronate
Aredia	Adriamycin
denosumab	daclizumab, daratumumab, dinutuximab, dupilumab, durvalumab
Evista	AVINza, Eovist
Fosamax	Flomax, Fosamax Plus D, fosinopril, Zithromax
Prolia	Udenyca
raloxifene	ospemifene, toremifene
Xgeva	Jevtana, Xofigo, Xtandi, Zytiga

Drugs that look like a similar drug are noted in the Summary Drug Tables of each chapter.

INTERACTIONS

The following interactions may occur when a bisphosphonate is administered with another agent:

Interacting Drug	Common Use	Effect of Interaction
Calcium supplements or antacids with magnesium and aluminum	Relief of gastric upset	Decreased effectiveness of bisphosphonates
Aspirin	Pain relief	Increased risk of GI bleeding
Theophylline	Alleviation of breathing problems	Increased risk of theophylline toxicity

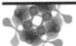 URIC ACID INHIBITORS

Gout is a type of arthritis in which uric acid accumulates in increased amounts in the blood and often is deposited in the joints. The deposit or collection of urate crystals in the joints causes the symptoms (pain, redness, swelling, joint deformity) of gout.

ACTIONS

Allopurinol (Zyloprim) reduces the production of uric acid, thereby decreasing serum uric acid levels and the deposit of urate crystals in joints. This probably accounts for its ability to relieve the severe pain of acute gout. Febuxostat (Uloric), a newer drug, is used to reduce serum uric acid levels, preventing gout attacks.

The exact mechanism of action of colchicine is unknown, but it does reduce the inflammation associated with the deposit of urate crystals in the joints. Colchicine has no effect on uric acid metabolism.

In people with gout, the serum uric acid level is usually elevated. In an acute attack, pegloticase, an IV infusion, may be used to decrease the amount of uric acid in the body. Probenecid works in the same manner and may be given alone or with colchicine as combination therapy when there are frequent, recurrent attacks of gout. Probenecid also has been used to prolong the plasma levels of penicillins and cephalosporins.

USES

Drugs indicated for treatment of gout may be used to manage acute attacks of gout or in preventing acute attacks of gout (prophylaxis).

ADVERSE REACTIONS

Gastrointestinal System Reactions
- Nausea, vomiting, diarrhea
- Abdominal pain

Other Reactions
- Headache
- Urinary frequency

One adverse reaction associated with allopurinol is skin rash, which in some cases has been followed by serious hypersensitivity reactions, such as exfoliative dermatitis and **Stevens–Johnson syndrome**. Colchicine administration may result in severe nausea, vomiting, and bone marrow depression; therefore, it is used as a second line of treatment when other drugs fail.

CONTRAINDICATIONS

The drugs used for gout are contraindicated in clients with known hypersensitivity. Colchicine is contraindicated in clients with serious GI, renal, hepatic, or cardiac disorders and those with blood dyscrasias. Probenecid is contraindicated in clients with blood dyscrasias or uric acid kidney stones and in children younger than 2 years. If clients are taking azathioprine (Imuran), mercaptopurine, or theophylline they should not be prescribed febuxostat.

PRECAUTIONS

Uric acid inhibitors are used cautiously in clients with renal impairment and during pregnancy; these agents are either pregnancy category B or C drugs. Allopurinol is used cautiously in clients with liver impairment. Probenecid is used cautiously in clients who are hypersensitive to sulfa drugs or have peptic ulcer disease. Colchicine is used with caution in older adults.

Anaphylactic reactions have been seen with pegloticase infusions; therefore, antihistamines and corticosteroids are used to premedicate clients.

LASA ALERT

The following drugs may sound alike; be sure to clarify when they are ordered:

Drug Name	Sounds Like
colchicine	Cortrosyn
probenecid	Procanbid

Drugs that look like a similar drug are noted in the Summary Drug Tables of each chapter.

INTERACTIONS

The following interactions may occur when a uric acid inhibitor is administered with another agent:

Interacting Drug	Common Use	Effect of Interaction
Allopurinol and Febuxostat		
Ampicillin	Anti-infective agent	Increased risk of rash
Theophylline	Alleviation of breathing problems	Increased risk of theophylline toxicity
Aluminum-based antacids	Relief of gastric upset	Decreased effectiveness of allopurinol
Probenecid		
Penicillins, cephalosporins, acyclovir, rifampin, and the sulfonamides	Anti-infective agent	Increased serum level of anti-infective
Barbiturates and benzodiazepines	Sedation	Increased serum level of sedative
NSAIDs	Pain relief	Increased serum level of NSAID
Salicylates	Pain relief	Decreased effectiveness of probenecid

Herbal Considerations

Glucosamine and chondroitin are used, in combination or alone, to treat arthritis, particularly osteoarthritis. Chondroitin acts as the flexible connecting matrix between the protein filaments in cartilage. Chondroitin can be produced in the laboratory or can come from natural sources (e.g., shark cartilage). Some studies suggest that if chondroitin is available to the cell matrix, synthesis of tissue can occur. For this reason, it is used to treat arthritis. Although there is little information on chondroitin's long-term effects, it is generally not considered to be harmful.

Glucosamine theoretically provides a building block for regeneration of damaged cartilage. The absorption of oral glucosamine is 90%–98%, making it widely accepted for use. Glucosamine is generally well tolerated, and no adverse reactions have been reported with its use (DerMarderosian & Beutler, 2003).

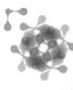

NURSING PROCESS: STEPS TO BUILDING CLINICAL JUDGMENT
Client Receiving a Drug for a Musculoskeletal Disorder

ASSESSMENT

Preadministration Assessment
Data gathering suggestions before the initial administration of the drug include:
Objective data

- Description of signs of immobility and effects or change in activities of daily living
- Description of the affected joints in the extremities (especially arthritis and gout diagnoses)—appearance of the skin over the joint, evidence of joint deformity, and signs of immobility of the affected joint
- Vital signs (temperature, pulse, respirations, and blood pressure) and weight
- Laboratory tests and bone scans to measure bone density
- TST (tuberculin skin test)—when biologic DMARDs are ordered

Subjective data

- Type and duration of symptoms (immobility, has it impacted ability to work?)
- Pain experience—onset, type (e.g., sharp, dull, squeezing), radiation, location, intensity, and duration (osteoporosis, particularly upper and lower back or hips)
- If preventative (such as the use of bisphosphonates), factors supporting client to use the drug and what might promote adherence over a long period of time

- Health history especially regarding immunocompromise or travel to areas with infectious diseases
- Remedies attempted before seeking care

NURSING ALERT

When bisphosphonates are administered, serum calcium levels are monitored before, during, and after therapy.

Ongoing Assessment
Periodic evaluation is an important part of therapy for musculoskeletal disorders. With some disorders, such as acute gout, the client can be expected to respond to therapy in hours. Therefore, it is important to inspect and document the joints involved every 1–2 hours to identify immediately a response or nonresponse to therapy. Also, question the client regarding the relief of pain, as well as adverse drug reactions.

In other disorders, response is gradual and may take days, weeks, and even months of treatment. Depending on the drug administered and the disorder being treated, the evaluation of therapy may be daily or yearly. These documented evaluations help the primary health care provider plan current and future therapy, including dosage changes, changes in the drug administered, and institution of physical therapy.

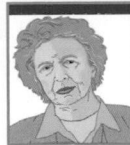

PHARMACOLOGY IN PRACTICE

ASSESSMENT

A long-term care client tells the nurse, "I have painful gout." What should the nurse assess to determine if the client has gout?

1. Appearance of skin for rash
2. Evidence of hearing loss
3. Pain in the abdomen
4. Mobility of affected joint

NURSING DIAGNOSES

Drug-specific nursing diagnoses include the following:

- **Readiness for enhanced fluid balance** related to need for increased fluid intake to promote excretion of urate crystals
- **Impaired comfort: gastric distress** related to irritation of gastric lining from medication administration
- **Injury risk** related to medication-induced drowsiness and associated risk for imbalance and falls
- **Allergic risk** related to response to substance trigger (drug allergy)

Nursing diagnoses related to drug administration are discussed in Chapter 4.

PLANNING

The expected outcomes for the client depend on the reason for administration but may include an optimal response to therapy, meeting client needs related to the management of adverse reactions, and confidence in an understanding of the medication regimen.

IMPLEMENTATION

Promoting an Optimal Response to Therapy

The client with a musculoskeletal disorder may have long-standing chronic pain, which can be just as difficult to tolerate as acute pain. Along with pain, there may be skeletal deformities, such as the joint deformities seen with advanced RA. For many musculoskeletal conditions, drug therapy is a major treatment modality. In addition to drug therapy, rest, physical therapy, and other measures may be part of treatment. Including drugs as a major part of the treatment plan may keep the disorder under control (e.g., therapy for gout), improve the client's ability to carry out activities of daily living, or make the pain and discomfort tolerable.

Clients with a musculoskeletal disorder may have negative or self-defeating feelings related to the symptoms and the chronicity of the disorder. In addition to physical care, these clients often require emotional support, especially when a disorder is disabling and chronic. Be encouraging as you explain to the client that therapy may take weeks or longer before any benefit is noted. When this is explained before therapy starts, the client is less likely to become discouraged over slow results.

It is important to be alert to reactions such as skin rash, fever, cough, or easy bruising. Listen carefully for specific client complaints that may seem unrelated to drug therapy, such as visual changes, tinnitus, or hearing loss. Be sure to immediately report these adverse reactions; the primary health care provider may need to change doses or even drugs. Particular attention is paid to visual changes because irreversible retinal damage may occur.

Administration of allopurinol may result in skin rash. A rash should be monitored carefully because it may precede a serious adverse reaction, such as Stevens–Johnson syndrome. Immediately report any rash to the primary health care provider.

Methotrexate is potentially toxic. Therefore, monitor laboratory test results closely for development of adverse reactions, such as thrombocytopenia and leukopenia. Hematology, liver, and renal function studies are monitored every 1–3 months with methotrexate therapy. Notify the primary health care provider of abnormal hematology, liver function, or kidney function findings.

Monitoring and Managing Client Needs

Readiness for Enhanced Fluid Balance

When the client is using the uric acid inhibitors, encourage liberal fluid intake. The client can tell if they are getting adequate fluids when the daily urine output is about 2 L. An increase in urinary output is necessary to excrete the urates (uric acid salts) and prevent urate acid stone formation in the genitourinary tract. Discuss ways to provide adequate fluids and remind the client frequently of the importance of increasing fluid intake. If the client fails to increase fluid intake, contact the primary health care provider. In some instances, it may be necessary to administer intravenous (IV) fluids to supplement the oral intake when the client fails to drink about 3000 mL of fluid per day.

Impaired Comfort: Gastric Distress

Adequate drug absorption and metabolism can depend on timing with meals. To facilitate delivery of the bone resorption inhibitor to the stomach and minimize adverse GI effects, instruct the client to take the drug upon arising in the morning, with 6–8 ounces of water, and remain in an upright position. The client is instructed to remain upright (avoid lying down) for at least 30 minutes after taking the drug. Helping the client to maintain a routine of being upright for 30 minutes after administration will reduce gastric distress and support adherence to the medication schedule (Fig. 29.2). Specific instructions to help clients remember the routine are provided in Client Teaching for Improved Outcomes: Taking Bisphosphonates for Best Results. Etidronate is not administered within 2 hours of food, vitamin and mineral supplements, or antacids.

Many bisphosphonates are available in both once-a-week and once-a-month dosing forms. Although there is a once-a-year drug, the client has to come to the ambulatory clinic for IV administration. DMARDs, uric acid inhibitors, and skeletal muscle relaxants are taken with, or immediately after, meals to minimize gastric distress.

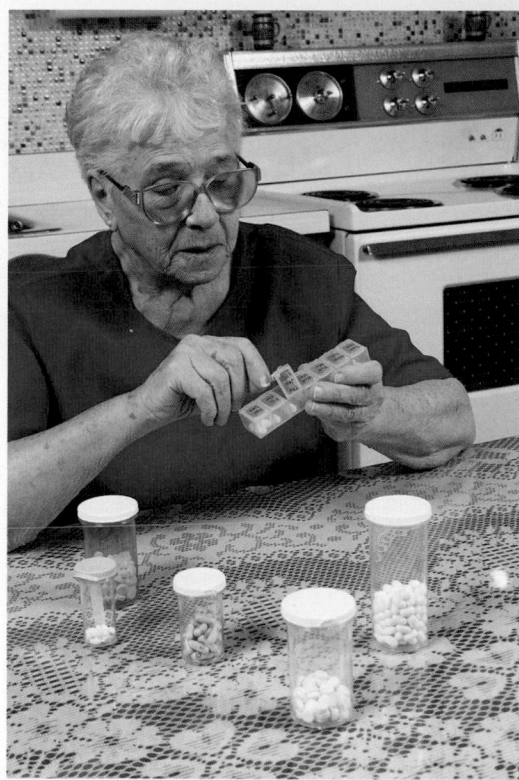

FIGURE 29.2 Adherence to specific routines when taking bisphosphonates will help reduce unpleasant adverse reactions.

Client Teaching for Improved Outcomes

Taking Bisphosphonates for Best Results
When you teach, make sure your client understands the following:

Bone resorption inhibitors work to not only build bone density but also prevent bone fractures (sometimes by as much as 50%). You may have heard both good and bad issues from friends and family taking these drugs. Here is how to learn what is best for you.

When to treat. Diagnosis for osteoporosis treatment is made by your T-score (from the bone mineral density scan). You may not be a candidate for treatment if you have gastroesophageal problems, kidney disease, or severe vitamin D deficiency. Some preparations are taken daily and others as infrequently as monthly. Research shows good results when taken for 5–10 years—so, correct administration is important.

Supplements. These drugs work by using the building blocks of bone formation. You need an intake of 1500 mg of calcium and 400–800 units of vitamin D daily. The drug you take may or may not have this supplement in the preparation. Check with your primary health care provider and follow the vitamin supplement recommended.

Specific drug administration routine. These drugs are absorbed slowly from the stomach and can cause severe irritation of the esophagus. You must take the pill with 6–8 ounces of plain water and cannot eat or drink for 30 minutes after taking the drug, and you must be in an upright position during that time. Here are suggestions to make taking this drug easier and build it into your weekly routine:

✔ Use a calendar or cell phone alert to remember your monthly dose.
✔ Do not prepare your coffee maker the night before you are to take the drug. This will prevent you from drinking your morning cup of coffee before you realize you should have taken the medication.
✔ Put the medication out the night before in a place you will see it when you first get up out of bed.
✔ Take your medication and then do a distracting activity, such as taking your morning shower or sitting in a chair and watching the morning news on television, listening to music on the radio, or looking at or answering e-mail.
✔ Make this morning's breakfast special with foods you especially like to eat; use breakfast as a reward for having taken your medication correctly!
✔ Make a habit of calling your primary health care provider at least every 6 months (if taking monthly) to talk about whether you are or are not having any GI changes (belching, pressure, heartburn)—it could be from the medication.

Injury Risk
Many of these drugs may cause drowsiness. In addition, pain or deformity may hamper mobility. These two factors place the client at risk of injury. Therefore, teach the family to monitor the client carefully before allowing the client to ambulate alone. If drowsiness does occur, assistance with ambulatory activities is necessary. If drowsiness is severe, instruct the client or family to contact the primary health care provider before the next dose is due.

The client with an arthritis disorder may experience much pain or discomfort and may require assistance with activities, such as ambulating, eating, and grooming. Clients on bed rest require position changes and skin care every 2 hours. Clients with osteoporosis may require a brace or corset when out of bed.

Allergic Risk
When first-line treatments for gout are not successful, sometimes drugs that are more toxic may be prescribed, such as the pegloticase infusion. During the infusion the client is closely monitored for the development of adverse reactions. Should an anaphylactic reaction occur, the infusion center staff members are prepared to start resuscitative measures as emergency personnel are notified.

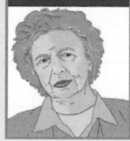

PHARMACOLOGY IN PRACTICE

MANAGING NEEDS
Which of the following nursing diagnoses is of greatest priority when a client is taking a bisphosphonate drug?
1. Readiness for enhanced fluid balance
2. Impaired comfort: gastric distress
3. Injury risk
4. Allergic risk

Educating the Client and Family

The dosing schedule for these drugs may be variable. Dosing schedules may require taking medications on alternate days, at specific times of the day, or weekly, or even monthly. The client may not see a therapeutic response until 3–6 weeks of therapy and become discouraged. In some cases, a client may stop treatment. To ensure adherence with the treatment regimen, the client must feel confident in understanding the importance of the prescribed therapy and taking the drug exactly as directed, to obtain the best results. To meet this goal, develop an effective plan of client and family teaching. The following points are included in the teaching plan:

- Explain carefully that treatment for the disorder includes drug therapy, as well as other medical management, such as diet, exercise, limitations or specifications of activity, and periodic physical therapy treatments.
- Teach the importance of asking the primary health care provider before taking any nonprescription drugs or supplements.
- Some drugs used for RA require self-administered subcutaneous injections. Teach the client and family proper injection and disposal techniques.
- Teach about site rotation, and have the client demonstrate proper injection technique before this becomes a self-administered procedure.
- Clients need to be taught how to manage the discomfort at the site of injection and to report redness, pain, and swelling to the primary health care provider.

When using drugs for muscle spasm and cramping:

- This drug may cause drowsiness. Do not drive or perform other hazardous tasks if drowsiness occurs.
- This drug is for short-term use. Do not use the drug for longer than 2–3 weeks.
  - Avoid alcohol or other CNS depressants while taking this drug.

When using drugs to treat RA:

- When taking methotrexate, use a calendar or some other memory device to remember to take the drug on the same day each week.
- Notify the primary health care provider immediately if any of the following occurs: sore mouth or sores in the mouth, diarrhea, fever, sore throat, easy bruising, rash, itching, or nausea and vomiting.
- Women of childbearing age should use an effective contraceptive during therapy with methotrexate and for 8 weeks after therapy.

When using drugs to treat gout:

- Drink at least 10 glasses of water a day until the acute attack has subsided.
- Take this drug with food to minimize GI upset.
- If drowsiness occurs, avoid driving or performing other hazardous tasks.
- Acute gout—notify the primary health care provider if pain is not relieved in a few days.
- Notify the primary health care provider if a skin rash occurs.

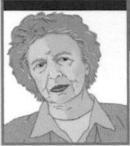

PHARMACOLOGY IN PRACTICE

TEACHING AND LEARNING

A client with rheumatic arthritis is administered a DMARD. What specific problem should the client be instructed to monitor for while taking an immunosuppressive drug?
1. Bleeding tendencies
2. Hypoglycemia
3. Infections
4. Epigastric distress

EVALUATION

- Therapeutic drug effect is achieved, pain is decreased, and mobility is improved or maintained.
- Adverse reactions are identified, reported to the primary health care provider, and managed using appropriate nursing interventions:
  - Client improves fluid balance.
  - GI comfort is maintained.
  - No evidence of injury is seen.
  - Allergic risk is minimized.
- Client and family express confidence and demonstrate an understanding of the drug regimen.

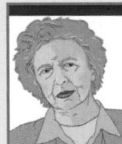

PHARMACOLOGY IN PRACTICE

USING CLINICAL REASONING

Based on your understanding of drugs to improve bone density and the requirements of these drugs, is Mrs. Moore an appropriate candidate for this medication?

KEY POINTS

■ Musculoskeletal disorders that use drug therapy include arthritis (both rheumatoid and osteoarthritis), increased uric acid causing gout, and bone diseases such as osteoporosis. These are chronic and require long-term therapy.

■ A variety of drugs are used to treat musculoskeletal injuries and disorders; they include DMARDs, bone resorption inhibitors, skeletal muscle relaxants, and uric acid inhibitors.

■ The most common adverse reactions include GI distress, hair loss, and drowsiness.

■ Clients using DMARDs should be monitored carefully for infection. Those taking bisphosphonates have specific drug routines to follow to prevent gastroesophageal irritation. When using uric acid inhibitors severe rashes should be monitored.

SUMMARY DRUG TABLE
Drugs Used to Treat Musculoskeletal, Bone, and Joint Disorders

Generic Name	Trade Name	Uses	Adverse Reactions	Dosage Ranges
Skeletal Muscle Relaxants				
baclofen BAK-loe-fen	Ozobax	Spasticity caused by multiple sclerosis, spinal cord injuries (intrathecal administration for severe spasticity)	Drowsiness, dizziness, nausea, weakness, hypotension	15–80 mg/day orally in divided doses
carisoprodol kar-eye-soe-PROE-dole	Soma	Relief of discomfort caused by acute, painful musculoskeletal conditions	Dizziness, drowsiness, tachycardia, nausea, vomiting	350 mg orally TID or QID
chlorzoxazone klor-ZOKS-a-zone	Lorzone	Same as carisoprodol	GI disturbances, drowsiness, dizziness, rash	250–750 mg orally TID or QID
cyclobenzaprine sye-kloe-BEN-za-preen	Amrix	Same as carisoprodol	Drowsiness, dizziness, dry mouth, nausea, constipation	10–60 mg/day orally in divided doses
dantrolene DAN-troe-leen	Dantrium	Spasticity caused by spinal cord injury, stroke, cerebral palsy, multiple sclerosis	Drowsiness, dizziness, weakness, constipation, tachycardia, malaise	Initial dose: 25 mg/day orally, then 50–400 mg/day orally in divided doses
diazePAM dye-AZ-e-pam	Valium	Relief of skeletal muscle spasm, spasticity caused by cerebral palsy, epilepsy, paraplegia, anxiety	Drowsiness, sedation, sleepiness, lethargy, constipation, diarrhea, bradycardia, tachycardia, rash	2–10 mg orally BID–QID; 2–20 mg IM, IV Sustained release: 15–29 mg/day orally
metaxalone me-TAKS-a-lone	Skelaxin	Same as carisoprodol	Drowsiness, dizziness, headache, nausea, rash	800 mg orally TID or QID
methocarbamol meth-oh-KAR-ba-mole	Robaxin	Relief of discomfort caused by musculoskeletal disorders	Drowsiness, dizziness, lightheadedness, confusion, headache, rash, blurred vision, GI upset	1–1.5 g QID orally; limit IM, IV dose to 3 g/day
orphenadrine or-FEN-a-dreen		Discomfort caused by musculoskeletal disorders	Drowsiness, dizziness, lightheadedness, confusion, headache, rash, blurred vision, GI upset	100 mg BID orally; 60 mg IV or IM q12hr
tiZANidine tye-ZAN-i-deen	Zanaflex	Spasticity caused by spinal cord injury, multiple sclerosis	Somnolence, fatigue, dizziness, dry mouth, urinary tract infections (UTIs)	4–8 mg orally up to TID
Disease-Modifying Antirheumatic Drugs (DMARDs)				
hydroxychloroquine hye-droks-ee-KLOR-oh-kwin	Plaquenil	RA, antimalarial	Irritability nervousness, retinal and corneal changes, anorexia, nausea, vomiting, hematologic effects	400–600 mg/day orally
leflunomide le-FLOO-noh-mide	Arava	RA	Hypertension, alopecia, rash, nausea, diarrhea	Initial dose: 100 mg for 3 days Maintenance dose: 20 mg/day orally
methotrexate meth-oh-TREKS-ate	Trexall, Xatmep, RediTrex	RA, psoriatic arthritis (PA), cancer chemotherapy	Nausea, stomatitis, alopecia	7.5–20.0 mg orally once weekly
sulfaSALAzine sul-fa-SAL-a-zeen	Azulfidine	RA, Crohn disease, ulcerative colitis	Nausea, emesis, abdominal pains, crystalluria, hematuria, Stevens–Johnson syndrome, rash, headache, drowsiness, diarrhea	2–4 g/day orally in divided doses

Continued

SUMMARY DRUG TABLE (continued)
Drugs Used to Treat Musculoskeletal, Bone, and Joint Disorders

Generic Name	Trade Name	Uses	Adverse Reactions	Dosage Ranges
Disease-Modifying Antirheumatic Drugs (DMARDs)—Biologics				
abatacept ab-a-TA-sept	Orencia	Arthritis—juvenile idiopathic, psoriatic, rheumatoid	Headache, nasal congestion, upper respiratory infection (URI) symptoms, nausea	500–750 mg IV every 4 weeks
adalimumab a-da-LIMyoo-mab	Humira	RA; other autoimmune disorders (e.g., Crohn disease)	Irritation at injection site, increased risk of infections	40 mg subcut every other week
anakinra an-a-KIN-ra	Kineret	RA	Headache, irritation at injection site, pancytopenia	100 mg subcut daily
baricitinib bar-i-SYE-ti-nib	Olumiant	RA, when refractory to (TNF) therapies	URI symptoms, rhinitis	2 mg orally daily
certolizumab cer-to-LIZ-u-mab	Cimzia	RA, Crohn disease	URI and UTI symptoms	400 mg subcut every 2 weeks or monthly
etanercept et-a-NER-sept	Enbrel	Arthritis—juvenile idiopathic, psoriatic, rheumatoid	Headache, rhinitis, irritation at injection site, increased risk of infections	25 mg subcut twice weekly, or 50 mg subcut weekly
golimumab goe-LIM-ue-mab	Simponi	Arthritis—psoriatic, rheumatoid, ulcerative colitis	URI symptoms, rhinitis, irritation at injection site, increased risk of infections	50 mg subcut weekly
inFLIXimab in-FLIKS-e-mab	Remicade	RA in combination with methotrexate, Crohn disease, ulcerative colitis	Fever, chills, headache	3–10 mg/kg IV infusion at specified weekly intervals
sarilumab sar-IL-ue-mab	Kevzara	RA	Increase liver enzymes, skin reactions	200 mg subcut every 2 weeks
tocilizumab toe-si-LIZ-oo-mab	Actemra	Arthritis—juvenile idiopathic, psoriatic, rheumatoid	Headache, nasal congestion, URI symptoms, increased blood pressure, elevated alanine aminotransferase (liver function)	4 mg/kg IV every 4 weeks
tofacitinib toe-fa-SYE-ti-nib	Xeljanz	RA, ulcerative colitis, PA	URI symptoms, rhinitis	5–11 mg orally, 1–2 times daily
upadacitinib ue-PAD-a-SYE-ti-nib	Rinvoq	RA	URI symptoms, rhinitis	15 mg orally once daily
Bone Resorption Inhibitors: Bisphosphonates				
alendronate a-LEN-droe-nate	Binosto, Fosamax	Treatment and prevention of postmenopausal osteoporosis, glucocorticoid-induced osteoporosis, osteoporosis in men, Paget disease	Abdominal pain, esophageal reflux	5–10 mg orally, in daily or (70-mg) weekly doses
ibandronate eye-BAN-droh-nate	Boniva	Postmenopausal osteoporosis	Abdominal pain, nausea, diarrhea	2.5 mg/day orally, available in 150-mg tablet taken once monthly; 3-mg IV form available for dose once every 3 months
pamidronate pa-mi-DROE-nate	Aredia	Hypercalcemia of malignancy, bone metastases, Paget disease	Anxiety, headache, insomnia, nausea, vomiting, diarrhea, constipation, dyspepsia, pancytopenia, fever, fatigue, bone pain	60–90 mg in a single IV dose infused over 2–24 hour

Generic Name	Trade Name	Uses	Adverse Reactions	Dosage Ranges
⊘ **risedronate** *ris-ED-roe-nate*	Actonel, Atelvia	Treatment and prevention of postmenopausal osteoporosis, glucocorticoid-induced osteoporosis, osteoporosis in men, Paget disease	Headache, abdominal pain, arthralgia, recurrent bone pain, nausea, diarrhea	5–75 mg orally, in daily or (75-mg) weekly doses
zoledronic acid *zole-le-DRON-ik*	Reclast	Postmenopausal osteoporosis, Paget disease	Hypotension, confusion, anxiety, agitation, nausea, diarrhea, constipation, fatigue	5 mg IV once per year
Bone Resorption Inhibitors: Non-Bisphosphonates				
denosumab *den-OH-sue-mab*	Prolia, Xgeva	Treatment postmenopausal osteoporosis, bone loss in men w/osteoporosis, prostate cancer, women with breast cancer	Skin rash, immune suppression, high dose—osteonecrotic jaw	60 mg subcut every 6 months
raloxifene *ral-OKS-i-feen*	Evista	Treatment and prevention of postmenopausal osteoporosis	Leg cramps, dizziness, blood clots	60 mg orally daily
teriparatide *ter-i-PAR-a-tidetyd*	Forteo	Treatment and prevention of high-risk postmenopausal osteoporosis	Leg cramps, dizziness, increased calcium levels	20 mcg subcut daily, max time is 2 years
Uric Acid Inhibitors				
allopurinol *al-oh-PURE-i-nole*	Zyloprim	Management of symptoms of gout	Rash, exfoliative dermatitis, Stevens–Johnson syndrome, nausea, vomiting, diarrhea, abdominal pain, hematologic changes	100–800 mg/day orally
colchicine *KOL-chi-seen*	Gloperba	Relief of acute attacks of gout, prevention of gout attacks	Nausea, vomiting, diarrhea, abdominal pain, bone marrow depression	Prophylaxis: 0.5–0.6 mg/day orally Acute attack: initial dose 0.5–1.2 mg orally or 2 mg IV, then 0.5–1.2 mg orally q1–2hr or 0.5 mg IV q6hr until attack is aborted or adverse effects occur
febuxostat *feb-UX-oh-stat*	Uloric	Hyperuricemia	Nausea, rash, arthralgia	40–80 mg orally daily
pegloticase *peg-LOE-ti-kase*	Krystexxa	Management of symptoms of gout	Disease flare-up, infusion reaction, nausea, bruising	8 mg IV every 2 weeks
probenecid *proe-BEN-e-sid*		Treatment of hyperuricemia of gout and gouty arthritis; adjuvant to antibiotics	Headache, anorexia, nausea, vomiting, urinary frequency, flushing, dizziness	0.25 g orally BID for 1 week, then 0.5 g orally BID

⊘ This drug should be administered at least 1 hour before or 2 hours after a meal.

CHAPTER REVIEW

Know Your Drugs

Clients sometimes know a medication by the brand (or trade) name and not the generic name. To help you recognize both names, match the brand name with the generic name of the same medication.

Generic Name	Brand Name
1. alendronate	A. Amrix
2. allopurinol	B. Enbrel
3. cyclobenzaprine	C. Fosamax
4. etanercept	D. Zyloprim

Calculate Medication Dosages

1. A client is to receive allopurinol 300 mg orally for gout. The nurse has 100-mg tablets available. How many tablets would the nurse administer?

2. The physician prescribes 1.5 g methocarbamol (Robaxin) orally for a musculoskeletal disorder. Available for administration are 500-mg tablets. The nurse administers _____.

Prepare for the NCLEX

RECALL THE FACTS

1. Bisphosphonates work by _____.
   1. inhibiting calcium digestion
   2. inhibiting abnormal bone resorption
   3. eliminating more phosphorus
   4. prohibiting vitamin D absorption

2. When administering a skeletal muscle relaxant, the nurse observes the client for the most common adverse reaction, which is _____.
   1. drowsiness
   2. GI bleeding
   3. vomiting
   4. constipation

3. When alendronate (Fosamax) is prescribed for osteoporosis, the nurse teaches the client to take the drug _____.
   1. with food or milk
   2. by injection
   3. 30 minutes before breakfast
   4. at bedtime

4. When allopurinol (Zyloprim) is used for treating gout, the nurse _____.
   1. administers the drug with juice or milk
   2. administers the drug after the evening meal
   3. restricts fluids during evening hours
   4. encourages liberal fluid intake

5. What teaching points would the nurse include when educating the client who will begin taking risedronate?
   1. The drug is administered once weekly.
   2. Take a daily laxative, because the drug will likely cause constipation.
   3. Take the drug with antacids to decrease gastric distress.
   4. After taking the drug, remain upright for at least 30 minutes.

ANALYZE THE FACTS

6. When giving one of the uric acid inhibitors, the nurse assesses the client for the most common adverse reactions, which are _____.
   1. related to the GI tract
   2. urinary retention
   3. hypertension
   4. related to the nervous system

7. When administering a DMARD subcutaneously, the nurse should:
   1. use a 5-mL syringe.
   2. inject tissue close to the umbilicus.
   3. massage the area to increase blood flow to the muscles.
   4. rotate sites to minimize tissue irritation.

8. Which of the following statements if made by the client would indicate that they understand how to take a bone resorption medication properly?
   1. "If I get sleepy after taking my medication, it is okay to lie down."
   2. "If I get a pain in the stomach, it means the medicine is working."
   3. "Take this until you get diarrhea."
   4. "I can take a nice shower after taking the med, before I eat."

ALTERNATE-FORMAT QUESTIONS

9. Identify which drugs are included in therapy for RA. **Select all that apply.**
   1. NSAIDs
   2. DMARDs
   3. anti-infectives
   4. corticosteroids
   5. immunosuppressives

10. A client weighs 63 kg. If tocilizumab 4 mg/kg is prescribed, what is the total dosage of tocilizumab for this client?

To check your answers, see Appendix F.

_____

'Indicates the question is directly linked to the NCLEX-PN test plan in Appendix G.

WANT TO KNOW MORE? A wide variety of resources are available to enhance your learning and understanding of this chapter.
- Visit the**Point** for resources such as:
  - NCLEX-Style Student Review Questions
  - Journal Articles
  - Dosage Calculations
  - Drug Monographs
  - Watch and Learn Videos
  - Concepts in Action Animations
- The *Study Guide to Accompany Introductory Clinical Pharmacology*, 12th edition, sold separately, will help you review and apply essential content.
- ✔**PrepU** is available to help students prepare for the NCLEX-PN examination.

UNIT 7
Drugs That Affect the Respiratory System

The respiratory system consists of the upper and lower airways, the lungs, and the thoracic cavity. It provides a mechanism for the exchange of oxygen and carbon dioxide in the lungs. Any change in a person's respiratory status has the potential to affect every other bodily system. This is because all cells need an adequate supply of oxygen for optimal functioning. Unit 7 focuses on drugs used to treat some of the more common disorders affecting the respiratory system. Drugs in this unit are presented in two groups: those that are used for upper respiratory problems and those used for lower respiratory problems.

Among the most common conditions of the upper respiratory system are infections, allergic rhinitis, coughs, the common cold, and congestion. Most conditions are allergen or viral (e.g., a cold virus), and comfort measures are used to tolerate the course of the illness. These measures include (1) intranasal steroids or antihistamines to relieve allergy symptoms; (2) decongestants to reduce nasal edema; and (3) antitussives, mucolytics, and expectorants to treat accompanying cough. Typically, upper respiratory infections are treated with an antibiotic only if bacteria are involved. These drugs are discussed in Chapter 30. Many of these drugs are available as nonprescription (over-the-counter) drugs, whereas, a few are available only by prescription.

Chapter 31 features disorders of the lower respiratory tract including asthma (chronic inflammatory disease of the airways), emphysema (lung disorder in which the alveoli become enlarged and plugged with mucus), and chronic bronchitis (chronic inflammation and possible infection of the bronchi). These conditions are collectively termed chronic obstructive pulmonary disease (COPD). COPD is a slowly progressive disease of the airways characterized by a gradual loss of lung function. The symptoms of COPD range from chronic cough and sputum production to severe, disabling shortness of breath. There is no known cure for COPD; the treatment is usually supportive and designed to relieve symptoms and improve quality of life.

Asthma is a chronic inflammatory condition of the lower airway with bronchospasm and bronchoconstriction. This condition and the drugs used to treat it are featured in Chapter 31. Clients with asthma may experience periods of exacerbation alternating with periods of normal lung function.

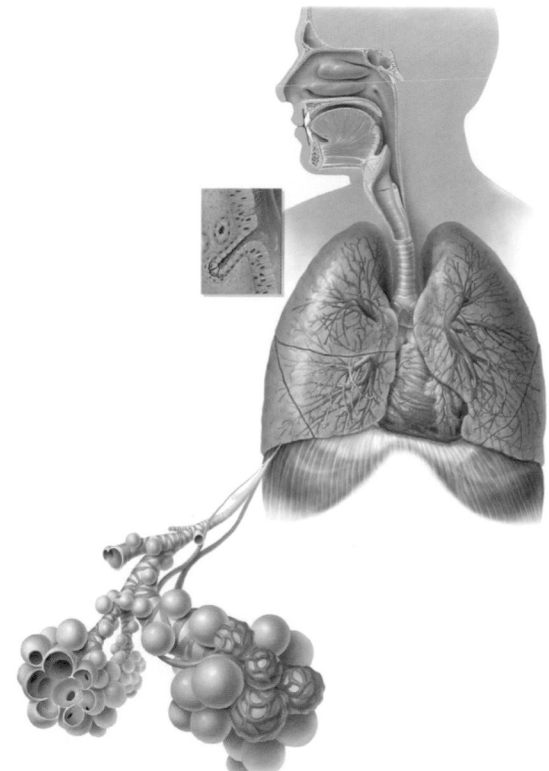

Environmental exposure to allergens, such as house dust mites, tobacco smoke, pets and pet dander, mold, cockroach wastes, and physical exercise, are "triggers" for an asthma attack. Anti-inflammatory drugs play an important role in treating individuals with asthma. These drugs prevent asthma attacks by decreasing the swelling and mucous production in the airways, thereby making the airways less sensitive to asthma triggers. Drug therapy for asthma is aimed at preventing attacks and reducing swelling and mucous production in the airways.

The drugs used to treat disorders of the lower respiratory tract are discussed in Chapter 31. These drugs include bronchodilating drugs, which are beta$_2$-adrenergic agonists (β_2-adrenergic agonists) (these have sympathomimetic properties) and xanthine derivatives. Along with bronchodilating drugs, the antiasthma drugs are featured and include corticosteroids, leukotriene modifiers, and mast cell stabilizers.

Upper Respiratory System Drugs

Key Terms

anticholinergic action blockage of parasympathetic nervous system

histamine substance found in various parts of the body (i.e., liver, lungs, intestines, and skin) and produced from the amino acid histidine in response to injury to trigger the inflammatory response

nonproductive cough dry, hacking cough that produces no secretions

productive cough cough by which secretions from the respiratory tract are expelled

rhinitis inflammation of the nasal passages

urticaria hives, itchy wheals on the skin resulting from contact with, or ingestion of, an allergenic substance or food

Learning Objectives

On completion of this chapter, the student will:

1. Compare and contrast the classes of medications used for upper respiratory system problems.
2. Explain the uses, general drug actions, adverse reactions, contraindications, precautions, and interactions of intranasal steroids, antitussives, mucolytics, expectorants, antihistamines, and decongestants.
3. Distinguish important preadministration and ongoing assessment activities that should be performed on the client receiving intranasal steroids, antitussive, mucolytic, expectorant, antihistamine, or decongestant.
4. List nursing diagnoses particular to a client taking intranasal steroids, antitussive, mucolytic, expectorant, antihistamine, or decongestant.
5. Examine ways to promote an optimal response to therapy, manage common adverse reactions, and educate the client about the use of intranasal steroids, antitussive, mucolytic, expectorant, antihistamine, or decongestant.

 Drug Classes

Intranasal steroid
Antihistamine
Decongestant
Antitussive
Expectorant
Mucolytic

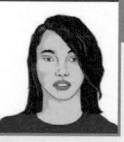

PHARMACOLOGY IN PRACTICE

Janna Wong, a 16-year-old gymnast, is experiencing nasal congestion. She has been prescribed a combination antihistamine and nasal decongestant. A number of antihistamines have anticholinergic effects. Think about the teaching points you will want to cover with Janna.

Acute **rhinitis**, or nasal inflammation, resulting in a variety of symptoms, is one of the most bothersome problems of the upper respiratory system. This condition is frequently caused by an allergen, and individuals typically seek self-treatment options for issues such as nasal congestion. Other symptoms for which individuals seek self-treatment include sneezing, postnasal drip, itchy and reddened eyes, sore throat, fatigue, and facial pressure. The drugs used to treat the discomfort associated with upper respiratory disorders include intranasal steroids, antihistamines, decongestants, antitussives, and expectorants. Many of these drugs are available as nonprescription (over-the-counter [OTC]) drugs, whereas others are available only by prescription. When seeing clients during a history assessment, ask about use of these drugs, which can affect other health conditions or prescription medications.

This chapter will also look at mucolytics—drugs used to treat the buildup of secretions in the lower respiratory system. These agents break down the thickness of the secretions for easier removal.

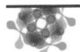 # INTRANASAL STEROIDS

USES AND ACTIONS

Intranasal steroids (INSs), also known as nasal glucocorticoids, are the first-line treatment for symptoms of allergic rhinitis. In addition, INSs are used to treat rhinitis caused by nonallergens, nasal polyps, and chronic sinusitis. The drugs exert anti-inflammatory action by inhibiting the response of a number of cells, including mast cells and white bloods cells such as neutrophils, eosinophils, and macrophages. These steroids also reduce mediators such as **histamine** and, in return, this reduces the inflammatory response. Because these agents are administered topically, the result occurs locally and produces minimal systemic adverse reactions.

ADVERSE REACTIONS

Adverse reactions are typically mild and include an unpleasant smell or taste. Drying of the nasal passages resulting in irritation and nose bleeds (epistaxis)—especially when the weather is dry—may occur. Discontinuation of INS drugs is recommended when epistaxis persists. Fungal infections (*Candida albicans*) of the nares are a rare reaction.

CONTRAINDICATIONS AND PRECAUTIONS

Those hypersensitive to steroids should not take INSs. INSs are pregnancy category C and should be used only when the benefit outweighs the risk to the fetus. INSs are used cautiously in clients taking systemic steroids. In study subjects, the blood level of budesonide was found to be twice that of an adult when also using systemically. This was thought to be attributed to weight differences. Some studies suggest there may be a slowing in growth rate of children using these products for extended periods (Lee et al., 2014).

INTERACTIONS

When cimetidine (used to reduce stomach acid) is taken with budesonide, the INS is less effective.

ANTIHISTAMINES

Histamine is produced in response to an allergic reaction or tissue injury. The release of histamine produces an inflammatory response. Dilation of small arterioles results in localized redness. An increase in the permeability of small blood vessels promotes an escape of fluid from these blood vessels into the surrounding tissues, which produces localized swelling. This reaction is illustrated in Figure 30.1. Histamine is also released from mast cells in allergic reactions or hypersensitivity reactions, such as anaphylactic shock.

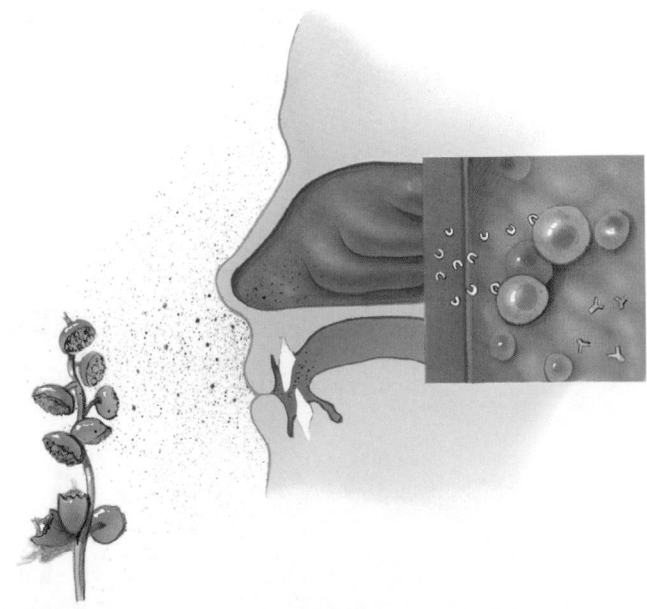

FIGURE 30.1 Allergens and upper respiratory system inflammation. (Courtesy of Anatomical Chart Co.)

ACTIONS

Antihistamines (or H₁ receptor antagonists) block most, but not all, of the effects of histamine. They do this by competing at the histamine receptor sites throughout the body, thereby preventing histamine from entering these receptor sites and producing an effect on body tissues. First-generation antihistamines bind *nonselectively* to central and peripheral H₁ receptors and may result in central nervous system (CNS) stimulation or depression. CNS depression usually occurs with higher doses and explains why some of these agents are used for sedation. Other first-generation drugs may have additional effects, such as antipruritic (anti-itching) or antiemetic (antinausea) effects. Second-generation antihistamines are selective for peripheral H₁ receptors and, as a group, are less sedating.

Desloratadine, loratadine, and fexofenadine minimally penetrate the blood–brain barrier, which means that little of the drug is distributed in the CNS so that fewer of the sedating effects are felt.

USES

The general uses of antihistamines include the following:

- Relief of the symptoms of seasonal and perennial allergies
- Allergic and vasomotor rhinitis
- Allergic conjunctivitis
- Mild and uncomplicated angioneurotic edema and urticaria
- Relief of allergic reactions to drugs, blood, or plasma
- Relief of coughs caused by colds or allergies
- Adjunctive therapy in anaphylactic shock
- Treatment of Parkinson-like symptoms
- Relief of nausea and vomiting
- Relief of motion sickness
- Sedation
- Adjuncts to analgesics

Each antihistamine may be used for one or more of these reasons. The more specific uses of the various antihistamine preparations are given in the Summary Drug Table: Upper Respiratory System Drugs.

ADVERSE REACTIONS

Central Nervous System Reactions

- Drowsiness or sedation
- Disturbed coordination

Respiratory System Reactions

Anticholinergic actions of antihistamines affect the respiratory system and include the following:

- Dryness of the mouth, nose, and throat
- Thickening of bronchial secretions

Second-generation preparations (e.g., loratadine) cause less drowsiness and fewer anticholinergic effects than some of the other antihistamines. Although these drugs are sometimes used to treat allergies, a drug allergy can occur with the use of an antihistamine. Symptoms that may indicate an allergy to these drugs include skin rash or **urticaria**.

CONTRAINDICATIONS

Although antihistamines are classified as pregnancy categories B (chlorpheniramine, cetirizine, dexchlorpheniramine, clemastine, diphenhydramine, and loratadine) and C (brompheniramine, desloratadine, fexofenadine, hydroxyzine, and promethazine), they are contraindicated during pregnancy and lactation.

First-generation antihistamine drugs are contraindicated in clients with known hypersensitivity to the drugs and in newborns, premature infants, and nursing mothers. These drugs are also contraindicated in individuals taking monoamine oxidase inhibitor (MAOI) antidepressants or who have one of the following conditions: angle-closure glaucoma, peptic ulcer, symptomatic prostatic hypertrophy, and bladder neck obstruction.

Second-generation antihistamines are contraindicated in clients with known hypersensitivity. Cetirizine is contraindicated in clients who are sensitive to hydroxyzine.

PRECAUTIONS

Antihistamines are used cautiously in clients with bronchial asthma, cardiovascular disease, narrow-angle glaucoma, hypertension, impaired kidney function, urinary retention, pyloroduodenal obstruction, and hyperthyroidism.

 Lifespan Considerations

Pediatric/Adolescents

In addition to offering the ability to connect with others, social media has the ability to engage a wide circle of individuals into daring each other to do silly and dangerous things. The *Benadryl Challenge* is one such opportunity individuals have to engage with others in behavior that can have a bad outcome. Not all blame the Internet, saying "The issue does not stem from being on 'the computer', rather it is the fact that the ability to interact is so easy" (Klass, 2019). With this encounter individuals are challenged to take large quantities of diphenhydramine (Benadryl) to produce a hallucinatory state. Primarily adolescents, on social media, encourage each other to take up to 12 tablets, for the euphoric effect. Consequently, individuals experience increased body temperature and heart rate, confusion, sedation, and delirium in addition to hallucination. Blurred vision, dizziness, constipation, urinary retention, and, for some, death (Forester, 2020). Large doses of diphenhydramine can also cause arrhythmia, seizure and cardiac arrest. One hospital in Texas had three cases in the pediatric emergency department (ED) in 1 month—one child had taken 14 tablets at once (Forster, 2020). A number of other pediatric EDs are claiming to see children at the point of near death due to the overdose of diphenhydramine. An important nursing role exists here, for the education of parents to talk to their children about web encounters and monitoring OTC products in their homes.

LASA ALERT

The following drugs may sound alike; be sure to clarify when they are ordered:

Drug Name	Sounds Like
cetirizine	levocetirizine
Chlor-Trimeton	Chloromycetin
Clarinex	Celebrex
fexofenadine	Fesoterodine
Sudafed	Sufenta
ZyRTEC	ZyPREXA

Drugs that look like a similar drug are noted in the Summary Drug Tables of each chapter.

INTERACTIONS

The following interactions may occur when an antihistamine is administered with another agent:

Interacting Drug	Common Use	Effect of Interaction
Rifampin	Antitubercular agent	May reduce the absorption of the antihistamine (e.g., fexofenadine)
MAOIs	Antidepressant agent	Increased anticholinergic and sedative effects of the antihistamine
CNS depressants (e.g., opioid analgesics or alcohol)	Pain relief	Possible additive CNS depressant effect
Beta blockers	Management of cardiovascular disease	Risk of increased cardiovascular effects (e.g., with diphenhydramine)
Aluminum- or magnesium-based antacids	Relief of gastrointestinal (GI) problems and upset	Decreased concentrations of drug in blood (e.g., fexofenadine)

DECONGESTANTS

A decongestant is a drug that works directly on blood vessels to reduce swelling of the nasal passages, which, in turn, opens clogged nasal passages and enhances drainage of the sinuses. These drugs are used for the temporary relief of nasal congestion caused by the common cold, hay fever, sinusitis, and other respiratory allergies.

ACTIONS

Nasal decongestants are sympathomimetic, in that they produce localized vasoconstriction of the small blood vessels of the nasal membranes similar to adrenergic drugs. Vasoconstriction reduces swelling in the nasal passages (decongestive activity). Nasal decongestants may be applied topically, and a few are available for oral use. They may be used in conjunction with INS to open nasal passages before administering the steroid. Examples of nasal decongestants include phenylephrine (Neo-Synephrine) and oxymetazoline (Afrin), both of which are available as nasal sprays or drops, and pseudoephedrine (Sudafed), which is taken orally. Additional nasal decongestants are listed in the Summary Drug Table: Upper Respiratory System Drugs.

USES

Decongestants are used to treat congestion associated with the following conditions:

- Common cold
- Hay fever
- Sinusitis
- Allergic rhinitis
- Congestion associated with rhinitis

ADVERSE REACTIONS

When used topically in prescribed doses, there are usually minimal systemic effects in most individuals. On occasion, nasal burning, stinging, and dryness may be seen. When the topical form is used frequently or if the liquid is swallowed, the same adverse reactions seen with the oral decongestants may occur. Use of oral decongestants may result in the following adverse reactions:

- Tachycardia and other cardiac arrhythmias
- Nervousness, restlessness, and insomnia
- Blurred vision
- Nausea and vomiting

CONTRAINDICATIONS

Decongestants are contraindicated in clients with known hypersensitivity and in clients taking MAOI antidepressants. Sustained-release pseudoephedrine is contraindicated in children younger than 12 years.

PRECAUTIONS

Decongestants are used cautiously in clients with the following:

- Thyroid disease
- Diabetes mellitus
- Cardiovascular disease

- Prostatic hypertrophy
- Coronary artery disease
- Peripheral vascular disease
- Hypertension
- Glaucoma

Clients with hypertension are cautioned to ask their health care provider which cough and cold products are best taken to reduce the chance of increasing blood pressure. Safe use of decongestants during pregnancy (pregnancy category C) and lactation has not been established. Pregnant women should consult with their primary health care provider (PHCP) before using these drugs.

INTERACTIONS

The following interactions may occur when a decongestant is administered with another agent:

Interacting Drug	Common Use	Effect of Interaction
MAOIs	Antidepressant	Severe headache, hypertension, and possibly hypertensive crisis
Beta-adrenergic blocking drugs	Management of cardiovascular disease	Initial hypertension episode followed by bradycardia

ANTITUSSIVES, EXPECTORANTS, AND MUCOLYTICS

Coughing is the forceful expulsion of air from the lungs. A cough may be productive or nonproductive. A **nonproductive cough** is a dry, hacking one that produces no secretions. An antitussive drug is used to relieve coughing.

With a **productive cough**, secretions are made in the respiratory tract. An expectorant is a drug that thins respiratory secretions to remove them more easily from the respiratory system. Many *cough and cold* preparations are a combination, such as an antihistamine and antitussive, and are sold OTC as a nonprescription cough medicine. Other antitussives, either alone or in combination with other drugs, are available by prescription only. A **mucolytic** is a drug that breaks down thick, tenacious mucus in the lower portions of the lungs for better elimination from the respiratory system.

ACTIONS

Most antitussives depress the cough center located in the medulla and are called centrally acting drugs.

Codeine and dextromethorphan are examples of centrally acting antitussives. Benzonatate (Tessalon) is an exception; it works peripherally by anesthetizing stretch receptors in the respiratory passages, thereby decreasing cough.

Expectorants increase the production of respiratory secretions, which in turn appear to decrease the viscosity of the mucus. This helps to raise secretions from the respiratory passages. An example of an expectorant is guaifenesin. Drugs with mucolytic activity reduce the viscosity (thickness) of respiratory secretions by direct action on the mucus. An example of a mucolytic drug is acetylcysteine. One other mucolytic drug is on the market, dornase alfa (Pulmozyme). This agent is used for the treatment of cystic fibrosis.

USES

Antitussives are used to relieve a nonproductive cough. Expectorants are used to help bring up respiratory secretions. The mucolytic acetylcysteine is used to treat the following:

- Acute bronchopulmonary disease (pneumonia, bronchitis, tracheobronchitis)
- Tracheostomy care
- Pulmonary complications of cystic fibrosis
- Pulmonary complications associated with surgery and during anesthesia
- Posttraumatic chest conditions
- Atelectasis because of mucous obstruction
- Acetaminophen overdosage

This drug is also used for diagnostic bronchial studies, such as bronchograms and bronchial wedge catheterizations. It is primarily given by nebulizer, but it may also be directly instilled into a tracheostomy to liquefy (thin) secretions.

ADVERSE REACTIONS

When used as directed, nonprescription cough medicines produce few adverse reactions. However, those that are combined with an antihistamine may cause:

- Lightheadedness
- Dizziness
- Drowsiness or sedation

CONTRAINDICATIONS

Antitussives, expectorants, and mucolytics are contraindicated in clients with known hypersensitivity to these drugs. Opioid antitussives (those with codeine) are contraindicated in premature infants or during labor when delivery of a premature infant is anticipated. Mucolytics are not recommended for use by clients with asthma. The expectorant potassium iodide is contraindicated during pregnancy (pregnancy category D).

PRECAUTIONS

Antitussives are given with caution to clients with a persistent or chronic cough or a cough accompanied by excessive secretions, a high fever, rash, persistent headache, and nausea or vomiting.

Antitussives containing codeine are used with caution during pregnancy (pregnancy category C) and labor (pregnancy category D) and in clients with chronic obstructive pulmonary disease, acute asthmatic attack, pre-existing respiratory disorders, acute abdominal conditions, head injury, increased intracranial pressure, convulsive disorders, hepatic or renal impairment, and prostatic hypertrophy.

Expectorants are used cautiously during pregnancy and lactation (guaifenesin is a pregnancy category C drug and acetylcysteine is a pregnancy category B drug); in clients with persistent cough, severe respiratory insufficiency, or asthma; and in older adults or debilitated clients.

 Lifespan Considerations

Pediatric/Adolescents
Dextromethorphan in high doses produces a hallucinogenic effect much like Ketamine or PCP (Prybys, 2017). Cough syrups containing dextromethorphan are readily available OTC, inexpensive, and perceived by many to be safe. All these factors make cough syrup products easily accessible for adolescent abuse. Triple-C (Coricidin Cough & Cold) or Robotripping (using Robitussin products) are references to the use of cough syrups for their intoxicating purposes. In addition to the above ingredients, many of these products also contain acetaminophen. Again, when the cough and cold product is taken in multiple doses for the high effect, too much acetaminophen is also taken and poisoning can occur.

INTERACTIONS

Other CNS depressants and alcohol may cause additive depressant effects when administered with antitussives containing codeine. When dextromethorphan is administered with the MAOI antidepressants (see Chapter 21), clients may experience hypotension, fever, nausea, jerking motions of the leg, and coma. No significant interactions have been reported when expectorants are used as directed. The exception is iodine products. If used concurrently with iodine products, lithium and other antithyroid drugs may potentiate the hypothyroid effects of these drugs. When potassium-containing medications and potassium-sparing diuretics are administered with iodine products, the client may experience hypokalemia, cardiac arrhythmias, or cardiac arrest. Thyroid function test results may also be altered by iodine.

 NURSING ALERT

Potassium iodide (SSKI), at one time, was added to liquids in minimal amounts to function as both an expectorant and to reduce the viscosity of secretions. This use fell out of favor. Instead, we see potassium iodide used as an emergency treatment for hyperthyroidism or radiation exposure. As people turn to homeopathic remedies, nurses may again see clients using SSKI as a cough expectorant.

Herbal Considerations

Eucalyptus is used as a decongestant and expectorant and is found as a component in OTC products used for the treatment of sinusitis and pharyngitis. The plant is grown throughout the world and the leaves and oil are used to treat various respiratory conditions, such as asthma and chronic bronchitis. Lozenges are useful to soothe sore throats and as cough drops. Eucalyptus can also be used as a vapor bath for asthma or other bronchial conditions. Scientific evidence is inconclusive regarding the respiratory benefit of the herb, yet people feel a sense of well-being from its use. The herb is available in many forms, including an essential oil, a fluid extract, and an aqueous solution in alcohol, as well as a component of various OTC products. Eucalyptus should not be used during pregnancy and lactation and in children younger than 2 years of age. Eucalyptus may be used topically on children and adults in combination with menthol and camphor. Individuals with hypersensitivity to eucalyptus should avoid its use (DerMarderosian & Beutler, 2003).

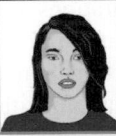 **PHARMACOLOGY IN PRACTICE**

PHYSIOLOGY
Given below, in random order, are the steps of the inflammatory response to injury. Arrange the steps of the inflammatory response in the order they likely occur in most situations.
1. Dilatation of arterioles
2. Increased capillary permeability
3. Release of histamine
4. Escape fluid from blood vessels
5. Localized redness
6. Localized swelling

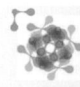

NURSING PROCESS—STEPS TO BUILDING CLINICAL JUDGMENT
Client Receiving an Upper Respiratory System Drug

ASSESSMENT

Preadministration Assessment

Clients most commonly self-prescribe what is frequently termed a *cough and cold* preparation (an antihistamine, decongestant, antitussive, and/or expectorant medication). For allergy relief, INSs can be purchased OTC and are preferred because sedative reactions are reduced.

Data gathering suggestions before the initial administration of the drug include:

Objective data

- Vital signs (temperature, pulse, respirations, and blood pressure)
- Weight (for peds, many preparations are prescribed according to weight)
- Auscultate breath sounds

Subjective data

- Type and duration of symptoms (sputum description, sinus pain, chest pains)
- Description of activity disruption by symptoms (inability to sleep, etc.)
- Health history especially regarding seasonal allergies or allergens in household
- Remedies attempted before seeking care

A hospitalized client may occasionally have one of these preparations prescribed, because of an existing respiratory disorder or if coughing prevents a surgical client from getting up and about or causes pain at the incisional site when coughing.

Ongoing Assessment

Effectiveness of the preparation is measured by the client's self-report of diminishing symptoms (e.g., ability to sleep better because of less coughing). If the client returns to the ambulatory setting or is monitored daily, lung sounds are auscultated and vital signs are taken periodically.

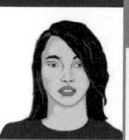

PHARMACOLOGY IN PRACTICE

ASSESSMENT

What information should be obtained from the client by the nurse and documented prior to the recommendation of an antitussive?

Select all that apply.
1. Type of cough
2. Presence of sputum
3. Color and amount of sputum
4. Home remedies used to treat the cough
5. Vital signs of the last PHCP visit

NURSING DIAGNOSES

Drug-specific nursing diagnoses include the following:

- **Injury risk** related to drowsiness, dizziness, or sedation
- **Ineffective airway clearance** related to pooling of or thick secretions

- **Impaired oral mucous membranes** related to dry mouth, nose, and throat

Nursing diagnoses related to drug administration are discussed in Chapter 4.

PLANNING

The expected outcomes for the client depend on the reason for administration but may include an optimal response to therapy, support of client needs related to managing adverse reactions, and confidence in an understanding of the medication regimen.

IMPLEMENTATION

Promoting an Optimal Response to Therapy

Problems can arise from the use of a nonprescription upper respiratory system medication for self-treatment of a chronic cough. Indiscriminate use of these products by the general public may prevent early diagnosis and treatment of serious disorders, such as lung cancer and emphysema. Clients should be advised that, if a cough lasts more than 10 days or is accompanied by fever, chest pain, severe headache, or skin rash, the client should consult the primary health care provider.

Monitor children taking INS for prolonged periods of time or routinely each year (e.g., 2 months of every year). Height and weight measurements should be taken and compared with growth charts for retardation of growth. Although retardation of growth is unlikely, it is important to discover this occurrence, especially when other forms of steroids may be taken.

When you do have contact with clients taking upper respiratory system medications, be sure to reinforce teaching points such as the following:

- Loratadine or other rapidly disintegrating tablets can be administered with or without water and are placed on the tongue, where the tablet dissolves almost instantly.
- Fexofenadine is not administered within 2 hours of an antacid.
- Chewing benzonatate tablets may result in a local anesthetic effect (oropharyngeal anesthesia) with possible choking as a result.
- Acetylcysteine has a distinctive, disagreeable odor. The medication may smell like "rotten eggs." Although this odor may be nauseating, the smell dissipates quickly.

Monitoring and Managing Client Needs

Injury Risk

If drowsiness is severe or if other problems such as dizziness or a disturbance in muscle coordination occur, the client may require assistance with ambulation and other activities. If the client is in an institution, ensure they are oriented to the surroundings, that pathways to the bathroom are free of equipment, and supervision is provided if there is a cognitive issue. Place call lights within easy reach and instruct the client to call before attempting to get out of bed or ambulate. When the drug is taken in the home environment, caution the client to refrain from activities that require a clear mind or operating equipment that requires attentive detail. Tell the client that this adverse reaction may decrease with continued use of the drug.

 Lifespan Considerations

Gerontology

Older adults are more likely to experience injury from dizziness because with age comes an increased risk for falls. Sensorimotor deficits, such as hearing loss, visual impairments, or balance problems, increase the older adult's risk for injury. Codeine may cause orthostatic hypotension when a client rises too quickly from a sitting or lying position. Clients should not take codeine preparations for persistent or chronic cough, such as occurs with smoking, asthma, or emphysema, or when the cough is accompanied by excessive secretions, except when under the supervision of a health care provider.

Ineffective Airway Clearance

One problem associated with the use of an antitussive is related to its drug action. Although not an adverse reaction, depression of the cough reflex can cause secretions to pool in the lungs. Pooling of the secretions that are normally removed by coughing may result in more serious problems, such as pneumonia and atelectasis. For this reason, using an antitussive for a *productive cough* is contraindicated in many situations. Clients should be encouraged to increase fluids and change position frequently to facilitate removal of secretions.

When the client is having difficulty coughing up secretions it is a good safety habit to have suction equipment available. Should the client need assistance, the nurse can assist in repositioning and removal of thick sputum from the oral cavity. On occasion the weak or debilitated client may find having a suction tip available to self-assist in sputum removal helpful.

For the client with thick sputum, encourage fluid intake of up to 2000 mL/day if this amount is not contraindicated by the client's condition or disease process. Instruction is provided to help the client with deep, diaphragmatic breathing. As sputum is expelled from the respiratory system, monitor color, amount, and consistency.

Overuse of the topical form of INSs, antihistamines, and decongestants can cause "rebound" nasal congestion. This means that the congestion becomes worse with the use of the drug. Although congestion may be relieved briefly after the drug is used, it

recurs within a short time, which prompts the client to use the drug at more frequent intervals, perpetuating the rebound congestion. Teach the client to take the drug exactly as prescribed. A simple but uncomfortable solution to rebound congestion is to withdraw completely from the topical medication. The primary health care provider may recommend an oral decongestant. An alternative method to minimize the occurrence of rebound nasal congestion is to discontinue the drug therapy gradually by initially discontinuing the medication in one nostril, followed by withdrawal from the other nostril. You may suggest saline irrigation of nasal passages using a "neti pot" in place of using a decongestant. A neti pot, originally from the yogic tradition and now a part of Ayurvedic medicine, is a container that is filled with distilled or sterile water (not tap water) for flushing out the nasal sinuses. These can often be purchased at natural or health food stores.

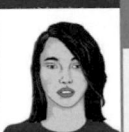 **PHARMACOLOGY IN PRACTICE**

MANAGING NEEDS

A nurse in a rehab care facility is caring for a client with a tracheostomy who has a severe cough. The PHCP has prescribed acetylcysteine for the client. What is typically the nurse's role when the drug is to be inserted into the tracheostomy?
1. Ensure that the client is not receiving any other drug therapy.
2. Ensure that suction equipment is at the client's bedside.
3. Ensure that the client gets continuous oxygen supply.
4. Ensure that the client keeps drinking warm water.

Impaired Oral Mucous Membranes

Dryness of the mouth, nose, and throat may occur when antihistamines are taken. Offer the client frequent sips of water or ice chips to relieve these symptoms. Sugarless gum or sugarless hard candy may also relieve these symptoms.

 Lifespan Considerations

Gerontology

Older adults are more likely to experience anticholinergic effects (e.g., dryness of the mouth, nose, and throat), dizziness, sedation, hypotension, and confusion from antihistamines.

Educating the Client and Family

During any client encounter, you can teach clients the proper use of OTC upper respiratory system medications, especially when coughing produces sputum. Advise the client to read the label carefully, follow the dosage recommendations, and consult the primary health care provider if the cough persists for more than 10 days, the color of sputum changes, or fever or chest pain occurs.

Acetylcysteine usually is administered in the hospital but may be prescribed for the client being discharged. Typically, the respiratory therapist gives the client or a family member full instruction in the use and maintenance of the equipment, as well as the technique of administration of acetylcysteine. As the nurse, your responsibility is to be sure the client or family member understands the instruction and has all questions addressed before use.

As you develop a teaching plan for the client or family member, include the following points:

- Do not exceed the recommended dose.
- Avoid irritants, such as cigarette smoke, dust, or fumes, to decrease irritation to the throat.
- Drink plenty of fluids (if not contraindicated by disease process). A fluid intake of 1500–2000 mL is recommended.
- If taking oral capsules, do not chew or break open the capsules; swallow them whole.
- If taking a lozenge, avoid drinking fluids for 31 min after use to avoid losing effectiveness of the drug.
- Antihistamines may cause dryness of the mouth and throat. Frequent sips of water, sucking on hard candy, or chewing gum (preferably sugarless) may relieve this problem.
- High doses of antihistamines can contribute to mental changes in vulnerable populations.
- Do not drive or perform other hazardous tasks if drowsiness occurs. This effect may diminish with continued use.
  - 🍷 Avoid the use of alcohol, as well as other drugs that cause sleepiness or drowsiness, while taking these drugs.
- Understand that overuse of topical nasal decongestants can make the symptoms worse, causing rebound congestion.

- Nasal burning and stinging may occur with the topical decongestants. This effect usually disappears with use. If burning or stinging becomes severe, discontinue use and discuss this problem with the primary health care provider, who may prescribe or recommend another drug.
- If using a spray, do not allow the tip of the container to touch the nasal mucosa and do not share the container with other people.
- Use of INS can result in a fungal infection of the nares. Contact the primary health care provider if the area becomes reddened, sore, or you can see white patches.
- If the cough is not relieved or becomes worse, contact the primary health care provider.
- If chills, fever, chest pain, or sputum production occurs, contact the primary health care provider as soon as possible.

EVALUATION

- Therapeutic response is achieved and coughing is relieved.
- Adverse reactions are identified, reported to the primary health care provider, and managed successfully with appropriate nursing interventions:
  - No evidence of injury is seen.
  - Client has a clear airway.
  - Mucous membranes are moist and intact.
- Client and family express confidence and demonstrate an understanding of the drug regimen.

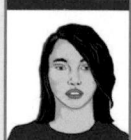

PHARMACOLOGY IN PRACTICE

USING CLINICAL REASONING

As her nurse, you know that Janna is an active teenager. Describe important teaching points that should be included in developing a teaching plan for her. What limitations might these drugs have on her activity? What other OTC products should she avoid?

KEY POINTS

■ Cough, cold, congestion, and allergies are common problems in the upper respiratory system.

■ INSs and antihistamines are used to reduce inflammation; decongestants are used to reduce edema and swelling; and antitussives are used to eliminate cough. When congestion produces secretions in either the respiratory passages or the lungs, expectorants or mucolytics are used, respectively.

■ Many of these products are obtained OTC, not requiring a prescription. Therefore, assessment of use and proper instruction are important nursing actions to remember because clients may not readily think to offer information about use.

■ Antihistamines can produce drowsiness; other medications typically do not have bothersome adverse reactions unless the effects are potentiated by interaction with prescription drugs (especially extrapyramidal symptoms).

SUMMARY DRUG TABLE
Upper Respiratory System Drugs

Generic Name	Trade Name	Uses	Adverse Reactions	Dosage Ranges
Intranasal Steroids (INSs)				
beclomethasone *be-kloe-METH-a-sone*	Beconase AQ, Qnasl	Nasal polyps and rhinitis (perennial, seasonal, and vasomotor)	Nasal irritation, headache	1–2 inhalations, BID
budesonide *byoo-DES-oh-nide*	Rhinocort	Rhinitis (perennial and seasonal)	Epistaxis	Up to 4 sprays per nare, once daily
ciclesonide *sye-KLES-oh-nide*	Omnaris, Zetonna	Same as budesonide	Epistaxis, nasal discomfort	2 sprays per nare up to 3 times daily
flunisolide *floo-NISS-oh-lide*		Same as budesonide	Nasal sting on administration	2 sprays per nare up to 3 times daily
fluticasone *floo-TIK-a-sone*	ClariSpray, Flonase	Same as budesonide	Epistaxis	2 sprays per nare once daily
mometasone *mo-MET-a-sone*	Nasonex	Nasal polyps, rhinitis (perennial and seasonal)	Epistaxis, cough	2 sprays per nare once daily
triamcinolone *trye-am-SIN-oh-lone*	Nasacort AQ and HFA	Rhinitis (perennial and seasonal)	Pharyngitis	2 sprays per nare once daily
azelastine/fluticasone *a-ZEL-as-teen/floo-TIK-a-sone*	Dymista	Rhinitis (seasonal)	Epistaxis, taste changes	1 spray per nare twice daily
First-Generation Antihistamines				
brompheniramine *brome-fen-IR-a-meen*	Ala-Hist, Veltane	Temporary relief of sneezing, itchy, watery eyes, itchy nose or throat, and runny nose caused by hay fever or other respiratory allergies; VaZol also used for symptoms of the common cold; treatment of allergic reactions to blood or plasma and anaphylactic reactions	Drowsiness, sedation, dizziness, disturbed coordination, hypotension, headache, blurred vision, thickening of bronchial secretions	Adults and children 12 years and older: 6–12 mg orally q12hr Sustained release: 8–12 mg orally q12hr Oral liquid: 4 mg QID
chlorpheniramine *klor-fen-IR-a-meen*	Aller-Chlor, Chlor-Trimeton	Temporary relief of sneezing, itchy, watery eyes, itchy throat, and runny nose caused by hay fever, other upper respiratory allergies, and the common cold	Drowsiness, sedation, hypotension, palpitations, blurred vision, dry mouth, urinary hesitancy	Adults and children 12 years and older: 4 mg q4–6hr, maximum dose 24 mg in 24 hours Extended release: 8–12 mg orally q8–12hr
clemastine *KLEM-as-teen*	Dayhist	Allergic rhinitis, urticaria, angioedema	Drowsiness, sedation, hypotension, palpitations, blurred vision, dry mouth, urinary hesitancy	Allergic rhinitis: 1.34 mg orally BID (not to exceed 8.04 mg/day for the syrup and 2.68 mg for the tablets) Urticaria and angioedema: 2.68 mg BID orally (not to exceed 4.02 mg/day)
diphenhydrAMINE *dye-fen-HYE-dra-meen*	Benadryl, Unisom	Allergic symptoms; hypersensitivity reactions, including anaphylaxis and transfusion reactions; motion sickness; sleep aid; antitussive and Parkinson-like effects	Drowsiness, dry mouth, anorexia, blurred vision, urinary frequency	25–50 mg orally every 4–6 hours, maximum daily dose 310 mg; 10–400 mg IM, IV

Generic Name	Trade Name	Uses	Adverse Reactions	Dosage Ranges
promethazine *proe-METH-a-zeen*		Antiemetic, hypersensitivity reactions, motion sickness, sedation	Excessive sedation, drowsiness, dry mouth, confusion, disorientation, dizziness, fatigue, blurred vision	Individualize dosage to smallest effective dose Allergy: 12.5–25 mg orally, 25 mg IM, IV Antiemetic: 12.5–25 mg orally, IM, IV Motion sickness: 25 mg BID Preoperative: 50 mg IM or orally the night before surgery
Second-Generation Antihistamines				
azelastine *ah-ZEL-as-teen*		Seasonal and vasomotor rhinitis	Dizziness, drowsiness, glossitis, nose bleeds	2 sprays per nare twice daily
cetirizine *se-TI-ra-zeen*	ZyrTEC	Seasonal or perennial rhinitis, chronic urticaria	Sedation, dry mouth, pharyngitis, somnolence, dizziness	5–10 mg/day orally; maximum dosage 20 mg/day
desloratadine *des-lor-AT-a-deen*	Clarinex	Seasonal or perennial allergic rhinitis	Headache; fatigue; drowsiness; dry mouth, nose, and throat; flu-like symptoms	Adults and children 12 years and older: 5 mg/day orally
fexofenadine *feks-oh-FEN-a-deen*	Allegra	Seasonal rhinitis, urticaria	Headache, nausea, drowsiness, dyspepsia, fatigue, back pain, upper respiratory infection	30–60 mg orally BID; maximum dosage 180 mg/day
levocetirizine *LEE-vo-se-TI-ra-zeen*	Xyzal	Allergic rhinitis, urticaria	Dizziness, drowsiness	5 mg orally in evening
loratadine *lor-AT-a-deen*	Claritin, Alavert	Allergic rhinitis	Dizziness, headache, tremors, insomnia, dry mouth, fatigue	10 mg/day orally
olopatadine *oh-la-PAT-a-deen*	Patanase	Seasonal rhinitis	Bitter taste, headache, epitaxis	Two sprays per nare twice daily
Decongestants				
epinephrine *ep-ih-nef'-rin*	Adrenalin	Nasal congestion	Anxiety, restlessness, anorexia, arrhythmias, nervousness	2–3 drops or spray in each nostril q4–6hr
fexofenadine and pseudoephedrine	Allegra-D	Allergic rhinitis and nasal congestion	See separate drugs	1 tablet every 12 hours
naphazoline *nah-faz'-oh-leen*	Privine	Nasal congestion	Same as epinephrine	1–2 drops or sprays in each nostril no more than q6hr
oxymetazoline *oks-i-met-AZ-oh-leen*	Afrin	Nasal congestion	Same as epinephrine	2–3 drops or sprays q10–12hr
phenylephrine *fen-il-EF-rin*	Neo-Synephrine	Nasal congestion	Same as epinephrine	2–3 sprays of 0%–25% solution q3–4hr
pseudoephedrine *soo-doe-e-FED-rin*	Sudafed	Nasal congestion	Anxiety, restlessness, anorexia, arrhythmias, nervousness, nausea, vomiting, blurred vision	60 mg orally q4–6hr
tetrahydrozoline *tet-ra-hye-DROZ-a-leen*		Nasal congestion	Same as pseudoephedrine	2–4 drops in each nostril or 3–4 sprays in each nostril q3hr
xylometazoline *zye-loe-met-AZ-oh-leen*	Sinutab Nasal Spray	Nasal congestion	Same as epinephrine	2–3 drops or sprays in each nostril q8–10hr

Continued

SUMMARY DRUG TABLE (continued)
Upper Respiratory System Drugs

Generic Name	Trade Name	Uses	Adverse Reactions	Dosage Ranges
Antitussives				
Opioid Antitussives				
codeine *KOE-deen*		Suppression of nonproductive cough, relief of mild to moderate pain	Sedation, nausea, vomiting, dizziness, constipation, CNS depression	10–20 mg orally q4–6hr; maximum dosage 120 mg/day
Nonopioid Antitussives				
benzonatate *ben-ZOE-na-tate*	Tessalon	Symptomatic relief of cough	Sedation, headache, mild dizziness, constipation, nausea, GI upset, pruritus, nasal congestion	Adults and children older than 10 years: 100–200 mg TID (up to 600 mg/day)
dextromethorphan *deks-troe-meth-OR-fan*	Robitussin	Symptomatic relief of cough	Drowsiness, dizziness, GI upset	Adults and children older than 12 years: 10–30 mg q4–8hr; sustained-release (SR) 60 mg q12hr orally Children 6–12 years: 5–10 mg q4hr or 15 mg q6–8hr; SR 30 mg q12hr orally Children 2–5 years: 2.5–7.5 mg q4–8hr; SR 15 mg q12hr orally
diphenhydrAMINE *dye-fen-HYE-dra-meen*	Nytol, ZzzQuil	Symptomatic relief of cough caused by colds, allergy, or bronchial irritation	Drowsiness, dizziness, GI upset	Adults: 25 mg q4hr orally, not to exceed 150 mg/day Children 6–12 years: 12.5 mg orally q4hr, not to exceed 75 mg/day Children 2–5 years: 6.25 mg q4hr, not to exceed 25 mg/day
Mucolytics				
acetylcysteine *a-se-teel-SIS-teen*		Reduction of viscosity of mucus in acute and chronic bronchopulmonary diseases and diagnostic bronchial studies, acetaminophen toxicity	Stomatitis, nausea, vomiting, fever, drowsiness, bronchospasm, irritation of the trachea and bronchi	1–10 mL of 20% solution by nebulization or 2–20 mL of 10% solution q2–6hr PRN Acetaminophen toxicity: initially 140 mg/kg orally, then 70 mg/kg orally q4hr for 17 doses (total)
Expectorants				
guaiFENesin *gwye-FEN-e-sin*	Mucinex	Relief of cough associated with respiratory tract infection (sinusitis, asthma, bronchitis, pharyngitis), especially when the cough is dry and nonproductive	Nausea, vomiting, dizziness, headache, rash	Adults and children 12 years and older: 200–400 mg orally q4hr Children 6–12 years: 100–200 mg q4hr orally Children 2–6 years: 50–100 mg q4hr

CHAPTER REVIEW

Know Your Drugs

Clients sometimes know a medication by the brand (or trade) name and not the generic name. To help you recognize both names, match the brand name with the generic name of the same medication.

Generic Name	Brand Name
1. dextromethorphan	A. Robitussin
2. diphenhydramine	B. Nasonex
3. loratadine	C. Claritin
4. mometasone	D. Benadryl

Calculate Medication Dosages

1. A client is prescribed 200 mg of guaifenesin syrup. The drug is available in syrup of 200 mg/5 mL. The nurse administers _____.
2. Loratadine 10 mg is prescribed. The drug is available in 5-mg tablets. The nurse instructs the client to take _____.

Prepare for the NCLEX

RECALL THE FACTS

1. Antitussives are medications that _____.
   1. loosen respiratory secretions
   2. depress the cough center in the brain
   3. increase production of mucous secretion
   4. fight microbial infections of the lungs
2. Which of these drugs is classified as an expectorant?
   1. guaifenesin
   2. codeine
   3. dextromethorphan
   4. diphenhydramine
3. Which of the following is a common adverse reaction seen when administering an antihistamine?
   1. sedation
   2. blurred vision
   3. headache
   4. hypertension
4. When antihistamines are administered to clients receiving CNS depressants, the nurse monitors the client for _____.
   1. an increase in anticholinergic effects
   2. excessive sedation
   3. seizure activity
   4. loss of hearing

5. A client receives a prescription for phenylephrine (Neo-Synephrine). The nurse explains that overuse of this drug may _____.
   1. result in hypotensive episodes
   2. decrease sinus drainage
   3. cause rebound nasal congestion
   4. dilate capillaries in the nasal mucosa

ANALYZE THE FACTS

6. Which of the following statements is appropriate for the nurse to include in discharge instructions for a client taking an antitussive?
   1. Increase the dosage if the drug does not relieve the cough.
   2. Limit fluids to less than 1000 mL each day.
   3. Expect the cough to worsen during the first few days of treatment.
   4. Frequent sips of water may diminish coughing.
7. The nurse is to administer a mucolytic agent. Which of the following nursing actions is appropriate to take to promote an effective airway?
   1. Increase fluid intake to 2000 mL/day
   2. Limit fluids to 200 mL/day
   3. Monitor intake and output every 8 hours
   4. Have the client take the mucolytic after each coughing episode
8. *Which of the following interactions would most likely occur when diphenhydramine is administered with a beta-blocker drug such as propranolol (Inderal)?
   1. increased risk for cardiovascular effects
   2. increased risk for seizures
   3. decreased risk for cardiovascular effects
   4. decreased risk for seizures

ALTERNATE-FORMAT QUESTIONS

9. Which of these drugs would mostly likely be used to bring up deep mucous plugs in the lungs of a client with a tracheostomy? **Select all that apply.**
   1. acetylcysteine
   2. guaifenesin
   3. benzonatate
   4. dextromethorphan

10. *A client with limited health literacy is prescribed an antihistamine for an upper respiratory tract allergy. You want to be sure the client does not use other cold remedies with antihistamines included. What is the best way to relay this information? **Select all that apply.**
    1. Tell the client which drugs not to use
    2. Give the client a list of medicines that include antihistamines
    3. Show the client where to look on the medicine label for the ingredients
    4. Make a poster for your clinic with drugs that contain antihistamines for teaching

To check your answers, see Appendix F.

_____

*Indicates the question is directly linked to the NCLEX-PN test plan in Appendix G.

WANT TO KNOW MORE? A wide variety of resources are available to enhance your learning and understanding of this chapter.
- Visit thePoint for resources such as:
  - NCLEX-Style Student Review Questions
  - Journal Articles
  - Dosage Calculations
  - Drug Monographs
  - Watch and Learn Videos
  - Concepts in Action Animations
- The *Study Guide to Accompany Introductory Clinical Pharmacology,* 12th edition, sold separately, will help you review and apply essential content.
- ✓*PrepU* is available to help students prepare for the NCLEX-PN examination.

Lower Respiratory System Drugs

Key Terms

asthma respiratory disorder characterized by bronchospasm and difficulty in breathing, especially exhaling

dyspnea feelings of shortness of breath, labored or difficult breathing

leukotrienes inflammatory substance that is released by mast cells during an asthma attack

nebulizer a device turning liquid into an aerosol mist to deliver medication into bronchial airway

tachypnea rapid breathing

theophyllinization delivery of a high enough dose of theophylline to bring blood levels to a therapeutic range more quickly than over several days

Learning Objectives

On completion of this chapter, the student will:

1. Explain the uses, general drug actions, general adverse reactions, contraindications, precautions, and interactions of the bronchodilators and antiasthma drugs.
2. Distinguish important preadministration and ongoing assessment activities the nurse should perform on the client taking a bronchodilator or an antiasthma drug.
3. List nursing diagnoses particular to a client taking a bronchodilator or an antiasthma drug.
4. Examine ways to promote an optimal response to therapy, how to manage common adverse reactions, and important points to keep in mind when educating a client about the use of bronchodilators or antiasthma drugs.

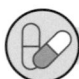 **Drug Classes**

Bronchodilators
- Short-acting beta$_2$ (β_2) (adrenergic) agonists (SABAs)
- Long-acting beta$_2$ (β_2) (adrenergic) agonists (LABAs)
- Xanthine derivative
- Cholinergic blocking (anticholinergic)

Antiasthma
- Inhaled corticosteroids (ICSs)
- Mast cell stabilizer
- Leukotriene modifier and immunomodulator

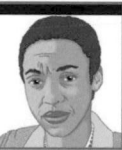

PHARMACOLOGY IN PRACTICE

Lillian Chase, a 36-year-old woman who had a breathing problem over the weekend, was seen in the emergency department of the local hospital. You are seeing her in the clinic for her follow-up visit. At the end of the chapter, review the medication order and compare it with the established guidelines for her self-management of asthma.

In this chapter, the drugs used to treat many of the conditions that present in the bronchi and alveoli of the lungs are discussed. The term *chronic obstructive pulmonary disease* (COPD) is used to describe the disorders of **asthma**, chronic bronchitis, chronic obstructive bronchitis, and emphysema, or a combination of these conditions. The client with COPD experiences **dyspnea** (difficulty breathing) with physical exertion, has difficulty inhaling and exhaling, and may have a chronic cough. All of these disorders interfere with the exchange of gases in the lung alveoli. The best way to learn about treatment strategies is to focus on one of the disorders. In this chapter, asthma is used as the condition to help you understand the drugs used for lower respiratory system conditions.

ASTHMA

More than 24 million Americans have asthma (CDC, 2020), which is a chronic inflammatory disease causing spasmodic constriction of the bronchi. It is one of the most common chronic diseases of childhood, affecting an estimated 6 million children.

Figure 31.1 illustrates what happens during an episode of the airway restriction of asthma. During the inflammatory process, a large amount of histamine is released from the mast cells of the respiratory tract. The lung bronchi constrict, becoming hyperresponsive to the bronchoconstriction, and edema results. With asthma, the airways become narrow, the muscles around the airways tighten, the inner lining of the bronchi swells, and extra mucus clogs the smaller airways. Characterized by recurrent attacks of dyspnea and wheezing, this breathlessness causes the client to experience anxiety.

Clients with asthma may experience periods of normal respiratory function alternating with exacerbation of respiratory symptoms. The period of exacerbation may appear to begin abruptly, often triggered by exercise or cold air, but it is usually preceded by increasing symptoms (which the client may or may not recognize) over a period of several days:

- Cough (worse at night or early morning)
- Generalized wheezing (a whistle or squeaking sound on inspiration or expiration)
- Generalized chest tightness (may feel like someone is sitting on the chest)
- Dyspnea (shortness of breath or feeling of breathlessness)
- **Tachypnea** (rapid breathing)

These symptoms are similar to those seen with stimulation of the sympathetic nervous system, the fight-or-flight response (as described in Chapter 23). This sympathetic response is the body's reaction to the inflammation occurring in the lungs.

Asthma medications are categorized into two major groups: (1) long-term control medications and (2) quick-relief medications used to treat acute air flow obstruction. The long-term management of asthma uses a stepwise approach (Box 31.1), meaning that medications and their

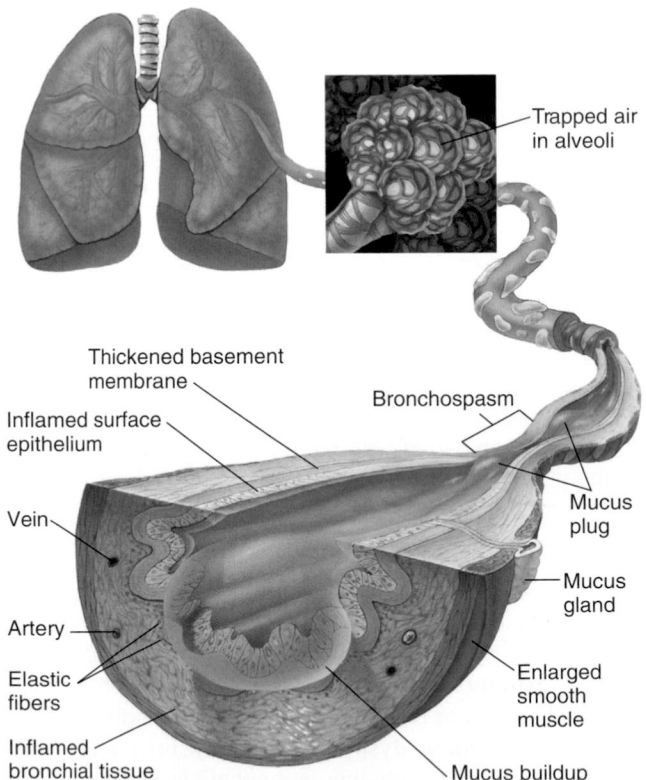

Thickened basement membrane
Bronchospasm
Inflamed surface epithelium
Vein
Mucus plug
Artery
Mucus gland
Elastic fibers
Enlarged smooth muscle
Inflamed bronchial tissue
Mucus buildup
Trapped air in alveoli

FIGURE 31.1 Bronchus airflow obstruction in asthma. (Courtesy of Anatomical Chart Co.)

	BOX 31.1	**Step Care Approach for Managing Asthma in Adults and Youth 12 Years and Older**	
Asthma Classification	**Daily Medications for Long-Term Management**	**Rescue Drugs**
Step 1: intermittent asthma	No daily medications	SABA
Step 2: mild persistent asthma	Low-dose ICS **Alternative:** cromolyn or LTRA or sustained-release theophylline; consider immunotherapy for persistent symptoms	SABA
Step 3: mild to moderate persistent asthma	Low-dose ICS *plus* LABA *or* medium-dose ICS **Alternative:** low-dose ICS and LTRA or theophylline or zileuton; consider immunotherapy for persistent symptoms	SABA
Step 4: moderate persistent asthma	Medium-dose ICS *plus* LABA **Alternative:** low-dose ICS and LTRA or theophylline or zileuton; consider immunotherapy for persistent symptoms	SABA
Step 5: moderately severe persistent asthma	Daily combined use of a high-dose ICS *and* LABA, and an immunomodulator	SABA
Step 6: severe persistent asthma	High-dose ICS *and* LABA *plus* oral corticosteroid, and consider immunomodulator	SABA

LTRA, leukotriene receptor antagonist.
Expert Panel Report 3: Guidelines for the Diagnosis and Management of Asthma, National Heart, Lung, and Blood Institute, 2007.

frequency of administration are adjusted according to the severity of the client's asthma. The most effective long-term control medications are those that reduce inflammation, with inhaled corticosteroids (ICSs) being the first-line intervention. Quick-relief medications include inhaled short-acting $beta_2$-adrenergic (β_2-adrenergic) agonists (SABAs) and oral steroids.

Bronchodilators are the mainstay of treatment for many chronic pulmonary disorders. SABA bronchodilators are drugs used to relieve bronchospasm associated with respiratory disorders, such as bronchial asthma, chronic bronchitis, and emphysema. These conditions are progressive disorders characterized by a decrease in the inspiratory and expiratory capacity of the lung. Examples of $beta_2$ (β_2)-agonist bronchodilators include albuterol (Ventolin), epinephrine (Adrenalin), salmeterol (Serevent), and terbutaline. Along with the bronchodilators, several types of drugs are effective in treating asthma. These include ICSs, mast cell stabilizers, **leukotriene** formation inhibitors, leukotriene receptor agonists, and immunomodulators.

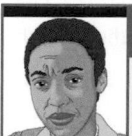

PHARMACOLOGY IN PRACTICE

DRUG RECOGNITION
A client has been prescribed a step care approach regimen for the treatment of asthma. Which of the following drugs may be given as adjuncts to bronchodilator therapy in such a case? Select all that apply.

1. Decongestants
2. Inhaled corticosteroids
3. Uricosuric agents
4. Mast cell stabilizers
5. Immunomodulators

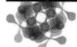 # BRONCHODILATORS

The two major types of bronchodilators are the $beta_2$-adrenergic agonists (or sympathomimetics) and the xanthine derivatives. The cholinergic blocking drug ipratropium bromide (Atrovent) is used for maintenance therapy to prevent bronchospasm associated with COPD, chronic bronchitis, and emphysema. When drugs such as ipratropium are used to manage bronchodilation in nonacute conditions, the drug blocks the release of acetylcholine in bronchial smooth muscle nerves, thus reducing airway constriction. When used once or twice daily, this drug helps to reduce breathing distress and increase lung function. Because the drugs are selective for M_3 muscarinic (cholinergic) receptors, they have less adverse reactions in other body systems (Buels & Fryer, 2012). See Chapter 26 for impact of the drug on other body systems.

ADRENERGIC BRONCHODILATORS

When alpha-adrenergic (α-adrenergic) receptors (the sympathetic peripheral nervous system) in the lungs are stimulated, bronchoconstriction results, and the client feels acute shortness of breath. The opposite, *bronchodilation,* occurs when beta-adrenergic (β-adrenergic) receptors are stimulated. Some theories propose that asthma is a lack of beta-adrenergic stimulation. Many of the adrenergics used as bronchodilators have the subclassification of beta$_2$-receptor (β_2-receptor) agonists, which are either *short acting* (e.g., albuterol and terbutaline) or *long acting* (e.g., salmeterol). Additional information concerning the various adrenergic drugs is given in the Summary Drug Table: Lower Respiratory System Drugs.

ACTIONS

When bronchospasm occurs, there is a decrease in the lumen (or inside diameter) of the bronchi, which decreases the amount of air taken into the lungs with each breath. A decrease in the amount of air taken into the lungs results in respiratory distress. Use of a bronchodilating drug opens the bronchi by relaxing the smooth muscles and allows more air to enter the lungs, which, in turn, completely or partially relieves respiratory distress.

USES

The beta$_2$-adrenergic drugs (which mimic the sympathetic nervous system) are used in the treatment of chronic respiratory problems caused by bronchoconstriction, such as:

• Bronchospasm associated with acute and chronic bronchial asthma
• Exercise-induced bronchospasm (EIB)
• Bronchitis
• Emphysema
• Bronchiectasis (chronic dilation of the bronchi and bronchioles)
• Other obstructive pulmonary diseases

ADVERSE REACTIONS

Cardiovascular System Reactions
• Tachycardia, palpitations, or cardiac arrhythmias
• Hypertension

Other Reactions
• Nervousness, anxiety
• Insomnia

When these drugs are taken by inhalation, excessive use (e.g., more than the recommended dose times) may result in paradoxical bronchospasm.

NURSING ALERT

Long-acting beta$_2$ (adrenergic) agonists (LABAs; e.g., salmeterol) may increase the risk of asthma-related death. ICSs should be considered first for long-term control of asthma.

CONTRAINDICATIONS

The adrenergic bronchodilators are contraindicated in clients with known hypersensitivity to the drug, cardiac arrhythmias associated with tachycardia, organic brain damage, cerebral arteriosclerosis, and narrow-angle glaucoma. Salmeterol is contraindicated during acute bronchospasm.

PRECAUTIONS

The adrenergics are used cautiously in clients with hypertension, cardiac dysfunction, hyperthyroidism, glaucoma, diabetes, prostatic hypertrophy, and a history of seizures. The adrenergic drugs are also used cautiously during pregnancy and lactation (all are in pregnancy category C, except terbutaline, which is a pregnancy category B drug).

LASA ALERT

The following drugs may sound alike; be sure to clarify when they are ordered:

Drug Name	*Sounds Like*
Metaproterenol	metipranolol, metoprolol

Drugs that look like a similar drug are noted in the Summary Drug Tables of each chapter.

INTERACTIONS

The following interactions may occur when an adrenergic drug is used concurrently with another agent:

Interacting Drug	Common Use	Effect of Interaction
Adrenergic drugs	Treatment of hypotension and shock	Possible additive adrenergic effects
Tricyclics	Treatment of depression	Possible hypotension
Beta-adrenergic blockers	Treatment of hypertension	Inhibition of the cardiac, bronchodilating, and vasodilating effects of the adrenergic
Methyldopa	Treatment of hypertension	Possible hypotension
Oxytocic drugs	Uterine stimulant	Possible severe hypotension
Theophylline	Treatment of asthma and COPD	Increased risk for cardiotoxicity

XANTHINE DERIVATIVE BRONCHODILATORS

Xanthine derivatives (also called *methylxanthines*) are a different class of drugs from the adrenergics and also have bronchodilating activity. Sometimes classified in the mast cell stabilizer group, they are included here separately because of their action and uses. Although these are not considered first-line drugs for asthma treatment, they may be used when clients are refractory to other medications. Client improvement needs to be measured against the monitoring and toxic side effects of the drugs (Simon, 2016). In some circumstances, the significantly lower cost of the drugs makes their use a good alternative for some populations. Examples are theophylline and aminophylline. Additional information concerning the xanthine derivatives is found in the Summary Drug Table: Lower Respiratory System Drugs.

ACTIONS

The xanthine derivatives are drugs that stimulate the central nervous system (CNS) to promote bronchodilation. They cause direct relaxation of the smooth muscles of the bronchi.

USES

The xanthine derivatives are used for the following:

- Symptomatic relief or prevention of bronchial asthma
- Treatment of reversible bronchospasm associated with chronic bronchitis and emphysema

ADVERSE REACTIONS

Central Nervous System Reactions
- Restlessness, irritability, headache
- Nervousness, tremors

Cardiac and Respiratory System Reactions
- Tachycardia
- Palpitations
- Electrocardiographic changes
- Increased respirations

Other Reactions
- Nausea, vomiting, fever
- Hyperglycemia, flushing, alopecia

CONTRAINDICATIONS

The xanthine derivatives are contraindicated in those with known hypersensitivity to the drugs, peptic ulcers, seizure disorders (unless well controlled with appropriate anticonvulsant medication), and serious uncontrolled arrhythmias.

PRECAUTIONS

The xanthine derivatives are used cautiously in clients with cardiac disease, hypoxemia, hypertension, congestive heart failure, and liver disease. They are also used cautiously in older adult clients and those who use alcohol habitually. Aminophylline, dyphylline, oxtriphylline, and theophylline are pregnancy category C drugs and are used cautiously during pregnancy and lactation.

INTERACTIONS

When taken with theophylline, the following agents have an effect on theophylline levels:

Decreased theophylline levels result when the drug is taken with the interacting drug noted below.

Theophylline Serum Level	Interacting Drug	Common Use
	Barbiturates	Sedation
	Charcoal (in large amounts)	Neutralize poisoning
	Hydantoins	Anticonvulsant
	Ketoconazole	Antifungal agent
	Rifampin	Antitubercular agent
	Nicotine (tobacco, nicotine gum, and patches)	Effect from smoking tobacco or to aid smoking cessation
	Adrenergic agents	Treatment of hypotension and shock
	Isoniazid	Antitubercular agent
	Loop diuretics	Treatment of hypertension

Increased theophylline levels result when the drug is taken with the interacting drug noted below.

Theophylline Serum Level	Interacting Drug	Common Use
	Allopurinol	Antigout agent
	Beta-adrenergic blockers	Treatment of hypertension
	Calcium channel blockers	Treatment of angina and hypertension
	Cimetidine	Treatment of gastrointestinal (GI) problems
	Oral contraceptives	Birth control
	Corticosteroids	Anti-inflammatory agents
	Influenza virus vaccine	Prevention of flu
	Macrolide, quinolone antibiotics	Treatment of infections
	Thyroid hormones	Treatment of hypothyroidism
	Isoniazid	Antitubercular agent
	Loop diuretics	Treatment of edema

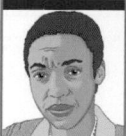

PHARMACOLOGY IN PRACTICE

SAFE DRUG ADMINISTRATION
A client was using a nicotine patch to stop smoking when they were started on theophylline for emphysema. After successfully stopping smoking and when ready to stop using the nicotine patch, which of following would be warranted?

1. Theophylline dose should be decreased
2. Theophylline should be discontinued
3. Theophylline dose should be increased
4. Theophylline dose should remain the same

ANTIASTHMA-SPECIFIC DRUGS

Long-term control medications are used daily to achieve and maintain control of persistent asthma. The most effective are those that reduce the underlying inflammation of asthma.

INHALED CORTICOSTEROIDS

ICSs are the most consistently effective long-term control medication at all steps of care for persistent asthma. ICS and LABA drugs may be combined to ease administration of the medications and produce positive outcomes in the management of asthma; these ICS/LABA combinations can be found in the Summary Drug Table: Lower Respiratory System Drugs.

ACTIONS

ICSs are anti-inflammatory medications that reduce airway hyperresponsiveness, reduce the number of mast cells in the airway, and block reaction to allergens. ICSs, such as beclomethasone (QVAR) or flunisolide (AeroBid), are given by inhalation and decrease the inflammatory process directly in the airways. In addition, the corticosteroids increase the sensitivity of the beta$_2$ receptors, which in turn increases the effectiveness of the beta$_2$-receptor agonist drugs.

USES

The ICSs are used in the management and prophylactic treatment of the inflammation associated with chronic asthma. In addition, a number of these preparations may be used intranasally for the treatment of nasal polyps and rhinitis (see Chapter 30). Special note—the brand names are different to reflect the difference in product use. See the Summary Drug Table in Chapter 30 for the intranasal steroids used for upper respiratory system conditions.

ADVERSE REACTIONS

When used to manage chronic asthma, the corticosteroids are most often given by inhalation. Systemic adverse reactions to the corticosteroids are less likely to occur when the drugs are given by inhalation rather than taken orally. Occasionally, clients may experience reactions.

Respiratory System Reactions
- Throat irritation
- Hoarseness
- Upper respiratory tract infection
- Fungal infection of the mouth and throat

See Chapter 41 for adverse reactions after oral administration of the corticosteroids. A more complete listing of the adverse reactions associated with the ICSs is found in the Summary Drug Table: Lower Respiratory System Drugs.

CONTRAINDICATIONS

The ICSs are contraindicated in clients with hypersensitivity to the corticosteroids, acute bronchospasm, status asthmaticus, or other acute episodes of asthma. Beclomethasone is contraindicated for the relief of symptoms that can be controlled by a bronchodilator and other nonsteroidal medications and in the treatment of nonasthmatic bronchitis.

PRECAUTIONS

The ICSs are used cautiously in clients with compromised immune systems, glaucoma, kidney disease, liver disease, convulsive disorders, and diabetes. Combining ICSs with systemic corticosteroids can increase the risk of hypothalamic–pituitary–adrenal (HPA) suppression, resulting in adrenal insufficiency. These drugs are also used with caution during pregnancy (pregnancy category C) and lactation (pregnancy category B—budesonide).

> **! NURSING ALERT**
>
> During periods of stress or a severe asthmatic attack, clients who have been withdrawn from systemic corticosteroids should be instructed to resume systemic steroids immediately and to contact the primary health care provider. Client deaths can result from adrenal insufficiency that may occur during and after transfer from systemic corticosteroids to ICSs.

INTERACTIONS

Ketoconazole may increase plasma levels of budesonide and fluticasone. To enhance client self-administration of different respiratory medications, a number have been formulated

TABLE 31.1 Examples of Respiratory Inhalant Combinations

GENERIC DRUG COMBINATIONS[a]	COMBINATION DRUG TRADE NAME
budesonide, formoterol	Symbicort
budesonide, formoterol, glycopyrrolate	Breztri Aerosphere
fluticasone, salmeterol	Advair, Airduo, Wixela
fluticasone, vilanterol	Breo Ellipta
fluticasone, vilanterol, umeclidinium	Trelegy Ellipta
formoterol, aclidinium	Duaklir Pressair
formoterol, glycopyrrolate	Bevespi Aerosphere
formoterol, mometasone	Dulera
glycopyrrolate, indacaterol	Utibron Neohaler
tiotropium, olodaterol	Stiolto Respimat
vilanterol, umeclidinium	Anoro Ellipta

[a]These drug combinations consist of two long-acting inhalants combined for additive therapeutic results to assist in the long-term management of airflow obstruction.

into combination products with both ICS and LABA in one inhaler (see Table 31.1 for examples).

MAST CELL STABILIZER

Cromolyn is a mast cell stabilizer. Other products are used for nasal and eye allergies.

ACTIONS

Although its action is not fully understood, this drug is thought to stabilize the mast cell membrane, possibly by preventing calcium ions from entering mast cells, thus preventing the release of inflammatory mediators such as histamine and leukotrienes.

USES

The mast cell stabilizer is used in combination with other drugs in the treatment of asthma and allergic disorders, including allergic rhinitis (nasal solution). It is also used to prevent EIB. They are typically used in step 2 care for chronic asthma (see Box 31.1).

ADVERSE REACTIONS

Respiratory System Reactions
- Throat irritation and dryness
- Unpleasant taste sensation
- Cough or wheeze

This drug may cause a nauseated feeling. A more complete listing of the adverse reactions associated with the mast cell stabilizer is found in the Summary Drug Table: Lower Respiratory System Drugs.

CONTRAINDICATIONS AND PRECAUTIONS

The mast cell stabilizer is contraindicated in clients with known hypersensitivity to the drugs and during attacks of acute asthma, because they may worsen bronchospasm during the acute asthma attack.

A mast cell stabilizer is used cautiously during pregnancy (pregnancy category B) and lactation and in clients with impaired renal or hepatic function.

INTERACTIONS

No significant drug interactions have been reported.

LEUKOTRIENE MODIFIERS AND IMMUNOMODULATORS

Leukotriene receptor antagonists include montelukast (Singulair) and zafirlukast (Accolate). Zileuton (Zyflo) is classified as a leukotriene formation inhibitor. Omalizumab (Xolair) is a monoclonal antibody used in the treatment of asthma; more information is provided about immunotherapy in Unit 12. Additional information concerning these drugs is found in the Summary Drug Table: Lower Respiratory System Drugs.

ACTIONS

Asthma attacks are often triggered by allergens or exercise. Inflammatory substances called *leukotrienes* are one of several substances that are released by mast cells during an asthma attack. Leukotrienes are primarily responsible for bronchoconstriction. When leukotriene production is inhibited, bronchodilation is facilitated. Zileuton (an inhibitor) acts by decreasing the formation of leukotrienes. Although the result is the same, montelukast and zafirlukast work in a manner slightly different from that of zileuton. Montelukast and zafirlukast are considered leukotriene receptor antagonists because they inhibit leukotriene receptor sites in the respiratory tract, preventing airway edema and facilitating bronchodilation. Omalizumab modulates the immune response by preventing the binding of immunoglobulin to the receptors on basophils and mast cells, thereby limiting the allergic reaction. The action of these drugs is illustrated in Figure 31.2, which shows how exposure to an allergen triggers the antibody response in the respiratory system.

USES

Leukotriene modifiers are used in the prophylaxis and treatment of chronic asthma in adults and children older than 12 years. Omalizumab is used as adjunctive therapy for clients 12 years of age and older who are sensitive to allergens (e.g., dust mites, cockroaches, cat or dog dander) and who require step 3 or higher care (see Box 31.1).

ADVERSE REACTIONS

- CNS reaction includes headache.
- Generalized body system reactions include flu-like symptoms.
- Immunomodulators may cause anaphylactic reactions.
- Emergency equipment should be available when administering this medication.

CONTRAINDICATIONS AND PRECAUTIONS

These drugs are contraindicated in clients with known hypersensitivity, bronchospasm in acute asthma attacks, or liver disease (zileuton). They should be used cautiously in pregnancy and not at all during lactation (zafirlukast, montelukast, and omalizumab are pregnancy category B drugs and zileuton is a pregnancy category C drug).

INTERACTIONS

The following interactions may occur when a leukotriene modifier is administered with another agent:

Interacting Drug	Common Use	Effect of Interaction
Aspirin	Pain relief	Increased plasma levels of zafirlukast
Warfarin	Anticoagulant	Increased anticoagulant effect
Theophylline	Treatment of asthma and COPD	Decreased level of zafirlukast; increased serum theophylline levels with zileuton use
Erythromycin	Treatment of bacterial infection	Decreased level of zafirlukast

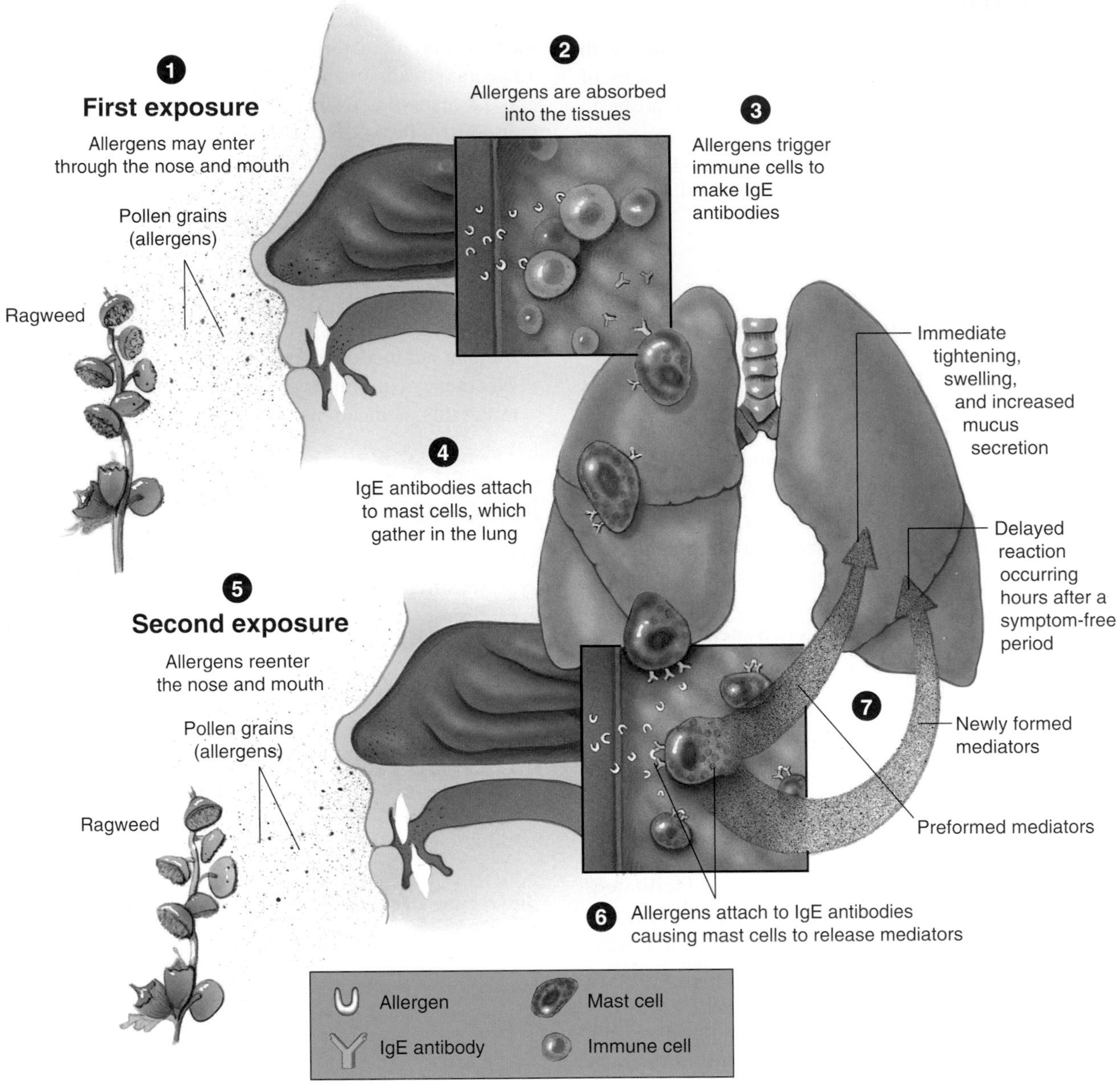

①
First exposure
Allergens may enter
through the nose and mouth

Pollen grains
(allergens)

Ragweed

②
Allergens are absorbed
into the tissues

③
Allergens trigger
immune cells to
make IgE
antibodies

④
IgE antibodies attach
to mast cells, which
gather in the lung

Immediate
tightening,
swelling,
and increased
mucus
secretion

Delayed
reaction
occurring
hours after a
symptom-free
period

⑤
Second exposure
Allergens reenter
the nose and mouth

Pollen grains
(allergens)

Ragweed

⑦

Newly formed
mediators

Preformed mediators

⑥
Allergens attach to IgE antibodies
causing mast cells to release mediators

∪ Allergen	Mast cell
Y IgE antibody	Immune cell

FIGURE 31.2   Exposure to allergen and immune response. (Courtesy of Anatomical Chart Co.)

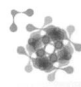

NURSING PROCESS: STEPS TO BUILDING CLINICAL JUDGMENT
Client Receiving a Lower Respiratory System Drug

ASSESSMENT

Preadministration Assessment

Because the bronchodilators or antiasthma drugs may be given for asthma, emphysema, or chronic bronchitis, the preadministration assessment of the client requires careful observation and documentation. Many respiratory problems are chronic conditions with acute exacerbations. Quick recognition and immediate action are essential in treating acute breathing problems. Long-term control of respiratory conditions consists of assessment and monitoring,

client education, environmental control, and medication management. Clients are encouraged to use asthma action plans for daily self-management and for acute respiratory exacerbations.

Action plans use a "traffic signal" approach to monitoring breathing status (Fig. 31.3). Clients are encouraged to monitor their own breathing and be alert for distress or by using a peak flow meter. Results are recorded on the plan in the green, yellow, and red zones, which signal an impending respiratory exacerbation,

ASTHMA ACTION PLAN

For: _____   Doctor: _____   Date: _____

Doctor's Phone Number: _____   Hospital/Emergency Department Phone Number: _____

GREEN ZONE

DOING WELL

- No cough, wheeze, chest tightness, or shortness of breath during the day or night
- Can do usual activities

And, if a peak flow meter is used,

Peak flow: more than _____
(80 percent or more of my best peak flow)

My best peak flow is: _____

Daily Medications

Medicine	How much to take	When to take it
_____	_____	_____
_____	_____	_____
_____	_____	_____
_____	_____	_____

Before exercise   ☐_____   ☐2 or ☐4 puffs   5 minutes before exercise

YELLOW ZONE

ASTHMA IS GETTING WORSE

- Cough, wheeze, chest tightness, or shortness of breath, or
- Waking at night due to asthma, or
- Can do some, but not all, usual activities

–Or–

Peak flow: _____ to _____
(50 to 79 percent of my best peak flow)

1st **Add: quick-relief medicine—and keep taking your GREEN ZONE medicine.**

_____   _____ Number of puffs   Can repeat every _____ minutes
(quick-relief medicine)   **or** ☐Nebulizer, once   up to maximum of _____ doses

2nd If your symptoms (and peak flow, if used) return to GREEN ZONE after 1 hour of above treatment:

☐Continue monitoring to be sure you stay in the green zone.

–Or–

If your symptoms (and peak flow, if used) do not return to GREEN ZONE after 1 hour of above treatment:

☐Take: _____   _____ Number of puffs **or** ☐Nebulizer
(quick-relief medicine)

☐Add: _____ mg per day For _____ (3–10) days
(oral steroid)

☐Call the doctor ☐before/ ☐within_____ hours after taking the oral steroid.

RED ZONE

MEDICAL ALERT!

- Very short of breath, or
- Quick-relief medicines have not helped, or
- Cannot do usual activities, or
- Symptoms are same or get worse after 24 hours in Yellow Zone

–Or–

Peak flow: less than _____
(50 percent of my best peak flow)

Take this medicine:

☐_____   _____ Number of puffs **or** ☐Nebulizer
(quick-relief medicine)

☐_____ mg
(oral steroid)

Then call your doctor NOW. Go to the hospital or call an ambulance if:

- You are still in the red zone after 15 minutes AND
- You have not reached your doctor.

DANGER SIGNS

- **Trouble walking and talking due to shortness of breath**
- **Lips or fingernails are blue**

➡ - Take _____ puffs of _____ (quick relief medicine) AND
- Go to the hospital or call for an ambulance _____ NOW!
(phone)

FIGURE 31.3 Example of Asthma Action Plan from the NHLBI, publication No. 20-HL-5251. (Adapted from National Heart, Lung and Blood Institute. (2020). *2020 Focused Updates to the Asthma Management Guidelines – Learn More, Breathe Better*. National Institutes of Health. https://www.nhlbi.nih.gov/health-topics/all-publications-and-resources/asthma-action-plan-2020)

depending on the color of the findings. Interventions for each section are listed using the stepwise approach as recommended by the primary health care provider.

Data gathering suggestions before the initial administration of the drug include:

Objective data

- Vital signs (temperature, pulse, respirations, and blood pressure)
- Pulse oximetry reading/peak flow meter readings if client has one
- Auscultate breath sounds (note any dyspnea, cough, wheezing, "noisy" respirations, or use of accessory muscles when breathing)
- Description of sputum (color, consistency, smell, blood)
- Signs of hypoxia (mental confusion, restlessness, anxiety)
- Cyanosis of skin or mucous membranes
- Laboratory tests—arterial blood gases or pulmonary function test

Subjective data

- Type and duration of symptoms (sputum description, chest pains)

- Description of any environmental triggers (see Fig. 31.4)
- Description of activity disruption by symptoms (activity changes)
- Health history especially regarding seasonal allergies or allergens in household
- Remedies attempted before seeking care

Pulse oximetry readings are dependent on the client's condition. A reading of 96% may indicate distress in a person without chronic disease, yet this may be the normal reading of a person with COPD.

When the client is able to talk comfortably, ask about possible triggers of the asthma attack causing the inability to breathe. Figure 31.4 illustrates common triggers of asthma. Has the client been around different environmental items, such as a new pet or changes in environmental temperature? Has the client been under undue stress either physically or emotionally? Has the client been monitoring lung function with a peak flow meter, and has a change been noted?

Ongoing Assessment

During an acute attack, assess the respiratory status about 30 min after a drug is administered or every 4 hr as the

Common Triggers of Asthma

Triggers are those factors that set off asthma symptoms. They may vary among asthmatics, making it important to identify which factors bring on an attack.

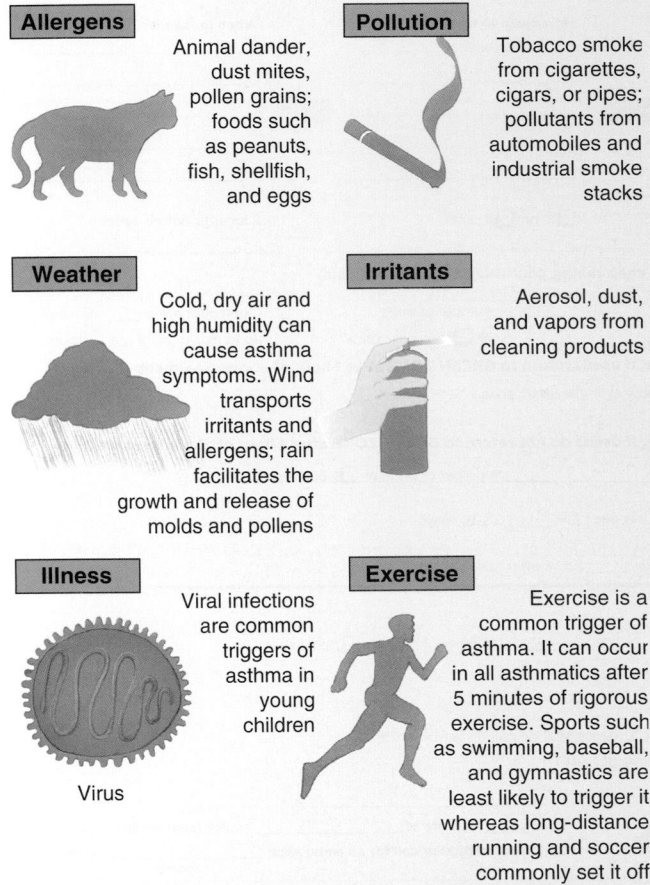

Allergens

Animal dander, dust mites, pollen grains; foods such as peanuts, fish, shellfish, and eggs

Pollution

Tobacco smoke from cigarettes, cigars, or pipes; pollutants from automobiles and industrial smoke stacks

Weather

Cold, dry air and high humidity can cause asthma symptoms. Wind transports irritants and allergens; rain facilitates the growth and release of molds and pollens

Irritants

Aerosol, dust, and vapors from cleaning products

Illness

Viral infections are common triggers of asthma in young children

Virus

Exercise

Exercise is a common trigger of asthma. It can occur in all asthmatics after 5 minutes of rigorous exercise. Sports such as swimming, baseball, and gymnastics are least likely to trigger it whereas long-distance running and soccer commonly set it off

FIGURE 31.4 Common triggers of asthma. (Courtesy of Anatomical Chart Co.)

client returns to a normal breathing pattern (or more often if needed). Note the respiratory rate, lung sounds, and use of accessory muscles in breathing. In addition, keep a careful record of the intake and output and report any imbalance, which may indicate a fluid overload or excessive diuresis.

During stable chronic phases the client assumes responsibility to monitor for changes. When an asthma action plan is used, the primary health care provider prescribes daily medications for the client as well as quick-relief medications. The client in turn monitors for symptoms such as wheezing and coughing, peak flow meter changes, and triggers that might be making the asthma worsen. During follow-up sessions ask the client about changes seen on the asthma action plan.

Has the client's condition stayed within the parameters of the green zone or has the client's status moved to the yellow or red zone? It is important to monitor any client with a history of cardiovascular problems for chest pain and changes in the electrocardiogram. The primary health care provider may order periodic pulmonary function tests, particularly for clients with emphysema or bronchitis, to help monitor respiratory status.

NURSING DIAGNOSES

Drug-specific nursing diagnoses include the following:

- **Anxiety** related to feelings of breathlessness
- **Ineffective airway clearance** related to bronchospasm
- **Impaired oral mucous membranes** related to dryness or irritation
- **Malnutrition risk: less than body requirements** related to decreased appetite caused by nausea, heartburn, or unpleasant taste

Nursing diagnoses related to drug administrations are discussed in Chapter 4.

PLANNING

The expected outcomes for the client depend on the specific reason for administering the drug but may include an optimal response to therapy, support of client needs related to managing adverse reactions, and confidence in an understanding of the medication regimen.

IMPLEMENTATION

Promoting an Optimal Response to Therapy

Nursing care of the client receiving a bronchodilating drug or an antiasthma drug requires careful monitoring of the client and instruction for proper administration of the various drugs. These drugs may be given orally, parenterally, or topically by inhalation or nebulization. Dosages are individualized for each client, which allows the smallest effective dose to be given.

Quick Relief for Acute Symptom Intervention

SABA bronchodilators are used to treat acute respiratory symptoms. Instruct the client to administer two to four puffs of the inhaled medication when acute distress occurs. Depending on the severity of the exacerbation, up to three treatments at 20-min intervals may be administered.

A **nebulizer** may be ordered to deliver the medication rather than an inhaler device (see Fig. 31.5). These devices are used when the inhaler is either difficult or ineffective. Often times in facilities or at home, nebulizers are used to help medications get directly to bronchial tissues

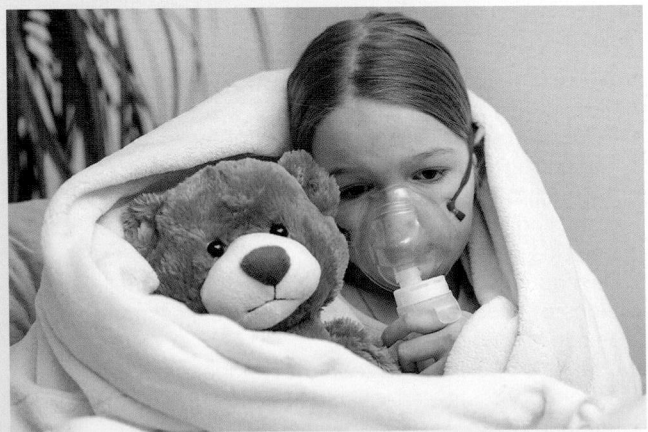

FIGURE 31.5 Nebulized medications may be more effective in vulnerable populations.

where they can have immediate effect. The following are examples of nebulizer use:

- ICS and SABA—to reduce inflammation and dilate bronchioles
- Racemic epinephrine—to relieve croup symptoms in children
- Antibiotics, mucolytics—treat lung infections or loosen secretions of clients with cystic fibrosis

 Lifespan Considerations

Gerontology

Older adults taking the adrenergic bronchodilators are at increased risk for adverse reactions related to both the cardiovascular system (tachycardia, arrhythmias, palpitations, and hypertension) and the CNS (restlessness, agitation, and insomnia).

If the client seeks care at an urgent or emergent facility, health care providers may administer epinephrine subcutaneously for an acute bronchospasm. Doses of drugs, such as epinephrine, are measured in tenths of a milliliter. Minimize distractions that may prevent you from reading the primary health care provider's order when preparing these drugs for administration to prevent error. Therapeutic effects occur within 5 min after administration and last as long as 4 hr. Anticholinergic medications or intravenous (IV) steroids may also be used when the situation is emergent.

Rapid **theophyllinization** using one of the xanthine derivatives may be required for acute respiratory symptoms. Clients are encouraged to use SABA inhalers as part of the Step Method to resolve acute respiratory symptoms, yet theophylline remains a low-cost effective alternative. Theophyllinization is accomplished by giving the client a higher initial dose, called a *loading dose,* to bring blood levels to a therapeutic range more quickly than waiting several days for the drug to exert a therapeutic effect. Typically this is achieved in an inpatient setting and the primary health care provider may prescribe loading doses to be administered orally or IV over 12–24 hr. It is important to monitor the client closely for signs of theophylline toxicity (Table 31.2). If a bronchodilator is given IV, it is administered through an infusion pump.

TABLE 31.2 Theophyllinization Process

Drug administered (IV or orally) over 12–24 hr		
Serum blood level measured 1–2 hr after dose (5–9 hr with sustained-release drug)		
Therapeutic range: 10–20 mcg/L	Monitor for toxicity: 15–20 mcg/L	Toxicity: +20 mcg/L
	Anorexia	Abdominal
	Nausea	cramping
	Vomiting	confusion
	Diarrhea	Restlessness
	Headache	Tachycardia
	Insomnia	Arrhythmias
		Seizures

Check the IV infusion site at frequent intervals, because these clients may be extremely restless and extravasation can occur.

Long-Term Control of Symptoms

Controlling respiratory mucosal inflammation is the goal of long-term medications. The stepwise method of self-care (see Box 31.1) is a guideline for clients and is the basis for an individualized plan made by the primary health care provider. Using the Step Method, clients manage the first step without daily medications. ICSs are used in the second step of the plan. It is important to remind the client to refrain from swallowing the medication and to rinse the mouth thoroughly after using the inhaler.

 Lifespan Considerations

Pediatric/Gerontology

When taking oral corticosteroids or higher doses of the inhalant form:

- Children are at risk for growth reduction. Document the client's growth record consistently, particularly during growth periods such as puberty and adolescence.
- For older adults at risk for osteoporosis, a calcium or vitamin D supplement may be prescribed.

Instruct the client to ensure confidence in understanding that the purpose of step care is a self-management program for worsening symptoms. Part of a step care program is to start the client on the lowest number and dosage of drugs that will treat the respiratory condition. As the client's breathing becomes distressed, doses are changed by the client, and different medications are added at each step. As the symptoms lessen, the client reduces medications, and the client's medication routine moves down a step. Providing emotional support and encouragement as the client makes adjustments in accordance with each step is a key factor to success.

The client learns to adjust according to daily experiences of breathing distress or peak expiratory flow readings. LABA bronchodilators are not administered more frequently than twice daily (morning and evening). LABA drugs, such as salmeterol or formoterol, do not replace the fast-acting inhalers for sudden symptoms, nor are they used to treat acute asthma symptoms. The drugs may be administered by a metered-dose inhaler (Box 31.2). If a dry-powder inhaler is used for administration, you should teach the client how to use it.

! NURSING ALERT

Formoterol (Foradil Aerolizer) comes in capsule form and is administered only by oral inhalation using the Aerolizer inhaler. Be sure to remind the client that this capsule is not to be taken orally.

The mast cell stabilizer cromolyn may be added to the client's existing treatment regimen (e.g., ICSs). If use of the mast cell stabilizer must be discontinued

BOX 31.2 Using a Metered-Dose Inhaler

How to Use an Inhaler

When a client is first diagnosed with asthma and prescribed inhalation therapy, they may need to learn how to use the inhaler that will deliver drug therapy. You may be the health care provider who supplies instructions such as these:

Metered-Dose Inhaler

1. When using a new inhaler, or one that has not been used in several days, point the inhaler away from you and prime the inhaler 1–2 times.
2. Hold the device upright and shake it.
3. Tilt the head back slightly.
4. Exhale and open mouth.
5. Position the inhaler in one of three ways:
   • Held 1–2 inches from the mouth (this is preferred)
   • Using a spacer
   • With the inhaler between the lips
6. Start to inhale slowly and press down on the inhaler to release the medication.
7. Breathe in for 3–5 seconds.

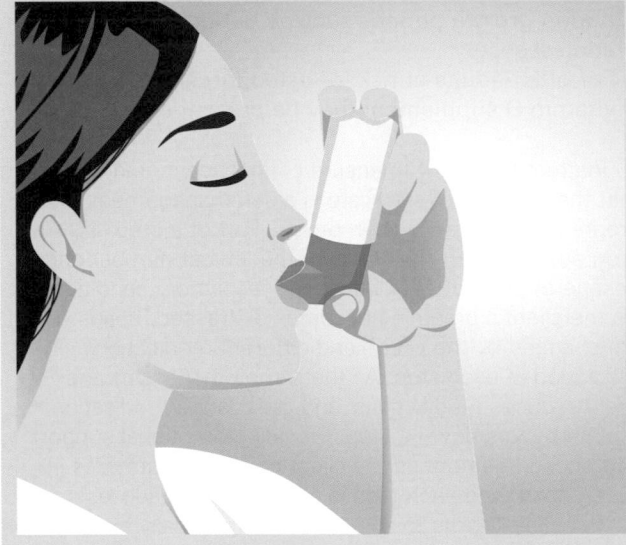

8. Hold your breath for 10 seconds to allow the drug to reach deep into the lungs.
9. Repeat for the ordered number of puffs, allowing 1 minute between each puff.

   Spacers are recommended for children, older adults, and anyone who has difficulty using a nebulizer alone. Spacers are indicated when using inhaled steroids.

Dry-Powder Inhaler

1. Prepare the medication for inhalation.
2. Place the mouthpiece to the lips.
3. Inhale quickly.
4. Hold your breath for 10 seconds to allow the drug to reach deep into the lungs.
5. Capsules for inhalation (such as those used in Foradil Aerolizer or Spiriva HaniHaler) must not be swallowed.
6. Do not place your device in water.

   When the client is prescribed more than one type of inhaler, instruct the client to use the bronchodilator first to open the air passages, and then use other prescribed medications.

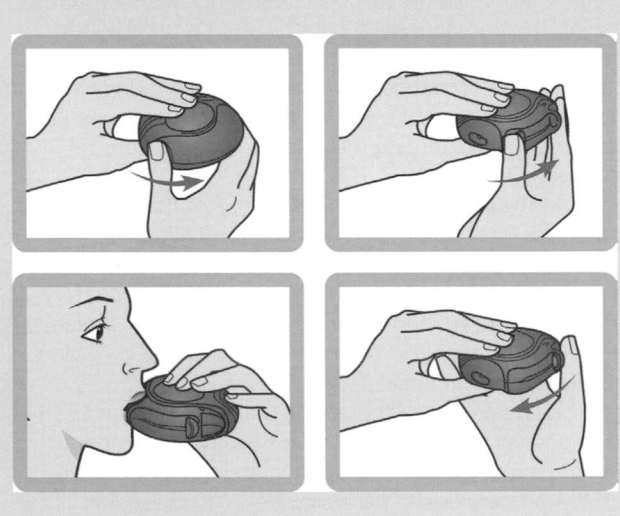

for any reason, the dosage is gradually tapered. When administered orally, cromolyn is given one-and-a-half hour before meals and at bedtime. The oral form of the drug comes in an ampule. The ampule is opened, and its contents are poured into a glass of water. The client or care provider stirs the mixture thoroughly. The client must drink all of the mixture. The drug may not be mixed with any other substance (e.g., fruit juice, milk, or foods).

Leukotriene receptor antagonists, leukotriene inhibitors, and immunomodulators are drugs used for managing asthma and are never administered during an acute asthma attack. If used during an acute attack, these drugs may worsen the attack. These drugs are administered orally.

Zileuton may cause liver damage. Because of the danger of liver toxicity, the primary health care provider may order hepatic aminotransferase levels at the beginning of treatment and during therapy. Clients are instructed to

immediately report any symptoms of liver dysfunction, such as upper right quadrant pain, nausea, fatigue, lethargy, pruritus, and jaundice. Clients may be hypersensitive to monoclonal antibodies (e.g., omalizumab), which are used to modulate the immune response. It is administered subcutaneously every 2–4 weeks (mepolizumab is administered monthly), typically in the clinic setting, where the client can be monitored after the injection for an anaphylactic reaction. Be sure to tell the client a reaction may occur up to 4 days following the injection and to have emergency contact information close at hand.

Monitoring and Managing Client Needs

Anxiety

Clients who have difficulty breathing and are receiving a bronchodilator or antiasthma drug may experience extreme anxiety, nervousness, and restlessness, which may be caused by their breathing difficulty or by the action of the drug. In these clients, it may be difficult for the primary health care provider to determine whether the client is having an adverse drug reaction or the problem is related to the respiratory disorder. Reassure the client that the drug being administered will most likely relieve the respiratory distress in a short time. Clients who are extremely apprehensive are observed more frequently until their respirations are near normal. Closely monitor the client's blood pressure and pulse during therapy and report any significant changes. If you remember to speak and act in a calm manner, this will help to decrease the anxiety or nervousness caused by the adrenergic drug. Explaining the effects of the drug may help the client to tolerate these uncomfortable adverse reactions.

Ineffective Airway Clearance

Occasionally the client may experience an acute bronchospasm either as a result of the disease, after exposure to an allergen, or as an adverse reaction to some antiasthma drugs, such as ICSs.

! NURSING ALERT

Acute bronchospasm causes severe respiratory distress and wheezing from the forceful expiration of air and is considered a medical emergency. Initiate medical intervention, or instruct the client and family to call emergency services if this happens at home.

During an acute bronchospasm, check the blood pressure, pulse, respiratory rate/pulse oximetry, and response to the drug every 5–15 min until the client's condition stabilizes and respiratory distress is relieved.

Impaired Oral Mucous Membranes

Inhalers, particularly the corticosteroid or mast cell aerosols, may cause throat irritation and promote infection with *Candida albicans*. Instruct the client to use strict oral hygiene, cleanse the inhaler as directed in the package directions, and use the proper technique when taking an inhalation. Using the ICS in conjunction with daily tooth brushing after treatment can also reduce the incidence of fungal infections. These interventions will decrease the incidence of candidiasis and help to soothe the throat. Occasionally an antifungal drug may be prescribed by the primary health care provider to manage the candidiasis.

Malnutrition Risk: Less Than Body Requirements

Some antiasthma drugs cause nausea. The client with nausea should be offered frequent smaller meals rather than three large meals. Meals should be followed by good mouth care. Limiting fluids with meals can help lessen nausea. Teach the family ways to provide a pleasant, relaxed atmosphere for meals.

The client taking theophylline may report heartburn, because the drug relaxes the lower esophageal sphincter, allowing gastroesophageal reflux. Heartburn is minimized if the client remains in an upright position and sleeps with the head of the bed elevated. Some antiasthma drugs may cause an unpleasant taste in the mouth. Asking the client

to take frequent sips of water, suck on sugarless candy, or chew gum helps to alleviate the problem.

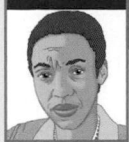

PHARMACOLOGY IN PRACTICE

MANAGING NEEDS

A client complains of nausea after receiving an antiasthma medication. Which of the following instructions should the nurse provide to alleviate the client's symptoms? Select all that apply.

1. Keep head end of bed elevated.
2. Eat frequent small meals.
3. Monitor blood pressure closely.
4. Limit fluids with meals.
5. Rinse mouth properly after eating.

Educating the Client and Family

Because of the chronic nature of respiratory illnesses, the nurse's role is to instruct the client and family in methods to monitor the condition, control triggers in the environment, and manage medications properly for optimal breathing.

Asthma action plans in multiple languages can be found on the Internet. You can provide websites to the client or demonstrate how to fill out the plans during a client teaching session. These can be printed, or the individual can fill out the information and use it to monitor daily asthma management and acute episodes.

Teach the client to monitor breathing status and regulate medications based on the asthma action plan. Demonstrate to the client how to fill in the medications prescribed to maintain optimal breathing. Then instruct the client to monitor their own breathing pattern based on zones defined by specific symptoms, peak flow meter readings, and corresponding adjusted medications as defined by the primary health care provider. A commonly used method to interpret breathing status is to relate it to the three colors of a traffic light: green, yellow, and red (see Fig. 31.3).

The client uses a peak flow meter at home to monitor breathing status and the effectiveness of the drug regimen. The client is taught how to use the peak flow meter and when to notify the primary health care provider (see Client Teaching for Improved Outcomes: Using a Peak Flow Meter). A majority of the medications prescribed will be delivered by inhalation. If the client is to use an aerosol inhaler for administration of the medication, provide thorough explanation of its use (see Box 31.2). Do not assume that the client understands how to use an aerosol inhaler correctly. Many different devices are on the market; these are used with specific medications and do not all work the same. Review the written instructions and examine the device with the client. Then have the client demonstrate the use of the inhaler to evaluate whether they are using the proper technique. It is important to review instructions at each follow-up visit.

Client Teaching for Improved Outcomes

Using a Peak Flow Meter

Clients receiving bronchodilators or antiasthma drugs often need to monitor their lung function at home with a peak flow meter. Doing so provides the client and the primary health care provider with valuable information about the status of the client's condition and the effectiveness of therapy. Often, trends in the readings can detect changes in the client's airway and airflow even before any signs and symptoms are experienced. This allows possible intervention before a major problem arises.

Because a variety of meters are commercially available, explain about the type of meter that will be used, how often the peak flow should be checked, and the ranges for the readings along with instructions on what to do for each range. Use the following steps to instruct the client on the use of the peak flow meter:

✔ Check to make sure that the indicator is at the lowest level of the scale.
✔ Stand upright to allow the best inhalation possible. (Be sure to remove gum or food from your mouth.)
✔ Inhale as deeply as you can and then place your lips around the mouthpiece, making sure you have a tight seal.
✔ Exhale as forcibly and as quickly as possible in one large "huff."
✔ Watch the indicator rise on the scale, noting where it stops. The number below the indicator's position is your *peak flow reading.*
✔ Repeat the procedure two more times.
✔ Compare the three readings. Record the highest reading on your action plan. Do not calculate an average.
✔ Bring the action plan with peak flow meter readings to your follow-up visits.
✔ Measure the peak flow rate close to the same time each day. (Your physician may provide you with a suggested time. Some clients measure the peak flow rate twice daily between 7 and 9 a.m and between 6 and 8 p.m. Others measure the peak flow rate before or after taking their medication.)
✔ Follow the medication instructions written on your action plan next to the zone color of your reading (see Fig. 31.3).
✔ Clean your meter with mild soap and hot water after use.

As the client becomes more confident in managing the asthma medications, you can begin to help the client assess the living environment. Box 31.3 describes ways to reduce or limit exposure to environmental triggers. Clients may be able to reduce asthma attacks if they feel they have control to modify exposure to the trigger elements.

As you develop a teaching plan for the client or family member, include the following points:

- Take the drug regularly as prescribed by the primary health care provider, even during symptom-free times. Long-acting medications are taken to prevent acute

BOX 31.3 Promoting Environmental Control for Asthma

You need to know what things bring on your asthma symptoms. Then do what you can to avoid or limit contact with these things.

- If animal dander is a problem for you, keep your pet out of the house or at least out of your bedroom, or find it a new home.
- Do not smoke or allow smoking in your home.
- If pollen is a problem for you, stay indoors with the air conditioner on, if possible, when the pollen count is high.
- To control dust mites, wash your sheets, blankets, pillows, and stuffed toys once a week in hot water. You can get special dust-proof covers for your mattress and pillows.
- If cold air bothers you, wear a scarf over your mouth and nose in the winter.
- If you have symptoms when you exercise or do routine physical activities like climbing stairs, work with your doctor to find ways to be active without having asthma symptoms. Physical activity is important.
- If you are allergic to sulfites, avoid foods (like dried fruit) or beverages (like wine) that contain them.

attacks and maintain a level of breathing—do not use to treat acute episodes of asthma.
- If symptoms become worse, increase the dose or frequency of use as directed to do so by the primary health care provider or as established in the action plan.
- Ask before using nonprescription drugs or herbal preparations. Some may contain similar drugs and may cause you to increase doses unknowingly.
- Check medications weekly to be sure you can reorder prescriptions and avoid running out of medication when stores are closed. Many inhalers have a counter on the back. Look to see how many treatments remain in the device.
- Do not chew or crush coated or sustained-release tablets.
- Be sure you understand how the inhaler unit is assembled, used, and cleaned.
- If LABAs are used for preventing EIB, the drug is administered at least 30 min before exercise. Additional doses are not to be given for at least 12 hr.
- *For clients using adrenergic bronchodilators*—these drugs may cause nervousness, insomnia, and restlessness. Contact the primary health care provider if the symptoms become severe.
- *For clients using xanthine derivatives*—follow your primary health care provider's instructions concerning monitoring of theophylline serum levels. Avoid foods that contain xanthine, such as colas, coffee, chocolate, and charcoal-prepared foods.
- *For clients using ICSs*—wear a medical alert item (e.g., bracelet) indicating the need for supplemental systemic steroids in the event of stress or severe asthmatic attack that is unresponsive to bronchodilators. Do not stop therapy abruptly.
- *For clients using immunomodulators*—be aware that an anaphylactic reaction can occur for up to a year after

dosing. Contact the primary health care provider should you begin itching or get hives, and seek emergent care if you have trouble breathing.

EVALUATION

- Therapeutic response is achieved and breathing is easier and more effective.
- Adverse reactions are identified, reported to the primary health care provider, and managed successfully with appropriate nursing interventions:
  - Anxiety is managed successfully.
  - Client has a clear patent airway.
  - Mucous membranes are moist and intact.
  - Nutrition is adequately maintained.
- Client and family express confidence and demonstrate an understanding of the drug regimen and use of both the peak flow meter and inhalator device.

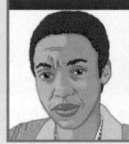

PHARMACOLOGY IN PRACTICE

USING CLINICAL REASONING

Mrs. Chase has been diagnosed with asthma by her primary care provider, and the following plan is established:
- Goal of peak flow meter should be 350.
- Asmanex Twisthaler 1 puff daily at bedtime.
- Albuterol inhaler, 2 puffs 30 min before exercise, or if peak flow reading is in yellow zone, or if feel short of breath.
- Call for medication changes if in red zone.

Mrs. Chase remarks that she does not want to use the inhaler because when her older mother used inhaled medication it smelled like rotten eggs.

KEY POINTS

■ COPD includes asthma, chronic bronchitis, obstructive bronchitis, and emphysema, or any combination of these conditions. Asthma is a chronic lung condition causing spasmodic constriction of the bronchi and lung inflammation. Many Americans suffer from the ailment, and it is one of the most common childhood chronic conditions.

■ Bronchodilators are used for clients with COPD who experience difficulty breathing (dyspnea) and an interference of gas exchange at the alveoli level in the lungs.

■ Antiasthma drugs are used for both long-term management and short-term breathing relief. Guidelines for medication use are called the Step Method. ICSs reduce inflammation, while bronchodilators relieve bronchospasm. Providers define parameters and help the client make an asthma action plan to help the client in self-management of the condition.

■ Common adverse reactions to the medications include nervousness and restlessness, nausea, anorexia, vomiting, and tachycardia, or the feeling of heart palpitations.

SUMMARY DRUG TABLE
Lower Respiratory System Drugs

Generic Name	Trade Name	Uses	Adverse Reactions	Dosage Ranges
Bronchodilators				
Short-Acting Beta₂ Agonists (SABAs—Adrenergics or Sympathomimetics Used for Acute Symptom Relief)				
albuterol *al-BYOO-ter-ole*	Proventil, Ventolin	Bronchospasm, prevention of EIB	Headache, palpitations, tachycardia, tremor, dizziness, shakiness, nervousness, hyperactivity	2–4 mg TID, QID orally; 1–2 inhalations q4–6hr; 2 inhalations before exercise; may also be given by nebulizer
EPHEDrine *e-FED-rin*		Asthma, bronchospasm	Precordial pain, urinary hesitancy	12.5–25 mg orally q3–4hr PRN; 25–50 mg IM, subcut, IV
EPINEPHrine *ep-i-NEF-rin*	Adrenalin	Asthma, bronchospasm	Palpitations, tremor, dizziness, drowsiness, vertigo, shakiness, nervousness, headache, nausea, vomiting, anxiety, fear, pallor	Inhalation aerosol: individualize dose Injection: solution 1:1000, 0.3–0.5 mL subcut, IM suspension (1:200), 0.1–0.3 mL subcut only
levalbuterol *leve-al-BYOO-ter-ole*	Xopenex	Treat and prevent bronchospasm	Tachycardia, nervousness, anxiety, pain, dizziness, rhinitis, cough, cardiac arrhythmias	0.63 mg TID, q6–8hr by nebulization; if no response, dose may be increased to 1.25 mg TID by nebulizer
metaproterenol *met-a-proe-TER-e-nol*		Asthma, bronchospasm	Tachycardia, tremor, nervousness, shakiness, nausea, vomiting	20 mg TID orally, aerosol 2–3 inhalations q3–4hr; do not exceed 12 inhalations
terbutaline *ter-BYOO-ta-leen*		Treat and prevent bronchospasm	Palpitations, tremor, dizziness, vertigo, shakiness, nervousness, drowsiness, headache, nausea, vomiting, GI upset	2.5–5 mg q6hr orally TID during waking hours; 0.25 mg subcut (may repeat once if needed)

Continued

SUMMARY DRUG TABLE (continued)
Lower Respiratory System Drugs

Generic Name	Trade Name	Uses	Adverse Reactions	Dosage Ranges
Long-Acting Beta₂ Agonists (LABAs—Adrenergics or Sympathomimetics Used for Long-Term Management)				
arformoterol ar-for-MOE-ter-ol	Brovana	Long-term treatment and prevention of bronchospasm in COPD	Nervousness, tremor, dizziness, headache, insomnia, nausea, vomiting, diarrhea, leg cramps, back pain	15-mcg inhalation BID morning and evening
formoterol for-MOH-te-rol	Perforomist	Long-term treatment and prevention of bronchospasm	Palpations, tachycardia, dizziness, nervousness	One 12-mg capsule q12hr using inhalation device, not for oral use; EIB use 15 min before exercise
indacaterol in-da-KA-ter-ol	Arcapta Neohaler	Long-term treatment and prevention of bronchospasm	Palpations, tachycardia, weakness, cramping, thirst, increased urination	One 75-mcg capsule daily
olodaterol oh-loe-DA-ter-ol	Striverdi Respimat	Long-term treatment of COPD, not approved for asthma	Nasopharyngitis	Two inhalations once daily
salmeterol sal-ME-te-role	Serevent Diskus	Long-term treatment and prevention of bronchospasm	Tremor, headache, cough	One inhalation BID morning and evening; inhalation powder, do not use spacer
Xanthine Derivatives				
aminophylline am-in-OFF-i-lin		Symptomatic relief or prevention of bronchial asthma and reversible bronchospasm of chronic bronchitis and emphysema	Nausea, vomiting, restlessness, nervousness, tachycardia, tremors, headache, palpitations, hyperglycemia, electrocardiographic changes, cardiac arrhythmias	Individualize dosage: base adjustments on clinical responses, monitor serum aminophylline levels, maintain therapeutic range of 10–20 mcg/mL; base dosage on lean body mass
dyphylline DYE-fi-lin	Lufyllin	Same as aminophylline	Same as aminophylline	Up to 15 mg/kg orally q6hr
theophylline thee-OFF-i-lin	Theochron	Same as aminophylline	Same as aminophylline	Initial dosing: 16 mg/kg/day or 400 mg/day
Cholinergic Blocking Drug (Anticholinergics Used for Long-Term Management)				
aclidinium a-kli-DIN-ee-um	Tudorza Pressair	Prevention of bronchospasm associated with COPD, chronic bronchitis and emphysema	Headache, cough, sinus irritation, vomiting, diarrhea, toothache, urinary tract infection	400-mcg inhalation twice daily
ipratropium i-pra-TROE-pee-um	Atrovent	Bronchospasm associated with COPD, chronic bronchitis and emphysema, rhinorrhea	Dryness of the oropharynx, nervousness, irritation from aerosol, dizziness, headache, GI distress, dry mouth, exacerbation of symptoms, nausea, palpitations	Aerosol: 2 inhalations QID, not to exceed 12 inhalations. Solution: 500 mg (1 unit dose vial) TID, QID by oral nebulization. Nasal spray: 2 sprays per nostril BID, TID of 0.03%, or 2 sprays per nostril TID, QID of 0.06%
revefenacin REV-e-FEN-a sin	Yupelri	Bronchospasm associated with COPD	Dryness of the oropharynx, nervousness, irritation from aerosol, dizziness, headache, increased blood pressure	One metered dose daily (175 mcg)
tiotropium ty-oh-TRO-pee-um	Spiriva	Same as ipratropium	Same as ipratropium, increased stroke potential	One capsule per day using inhalation device, not for oral use
umeclidinium ue-me-kli-DIN-ee-um	Incruse Ellipta	Prevention of bronchospasm associated with COPD, chronic bronchitis and emphysema	Stuffy nose, cough, sore throat, muscle–joint–tooth pain, rapid heartbeat	62.5-mcg inhalation once daily

Generic Name	Trade Name	Uses	Adverse Reactions	Dosage Ranges
Antiasthma Drugs				
Inhaled Corticosteroids				
beclomethasone *be-kloe-METH-a-sone*	QVAR	Maintenance treatment of asthma	Oral, laryngeal, pharyngeal irritation; fungal infections; suppression of HPA function	Starting dose used with bronchodilators alone: 40–80 mcg BID; when used with ICSs: 40–160 mcg BID; maximum 310 mcg BID Children 5–12 years: 40 mcg BID when used with bronchodilators alone or with ICSs
budesonide *byoo-DES-oh-nide*	Pulmicort	Maintenance treatment of asthma	Same as beclomethasone	Individualized dosage by oral inhalation Adults: 200–800 mcg BID Children 6 years and older: 200–400 mcg BID Children 12 months–8 years: 0.5–1 mcg total daily dose administered once or twice daily in divided doses
ciclesonide *sye-KLES-oh-nide*	Alvesco	Prophylactic maintenance and treatment of asthma	Same as beclomethasone	Up to 320 mcg twice daily inhaled
flunisolide *floo-NISS-oh-lide*		Maintenance treatment of asthma, especially those on systemic corticosteroid therapy	Same as beclomethasone	Adults: 2 inhalations BID; maximum dose, 4 inhalations BID Children 6–15 years: 2 inhalations BID
fluticasone *floo-TIK-a-sone*	Flovent HFA, Flovent Diskus	Prophylactic maintenance and treatment of asthma	Same as beclomethasone	88–880 mcg BID
mometasone *mo-MET-a-sone*	Asmanex	Maintenance treatment of asthma	Same as beclomethasone	One inhalation (220 mcg) QD in the evening for clients previously maintained on bronchodilators alone or ICSs; 2 inhalations (440 mcg) BID for clients previously maintained on oral corticosteroids
Mast Cell Stabilizer				
cromolyn *KROE-moe-lin*	Gastrocrom	Bronchial asthma, prevention of bronchospasm, prevention of EIB Nasal preparations: prevention and treatment of allergic rhinitis	Cough, wheeze, unusual taste, dizziness, headache, nausea, dry and irritated throat, rash, joint swelling, and pain	Inhalation solution: 20 mg (1 ampule/vial) administered by nebulizer QID Aerosol: adults and children 5 years and older: 2 metered sprays QID EIB: 2 metered sprays shortly (10–15 min but not more than 60 min) before exposure to the precipitating factor Nasal solution: 1 spray each nostril 3–6 times/day Oral: adults and children 13 years and older: 2 ampules QID 30 min before meals and at bedtime Children 2–12 years: 1 ampule QID before meals and at bedtime; do not exceed 40 mg/kg/day

Continued

SUMMARY DRUG TABLE (continued)
Lower Respiratory System Drugs

Generic Name	Trade Name	Uses	Adverse Reactions	Dosage Ranges
Leukotriene Modifiers and Immunomodulators				
benralizumab *ben-ra-LIZ-ue-mab*	Fasenra	Adjunct for severe asthma	Headache, pharyngitis, antibody development	30 mg subcut every 4 weeks for 3 doses, then every 8 weeks
dupilumab *doo-PIL-ue-mab*	Dupixent	Adjunct for severe asthma	Eye irritation, injection site irritation, antibody development	100 mg subcut every 2 weeks
mepolizumab *me-poe-LIZ-ue-mab*	Nucala	Adjunct for severe asthma	Headache, injection site irritation, antibody development	100 mg subcut once a month
montelukast *mon-te-LOO-kast*	Singulair	Prophylaxis and treatment of chronic asthma in adults and pediatric clients 12 months and older, seasonal allergic rhinitis in adults and pediatric clients 2 years and older	Headache, influenza-like symptoms	Adults and children older than 15 years: 10 mg orally in the evening Children 6–14 years: one 5-mg chewable tablet daily, in the evening Children 1–5 years: one 4-mg chewable tablet daily, in the evening, or one 4-mg oral granule packet daily
omalizumab *oh-mah-lye-ZOO-mab*	Xolair	Moderate to severe persistent asthma	Injection site reaction, anaphylaxis	150–375 mg subcut every 2–4 weeks
reslizumab *res-LIZ-ue-mab*	Cinqair	Adjunct for severe asthma	Increased creatine, antibody development	3 mg/kg IV every 4 weeks
roflumilast *roe-FLUE-mi-last*	Daliresp	Severe COPD—phosphodiesterase inhibitor	Diarrhea	500 mcg orally daily
zafirlukast *za-FIR-loo-kast*	Accolate	Prophylaxis and treatment of chronic asthma in adults and children 5 years or older	Same as montelukast	Adults and children older than 12 years: 20 mg orally BID Children 5–11 years: 10 mg orally BID
zileuton *zye-LOO-ton*	Zyflo	Prophylaxis and treatment of chronic asthma in adults and children 12 years or older	Dyspepsia, nausea, headache	600 mg orally QID

CHAPTER REVIEW

Know Your Drugs

Clients sometimes know a medication by the brand (or trade) name and not the generic name. To help you recognize both names, match the brand name with the generic name of the same medication.

Generic Name	Brand Name
1. albuterol	A. Asmanex
2. mometasone	B. Proventil
3. montelukast	C. Singulair
4. tiotropium	D. Spiriva

Calculate Medication Dosages

1. A client is prescribed 0.25 mg of terbutaline subcutaneously. The drug is available for injection in a solution of 1 mg/mL. The nurse administers _____.

2. The client is prescribed zafirlukast 20 mg orally BID. The drug is available in 10-mg tablets. The nurse administers _____. How many milligrams of zafirlukast will the client receive each day?

Prepare for the NCLEX

RECALL THE FACTS

1. COPD does not include which of the following conditions?
   1. Acute asthma
   2. Acute pneumonia
   3. Chronic bronchitis
   4. Emphysema
2. Which of the following actions are accomplished when using bronchodilators?
   1. Reduce inflammatory response
   2. Promote mucus removal

3. Reverse bronchoconstriction

4. Remove fluid from the lungs

3. When the SABA drugs are administered to older adults, there is a greater increased risk of _____.
   1. GI effects
   2. nephrotoxic effects
   3. neurotoxic effects
   4. cardiovascular effects

4. When administering aminophylline, a xanthine derivative bronchodilating drug, the nurse monitors the client for adverse reactions, which include _____.
   1. restlessness and nervousness
   2. hypoglycemia and hypothyroidism
   3. bradycardia and bronchospasm
   4. somnolence and lethargy

5. The nurse correctly administers montelukast (Singulair) _____.
   1. once daily in the evening
   2. twice daily in the morning and evening
   3. three times a day with meals
   4. once daily in the morning

ANALYZE THE FACTS

6. *Which of the following laboratory tests would the nurse expect to be ordered for a client taking Theolair?
   1. Thyroid hormone levels
   2. Alanine aminotransferase
   3. Sodium electrolytes
   4. Serum theophylline levels

7. The body reacts to a trigger and stimulates the sympathetic branch of the nervous system causing bronchoconstriction and inflammation. Which neurotransmitter is stimulated?
   1. Serotonin
   2. Norepinephrine
   3. Dopamine
   4. Acetylcholine

8. The following statement indicates that the client understands the purpose of the peak flow meter.
   1. "I use the peak flow meter when I am short of breath."
   2. "I must wash the peak flow meter after every use."
   3. "I should measure my peak flow every day."
   4. "I put the medicine in the peak flow meter."

ALTERNATE-FORMAT QUESTIONS

9. The drug Advair is a combination of different medications. Which drugs are in this inhaler? **Select all that apply.**
   1. Fluticasone
   2. Omalizumab
   3. Salmeterol
   4. Zafirlukast

10. The drug Advair is a combination of which drug categories? **Select all that apply.**
    1. Corticosteroids
    2. Immunomodulators
    3. Long-acting beta$_2$ agonists
    4. Xanthine derivatives

To check your answers, see Appendix F.

_____

*Indicates the question is directly linked to the NCLEX-PN test plan in Appendix G.

WANT TO KNOW MORE? A wide variety of resources are available to enhance your learning and understanding of this chapter.

- Visit the**Point** for resources such as:
  - NCLEX-Style Student Review Questions
  - Journal Articles
  - Dosage Calculations
  - Drug Monographs
  - Watch and Learn Videos
  - Concepts in Action Animations
- The *Study Guide to Accompany Introductory Clinical Pharmacology*, 12th edition, sold separately, will help you review and apply essential content.
- ✓**PrepU** is available to help students prepare for the NCLEX-PN examination.

UNIT 8
Drugs That Affect the Cardiovascular System

The cardiovascular system includes the heart and all the blood vessels of the body, down to the tiniest capillaries, both arterial and venous. The circulatory system brings nutrients to the body tissues and takes away waste products from those same cells. Thus, our bodies can work properly when the heart pumps effectively and the blood vessels move fluid without blockage or restriction.

Cardiovascular disease (CVD) is one condition that hampers this process. One out of every three deaths in the United States is due to heart-associated causes (Virani et al., 2020). Coronary heart disease (CHD) is the single largest killer of both men and women in the United States. These seem like high numbers, yet the death rate from CHD and stroke has decreased by 68% from 1969 to 2013 (American Heart Association, 2016). This is due in part to advances in diagnosis, treatment, and changes in lifestyle. In this unit, you will learn how drugs continue to play an important role in all stages of heart health or disease. The drugs discussed in this unit range from those used early in treatment (such as diuretics) to drugs used in critical care units when advanced disease is present.

In this unit, the first few chapters discuss drugs used to reduce risk of CVDs. Individuals at risk for hypertension require health-promoting lifestyle modifications to prevent CVD. When these efforts are not enough, the addition of some medications may support risk reduction of CVD. Chapter 32 discusses the use of diuretics. These drugs make the kidneys filter more effectively and remove fluid as well as waste products from the body. Although the kidney is the target organ of these drugs, fluid removal is necessary for some clients to promote cardiac function. Sometimes, reducing fluid, along with lifestyle changes, is all that is necessary to reduce blood pressure.

Another heart health concern is cholesterol. Chapter 33 features the cholesterol-lowering drugs or antihyperlipidemic drugs. As blood cholesterol levels increase, so does the risk of CHD. In general, the higher the low-density lipoprotein (LDL) level and the more risk factors involved, the greater the risk for heart disease. Atherosclerosis is a condition characterized by deposits of fatty plaques on the inner walls of arteries. Lowering blood cholesterol levels can arrest or reverse atherosclerosis in the vessels and can significantly decrease the incidence of heart disease.

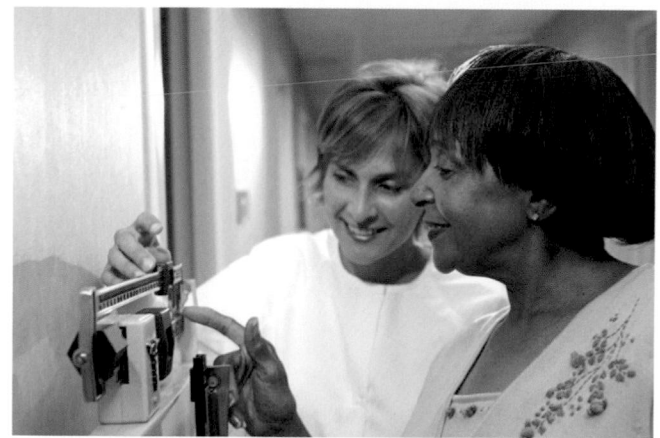

Diuretics alone do not always reduce blood pressure sufficiently. Chapter 34 introduces specific drugs used to treat hypertension when diuretics alone do not work to reduce blood pressure. Some of those include adrenergic-blocking drugs, angiotensin-converting enzyme (ACE) inhibitors, calcium channel blockers, and other inhibitors or antagonists. Hypertension, if untreated, can lead to dysfunction not only in the cardiovascular system but also in other systems such as the renal and respiratory systems. In individuals between the ages of 40 and 70 years, every increase of 20 mm Hg in systolic pressure or every increase of 10 mm Hg in diastolic pressure doubles the risk of CVD (Virani, 2020).

Treating hypertension early reduces the risk for CVD and death. Additionally, medications can protect against hypertension-related complications such as stroke, heart failure (HF), and kidney disease. Chapter 35 discusses the antianginal drugs whose primary purpose is to increase blood supply to an area by dilating blood vessels. Sharp pains in the chest, jaw, or arm may be one of the first times a person will stop and consider their cardiac status. This is because the narrowing of the arteries (due to disease) results in pain when tissues are denied oxygen.

Blockage of the vessels in the form of blood clots can occur in the cardiovascular system. Drug therapy for vascular diseases may include drugs that dilate blood vessels and thereby increase blood supply to an area. Chapter 36 discusses drugs used to prevent (anticoagulants or antiplatelets) and drugs used to remove (thrombolytics) blood clots from the blood vessels.

When tissues become more compromised, other diseases occur. Almost 6.2 million Americans have heart failure (HF) (previously referred to as *congestive HF*). It is the most frequent cause of hospitalization for individuals older than 65 years. African Americans and obese individuals are at the highest risk for HF (Virani, 2020). With treatment, some clients may lead nearly normal lives, although more than 380,000 individuals with HF die each year (Virani, 2020). The ACE inhibitors are considered the first-choice treatment and are the cornerstones of HF drug therapy. These drugs are discussed in terms of their ability to reduce hypertension. Digoxin (a cardiotonic drug) is prescribed for clients with HF who do not respond to the ACE inhibitors and diuretics. Many older adults may continue to use a cardiotonic, for example, digoxin, discussed in Chapter 37. Because HF and cardiac arrhythmias are found together clinically, this chapter includes the antiarrhythmic drugs.

As you progress through this unit, you will notice that some of the drug classes may be repeated in multiple chapters. This is because their use effectively reduces death from heart disease, the reason we administer these medications to our clients.

32

Diuretics

Key Terms

anuria   cessation of urine production

azotemia   absence of urine production

diuresis   production of urine

edema   accumulation of excess water in the body

gynecomastia   male breast enlargement

hyperkalemia   increase in potassium levels in the blood

hypokalemia   low blood potassium level

Learning Objectives

On completion of this chapter, the student will:

1. List the five general types of diuretics.
2. Explain the uses, general drug actions, adverse reactions, contraindications, precautions, and interactions of the diuretics.
3. Distinguish important preadministration and ongoing assessment activities that the nurse should perform on the client taking a diuretic.
4. List nursing diagnoses particular to a client taking a diuretic.
5. Examine ways to promote an optimal response to therapy, how to manage common adverse reactions, and important points to keep in mind when educating clients about the use of diuretics.

 Drug Classes

Loop diuretics	Osmotic diuretics
Thiazides and related diuretics	Carbonic anhydrase inhibitors
Potassium-sparing diuretics	

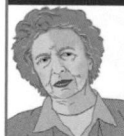 **PHARMACOLOGY IN PRACTICE**

You are concerned about Mrs. Moore because of the increase in calls from her out-of-town daughter. It is time to do a medication reconciliation. When she brings in a bag of pills, you find that a prescription bottle for a daily diuretic filled 3 weeks ago is almost full. As you read on see if you can determine what questions to ask Mrs. Moore.

When studying about cardiac conditions, you may wonder what a drug that affects the kidney has to do with the heart. Hypertension, a cardiac condition, is often initially treated by reducing body fluids using a diuretic, or what many clients call "a water pill." Therefore, we start the cardiac unit with a group of drugs whose site of action is the kidneys—the diuretics.

Many conditions or diseases, such as heart failure (HF), endocrine disturbances, and kidney and liver diseases, can cause fluid overload or **edema** (retention of excess fluid). When the client shows signs of excess fluid retention, the primary health care provider (PHCP) may prescribe a diuretic to reduce the increased fluid. A diuretic is a drug that increases the excretion of urine (i.e., water, electrolytes, and waste products) by the kidneys. There are various types of diuretic drugs, and the PHCP selects the one that best suits the client's needs and effectively reduces the amount of excess fluid in body tissues.

Because hypertension and other cardiac conditions require reduction of circulatory volume (or fluid), we frequently prescribe the administration of an antihypertensive drug and a diuretic. The diuretics used for this combination therapy include the loop diuretics and the thiazides. The specific uses of each type of diuretic drug are discussed in the following sections.

ACTIONS

Diuretics work by altering the excretion or reabsorption of electrolytes (sodium and chloride) in the kidney. In turn, this determines the amount of water that is reabsorbed in the kidney or the amount that becomes urine and is eliminated in the genitourinary system. Refer to the illustration of the nephron in the kidney (Fig. 32.1) for a better understanding of the actions as you read about the diuretics.

- *Loop diuretics* inhibit reabsorption of sodium and chloride in the ascending portion of the loop of Henle. A high percentage of sodium is typically reabsorbed here as is fluid. By blocking this action, this group of drugs is very effective as diuretics.
- *Thiazide and related diuretics* inhibit the reabsorption of sodium and chloride ions in the early distal tubule of the nephron. This action results in the excretion of sodium, chloride, and water. Thiazides are often the first drug used in the treatment of hypertension (Mayo Clinic, 2019).

Both these diuretic groups will also cause the electrolyte potassium to be excreted in urine, thus resulting in the potential of causing the client to become hypokalemic. If there is an issue of maintaining potassium in the body, another type of diuretic may be used.

- *Potassium-sparing diuretics* (or potassium saving) reduce the excretion of potassium from the kidney. Potassium-sparing diuretics work by blocking the reabsorption of sodium in the collecting tubules, thereby increasing sodium and water in the urine; this reduces the excretion of potassium. Spironolactone (Aldactone) works to antagonize the action of aldosterone. Aldosterone, a hormone produced by the adrenal cortex, enhances the reabsorption of sodium in the distal convoluted tubules of the kidney. When this is blocked by the drug, sodium (but not potassium) and water are excreted.
- *Osmotic diuretics* increase the density of the filtrate in the glomerulus. This prevents selective reabsorption of water, and it passes out as urine. Sodium and chloride excretion is also increased.
- *Carbonic anhydrase inhibitors* are sulfonamides, without bacteriostatic action, that inhibit the enzyme carbonic anhydrase. Carbonic anhydrase inhibition results in the excretion of sodium, potassium, bicarbonate, and water.

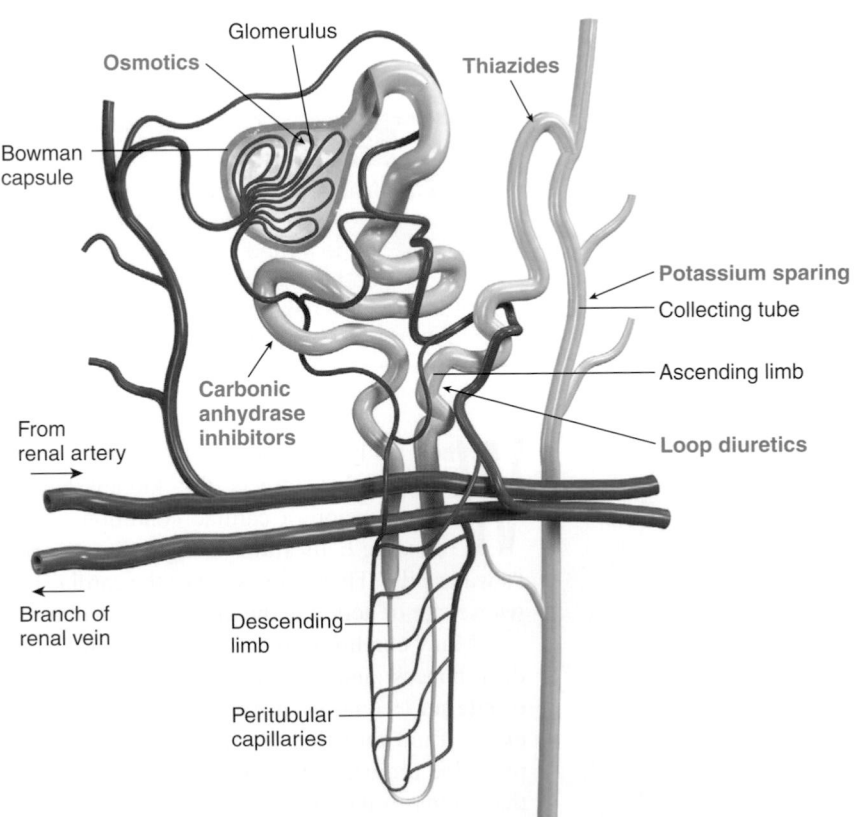

FIGURE 32.1 The nephron is the functional unit of the kidney. Note where the various diuretic drug classes work on the various tubules of the kidney nephron.

TABLE 32.1 Diuretic Combination Drugs

GENERIC DRUGS[a]	COMBINATION DRUG TRADE NAME
hydrochlorothiazide/amiloride hydrochloride	
hydrochlorothiazide/spironolactone	Aldactazide
hydrochlorothiazide/triamterene	Dyazide, Maxide

[a]These drug combinations consist of a diuretic and other agent or two diuretics combined to treat specific types of fluid retention or buildup.

USES

Diuretic drugs are used in the treatment of the following:

- Hypertension.
- Edema (fluid retention) associated with HF, corticosteroid/estrogen therapy, and cirrhosis of the liver.
- Renal disease (acute failure, renal insufficiency, and nephrotic syndrome).
- Cerebral edema.
- Seizures and altitude sickness.
- Spironolactone is used for male-to-female hormonal therapy for gender dysphoria.
- Infrequently for acute glaucoma (topically) and increased intraocular pressure (IOP; before and after eye surgery).

Ethacrynic acid (a loop diuretic) is also used for the short-term management of ascites caused by malignancy, idiopathic edema, or lymphedema. When clients are at risk for potassium loss, the potassium-sparing diuretics may be used with or in place of other categories of diuretics. Combination drugs have been developed to help reduce fluid, when one agent is not sufficient for fluid reduction and may be ordered for specific situations, see Table 32.1. These drugs are useful in treating clients who may be more likely to become hypokalemic or have severe edema from HF, cirrhosis, or nephrotic syndrome. Typically these drugs are not used initially to treat hypertension.

 NURSING ALERT

Nonprescription diuretics (e.g., Aqua-Ban) may be taken to relieve premenstrual bloating. These products typically are composed of caffeine and ammonium chloride. Be aware, people may use these drugs for weight loss, causing electrolyte imbalances.

ADVERSE REACTIONS

Adverse reactions associated with any category of diuretics involve various body systems.

Neuromuscular System Reactions
- Dizziness, lightheadedness, headache
- Weakness, fatigue

Cardiovascular System Reactions
- Orthostatic hypotension
- Electrolyte imbalances, glycosuria

Gastrointestinal System Reactions
- Anorexia
- Nausea, vomiting

Other System Reactions

Dermatologic reactions include rash and photosensitivity. Extremity paresthesias (numbness or tingling) or flaccid muscles may indicate **hypokalemia** (low blood potassium levels). **Hyperkalemia** (an increase in potassium level in the blood), a serious event, may occur with the administration of potassium-sparing diuretics. Hyperkalemia is most likely to occur in clients with an inadequate fluid intake and urine output, those with diabetes or renal disease, older adults, and those who are severely ill.

In male clients taking spironolactone, **gynecomastia** (breast enlargement) may occur. This reaction appears to be related to both dosage and the duration of therapy. The gynecomastia is usually reversible when therapy is discontinued, but in rare instances, some breast enlargement may remain.

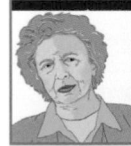 **Lifespan Considerations**

Transgender
Spironolactone inhibits the secretion of testosterone and is used in feminizing hormonal therapy during male-to-female (MTF) gender reassignment (Fisher & Maggi, 2015).

Additional adverse reactions of these drugs are listed in the section Summary Drug Table: Diuretics. When a potassium-sparing diuretic and another diuretic are given together, the adverse reactions associated with both drugs may be greater.

PHARMACOLOGY IN PRACTICE

ASSESSMENT
A nurse is caring for a client with edema due to HF. The PHCP has prescribed spironolactone for the client. Which of the following adverse reactions to the drug should the nurse monitor for in the client?

1. Vertigo
2. Paresthesias
3. Hyperkalemia
4. Anorexia

CONTRAINDICATIONS

Diuretics are contraindicated in clients with known hyper-sensitivity to the drugs, electrolyte imbalances, severe kidney or liver dysfunction, and **anuria** (cessation of urine production). Mannitol (an osmotic diuretic) is contraindi-cated in clients with active intracranial bleeding (except during craniotomy). The potassium-sparing diuretics are contraindicated in clients with hyperkalemia and are not recommended for pediatric clients.

PRECAUTIONS

Diuretics are used cautiously in clients with renal dysfunc-tion. Most of the diuretics are pregnancy category C drugs (although ethacrynic acid, torsemide, isosorbide, amiloride, and triamterene are in pregnancy category B) and must be used cautiously during pregnancy and lactation. All the thiazide diuretics are pregnancy category B drugs, with the exception of benzthiazide and methyclothiazide, which are pregnancy category C drugs. The safety of these drugs for use during pregnancy and lactation has not been established, so they should be used only when the drug is clearly needed and when the potential benefits to the client outweigh the potential hazards to the fetus.

LASA ALERT

The following drugs may sound alike; be sure to clarify when they are ordered:

Drug Name	Sounds Like
acetaZOLAMIDE	acetaminophen
Aldactone	Aldactazide
AMILoride	amiodarone, amLODIPine, inamrinone
bumetanide	Buminate
Bumex	Brevibloc, Buprenex
Dyrenium	Pyridium
Edecrin	Eulexin, Ecotrin
furosemide	famotidine, finasteride, fluconazole, FLUoxetine, fosinopril, loperamide, torsemide
hydroCHLORO-thiazide	hydrALAZINE, hydrocortisone, hydrOXYzine, Viskazide
indapamide	Iopidine
Lasix	Lanoxin, Lidex, Lomotil, Lovenox, Luvox, Luxiq, Wakix
metOLazone	metaxalone, methadone, methazolAMIDE, methIMAzole, methotrexate, metoclopramide, metoprolol, minoxidil
Osmitrol	esmolol
torsemide	furosemide
triamterene	trimipramine

Drugs that look like a similar drug are noted in the Summary Drug Tables of each chapter.

The thiazide and loop diuretics are used cautiously in clients with gout, liver disease, diabetes, systemic lupus erythematosus (may exacerbate or activate the disease), or diarrhea. A cross-sensitivity reaction may occur with the thiazides and sulfonamides. Some of the thiazide diuretics contain tartrazine (a yellow food dye), which may cause allergic-type reactions or bronchial asthma in individuals sensitive to tartrazine. Clients with sensitivity to sulfon-amides may show allergic reactions to loop diuretics (furo-semide, torsemide, or bumetanide). The potassium-sparing diuretics should be used cautiously in clients with liver disease or diabetes.

INTERACTIONS

All the diuretics may cause an increased risk of hypotension when taken with antihypertensive drugs. The interactions for specific diuretic categories are listed here.

Interacting Drug	Common Use	Effect of Interaction
Carbonic Anhydrase Inhibitors		
Primidone	Treatment of seizure activity	Decreased effectiveness
Loop Diuretics		
Cisplatin and aminoglycosides	Cancer treatment and anti-infective, respectively	Increased risk of ototoxicity
Anticoagulants or thrombolytics	Blood thinner	Increased risk of bleeding
Digitalis	Cardiac problems	Increased risk of arrhythmias
Lithium	Psychotic symptoms	Increased risk of lithium toxicity
Hydantoins	Treatment of seizure activity	Decreased diuretic effectiveness
NSAIDs and salicylates	Pain relief	Decreased diuretic effectiveness
Potassium-Sparing Diuretics		
ACE inhibitors or potassium supplements	Cardiovascular problems	Increased risk of hyperkalemia
NSAIDs and salicylates, and anticoagulants	Pain relief and blood thinner, respectively	Decreased diuretic effectiveness
Thiazides and Related Diuretics		
Allopurinol	Treatment of gout	Increased risk of hypersensitivity to allopurinol
Anesthetics	Surgical anesthesia	Increased anesthetic effectiveness
Antineoplastic drugs	Cancer treatment	Extended leukopenia
Antidiabetic drugs	Control of diabetes	Hyperglycemia

Herbal Considerations

Numerous herbal diuretics are available as over-the-counter (OTC) products. Most plant and herbal extracts available as OTC diuretics are nontoxic. The following herbals are believed to possess diuretic activity: celery, chicory, sassafras, juniper berries, St. John's wort, foxglove, horsetail, licorice, dandelion, digitalis purpurea, ephedra, hibiscus, parsley, and elderberry. However, most are either ineffective or no more effective than caffeine. There is very little scientific evidence to justify the use of these plants as diuretics. For example, dandelion root was once believed to be a strong diuretic. However, research has found dandelion root to be safe but ineffective as a diuretic. No herbal diuretic should be taken without discussing with your PHCP. Diuretic teas such as juniper berries and shave grass or horsetail are contraindicated. Juniper berries have been associated with renal damage, and horsetail contains severely toxic compounds. Teas with ephedrine should be avoided, especially by individuals with hypertension (DerMarderosian, 2003).

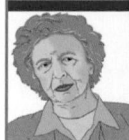
PHARMACOLOGY IN PRACTICE
SAFE DRUG ADMINISTRATION
A PHCP has prescribed treatment with an antihypertensive drug along with a diuretic to a client as a treatment for hypertension. The client informs the nurse about their preference for herbal extracts over medical drugs. What information regarding herbal extracts should the nurse provide to the client? Select all that apply.

1. No herbal diuretic should be taken unless approved by the PHCP.
2. Some herbal extracts have been associated with renal damage.
3. Herbal extracts are more effective than caffeine.
4. Most plant and herbal extracts available as diuretics are nontoxic.
5. Consume diuretic teas such as juniper berries.

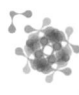
NURSING PROCESS: STEPS TO BUILD CLINICAL JUDGMENT
Client Receiving a Diuretic

ASSESSMENT
Preadministration Assessment
Data gathering suggestions before the initial administration of a diuretic include the following.
Objective data
- Vital signs (temperature, pulse, respirations, and blood pressure).
- Weight (best method to measure water loss).
- Description of edema and skin turgor.
- Description of lung sounds and effortful breathing.
- Body circumference measurements for peripheral edema on extremities.
- Initiate input and output if not already done.
- Laboratory tests—serum electrolytes and hepatic and renal function tests (blood urea nitrogen [BUN] and creatinine clearance).

Subjective data
- Ability to engage in toilet activities with increased urination, such as ambulation difficulty.
- Medical history of fluid status conditions.
- Family history of diseases affecting fluid (cardiac, hepatic, renal).
- Drug therapy (list of all current drugs, use of diuretics in the past).

Ongoing Assessment
The type of assessment depends on factors such as the reason for the administration of the diuretic, the type of diuretic administered, the route of administration, and the condition of the client. When the client is institutionalized measure and record fluid intake and output and report to the PHCP about any marked decrease in the output. Report fluid loss as measured by weighing the client at the same time daily, making certain that the client is wearing the same amount or type of clothing. Depending on the specific diuretic, frequent serum electrolyte, uric acid, and liver and kidney function test results may be performed during the first few months of therapy and periodically thereafter. When clients take diuretics on an outpatient basis, it is your responsibility to instruct clients or caregivers regarding the observations to be made, such as weighing the client, and when to contact the PHCP about weights outside an established parameter.

NURSING DIAGNOSES
Drug-specific nursing diagnoses include the following:
- **Increased urinary frequency** related to action of the diuretics causing increased bladder filling.
- **Hypovolemia/dehydration** related to excessive diuresis secondary to administration of a diuretic.
- **Injury risk** related to lightheadedness, dizziness, or cardiac arrhythmias.

Nursing diagnoses related to drug administration are discussed in Chapter 4.

PLANNING
The expected outcomes for the client depend on the reason for administration of the diuretic but may include an optimal response to drug therapy, support of client needs related to adverse drug reactions, and confidence in an understanding of the medication regimen.

IMPLEMENTATION

Promoting an Optimal Response to Therapy

Diuretics are used to treat many different types of conditions. Therefore promoting an optimal response to therapy for clients taking diuretics often depends on the specific diuretic and the client's condition.

Client With Hypertension

Teach the hypertensive client how to monitor their own blood pressure and pulse rate when receiving a diuretic or a diuretic along with an antihypertensive drug. Clients can monitor their own vital signs easily when going to the grocery store or pharmacy; many of these places have access for free monitoring. For those who wish to use technology, many devices will monitor pulse and blood pressure, as well as activity.

Vital signs, including respiratory rate, are more frequently monitored when the client is critically ill or the blood pressure is excessively high.

Client With Edema

Clients with edema caused by HF or other conditions are weighed daily or as ordered by the PHCP. Parenteral (intravenous [IV]) loop diuretics are typically used in the hospital for rapid fluid loss when it interferes with cardiac function (Albert, 2012). Weight loss of about 0.9 kg (2 lb) daily is desirable to manage fluid loss and prevent dehydration and electrolyte imbalances. Every 8 hours, carefully measure and document the fluid intake and output. The critically ill client or the client with renal disease may require more frequent measurements of urinary output. The blood pressure, pulse, and respiratory rate are assessed every 4 hours or as ordered by the PHCP. An acutely ill client may require more frequent monitoring of the vital signs.

Areas of edema are examined daily to evaluate the effectiveness of drug therapy. Note the client's general appearance and condition daily or more often if the client is acutely ill.

Client With Increased Intracranial Pressure

Mannitol is administered only by the IV route. Mannitol solution may crystallize when exposed to low temperatures, so inspect the solution before administration. If this happens, return the solution to the pharmacy and request another dose. The rate of administration and concentration of the drug is individualized to maintain a urine flow of at least 30–50 mL/hour.

When a client is receiving the osmotic diuretic mannitol for treatment of increased intracranial pressure caused by cerebral edema perform neurologic assessments (response of the pupils to light, level of consciousness, or response to a painful stimulus), in addition to checking vital signs, at the time intervals ordered by the PHCP.

Client With Renal Compromise

When thiazide diuretics are administered, renal function should be monitored periodically. These drugs may cause **azotemia** (accumulation of nitrogenous waste in the blood). If nonprotein nitrogen (NPN) or BUN level increases, the PHCP may consider withholding the drug or discontinuing its use. In addition, serum uric acid concentrations are monitored periodically during treatment with thiazide diuretics because these drugs may cause an acute attack of gout; therefore be alert to client complaints of joint pain or discomfort. Insulin or oral antidiabetic drug dosages may require alterations because of hyperglycemia; therefore serum glucose concentrations are monitored periodically.

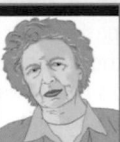

PHARMACOLOGY IN PRACTICE

MANAGING NEEDS

A nurse is caring for a client with renal dysfunction. The PHCP has prescribed a metolazone drug for the client. What should the nurse monitor in the client before administering the drug? Select all that apply.
1. Serum cholesterol levels
2. Levels of serum electrolytes
3. Fluid loss every hour
4. Creatinine clearance levels
5. BUN level

Client at Risk for Electrolyte Imbalances

As fluids and electrolytes shift in the body be alert for imbalances. Signs and symptoms of common imbalances are listed in Box 32.1. One of the primary imbalances to monitor is potassium. Clients who experience cardiac arrhythmias or who are being "digitalized" (initiating digoxin therapy) may be more susceptible to significant potassium loss when taking diuretics. The potassium-sparing diuretics are recommended for these clients.

Monitor clients taking potassium-sparing diuretics because they are at risk for *hyperkalemia*. If the serum potassium levels exceed 5.3 mEq/mL, the diuretic is stopped and the PHCP is notified immediately. Treatment to reduce the potassium levels can include administration of IV bicarbonate (if the client is acidotic) or oral or parenteral glucose with rapid-acting insulin. Persistent hyperkalemia may require dialysis. Serum potassium levels are monitored frequently, particularly during initial treatment.

Monitoring and Managing Client Needs

Increased Urinary Frequency

Because many of the conditions treated with diuretics are cardiac in nature explain to the client how eliminating fluids helps the heart and blood vessels work more efficiently. This is hard for some clients to understand and can impact their decisions to stop taking a drug they find unpleasant. Researchers show that when clients with HF experience urinary incontinence, they stop or reduce the diuretic drug (Hwang, 2013). Therefore it is important for clients to understand how quickly some of these drugs work and how they cause increased urination. Before a diuretic is given explain to the client when **diuresis** may be expected to occur and how long diuresis will last (Table 32.2). These drugs are taken early in the day to prevent any nighttime sleep disturbance caused by increased urination.

BOX 32.1 Signs and Symptoms of Common Fluid and Electrolyte Imbalance Associated With Diuretic Therapy

Dehydration (Excessive Water Loss)
- Thirst
- Poor skin turgor
- Dry mucous membranes
- Weakness
- Dizziness
- Fever
- Low urine output

Hyponatremia (Excessive Loss of Sodium)
Note: Normal laboratory value of sodium is 132–145 mEq/L
- Cold, clammy skin
- Decreased skin turgor
- Confusion
- Hypotension
- Irritability
- Tachycardia

Hypomagnesemia (Low Levels of Magnesium)
Note: Normal laboratory value of magnesium is 1.5–2.5 mEq/L or 1.8–3 mg/dL
- Leg and foot cramps
- Hypertension
- Tachycardia
- Neuromuscular irritability
- Tremor
- Hyperactive deep tendon reflexes
- Confusion
- Visual or auditory hallucinations
- Paresthesias

Hypokalemia (Low Blood Potassium)
Note: Normal laboratory value of potassium is 3.5–5 mEq/L
- Anorexia
- Nausea and vomiting
- Muscle *twitching*
- Depression
- Confusion
- Bradycardia
- Impaired thought processes
- Drowsiness

Hyperkalemia (High Blood Potassium)
- Irritability
- Anxiety
- Confusion
- Muscle *cramps*
- Numbness or tingling sensation
- Nausea
- Diarrhea
- Cardiac arrhythmias
- Flaccid paralysis

TABLE 32.2 Examples of Onset and Duration of Activity of Diuretics

DRUG	ONSET	DURATION OF ACTIVITY
Acetazolamide tablets	1–1.5 hours	8–12 hours
Sustained-release capsules	2 hours	18–24 hours
IV route	2 minutes	4–5 hours
Amiloride	2 hours	24 hours
Bumetanide oral	30–60 minutes	4–6 hours
IV route	Within a few minutes	Less than 1 hour
Ethacrynic acid oral	Within 30 minutes	6–8 hours
IV route	Within 5 minutes	2 hours
Furosemide oral	Within 1 hour	6–8 hours
IV route	Within 5 minutes	2 hours
Mannitol (IV route)	30–60 minutes	6–8 hours
Spironolactone	24–48 hours	48–72 hours
Thiazides and related diuretics	1–2 hours	Varies[a]
Triamterene	2–4 hours	12–16 hours

[a]Duration varies with drug used. Average duration is 12–24 hours. Indapamide has a duration of more than 24 hours.

Some clients may become worried or anxious because it is necessary to urinate at frequent intervals and they may experience incontinence if their need is not responded to quickly. As illustrated in Figure 32.2 reassure the client on bed rest with prompt responses to a call light and, when necessary, have a bedpan or urinal within easy reach. Teach the client using the drug at home to take it early in the day so that nighttime sleep will not be interrupted. Also help plan activities so that onset (less than 60 min) and peak (1–4 hours) actions of the diuretic do not occur while in a car or when taking a walk and bathroom access is not readily available. Although the duration of action of most diuretics is about 8 hours or less, some diuretics have a longer activity, which may result in a need to urinate during nighttime hours. This is especially true early in therapy.

Hypovolemia/Dehydration
The most common adverse reaction associated with the administration of a diuretic is the loss of fluid and electrolytes (see Box 32.1), especially during initial therapy with the drug. In some clients the diuretic effect is moderate, whereas in others a large volume of fluid is lost. Regardless of the amount of fluid lost, there is always the possibility of excessive electrolyte loss, which is potentially serious.

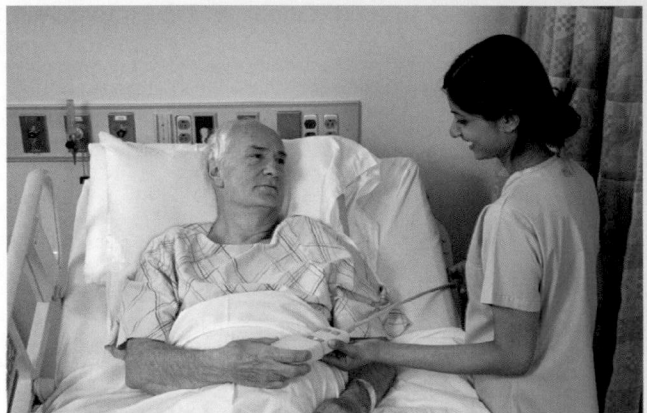

FIGURE 32.2 Reduce fear of incontinence by providing urinals or bedpans and answering call lights promptly for clients taking diuretics.

The most common imbalances are loss of potassium and water. Other electrolytes, particularly magnesium, sodium, and chloride, are also lost. When too much potassium is lost, hypokalemia occurs (see Client Teaching for Improved Outcomes: Preventing Potassium Imbalances). In certain clients, such as those also receiving a digitalis glycoside or those who currently have a cardiac arrhythmia, hypokalemia has the potential to create a more serious arrhythmia.

Hypokalemia is treated with potassium supplements or foods with high potassium content or by changing the diuretic to a potassium-sparing diuretic. In addition to hypokalemia, clients taking the loop diuretics are prone to magnesium deficiency (see Box 32.1). Whether a fluid or electrolyte imbalance occurs depends on the amount of fluid and electrolytes lost and the ability of the individual to replace them. For example, if a client receiving a diuretic eats poorly and does not drink extra fluids, an electrolyte and water imbalance is likely to occur. However, preventive treatment is not always a guarantee; even when a client drinks adequate amounts of fluid and eats a balanced diet, an electrolyte imbalance may still occur and require electrolyte replacement (see Chapter 54 for additional discussion of fluid and electrolyte imbalances).

 Lifespan Considerations

Gerontology
Older adults are particularly prone to fluid volume deficit and electrolyte imbalances while taking diuretics. Dehydration can occur if the client reduces fluid intake because of fear of incontinence.

Encourage oral fluids at frequent intervals during waking hours to prevent a fluid volume deficit. A balanced diet may help prevent electrolyte imbalances. Encourage potassium-

Client Teaching for Improved Outcomes

Preventing Potassium Imbalances
Diuretics increase the excretion of water and sodium. Some of these drugs also increase the excretion of potassium, which places the client at risk for *hypokalemia,* a possibly life-threatening condition. Clients can reduce their risk of hypokalemia by eating foods rich in potassium, which will replace the loss caused by the diuretic.

When you teach, make sure your client understands the following:

Potassium can be replenished by diet; take supplements only when instructed to do so by your PHCP. The following foods have higher levels of potassium than other foods:

✔ **Top 10 foods** with the highest amount of potassium per serving: white beans, dark leafy greens, baked potatoes with skin on, dried apricots, acorn squash, plain low-fat yogurt, salmon, avocado, mushrooms, and bananas.
✔ **Fruits (10 highest):** apricots, prunes, dried currants/raisins, dates, figs, dried coconut, avocado, bananas, oranges, nectarines, and peaches.
✔ **Vegetables (10 highest):** sun-dried tomatoes, spinach, Swiss chard, mushrooms, sweet potato, kale, brussels sprouts, zucchini, green beans, and asparagus.
✔ **Other sources:** chocolate, molasses, nuts, and nut butters (http://www.myfooddata.com).

rich snacks between meals and in the evening (when allowed). Monitor the fluid intake and output and notify the PHCP if the client fails to drink an adequate amount of fluid, if the urinary output is low, if the urine appears concentrated, if the client appears dehydrated, or if signs and symptoms of an electrolyte imbalance are apparent.

⚠ NURSING ALERT

Warning signs of a fluid and electrolyte imbalance include dry mouth, thirst, weakness, lethargy, drowsiness, restlessness, muscle pains or cramps, confusion, gastrointestinal (GI) disturbances, hypotension, oliguria, tachycardia, and seizures.

Injury Risk
Clients receiving a diuretic (particularly a loop or thiazide diuretic) and a digitalis glycoside concurrently require frequent monitoring of the pulse rate and rhythm because of the possibility of cardiac arrhythmias. Any significant changes in the pulse rate and rhythm are immediately reported to the PHCP.

Some clients experience dizziness or lightheadedness, especially during the first few days of therapy or when a rapid diuresis has occurred. Clients who are dizzy but who are allowed out of bed are assisted with ambulatory activities until these adverse drug effects disappear.

Educating the Client and Family

The client and the family may modify drug administration because of the excessive amount of urination or when the diuretic works at inappropriate times for client activity. To ensure adherence to the prescribed drug regimen be sure the client is taking the drug correctly. Emphasize the importance of diuretic therapy in treating the client's disorder. As you develop a teaching plan include the following information:

- Do not stop taking the drug or omit doses, except on the advice of a PHCP.
- If GI upset occurs, then take the drug with food or milk.
- Take the drug early in the morning (once-a-day dosage) unless directed otherwise to minimize the effects on nighttime sleep. Twice-a-day dosing should be administered early in the morning (e.g., 7 a.m.) and early afternoon (e.g., 2 p.m.) or as directed by the PHCP.
- Do not reduce fluid intake to reduce the need to urinate. Be sure to continue the fluid intake recommended by the PHCP.

  🍷 Avoid alcohol and nonprescription drugs unless approved by the PHCP. Hypertensive clients should be careful to avoid medications that increase blood pressure, such as OTC drugs for appetite suppression and cold symptoms.

- Notify the PHCP if any of the following occur: muscle cramps or weakness, dizziness, nausea, vomiting, diarrhea, restlessness, excessive thirst, general weakness, rapid pulse, increased heart rate or pulse, or GI distress.
- If dizziness or weakness occurs, then observe caution while driving or performing hazardous tasks, rise slowly from a sitting or lying position, and avoid standing in one place for an extended time.
- Weigh yourself weekly or as recommended by the PHCP. Keep a record of these weekly weights and contact the PHCP if weight loss or gain exceeds 1.3–2.2 kg (3–5 lb) a week.
- If foods or fluids high in potassium are recommended by the PHCP, then eat the amount recommended. Do not exceed this amount or eliminate these foods from the diet for more than 1 day, except when told to do so by the PHCP (see Client Teaching for Improved Outcomes: Preventing Potassium Imbalances).
- After a time, the diuretic effect of the drug may be minimal because most of the body's excess fluid has been removed. Continue therapy to prevent further accumulation of fluid.
- If taking thiazide or related diuretics, loop diuretics, potassium-sparing diuretics, carbonic anhydrase inhibitors, or triamterene, then avoid exposure to sunlight or ultraviolet light (sunlamps, tanning beds) because exposure may cause exaggerated sunburn (a photosensitivity reaction). Wear sunscreen and protective clothing until tolerance is determined.
- *For clients who have diabetes mellitus and who take loop or thiazide diuretics* know that blood glucometer test results for glucose may be elevated. Contact the PHCP if home-tested blood glucose levels increase.
- *For clients who take potassium-sparing diuretics* avoid eating foods high in potassium and avoid the use of salt substitutes containing potassium. Read food labels carefully. Do not use a salt substitute unless a particular brand has been approved by the PHCP. Also avoid the use of potassium supplements. Male clients who take spironolactone may experience gynecomastia. This is usually reversible when therapy is discontinued.
- *For clients who take thiazide diuretics,* these agents may cause gout attacks. Contact the PHCP if significant, sudden joint pain occurs.
- *For clients who take carbonic anhydrase inhibitors,* during treatment for glaucoma, contact the PHCP immediately if eye pain is not relieved or if it increases. When a client with epilepsy is being treated for seizures, a family member of the client should keep a record of all seizures witnessed and bring this to the PHCP at the time of the next visit. Contact the PHCP immediately if the number of seizures increases.

EVALUATION

- Therapeutic effect is achieved and diuresis occurs.
- Adverse reactions are identified, reported to the PHCP, and managed successfully through appropriate nursing interventions.

  - Urinary elimination occurs without incident.
  - Fluid volume problems are corrected.
  - No injury is evident.

- Client and family express confidence and demonstrate an understanding of the drug regimen.

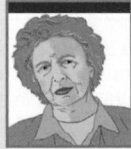

PHARMACOLOGY IN PRACTICE

USING CLINICAL REASONING

When you question Mrs. Moore, she tells you the water pills just do not do the job and she needs to go out of the house too frequently to take them on a regular basis. Based on your understanding of diuretic medications, why do you think Mrs. Moore has decided not to take the medications as prescribed?

KEY POINTS

■ Excessive fluid is involved in many conditions such as HF, endocrine disturbances, and kidney and liver diseases. Pressure of fluid in the blood vessels contributes to hypertension. Diuretics are drugs that reduce body fluid by increasing production of urine by altering the excretion or reabsorption of electrolytes in the kidney.

■ Loop, thiazide, and potassium-sparing diuretics are used to treat HF, endocrine disturbances, and kidney and liver diseases. Osmotic and carbonic anhydrase inhibitors are used in the treatment of cerebral edema and seizures, IOP, and altitude sickness.

■ Fluid loss is monitored by vital signs and weight reduction, as well as measured fluid intake and output. Some people may be reluctant to take diuretics for fear of incontinence. Others may reduce fluid intake for the same reason. Dehydration and electrolyte imbalances are more likely to occur when clients engage in these behaviors.

■ Common adverse reactions to the medications include dizziness, headache, weakness, anorexia, nausea, and vomiting. Rashes and photosensitivity may occur with sun exposure. Again, clients should be monitored for electrolyte imbalances to reduce these adverse reactions.

SUMMARY DRUG TABLE
Diuretics

Generic Name	Trade Name	Uses	Adverse Reactions	Dosage Ranges
Loop Diuretics				
bumetanide *byoo-MET-a-nide*	Bumex	Edema caused by HF, cirrhosis of the liver, renal disease, acute pulmonary edema	Electrolyte and hematologic imbalances, anorexia, nausea, vomiting, dizziness, rash, photosensitivity, orthostatic hypotension, glycosuria	0.5–10 mg/day orally, IV, IM
ethacrynic acid *eth-a-KRIN-ik*	Edecrin	Same as bumetanide plus ascites caused by malignancy, idiopathic edema, lymphedema	Same as bumetanide, plus diarrhea	50–200 mg/day orally, IV
furosemide *fur-OH-se-mide*	Lasix	Same as bumetanide plus hypertension	Same as bumetanide	Edema: 20–80 mg/day, may go up to 600 mg/day for severe edema Hypertension: 40 mg orally BID HF/renal failure: up to 2.5 g/day
torsemide *TORE-se-mide*		Same as bumetanide plus hypertension	Same as bumetanide plus headache	HF/renal failure: 10–20 mg/day orally, IV Cirrhosis/hypertension: 5–10 mg/day orally, IV
Potassium-Sparing Diuretics				
AMILoride *a-MIL-oh-ride*		HF, hypertension, prevention of hypokalemia in at-risk clients, polyuria prevention with lithium use	Headache, dizziness, nausea, anorexia, diarrhea, vomiting, weakness, fatigue, rash, hypotension	5–20 mg/day orally
spironolactone *speer-on-oh-LAK-tone*	Aldactone	Hypertension, edema caused by HF, cirrhosis, renal disease; hypokalemia, prophylaxis of hypokalemia in at-risk clients, hyperaldosteronism, MTF hormone therapy	Headache, diarrhea, drowsiness, lethargy, hyperkalemia, cramping, gastritis, erectile dysfunction, gynecomastia	Up to 400 mg/day orally in single dose or divided doses
triamterene *trye-AM-ter-een*	Dyrenium	Prevention of hypokalemia, edema caused by HF, cirrhosis, renal disease, hyperaldosteronism	Diarrhea, nausea, vomiting, hyperkalemia, photosensitivity	Up to 300 mg/day orally in divided doses

Generic Name	Trade Name	Uses	Adverse Reactions	Dosage Ranges
Thiazides and Related Diuretics				
chlorothiazide *klor-oh-THYE-a-zide*	Diuril	Hypertension, edema caused by HF, cirrhosis, corticosteroid, and estrogen therapy	Orthostatic hypotension, dizziness, vertigo, lightheadedness, weakness, anorexia, gastric distress, nausea, diarrhea, constipation, hematologic changes, rash, photosensitivity reactions, hyperglycemia, fluid and electrolyte imbalance, reduced libido	0.5–2 g orally or IV, QID or BID
chlorthalidone *klor-THAL-i-done*		Same as chlorothiazide	Same as chlorothiazide	Edema: 50–120 mg/day orally Hypertension: 25–100 mg/day orally
hydroCHLOROthiazide *hye-droe-klor-oh-THYE-a-zide*		Same as chlorothiazide	Same as chlorothiazide	Edema: 25–200 mg/day orally Hypertension: 12.5–50 mg/day orally
indapamide *in-DAP-a-mide*		Hypertension, edema caused by HF	Same as chlorothiazide	Edema: 2.5–5 mg/day orally Hypertension: 1.25–5 mg/day orally
metOLazone *me-TOLL-a-zone*		Edema in HF, cirrhosis, corticosteroids, estrogen therapy, renal dysfunction	Same as chlorothiazide	2.5–20 mg/day orally
methyclothiazide *meth-i-kloe-THYE-a-zide*		Same as chlorothiazide	Same as chlorothiazide	Edema: 2.5–10 mg/day orally Hypertension: 2.5–5 mg/day orally
Carbonic Anhydrase Inhibitors				
acetaZOLAMIDE *a-set-a-ZOLE-a-mide*		Altitude sickness (acute), edema caused by HF, drug-induced edema, centrencephalic epilepsy	Weakness, fatigue, anorexia, nausea, vomiting, rash, paresthesias, photosensitivity	Altitude sickness: up to 1 g/day orally in divided doses before ascent Epilepsy: 8–30 mg/kg/day in divided doses HF and edema: 250–375 mg/day orally
dichlorphenamide *dye-klor-FEN-a-mide*	Keveyis	Hyperkalemic paralysis	Confusion, paresthesia, taste changes, fatigue	50–200 mg daily orally
Osmotic Diuretics				
mannitol *MAN-i-tole*	Osmitrol	To promote diuresis in acute renal failure, reduction of IOP, treatment of cerebral edema, irrigation solution in prostate surgical procedures	Edema, fluid and electrolyte imbalance, headache, blurred vision, nausea, vomiting, diarrhea, urinary retention	Diuresis: 50–200 g/24 hr IV IOP: 1.5–2 g/kg IV

CHAPTER REVIEW

Know Your Drugs

Clients sometimes know a medication by the brand (or trade) name and not the generic name. To recognize both names match the brand name with the generic name of the same medication.

Generic Name	Brand Name
1. chlorothiazide	A. Aldactone
2. furosemide	B. Diuril
3. dichlorphenamide	C. Lasix
4. spironolactone	D. Keveyis

Calculate Medication Dosages

1. The PHCP prescribes spironolactone (Aldactone) 100 mg orally. The drug is available in 50-mg tablets. The nurse administers _____.
2. Furosemide (Lasix) 20-mg oral solution is prescribed. The oral solution is available in a concentration of 40 mg/5 mL. The nurse administers into the nasogastric tube _____.

Prepare for the NCLEX

RECALL THE FACTS

1. The best description of how diuretic medications work is that they:
   1. promote retention of fluid in the kidney.
   2. achieve acid balance in the lungs.
   3. increase the removal of potassium from the blood.
   4. inhibit reabsorption of sodium in the nephron.
2. When ordered two times daily, the best schedule for taking furosemide would be _____.
   1. 9 a.m. and 9 p.m.
   2. 7 a.m. and 9 a.m.
   3. 6 a.m. and 7 p.m.
   4. 8 a.m. and 2 p.m.
3. When evaluating the effectiveness of chlorothiazide, the nurse questions the client about _____.
   1. the number of times voiding
   2. relief of eye pain
   3. amount of fluids drank
   4. daily weight
4. When administering spironolactone (Aldactone), the nurse monitors the client for which of the following electrolyte imbalances?
   1. Hypernatremia
   2. Hyponatremia
   3. Hyperkalemia
   4. Hypokalemia
5. Which electrolyte imbalance would the client taking a loop or thiazide diuretic most likely develop?
   1. Hypernatremia
   2. Hyponatremia
   3. Hyperkalemia
   4. Hypokalemia

ANALYZE THE FACTS

6. *The nurse is seeing a client in the clinic 1 week after the client began taking a diuretic. Which finding would make you suspect that the client is not taking the diuretic?
   1. Serum potassium of 3.0 mEq/mL
   2. Urine output of 200 mL for the past 2 hr
   3. Blood pressure of 130/90 mm Hg
   4. Weight gain of 1.8 kg (4 lb) since the past week

7. *When a client is given mannitol for increased intracranial pressure, which of the following findings would be most important for the nurse to report?
   1. Serum potassium of 3.5 mEq/mL
   2. Urine output of 20 mL for the past 2 hr
   3. Blood pressure of 140/80 mm Hg
   4. Heart rate of 72 bpm
8. When a diuretic is being administered for HF, which of the following would be most indicative of an effective response to diuretic therapy?
   1. Output of 30 mL/hr
   2. Daily weight loss of 2 lb
   3. Increase in blood pressure
   4. Increasing edema of the lower extremities

ALTERNATE-FORMAT QUESTIONS

9. Which of the following foods would the nurse most likely recommend the client to include in the daily diet to prevent hypokalemia? **Select all that apply.**
   1. Potatoes
   2. Apricots
   3. Bananas
   4. Corn
10. Match the diuretic with its use:

1. Reduces cerebral edema	A. acetazolamide
2. Reduces hypertension	B. Lasix
3. Removes fluid, spare potassium	C. mannitol
4. Treats altitude sickness	D. spironolactone
	E. metolazone

To check your answers, see Appendix F.

*Indicates the question is directly linked to the NCLEX-PN test plan in Appendix G.

WANT TO KNOW MORE? A wide variety of resources are available to enhance your learning and understanding of this chapter.

- Visit the**Point** for resources such as
  - NCLEX-Style Student Review Questions
  - Journal Articles
  - Dosage Calculations
  - Drug Monographs
  - Watch and Learn Videos
  - Concepts in Action Animations
- The *Study Guide to Accompany Introductory Clinical Pharmacology*, 12th edition, sold separately, will help you review and apply essential content.
- ✓**PrepU** is available to help students prepare for the NCLEX-PN examination.

33

Antihyperlipidemic Drugs

Key Terms

atherosclerosis disease characterized by deposits of fatty plaques on the inner walls of arteries

catalyst substance that accelerates a chemical reaction without itself undergoing a change

cholecystitis inflammation of the gallbladder

cholelithiasis stones in the gallbladder

cholesterol fat-like substance produced mostly in the liver of animals

high-density lipoproteins (HDLs) macro (big) molecules that carry cholesterol from the body cells to the liver to be excreted

hyperlipidemia increase in the lipids in the blood

lipid group of fats or fat-like substances

lipoprotein macromolecule consisting of lipid (fat) and protein; how fats are transported in the blood

low-density lipoproteins (LDLs) macromolecules that carry cholesterol from the liver to the body cells

orphan drug status medication that is used for a low number of clients, or may not recover the expense of research and development. Status gives incentive to manufacture the drug

Risk Evaluation and Mitigation Strategies (REMS) A program of the FDA designed to monitor drugs that have a high risk compared with benefit ratio

rhabdomyolysis condition in which muscle damage results in the release of muscle cell contents into the bloodstream

statins (HMG-CoA reductase inhibitors) common name for drugs that inhibit the manufacture or promote breakdown of cholesterol

triglycerides types of lipids that circulate in the blood

xanthomas yellow deposits of cholesterol in tendons and soft tissues

Learning Objectives

On completion of this chapter, the student will:

1. Compare and contrast cholesterol, high-density lipoprotein (HDL), low-density lipoprotein (LDL), and triglyceride levels and how they contribute to the development of heart disease.
2. Define therapeutic life changes (TLCs) and how they affect cholesterol levels.
3. Explain the uses, general drug actions, general adverse reactions, contraindications, precautions, and interactions of antihyperlipidemic drugs.
4. Distinguish important preadministration and ongoing assessment activities the nurse should perform on the client taking an antihyperlipidemic drug.
5. List nursing diagnoses particular to a client taking an antihyperlipidemic drug.
6. Examine ways to promote an optimal response to therapy, how to manage common adverse reactions, and important points to keep in mind when educating clients about the use of antihyperlipidemic drugs.

 ## Drug Classes

HMG-CoA reductase inhibitors (statins)
Bile acid resins
Fibric acid derivatives
Niacin

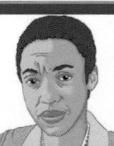 ### PHARMACOLOGY IN PRACTICE

Lillian Chase is taking cholestyramine for hyperlipidemia. The primary health care provider has prescribed therapeutic life changes (TLCs) for the client, who is on a low-fat diet and walks short distances daily for exercise. Her major complaint at this visit is constipation, which is very bothersome to her. She feels depressed and has started smoking again. She tells you the medicine is not working and wants to stop taking it. As you read about medications in this chapter, think about Lillian's concerns.

Prevention as a means of treatment is a concept used in cardiac health. By reducing lipid levels in the circulation of asymptomatic populations, we can reduce the need for more aggressive medications and interventions later on. When therapeutic lifestyle interventions are not enough, the use of antihyperlipidemic drugs is one of these prevention tactics available in our health care system.

LIPID CONTROL

Atherosclerosis is considered to be a major contributor in the development of heart disease, particularly heart attacks and stroke. It is a disorder in which **lipid** (fat or fat-like substance) deposits accumulate on the lining of the blood vessels, eventually producing degenerative changes and obstructing blood flow. The two lipids in our blood are **cholesterol** and the **triglycerides**. Serum cholesterol levels above 240 mg/dL and triglyceride levels above 150 mg/dL are known as **hyperlipidemia** and are associated with atherosclerosis.

Triglycerides and cholesterol are fats that are insoluble in water. For these fats to be transported throughout the body, they must be bound to a lipid-containing protein (**lipoprotein**) (Fig. 33.1). Although several lipoproteins are found in the blood, this chapter focuses on drugs used to regulate the low-density lipoproteins (LDLs), the high-density lipoproteins (HDLs), and cholesterol.

LIPOPROTEINS

Low-density lipoproteins (LDLs) transport cholesterol to the peripheral cells. When the cells have all the cholesterol they need, the excess cholesterol is discarded into the blood (see Fig. 33.1). This excess penetrates the walls of the arteries, resulting in atherosclerotic plaque formation. Elevation of the LDL level increases the risk for heart disease. On the other hand, **high-density lipoproteins** (HDLs) take cholesterol from the peripheral cells and transport it to the liver, where it is metabolized and

excreted; the higher the HDL level, the lower the risk for development of atherosclerosis. Therefore, it is desirable to see an increase in the HDL (the "good" lipoprotein) level, because of the protective nature of its properties against the development of atherosclerosis and a decrease in the LDL level. A laboratory examination of blood lipids, called a *lipoprotein profile,* provides valuable information on the important cholesterol levels, such as:

- Total cholesterol
- LDL (the harmful lipoprotein)
- HDL (the protective lipoprotein)
- Triglycerides

Table 33.1 provides an analysis of cholesterol levels.

CHOLESTEROL LEVELS

HDL cholesterol protects against heart disease, so the higher its numbers (i.e., blood level) the better. An HDL level less than 40 mg/dL is low and considered a major risk factor for heart disease. Triglyceride levels that are borderline (150 to 190 mg/dL) or high (above 190 mg/dL) may need treatment in some individuals.

In general, the higher the LDL level and the more risk factors involved, the greater the risk for heart disease. Other

TABLE 33.1 Cholesterol Level Analysis

LEVEL	CATEGORY
***Total Cholesterol*[a]**	
Less than 200 mg/dL	Desirable
200–239 mg/dL	Borderline
240 mg/dL and above	High
***LDL Cholesterol*[a]**	
Less than 100 mg/dL	Optimal
100–129 mg/dL	Near optimal/above optimal
130–159 mg/dL	Borderline
160–189 mg/dL	High
190 mg/dL and above	Very high
***HDL Cholesterol*[a]**	
Less than 40 mg/dL	Low
60 mg/dL and above	High
***Triglycerides*[a]**	
Less than 150 mg/dL	Normal
151–199 mg/dL	Borderline high
200–499 mg/dL	High
500 mg/dL or higher	Very high

[a]Cholesterol and triglyceride levels are measured in milligrams (mg) of cholesterol per deciliter (dL) of blood.
From 2019 ACC/AHA Prevention Guidelines.

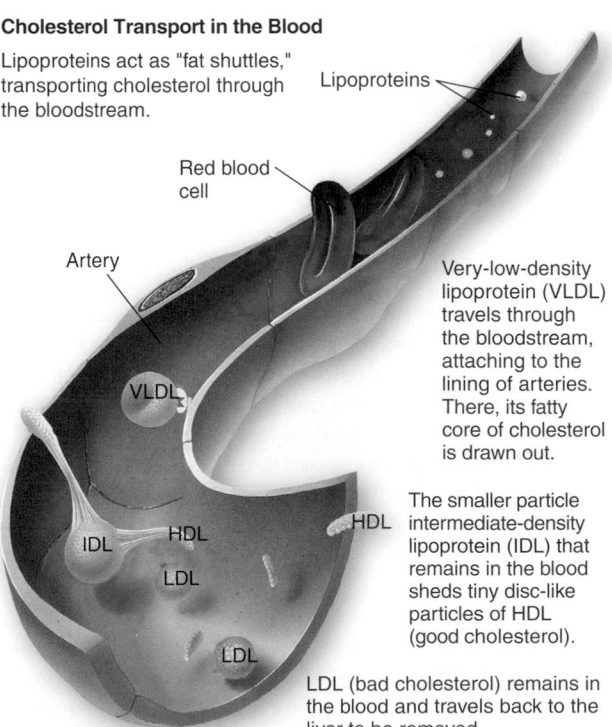

Cholesterol Transport in the Blood

Lipoproteins act as "fat shuttles," transporting cholesterol through the bloodstream.

Lipoproteins

Red blood cell

Artery

VLDL

IDL

HDL

LDL

HDL

LDL

Very-low-density lipoprotein (VLDL) travels through the bloodstream, attaching to the lining of arteries. There, its fatty core of cholesterol is drawn out.

The smaller particle intermediate-density lipoprotein (IDL) that remains in the blood sheds tiny disc-like particles of HDL (good cholesterol).

LDL (bad cholesterol) remains in the blood and travels back to the liver to be removed.

FIGURE 33.1 Cholesterol transport in the blood. (Courtesy of Anatomical Chart Co.)

risk factors, besides elevated cholesterol levels, that play a role in the development of *hyperlipidemia* are listed here. Uncontrollable risk factors include:

- Age (men older than 45 years and women older than 55 years)
- Gender (in women after menopause, LDL cholesterol levels increase)
- Family history of early heart disease (father/brother before age 55 years and mother/sister before age 65 years)

Those factors a person *can* control or modify include:

- Diet (saturated fat and cholesterol in food raise total and LDL cholesterol levels)
- Weight (increased weight can make LDL cholesterol level go up and HDL level go down)
- Physical inactivity (increased physical activity helps to lower LDL cholesterol and raise HDL cholesterol levels)
- Tobacco use

The main goal of treatment in clients with hyperlipidemia is to lower the LDLs to a level that will reduce the risk of heart disease.

The primary health care provider may initially seek to control the cholesterol level by encouraging *therapeutic life changes* (TLCs). This includes a cholesterol-lowering diet (the TLC diet), physical activity, smoking cessation (if applicable), and weight management. The TLC diet is a low-saturated fat and low-cholesterol eating plan that includes less than 200 mg of dietary cholesterol per day.

In addition, 30 minutes of physical activity each day is recommended for the TLC plan. Walking at a brisk pace for 30 minutes a day 5 to 7 days a week can help raise the HDL and lower the LDL levels. Added benefits of a healthy diet and exercise program include a reduction of body weight. If TLCs do not result in bringing blood lipids to therapeutic levels, the primary health care provider may add one of the antihyperlipidemic drugs to the treatment plan. TLCs are continued along with the drug regimen.

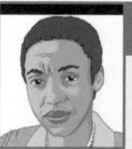

PHARMACOLOGY IN PRACTICE

TEACHING AND LEARNING

Which of the following are examples of modifiable risk factors for hyperlipidemia? Select all that apply.

1. Weight
2. Diet
3. Postmenopausal
4. Age older than 55 years (women)
5. Age older than 45 years (men)

In addition to reduction of dietary fat, particularly saturated fatty acids, antihyperlipidemic drug therapy is used to

TABLE 33.2 Antihyperlipidemia Combination Drugs

GENERIC DRUGS[a]	COMBINATION DRUG TRADE NAME
amlodipine/atorvastatin	Caduet
ezetimibe/simvastatin	Vytorin
bempedoic acid/ezetimibe	Nexlizet

[a]These drug combinations consist of two different drugs that target lipid reduction differently.

lower serum levels of cholesterol and triglycerides. HMG-CoA reductase inhibitors (frequently called statins) are the first-line drug of choice to lower lipid levels (Arnett, 2019). The target LDL level is less than 130 mg/dL. If the response to behavior modification and drug treatment is adequate, lipid levels are monitored every 4 months. If the response is inadequate, another drug or a combination of two drugs is used. See Table 33.2 for combination drugs currently marketed to treat hyperlipidemia.

Three classes of antihyperlipidemic drugs are currently in use, as well as a few miscellaneous antihyperlipidemic drugs (see Summary Drug Table: Antihyperlipidemic Drugs for a complete listing of the drugs). The various antihyperlipidemic drugs decrease cholesterol and triglyceride levels in several ways. Although the end result is a lower lipid blood level, each has a slightly different action.

HMG-COA REDUCTASE INHIBITORS

ACTIONS

The antihyperlipidemic drugs, HMG-CoA reductase inhibitors, are typically referred to as **statins**. This "nickname" comes from the fact that the generic drugs in this category all end in *-statin*, thus they are referred to as statins. HMG-CoA (3-hydroxy-3-methyglutaryl coenzyme A) reductase is an enzyme that is a **catalyst** (a substance that accelerates a chemical reaction without itself undergoing a change) in the manufacture of cholesterol. These drugs appear to have one of two activities, namely, inhibiting the manufacture of cholesterol or promoting the breakdown of cholesterol. Either drug activity lowers the blood levels of cholesterol, LDLs, and serum triglycerides. Examples of these drugs can be found in the Summary Drug Table: Antihyperlipidemic Drugs.

USES

Statin drugs, along with a diet restricted in saturated fat and cholesterol, are used for the following:

- Treatment of hyperlipidemia

- Primary prevention of coronary events (in clients with hyperlipidemia without clinically evident coronary heart disease to reduce the risk of myocardial infarction and death from other cardiovascular events, including strokes, transient ischemic attacks, and cardiac revascularization procedures)
- Secondary prevention of cardiovascular events (in clients with hyperlipidemia with evident coronary heart disease to reduce the risk of coronary death, slow the progression of coronary atherosclerosis, and reduce risk of death from stroke/transient ischemic attack and in those undergoing myocardial revascularization procedures)

ADVERSE REACTIONS

The statins are usually well tolerated. Adverse reactions, when they do occur, are often mild and transient and do not require discontinuing therapy. These reactions may include the following.

Central Nervous System Reactions
- Headache
- Dizziness
- Insomnia
- Memory and cognitive impairment

Gastrointestinal System Reactions
- Flatulence, abdominal pain, cramping
- Constipation, nausea
- Hyperglycemia in nondiabetic clients

Clients may experience leg pain or cramping. This can be an indication of a more serious condition—rhabdomyolysis.

> ### ⓘ NURSING ALERT
> The drug rosuvastatin in higher doses is linked to risks for serious muscle toxicity (myopathy/rhabdomyolysis) in certain populations. These include clients taking cyclosporine, Asian clients, and clients with severe renal insufficiency. A 5-mg dose is available as a starting dose for those individuals who do not require aggressive cholesterol reductions or who have predisposing factors for myopathy.

CONTRAINDICATIONS AND PRECAUTIONS

The statins are contraindicated in individuals with hypersensitivity to the drugs or serious liver disorders, and during pregnancy (pregnancy category X) and lactation. In some individuals with diabetes risk factors, statin drugs may elevate serum glucose and HbA$_{1c}$ levels.

These drugs are used cautiously in clients with a history of alcoholism, non–alcohol-related liver disease, acute infection, hypotension, trauma, endocrine disorders, visual disturbances, and myopathy.

LASA ALERT

The following drugs may sound alike; be sure to clarify when they are ordered:

Drug Name	Sounds Like
atorvaSTATin	atoMOXetine, lovastatin, nystatin, pitavastatin, pravastatin, rosuvastatin, simvastatin
fluvastatin	fluoxetine, nystatin, pitavastatin
Lipitor	labetalol, Levatol, lisinopril, Loniten, Lopid, Mevacor, Zocor, ZyrTEC
lovastatin	atorvaSTATin, Leustatin, Livostin, Lotensin, nystatin, pitavastatin
pitavastatin	atorvaSTATin, fluvastatin, lovastatin, nystatin, pravastatin, rosuvastatin, simvastatin
Pravachol	atorvaSTATin, Prevacid, Prinivil, propranolol
Zocor	Cozaar, Lipitor, Zoloft, ZyrTEC

Drugs that look like a similar drug are noted in the Summary Drug Tables of each chapter.

INTERACTIONS

The following interactions may occur when the statin drugs are administered with another agent:

Interacting Drug	Common Use	Effect of Interaction
Macrolides, erythromycin, clarithromycin	Treatment of infections	Increased risk of severe myopathy or rhabdomyolysis
Amiodarone	Cardiovascular problems	Increased risk of myopathy
Niacin	Used to lower elevated cholesterol	Increased risk of severe myopathy or rhabdomyolysis
Protease inhibitors	Treatment of human immunodeficiency virus (HIV) infection and acquired immunodeficiency syndrome (AIDS)	Elevated plasma levels of statins
Verapamil	Treatment of cardiovascular problems and hypertension	Increased risk of myopathy
Warfarin	Blood thinner (anticoagulant)	Increased anticoagulant effect

The statin drugs have an additive effect when used with the bile acid resins, which may provide an added benefit in treating hypercholesterolemia that does not respond to a single-drug regimen. Because of a specific synergistic enzyme reaction, grapefruit or its juice should not be taken if the client is on a statin drug.

Herbal Considerations

Red yeast is a traditional Chinese medicine currently sold as a supplement to lower cholesterol. It comes from an extract of fermented yeast (*Monascus purpureus*) grown on rice. Its use as an aid for gastric (indigestion, diarrhea, stomach, and spleen) ailments and blood circulation enhancement dates back to 800 AD in China. It is also used as the red food coloring additive seen in Chinese meats and poultry dishes.

The red yeast naturally contains ingredients that help to control cholesterol levels; these include "healthy fats" and monacolin—the ingredient used in the drug lovastatin (http://nccam.nih.gov/health/redyeastrice). Therefore, the supplement would have all the adverse reactions and drug interactions of the statin drugs. Taking this supplement with statin antihyperlipidemic drugs can increase the chance of serious reactions, notably liver or muscle damage (Lapi et al., 2008).

Clients may not volunteer information regarding their use of alternative or complementary remedies. You should always inquire about use of herbal products, especially niacin (purchased as a supplement) or red yeast. Be aware that a possible interaction with St. John's wort, used to relieve depression, causes a decrease in statin effectiveness.

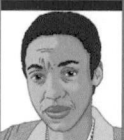

PHARMACOLOGY IN PRACTICE

ASSESSMENT
A client is prescribed atorvastatin for hyperlipidemia. The nurse checks the client's medical history for which of the following contraindicated conditions?
1. Visual disturbances
2. Biliary obstruction
3. Serious liver disorders
4. Renal dysfunction

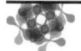 ## PCSK9 INHIBITORS

Proprotein convertase subtilisin/kexin type 9 (PCSK9) inhibitors are a class of LDL-lowering drugs used for clients who have genetic familial hyperlipidemia or are at very high risk for cardiovascular disease (Myerson, 2016).

Therapy for genetic familial hyperlipidemia begins with diet modification and statin drugs. If this is not successful, then the drug is changed to a PCSK9 inhibitor. PCSK9 is an enzyme that binds with LDL and prevents it from being removed from the blood. These inhibitor drugs are monoclonal antibodies that block the enzyme process and lower LDL cholesterol. Two drugs, alirocumab (Praluent) and evolocumab (Repatha), are approved for this treatment option.

These drugs, which are administered subcutaneously only once or twice monthly, are successful in lowering LDL cholesterol, yet are expensive (over $14,000 annually). This is compared with the yearly cost of a statin drug at approximately $250/year (Santye, 2017). In addition, there is concern regarding these drugs and a possibility of cognitive adverse reactions.

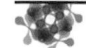 ## BILE ACID RESINS

ACTIONS

Bile, which is manufactured and secreted by the liver and stored in the gallbladder, emulsifies fat and lipids as these products pass through the intestine. Once emulsified, fats and lipids are readily absorbed in the intestine. The bile acid resins bind to bile acids to form an insoluble substance that cannot be absorbed by the intestine, so it is excreted in the feces. With increased loss of bile acids, the liver uses cholesterol to manufacture more bile. This is followed by a decrease in cholesterol levels.

USES

The bile acid resins are used to treat the following:

- Hyperlipidemia (in clients who do not have an adequate response to a diet and exercise program)
- Gallstone dissolution in clients where surgery (cholecystectomy) is not recommended
- Pruritus associated with partial biliary obstruction (cholestyramine only)

ADVERSE REACTIONS

- Constipation (may be severe and occasionally result in fecal impaction), aggravation of hemorrhoids, abdominal cramps, flatulence, nausea
- Increased bleeding tendencies related to vitamin K malabsorption, and vitamin A and D deficiencies

CONTRAINDICATIONS AND PRECAUTIONS

The bile acid resins are contraindicated in clients with known hypersensitivity to the drugs. Bile acid resins are also contraindicated in those with complete biliary obstruction.

These drugs are used cautiously in clients with diabetes, liver, peptic ulcer, or kidney disease. Bile acid resins should be used cautiously during pregnancy (pregnancy category C) and lactation (decreased absorption of vitamins may affect the infant).

INTERACTIONS

The following interactions may occur when the bile acid resins are administered with another agent:

Interacting Drug	Common Use	Effect of Interaction
Anticoagulants	Blood thinners	Decreased effect of the anticoagulant (cholestyramine)
Thyroid hormone	Treatment of hypothyroidism	Loss of efficacy of thyroid; also hypothyroidism (particularly with cholestyramine)
Fat-soluble vitamins (A, D, E, K) and folic acid	Nutritional supplements	Reduced absorption of vitamins

When administered with the bile acid resins, a decreased serum level or decreased gastrointestinal (GI) absorption of the following drugs may occur:

- nonsteroidal anti-inflammatory drugs (used to treat pain)
- penicillin G and tetracycline (used to treat infection)
- niacin (used to treat elevated cholesterol levels)
- digitalis glycosides (used to treat heart failure)
- furosemide and thiazide diuretics (used to treat edema)
- glipizide (used to treat diabetes)
- hydrocortisone (used to treat inflammation)
- methyldopa and propranolol (used to treat hypertension and cardiovascular problems, respectively)

Because the bile acid resins, particularly cholestyramine, can decrease the absorption of numerous drugs, the bile acid resins should be administered alone and other drugs given at least 1 hour before or 4 hours after administration of the bile acid resins.

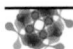 # FIBRIC ACID DERIVATIVES

ACTIONS

Fibric acid derivatives, also known as fibrates, are the third group of antihyperlipidemic drugs and work in a variety of ways. Fenofibrate acts by reducing **very-low-density lipoproteins** (VLDLs) and stimulating the catabolism of triglyceride-rich lipoproteins, resulting in a decrease in plasma triglycerides and cholesterol. Gemfibrozil increases the excretion of cholesterol in the feces and reduces the production of triglycerides by the liver, thus lowering serum lipid levels.

USES

Although the fibric acid derivatives have antihyperlipidemic effects, their use varies depending on the drug. For example, gemfibrozil is used to treat individuals with very high serum triglyceride levels who are at risk for abdominal pain and pancreatitis and who do not experience a response to dietary modifications. Fenofibrate is used as adjunctive treatment for reducing LDLs, total cholesterol, and triglycerides in clients with hyperlipidemia.

ADVERSE REACTIONS

The adverse reactions associated with fibric acid derivatives include the following:

- Nausea, vomiting, and GI upset
- Diarrhea
- **Cholelithiasis** (stones in the gallbladder) or **cholecystitis** (inflammation of the gallbladder)

If cholelithiasis is found, the primary health care provider may discontinue the drug. See the Summary Drug Table: Antihyperlipidemic Drugs for additional adverse reactions.

CONTRAINDICATIONS AND PRECAUTIONS

The fibric acid derivatives are contraindicated in clients with hypersensitivity to the drugs and in those with significant hepatic or renal dysfunction or primary biliary cirrhosis because these drugs may increase the already elevated cholesterol. The drugs are used cautiously during pregnancy (pregnancy category C) and not during lactation.

INTERACTIONS

The following interactions may occur when the fibric acid derivatives are administered with another agent:

Interacting Drug	Common Use	Effect of Interaction
Anticoagulants	Blood thinners	Enhanced effects of the anticoagulants
Cyclosporine	Immunosuppression after organ transplantation	Decreased effects of cyclosporine (particularly with gemfibrozil)
HMG-CoA reductase inhibitors (statins)	Treatment of elevated blood cholesterol levels	Increased risk of rhabdomyolysis
Sulfonylureas	Treatment of diabetes	Increased hypoglycemic effects (particularly with gemfibrozil)

MISCELLANEOUS ANTIHYPERLIPIDEMIC DRUGS

Miscellaneous antihyperlipidemic drugs include niacin, bempedoic acid, and ezetimibe.

ACTIONS

The mechanism by which niacin (nicotinic acid) lowers blood lipid levels is not fully understood. Bempedoic acid inhibits the synthesis of cholesterol in the liver. Finally, ezetimibe inhibits the absorption of cholesterol in the small intestine, leading to a decrease in cholesterol in the liver.

USES

Niacin is used as adjunctive therapy for lowering very high serum triglyceride levels in clients who are at risk for pancreatitis (inflammation of the pancreas) and whose response to dietary control is inadequate. Bempedoic acid and ezetimibe are typically used in combinations with other antihyperlipidemics in lipid-lowering treatments.

ADVERSE REACTIONS

Gastrointestinal System Reactions
- Nausea, vomiting, abdominal pain
- Diarrhea

Other Reactions
- Severe, generalized flushing of the skin; sensation of warmth
- Severe itching or tingling
- Generalized muscle aches and flu-like symptoms

CONTRAINDICATIONS, PRECAUTIONS, AND INTERACTIONS

Niacin is contraindicated in clients with known hypersensitivity to niacin, active peptic ulcer, hepatic dysfunction, and arterial bleeding. The drug is used cautiously in clients with renal dysfunction, high alcohol consumption, unstable angina, gout, and pregnancy (pregnancy category C). Increased uric acid levels and possible risk of tendon rupture can occur with the use of bempedoic acid. Pregnant and lactating women should not use bempedoic acid or ezetimibe.

LASA ALERT

The following drugs may sound alike; be sure to clarify when they are ordered:

Drug Name	Sounds Like
Ezetimibe	Ezogabine
Zetia	Zebeta, Zestril

Drugs that look like a similar drug are noted in the Summary Drug Tables of each chapter.

GENETIC HYPERCHOLESTEROLEMIA

Approximately 1 of every 200 individuals has familial hypercholesterolemia, an inherited genetic disorder, resulting in extreme elevation in the LDL cholesterol level (Santos & Watts, 2015). These clients have a 20 times greater risk of developing coronary heart disease (CHD) than the general population (Siskey & Deyo, 2014). Worldwide, 1 in 160,000 will inherit the genetic mutation from both parents, which results in homozygous familial hypercholesterolemia (HoFH). Mipomersen (Kynamro) and lomitapide (Juxtapid) are considered **orphan drugs status** (designation for production purposes), which are available when TLC, statins, and adjuvant drugs do not lower LDL levels sufficiently in this small, specific population with HoFH. These drugs inhibit cellular actions resulting in decreasing LDL yet carry severe adverse reactions primarily to liver tissue. Because mipomersen and lomitapide have severe hepatotoxic risk, they are only prescribed as part of the **Risk Evaluation and Mitigation Strategies (REMS)** program. The REMS program is designed to assess risk and administer and monitor drugs that have high risk compared with benefit (see Chapter 1 for explanation of this program). Restrictions placed upon these drugs (or any drug in a REMS program) are available on the website of the brand name drug.

Herbal Considerations

Garlic has been used for many years throughout the world. The benefits of garlic on cardiovascular health are the best known and most extensively researched benefits of the herb. Its benefits include lowering serum cholesterol and triglyceride levels, improving the ratio of HDL to LDL cholesterol, lowering blood pressure, and helping to prevent the development of atherosclerosis. The recommended dosages of garlic are 600–900 mg/day of the garlic powder tablets, 10 mg of garlic oil "perles,"

or one moderate-sized fresh clove of garlic a day. Adverse reactions include mild stomach upset or irritation that can usually be alleviated by taking garlic supplements with food. There is an increased risk of bleeding when garlic is taken with warfarin. Although no serious reactions have occurred in pregnant women taking garlic, its use is not recommended. Garlic is excreted in breast milk and may cause colic in some infants. As with all herbal therapy, when garlic is used for therapeutic purposes, the primary health care provider should be aware of its use (DerMarderosian & Beutler, 2003).

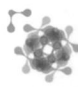

NURSING PROCESS—STEPS TO BUILDING CLINICAL JUDGMENT
Client Receiving an Antihyperlipidemic Drug

ASSESSMENT

Preadministration Assessment
Many individuals with hyperlipidemia have no symptoms, and the disorder is not discovered until laboratory tests reveal elevated cholesterol and triglyceride levels, elevated LDL levels, and decreased HDL levels. Often, these drugs are initially prescribed on an outpatient basis, but initial administration may occur in the client hospitalized for cardiac symptoms and laboratory work shows elevated cholesterol results.

Data gathering suggestions before the initial administration of a hyperlipidemia drug include:
Objective data

- Vital signs (temperature, pulse, respirations, and blood pressure)
- Weight
- Inspect skin and eyelids for evidence of **xanthomas** (flat or elevated yellowish deposit, see Figure 33.2)
- Laboratory tests—lipid profile (serum cholesterol) and other tests for specific client populations (liver function, blood glucose, and HbA$_{1c}$)

Subjective data

- Dietary history (1–3 days diet recording of normal food intake)

- Medical/family history of cholesterol/cardiac issues
- Drug therapy (list of all current drugs and supplements taken)

Ongoing Assessment
Clients usually take antihyperlipidemic drugs on an outpatient basis and come to the clinic or the primary health care provider's office for periodic monitoring of blood cholesterol and triglyceride levels. Liver monitoring should occur when doses are changed or if the client shows signs or symptoms of liver disease (jaundice, nausea, or abdominal pain). One of the best measurements for statin-caused liver compromise is fractionated (indirect) bilirubin levels. Your responsibility is to monitor these levels and report any increase to the primary health care provider. If aspartate aminotransferase levels increase to three times normal, the primary health care provider may discontinue drug therapy. Because the maximum effects of these drugs are usually evident within 4 weeks, periodic lipid profiles are ordered to determine the therapeutic effect of the drug regimen. The dose may be increased, another antihyperlipidemic drug added, or drug therapy discontinued, depending on the client's response.

NURSING ALERT
Sometimes a paradoxical elevation of blood lipid levels occurs. Should this happen, bring this to the attention of the primary health care provider because they may prescribe a different antihyperlipidemic drug.

During the ongoing assessment, check vital signs and assess bowel functioning because an adverse reaction to these drugs is constipation. Constipation may become serious if not treated early in the medication regimen.

NURSING DIAGNOSES
Drug-specific nursing diagnoses include the following:

- **Constipation** related to antihyperlipidemic drugs
- **Malnutrition risk** related to malabsorption of vitamins
- **Altered skin integrity risk** related to rash and flushing

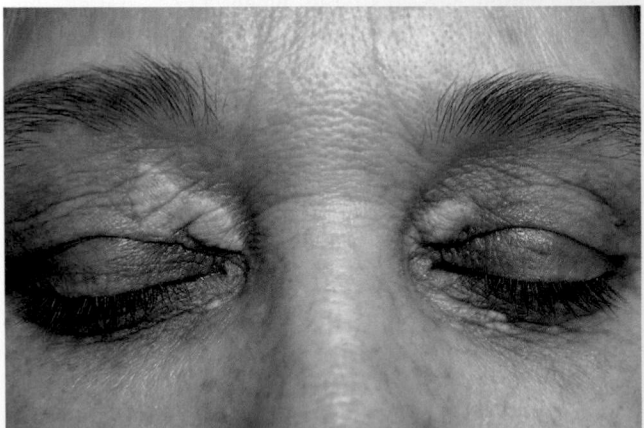

FIGURE 33.2 Xanthomas—fatty deposits in skin of eyelids.

- **Nausea** related to antihyperlipidemic drugs
- **Injury risk** related to dizziness

Nursing diagnoses related to drug administration are discussed in depth in Chapter 4.

PLANNING

The expected outcomes of the client depend on the specific reason for administering the drug but may include an optimal response to therapy, support of client needs related to the management of adverse reactions, and confidence in an understanding of the medication regimen.

IMPLEMENTATION

Promoting an Optimal Response to Therapy

Because hyperlipidemia is often treated on an outpatient basis, it is your responsibility to explain the drug regimen and possible adverse reactions. If printed dietary guidelines are given to the client, utilize language-appropriate printed materials to emphasize the importance of following these recommendations. Drug therapy usually is changed if the antihyperlipidemic drug is not effective after 3 months of treatment.

Statin drugs do not absorb well when administered close to a high-fat meal. Therefore, it is a good idea to take these drugs at bedtime. Discuss with the client minimizing high-fat bedtime snacks such as ice cream to ensure the effectiveness of the drug.

Monitoring and Managing Client Needs

Constipation
Clients taking the antihyperlipidemic drugs, particularly the bile acid resins, may experience constipation. The drugs can produce or severely worsen pre-existing constipation. Instruct the client to increase fluid intake, eat foods high in dietary fiber, and exercise daily to help prevent constipation. If the problem persists or becomes severe, a stool softener or laxative may be required. Some clients require decreased dosage or discontinuation of the drug therapy.

 Lifespan Consideration

Gerontology

Older adults are particularly prone to constipation when taking the bile acid resins. Question older adults about hard, dry stools; difficulty passing stools; and any complaints of constipation. Early intervention with stool softeners or laxatives may improve adherence.

Malnutrition Risk
Bile acid resins may interfere with the digestion of fats and prevent the absorption of the fat-soluble vitamins (vitamins A, D, E, and K) and folic acid. When the bile acid resins are used for long-term therapy, vitamins A and D may be given in a water-soluble form or administered parenterally.

Altered Skin Integrity Risk
Clients taking nicotinic acid (niacin) may experience moderate to severe, generalized flushing of the skin; a sensation of warmth; and severe itching or tingling. They may also complain of ringing in the ears. Although these reactions are most often seen at higher dose levels, some clients may experience them even when small doses of nicotinic acid are administered. The sudden appearance of these reactions may frighten the client.

🛈 **NURSING ALERT**

Advise the client taking niacin to contact the primary health care provider if the skin reactions are severe or cause extreme discomfort. Aspirin may be recommended before taking niacin preparations to reduce adverse reactions.

Nausea
Some antihyperlipidemic drugs cause nausea. If nausea occurs, the drug should be taken with meals or with food such as crackers. Other measures to help alleviate the nausea include providing a relaxed atmosphere for eating with no unpleasant odors or sights. Teach the client to eat several small meals rather than three large meals. If nausea is severe or vomiting occurs, the primary health care provider is notified.

Injury Risk
Injury can occur when the client falls as the result of dizziness as an adverse reaction from the fibrates or statins. Monitor the hospitalized client starting this medication carefully, placing the call light within easy reach. The client may require assistance with ambulation until the effects of the medication are known, especially with the initial doses of the antihyperlipidemic.

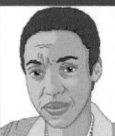 **PHARMACOLOGY IN PRACTICE**

MANAGING NEEDS
A nurse is caring for an older client using bile acid sequestrants. What should the nurse monitor for in the client? Select all that apply.
1. Difficulty in passing stools
2. Hard, dry stools
3. Constipation
4. Mouth dryness
5. Urinary hesitancy

Potential Medical Complication: Vitamin K Deficiency
To prevent deficiency, the client is encouraged to include foods high in vitamin K in the diet, such as asparagus, broccoli, green beans, lettuce, turnip greens, beef liver, collard greens, green tea, and spinach. Teach the client to check for bruises over the body as an indication of vitamin K deficiency. If bruising is observed or if bleeding tendencies occur, instruct the client to contact the primary health care provider immediately. Parenteral vitamin K

may be prescribed by the primary health care provider for immediate treatment and oral vitamin K for preventing a deficiency in the future.

Potential Medical Complication: Rhabdomyolysis
Antihyperlipidemic drugs, particularly the statin drugs, have been associated with skeletal muscle effects leading to rhabdomyolysis. **Rhabdomyolysis** is a rare condition in which muscle damage results in the release of muscle cell contents into the bloodstream. Rhabdomyolysis may precipitate renal dysfunction or acute renal failure. Be alert for complaints of unexplained muscle pain, muscle tenderness, or weakness, especially if accompanied by malaise or fever. This reaction is more likely in Asian clients; therefore, a lower starting dose of the statin rosuvastatin is recommended (Naito et al., 2017). These symptoms should be reported to the primary health care provider because the drug may need to be discontinued.

Educating the Client and Family
Many of the circulatory-related ailments require lifestyle changes. Diet is an important aspect of cholesterol management for the client. Emphasize the importance of following the diet recommended by the primary health care provider because drug therapy alone will not significantly lower cholesterol and triglyceride levels. Contact the client periodically to see how they are handling a new eating plan; in addition, provide a copy of the recommended diet. Learn about your resources and refer the client or family member to a clinical dietitian, a cardiovascular dietary health workshop, Internet websites, or a lecture/workshop provided by a hospital or community agency (see Client Teaching for Improved Outcomes: Using Self-Management Skills to Control Blood Cholesterol Levels). As you develop a teaching plan include the following information:

Statins (HMG-CoA Reductase Inhibitors)
- Usually statins are taken in the evening or at bedtime.
- Choose juices other than grapefruit juice because of an enzyme reaction.
- Antacids should be taken at least 2 hours after rosuvastatin.
- When fluvastatin or pravastatin is prescribed with a bile acid resin, the statin should be taken 2 hours before the bile acid resin or at least 4 hours afterward.
- These drugs may cause photosensitivity; avoid exposure to the sun and wear both sunscreen and protective clothing.
- These drugs cannot be used during pregnancy (pregnancy category X). Use a barrier contraceptive while taking these drugs. If the client wishes to become pregnant while taking these drugs, the primary health care provider should be consulted before efforts at conception.
- Advise the client to contact the primary health care provider as soon as possible if muscle pain, tenderness, or weakness occurs.

Client Teaching for Improved Outcomes

Using Self-Management Skills to Control Blood Cholesterol Levels
Feeling you personally have control makes adherence to long-term medical management of chronic conditions such as hyperlipidemia or hypertension more successful. As the nurse, you can empower clients by supporting efforts rather than telling them to participate in strategies for self-care.

Encourage clients to participate in managing their abilities to reduce cardiovascular risk by accessing interactive tools on the Internet. Various sites use information from the Framingham Heart Study to predict heart attack risk (see example at National Heart, Lung, and Blood Institute website). To use most interactive sites, the following data are entered into the cardiovascular risk calculator:
- Age
- Gender
- Cholesterol laboratory value
- Blood pressure reading

A prediction for heart attack risk in the next 10 years is calculated. By reviewing these notations periodically, adherence to treatment recommendations will be reinforced as the client sees risk reduction over time.

Bile Acid Resins
- Take the drug before meals unless the primary health care provider directs otherwise.
- Cholestyramine powder: The prescribed dose must be mixed in 2–6 fluid ounces of water or noncarbonated beverage and shaken vigorously. The powder can also be mixed with highly fluid soups or pulpy fruits (e.g., applesauce, crushed pineapple). The powder should not be ingested in the dry form. Other drugs are taken 1 hour before or 4–6 hours after cholestyramine. Cholestyramine is available combined with the artificial sweetener aspartame for clients with diabetes or those who are concerned about weight gain.
- Colestipol granules: The prescribed dose must be mixed in liquids, soup, cereals, carbonated beverages, or pulpy fruits. Use approximately 90 mL of liquid and, when mixing with a liquid, slowly stir the preparation until ready to drink. The granules will not dissolve. Take the entire drug, rinse the glass with a small amount of water, and drink to ensure that all the medication is taken.
- Colestipol tablets: Tablets should be swallowed whole, one at a time, with a full glass of water or other fluid—not chewed, cut, or crushed.
- Sipping or holding the liquid preparations in the mouth can cause tooth discoloration or enamel decay.
- Constipation, nausea, abdominal pain, and distention may occur and may subside with continued therapy. Contact the primary health care provider if these effects become bothersome or if unusual bleeding or bruising occurs.

Fibric Acid Derivatives
- Gemfibrozil may cause dizziness or blurred vision. Observe caution when driving or performing hazardous tasks. Notify the primary health care provider if epigastric pain, diarrhea, nausea, or vomiting occurs.

Miscellaneous Preparations
- Nicotinic acid (niacin): Take this drug with meals. This drug may cause mild to severe facial flushing, a sensation of warmth, severe itching, or headache. These symptoms usually subside with continued therapy, but contact the primary health care provider as soon as possible if symptoms are severe. The primary health care provider may prescribe aspirin (325 mg) to be taken about 30 minutes before nicotinic acid to decrease the flushing reaction. If dizziness occurs, avoid sudden changes in posture.
- Ezetimibe: this drug should be taken at least 2 hours before or 4 hours after a bile acid sequestrant. Report unusual muscle pain, weakness or tenderness, severe diarrhea, or respiratory infections.

EVALUATION
- Therapeutic response is achieved and serum lipid levels are decreased.

- Adverse reactions are identified, reported to the primary health care provider, and managed successfully with appropriate nursing interventions:
  - Client reports adequate bowel movements.
  - Client maintains an adequate nutritional status.
  - Skin remains intact.
  - Nausea is controlled.
  - No evidence of injury is seen.
- Client and family express confidence and demonstrate an understanding of the drug regimen.

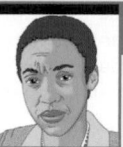

PHARMACOLOGY IN PRACTICE

USING CLINICAL REASONING

Lillian's first visit to the clinic was a year ago. Her blood pressure was 156/98 and laboratory work drawn that day was cholesterol = 320, LDL = 178, and HDL = 20.

The following information from her medical record today shows that T = 98.6 °F, P = 104, R = 18, and BP = 136/92. Laboratory work drawn had the following values: cholesterol = 256, LDL = 160, and HDL = 36. How can you use this information to help encourage Mrs. Chase to continue her medication? What information would you give the client concerning her constipation?

KEY POINTS

■ Atherosclerosis is a disorder in which lipid deposits accumulate on the lining of blood vessels. Cholesterol and triglycerides are two lipids in our blood; elevation of one or both is termed hyperlipidemia.

■ Antihyperlipidemic drugs decrease cholesterol and triglycerides in the blood. When included with lifestyle changes such as diet modifications, physical activity, smoking cessation, and weight management, the risk of coronary heart disease is lessened.

■ HMG-CoA reductase inhibitors are frequently called "statin" drugs. These drugs lower the blood level of LDL cholesterol and triglycerides. Bile acid resins and fibric acid derivatives act in a similar manner to reduce cholesterol by binding with bile so the liver will use more, putting less in the system.

■ Common adverse reactions include headache, dizziness, insomnia, and GI complaints such as increased flatulence and constipation. Clients taking bile acid resins need to be alert for bleeding tendencies. Those taking niacin have experienced a sensation of warmth, flushing, and itching; a reduction in dose diminishes the reactions.

SUMMARY DRUG TABLE
Antihyperlipidemic Drugs

Generic Name	Trade Name	Uses	Adverse Reactions	Dosage Ranges
HMG-CoA Reductase Inhibitors (Statins)				
atorvaSTATin a-TORE-va-sta-tin	Lipitor	Reduce risk of CHD events, hyperlipidemia, familial hypercholesterolemia	Headache, diarrhea, sinusitis	10–80 mg/day orally
fluvastatin FLOO-va-sta-tin	Lescol XL	Atherosclerosis, hyperlipidemia, familial hypercholesterolemia	Headache, back pain, upper respiratory infection, flu-like syndrome	20–80 mg/day orally

Continued

SUMMARY DRUG TABLE (continued)
Antihyperlipidemic Drugs

Generic Name	Trade Name	Uses	Adverse Reactions	Dosage Ranges
lovastatin *LOE-va-sta-tin*	Altoprev	Reduce risk of CHD events, atherosclerosis, hyperlipidemia, familial hypercholesterolemia	Headache, flatulence, infection	10–80 mg/day orally in single or divided doses Adolescents: 10–40 mg/day orally
pitavastatin *pi-TA-va-sta-tin*	Livalo, Zypitamag	Hyperlipidemia	Constipation, diarrhea, confusion, back pain	2–4 mg/day orally
pravastatin *prav-a-STAT-in*	Pravachol	Reduce risk of CHD events, atherosclerosis, hyperlipidemia, familial hypercholesterolemia	Headache, nausea, vomiting, diarrhea, localized pain, cold symptoms	40–80 mg/day orally Children 8–13 years: 20 mg/day orally Adolescents 14–18 years: 40 mg/day orally
rosuvastatin *roe-soo-va-STAT-in*	Crestor, Ezallor Sprinkle	Hyperlipidemia, lipid management. post solid organ transplant	Headache	5–40 mg/day orally
simvastatin *sim-va-STAT-in*	FloLipid, Zocor	Reduce risk of CHD events, hyperlipidemia, familial hypercholesterolemia	Constipation	5–80 mg/day orally
PCSK9 Inhibitors				
alirocumab *al-i-ROK-ue-mab*	Praluent	Adjunctive treatment for familial hyperlipidemia	Diarrhea, flu-like symptoms injection site reaction	75–150 mg subcut every 2 weeks
evolocumab *e-voe-LOK-ue-mab*	Repatha	Adjunctive treatment for familial hyperlipidemia	Dizziness, flu-like symptoms, arthralgia	420 mg subcut monthly
Bile Acid Resins				
cholestyramine *koe-LES-teer-a-meen*	Prevalite, Questran	Hyperlipidemia, relief of pruritus associated with partial biliary obstruction	Constipation (may lead to fecal impaction), exacerbation of hemorrhoids, abdominal pain, distention and cramping, nausea, increased bleeding related to vitamin K malabsorption, vitamin A and D deficiencies	4 g orally 1–6 times/day; individualize dosage based on response
colestipol *koe-LES-ti-pole*	Colestid	Hyperlipidemia	Same as cholestyramine	Granules: 5–30 g/day orally in divided doses Tablets: 2–16 g/day
colesevelam *koe-le-SEV-a-lam*	Welchol	Hyperlipidemia, adjuvant in type 2 diabetes	Same as cholestyramine	3–7 tablets/day orally
Fibric Acid Derivatives (Fibrates)				
fenofibrate *fen-oh-FYE-brate*	TriCor, Triglide, Trilipix, Antara, Lipofen	Hyperlipidemia, hypertriglyceridemia	Abnormal liver function test results, respiratory problems, abdominal pain	Tablet: 48–145 mg/day orally
gemfibrozil *jem-FI-broe-zil*	Lopid	Reduce risk of CHD events, hypertriglyceridemia	Dyspepsia, abdominal pain, diarrhea, nausea, vomiting, fatigue	1200 mg/day orally in two divided doses 30 minutes before morning and evening meals
Miscellaneous Preparations				
ezetimibe *ez-ET-i-mibe*	Zetia	Primary hypercholesterolemia	Diarrhea, back pain, sinusitis, dizziness, abdominal pain, arthralgia, coughing, fatigue	10 mg/day orally

Generic Name	Trade Name	Uses	Adverse Reactions	Dosage Ranges
niacin (nicotinic acid) NYE-a-sin	Niaspan, Niacor	Adjunctive treatment for hyperlipidemia	Generalized flushing, sensation of warmth, severe itching and tingling, nausea, vomiting, abdominal pain	Immediate release: 1–2 g orally BID, TID Extended release: 500–2000 mg/day orally
bempedoic acid BEM-pe-DOE-ik	Nexletol	Familial hypercholesterolemia, CAD	Gout, hyperuricemia	180 mg orally daily with "statin"
Antihyperlipidemia Agents Offered Only Through REMS Program				
lomitapide loe-MI-ta-pide	Juxtapid	Familial hypercholesterolemia	Nausea, vomiting, diarrhea, chest/abdominal pain, fatigue, fatty lever	60 mg/day orally
mipomersen mi-poe-MER-sen		Familial hypercholesterolemia	Fatigue, headache, antibody development, fatty liver	200 mg subcut weekly

CHAPTER REVIEW

Know Your Drugs

Clients sometimes know a medication by the brand (or trade) name and not the generic name. To help you recognize both names, match the brand name with the generic name of the same medication.

Generic Name	Brand Name
1. atorvastatin	A. Crestor
2. lovastatin	B. Lipitor
3. rosuvastatin	C. Altoprev
4. simvastatin	D. Zocor

Calculate Medication Dosages

1. A client is prescribed 10 mg simvastatin orally daily for high cholesterol. The drug is available in 5-mg tablets. The nurse administers _____.
2. Lipitor comes in both 20- and 40-mg tablets. To use the least number of pills, what strength of tablet should be used for a client prescribed 80 mg orally daily?

Prepare for the NCLEX

RECALL THE FACTS

1. Which of the following blood elements has a protective property for heart disease?
   1. Cholesterol
   2. Low-density lipoproteins
   3. High-density lipoproteins
   4. Triglycerides
2. Antihyperlipidemia drugs work to:
   1. reduce fat in dietary intake.
   2. decrease cholesterol and triglycerides.
   3. remove plaque from arterioles.
   4. lessen gallbladder stones.

3. Select the most common adverse reaction in a client taking a bile acid resin:
   1. anorexia
   2. vomiting
   3. constipation
   4. headache
4. Lovastatin is best taken _____.
   1. once daily, preferably with the evening meal
   2. three times daily with meals
   3. at least 1 hour before or 2 hours after meals
   4. twice daily without regard to meals
5. A client taking niacin reports flushing after each dose of the niacin. Which of the following drugs would the nurse expect to be prescribed to help alleviate the flushing?
   1. meperidine (Demerol)
   2. aspirin
   3. vitamin K
   4. diphenhydramine (Benadryl)

ANALYZE THE FACTS

6. When assessing a client taking cholestyramine for vitamin K deficiency, the nurse would _____.
   1. check the client for bruising
   2. keep a record of the client's intake and output
   3. monitor the client for myalgia
   4. keep a dietary record of foods eaten
7. *Which of the following points is important for the nurse to tell the client when teaching about drug and diet therapy for hyperlipidemia?
   1. Fluids are taken in limited amounts when eating a low-fat diet.
   2. The medication should be taken at least 1 hour before meals.
   3. Medication alone will not lower cholesterol.
   4. Meat is not allowed on a low-fat diet.

8. As the client makes breakfast selections for tomorrow, which of the following items should the nurse recognize as a potential problem food?
   1. Scrambled eggs
   2. Oatmeal with cream and sugar
   3. Stewed prunes
   4. Grapefruit juice

ALTERNATE-FORMAT QUESTIONS

9. A client taking bile acid resins can become vitamin deficient in which of the following? **Select all that apply.**
   1. Vitamin A
   2. Vitamin B
   3. Vitamin C
   4. Vitamin D
   5. Vitamin E

10. The primary health care provider prescribes fenofibrate for the treatment of hypertriglyceridemia. The client is now taking 200 mg/day orally. Is this an appropriate dosage? If not, what action would you take? If the dose is appropriate, how many capsules would you administer if the drug is available in 67-mg capsules?

To check your answers, see Appendix F.

---

*Indicates the question is directly linked to the NCLEX-PN test plan in Appendix G.

WANT TO KNOW MORE? A wide variety of resources are available to enhance your learning and understanding of this chapter.

- Visit the Point for resources such as:
  - NCLEX-Style Student Review Questions
  - Journal Articles
  - Dosage Calculations
  - Drug Monographs
  - Watch and Learn Videos
  - Concepts in Action Animations
- The *Study Guide to Accompany Introductory Clinical Pharmacology*, 12th edition, sold separately, will help you review and apply essential content.
- ✓**PrepU** is available to help students prepare for the NCLEX-PN examination.

34

Antihypertensive Drugs

Key Terms

angioedema localized wheals or swellings in subcutaneous tissues or mucous membranes, which may be because of an allergic response; also called angioneurotic edema

blood pressure force of blood against artery walls

endogenous pertaining to something that normally occurs or is produced within the organism

hyperkalemia increase in potassium levels in the blood

hypertension high blood pressure that stays elevated over time

hypertensive emergency extremely high blood pressure that must be lowered immediately to prevent damage to target organs (i.e., heart, kidneys, eyes)

hypokalemia low blood potassium level

hyponatremia low blood sodium level

isolated systolic hypertension systolic blood pressure over 140 mm Hg with diastolic blood pressure under 90 mm Hg

lumen inner diameter of a tube; the space or opening within an artery

orthostatic hypotension decrease in blood pressure occurring after standing in one place for an extended period

prehypertension (or elevated) blood pressure readings which indicate lifestyle modifications should be initiated to return pressures to normal levels

primary hypertension hypertension that has no known cause; also known as essential or idiopathic hypertension

secondary hypertension hypertension with a known cause, such as kidney disease

vasodilation increase in the diameter of the blood vessels that, when widespread, results in a drop in blood pressure

Learning Objectives

On completion of this chapter, the student will:

1. Compare and contrast the various types of hypertension and risk factors involved.
2. Identify normal and abnormal blood pressure levels for adults.
3. List the various types of drugs used to treat hypertension.
4. Explain the general drug actions, uses, adverse reactions, contraindications, precautions, and interactions of the antihypertensive drugs.
5. Distinguish important preadministration and ongoing assessment activities the nurse should perform for the client taking an antihypertensive drug.
6. Explain why blood pressure determinations are important during therapy with an antihypertensive drug.
7. List nursing diagnoses particular to a client taking an antihypertensive drug.
8. Examine ways to promote an optimal response to therapy, how to manage adverse reactions, and important points to keep in mind when educating clients about the use of an antihypertensive drug.

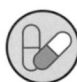 **Drug Classes**

Beta-adrenergic (β-adrenergic) blocking drugs
Alpha/beta-antiadrenergic (α/β-antiadrenergic) drugs (centrally and peripherally acting)
Calcium channel blocking drugs
Angiotensin-converting enzyme (ACE) inhibitors (ACEIs)
Angiotensin II receptor antagonists
Vasodilators.

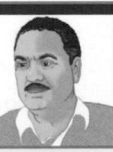 **PHARMACOLOGY IN PRACTICE**

Mr. Alfredo Garcia was in the clinic a month ago for a respiratory infection. At that time his blood pressure was 210/120 mm Hg. He was prescribed a beta-blocking drug. When he returns today, his weight is down 15 lb and his blood pressure is 170/95 mm Hg. Read about the different drugs in this chapter to see if any changes should be made.

What is meant by the term—**blood pressure**? It is simply the force of the blood against the walls of the arteries. Blood pressure increases and decreases throughout the day. The condition in which blood pressure stays elevated over time is known as

Blood pressure categories

	Systolic mmHg (Upper number)		Diastolic mmHg (Lower number)
Normal	**Below 120**	**and**	**Below 80**
Elevated (Pre hypertension)	**120 - 129**	**and**	**Below 80**
Hypertension stage 1	**130 - 139**	**or**	**80 - 89**
Hypertension stage 2	**140 or higher**	**or**	**90 or higher**
Hypertensive crisis	**Above 180**	**and/or**	**Above 120**

FIGURE 34.1 Classification of blood pressure categories.

hypertension. The term *silent killer* is sometimes used to describe hypertension. This is because there are few symptoms seen or felt by the client who has increased blood pressure, yet it can have devastating effects on the body. Hypertension leads to many problems that we do not even associate with the heart such as stroke, kidney damage, and vision loss. This is why understanding hypertension is critical. In fact, 103 million Americans have high blood pressure; this is almost 1 in every 2 adults. African Americans are twice as likely as Caucasians to experience hypertension. After age 65, African-American women have the highest incidence of hypertension (AHA, 2020).

Hypertension is defined as a blood pressure of 130/30 mm Hg or higher. A systolic blood pressure less than 120 mm Hg and a diastolic blood pressure less than 80 mm Hg (120/80) are considered normal. **Prehypertension** or elevated pressure occurs when the systolic pressure falls between 120 and 129 mm Hg and the diastolic pressure remains below 80 mm Hg. Individuals with prehypertensive blood pressure readings are at risk for developing hypertension and should begin health-promoting lifestyle modifications. Figure 34.1 identifies current blood pressure classifications.

RISKS FACTORS FOR HYPERTENSION

Hypertension is a serious condition, because it causes the heart to work too hard and contributes to atherosclerosis. Yet, most cases of hypertension have no known cause and is termed **primary hypertension**. Although the cause may be unknown, certain risk factors, such as diet and lifestyle, can influence primary hypertension. Box 34.1 identifies the risk factors associated with hypertension.

Primary hypertension cannot be cured but it can be controlled. Although hypertension is not a part of healthy aging, many individuals experience hypertension as they

---

BOX 34.1   Risk Factors for Hypertension

Nonmodifiable
- Age and sex (women older than 55 years and men older than 45 years of age)
- Family history of high blood pressure and/or cardiovascular disease, diabetes, persistent stress
- Race (African Americans have higher rates than Asian, Caucasian, or Hispanic individuals)

Modifiable
- Obesity[a]
- Excessive dietary intake of salt and too little intake of potassium
- Chronic alcohol consumption
- Lack of physical activity
- Cigarette smoking
  [a]Overweight in youth younger than 18 years has become a risk factor for prehypertension in teens.

grow older. For many older individuals, the *systolic* pressure gives the most accurate diagnosis of hypertension (Uribe & Oji, 2018).

 Lifespan Considerations

Gerontology
Individuals with only an elevated systolic pressure have a condition known as **isolated systolic hypertension** (ISH). When the systolic pressure is high, blood vessels become less flexible and stiffen, leading to cardiovascular disease and kidney damage. Often ISH is a condition of aging. Research indicates that treating ISH saves lives and reduces illness. The treatment is the same for ISH as for other forms of hypertension. Diastolic pressure should not be reduced lower than 70 mm Hg. Therefore, caution is advised in treating those with ISH and existing heart disease (Duprez, 2012).

NONPHARMACOLOGIC MANAGEMENT FOR HYPERTENSION

Once primary hypertension develops, management of the disorder becomes a lifetime task. On the other hand, when a direct cause of the hypertension can be identified, the condition is described as secondary hypertension. Among the known causes of **secondary hypertension** kidney disease ranks first (often caused by diabetes), with tumors or other abnormalities of the adrenal glands following. Most primary health care providers prescribe lifestyle changes to reduce risk factors before prescribing drugs. The primary health care provider may recommend measures such as:

- Weight loss (if the client is overweight)
- Stress reduction (e.g., relaxation techniques, meditation, and yoga)
- Regular aerobic exercise
- Smoking cessation (if applicable)
- Moderation of alcohol consumption
- Dietary changes, such as a decrease in sodium (salt) intake

Many people with hypertension are "salt sensitive," in that any salt or sodium more than the minimum need is too much for them and leads to an increase in blood pressure. Dietitians usually recommend the Dietary Approaches to Stop Hypertension (DASH) diet. Studies indicate that blood pressure can be reduced by eating a diet low in saturated fat, total fat, and cholesterol and rich in fruits, vegetables, and low-fat dairy foods. The DASH diet includes whole grains, poultry, fish, and nuts and has reduced amounts of fats, red meats, sweets, and sugared beverages.

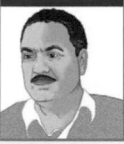

PHARMACOLOGY IN PRACTICE

TEACHING AND LEARNING

A nurse is presenting an educational session to clients on the consequences of untreated hypertension. Which of the following may develop if hypertension is not treated? Select all that apply.
1. Adrenal tumor
2. Blindness
3. Stroke
4. Heart disease
5. Obesity

DRUG THERAPY FOR HYPERTENSION

When nonpharmacologic measures do not control high blood pressure, drug therapy usually begins, and the primary health care provider may first prescribe a thiazide type diuretic (see Chapter 32) with or without a beta-adrenergic (β-adrenergic) blocker (see Chapter 24) (Wright et al., 2018). If this combination does not prove to be effective, therapy may be switched to one of the other hypertensive categories listed below.

The types of drugs used for the treatment of hypertension include the following:

- Diuretics—for example, furosemide and hydrochlorothiazide
- Beta-adrenergic blocking drugs—for example, atenolol and propranolol
- Antiadrenergic drugs (centrally acting)—for example, clonidine and methyldopa
- Antiadrenergic drugs (peripherally acting)—for example, doxazosin and prazosin
- Calcium channel blocking drugs—for example, amlodipine and diltiazem
- ACEIs—for example, captopril and enalapril
- Angiotensin II receptor antagonists—for example, irbesartan and losartan
- Vasodilating drugs—for example, hydralazine and minoxidil

Two drug types are relatively new—direct renin inhibitors (aliskiren) and selective aldosterone receptor antagonists (SARAs; eplerenone). Aliskiren inhibits renin and subsequently prevents the angiotensin conversion process. Eplerenone also blocks the angiotensin process by binding with aldosterone. Additionally, vasodilating drugs used in urgent situations to reduce blood pressure are listed in the Summary Drug Table.

However, as in many other diseases and conditions, there is no "best" single agent, drug combination, or medical regimen for treatment of hypertension. Clients may be initially started on one of the other hypertensive drugs listed above due to concurrent disease (such as diabetes) or familial history. Figure 34.2 illustrates the recommendations of the National Heart, Lung, and Blood Institute's eighth report on hypertension displayed as an algorithm for the treatment of hypertension which are slightly different than Wright's findings (Wright, 2018).

The primary health care provider also recommends that the client continue with stress reduction, dietary modifications, and other lifestyle modifications needed for controlling hypertension.

For additional information concerning the antiadrenergic drugs (both centrally and peripherally acting), and the alpha- and beta-adrenergic blocking drugs, see Chapter 24. Information on the vasodilating drugs and the diuretics can be found in Chapters 35 and 32, respectively. In addition to these antihypertensive drugs, many antihypertensive combinations are available, such as Aldoril, or Lopressor HCT (Table 34.1). Most combination antihypertensive drugs combine antihypertensive and diuretic agents. A few combination drugs include an antihypertensive and another drug for ease of administration, those are noted in Table 34.1.

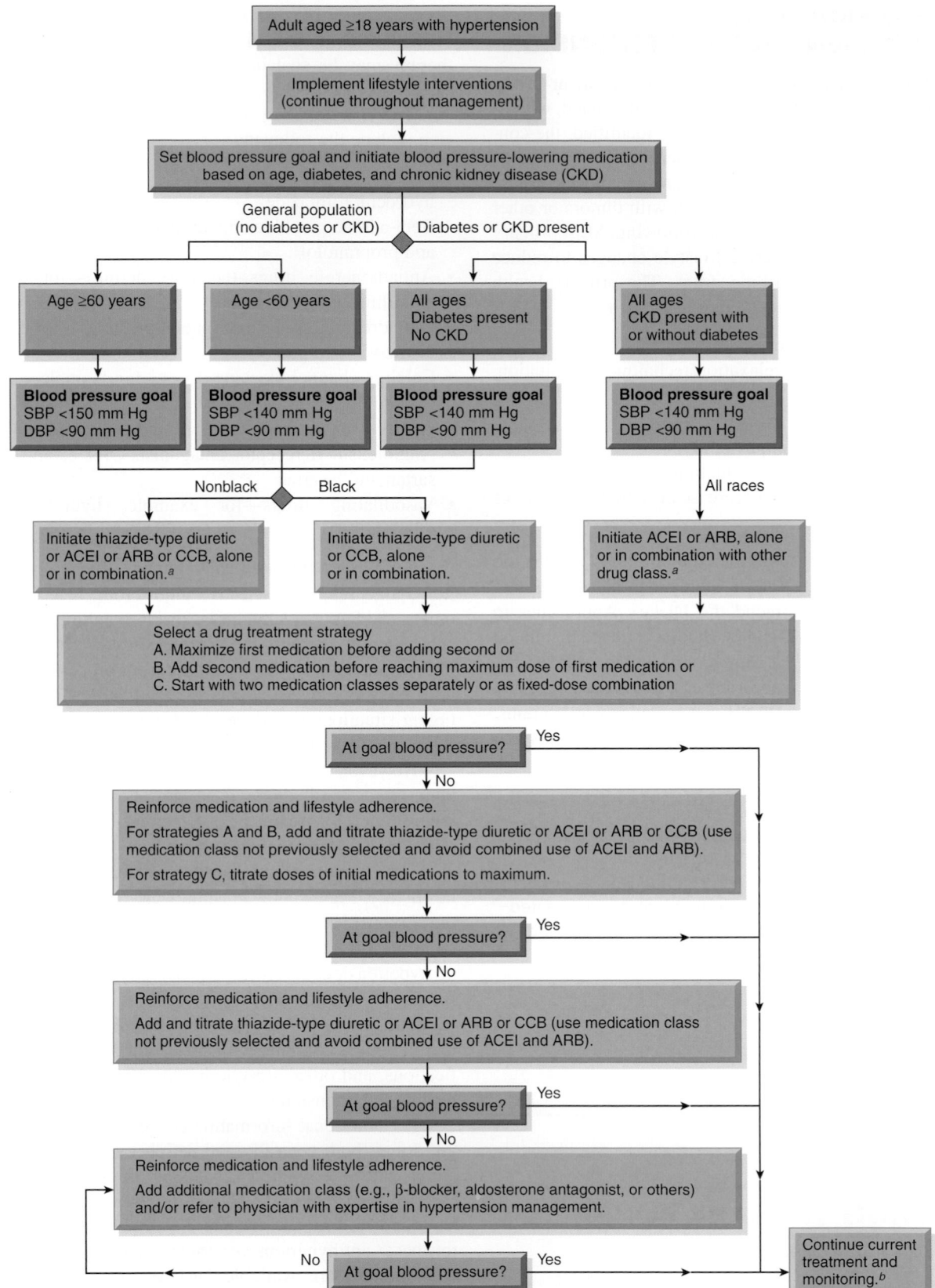

FIGURE 34.2 Algorithm for treatment of hypertension. (Adapted from National Heart, Lung and Blood Institute. (2014). *The eighth report of the Joint National Committee on Prevention, Detection, Evaluation, and Treatment of High Blood Pressure. National Institutes of Health.* http://www.nhlbi.nih.gov/guidelines/hypertension/)

TABLE 34.1 Examples of Antihypertensive Combinations

COMBINATION TYPE	GENERIC DRUG COMBINATIONS[a,b]	COMBINATION DRUG TRADE NAME
ACEIs and CCBs	amlodipine-benazepril	Lotrel
	amlodipine-perindopril	Prestalia
	trandolapril-verapamil	Tarka
ACEIs and diuretics	benazepril-hydrochlorothiazide	Lotensin HCT *generic only*
	captopril-hydrochlorothiazide	Vaseretic *generic only*
	enalapril-hydrochlorothiazide	Zestoretic *generic only*
	fosinopril-hydrochlorothiazide	Accuretic
	lisinopril-hydrochlorothiazide	
	moexipril-hydrochlorothiazide	
	quinapril-hydrochlorothiazide	
ARBs and CCBs	amlodipine-olmesartan	Azor
	amlodipine-olmesartan-hydrochlorothiazide	Tribenzor
	amlodipine-telmisartan	Twynsta
ARBs and diuretics	azilsartan-chlorthalidone	Edarbyclor
	candesartan-hydrochlorothiazide	Atacand HCT *generic only*
	eprosartan-hydrochlorothiazide	Avalide
	irbesartan-hydrochlorothiazide	Hyzaar
	losartan-hydrochlorothiazide	Benicar HCT
	olmesartan-hydrochlorothiazide	Micardis HCT
	telmisartan-hydrochlorothiazide	Exforge HCT
	amlodipine-valsartan-hydrochlorothiazide	
BBs and diuretics	atenolol-chlorthalidone	Tenoretic 50
	bisoprolol-hydrochlorothiazide	Ziac
	metoprolol-hydrochlorothiazide	Lopressor HCT *generic only*
	nadolol-bendroflumethiazide	*generic only*
	propranolol-hydrochlorothiazide	
Misc. and diuretic	aliskiren-hydrochlorothiazide	Tekturna HCT *generic only*
	clonidine-chlorthalidone	*generic only*
	methyldopa-hydrochlorothiazide	
Diuretic and diuretic	spironolactone-hydrochlorothiazide	Aldactazide
	triamterene-hydrochlorothiazide	Dyazide, Maxzide
CCB and Cox-2 (hypertension/osteoarthritis)	amlodipine-celecoxib	Consensi
ARB and NI (hypertension/heart failure)	valsartan-sacubitril	Entresto

ACEI, angiotensin-converting enzyme inhibitor; ARB, angiotensin receptor blocker; BB, beta-blocker; CCB, calcium channel blocker; NI, neprilysin inhibitor.
[a]Some drug combinations are available in multiple fixed doses.
[b]These Drug Combinations Consist of an Antihypertensive and Another Drug (Typically a diuretic) Combined for Additive Therapeutic Results or when Other Chronic Conditions Require Medications and this Reduces the Number of Doses for Intended Outcome

NURSING ALERT

Some combination drugs which include hydrochlorothiazide have "HCT" as the ending of the drug brand name, such as with *Lopressor HCT*. Note, not all combination drugs are like this—the combination of irbesartan and hydrochlorothiazide is marketed as the brand name drug—*Avalide*.

ACTIONS

Many antihypertensive drugs lower the blood pressure by dilating or increasing the size of the arterial blood vessels (**vasodilation**). Vasodilation creates an increase in the **lumen** (the space or opening within a blood vessel) of the arterial blood vessels, which in turn increases the amount of space available for the blood to circulate. Because blood volume (the amount of blood) remains relatively constant, an increase in the space in which the blood circulates (i.e., the blood vessels) lowers the pressure of the fluid (measured as blood pressure) in the blood vessels. Although the method by which antihypertensive drugs dilate blood vessels varies, the result remains basically the same. Figure 34.3 shows the organs affected by the different classes of antihypertensive drugs.

Antihypertensive drugs with vasodilating activity include the adrenergic blocking and calcium channel blocking drugs. Diuretics (Chapter 32) are also considered antihypertensive drugs. The mechanism by which the diuretics reduce elevated blood pressure is not

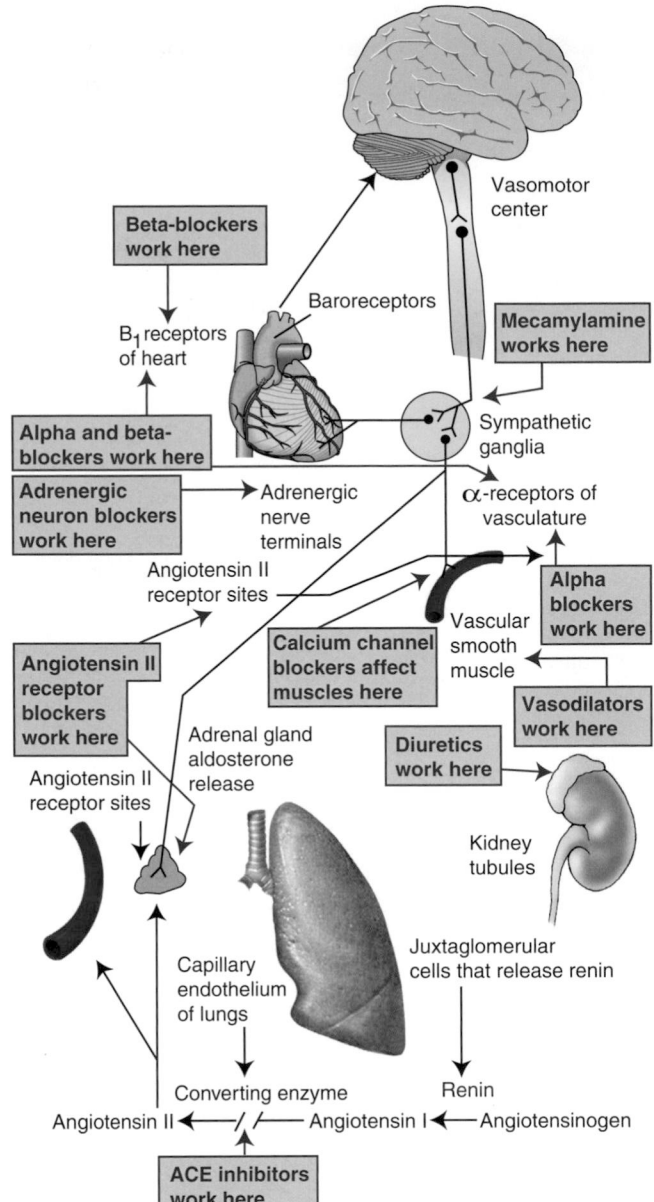

FIGURE 34.3 Sites of action of antihypertensive drugs. ACE, angiotensin-converting enzyme.

completely understood, but it is thought to be based, in part, on their ability to increase the excretion of sodium from the body.

Action of Angiotensin-Converting Enzyme Inhibitors

The ACEIs appear to act primarily through suppression of the renin–angiotensin–aldosterone system. These drugs prevent (or inhibit) the activity of ACE, which converts angiotensin I to angiotensin II, a powerful vasoconstrictor. Both angiotensin I and ACE normally are manufactured by the body and are called **endogenous** substances. The vasoconstricting activity of angiotensin II stimulates the secretion of the endogenous hormone aldosterone by the adrenal cortex. Aldosterone promotes the retention of sodium and

water, which may contribute to a rise in blood pressure. By preventing the conversion of angiotensin I to angiotensin II, this chain of events is interrupted, sodium and water are not retained, and blood pressure decreases.

Action of Calcium Channel Blockers

Systemic and coronary arteries are influenced by movement of calcium across cell membranes of vascular smooth muscle. The contractions of cardiac and vascular smooth muscle depend on movement of extracellular calcium ions into these walls through specific ion channels.

Calcium channel blockers act by inhibiting the movement of calcium ions across cell membranes of cardiac and arterial muscle cells. This results in less calcium available for the transmission of nerve impulses. As a result, these drugs relax blood vessels, increase the supply of oxygen to the heart, and reduce the heart's workload.

Action of Angiotensin II Receptor Antagonists

These drugs act to block the binding of angiotensin II at various receptor sites in the vascular smooth muscle and adrenal gland, which blocks the vasoconstrictive effect of the renin–angiotensin system and the release of aldosterone, resulting in a lowering of the blood pressure.

> **⓵ NURSING ALERT**
>
> In 2019, a number of angiotensin II receptor antagonists were recalled due to the finding of a cancer-causing substance in the medication (Patel & Shah, 2019). The issue was not with the antihypertensive but with a filling agent in the oral medication. Clients may ask you about this when an antihypertensive is prescribed. Reassure them that they should not stop taking their drugs, rather inquire with the clinical pharmacist if the drug they take was in the recall batches and if they are safe to take now, or should another drug category be substituted.

USES

Antihypertensive drugs are used in the treatment of hypertension. Although many antihypertensive drugs are available, not all drugs work equally well for a given client (Wright, 2018). In some instances, the primary health care provider may find it necessary to prescribe a different antihypertensive drug when the client does not experience a response to therapy. Some antihypertensive drugs are used only in severe cases of hypertension and when other less potent drugs fail to lower the blood pressure. At times, two antihypertensive drugs may be given together to achieve a better response.

Because of the narrow therapeutic index (range when a drug works vs. produces toxic reactions) of cardiotonics, hypertensive agents have become the mainstay of treatment for heart failure (HF) (see Chapter 37). The most frequently used drug categories include ACE inhibitors, angiotensin receptor blockers (ARB), diuretics, and beta-blockers.

Combining the drug sacubitril (neprilysin inhibitor) with valsartan (ACEI) significantly reduces mortality and hospitalization due to HF compared to the use of ARB or ACEI drugs alone (Januzzi, 2016). This combination is manufactured under the brand name Entresto; solitary agents need to be discontinued 36 hr before this combination drug is initiated.

Nitroprusside (Nitropress) is an example of an intravenous (IV) drug that may be used to treat hypertensive emergencies. A hypertensive emergency is a case of extremely high blood pressure in which blood pressure must be lowered immediately to prevent damage to the target organs. Target organs of hypertension include the heart, kidney, and eyes (retinopathy). Additional uses of the antihypertensive drugs are given in the Summary Drug Table: Antihypertensive Drugs.

ADVERSE REACTIONS

When any antihypertensive drug is given, orthostatic (or postural) hypotension may result in some clients, especially early in therapy. Orthostatic hypotension occurs when the individual has a significant drop in blood pressure (usually 10 mm Hg systolic or more) when assuming an upright position. The client can become dizzy and may fall, resulting in an injury. Butt et al. (2012) reported that the risk of hip fracture is increased by almost 50% for those older than 66 when they are started on antihypertensives. This is thought to be from fainting and falling related to orthostatic hypotension.

Central Nervous System Reactions
• Fatigue, depression, dizziness, headache, and syncope

Respiratory System Reactions
• Upper respiratory infections (URIs) and cough

Gastrointestinal System Reactions
• Abdominal pain, nausea, diarrhea, constipation, gastric irritation, and anorexia

Other Reactions
• Rash, pruritus, dry mouth, tachycardia, hypotension, proteinuria, and neutropenia

Additional adverse reactions that may occur when an antihypertensive drug is administered are listed in the Summary Drug Table: Antihypertensive Drugs. For the adverse reactions that may result when a diuretic is used as an antihypertensive drug, see the Summary Drug Table: Diuretics in Chapter 32.

CONTRAINDICATIONS

Antihypertensive drugs are contraindicated in clients with known hypersensitivity to the individual drugs.

The ACEIs and angiotensin II receptor blockers are contraindicated if the client has impaired renal function, salt or volume depletion, bilateral stenosis, or angioedema. They are also contraindicated during pregnancy (pregnancy category C during first trimester and pregnancy category D in the second and third trimesters) or during lactation. Use of the ACEIs and the angiotensin II receptor blockers during the second and third trimesters of pregnancy is contraindicated, because use may cause fetal and neonatal injury or death.

 Lifespan Considerations

Women of Childbearing Age
Because of the risk for fetal toxicity, always do a pregnancy test before prescribing ACEIs to women.

Calcium channel blockers are contraindicated in clients who are hypersensitive to the drugs and those with sick sinus syndrome, second- or third-degree atrioventricular (AV) block (except with a functioning pacemaker), hypotension (systolic pressure less than 90 mm Hg), ventricular dysfunction, or cardiogenic shock.

Precautions
Antihypertensive drugs are used cautiously in clients with renal or hepatic impairment or electrolyte imbalances, during lactation and pregnancy, and in older clients. The calcium channel blockers are used cautiously in clients with HF or renal or hepatic impairment. The calcium channel blockers are used cautiously during pregnancy (pregnancy category C) and lactation. ACEIs are used cautiously in clients with sodium depletion, hypovolemia, or coronary or cerebrovascular insufficiency, and in those receiving diuretic therapy or dialysis. The angiotensin II receptor agonists are used cautiously in clients with renal or hepatic dysfunction, hypovolemia, or volume or salt depletion, and in clients receiving high doses of diuretics.

LASA ALERT

The following drugs may sound alike; be sure to clarify when they are ordered:

Drug Name	Sounds Like
Altace	alteplase, Amaryl, Amerge, Artane
AmLODIPine	aMILoride
Atacand	Antacid
Avapro	Anaprox
benazepril	Benadryl
Benicar	Mevacor
captopril	calcitriol, Capitrol, carvedilol
Cardene	Cardizem, Cardura, codeine
Cardizem	Cardene, Cardene SR, Cardizem CD, Cardizem SR, cortisone
Cartia XT	Procardia XL
clevidipine	cladribine, clofarabine, clomiPRAMINE
Cleviprex	Claravis
Cozaar	Colace, Coreg, Hyzaar, Zocor
dilTIAZem	Calan, diazePAM, Dilantin
Diovan	Zyban

Drug Name	Sounds Like
enalapril	Anafranil, Elavil, Eldepryl, ramipril
fosinopril	FLUoxetine, Fosamax, furosemide, lisinopril
Inspra	Spiriva
lisinopril	fosinopril, Lioresal, Lipitor, RisperDAL
losartan	lorcaserin, valsartan
Lotensin	Lioresal, lorcaserin, lovastatin
moexipril	Monopril
niCARdipine	niacinamide, NIFEdipine, niMODipine
Norvasc	Navane, Norvir, Vascor
Prinivil	Plendil, Pravachol, Prevacid, PriLOSEC, Proventil
ramipril	enalapril, Monopril, Amaryl
Tekturna	Valturna
Tiazac	Tigan, Ziac
valsartan	losartan, Valstar, Valturna
Zestril	Desyrel, Restoril, Vistaril, Zegerid, Zerit, Zetia, Zostrix, ZyPREXA

Drugs that look like a similar drug are noted in the Summary Drug Tables of each chapter.

INTERACTIONS

The hypotensive effects of most antihypertensive drugs are increased when administered with diuretics and other antihypertensives. Many drugs can interact with the antihypertensive drugs and decrease their effectiveness (e.g., monoamine oxidase inhibitor antidepressants, antihistamines, and sympathomimetic bronchodilators).

The following interactions may occur when ACEI drugs are administered with another agent:

Interacting Drug	Common Use	Effect of Interaction
Nonsteroidal anti-inflammatory drugs (NSAIDs)	Relief of pain and inflammation	Reduced hypotensive effects of the ACEIs
Rifampin	Antitubercular agent	Decreased pharmacologic effect of ACEIs (particularly of enalapril)
Allopurinol	Antigout agent	Higher risk of hypersensitivity reaction
Digoxin	Management of HF	Increased or decreased plasma digoxin levels
Loop diuretics	Reduce/eliminate edema	Decreased diuretic effects
Lithium	Management of bipolar disorder	Increased serum lithium levels, possible lithium toxicity
Hypoglycemic agents and insulin	Management of diabetes	Increased risk of hypoglycemia

Interacting Drug	Common Use	Effect of Interaction
Potassium-sparing diuretics or potassium preparations	Diuretics: reduce blood pressure and edema. Potassium preparations: control of low serum potassium levels	Elevated serum potassium level

The following interactions may occur when the calcium channel blockers are used with another agent:

Interacting Drug	Common Use	Effect of Interaction
Cimetidine or ranitidine	Gastrointestinal (GI) disorders	Increased effects of calcium channel blockers
Theophylline	Control of asthma and chronic obstructive pulmonary disease	Increased pharmacologic and toxic effects of theophylline
Digoxin	HF	Increased risk for digitalis toxicity
Rifampin	Antitubercular agent	Decreased effect of calcium channel blocker

The following interactions may occur when angiotensin II receptor antagonists are administered with other agents:

Interacting Drug	Common Use	Effect of Interaction
Fluconazole	Antifungal agent	Increased antihypertensive and adverse effects (particularly with losartan)
Indomethacin	Pain relief	Decreased hypotensive effect (particularly with losartan)

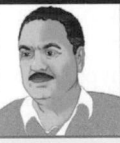

PHARMACOLOGY IN PRACTICE

SAFE DRUG ADMINISTRATION
A client with diabetes mellitus and hypertension is on insulin and enalapril for the hypertension. Which of the following interactions would occur with the combined administration of both drugs?
1. Increased risk of hypersensitivity reaction
2. Increased risk of electrolyte imbalance
3. Increased risk of hypoglycemia
4. Increased risk of hypotensive effect

Herbal Considerations

Flaxseed

Evidence suggests blood pressure can be improved with diet modifications which include lower amounts of fat, more fruits, vegetables and fiber. Blood pressure improves when dietary fiber is increased through secondary results of improving a person's lipid profile, reducing insulin resistance for those predisposed to type 2 diabetes and generally improving the intestinal gut flora (Khalesi et al., 2015).

One study (Khalesi et al., 2015) found that consumption of flaxseed for a duration of 3–48 weeks may reduce blood pressure readings. Flax or *Linum usitatissimum* L., is a plant typically associated with textiles (linen) or oil (linseed oil). The seeds of the plant, flaxseeds, are a yellow or reddish-brown color and have a nutty flavor. Flaxseed is one of the richest sources of dietary fiber and is believed to have anti-inflammatory and antioxidant properties as well.

Flaxseeds are small and typically eaten whole. They may be used to enhance salads, or soups and as additional fiber in meat loaf, muffins, or smoothies. It can also be used ground, yet the shelf life of ground flax seed it less than when kept whole.

Because increasing fiber can cause intestinal discomfort in some people, it is recommended to start with 1 tablespoon of ground flaxseed per day. People should increase water consumption to 8–10 glasses per day to help facilitate bowel transit of the additional fiber. Individuals can consume 2–4 tablespoons of flaxseed daily without issue.

Clients may not volunteer information regarding their use of complementary and alternative remedies. Always inquire about use of herbal products. Medical reports indicate a possible interaction with St. John's wort, used to relieve depression, causing a decrease in serum levels of calcium channel blockers. Because of a specific enzyme reaction, grapefruit or its juice should not be taken if a client is prescribed a calcium channel blocker.

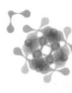

NURSING PROCESS: STEPS TO BUILDING CLINICAL JUDGMENT
Client Receiving an Antihypertensive Drug

ASSESSMENT

Preadministration Assessment
Data gathering suggestions before the initial administration of an antihypertensive include:
Objective data

- Vital signs (temperature, pulse, respirations)
- Specific blood pressure readings (bilateral arms with the client in standing, sitting, and lying positions. Correctly label the readings for each extremity and position)
- Weight
- Laboratory tests—lipid profile (serum cholesterol) and possible pregnancy testing (female clients of childbearing age using ACEIs, angiotensin antagonists, or renin inhibitors)

Subjective data

- Medical/family/dietary history of hypertension and modifiable factors (see Box 34.1)
- Drug therapy (list of all current drugs and supplements taken)

Lifespan Considerations

Menopause
Women experiencing the start of menopause may have irregular ovulation and periods. Some women are reluctant to use birth control as they age because they feel they are not capable of becoming pregnant. Because the ACEIs and angiotensin II receptor antagonists can cause injury and death to a developing fetus, it is important to teach the hypertensive woman who is entering menopause that pregnancy

can still occur. Birth control measures should be discussed. Should a woman taking the aforementioned hypertensive medicines become pregnant, medications should be discontinued immediately.

Ongoing Assessment
Monitoring and recording the blood pressure is an important part of the ongoing assessment, especially early in therapy. The primary health care provider may need to adjust the dose of the drug upward or downward, try a different drug, or add another drug to the therapeutic regimen if the client's response to drug therapy is inadequate.

Each time the blood pressure is measured, use the same arm with the client in the same position (e.g., standing, sitting, or lying down). In some instances, the primary health care provider may order the blood pressure taken in one or more positions, such as standing and lying down (Fig. 34.4). When the client has severe hypertension, or does not have the expected response to drug therapy, or is critically ill, continuous monitoring is performed.

⚠ NURSING ALERT
The blood pressure is taken before each administration of an antihypertensive drug when therapy is started in the inpatient setting. Electronic medication administration records (eMARs) will indicate a place to document the reading. If the blood pressure is significantly decreased from baseline values, do not give the drug but notify the primary health care provider. In addition, the primary health care provider is notified if there is a significant increase in the blood pressure.

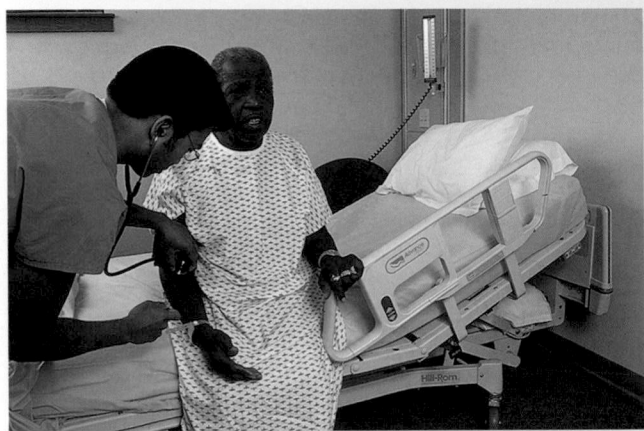

FIGURE 34.4 Nurse shown taking the client's blood pressure before standing while monitoring for orthostatic hypotension when an antihypertensive drug is being started.

Clients taking an antihypertensive drug occasionally retain sodium and water, resulting in edema and weight gain. Assess the client's weight and examine the extremities for edema daily when the client is an inpatient. Report a weight gain of 0.9 kg (2 lb) or more per day and any evidence of edema in the hands, fingers, feet, legs, or sacral area. The client is also weighed at regular intervals if a weight reduction diet is used to lower the blood pressure or if the client is receiving a thiazide or related diuretic as part of antihypertensive therapy.

In the ambulatory setting, help the client to plan a schedule of regular self-monitoring of weight and blood pressure. Teach the client to record weight and blood pressure readings and to find local resources for taking blood pressures in the community. The client is instructed to bring these records in to the primary care provider at each appointment.

NURSING DIAGNOSES

Drug-specific nursing diagnoses include the following:

- **Dehydration** related to excessive diuresis secondary to administration of a diuretic
- **Injury risk** related to dizziness or lightheadedness secondary to postural or orthostatic hypotensive episodes
- **Impaired sexual functioning** related to impotence secondary to effects of antihypertensive drugs
- **Activity intolerance** related to fatigue and weakness
- **Acute pain** (acute headache) related to antihypertensive drugs

Nursing diagnoses related to drug administration are discussed in Chapter 4.

PLANNING

The expected outcomes for the client may include an optimal response to therapy (blood pressure maintained in an acceptable range), support of client needs related to managing adverse reactions, and confidence in an understanding of the medication regimen.

IMPLEMENTATION

Promoting an Optimal Response to Therapy

Most of the antihypertensive drugs can be taken without regard to meals. If GI upset occurs, the drug should be taken with meals. The ACEIs, captopril and moexipril, should be taken 1 hr before or 2 hr after meals to enhance absorption. The drugs are sustained-release capsules that should not be crushed, opened, or chewed. Increased serum potassium, or **hyperkalemia**, can occur with direct renin inhibitor medications; therefore, teach the client to refrain from using potassium-based salt substitutes in the preparation of foods.

Some clients taking an ACEI experience a dry cough that does not subside until the drug therapy is discontinued. This reaction may need to be tolerated. A variety of mechanisms of action are possible for causing the dry cough (from bradykinin stimulation of the vagal nerve to increased prostaglandins), yet there are no conclusive findings. Suggested remedies include treating the cough locally in the respiratory system using cromolyn, baclofen, or a local anesthetic. Some studies (Dykewicz, 2004) recommend that sulindac and aspirin 500 mg or even an iron supplement may work to treat the underlying cause of the cough. If the cough becomes too bothersome, the primary health care provider may change to a different antihypertensive drug. The ACEIs may cause a significant drop in blood pressure after the first dose. This effect can be minimized if the primary health care provider discontinues the diuretic therapy (if the client is taking a diuretic) or begins treatment with small doses.

Clonidine is available as an oral tablet (Catapres) and transdermal patch (Catapres-TTS). If using the transdermal patch, apply it to a hairless area of intact skin on the upper arm or torso; the patch is kept in place for 7 days. The adhesive overlay is applied directly over the system to ensure the patch remains in place for the required time. A different body area is selected for each application. If the patch loosens before 7 days, the edges can be reinforced with nonallergenic tape. The date the patch was placed and the date the patch is to be removed can be written on the surface of the patch with a fiber-tipped pen.

> ### ⚠ NURSING ALERT
>
> Advise clients that **angioedema** (see Fig. 34.5) may occur at any time when taking aliskiren. If the client experiences swelling of the face, throat, or extremities, they should hold the next dose of medication and immediately call the primary health care provider to report symptoms and get instruction regarding antihypertensive treatment.

Nitroprusside, a vasodilator, is used to treat clients with a hypertensive emergency (see SDT in Chapter 35). When vasodilators are used, hemodynamic monitoring of the client's blood pressure and cardiovascular status is required throughout the course of therapy.

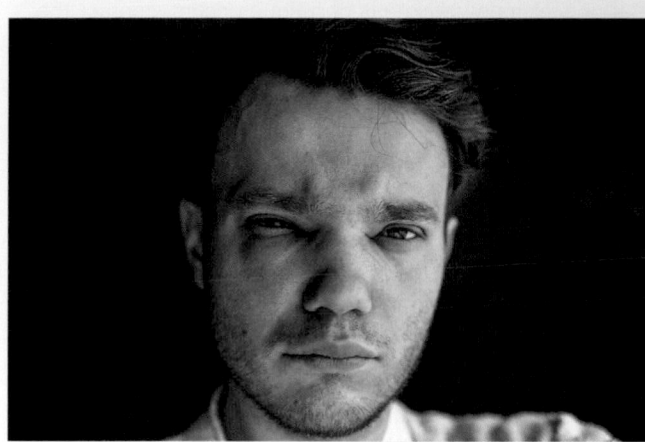

FIGURE 34.5 Facial angioedema should be brought to the health care provider's attention immediately.

 Lifespan Considerations

Gerontology

Older adults are particularly sensitive to the hypotensive effects of nitroprusside. To minimize hypotensive effects, the drug is initially given in lower dosages. Older adults require more frequent monitoring during the administration of nitroprusside.

Monitoring and Managing Client Needs

Observe the client for adverse drug reactions, because their occurrence may require a change in the dose of the drug. In some instances, the client may have to tolerate mild adverse reactions, such as dry mouth or mild anorexia. Contact the primary health care provider to determine if the medication should be changed or the reactions tolerated.

⚠ NURSING ALERT

If it becomes necessary to discontinue antihypertensive therapy, never discontinue use of the drug abruptly. The primary health care provider will prescribe the parameters by which the dosage is to be discontinued. The dosage is usually gradually reduced over 2 to 4 days to avoid rebound hypertension (a rapid rise in blood pressure).

Dehydration

The client receiving a diuretic is observed for dehydration and electrolyte imbalances. A fluid volume deficit is most likely to occur if the client fails to drink a sufficient amount of fluid. This is especially true in the older or confused client. To prevent a fluid volume deficit, encourage clients to drink adequate oral fluids (up to 2000 mL/day, unless contraindicated because of a medical condition). This is especially important when a person excessively perspires or has episodes of vomiting or diarrhea.

Electrolyte imbalances that may occur during therapy with a diuretic include **hyponatremia** (low blood sodium level) and **hypokalemia** (low blood potassium level), although other imbalances may also be seen (see Chapters 32 and 54 for the signs and symptoms of electrolyte

imbalances). When administering aliskiren or eplerenone, monitor for hyperkalemia. The primary health care provider is notified if any signs or symptoms of an electrolyte imbalance occur.

Injury Risk

Dizziness or weakness along with orthostatic hypotension can occur with the administration of antihypertensive drugs. If orthostatic hypotension occurs, instruct the client to rise slowly from a sitting or lying position. Explain how to rise from a lying position, by sitting on the edge of the bed for 1 or 2 min, which often minimizes these symptoms. In addition, rising slowly from a chair and then standing for 1–2 min also minimizes the symptoms of orthostatic hypotension. When symptoms of orthostatic hypotension, dizziness, or weakness do occur, teach the client to call for assistance in getting out of bed or a chair and with ambulatory activities.

Impaired Sexual Functioning

Antihypertensive drugs can cause sexual dysfunction ranging from impotence to inhibition of ejaculation. Provide an open and understanding atmosphere when discussing sexuality. You can get literature in different languages explaining potential problems with sexual patterns that can occur with these drugs. If sexual patterns are affected negatively, suggest that the partners use other means of expressing caring, such as touching, massage, and personal closeness. Allow the client time to express feelings and concerns and encourage the client and partner to discuss ways to satisfy intimacy needs. You may suggest that the client discuss the use of drugs for erectile dysfunction (ED) with the primary care provider. Many ED medications are safe to take with antihypertensives when the dose is modified.

Activity Intolerance

Some clients on the antihypertensive drugs have decreased exercise tolerance and feel fatigued, weak, and lethargic. In addition, clients with hypertension may have other health problems (either cardiovascular or respiratory problems) that may affect their ability to perform activities. The client is encouraged to walk and ambulate as they can tolerate. Assistive devices may be used if needed. Gradually increase tolerance by increasing the daily amount of activity. Plan rest periods according to the individual's tolerance. Rest can take many forms, such as sitting in a chair, napping, watching television, or sitting with legs elevated. Reassure the client that often the fatigue diminishes after 4–6 weeks of therapy.

Acute Pain

Clients taking the antihypertensive drugs may complain of a headache that could be an adverse reaction to the drugs, particularly antiadrenergics or the angiotensin II receptor blocking drugs. If the headache is acute, the client may need to remain in bed with a cool cloth on the forehead, or offer the client a back and neck rub. Relaxation techniques such as guided imagery or progressive body relaxation may prove helpful. If nursing measures are not successful, the primary health care provider is notified, because an analgesic may be required.

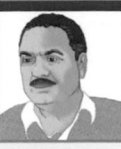

PHARMACOLOGY IN PRACTICE

MANAGING NEEDS

A client has developed a headache following the use of prazosin for hypertension. Which of the following instructions should the nurse provide the client receiving prazosin? Select all that apply.
1. Lie down and elevate legs above head level.
2. Withhold administration of prazosin.
3. Apply a cool cloth over the forehead.
4. Engage in progressive body relaxation.
5. Take an analgesic drug for the pain.

Educating the Client and Family

Educate all clients on the importance of having their blood pressure checked at periodic intervals. This includes people of all ages, because hypertension is not a disease that affects only older individuals. Once hypertension is detected, client teaching becomes an important factor in successfully returning the blood pressure to normal or near-normal levels.

To ensure lifetime adherence to the prescribed therapeutic regimen, emphasize the importance of drug therapy, as well as other treatments recommended by the primary health care provider. Educate the client by describing the adverse reactions from a particular antihypertensive drug and advise the client to contact the primary health care provider if any should occur.

The primary health care provider will want the client or family to monitor blood pressure during therapy. If the client purchases equipment, have them bring it in and teach the technique of taking blood pressure and pulse rate to the client or family member, allowing sufficient time for supervised practice. If the client or family is unable to do this, provide information on community resources where blood pressures are checked, such as local pharmacies or fire stations. Show the client how to keep a record of the blood pressure and to bring this record to each visit to the primary health care provider's office or clinic. A wallet-sized card can be obtained for use from the National Institutes of Health. As you develop a teaching plan include the following information:

- Never discontinue use of this drug except on the advice of the primary health care provider. These drugs control but do not cure hypertension. Skipping doses of the drug or voluntarily discontinuing the drug may cause severe rebound hypertension.
- Avoid the use of any nonprescription drugs (some may contain drugs that can increase the blood pressure) unless approved by the primary health care provider. Avoid alcohol unless its use has been approved by the primary health care provider.
- This drug may produce dizziness or lightheadedness when rising suddenly from a sitting or lying position. To avoid these effects, rise slowly from a sitting or lying position (see Client Teaching for Improved Outcomes: Preventing Injury from Orthostatic Hypotension).
- If the drug causes drowsiness, avoid hazardous tasks such as driving or performing tasks that require alertness. Drowsiness may disappear with time.

- If unexplained weakness or fatigue occurs, contact the primary health care provider.
- Follow the diet restrictions recommended by the primary health care provider. Do not use salt substitutes unless a particular brand of salt substitute is approved by the primary health care provider.
- Notify the primary health care provider if the diastolic pressure suddenly increases to 130 mm Hg or higher; this may signal a hypertensive emergency.

Client Teaching for Improved Outcomes

Preventing Injury From Orthostatic Hypotension
Many clients receiving antihypertensive therapy commonly receive more than one drug, placing them at risk for orthostatic hypotension. If it occurs, the client may fall and be injured. Teach the following measures to follow while in the acute care facility and at home:
- ✔ Place items close to the bed at night such as the cell phone to reduce need to sit up suddenly.
- ✔ Change your position slowly, and sleep with the head of the bed slightly elevated.
- ✔ Exercise calf muscles before getting out of bed or going from a sitting to standing position.
- ✔ Sit at the edge of the bed or chair for a few minutes before standing up.
- ✔ Stand for a few minutes before starting to walk.
- ✔ Avoid bending at the waist; use implements to reach items on the floor.
- ✔ Ask for assistance when necessary.
- ✔ If you feel dizzy or lightheaded, sit or lie down immediately.
- ✔ Make sure to drink adequate amounts of fluid throughout the day.

EVALUATION

- Therapeutic response is achieved and blood pressure is controlled.
- Adverse reactions are identified, reported to the primary health care provider, and managed successfully with appropriate nursing interventions:
  - No evidence of dehydration is seen.
  - No evidence of injury is seen.
  - Client is satisfied with sexual activity.
  - Client engages in activity as able.
  - Client is free of headache pain.
- Client and family express confidence and demonstrate an understanding of the drug regimen.

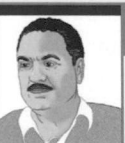

PHARMACOLOGY IN PRACTICE

USING CLINICAL REASONING

The primary health care provider asks you to explain to Mr. Alfredo Garcia how and where to monitor blood pressure readings on a weekly basis. As you compliment Mr. Garcia on his weight loss, he tells you nothing tastes good anymore. How will you educate a person with limited English proficiency about both diet and blood pressure measurement?

KEY POINTS

■ Hypertension is defined by a blood pressure of 130/80 mm Hg or greater. Unchecked, it can lead to heart and kidney disease, HF, or stroke.

■ Prehypertension exists when the blood pressure is 120/80–129/80 mm Hg, and the client should engage in lifestyle modifications to reduce risk factors for the diseases mentioned.

■ "Primary hypertension" is the term used when a direct cause is not established. When lifestyle changes do not reduce the pressures measured, then antihypertensive drugs are used to lower the blood pressure.

■ Various drugs are used alone or in combinations to cause vasodilation and reduce the pressure in the circulatory system. This may be done through a direct effect on blood vessels or the various hormonal/glandular processes that impact blood pressure in the body.

■ Common adverse reactions include headache, dizziness, and GI complaints. Also, those older than 66 years are at a greater risk of hip fracture because of orthostatic hypotension.

■ Many of the drug classes used can injure a developing fetus, so it is important to check for pregnancy in women and discuss birth control.

SUMMARY DRUG TABLE
Antihypertensive Drugs

Generic Name	Trade Name	Uses	Adverse Reactions	Dosage Ranges
Beta-Adrenergic Blocking Drugs (Beta-Blockers)				
acebutolol *a-se-BYOO-toe-lole*		Hypertension, ventricular arrhythmias	Bradycardia, dizziness, weakness, hypotension, nausea, vomiting, diarrhea, nervousness	Hypertension: 400 mg orally in 1–2 doses
atenolol *a-TEN-oh-lole*	Tenormin	Hypertension, angina, acute myocardial infarction (MI)	Bradycardia, dizziness, fatigue, weakness, hypotension, nausea, vomiting, diarrhea, nervousness	Hypertension/angina: 50–200 mg/day orally
betaxolol *be-TAKS-oh-lol*		Hypertension	Same as acebutolol	10–40 mg orally daily
bisoprolol *bis-OH-proe-lol*		Hypertension	Same as acebutolol	2.5–10 mg orally daily; maximum dose, 20 mg orally daily
metoprolol *me-toe-PROE-lol*	Lopressor, Toprol XL	Hypertension, angina, MI, HF	Dizziness, hypotension, HF, cardiac arrhythmia, nausea, vomiting, diarrhea	Hypertension/angina: 100–450 mg/day orally. Extended release: 50–100 mg/day orally
nadolol *NAY-doe-lol*	Corgard	Hypertension, angina	Dizziness, hypotension, nausea, vomiting, diarrhea, HF, cardiac arrhythmia	Hypertension: 40–80 mg/day orally
nebivolol *ne-BIV-oh-lol*	Bystolic	Hypertension	Dizziness, headache, nausea, diarrhea, tingling extremities	5–40 mg/daily
pindolol *PIN-doe-lole*		Hypertension	Bradycardia, dizziness, hypotension, nausea, vomiting, diarrhea	5–60 mg/day orally BID
propranolol *proe-PRAN-oh-lole*	Inderal	Cardiac arrhythmias, MI, angina, hypertension, migraine prophylaxis, hypertrophic subaortic stenosis, pheochromocytoma, primary tremor	Bradycardia, dizziness, hypotension, nausea, vomiting, diarrhea, bronchospasm, hyperglycemia, pulmonary edema	Hypertension: 120–240 mg/day orally in divided doses
timolol *TIM-oh-lole*		Hypertension, MI, migraine prophylaxis	Dizziness, hypotension, nausea, vomiting, diarrhea, pulmonary edema	Hypertension: 10–40 mg/day orally in divided doses. MI: 10 mg orally BID

Continued

SUMMARY DRUG TABLE (continued)
Antihypertensive Drugs

Generic Name	Trade Name	Uses	Adverse Reactions	Dosage Ranges
Antiadrenergic Drugs: Centrally Acting				
cloNIDine *KLON-i-deen*	Catapres, Catapres-TTS (transdermal)	Hypertension, ADHD, severe pain in clients with cancer, opiate withdrawal (supervised only)	Drowsiness, dizziness, sedation, dry mouth, constipation, syncope, dreams, rash	100–600 mcg/day orally Transdermal: release rate 0.1–0.3 mg/24 hr
guanFACINE *GWAHN-fa-seen*	Intuniv	Hypertension, ADHD	Dry mouth, somnolence, asthenia, dizziness, headache, constipation, fatigue	1–3 mg/day orally at bedtime
methyldopa *meth-il-DOE-pa*		Hypertension, hypertensive crisis	Bradycardia, aggravation of angina pectoris, HF, sedation, headache, rash, nausea, vomiting, nasal congestion	250 mg orally BID or TID; maintenance dose, 2 g/day; 250–500 mg q6hr IV
Antiadrenergic Drugs: Peripherally Acting				
doxazosin *doks-AY-zoe-sin*	Cardura	Hypertension, benign prostatic hyperplasia (BPH)	Headache, dizziness, fatigue	Hypertension: 1–8 mg orally daily BPH: 1–16 mg orally daily
prazosin *PRAZ-oh-sin*	Minipress	Hypertension	Dizziness, postural hypotension, drowsiness, headache, loss of strength, palpitation, nausea	1–20 mg orally daily in divided doses
terazosin *ter-AY-zoe-sin*		Hypertension, BPH, dislodge ureteral stones	Dizziness, postural hypotension, headache, dyspnea, nasal congestion	Hypertension: 1–20 mg orally daily BPH: 1–10 mg orally daily
Alpha/Beta-Adrenergic Blocking Drugs				
carvedilol *KAR-ve-dil-ole*	Coreg	Hypertension, HF, left ventricular dysfunction (LVD)	Bradycardia, hypotension, cardiac insufficiency, fatigue, dizziness, diarrhea	6.25–25 mg orally BID
labetalol *la-BET-a-lole*		Hypertension (severe incl. preeclampsia)	Fatigue, drowsiness, insomnia, hypotension, impotence, diarrhea	200–400 mg/day orally in divided doses IV: 20 mg over 2 min with blood pressure monitoring, may repeat
Calcium Channel Blockers				
amLODIPine *am-LOE-di-peen*	Norvasc	Hypertension, chronic stable angina, vasospastic angina (Prinzmetal angina)	Headache	Individualize dosage; 5–10 mg/day orally
clevidipine *klev-ID-i-peen*	Cleviprex	Hypertension	Rebound hypertension	IV only when unable to provide oral therapy
dilTIAZem *dil-TYE-a-zem*	Cardizem, Cardizem CD, Tiazac	Hypertension, chronic stable angina, atrial fibrillation/flutter, paroxysmal superventricular tachycardia	Headache, dizziness, AV block, bradycardia, edema, dyspnea, rhinitis	Extended-release tablets/capsules—hypertension: 120–540 mg/day
felodipine *fe-LOE-di-peen*		Hypertension	Headache, dizziness	2.5–10 mg/day orally
isradipine *iz-RA-di-peen*		Hypertension	Headache, edema	5–10 mg/day orally
levamlodipine *lev-am-LOE-di-peen*	Conjupri	Hypertension	Edema, palpations	1.25–5 mg/day orally
niCARdipine *nye-KAR-de-peen*	Cardene, Cardene IV, Cardene SR	Hypertension, chronic stable angina	Headache	Hypertension: immediate release 20–40 mg/TID; extended release 30–60 mg/BID

Generic Name	Trade Name	Uses	Adverse Reactions	Dosage Ranges
NIFEdipine *nye-FED-i-peen*	Procardia, Procardia XL	Hypertension (sustained release only), vasospastic angina, chronic stable angina	Headache, dizziness, weakness, edema, nausea, muscle cramps, cough, nasal congestion, wheezing	10–20 mg TID orally; may increase to 120 mg/day Sustained release: 30–60 mg/day orally; may increase to 120 mg/day
nisoldipine *nye-SOL-di-peen*	Sular	Hypertension	Headache, edema	20–40 mg/day orally
verapamil *ver-AP-a-mill*	Calan SR, Verelan	Hypertension, chronic stable angina, vasospastic angina, chronic atrial flutter, paroxysmal superventricular tachycardia	Headache, constipation	Individualize dosage; do not exceed 480 mg/day orally in divided doses Sustained release: 120–180 mg/day orally; maximum dose, 480 mg Extended release: 120–180 mg/day orally, maximum dose, 480 mg/day

Angiotensin-Converting Enzyme Inhibitors (ACE Inhibitors)

Generic Name	Trade Name	Uses	Adverse Reactions	Dosage Ranges
benazepril *ben-AY-ze-pril*	Lotensin	Hypertension	Headache, dizziness, fatigue	10–40 mg/day orally in single dose or two divided doses, maximum dose 80 mg
⊘ **captopril** *KAP-toe-pril*		Hypertension, HF, LVD after MI, diabetic nephropathy	Rash	Hypertension: 25–100 mg/day orally in divided doses, not to exceed 450 mg/day
enalapril *e-NAL-a-pril*	Vasotec, Epaned	Hypertension, HF, asymptomatic LVD	Headache, dizziness	Hypertension: 5–40 mg/day orally as a single dose or in two divided doses CHF: 2.5–20 mg BID
fosinopril *foe-SIN-oh-pril*		Hypertension, HF	Dizziness, cough	10–40 mg/day orally ,in a single dose or two divided doses
lisinopril *lyse-IN-oh-pril*	Prinivil, Qbrelis, Zestril	Hypertension, HF, post-MI	Headache, dizziness, diarrhea, orthostatic hypotension, cough	Hypertension: 10–40 mg/day orally as a single dose
⊘ **moexipril** *mo-EKS-i-pril*		Hypertension	Dizziness, cough, bronchospasm	7.5–30 mg orally as a single dose or two divided doses
⊘ **perindopril** *per-IN-doe-pril*		Hypertension	Dizziness, headache, cough, URI symptoms, asthenia	4–8 mg/day orally, maximum dose 16 mg
quinapril *KWIN-a-pril*	Accupril	Hypertension, HF	Dizziness	Hypertension: 10–80 mg/day orally as a single dose or two divided doses
ramipril *RA-mi-pril*	Altace	Hypertension, HF, decrease risk of cardiovascular disease, coronary artery disease	Dizziness, cough	Hypertension: 2.5–20 mg/day orally as a single dose or two divided doses
trandolapril *tran-DOE-la-pril*		Hypertension, clients post-MI with symptoms of HF and LVD	Dizziness, cough	Hypertension: 1–4 mg/day orally

Angiotensin II Receptor Antagonists

Generic Name	Trade Name	Uses	Adverse Reactions	Dosage Ranges
azilsartan *ay-zil-SAR-tan*	Edarbi	Hypertension	Dizziness, fainting, diarrhea	80 mg orally daily
candesartan *can-de-SAR-tan*	Atacand	Hypertension, HF	Dizziness, URI symptoms	8–32 mg/day orally in divided doses
eprosartan *ep-roe-SAR-tan*		Hypertension	Cough, URI, and urinary tract infection symptoms	400–800 mg/day orally in two divided doses

Continued

SUMMARY DRUG TABLE (continued)
Antihypertensive Drugs

Generic Name	Trade Name	Uses	Adverse Reactions	Dosage Ranges
irbesartan *ir-be-SAR-tan*	Avapro	Hypertension, nephropathy in type 2 diabetes	Headache, URI symptoms	150–300 mg/day orally as one dose
losartan *loe-SAR-tan*	Cozaar	Hypertension, hypertension in clients with LVD, diabetic nephropathy in type 2 diabetes	Dizziness, URI symptoms	Hypertension: 25–100 mg/day orally in one or two doses
olmesartan *ole-me-SAR-tan*	Benicar	Hypertension	Dizziness	20–40 mg/day orally
telmisartan *tell-mi-SAR-tan*	Micardis	Hypertension	Diarrhea, URI symptoms, sinusitis	40–80 mg/day orally
valsartan *val-SAR-tan*	Diovan	Hypertension, HF, post-MI	Viral infections	Hypertension: 80–320 mg/day orally
Direct Renin Inhibitors				
aliskiren *a-lis-KYE-ren*	Tekturna	Hypertension	Diarrhea, URI symptoms	150 mg/day orally, may increase to 300 mg/day
Selective Aldosterone Receptor Antagonists				
eplerenone *e-PLER-en-one*	Inspra	Hypertension, HF	Hyperkalemia	50 mg/day orally, may increase to 100 mg/day
Vasodilators used in urgent hypertensive situations				
hydrALAZINE *hye-DRAL-a-zeen*		Primary hypertension (oral); when need to lower blood pressure is urgent (parenteral)	Dizziness, palpitations, tachycardia, numbness/tingling in legs, nasal congestion	10–50 mg QID orally, up to 300 mg/day; 20–40 mg IM or IV
minoxidil *mi-NOKS-i-dill*		Severe hypertension	Dizziness, hypotension, electrocardiogram changes, tachycardia, sodium and water retention, gynecomastia, hair growth	5–100 mg/day orally; dose greater than 5 mg given in divided doses
nitroprusside *nye-troe-PRUS-ide*	Nitropress	Hypertensive crisis	Apprehension, headache, restlessness, nausea, vomiting, palpitations, diaphoresis	3 mcg/kg/min, not to exceed infusion rate of 10 mcg/min (if blood pressure is not reduced within 10 min, discontinue administration)

 This drug should be administered at least 1 hr before or 2 hr after a meal.

CHAPTER REVIEW

Know Your Drugs

Clients sometimes know a medication by the brand (or trade) name and not the generic name. To help you recognize both names, match the brand name with the generic name of the same medication.

Generic Name	Brand Name
1. lisinopril	A. Altace
2. propranolol	B. Minipress
3. ramipril	C. Prinivil
4. prazosin	D. Inderal

Calculate Medication Dosages

1. Oral nadolol 80 mg is prescribed. The drug is available in 40-mg tablets. The nurse administers _____.
2. Nifedipine 10-mg capsules are available. How many capsules will the client be instructed to take when the dose is 30 mg?

Prepare for the NCLEX

RECALL THE FACTS

1. The best description of how antihypertensives work is that they:
   1. promote workload of the heart.
   2. vasodilate vessels to reduce pressure.
   3. increase angiotensin production.
   4. increase reabsorption of sodium in the nephron.
2. Which of the following pressures is considered prehypertension?
   1. 110/80
   2. 120/70
   3. 126/79
   4. 145/92
3. The nurse instructs the client using the transdermal system Catapres-TTS to _____.
   1. place the patch on the torso and keep it in place for 24 hr
   2. change placement of the patch every day after bathing
   3. place the patch on the upper arm or torso and keep it in place for 7 days
   4. avoid getting the patch wet because it might detach from the skin
4. To avoid symptoms associated with orthostatic hypotension, the nurse advises the client to _____.
   1. sleep in a side-lying position
   2. avoid sitting for prolonged periods
   3. change position slowly
   4. get up from a sitting position quickly
5. During the preadministration assessment of a client prescribed an antihypertensive drug, the nurse _____.
   1. places the client in a high Fowler position
   2. places the client in a supine position
   3. darkens the room to decrease stimuli
   4. takes the client's blood pressure

ANALYZE THE FACTS

6. Before the first dose of an ACEI, the nurse assesses a female client for _____.
   1. elevated cardiac enzymes
   2. positive pregnancy test
   3. low–serum sodium
   4. complete blood count

7. The nurse gives the following instruction to the client when discontinuing use of an antihypertensive drug:
   1. Monitor the blood pressure every hour for 8 hr after the drug therapy is discontinued.
   2. Gradually decrease the medication over a period of 2–4 days to avoid rebound hypertension.
   3. Check the blood pressure and pulse every 30 min after discontinuing the drug therapy.
   4. Expect to taper the dosage of the drug over a period of 2 weeks to avoid a return of hypertension.
8. *Nifedipine extended-release tablets are prescribed. A nasogastric (NG) tube has recently been placed in the client. The nurse should:
   1. give the drug as ordered orally.
   2. crush the tablet and give via the NG tube.
   3. contact the primary health care provider for a new order.
   4. return the medication unused to the pharmacy.

ALTERNATE-FORMAT QUESTIONS

9. Which of the following drugs should not be taken with food? **Select all that apply.**
   1. Captopril
   2. Fosinopril
   3. Moexipril
   4. Ramipril
10. Diltiazem 180 mg is prescribed. The drug is available in 60-mg, 90-mg, and 120-mg tablets. Which tablet should you select as it is least likely to cause drug errors? How many tablets would you administer?

To check your answers, see Appendix F.

---

*Indicates the question is directly linked to the NCLEX-PN test plan in Appendix G.

WANT TO KNOW MORE? A wide variety of resources are available to enhance your learning and understanding of this chapter.
- Visit the**Point** for resources such as:
  - NCLEX-Style Student Review Questions
  - Journal Articles
  - Dosage Calculations
  - Drug Monographs
  - Watch and Learn Videos
  - Concepts in Action Animations
- The *Study Guide to Accompany Introductory Clinical Pharmacology*, 12th edition, sold separately, will help you review and apply essential content.
- ✔**PrepU** is available to help students prepare for the NCLEX-PN examination.

35

Antianginal and Vasodilating Drugs

Key Terms

angina acute pain in the chest resulting from decreased blood supply to the heart muscle

buccal space in the mouth between the gum and the cheek in either the upper or lower jaw

prophylaxis prevention

pulmonary arterial hypertension (PAH) high blood pressure in the pulmonary artery (heart to lungs), which can result in heart failure (HF) if not treated

sublingual under the tongue

topical pertaining to a substance applied directly to the skin by patch, ointment, gel, or other formulation

transdermal system drug delivery system by which the drug is applied to and absorbed through the skin

Learning Objectives

On completion of this chapter, the student will:

1. Describe the two types of antianginal drugs.
2. Explain the general actions, uses, adverse reactions, contraindications, precautions, and interactions of antianginal and vasodilating drugs.
3. Distinguish important preadministration and ongoing assessment activities the nurse should perform on the client taking an antianginal or vasodilating drug.
4. List nursing diagnoses particular to a client taking an antianginal or vasodilating drug.
5. Examine ways to promote an optimal response to therapy, how to manage common adverse reactions, and important points to keep in mind when educating clients about the use of antianginal or vasodilating drugs.

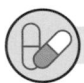 **Drug Classes**

Nitrates
Beta-blockers (anti-adrenergic)
Calcium channel blockers
Pulmonary arterial hypertensive agents

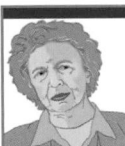 **PHARMACOLOGY IN PRACTICE**

Mrs. Moore was hospitalized with severe chest pain and a possible myocardial infarction (MI). After tests were completed, her primary health care provider prescribed sublingual nitroglycerin for her angina. Her daughter is calling about severe pain. As you assess the situation you find out it is not her heart but what the daughter calls "severe migraine headaches." As you read this chapter determine if this pain is related to cardiac function or medications.

Diseases of the arteries—coronary artery disease, cerebral vascular disease, and peripheral vascular disease—are caused by narrowing of the arteries and may result in pain when tissues are denied oxygen. As was learned in Chapter 33, the narrowing is frequently caused by atherosclerotic plaques which form and block the vessel, subsequently reducing oxygen and nutrients to the tissues on the distal side of the narrowing. This is also one of the ways hypertension develops.

Angina is a term given for the condition described when plaque formation occurs in the coronary arteries. The oxygen supply to the heart muscle decreases and results in a client experiencing chest pain

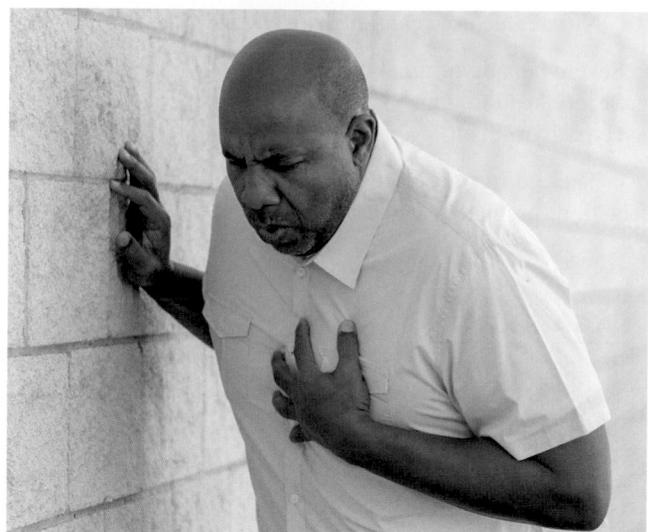

FIGURE 35.1 Activity increases cardiac workload and angina which may present as pressure or discomfort as well as a sharp pain.

or pressure. Activity that increases the workload of the heart, such as exercise or simply climbing stairs, can precipitate a painful angina attack (Fig. 35.1).

Antianginal drugs relieve chest pain or pressure by dilating coronary arteries, which increases the blood supply to the myocardium. First-line treatment to prevent anginal attacks includes beta-blockers (anti-adrenergic) and calcium channel blockers (Fogoros, 2020). Both groups used in the treatment of hypertension. These drugs are listed in the summary drug table and you can read about these categories of drugs in Chapters 24 and 34, respectively. In this chapter those taken immediately during an attack (Nitrates) are highlighted.

When a client mentions chest pain, we typically think of angina. Chest pain can also be a symptom of another issue: **pulmonary arterial hypertension**. This is different than regular hypertension. PAH is a condition where the pulmonary artery (from the heart to the lungs) has too much pressure. As a result, the right side of the heart has to work harder and it can result in HF if not treated.

Although this is a rare condition, it has demonstrated more prominence when PAH was linked to a number of weight-loss drugs which were removed from the market in 1997 (NORD, 2020). Typically, the client feels short of breath, yet chest pain, fatigue, and edema can all be indicators of PAH. Twenty percent of clients are found to have an inheritable form and there is a correlation between the autoimmune disorder scleroderma and PAH (York, 2011). To help reduce occurrence, clients with scleroderma should be evaluated for PAH. This disease is highlighted in this chapter because a number of drugs are now on the market to reduce pressure in the lungs and keep PAH stable. These vasodilating drugs relax the smooth muscle layer of arterial blood vessels, which results in vasodilation, an increase in the size of blood vessels, primarily small arteries and arterioles thus reducing pressure on the vessels. They are included in the Summary Drug Table of this chapter.

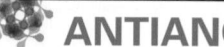 **ANTIANGINALS**

ACTIONS

Beta-blockers reduce heart rate and contractility (Wee, 2015). Both of these effects reduce the amount of oxygen needed by the heart muscle, and angina is prevented as a result. Additionally, in clients with angina who have had a myocardial infarction (MI), beta-blockers have been shown to reduce the risk of having another MI.

Calcium channel blockers act by inhibiting the movement of calcium ions across cell membranes of cardiac muscle cells. This results in less calcium available for the transmission of nerve impulses. As a result, these drugs relax blood vessels, increase the supply of oxygen to the heart, and reduce the heart's workload. Again, preventing anginal pain episodes.

The *nitrates* act by relaxing the smooth muscle layer of blood vessels, increasing the lumen of the artery or arteriole, and increasing the amount of blood flowing through the vessels.

USES

The antianginal drugs are used in the treatment of cardiac disease to:

- Relieve pain of acute anginal attacks
- Prevent angina attacks (**prophylaxis**)
- Treat chronic stable angina pectoris

Typically the nitrate group of drugs is used to relieve symptoms when an anginal attack happens, as opposed to the use of the "blocking" drugs to prevent angina from occurring by taking the drug on a regular basis.

Intravenous (IV) nitroglycerin may be used to control perioperative hypertension associated with surgical procedures. Beta-blockers and calcium channel blocking drugs are also used to treat hypertension (see Chapter 34) and other cardiac conditions. For example, verapamil affects the conduction system of the heart and is used to treat cardiac arrhythmias (Chapter 37). See the Summary Drug Table: Antianginal and Vasodilating Drugs for additional drugs.

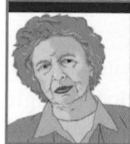 **PHARMACOLOGY IN PRACTICE**

PHYSIOLOGY
Which of the following statements are true in regards to nitrates? Select all that apply.
1. Relax the smooth muscle layer of blood vessels
2. Increase the lumen of the artery or arteriole
3. Slow the conduction velocity of the cardiac impulse
4. Depress myocardial contractility
5. Increase the amount of blood flowing through the vessel

ADVERSE REACTIONS

Adverse reactions to the blocking drugs used for prophylaxis, usually are not serious and rarely require discontinuation of the drug therapy (see Chapter 34 for specifics).

Adverse reactions associated with the nitrates include the following:

- Central nervous system (CNS) reactions, such as headache (may be severe and persistent), dizziness, weakness, and restlessness
- Other body system reactions, such as hypotension, flushing (caused by dilation of small capillaries near the surface of the skin), and rash

The nitrates are available in various forms (e.g., **sublingual**, translingual spray, transdermal, and parenteral). Some adverse reactions are a result of the method of administration. For example, sublingual nitroglycerin may cause a local burning or tingling in the oral cavity. However, the client must be aware that an absence of this effect does not indicate a decrease in the drug's potency. Contact dermatitis may occur from use of the transdermal delivery system.

In many instances, the adverse reactions associated with the nitrates lessen and often disappear with prolonged use of the drug. However, for some clients, these adverse reactions become severe, and the primary health care provider may lower the dose until symptoms subside. The dose may then be slowly increased if the lower dosage does not provide relief from the symptoms of angina. See the Summary Drug Table: Antianginal and Vasodilating Drugs for more information.

CONTRAINDICATIONS AND PRECAUTIONS

Beta- and calcium channel blockers are contraindicated in clients who are hypersensitive to the drugs and those with sick sinus syndrome, second- or third-degree atrioventricular block (except with a functioning pacemaker) or hypotension (systolic pressure less than 90 mm Hg). Beta-blockers are contraindicated in clients with asthma or emphysema. When discontinuing the drug, beta-blockers should always be tapered slowly, not abruptly stopped. The calcium channel blockers are used cautiously during pregnancy (pregnancy category C) and lactation.

Nitrates are contraindicated in clients with known hypersensitivity to the drugs, severe anemia, closed-angle glaucoma, postural hypertension, early MI (sublingual form), head trauma, cerebral hemorrhage (may increase intracranial hemorrhage), allergy to adhesive (transdermal system), or constrictive pericarditis. Clients taking phosphodiesterase inhibitors (drugs for erectile dysfunction [ED]) should not use nitrates.

Nitrates are used cautiously in clients with the following:

- Severe hepatic or renal disease
- Severe head trauma
- Hypothyroidism

These drugs are used cautiously during pregnancy and lactation (pregnancy category C).

LASA ALERT

The following drugs may sound alike; be sure to clarify when they are ordered:

Drug Name	Sounds Like
AmLODIPine	aMILoride
Cardene	Cardizem, Cardura, codeine
Cardizem	Cardene, Cardene SR, Cardizem CD, Cardizem SR, cortisone
dilTIAZem	Calan, diazePAM, Dilantin
niCARdipine	niacinamide, NIFEdipine, niMODipine, nisoldipine
nitroglycerin	nitrofurantoin, nitroprusside
Nitrostat	Nilstat, nystatin
Norvasc	Navane, Norvir, Vascor

Drugs that look like a similar drug are noted in the Summary Drug Tables of each chapter.

INTERACTIONS

The following interactions may occur when the nitrates are used with another agent:

Interacting Drug	Common Use	Effect of Interaction
Aspirin	Pain reliever	Increased nitrate serum concentrations and action may occur
Calcium channel blockers	Treatment of angina	Increased symptomatic orthostatic hypotension
Dihydroergotamine	Migraine headache treatment	Increased risk of hypertension and decreased antianginal effect
Heparin	Anticoagulant	Decreased effect of heparin
Phosphodiesterase inhibitors	Erectile dysfunction (ED)	Severe hypotension and cardiovascular collapse may occur
Alcohol	Relaxation and enjoyment of social situations	Severe hypotension and cardiovascular collapse may occur

The following interactions may occur when the calcium channel blockers are used with another agent:

Interacting Drug	Common Use	Effect of Interaction
Cimetidine or ranitidine	Gastrointestinal (GI) disorders	Increased effects of calcium channel blockers
Theophylline	Control of asthma and chronic obstructive pulmonary disease	Increased pharmacologic and toxic effects of theophylline
Digoxin	HF	Increased risk for digitalis toxicity
Rifampin	Antitubercular agent	Decreased effect of calcium channel blocker

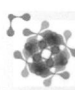

DRUGS FOR PAH

Many of the drugs used to treat PAH are considered orphan drugs (those made for rare conditions). Some are taken orally, by inhalation, subcutaneously, or as with epoprostenol—which is a continuous IV infusion drug. The different routes of administration also have different mechanisms of action, yet all drugs primarily work by blocking receptors in pulmonary smooth muscles allowing vasodilation and as a result better oxygenation.

Another group of drugs used to treat PAH are the phosphodiesterase type 5 inhibitors, most commonly used for ED.

The drugs are known to cause relaxation in the smooth muscles of pulmonary tissue and vasodilation of pulmonary capillaries. Specific brands are used for PAH as opposed to ED.

Common adverse reactions are similar to those of other hypertensive agents such as headache, flushing, and nausea. Drugs taken orally for PAH have been associated with fetal defects and hepatotoxicity.

 Lifespan Considerations

Women of Childbearing Age
Some of the vasodilating drugs (used for PAH) may cause severe birth defects if taken when pregnant. Women are instructed to use two forms of birth control and are counseled to undergo monthly pregnancy testing while taking any of the following: ambrisentan, bosentan, macitentan, or riociguat.

LASA ALERT

The following drugs may sound alike; be sure to clarify when they are ordered:

Drug Name	Sounds Like
Revatio	ReVia, Revonto
sildenafil	sirolimus, silodosin
tadalafil	avanafil, sildenafil, vardenafil
Tracleer	TriCor

Drugs that look like a similar drug are noted in the Summary Drug Tables of each chapter.

NURSING PROCESS: STEPS TO BUILDING CLINICAL JUDGMENT
Client Receiving an Antianginal Drug

ASSESSMENT

Preadministration Assessment
The person using an antianginal drug for episodic, immediate pain is typically an outpatient; therefore, instruction about use is an essential intervention. Typically, the client will not actively be in pain and conducive to teaching.

Data gathering suggestions before the initial administration of an antianginal drug include:
Objective data
- Vital signs (temperature, pulse, respirations, and blood pressure)
- Inspect physical appearance, noting skin color and any lesions

- Auscultate lungs for adventitious sounds
- Weight
- Laboratory tests—electrocardiogram, stress test, chest x-ray, and laboratory panels and possible pregnancy testing (female clients of childbearing age using PAH drugs)

Subjective data
- Pain assessment (see Box 35.1 for specific cardiac episodes)
- Client's ideas regarding cause of pain and remedies used
- Medical/family/dietary history of hypertension and modifiable factors
- Drug therapy (list of all current drugs and supplements taken)

BOX 35.1 Angina-Specific Pain Assessment

History

- Describe the pain (e.g., tightness, pressure, sharp, stabbing).
- Location—is it in a specific place or generalized?
- Does the pain spread and where does it spread?
- Does it start suddenly or is it gradual? How long does it last?
- What events tend to cause anginal pain (e.g., exercise, emotion, other triggers)?
- What makes it feel worse (e.g., movement, breathing, activity)?
- What seems to relieve the pain (e.g., resting, position change)?

Ongoing Assessment

As a part of the ongoing assessment, monitor the client for the frequency and severity of any episodes of anginal pain. This assessment may be conducted by telephone for the client at home. With treatment, the client may expect that, episodes of angina should be eliminated or decrease in frequency and severity. Instruct the client to call for emergency assistance if the chest pain does not respond to three doses of nitroglycerin given every 5 minutes for 15 minutes.

Teach the client or caregiver to monitor vital signs frequently during administration of the antianginals. If the client's heart rate falls below 50 bpm or the systolic blood pressure drops below 90 mm Hg, hold the drug and notify the primary health care provider. A dosage adjustment may be necessary. For the client at home, instruct the client or the caregiver to also call the primary health care provider and ask if the drug should be given for the next episode of heart-related pain.

Assess clients receiving the beta- or calcium channel blockers for signs of HF: dyspnea, weight gain, peripheral edema, abnormal lung sounds (crackles/rales), and jugular vein distention. Any symptoms of HF are reported promptly to the primary health care provider. The dosage may be increased more rapidly in hospitalized clients under close supervision. When the drug is being titrated to a therapeutic dose, the client is typically monitored by telemetry.

NURSING DIAGNOSES

Drug-specific nursing diagnoses include the following:

- **Injury risk** related to hypotension, dizziness, lightheadedness
- **Pain** related to narrowing of peripheral arteries decreased blood supply to the extremities

Nursing diagnoses related to drug administration are discussed in Chapter 4.

PLANNING

The expected outcomes of the client depend on the specific reason for administering the drug but may include an optimal response to therapy, support of client needs related to the management of adverse reactions, and confidence in an understanding of the medication regimen.

IMPLEMENTATION

Promoting an Optimal Response to Therapy

Beta- and Calcium Channel Blockers—Preventing an Attack

With a few exceptions, the blockers may be taken without regard to meals. If gastrointestinal upset occurs, the drug may be taken with meals. Verapamil frequently causes gastric upset and should routinely be given with meals. Verapamil tablets may be opened and sprinkled on foods or mixed in liquids. Sometimes the tablet coverings of verapamil are expelled in the stool. This causes no change in the effect of the drug and need not cause the client concern. For clients who have difficulty swallowing diltiazem tablets can be crushed and mixed with food or liquids.

Nitrates—Stopping a Pain Attack

Nitrates may be administered by the sublingual (under the tongue), **buccal** (between the cheek and gum), oral, IV, or transdermal route. If the buccal form of nitroglycerin has been prescribed, you may want to show the client how and where to place the tablet in the mouth by using a small sugarless candy. Be sure the client understands that absorption of sublingual and buccal forms depends on salivary secretion and a dry mouth may decrease the effect.

Nitroglycerin may also be administered by a metered spray canister that is used to stop an acute anginal attack. Be sure the client understands that the spray is directed from the canister onto or under the tongue. Each dose is metered so that when the canister top is depressed, the same dose is delivered each time. Instruct the client not to shake the canister or inhale the spray. For some individuals, this is more convenient than placing small tablets under the tongue.

ⓘ NURSING ALERT

The dose of sublingual nitroglycerin may be repeated every 5 minutes until pain is relieved or until the client has received three doses in a 15-minute period. One to two sprays of translingual nitroglycerin may be used to relieve angina, but no more than three metered doses are recommended within a 15-minute period.

When the pain is not relieved or worsens or the frequency of attacks increases in the inpatient setting, the primary health care provider is notified because a change in the dosage of the drug or morphine may be ordered for pain relief.

ADMINISTERING ORAL NITRATES. Nitrates are also available as oral tablets that are swallowed. The sustained-release preparation must not be crushed or chewed.

ADMINISTERING NITROGLYCERIN OINTMENT. The dose of **topical** (ointment) nitroglycerin is measured in inches or millimeters. Check the vital signs frequently, and if the blood pressure is appreciably lower or the pulse rate higher than the client's baseline, contact the primary health care provider before applying the drug. The first step in application is to remove the paper from the previous application, fold the paper so no one can touch the drug, dispose, and cleanse the area. Applicator paper is supplied with the drug; one paper is used for each application. Wear disposable gloves to prevent contact with the ointment. While holding the paper, express the prescribed amount of ointment from the tube onto the paper. Use the applicator or dose-measured paper to gently spread a thin uniform layer over at least a 2¼- by 3½-in area. The ointment is usually applied to the chest or back. Application sites are rotated to prevent inflammation of the skin. Areas that may be used for application include the chest (front and back), abdomen, and upper arms and legs. After application of the ointment, you may secure the paper with nonallergenic tape.

Nitroglycerin ointment is also used to treat anal fissures. A small drop is applied around the anal opening, using the same technique as described above. The ointment reduces pressure on the internal anal sphincter and increases blood flow to promote healing. The product, Rectiv, is made especially for this purpose. Lower-dose nitroglycerin is typically compounded by a local pharmacy.

! NURSING ALERT

Do not rub the nitroglycerin ointment into the client's skin, because this will immediately deliver a large amount of the drug through the skin. Exercise care in applying topical nitroglycerin and do not allow the ointment to come in contact with your fingers or hands while measuring or applying the ointment, because the drug will be absorbed through your skin, causing a severe headache.

ADMINISTERING TRANSDERMAL NITROGLYCERIN. For most people, nitroglycerin **transdermal systems** are more convenient and easier to use because the drug is absorbed through the skin. A transdermal system has the drug imbedded in a pad. The primary health care provider may prescribe the system to be applied to the skin once a day for 10–12 hours. Tolerance to the vascular and antianginal effects of the nitrates may develop, particularly in clients taking higher dosages, those who are prescribed longer-acting products, or those who are on more frequent dosing schedules. Clients using the transdermal nitroglycerin patches are particularly prone to tolerance, because the nitroglycerin is released at a constant rate, and steady plasma concentrations are maintained. Applying the patch in the morning and leaving it in place for 10–12 hours, followed by leaving the patch off for 10–12 hours, typically yields better results and delays tolerance to the drug.

When applying the transdermal system, inspect the skin site to be sure it is dry, free of hair, and not subject to excessive rubbing or movement. If needed, shave the application site. The transdermal system should be applied at the same time each day and the placement sites should be rotated. Optimal sites include the chest, abdomen, and thighs. The system is not applied to distal extremities. The best time to apply the transdermal system is after daily care (bed bath, shower, tub bath) because it is important that the skin be clean and thoroughly dry before applying the system. When removing the system, fold the adhesive

side onto itself to prevent adhesion to another person or pet. To avoid errors in applying and removing the patch, the person applying the patch uses a fiber-tipped pen to write their name (or initials), date, and time of application on the top side of the patch; also documents location in the record. Patches should be removed before cardioversion or defibrillation to prevent client burns.

ADMINISTERING IV NITROGLYCERIN. IV nitroglycerin is diluted in normal saline solution or 5% dextrose in water (D_5W) for continuous infusion using an infusion pump to ensure an accurate rate. Because nitroglycerin can be absorbed by plastic, the drug comes in glass IV bottles and special infusion sets provided by the manufacturer. Nurses regulate the dosage according to the client's response and the cardiologist's instructions. Nitroglycerin solutions should not be mixed with any other drugs or blood products.

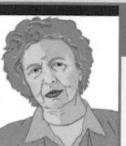

PHARMACOLOGY IN PRACTICE

SAFE DRUG ADMINISTRATION

A nurse is caring for a client in the intensive care unit with an IV nitroglycerin drip. The student nurse asks why there is special tubing with this IV. What is the correct rationale?
1. The drug is light-sensitive.
2. The hospital is switching IV products.
3. Nitroglycerin reacts with plastic tubing.
4. The IV does not need special tubing.

Monitoring and Managing Client Needs
Carefully monitor clients receiving these drugs for adverse reactions. Hypotension may be accompanied by paradoxical bradycardia and increased angina. Adverse reactions such as headache, flushing, and postural hypotension that are seen with the administration of the antianginal drugs often become less severe or even disappear after a period of time.

 Lifespan Considerations

Men
Quality of life has been enhanced for some clients with the advent of drugs for erectile dysfunction (phosphodiesterase inhibitors). When taken with nitrates, severe hypotension can occur; their use is contraindicated. Always assess for and discuss the use of ED drugs when a male client is prescribed a nitrate preparation.

Injury Risk
When postural hypotension is suspected, be sure to offer assistance with all ambulatory activities. Instruct those with episodes of postural hypotension to take the drug in a sitting or supine position and to remain in that position until symptoms disappear. The blood pressure should be frequently monitored in the client with dizziness or lightheadedness.

Lifespan Considerations

Adolescents and Young Adults

"Poppers" (alkyl nitrite, amyl nitrite, butyl nitrite, and isobutyl nitrite) are popular among men having sex with men (MSM) and young people at clubs and raves. The head rush, euphoria, uncontrollable laughter or giggling, and other sensations that result from the blood pressure drop are often felt to increase sexual arousal and desire. Historically, amyl nitrite was used to treat angina. Amyl nitrite and several other alkyl nitrites used in over-the-counter products such as air fresheners and video head cleaners are also inhaled to enhance sexual pleasure. The reduction in blood pressure can result in loss of balance and fainting, especially if people are involved in physical activity like dancing. The likelihood of accidents can increase, and people with heart conditions or high blood pressure are at greater risk. Another product to be aware of containing ethyl chloride and known as "huffers" (inhaled from a bag or rag) can cause heart arrhythmias (Hall, 2015). Inquire about popper use when injury and low blood pressure are presenting symptoms in the urgent care or emergency department.

Pain

In some clients, the anginal pain may be entirely relieved, whereas in others, it may be less intense or less frequent or may occur only with prolonged exercise. Document all information in the client's record, because this helps the primary health care provider plan future therapy as well as make dosage adjustments if required.

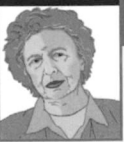

PHARMACOLOGY IN PRACTICE

MANAGING NEEDS

A client is being seen at an urgent care facility for the treatment of severe acute angina. A nurse is administering sublingual nitroglycerin to the client every 5 minutes. What is the maximum number of doses of nitroglycerin the nurse should administer before reporting no improvement to the primary health care provider?

1. 3 doses in a 15-minute period
2. 5 doses in a 30-minute period
3. 7 doses in a 30-minute period
4. 9 doses in a 60-minute period

Educating the Client and Family

The client and family should have a thorough understanding of the treatment of chest pain with an antianginal drug. These drugs are used either to prevent angina from occurring or to relieve the pain of angina during an attack. Explain the therapeutic regimen (dose, time of day the drug is taken, how often to take the drug, how to take or apply the drug) to the client. Include the following general areas, as well as those points relevant to specific routes of administration of the drug, in a teaching plan:

* Avoid the use of alcohol unless use has been permitted by the primary health care provider.
* Keep this medication isolated from other drugs and not in a container where pills can touch each other.
* Notify your emergency response providers if the drug does not relieve pain or if pain becomes more intense despite use of this drug.
* Follow the recommendations of the primary health care provider regarding frequency of use.
* Keep an adequate supply of the drug on hand for events, such as vacations, bad weather conditions, and holidays.
* Keep a record of the frequency of acute anginal attacks (date, time of the attack, drug, and dose used to relieve the acute pain), and bring this record to each primary health care provider or clinic visit.

For more teaching points related specifically to administration routes of nitrates, see the Client Teaching for Improved Outcomes: Directions for Administering Nitrates.

Client Teaching for Improved Outcomes

Directions for Administering Nitrates

General Instructions

✔ Headaches result from vasodilation and are an uncomfortable adverse reaction. If headache persists or becomes severe, notify the primary health care provider, because a change in dosage may be needed. Do not try to avoid headaches by altering the treatment schedule or dose. Ask about aspirin or acetaminophen for headache relief before you take it.

✔ Sit or lie down when you take your nitroglycerin. To relieve severe lightheadedness or dizziness, lie down, elevate the extremities, move the extremities, and breathe deeply.

✔ Store capsules and tablets in their original containers, because nitroglycerin must be kept in a dark container and protected from exposure to light. Never mix this drug with any other drug in a container. Nitroglycerin will lose its potency if stored in containers made of plastic or if mixed with other drugs.

✔ Always replace the cover or cap of the container as soon as the oral drug or ointment is removed from the container or tube. Replace caps or covers tightly, because the drug deteriorates on contact with air.

✔ Seek prompt medical attention if chest pain persists, changes character, increases in severity, or is not relieved by following the recommended dosing regimen.

✔ Do not use ED drugs while taking nitrates.

Oral Nitrates

✔ The drug works best on an empty stomach; if nausea occurs take the preparation with food.

Sublingual or Buccal Nitrates

✔ Do not handle the tablets any more than necessary. Perform thorough hand hygiene after use.

✔ Place the buccal tablet between the cheek and gum or between the upper lip and gum above the incisors. If you wear dentures, remove or place drug above denture line.

✔ Do not swallow or chew sublingual or transmucosal tablets; allow them to dissolve slowly. The tablet may cause a burning or tingling in the mouth. Absence of this effect does not indicate a decrease in potency. A dry mouth lessens absorption; you may want to rinse with water *before* placing the tablet in your cheek.

Translingual (Aerosol Spray) Nitrates

✔ Directions for use of translingual nitroglycerin are supplied with the product. Follow the instructions regarding using and cleaning the canister.

- This drug may be used prophylactically 5–10 minutes before engaging in activities that precipitate an anginal attack.
- Do not shake the canister before use.
- It is not an inhaler device, do not inhale the spray into your lungs.

✔ At the onset of an anginal attack, spray 1–2 metered doses onto or under the tongue. Do not exceed 3 metered doses within 15 minutes.

Topical Ointment or Transdermal System

✔ Instructions for application of the topical ointment or transdermal system are available with the product. Read these instructions carefully.

✔ Apply the topical ointment or topical transdermal system at approximately the same time each day.

✔ Remove the old system and inspect the body to be sure no other papers or systems have been missed.

✔ Be sure the area is clean and thoroughly dry before applying the topical ointment or transdermal system, and rotate the application sites. Apply the transdermal system to the chest (front and back), abdomen, and upper legs. Firmly press the patch to ensure contact with the skin. If the transdermal system comes off or becomes loose, apply a new system. Apply the topical ointment to the front or the back of the chest. If applying to the back, another person should apply the ointment.

✔ When using the topical ointment form or transdermal system, cleanse old application sites with soap and warm water as soon as the ointment or transdermal system is removed. Fold the old patch in half to prevent adherence to others.

✔ To use the topical ointment, apply a thin layer on the skin using the paper applicator (the client or family member may need practice regarding this technique). Avoid finger contact with the ointment.

✔ Wear disposable gloves when applying the ointment.

✔ Notify the primary health care provider if any of the following occurs: increased severity of chest pain or discomfort, irregular heartbeat, palpitations, nausea, shortness of breath, swelling of the hands or feet, or severe and prolonged episodes of lightheadedness and dizziness.

✔ Make position changes slowly to minimize hypotensive effects.

✔ Because these drugs can cause dizziness or drowsiness, do not drive or engage in hazardous activities until response to the drug is known.

EVALUATION

- Therapeutic response is achieved.
- Adverse reactions are identified, reported to the primary health care provider, and managed successfully with appropriate nursing interventions:
  - No evidence of injury is seen.
  - Pain is relieved.
- Client and family express confidence and demonstrate an understanding of the drug regimen.

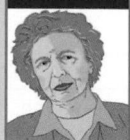

PHARMACOLOGY IN PRACTICE

USING CLINICAL REASONING

What you have discovered in your phone conversation is that Mrs. Moore is actually chewing the sublingual tablets, which is causing the vasodilation of cerebral arteries and headache. After reading this chapter, what do you think would be a better alternative?

KEY POINTS

■ When the fatty deposits of atherosclerosis involve the coronary vessels supplying the heart, anginal pain can occur. Other diseases of the arteries can cause serious problems: coronary artery disease, cerebral vascular disease, and peripheral vascular disease.

■ Antianginal drugs vasodilate and relax the smooth muscle of arterioles around the heart; this promotes blood flow and reduces pain. Some drugs are used for immediate relief of pain; others are used routinely to prevent painful episodes. These drugs are administered in multiple ways, from different oral to topical preparations.

■ Because the purpose of these drugs is to vasodilate, that is also a concern with the adverse reactions. Headache, from rapid vasodilation of cerebral arteries, is a very unpleasant reaction. Also, men taking antianginals need to be assessed and cautioned for use of ED medications because these drugs also cause vasodilation.

■ Some PAH drugs have teratogenic effects and possible pregnancy needs to be ruled out before, and during, use.

SUMMARY DRUG TABLE
Antianginal and Vasodilating Drugs

Generic Name	Trade Name	Uses	Adverse Reactions	Dosage Ranges
Nitrates				
isosorbide *eye-soe-SOR-bide*	Isordil, Dilatrate SR, Monoket	Treatment and prevention of angina	Headache, hypotension, dizziness, weakness, flushing, restlessness, rash	Initial dose 5–20 mg orally; maintenance dose 10–40 mg BID, TID orally Sublingually: 2.5–5 mg Prevention: 5–10 mg sublingually, 5 mg chewable
nitroglycerin, parenteral form *nye-troe-GLI-ser-in*		Angina, heart failure (HF), perioperative hypertension, induce intraoperative hypotension	Same as isosorbide	Initially 5 mcg/minute by IV infusion pump; may increase to 20 mcg/minute postoperative period
nitroglycerin, oral	Nitrostat (sublingual) Nitrolingual pump spray, NitroMist (aerosol used sublingually)	Acute relief of an attack or prophylaxis of angina	Same as isosorbide	One tablet under tongue or in buccal pouch at first sign of an acute anginal attack—may repeat every 5 minutes until relief or three tablets have been taken Pump spray: 1–2 metered doses onto or under the tongue; maximum of 3 metered doses in 15 minutes
nitroglycerin, ointment	Minitran, Nitro-Dur	Prevention and treatment of angina	Same as isosorbide	Used supplied ruled papers to give ½–2 in twice daily
nitroglycerin transdermal systems	Minitran, Nitro-Dur	Prevention of angina	Same as isosorbide	One system daily, 0.2–0.8 mg/hour
Miscellaneous Antianginal Agents				
ivabradine *eye-VAB-ra-deen*	Corlanor	Stable heart failure, when beta-blockers are contraindicated	Heart block, bradycardia	2.5–5 mg orally BID
ranolazine *ra-NOE-la-zeen*	Ranexa	Chronic angina	Dizziness, constipation	1000 mg orally BID
Beta-Adrenergic Blockers Used for Anginal Issues				
atenolol *a-TEN-oh-lole*	Tenormin	Hypertension, angina, acute myocardial infarction (MI)	Bradycardia, dizziness, fatigue, weakness, hypotension, nausea, vomiting, diarrhea, nervousness	Hypertension/angina: 50–200 mg/day orally Acute MI: 5 mg IV over 5 minutes, may be repeated
metoprolol *me-toe-PROE-lole*	Lopressor, Toprol-XL	Hypertension, angina, MI, HF	Dizziness, hypotension, HF, cardiac arrhythmia, nausea, vomiting, diarrhea	Hypertension/angina: 100–450 mg/day orally Extended-release: 50–100 mg/day orally HF: 25–200 mg/day orally Acute MI: 3 bolus doses of 5 mg IV
nadolol *NAY-doe-lole*	Corgard	Hypertension, angina	Dizziness, hypotension, nausea, vomiting, diarrhea, HF, cardiac arrhythmia	Hypertension: 40–80 mg/day orally Angina: 40–80, may go to 240 mg/day orally

Generic Name	Trade Name	Uses	Adverse Reactions	Dosage Ranges
propranolol *proe-PRAN-oh-lole*	Inderal	Cardiac arrhythmias, MI, angina, hypertension, migraine prophylaxis, hypertrophic subaortic stenosis, pheochromocytoma, essential tremor	Bradycardia, dizziness, hypotension, nausea, vomiting, diarrhea, bronchospasm, hyperglycemia, pulmonary edema	Arrhythmias: 10–30 mg orally TID, QID Hypertension: 120–240 mg/day orally in divided doses Angina: 80–320 mg/day orally in divided doses Migraine: 160–240 mg/day orally in divided doses
Calcium Channel Blockers Used for Anginal Issues				
amLODIPine *am-LOE-di-peen*	Norvasc	Hypertension, chronic stable angina, vasospastic angina (Prinzmetal angina)	Headache	Individualize dosage; 5–10 mg/day orally
dilTIAZem *dil-TYE-a-zem*	Cardizem, Cardizem CD, Tiazac	Hypertension, chronic stable angina, atrial fibrillation/flutter, paroxysmal supraventricular tachycardia	Headache, dizziness, atrioventricular block, bradycardia, edema, dyspnea, rhinitis	Extended-release tablets/capsules: Angina: 120–580 mg/day Exertional angina—immediate-release tablets: 30 mg/QID Heart arrhythmias—injection: 0.25 mg/kg over 2 minutes, then titrated continuous infusion
niCARdipine *nye-KAR-de-peen*	Cardene, Cardene IV, Cardene SR	Hypertension, chronic stable angina	Headache	Angina: individualize dosage; immediate release only, 20–40 mg TID orally
NIFEdipine *nye-FED-i-peen*	Procardia, Procardia XL	Vasospastic angina (Prinzmetal variant angina), chronic stable angina, hypertension (sustained-release only)	Headache, dizziness, weakness, edema, nausea, muscle cramps, cough, nasal congestion, wheezing	10–20 mg TID orally; may increase to 120 mg/day Sustained-release: 30–60 mg/day orally; may increase to 120 mg/day
niMODipine *nye-MOE-di-peen*	Nymalize	Subarachnoid hemorrhage	Headache, hypotension, diarrhea	60 mg every 4 hours orally
verapamil *ver-AP-a-mill*	Calan, Calan SR, Verelan	Hypertension, chronic stable angina, vasospastic angina (Prinzmetal variant angina), chronic atrial flutter, paroxysmal supraventricular tachycardia	Headache, constipation	Individualize dosage; do not exceed 480 mg/day orally in divided doses Sustained-release: 120–180 mg/day orally; maximum dose, 480 mg Extended-release: 120–180 mg/day orally, maximum dose, 480 mg/day Parenteral: 5–10 mg IV over 2 minutes
Agents Used for Pulmonary Arterial Hypertension (PAH)				
[a]**ambrisentan** *am-bri-SEN-tan*	Letairis	PAH	Headache, peripheral edema, nasal congestion	5–10 mg orally daily
[a]**bosentan** *boe-SEN-tan*	Tracleer	PAH	Headache, edema, respiratory infections	62.5–125 mg orally BID
epoprostenol *e-poe-PROST-en-ole*	Flolan, Veletri	PAH	Headache, nausea, flushing	Infused via central venous catheter line over time with pump
iloprost *EYE-loe-prost*	Ventavis	PAH	Headache, nausea, flushing, cough	Maximum dose of 45 mcg/day via inhaler device

Continued

SUMMARY DRUG TABLE (continued)
Antianginal and Vasodilating Drugs

Generic Name	Trade Name	Uses	Adverse Reactions	Dosage Ranges
ªmacitentan *ma-si-TEN-tan*	Opsumit	PAH	Headache, nasal congestion, fatigue	10 mg orally daily
ªriociguat *rye-oh-SIG-ue-at*	Adempas	PAH	Headache, dizziness, dyspepsia	0.5–1 mg orally TID
selexipag *Se-LEX-i-pag*	Uptravi	PAH	Headache, nausea, vomiting, diarrhea, jaw/limb pain, flushing, rash	1600 mcg orally twice daily
treprostinil *tre-PROST-in-il*	Orenitram (oral), Remodulin(parental), Tyvaso (nasal)	PAH	Headache, nausea, diarrhea, irritation at injection site	1.25 mg/kg/minute infused via subcut or central venous catheter line over time with pump
PD5E Inhibitors				
sildenafil *sil-DEN-a-fil*	Revatio, (Viagra for erectile dysfunction [ED] only)	Pulmonary arterial hypertension, altitude sickness	Headache, flushing, dyspepsia, nasal congestion	20 mg orally 3 times daily
tadalafil *tah-DA-la-fil*	Adcirca, Alyq, (Cialis for ED only)	Pulmonary arterial hypertension	Headache, dyspepsia, nasal congestion, back pain	40 mg orally daily given in a single dose

ªAdministered through REMS program.

CHAPTER REVIEW

Know Your Drugs

Clients sometimes know a medication by the brand (or trade) name and not the generic name. To help you recognize both names, match the brand name with the generic name of the same medication.

Generic Name	Brand Name
1. amlodipine	A. Isordil
2. isosorbide	B. Norvasc
3. nifedipine	C. Procardia
4. ranolazine	D. Ranexa

Calculate Medication Dosages

1. The primary care provider prescribed verapamil (Calan) 120 mg TID orally. The drug is available in 40-mg tablets. The nurse administers _____.
2. The client is prescribed isosorbide (Isordil) 40 mg orally BID. The drug form available is 20-mg tablets. The nurse administers _____.

Prepare for the NCLEX

RECALL THE FACTS

1. The nitrates for anginal pain are used to dilate which of the following vessels?
   1. Cerebral arteries
   2. Coronary arteries
   3. Peripheral veins
   4. Coronary veins

2. Which class of drug is used for the *prevention* of anginal pain?
   1. Calcium channel blockers
   2. Nitrates
   3. Alpha-adrenergics
   4. Phosphodiesterase inhibitors

3. When administering the nitrates for angina, the nurse monitors the client for which common adverse reaction?
   1. Hyperglycemia
   2. Headache
   3. Fever
   4. Anorexia

4. When teaching a client about prescribed sublingual nitroglycerin, the nurse informs the client that if pain is not relieved, the dose can be repeated in _____ minute(s).
   1. 1
   2. 5
   3. 15
   4. 30

5. When administering nitroglycerin ointment, the nurse _____.
   1. rubs the ointment into the skin
   2. applies the ointment every hour or until the angina is relieved
   3. applies the ointment to a clean, dry area
   4. rubs the ointment between their palms and then spreads it evenly onto the client's chest

ANALYZE THE FACTS

6. A client taking a calcium channel blocker experiences orthostatic hypotension. The nurse instructs the client with orthostatic hypotension to _____.
   1. remain in a supine position until the effects subside
   2. make position changes slowly to minimize hypotensive effects
   3. increase the dosage of the calcium channel blocker
   4. discontinue use of the calcium channel blocker until the hypotensive effects diminish

7. *A client has seen their primary health care provider for their heart condition. The provider gives you the prescription for sublingual nitrate to fax to the pharmacy. The client hands you more prescriptions from another provider to refill. Which one should you review with the primary health care provider first?
   1. Cimetidine
   2. Ibuprofen
   3. Lisinopril
   4. Sildenafil

8. Which of the following statements if made by the client taking a nitrate would indicate that he needs to be seen immediately by an urgent response team?
   1. "I had some chest pressure a week ago."
   2. "My wife had chest pain so I gave her one of my pills."
   3. "I woke this morning with swollen legs."
   4. "My heart feels worse after putting three of those little heart pills under my tongue."

ALTERNATE-FORMAT QUESTIONS

9. Best placement of a nitroglycerin transdermal system would be _____. **Select all that apply.**
   1. abdomen
   2. thigh
   3. chest
   4. forearm

10. The client has just been discharged with sublingual nitrate. He is experiencing chest tightness and has taken one tablet 4 minutes ago with minimal relief. He is calling confused about taking two more doses. When can he take those two additional doses?

To check your answers, see Appendix F.

_____

*Indicates the question is directly linked to the NCLEX-PN test plan in Appendix G.

WANT TO KNOW MORE? A wide variety of resources are available to enhance your learning and understanding of this chapter.
- Visit thePoint for resources such as:
  • NCLEX-Style Student Review Questions
  • Journal Articles
  • Dosage Calculations
  • Drug Monographs
  • Watch and Learn Videos
  • Concepts in Action Animations
- The *Study Guide to Accompany Introductory Clinical Pharmacology*, 12th edition, sold separately, will help you review and apply essential content.
- ✓**PrepU** is available to help students prepare for the NCLEX-PN examination.

36

Anticoagulant and Thrombolytic Drugs

Key Terms

aggregate clumping of blood elements

embolus thrombus that detaches from a blood vessel wall and travels through the bloodstream

fibrinolytic drug that dissolves clots already formed within blood vessel walls

hemostasis complex process by which fibrin forms and blood clots

lysis dissolution or destruction of cells

petechiae pinpoint-sized red hemorrhagic spots on the skin

prothrombin substance that is essential for the clotting of blood; clotting factor II

thrombolytic drug that helps to eliminate blood clots

thrombosis formation of a blood clot

thrombus blood clot attached to a vessel wall in the circulatory system (pl. thrombi)

Learning Objectives

On completion of this chapter, the student will:

1. Describe hemostasis and thrombosis.
2. Explain the uses, general drug actions, adverse reactions, contraindications, precautions, and interactions of anticoagulant, antiplatelet, and thrombolytic drugs.
3. Distinguish important preadministration and ongoing assessment activities the nurse should perform on the client taking an anticoagulant, antiplatelet, or thrombolytic drug.
4. List nursing diagnoses particular to a client taking an anticoagulant, antiplatelet, or thrombolytic drug.
5. Examine ways to promote an optimal response to therapy, how to manage common adverse reactions, and important points to keep in mind when educating clients about the use of anticoagulant, antiplatelet, and thrombolytic drugs.

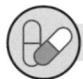 **Drug Classes**

Anticoagulants	Antiplatelets	Thrombolytics

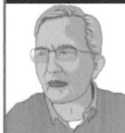 **PHARMACOLOGY IN PRACTICE**

Mr. Phillip is a widower and lives alone. He had not been seen in a number of years, and his physical examination shows that he has atrial fibrillation, for which he was prescribed warfarin to take at home. The clinical pharmacist asks you about Mr. Phillip's mental status. It seems that the weekly laboratory work for Mr. Phillip fluctuates considerably despite weekly teaching. After you read about these drugs, think about what action could be taken.

Clotting is an essential body mechanism. When a blood vessel is injured, a series of events occur to form a clot and stop the bleeding. This process is called **hemostasis**. It involves a complex process also called the *coagulation cascade*. The blood clotting or coagulation cascade is so named because as each factor is activated, it acts as a catalyst that enhances (or *cascades to*) the next reaction, with the net result being a large collection of fibrin (the clot) that forms a plug in the vessel, thus stopping the bleeding, resulting in the formation of a stable fibrin clot. Clotting factors exist in the blood in an inactive form and must be converted to an active form before the next step in the clotting pathway can occur. Clot formation in the intrinsic pathway is initiated by factor XII, with all of the components necessary for clot formation in

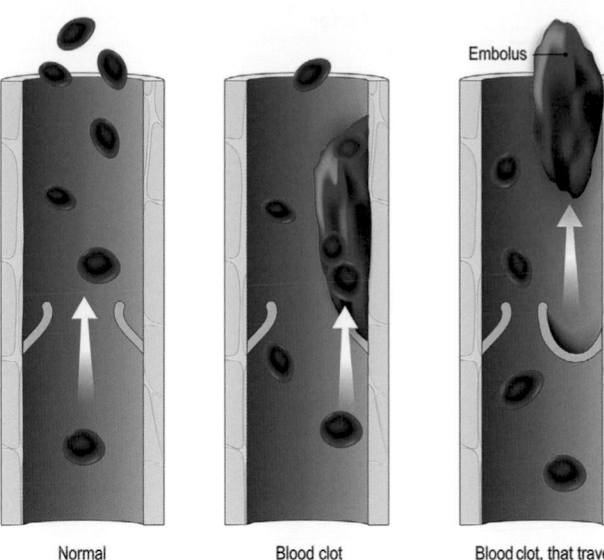

Normal blood flow · Blood clot formation · Embolus · Blood clot, that travels through the bloodstream

FIGURE 36.1 Process of thrombosis and emboli formation.

the circulating blood. In the extrinsic pathway, once vessel damage has happened, tissue thromboplastin, a factor not found in circulating blood, is released and factors VII and X are activated (Chaudhry, 2020). As complex as this sounds, it is a normal event, taking a few minutes, that happens daily in response to tears and leaks in blood vessels throughout the body. This concept is demonstrated later in the chapter.

Clotting can also cause damage to both blood vessels and the tissues nourished by those vessels. **Thrombosis** is the formation of a blood clot or **thrombus**. As illustrated in Figure 36.1, a thrombus may form in any vessel (artery or vein) and in turn impedes blood flow. For example, a venous thrombus can develop as the result of venous stasis (decreased blood flow or movement), injury to the vessel wall, or altered blood coagulation. Venous thrombosis most often occurs in the lower extremities and is associated with venous stasis. *Deep vein thrombosis* (DVT) occurs in the lower extremities and is the most common type of venous thrombosis.

Arterial thrombosis can occur because of atherosclerosis or arrhythmias, such as *atrial fibrillation*. The thrombus may begin small, but fibrin, platelets, and red blood cells attach to the thrombus, increasing its size. When a thrombus detaches itself from the wall of the vessel and is carried along through the bloodstream, it becomes an **embolus** (see Fig. 36.1). The embolus travels until it reaches a vessel that is too small to permit its passage. If the embolus goes to the lung and obstructs a pulmonary vessel, it is called a *pulmonary embolism* (PE). Similarly, if the embolus detaches and occludes a vessel supplying blood to the heart, it can cause a *myocardial infarction* (MI).

The types of drugs discussed in this chapter include drugs that prevent the formation of blood clots (anticoagulants), drugs that suppress platelet aggregation (antiplatelets), and drugs that help to eliminate the clot (thrombolytics). For more information about specific drugs,

see the Drug Summary Table: Anticoagulant, Antiplatelet, and Thrombolytic Agents.

ORAL AND PARENTERAL ANTICOAGULANTS

Anticoagulants prevent the formation and extension of a thrombus and are used prophylactically in clients who are at high risk for clot formation. Anticoagulants have no direct effect on an existing thrombus and do not reverse damage caused from the thrombus. However, once the presence of a thrombus has been established, anticoagulant therapy can prevent additional clots from forming.

Although they do not thin the blood, they are commonly called *blood thinners* by clients. The original anticoagulant group of drugs included warfarin and fractionated and unfractionated heparin. Recently, a number of direct-acting oral anticoagulants (DAOCs) have been developed (Gomez-Outes, 2015). Because of their performance and safety, they have become the first choice in anticoagulant therapy (Ballestri, 2020).

Warfarin is a commonly prescribed oral anticoagulant, primarily because of its low cost. Peak activity is reached 1.5–3 days after therapy is initiated. Although primarily given by the oral route, warfarin is also available for parenteral administration.

Heparin preparations are available as heparin sodium and the low–molecular-weight heparins (LMWHs; fractionated heparins). Heparin is not a single drug, but rather a mixture of high– and low–molecular-weight drugs. Examples of LMWH include dalteparin (Fragmin) and enoxaparin (Lovenox). LMWHs produce very stable responses when administered at recommended dosages. Because of this stability, frequent laboratory monitoring (as is done with heparin), is not necessary. In addition, bleeding is less likely to occur with LMWHs than with heparin.

The DAOCs include direct thrombin inhibitors (DTIs) that do not have the difficult management properties of warfarin or the heparins. These include the oral form, dabigatran (Pradaxa), and the parenteral drugs, argatroban, and bivalirudin.

Other anticoagulants include the factor X inhibitors—DAOCs apixaban (Eliquis), edoxaban (Savaysa), and rivaroxaban (Xarelto) as well as the parenteral drug, fondaparinux (Arixtra). These drugs are anticoagulating drugs that inhibit portions of the coagulation cascade. They are used to prevent DVT in clients undergoing hip, knee, or abdominal surgeries.

ACTIONS

All anticoagulants interfere with the clotting mechanism of the blood as illustrated in Figure 36.2. Warfarin interferes at many levels of the coagulation cascade, by the

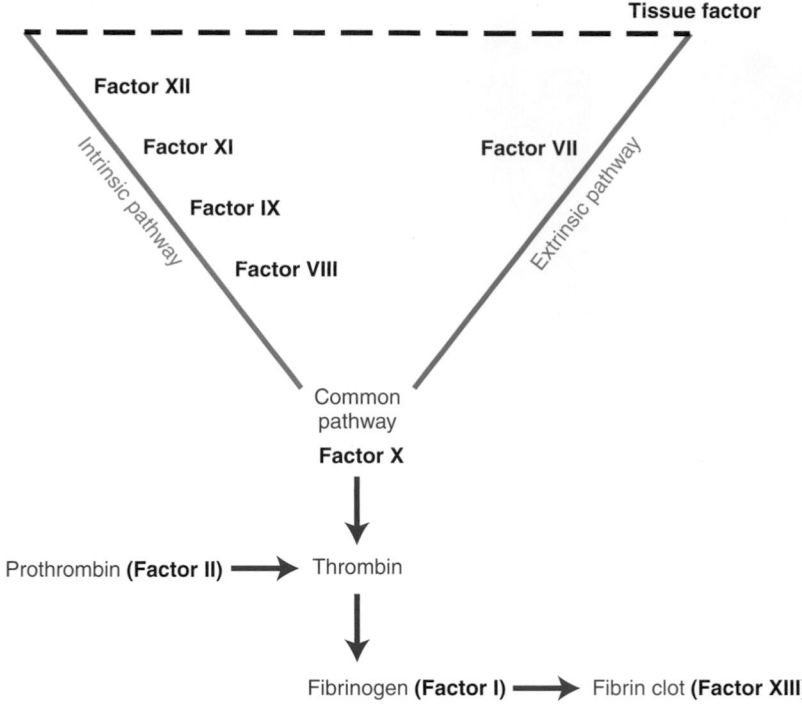

FIGURE 36.2 Coagulation cascade.

manufacturing of vitamin K–dependent clotting factors in the liver. This results in the depletion of clotting factors II (prothrombin), VII, IX, and X. It is the depletion of prothrombin (see Fig. 36.2), a substance that is essential for the clotting of blood, that accounts for most of the action of warfarin.

By contrast, heparin inhibits the formation of fibrin clots and inactivates several of the factors necessary for the clotting of blood. Heparin cannot be taken orally, because it is inactivated by gastric acid in the stomach; therefore, it must be given by injection. The LMWHs act to inhibit the synthesis of factor X and the formation of thrombin. These drugs have no effect on clots that have already formed and aid only in preventing the formation of new blood clots.

DAOCs are rapidly absorbed and have a short half-life. They target specific portions of the coagulation cascade (inhibit thrombin or factor X) making them safer than warfarin (Gomez-Outes, 2015). Because of their sites of action, these drugs do not have the same drug or food interactions, nor do they require the frequent monitoring of blood levels.

USES

Anticoagulants are used for the following:

- Prevention (prophylaxis) and treatment of DVT
- Prevention and treatment of atrial fibrillation with embolization
- Prevention and treatment of PE
- Adjuvant treatment of MI
- Prevention of thrombus formation after valve replacement surgery

Parenteral anticoagulants are used specifically for the following:

- Prevention of postoperative DVT and PE in certain clients undergoing surgical procedures, such as major abdominal surgery
- Prevention of clotting in arterial and heart surgery, in the equipment used for extracorporeal (occurring outside the body) circulation (e.g., in dialysis procedures), in blood transfusions, and in blood samples for laboratory purposes
- Prevention of a repeat cerebral thrombosis in some clients who have experienced a stroke
- Treatment of coronary occlusion, acute MI, and peripheral arterial embolism
- Diagnosis and treatment of disseminated intravascular coagulation (DIC), a severe hemorrhagic disorder
- Maintaining patency of intravenous (IV) catheters (very low doses of 10–100 units)

⚠ NURSING ALERT

Warfarin is the most commonly prescribed oral anticoagulant. Even when used at therapeutic doses, warfarin has a narrow therapeutic window and carries significant risk of hemorrhage. DAOCs have the advantage of less risk of hemorrhage and do not need frequent laboratory monitoring (Mureebe, 2007).

ADVERSE REACTIONS

The principal adverse reaction associated with anticoagulants is bleeding, which may range from very mild to severe. Bleeding may be seen in many areas of the body, such as the skin (bruising and petechiae), bladder, bowel, stomach, uterus, and mucous membranes. Other adverse reactions are rare but may include the following:

- Nausea, vomiting, abdominal cramping, diarrhea
- Alopecia (loss of hair)
- Rash or urticaria (hives)
- Hepatitis (inflammation of the liver), jaundice (yellowish discoloration of the skin and mucous membranes), thrombocytopenia (low platelet count), and blood dyscrasias (disorders)

Additional adverse reactions include local irritation when heparin is given by the subcutaneous (subcut) route. Hypersensitivity reactions may also occur with any route of administration and include fever and chills. More serious hypersensitivity reactions include an asthma-like reaction and an anaphylactic reaction. See the Summary Drug Table: Anticoagulant, Antiplatelet, and Thrombolytic Agents for additional adverse reactions.

CONTRAINDICATIONS

Anticoagulants are contraindicated in clients with known hypersensitivity to the drugs, active bleeding (except when caused by DIC), hemorrhagic disease, tuberculosis, leukemia, uncontrolled hypertension, gastrointestinal (GI) ulcers, recent surgery of the eye or central nervous system, aneurysms, or severe renal or hepatic disease, and during lactation. Use during pregnancy can cause fetal death (oral agents are in pregnancy category X and parenteral agents are in pregnancy category C). The LMWHs are also contraindicated in clients with a hypersensitivity to pork products.

 Lifespan Considerations

Jewish/Muslim Cultural Practices
Use of pork or porcine products is prohibited by some religious groups, and heparin is a pork derived product. Alert the primary health care provider if the client notes a Jewish or Muslim religious preference and is likely to undergo anticoagulant therapy. The DAOCs and the drug fondaparinux (Arixtra) are artificially produced and do not contain pork products; this may be used as a substitute for one of the pork derivative heparin products.

PRECAUTIONS

Anticoagulants are used cautiously in clients with fever, heart failure, diarrhea, diabetes, malignancy, hypertension, renal or hepatic disease, psychoses, or depression. Warfarin is used over DAOCs in clients with mechanical heart valves when on anticoagulant therapy. Some clients may have a genetic variation, making them more sensitive to warfarin (see Box 36.1). Although DAOCs are frequently used, warfarin may be chosen over these for clients also taking antiepileptics or HIV antiretrovirals. Apixaban is monitored by the Risk Evaluation

Clients with a specific gene duplication (CYP2C9 and VKORC1) are more likely to bleed when taking the average dose of the drug—warfarin. This is an example of how genetic make-up can impact drug administration. The genetic variation makes drug metabolism take longer, which means the drug stays active in the body longer—requiring lower dosing than what is normally prescribed (Johnson, 2011).

Clients who are warfarin sensitive, are more at risk of drug overdose leading to abnormal bleeding in the brain, GI tract, and other tissues. This increase in bleeding can lead to more serious problems or even death.

Although the occurrence of this gene duplication is unknown, approximately 25% of warfarin users are seen on an emergent basis yearly as a result of warfarin-related adverse drug reactions (Saleh, 2016).

and Mitigation Strategy (REMS) program for administration because of the greater chance of stroke when discontinued. Women of childbearing age must use a reliable contraceptive to prevent pregnancy. These drugs are used with caution in all clients with a potential site for bleeding or hemorrhage.

NURSING ALERT

Anticoagulant treated clients undergoing epidural or spinal anesthesia have a greater risk of hematoma at the site of injection. This risk is increased even more when other drugs such as NSAIDs or aspirin are taken.

LASA ALERT

The following drugs may sound alike; be sure to clarify when they are ordered:

Drug Name	Sounds Like
apixaban	axitinib
argatroban	Aggrastat, Organ
heparin	Hespan
Lovenox	Lasix, Levaquin, Levemir, Lotronex, Protonix

Drugs that look like a similar drug are noted in the Summary Drug Tables of each chapter.

INTERACTIONS

The following interactions may occur when an anticoagulant is administered with another agent:

Interacting Drug	Common Use	Effect of Interaction
Aspirin, acetaminophen, nonsteroidal anti-inflammatory drugs (NSAIDs), and chloral hydrate	Pain relief and sedation	Increased risk for bleeding

Interacting Drug	Common Use	Effect of Interaction
Penicillin, aminoglycosides, isoniazid, tetracyclines, and cephalosporins	Anti-infective agents	Increased risk for bleeding
Beta-blockers and loop diuretics	Treatment of cardiac problems	Increased risk for bleeding
Disulfiram and cimetidine	Management of GI distress	Increased risk for bleeding
Oral contraceptives, barbiturates, diuretics, and vitamin K	Birth control, sedation, treatment of cardiac problems, and treatment of bleeding disorders, respectively	Decreased effectiveness of the anticoagulant

Grapefruit and its juice will increase serum levels of apixaban and rivaroxaban.

Herbal Considerations

Any herbal remedy should be used with caution in clients taking warfarin. Warfarin, a drug with a narrow therapeutic index, has the potential to interact with many herbal remedies. For example, warfarin should not be combined with any of the following substances because they may have additive or synergistic activity and increase the risk for bleeding: celery, chamomile, clove, dong quai, feverfew, garlic, ginger, ginkgo biloba, ginseng, green tea, onion, passionflower, red clover, St. John's wort, and turmeric.

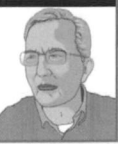

PHARMACOLOGY IN PRACTICE

ASSESSMENT

A nurse will initiate anticoagulant drug therapy with a client. In which of the following client conditions is an anticoagulant contraindicated? Select all that apply.
1. Diabetic retinopathy
2. Tuberculosis
3. GI bleeding
4. Leukemia
5. Hemorrhagic disease

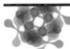

ANTIPLATELET DRUGS

Anticoagulant drugs prevent thrombosis in the *venous* system, and the antiplatelet drugs are used to prevent thrombus formation in the *arterial* system. Thrombi forming in the venous system are composed primarily of fibrin and red blood cells. In contrast, it is believed that arterial thrombosis formation is because of clumping of platelet aggregates; therefore, the platelets are the target rather than clotting

factors when the issue is arterial in nature. In addition to aspirin therapy, the antiplatelet drugs include adenosine diphosphate (ADP) receptor blockers and glycoprotein receptor blockers.

ACTIONS AND USES

These drugs work by decreasing the platelets' ability to stick together (**aggregate**) in the blood, thus forming a clot. Aspirin works by prohibiting the aggregation of the platelets for the lifetime of the platelet. The ADP blockers alter the platelet cell membrane, preventing aggregation. Glycoprotein receptor blockers work to prevent enzyme production, again inhibiting platelet aggregation. Antiplatelet drug therapy is designed primarily to treat clients at risk for acute coronary syndrome, MI, stroke, and intermittent claudication.

ADVERSE REACTIONS

Some of the more common adverse reactions include the following:

- Heart palpitations
- Bleeding
- Dizziness and headache
- Nausea, diarrhea, constipation, dyspepsia

CONTRAINDICATIONS AND PRECAUTIONS

Antiplatelet drugs are contraindicated in pregnant or lactating clients and those with known hypersensitivity to the drugs, congestive heart failure, active bleeding, or thrombotic thrombocytopenic purpura (TTP). These drugs are to be used cautiously in older adult clients, pancytopenic clients, or those with renal or hepatic impairment. If TTP is diagnosed, the antiplatelet treatment should be stopped immediately. Clopidogrel is a pregnancy category B and the others are pregnancy category C; none of these drugs have been well studied in humans. Antiplatelet drugs should be discontinued 1 week before any surgical procedure.

LASA ALERT

The following drugs may sound alike; be sure to clarify when they are ordered:

Drug Name	Sounds Like
Aggrastat	Aggrenox, argatroban
anagrelide	anastrozole
Brilinta	Brintellix
dipyridamole	disopyramide
Plavix	Elavil, Paxil, Pradaxa
prasugrel	pravastatin, propranolol

Drugs that look like a similar drug are noted in the Summary Drug Tables of each chapter.

INTERACTIONS

The following interactions may occur when an antiplatelet is administered with another agent:

Interacting Drug	Common Use	Effect of Interaction
Aspirin and NSAIDs	Pain relief	Increased risk of bleeding
Macrolide antibiotics	Anti-infective agents	Increased effectiveness of anti-infective
Digoxin	Management of cardiac problems	Decreased digoxin serum levels
Phenytoin	Control of seizure activity	Increased phenytoin serum levels

Although these agents produce strong anticoagulant effects, their mechanism of action is distinct from that of heparins; thus, these agents should be used carefully using specific guidelines provided for each product.

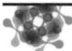 THROMBOLYTIC DRUGS

Whereas the anticoagulant agents prevent thrombus formation, the thrombolytic class of drugs dissolves blood clots that have already formed within the walls of a blood vessel. These drugs reopen blood vessels after they become occluded. Another term used to describe the thrombolytic drugs is "fibrinolytic". Examples of the thrombolytics include alteplase recombinant (Activase) and tenecteplase (TNKase).

> **! NURSING ALERT**
>
> Medication errors have occurred when the abbreviation—tPA is used when ordering thrombolytic drugs. The abbreviation can easily be misinterpreted as TPN (total parenteral nutrition).

ACTIONS

Although the exact action of each of the thrombolytic drugs is slightly different, these drugs break down fibrin clots by converting plasminogen to plasmin. Plasmin is an enzyme that breaks down the fibrin of a blood clot. This reopens blood vessels after their occlusion and prevents tissue necrosis. Because thrombolytic drugs dissolve all clots encountered (both occlusive and those repairing vessel leaks), bleeding is a great concern when using these agents. Before these drugs are used, their potential benefits must be weighed carefully against the potential dangers of bleeding.

USES

These drugs are used to treat the following:

- Acute stroke or MI by **lysis** (breaking up) of blood clots in the coronary arteries

- Blood clots causing pulmonary emboli and DVT
- Suspected occlusions in central venous catheters

See the Summary Drug Table: Anticoagulant, Antiplatelet, and Thrombolytic Agents for a more complete listing of the use of these drugs.

ADVERSE REACTIONS

Bleeding is the most common adverse reaction seen with the use of these drugs. Bleeding may be internal and involve areas such as the GI tract, genitourinary (GU) tract, and brain. Bleeding may also be external (superficial) and seen at areas of broken skin, such as venipuncture sites and recent surgical wounds. Allergic reactions may also be seen.

CONTRAINDICATIONS AND PRECAUTIONS

Thrombolytic drugs are contraindicated in a client with known hypersensitivity to the drugs, active bleeding, and history of stroke, aneurysm, and recent intracranial surgery.

These drugs are used cautiously in clients who have recently undergone major surgery (within 10 days), such as coronary artery bypass grafting; who experienced stroke, trauma, vaginal or cesarean section delivery, GI bleeding, or trauma within the last 10 days; who have hypertension, diabetic retinopathy, or any condition in which bleeding is a significant possibility; or who are currently receiving oral anticoagulants. All of the thrombolytic drugs discussed in this chapter are classified in pregnancy category C, with the exception of urokinase, which is a pregnancy category B drug.

> **LASA ALERT**
>
> The following drugs may sound alike; be sure to clarify when they are ordered:
>
> | Drug Name | Sounds Like |
> |---|---|
> | Activase | TNKase |
> | alteplase | Altace |
>
> Drugs that look like a similar drug are noted in the Summary Drug Tables of each chapter.

INTERACTIONS

When a thrombolytic is administered with medications that prevent blood clots, such as aspirin, dipyridamole, or an anticoagulant, the client is at increased risk for bleeding.

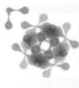

NURSING PROCESS: STEPS TO BUILDING CLINICAL JUDGMENT
Client Receiving an Anticoagulant, Antiplatelet, or Thrombolytic Drug

ASSESSMENT

Preadministration Assessment
When immobilization is anticipated, clients are often started on preventative anticoagulant therapy.

Data gathering suggestions before the initial administration of an anticoagulant or thrombolytic drug include:

Objective data

- Vital signs (temperature, pulse, respirations, and blood pressure)
- Inspect physical appearance, noting skin color, temperature and pain, differences bilaterally
- Palpate for pedal pulses, noting rate and strength if lower limb is involved
- Test for a positive Homans sign (pain in the calf when the foot is dorsiflexed), a positive finding suggests DVT
- Laboratory tests—baseline prothrombin time (PT) and the international normalized ratio (INR) and activated partial thromboplastin time (aPTT) if heparin is being administered
- Thrombolytic agent use—complete blood count and radiologic testing such as a computed tomography (CT) scan may be performed

Subjective data

- History of and reason for clotting experience, pain assessment if experiencing pain
- Medical/family history
- Drug therapy (list of all current drugs and supplements taken—specifically in last 3 weeks)

Most clients receiving a thrombolytic agent are admitted or transferred to an intensive care unit, because close monitoring is necessary for 48 hr or more after therapy.

Ongoing Assessment
In the ongoing assessment, a client receiving an anticoagulant, antiplatelet, or thrombolytic drug requires close observation and careful monitoring. During the course of therapy for both oral and parenteral drugs, continually assess the client for any signs of bleeding and hemorrhage. Areas of assessment include the gums, nose, stools, urine, or nasogastric drainage. Level of consciousness should be assessed on a routine basis to monitor for intracranial bleeding.

Clients receiving warfarin for the first time often require daily adjustment of the dose, which is based on the daily PT/INR results. In settings such as long-term care or rehabilitation, this may be done with an INR monitor, similar to the glucometers used for monitoring blood glucose. If the PT exceeds 1.2–1.5 times the control value or the INR ratio exceeds 3, the primary health care provider is notified before the drug is given. A daily PT/INR is performed until it stabilizes and when any other drug is added to or removed from the client's drug regimen. After the INR has stabilized, it is monitored every 4–6 weeks. See Box 36.2 for more information on the laboratory tests for monitoring warfarin.

BOX 36.2 Understanding Prothrombin Time and International Normalized Ratio

Prothrombin time (also called pro-time or abbreviated as "PT") and the *international normalized ratio* (INR) are used to monitor the client's response to warfarin therapy. The daily dose of the oral anticoagulant is based on the client's daily PT/INR. The therapeutic range of the PT is 1.2–1.5 times the control value. Studies indicate that levels greater than two times the control value do not provide additional therapeutic effects in most clients and are associated with a higher incidence of bleeding.

Laboratories report results for the INR along with the client's PT and the control value. The INR "corrects" the routine PT results from different laboratories. By measuring against a known standard, the INR gives a more consistent value. The INR is maintained between values 2 and 3. Values above 5 can be dangerous, and values below 1 are ineffective.

The dosage of heparin is adjusted according to daily aPTT monitoring. A therapeutic dosage is attained when the aPTT is 1.5–2.5 times the normal. The LMWHs have little or no effect on the aPTT values. Special monitoring of clotting times is not necessary when administering the DTI drugs. Periodic platelet counts, hematocrit, and tests for occult blood in the stool should be performed throughout the course of heparin therapy.

! NURSING ALERT
Blood coagulation tests for those receiving heparin by continuous IV infusion are taken at periodic intervals (usually every 4 hr) determined by the primary health care provider. If the client is receiving long-term heparin therapy, blood coagulation tests may be performed at less frequent intervals.

Remember to monitor for any indication of hypersensitivity reaction. Report reactions such as chills, fever, or hives to the primary health care provider. Examine the skin temperature and color in the client with a DVT for signs of improvement. Check and document vital signs every 4 hr or more frequently, if needed. When heparin is given to prevent the formation of a thrombus, observe the client for signs of thrombus formation every 2–4 hr. Because the signs and symptoms of thrombus formation vary and depend on the area or organ involved, evaluate and report any complaint the client may have or any change in the client's condition to the primary health care provider.

NURSING DIAGNOSES
Drug-specific nursing diagnoses include the following:

- **Injury risk** related to excessive bleeding because of drug therapy
- **Altered health seeking behavior** related to preparing to communicate drug use if incapacitated

- **Anxiety** related to fear of atypical bleeding during thrombolytic drug therapy

Nursing diagnoses related to drug administration are discussed in depth in Chapter 4.

PLANNING

The expected outcomes for the client may include an optimal response to therapy, support of client needs related to the management of adverse reactions, and confidence in an understanding of the medication regimen.

IMPLEMENTATION

Promoting an Optimal Response to Therapy

Oral Administration of Anticoagulants
DAOCs have a fixed dose, less dietary restrictions, and shorter half-life in the client. Additionally, blood level monitoring is not required as noted below for warfarin use.

DOSING WARFARIN. To hasten the onset of the therapeutic effect of warfarin, a higher dosage (loading dose) may be prescribed for 2–4 days, followed by a maintenance dosage adjusted according to the daily PT/INR. Otherwise, the drug takes 3–5 days to reach therapeutic levels. When rapid anticoagulation is required, heparin is preferred as a loading dose, followed by maintenance dose of warfarin based on the PT or INR. The dose is typically given in the evening at a specified time. This prevents errors in administration of doses too high or too low by providing ample time to allow time for adjustments based on laboratory results.

Optimal therapeutic results are obtained when the client's PT is 1.2–1.5 times the control value. In certain instances, such as in recurrent systemic embolism, a PT of 1.5–2 may be prescribed. Studies indicate that diet can influence the PT/INR values. A study at the Massachusetts General Hospital in Boston looked at the effect of varying dietary vitamin K intake on the INR in clients receiving anticoagulation therapy with warfarin. As vitamin K intake increased, INR became more consistent and stable. By contrast, as vitamin K intake decreased, INR became more variable and fluctuated to a greater extent. The key to vitamin K management for clients receiving warfarin is maintaining a consistent daily intake of vitamin K.

Parenteral Administration of Anticoagulants
Heparin preparations, unlike warfarin, must be given by the parenteral route, preferably subcut or IV. The onset of anticoagulation is almost immediate after a single dose. Maximum effects occur within 10 min of administration. Clotting time returns to normal within 4 hr unless subsequent doses are given. Although warfarin is most often administered orally, an injectable form may be used as an alternative route for clients who are unable to receive oral drugs.

Heparin may be given by intermittent IV administration, continuous IV infusion, and the subcut route. Intramuscular (IM) administration is avoided because of the possibility of the development of local irritation, pain, or hematoma (a collection of blood in the tissue). The dosage of heparin is measured in units and is available in various dosage strengths as units per milliliter (e.g., 10,000 units/mL). When selecting the strength used for administration,

choose the strength closest to the prescribed dose. For example, if 5000 units are ordered and the available strengths are 1000, 5000, 7500, 20,000, and 40,000 units/mL, use 1 mL of the 5000 units/mL for administration.

NURSING ALERT
Errors have been made by misreading the numbers on the bottles of heparin. Doses of 10,000 units have been misread as 100 units; as a result, clients have been put at risk for hemorrhage when receiving these higher doses. It is important for the nurse to prepare medications without distraction to minimize risk to clients.

To ensure safe administration when continuous infusion (IV) heparin is ordered, an infusion pump must be used. The infusion pump is checked every 1–2 hr to ensure that it is working properly. The needle site is inspected for signs of inflammation, pain, and tenderness along the pathway of the vein. If these occur, the infusion is discontinued and restarted in another vein.

When heparin or other anticoagulants are given by the subcut route, administration sites are rotated and the site used is documented on the client's chart. The recommended sites of administration are those on the abdomen, but areas within 2 in of the umbilicus are avoided because of the increased vascularity of that area. Other areas of administration of heparin are the buttocks, lateral thighs, and upper arms (Fig. 36.3). No fluctuation in absorption has been found by using the arms and legs. The application of firm pressure after the injection helps to prevent hematoma formation. Each time heparin is given by this route, inspect all recent injection sites for signs of inflammation (redness, swelling, tenderness) and hematoma formation.

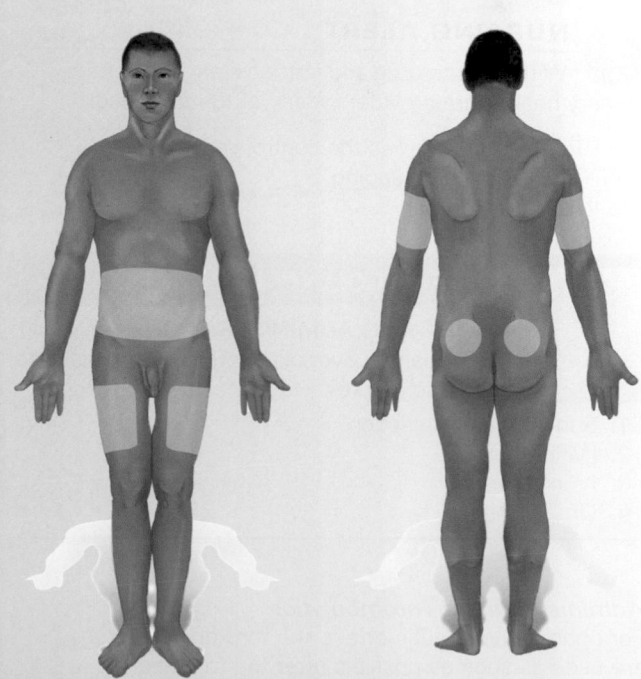

FIGURE 36.3 Sites for subcutaneous anticoagulant parenteral injection. (Adapted from Timby, B. K. (2017). *Fundamental nursing skills and concepts* (11th ed.). Wolters Kluwer, Lippincott Williams & Wilkins.)

Drugs for DVT prevention are available in prefilled syringes; do not expel the air bubble. They are administered deep in subcut tissue by pinching a fold of skin. Insert the needle into the tissue at a 90° angle so the air bubble is injected last. It is not necessary to aspirate before injecting the drug; this may activate the needle guard. Be careful not to let go of the plunger until the syringe is empty and pulled out of the skin; letting go causes the needle to withdraw into the barrel of the syringe, thus preventing injury from a needle stick following the injection.

Blood coagulation tests are usually ordered before and during heparin therapy, and the dose of heparin is adjusted to the test results. Coagulation tests are usually performed 30 min before the scheduled dose and from the extremity opposite the infusion site. When administering heparin by the subcut route, an aPTT test is performed 4–6 hr after the injection. Optimal results of therapy are obtained when the aPTT is 1.5–2.5 times the control value. The LMWHs and the DTIs do not require close monitoring of blood coagulation tests.

A complete blood count, platelet count, and stool analysis for occult blood may be ordered periodically throughout therapy. Thrombocytopenia may occur during heparin or antiplatelet administration. A mild, transient thrombocytopenia may occur 2–3 days after heparin therapy is begun. This early development of thrombocytopenia tends to resolve itself despite continued therapy. As you check periodic laboratory reports, a platelet count of less than 100,000 mm³ should be brought to the attention of the primary health care provider, who may choose to discontinue the heparin therapy. Overdose of antiplatelet drugs is typically managed by withholding treatment or by infusion of platelets.

! NURSING ALERT

Withhold the drug and immediately contact the primary health care provider for any of the following:

The PT exceeds 1.5 times the control value.
There is evidence of bleeding.
The INR is greater than 3.

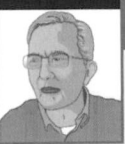

PHARMACOLOGY IN PRACTICE

SAFE DRUG ADMINISTRATION
Enoxaparin (Lovenox) should be administered via which route?

1. Subcutaneous injection
2. IM injection
3. IV infusion
4. Orally

Administration of Thrombolytics

For optimal therapeutic effect, the thrombolytic drugs are used as soon as possible after the formation of a thrombus, preferably within 4–6 hr or as soon as possible after the symptoms are identified. The greatest chance of recovery from an ischemic stroke is when the thrombolytic drug is administered within 3 hr. Benefit follows from drug administration within 4.5 hr, but significant benefits from occlusion of larger arteries may require mechanical removal using a wire cage device (AHA, 2016). Timing of the onset of symptoms is important. Here, you can help the family or person coming with the client to remember the situation and get estimates of the timing of symptoms.

Assess the client for bleeding every 15 min during the first 60 min of therapy, every 15–30 min for the next 8 hr and at least every 4 hr until therapy is completed. Vital signs are monitored continuously. If pain is present, the primary health care provider may order an opioid analgesic. Once the clot dissolves and blood flows freely through the obstructed blood vessel, severe pain usually decreases.

Monitoring and Managing Client Needs

Injury Risk

Bleeding can occur any time during therapy with warfarin or the heparin preparations, even when the INR appears to be within a safe limit (e.g., 2–3). All nursing personnel and medical team members should be made aware of any client receiving warfarin and the observations necessary with administration. If bleeding should occur, the primary health care provider may decrease the dose, discontinue the heparin therapy for a time, or order the administration of protamine sulfate. *Be alert to the following indicators of bleeding:*

- If a decided drop in blood pressure or rise in the pulse rate occurs, notify the primary health care provider, because this may indicate internal bleeding. Hemorrhage can begin as a slight bleeding or bruising tendency; frequently observe the client for these occurrences. Sometimes, hemorrhage occurs without warning.
- Urinal, bedpan, catheter drainage unit—inspect the urine for a pink to red color and the stool for signs of GI bleeding (bright red to black stools). Visually check the catheter drainage every 2–4 hr and when the unit is emptied. Oral anticoagulants may impart a red-orange color to alkaline urine, making hematuria difficult to detect visually. A urinalysis may be necessary to determine if blood is in the urine.
- Emesis basin, nasogastric suction units—visually check the nasogastric suction unit every 2–4 hr and when the unit is emptied. Check the emesis basin each time it is emptied.
- Skin, mucous membranes—inspect the client's skin daily for evidence of easy bruising or bleeding. Be alert for bleeding from minor cuts and scratches, nosebleeds, or excessive bleeding after IM, subcut, or IV injections. or after a venipuncture. After oral care, check the toothbrush and gums for signs of bleeding.

! NURSING ALERT

When clients using anticoagulants have spinal anesthesia or undergo spinal punctures, they are at risk for potential spinal or epidural hematoma formation, which can lead to long-term or permanent paralysis. These clients should be frequently monitored for signs and symptoms of neurologic impairment.

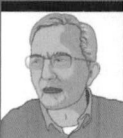

PHARMACOLOGY IN PRACTICE

MANAGING NEEDS

A nurse is caring for a client who has been administered heparin following the administration of a thrombolytic drug to prevent another thrombus from forming. What should the nurse monitor for in the client after the administration of heparin?

1. Internal bleeding
2. Difficulty in breathing
3. Excessive perspiration
4. Skin rash

Altered Health Seeking Behavior

The client needs to be aware of the many food and drug interactions that can cause a higher risk for bleeding when taking anticoagulants, or make the drugs less effective. A medical alert bracelet and list of drugs being taken should be on the client at all times in case the client becomes incapacitated by accident or illness, because other care providers need to know that anticoagulant or antiplatelet drugs are being taken.

The client is instructed to notify all health care providers of the anticoagulant or antiplatelet therapy when diagnostic tests or other treatments are performed. When the skin is pierced during procedures, explain why you must apply prolonged pressure to needle or catheter sites after venipuncture, removal of central or peripheral IV lines, and IM and subcut injections. Laboratory personnel or those responsible for drawing blood for laboratory tests are made aware of anticoagulant therapy, because prolonged pressure on the venipuncture site is necessary. All laboratory requests should be flagged that the client is receiving anticoagulant therapy.

Anxiety

Bleeding is the most common adverse reaction when thrombolytic drugs are administered. Conditions requiring thrombolytic treatment are typically of an urgent nature, and treatment occurs in special care units of the hospital such as the intensive care unit or operating room. Combined with the potential for bleeding, all this can be frightening and cause anxiety to the client and any family members present. As you monitor the client's status, it is important to reassure the client and communicate with family members that measures are being taken to diagnose and intervene early for any adverse reactions.

Throughout administration of the thrombolytic drug, assess for signs of bleeding and hemorrhage. Internal bleeding may involve the GI tract, GU tract, intracranial sites, or respiratory tract. Signs and symptoms of internal bleeding may include abdominal pain; coffee ground emesis; black, tarry stools; hematuria; joint pain; and spitting or coughing up blood.

Superficial bleeding may occur at venous or arterial puncture sites or recent surgical incision sites. Again, this can be disturbing to the client and family, and they may become anxious. Because fibrin is lysed during therapy, bleeding from recent injection sites may occur. Carefully monitor all potential bleeding sites (including catheter insertion sites, arterial and venous puncture sites, cutdown sites, and needle puncture sites). Reassure the client that bleeding will be reported to the primary health care provider and steps taken to minimize the bleeding. Minor bleeding at a puncture site can usually be controlled by applying pressure for at least 30 min at the site, followed by the application of a pressure dressing. The puncture site is checked frequently for evidence of further bleeding. IM injections and nonessential handling of the client are avoided during treatment. Venipunctures are done only when absolutely necessary.

NURSING ALERT

Heparin may be given along with or after administration of a thrombolytic drug to prevent another thrombus from forming. However, administration of an anticoagulant increases the risk for bleeding. The client must be monitored closely for internal and external bleeding.

If uncontrolled bleeding is noted or the bleeding appears to be internal, stop the drug and immediately contact the primary health care provider, because whole blood, packed red cells, or fresh frozen plasma may be required. Continuous monitoring of vital signs for at least 48 hr after the drug is discontinued should occur. Contact the primary health care provider if there is a marked change in one or more of the vital signs. Any signs of an allergic (hypersensitivity) reaction, such as difficulty breathing, wheezing, hives, skin rash, and hypotension, are reported immediately to the primary health care provider.

Managing Anticoagulant Overdosage

ORAL ANTICOAGULANTS. Symptoms of warfarin overdosage include blood in the stool (melena); **petechiae** (pinpoint-sized red hemorrhagic spots on the skin); oozing from superficial injuries, such as cuts from shaving or bleeding from the gums after brushing the teeth; or excessive menstrual bleeding. Immediately report any of these adverse reactions or evidence of bleeding to the primary health care provider.

If bleeding occurs, the PT exceeds 1.5 times the control value, or the INR exceeds 3, the primary health care provider may either discontinue the anticoagulant therapy for a few days or order vitamin K (phytonadione), an oral anticoagulant antagonist, which should be readily available when a client is receiving warfarin. Because warfarin interferes with the synthesis of vitamin K–dependent clotting factors, the administration of vitamin K reverses the effects of warfarin by providing the necessary ingredient to enhance clot formation and stop bleeding. However, withholding one or two doses of warfarin may quickly bring the PT to an acceptable level. The drug—idarucizumab is used to reverse the DTI—dabigatran.

Assess the client for additional evidence of bleeding until the PT is below 1.5 times the control value or until the bleeding episodes cease. The PT usually returns to a safe level within 6 hr of administration of vitamin K. Administration of whole blood or plasma may be necessary if severe bleeding occurs because of the delayed onset of action of vitamin K.

PARENTERAL ANTICOAGULANTS. In most instances, discontinuation of the drug is sufficient to correct overdosage because the duration of action of heparin is brief. However, if hemorrhaging is severe, the primary health care provider may order protamine, the specific heparin antagonist or antidote. Protamine is also used to treat overdosage of the LMWHs. Protamine has an immediate onset of action and a duration of 2 hr. It counteracts the effects of heparin and brings blood coagulation test results to within normal limits. The drug is given slowly by the IV route over a period of 10 min.

If administration of this drug is necessary, monitor the client's blood pressure and pulse rate every 15–30 min for 2 hr or more after administration of the heparin antagonist. Immediately report to the primary health care provider any sudden decrease in blood pressure or increase in the pulse rate. Observe the client for new evidence of bleeding until blood coagulation test results are within normal limits. To replace blood loss, the primary health care provider may order blood transfusions or fresh frozen plasma.

Educating the Client and Family

In many facilities, the clinical pharmacist is responsible for anticoagulant teaching. A thorough review of the dosage regimen, possible adverse drug reactions, and early signs of bleeding tendencies help the client cooperate with the prescribed therapy. You can provide further explanation or validate learning on the part of the client and family. Validate understanding of the following points in a client and family teaching plan:

- Follow the dosage schedule prescribed by the primary health care provider, and report any signs of active bleeding immediately.
- The INR will be monitored periodically. Keep all primary health care provider and laboratory appointments, because dosage changes may be necessary during therapy.
- Do not take or stop taking other drugs except on the advice of the primary health care provider. This includes nonprescription drugs, as well as those prescribed by a primary health care provider or dentist.
- Inform the dentist or other primary health care providers of therapy with this drug before any treatment or procedure is started or drugs are prescribed.
- Take the drug at the same time each day.
- Do not change brands of anticoagulants without consulting a physician or pharmacist.

- Avoid alcohol unless use has been approved by the primary health care provider.
- Be aware of foods high in vitamin K, such as leafy green vegetables, beans, broccoli, cabbage, cauliflower, cheese, fish, and yogurt. Maintaining a healthy diet including these foods may help maintain a consistent INR value.
- Keep in mind that antiplatelet drugs can lower all blood counts, including the white cell count. Clients may be at greater risk of infection during the first 3 months of treatment.
- If evidence of bleeding occurs, such as unusual bleeding or bruising, bleeding gums, blood in the urine or stool, black stool, or diarrhea, omit the next dose of the drug and contact the primary health care provider immediately.
- Use a soft toothbrush and consult a dentist regarding routine oral hygiene, including the use of dental floss. Use an electric razor when possible to avoid small skin cuts.
- Women of childbearing age should use a reliable contraceptive to prevent pregnancy.
- Wear or carry medical identification, such as a MedicAlert bracelet, to inform medical personnel and others of therapy with this drug.

EVALUATION

- Therapeutic response is achieved and blood coagulation is controlled.
- Adverse reactions are identified, reported to the primary health care provider, and managed successfully with appropriate nursing interventions:
  - No evidence of injury is seen.
  - Client enhances health behavior effectively.
  - Anxiety is managed successfully.
- Client and family express confidence and demonstrate an understanding of the drug regimen.

PHARMACOLOGY IN PRACTICE

USING CLINICAL REASONING

Mr. Phillip's last INR was 2.9; the week before it was 1.5. You ask him to bring in his medication and find seven different bottles and four different strengths of warfarin. When asked he tells you he has a weekly calendar and takes as many tablets as it says on the sheet. You know that warfarin pills come in strengths from 1 to 10 mg. When you ask about the bottles, he states, "They are all green, so they must be the same." What action would you take next?

KEY POINTS

■ Hemostasis is the process of clotting; this is beneficial when injury tears a vessel. A thrombus is a clot that forms in a vessel and impedes blood flow.

■ Anticoagulants are used to prevent the formation or extension of a thrombus (or blood clot). These drugs do not

affect existing clots, nor do they reverse damage already done by a clot. These drugs are used to prevent further clot development. Although they do not thin the blood, they are commonly called blood thinners.

■ Antiplatelet drugs decrease the platelets' ability to aggregate (or stick together). This reduces the chance of thrombus formation in the arterial circulation for conditions such as acute coronary syndrome, MI, and stroke.

■ Thrombolytic drugs are used to dissolve blood clots that have already formed within the walls of a blood vessel.

■ Many of these drugs are monitored with frequent laboratory tests because bleeding is an adverse reaction of all these drugs. The GI system, mental status, and pain should be monitored for signs of internal bleeding. Precautions with laboratory draws and previous skin punctures and monitoring of the skin can detect superficial bleeding.

SUMMARY DRUG TABLE
Anticoagulant, Antiplatelet, and Thrombolytic Agents

Generic Name	Trade Name	Uses	Adverse Reactions	Dosage Ranges
Anticoagulants				
Oral Anticoagulants				
warfarin *WAR-far-in*	Jantoven	Prophylaxis/treatment of venous thrombosis	Bleeding, fatigue, dizziness, abdominal cramping	2–10 mg/day orally, individualized dose based on PT or INR: IV form for injection
Direct-Acting Oral Anticoagulant				
DIRECT THROMBIN INHIBITORI				
dabigatran *da-BIG-a-tran*	Pradaxa	Stroke and embolism prevention	Bleeding, nausea, diarrhea	150 mg orally BID
FACTOR XA INHIBITORS				
apixaban *a-PIX-a-ban*	Eliquis	Stroke and embolism prevention nonvalve atrial fibrillation, post hip/knee replacement	Bleeding	2.5–10 orally BID
edoxaban *e-DOX-a-ban*	Savaysa	Stroke and embolism prevention nonvalve atrial fibrillation	Dizziness, fatigue, rash	30–60 mg orally daily
rivaroxaban *riv-a-ROX-a-ban*	Xarelto	DVT prophylaxis and stroke prevention	Bleeding	10–10 mg orally daily
PARENTERAL ANTICOAGULANTS				
heparin *HEP-a-rin*		Thrombosis/embolism, diagnosis and treatment of DIC, prophylaxis of DVT, clotting prevention	Bleeding, chills, fever, urticaria, local irritation, erythema, mild pain, hematoma, or bruising at the injection site (subcut)	10,000–20,000 units subcut in divided doses q 8–12 hr; 5000–10,000 units q 4–6 hr intermittent IV; 5000–40,000 units/day IV infusion
heparin sodium lock flush solution		Clearing intermittent infusion lines (heparin lock) to prevent clot formation at site	None significant	10–100 units/mL heparin solution
PARENTERAL ANTICOAGULANTS: LOW–MOLECULAR-WEIGHT HEPARINS				
dalteparin *dal-TE-pa-rin*	Fragmin	Unstable angina/non–Q-wave MI, DVT prophylaxis	Bleeding, bruising, rash, fever, erythema, and irritation at site of injection	Angina/MI: 120 units/kg subcut q 12 hr with concurrent oral aspirin; DVT: 2500 units/day subcut
enoxaparin *e-noks-a-PA-rin*	Lovenox	DVT and presurgical prophylaxis, PE treatment, unstable angina/non–Q-wave MI	Same as dalteparin	DVT prophylaxis: 30–40 mg subcut q 12 hr Treatment: 1 mg/kg subcut q 12 hr
DIRECT THROMBIN INHIBITOR—PARENTERAL				
argatroban *ar-GA-troh-ban*		Anticoagulation during procedures (angioplasty), heparin-induced thrombocytopenia	Hypotension, GU bleeding	10 mcg/kg/min IV

Continued

SUMMARY DRUG TABLE (continued)
Anticoagulant, Antiplatelet, and Thrombolytic Agents

Generic Name	Trade Name	Uses	Adverse Reactions	Dosage Ranges
bivalirudin *bye-VAL-i-roo-din*		Anticoagulation during procedures (angioplasty)	Bleeding (at injection site)	Dictated by procedure
FACTOR XA INHIBITORS —PARENTERAL				
fondaparinux *fon-da-PARE-i-nuks*	Arixtra	DVT prophylaxis	Bleeding (at injection site)	2.5 mg subcut 6–8 hr following surgery, then daily for 5–9 days postoperatively
Antiplatelet Agents				
abciximab *ab-SIK-si-mab*		Adjunct in coronary angioplasty	Bleeding, pain	0.125 mcg/kg/min IV during procedure
anagrelide *an-AG-gre-lide*	Agrylin	Thrombocythemia	Heart palpitations, dizziness, headache, nausea, abdominal pain, diarrhea, edema	1 mg orally BID
cangrelor *KAN-grel-or*	Kengreal	Adjunct in coronary angioplasty	Bleeding	IV infusion during procedure
cilostazol *sil-OH-sta-zol*		Intermittent claudication	Heart palpitations, dizziness, diarrhea, headache, rhinitis	100 mg orally BID
clopidogrel *kloh-PID-oh-grel*	Plavix	Recent MI, stroke, and acute coronary syndrome	Dizziness, skin rash, chest pain, constipation	Single loading dose: 300 mg; 75 mg/day orally
dipyridamole *dye-peer-ID-a-mole*		Postoperative thromboembolic prevention in valve replacement	Dizziness, abdominal distress	75–100 mg orally QID
eptifibatide *ep-TIF-i-ba-tide*	Integrilin	Adjunct in coronary angioplasty, acute coronary syndrome	Bleeding, pain	1 mcg/kg/min IV infusion
prasugrel *PRA-soo-grel*	Effient	Acute coronary syndrome	Bleeding, anemia	5–10 mg orally daily
ticagrelor *tye-KA-grel-or*	Brilinta	Acute coronary syndrome	Bleeding	90–180 mg orally daily
tirofiban *tye-roe-FYE-ban*	Aggrastat	Acute coronary syndrome	Bleeding, pain	0.4–0.1 mcg/kg/min IV infusion
vorapaxar *vor-a-PAX-ar*	Zontivity	Reduce risk of thrombus formation in legs, heart, or stroke	Fatigue, cool extremities	2.08 mg orally daily
Thrombolytics				
alteplase *AL-te-plase*	Activase, Cathflo Activase (for IV catheter occlusions only)	Acute MI, acute ischemic stroke, PE, IV catheter clearance	Bleeding (GU, gingival, intracranial) and epistaxis, ecchymosis	Total dose of 90–100 mg IV, given as a 2- to 3-hr infusion
reteplase *RE-ta-plase*	Retavase	Acute MI	Bleeding (GI, GU, or at injection site), intracranial hemorrhage, anemia	Prepackaged: 2- to 10-unit IV bolus injections
tenecteplase *ten-EK-te-plase*	TNKase	Acute MI	Bleeding (GI, GU, or at injection site), intracranial hemorrhage, anemia	Dosage based on weight, not to exceed 50 mg IV
Anticoagulant Antagonists				
phytonadione (vitamin K) *fye-toe-na-DYE-one*	Mephyton, Aqua-K	Treatment of warfarin overdosage, prophylaxis of Vitamin K deficiency of newborns	Gastric upset, unusual taste, flushing, rash, urticaria, erythema, pain and/or swelling at injection site	2.5–10 mg orally, IM, may repeat orally in 12–48 hr or in 6–8 hr after parenteral dose
protamine *PROE-ta-meen*		Treatment of heparin overdose	Flushing and warm feeling, dyspnea, bradycardia, hypotension	Dose is determined by amount of heparin to be neutralized; generally, 1 mg IV neutralizes 100 units of heparin

Generic Name	Trade Name	Uses	Adverse Reactions	Dosage Ranges
idaruCIZUmab *eye-da-roo-SIZ-uh-mab*	Praxbind	Treatment to reverse dabigatran	Delirium, constipation	Dose is determined by amount of drug to be neutralized
andexanet alfa *an-DEX-a-net*	Andexxa	Treatment to reverse apixaban, rivaroxaban, off label for betrixaban/edoxaban	Infusion reaction	Dose is determined by amount of drug to be neutralized

CHAPTER REVIEW

Know Your Drugs

Clients sometimes know a medication by the brand (or trade) name and not the generic name. To help you recognize both names, match the brand name with the generic name of the same medication.

Generic Name	Brand Name
1. clopidogrel	A. Brilinta
2. dalteparin	B. Lovenox
3. ticagrelor	C. Fragmin
4. enoxaparin	D. Plavix

Calculate Medication Dosages

1. The client is prescribed 5000 units of heparin. The drug is available as a solution of 2500 units/mL. The nurse administers _____.
2. Oral warfarin 5 mg is prescribed. On hand are 2.5-mg tablets. The nurse administers _____.

Prepare for the NCLEX

RECALL THE FACTS

1. Hemostasis is best defined as _____.
   1. thinning the blood for better flow in the vessels
   2. stopping all evidence of bleeding
   3. events forming a clot, stopping bleeding
   4. formation of a thrombus in the venous circulation
2. When a clot detaches from the vessel wall and begins to travel, this is termed _____.
   1. thrombus
   2. aggregation
   3. hemostasis
   4. embolus
3. Optimal INR during therapy is _____.
   1. more than 5
   2. less than 1
   3. between 1.8 and 2
   4. between 2 and 3

4. There is an increased risk for bleeding when the client receiving heparin is also taking _____.
   1. allopurinol
   2. NSAIDs
   3. digoxin
   4. furosemide
5. In which of the following situations would the nurse expect dalteparin to be prescribed?
   1. To prevent a DVT
   2. For a client with DIC
   3. To prevent hemorrhage
   4. For a client with atrial fibrillation

ANALYZE THE FACTS

6. The client is to begin oral anticoagulant drug therapy. Before administering the drug, the nurse _____.
   1. administers a loading dose of heparin
   2. has the laboratory draw blood for a serum potassium level
   3. takes the apical pulse
   4. sees that blood has been drawn for a baseline PT evaluation
7. If bleeding is noted while a client is receiving a thrombolytic drug, the client may receive _____.
   1. heparin
   2. whole blood or fresh frozen plasma
   3. a diuretic
   4. protamine sulfate
8. *The clinic nurse prepares teaching materials to give a client using warfarin. Which statement would cause them to contact the primary health care provider immediately?
   1. "I noticed my bowel movements were black yesterday."
   2. "I ordered a medical alert bracelet."
   3. "My mother died of a stroke."
   4. "A nutritious meal will make my blood better."

ALTERNATE-FORMAT QUESTIONS

To check your answers, see Appendix F.

*Indicates the question is directly linked to the NCLEX-PN test plan in Appendix G.

9. Clients on blood-thinning medications should be monitored for bleeding. Which of the following may indicate internal bleeding? **Select all that apply.**
   1. Sudden decrease in blood pressure
   2. INR of 1.5
   3. Cloudy, amber urine
   4. Multiple red spots on skin
   5. Black, tarry stool

10. Match the drug class with its function.

   1. Anticoagulant   A. Prevents cell aggregation
   2. Antiplatelet   B. Dissolves existing thrombi
   3. Thrombolytic   C. Prevents formation of new thrombi

WANT TO KNOW MORE? A wide variety of resources are available to enhance your learning and understanding of this chapter.

- Visit thePoint for resources such as:
  - NCLEX-Style Student Review Questions
  - Journal Articles
  - Dosage Calculations
  - Drug Monographs
  - Watch and Learn Videos
  - Concepts in Action Animations
- The *Study Guide to Accompany Introductory Clinical Pharmacology,* 12th edition, sold separately, will help you review and apply essential content.
- ✓*PrepU* is available to help students prepare for the NCLEX-PN examination.

Cardiotonic and Antiarrhythmic Drugs

Key Terms

action potential   electrical impulse that passes from cell to cell in the myocardium of the heart and stimulates the fibers to shorten, causing the heart muscle to contract

arrhythmia   abnormal heart rate or rhythm; also called *dysrhythmia*

atrial fibrillation   quivering of the atria of the heart

bradycardia   slow heart rate, usually below 60 bpm

cardiac output   volume of blood discharged from the left or right ventricle per minute

digitalis toxicity   toxic drug effects from the administration of digoxin

heart failure   condition in which the heart cannot pump enough blood to meet the tissue needs of the body; commonly called congestive heart failure

left ventricular dysfunction   condition in which fluids back up previous to the left ventricle of the heart and is characterized by shortness of breath and moist cough in heart failure

myocardium   the striated, muscle tissue of the heart

neurohormonal activity   in heart failure, increased secretions of epinephrine and norepinephrine result in arteriolar vasoconstriction, tachycardia, and myocardial contractility, leading to a worsening of heart failure and reduced ability of the heart to contract effectively

positive inotropic activity   increase in the force of cardiac contraction

refractory period   a quiet period between the transmission of nerve impulses along a nerve fiber

repolarization   return of positive and negative ions to their original place on the nerve cell after an impulse has passed along the nerve fiber (see *polarization*)

(continued)

Learning Objectives

On completion of this chapter, the student will:

1. Compare and contrast heart failure in relationship to left ventricular failure, right ventricular failure, neurohormonal activity, and treatment options.
2. Describe the different types of cardiac arrhythmias.
3. Explain the uses, general drug actions, general adverse reactions, contraindications, precautions, and interactions of the cardiotonic and antiarrhythmic drugs.
4. Discuss the use of other drugs with positive inotropic action.
5. Distinguish important preadministration and ongoing assessment activities the nurse should perform on the client taking a cardiotonic or antiarrhythmic drug.
6. List nursing diagnoses particular to a client taking a cardiotonic or antiarrhythmic drug.
7. Identify the symptoms of digitalis toxicity.
8. Examine ways to promote an optimal response to therapy, how to manage common adverse reactions, and important points to keep in mind when administering cardiotonic and antiarrhythmic drugs.

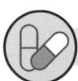 **Drug Classes**

- Cardiotonics
- Antiarrhythmics
  - Class I—sodium channel blockers
  - Class II—beta-adrenergic (β-adrenergic) blockers
  - Class III—potassium channel blockers
  - Class IV—calcium channel blockers
  - Class V—other antiarrhythmics

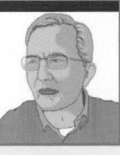 **PHARMACOLOGY IN PRACTICE**

Mr. Phillip was recently diagnosed with atrial fibrillation and prescribed both propranolol and Coumadin to take at home. When he comes in for weekly laboratory work, the phlebotomist tells you that Mr. Phillip is very dizzy and they are concerned about his safety. Read about the antiarrhythmic drugs and determine what should happen next.

Heart failure (HF) predisposes an individual to atrial fibrillation (AF), and AF may worsen the prognosis of a person with HF (Ehrlich et al., 2002). These two heart ailments are different and have independent causes, yet these conditions are occurring more frequently together and increase both the morbidity and mortality of clients as they age (Xiao, 2011).

Many of the drugs used in the treatment of arrhythmias and HF have been introduced and discussed in Chapters 32–36 of Unit 8—Drugs that affect the cardiovascular system. In this chapter the conditions warranting the use of cardiotonic and antiarrhythmic drugs are discussed. In this chapter, familiar drug names and classes, along with some new ones, will be studied in the categories of cardiotonic and antiarrhythmic drugs. Drugs are presented in the Drug Summary Tables for you to compare with other chapters and come to realize that a single drug can be used to treat many conditions of a cardiovascular nature.

HEART FAILURE

Heart failure is a complex clinical syndrome that can result from any number of cardiac or metabolic disorders, such as ischemic heart disease, hypertension, or hyperthyroidism. Any condition that impairs the ability of the ventricle to pump blood can lead to HF. During HF, the heart fails in its ability to pump enough blood to meet the needs of the body or can do so only with an elevated filling pressure. Although the term *congestive heart failure* is commonly used by both clients and providers, a more accurate term is simply *heart failure*.

HF causes a number of neurohormonal changes as the body tries to compensate for the increased workload of the heart. As noted in Box 37.1, a series of mechanisms occur that result in HF. First, the sympathetic nervous system increases the secretion of the catecholamines (the neurohormones, epinephrine and norepinephrine), which results in increased heart rate and vasoconstriction.

Second, activation of the renin-angiotensin-aldosterone (RAA) system occurs because of decreased perfusion to the kidneys. As the RAA system is activated, angiotensin II and aldosterone levels increase, which increases the blood pressure, adding to the workload of the heart.

As a result, these increases in **neurohormonal activity** cause a remodeling (restructuring) of the cardiac muscle cells, leading to hypertrophy (enlargement) of the heart, increased need for oxygen, and cardiac necrosis, which worsens the HF. The tissue of the heart is changed such that there is an increase in the cellular mass of cardiac tissue, the shape of the ventricle(s) is changed, and the heart's ability to contract effectively is reduced.

 Concept Mastery Alert

Peripheral edema, neck vein distention, and nocturia are most likely to be present in a client with right ventricular dysfunction. Most heart failure seen clinically is a mix of both right and left ventricular failures. If the two types of failure are considered separately, orthopnea is much more likely in left ventricular failure.

HF is best described by denoting the area of initial ventricular dysfunction: left-sided (left ventricular) dysfunction or right-sided (right ventricular) dysfunction. **Left ventricular dysfunction** causes a backup of fluid in the lungs and leads to pulmonary symptoms, such as dyspnea and moist cough with the production of frothy, pink (blood-tinged) sputum. **Right ventricular dysfunction** causes a backup in the peripheral venous system and leads to neck vein distention, peripheral edema, weight gain, and hepatic engorgement. Because both sides of the heart work together, ultimately both sides are affected in HF. Typically, the left side of the heart is affected first, followed by right ventricular involvement. The most common symptoms associated with HF include the following:

Left ventricular dysfunction
- Shortness of breath with exercise
- Dry, hacking cough or wheezing
- Orthopnea (difficulty breathing while lying flat)
- Restlessness and anxiety

Right ventricular dysfunction
- Swollen ankles, legs, or abdomen, leading to pitting edema
- Anorexia
- Nausea
- Nocturia (the need to urinate frequently at night)
- Weakness
- Weight gain as a result of fluid retention.

Other symptoms include
- Palpitations, fatigue, or pain when performing normal activities

---

BOX 37.1 Neurohormonal Responses Affecting Heart Failure

The body activates the neurohormonal compensatory mechanisms, which result in:
- Increased secretion of the neurohormones by the sympathetic nervous system,
- Activation of the renin-angiotensin-aldosterone (RAA) system,
- Remodeling of the cardiac tissue.

- Tachycardia or irregular heart rate
- Dizziness or confusion.

Left ventricular dysfunction, also called left ventricular systolic dysfunction, is the most common form of HF and results in decreased **cardiac output** and decreased ejection fraction (the amount of blood that the ventricle ejects per beat in relationship to the amount of blood available to eject). For your client to understand this concept, you can explain that cardiac output is a description of how much blood gets pumped out of the heart and to the body. Typically, the ejection fraction should be between 50% and 70% (AHA, 2016). With left ventricular systolic dysfunction, the ejection fraction is less than 40% and the heart is enlarged and dilated, which may be evidence of cardiomyopathy.

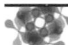 CARDIOTONICS

Cardiotonics are a class of drugs used to increase the efficiency and improve the contraction of the heart muscle, which leads to improved blood flow to all tissues of the body. In the past, specific cardiotonic drugs were the mainstay in HF treatment; currently, however, they are used in the treatment of clients who continue to experience symptoms *after* using the medications commonly prescribed for hypertension, such as angiotensin-converting enzyme (ACE) inhibitors, diuretics, and β-blockers.

Digoxin (Lanoxin) was the mainstay of oral cardiotonic drugs in use and provided the origin of naming this category of drug agents. This is because the original form of medication, i.e., digitoxin, was obtained from the leaves of the foxglove plant (*Digitalis purpurea* and *Digitalis lanata*) (see Fig. 37.1). Other terms used to identify the cardiotonics are cardiac glycosides or digitalis glycosides.

However, digoxin use continues for:

- Older clients maintained on the drug for many years
- Clients experiencing symptoms *after* unsuccessful trial of the first-choice drugs
- Some cases of atrial fibrillation (Freeman et al., 2015).

Ivabradine (Corlanor) is a newer cardiotonic replacing digoxin to treat HF. When used with a β-blocker drug (Chapter 24), ivabradine is shown to significantly reduce the repeated hospitalization associated with chronic HF. Another drug with positive inotropic action is milrinone, a nonglycoside, intravenous (IV) drug used in the short-term, acute management of HF.

Cardiotonics may be used in acute situations for HF, yet research shows there is no consistency in the use of these drugs over dopamine or dobutamine alone (Allen et al., 2014). Furthermore, with newer drugs on the market, use of digoxin to treat AF is also decreasing (Freeman, 2014). Although their use is diminishing, they remain a low-cost option for therapy and at the same time have adverse reactions, which are important to recognize in the clinical

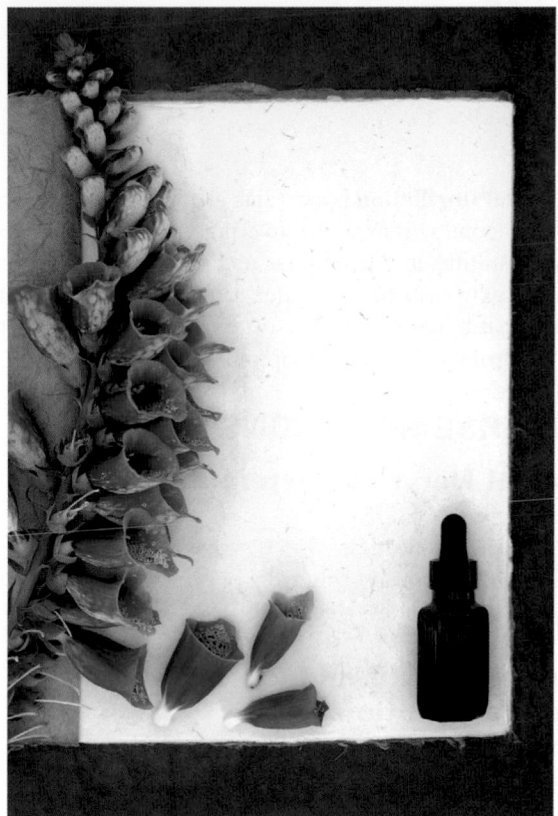

FIGURE 37.1 Digoxin origin is the foxglove plant *Digitalis purpurea.*

setting. See the Summary Drug Table: Cardiotonic Drugs for information concerning these drugs.

PRACTICE CONSIDERATIONS

Although not a cardiotonic, the drug sacubitril (neprilysin inhibitor) with valsartan (angiotensin-converting enzyme inhibitor [ACEI]) significantly reduces mortality and hospitalization in clients with HF. (Januzzi et al., 2016). This combination is manufactured under the brand name Entresto; solitary agents need to be discontinued 36 hr before this combination drug is initiated.

ACTIONS

Cardiotonics increase cardiac output through **positive inotropic activity** (an increase in the force of the contraction). They slow the conduction velocity through the atrioventricular (AV) node in the heart and decrease the heart rate through a negative chronotropic effect. Ivabradine blocks the I_f (funny) channel and inhibits the pacing of the sinoatrial (SA) node of the heart. This in turn slows the heart rate and allows blood to fill the heart chamber. Milrinone has inotropic action and is used in the short-term management of severe HF that is not controlled by the digitalis preparation.

USES

The cardiotonics are used to treat the following:

- HF
- AF

Atrial fibrillation is a cardiac arrhythmia characterized by rapid contractions and quivering of the atrial myocardium, resulting in an irregular and often rapid ventricular rate. Digoxin may be used after primary drugs are deemed unsuccessful. The cardiotonic drugs do not cure HF; rather, they control its signs and symptoms.

ADVERSE REACTIONS

Central Nervous System Reactions
- Headache
- Weakness, drowsiness
- Visual disturbances (blurring or yellow halo—digoxin; increased brightness—ivabradine)

Cardiovascular and Gastrointestinal System Reactions
- Arrhythmias
- Nausea and anorexia

Because some clients are more sensitive to the side effects of digoxin, dosage is calculated carefully and adjusted as the clinical condition indicates. There is a narrow margin of safety between the full therapeutic effects and the toxic effects of cardiotonic drugs. Even normal doses of a cardiotonic drug can cause toxic drug effects. Because substantial individual variations may occur, it is important to individualize the dosage. The term **digitalis toxicity** (or *digitalis intoxication*) is used to describe toxic drug effects that occur when digoxin is administered.

CONTRAINDICATIONS AND PRECAUTIONS

The cardiotonics are contraindicated in the presence of digitalis toxicity and in clients with known hypersensitivity, ventricular failure, ventricular tachycardia, cardiac tamponade, restrictive cardiomyopathy, or AV block.

The cardiotonics are given cautiously to clients with electrolyte imbalance (especially hypokalemia, hypocalcemia, and hypomagnesemia), thyroid disorders, severe carditis, heart block, myocardial infarction, severe pulmonary disease, acute glomerulonephritis, and impaired renal or hepatic function.

Digoxin is classified as a pregnancy category C drug and is used cautiously during pregnancy and lactation. Exposure to digoxin in a nursing infant is typically below an infant maintenance dose, yet caution should be exercised when digoxin is taken by a nursing woman. Ivabradine should not be used by women who are pregnant or lactating. Effective birth control methods must be used, and this drug use should be discontinued before a woman attempts to conceive a child.

 Chronic Care Considerations

Digoxin is less effective in African Americans than in Caucasians for the treatment of HF. When digoxin/ivabradine is being considered, the combination of hydralazine and isosorbide is found to be more efficacious for this population of clients (Sharma et al., 2014).

LASA ALERT

The following drugs may sound alike; so be sure to clarify when they are ordered:

Drug Name	Sounds Like
digoxin	Desoxyn, doxepin
Lanoxin	Lasix, levothyroxine, Levoxyl, Levsinex, Lomotil, Mefoxin, naloxone, Xanax

Drugs that look like a similar drug are noted in the Summary Drug Tables of each chapter.

INTERACTIONS

When the cardiotonics are taken with food, absorption is slowed, but the amount absorbed is the same. However, if taken with high-fiber meals, absorption of the cardiotonics may be decreased. The following interactions may occur with the cardiac glycosides:

Interacting Drug	Common Use	Effect of Interaction
Thyroid hormones	Treatment of hypothyroidism	Decreased effectiveness of digitalis glycosides, requiring a larger dosage of digoxin
Thiazide and loop diuretics	Management of edema and hypertension	Increased diuretic-induced electrolyte disturbances, predisposing the client to digitalis-induced arrhythmias

Clients may not always volunteer information regarding their use of complementary and alternative remedies. Be sure to inquire about use of herbal products. St. John's wort (used to relieve depression) causes a decrease in serum digitalis levels.

Certain drugs may increase or decrease serum digitalis levels as follows:

Interacting Drug	Common Use	Effect of Interaction
Amiodarone	Cardiac problems	Increased serum digitalis levels leading to toxicity
Benzodiazepines (alprazolam, diazepam)	Treatment of seizures and anxiety	
Indomethacin	Pain relief	
Itraconazole	Fungal Infections	
Macrolides (erythromycin, clarithromycin)	Infections	
Propafenone	Cardiac problems	
Quinidine	Cardiac problems	
Spironolactone	Edema	
Tetracyclines, macrolides	Infectios	
Verapamil	Cardiac problems	
Oral aminoglycoside	Infections	

Interacting Drug	Common Use	Effect of Interaction
Antacids	GI problems	Decreased serum digitalis levels
Antineoplastics (bleomycin, carmustine, cyclophosphamide, methotrexate, and vincristine)	Anticancer agents	
Activated charcoal	Antidote to poisoning with certain toxic substances	
Cholestyramine	Agent to lower high blood cholesterol levels	
Colestipol	Agent to lower high blood cholesterol levels	
Neomycin	Agent to suppress GI bacteria before surgery	
Rifampin	Antitubercular agent	

GI, gastrointestinal.

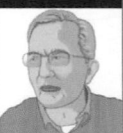

PHARMACOLOGY IN PRACTICE

SAFE DRUG ADMINISTRATION
A client is diagnosed with HF and is started on digoxin. The client informs the nurse that he is taking a benzodiazepine for anxiety. Which of the following interventions should the nurse implement?
1. Increase the dosage of digoxin.
2. Monitor for signs of digoxin toxicity.
3. Increase the dosage of benzodiazepine.
4. Monitor for signs of reduced effectiveness of digoxin.

ANTIARRHYTHMIC AGENTS

A cardiac **arrhythmia** (also referred to as a dysrhythmia or irregular heartbeat) is an electrical disturbance or irregularity in the rate or rhythm of the heart. This electrical disturbance makes the blood pumping action inefficient because the heart beats too fast (tachycardia) or too slow (bradycardia). Table 37.1 describes some examples of conduction problems known as arrhythmias.

Problems occur as a result of heart disease or from a disorder that affects cardiovascular function. Conditions such as emotional stress, hypoxia, and electrolyte imbalance may also trigger an arrhythmia. Some arrhythmias do not require treatment, whereas others require immediate treatment because they are potentially fatal. The goal of antiarrhythmic drug therapy is to restore normal cardiac function and prevent life-threatening conduction problems. Although these drugs are used to treat arrhythmia, they are also capable of causing or worsening an arrhythmia. The benefits of treatment must be carefully weighed by the primary health care provider against the risks of treatment with the antiarrhythmic drug.

ACTIONS

The cardiac muscle (**myocardium**) has both nerve and muscle tissues and therefore has the properties of both. Figure 37.2 illustrates where the electrical impulses are generated throughout the heart. Typically, the electrical impulse signals the heart muscle to contract (the heartbeat) in a regular, steady pattern. Some cardiac arrhythmias are caused by the generation of an abnormal number of electrical impulses (stimuli). These abnormal impulses may come from the SA node or may be generated in other areas of the myocardium. The antiarrhythmic drugs are classified according to their effects on what is termed the **action potential** (see Box 37.2 for a description). The pathophysiology of the cardiac condition guides the use of drugs to treat these conduction problems. The drugs used include five basic classes and several subclasses. Drugs in each group, or class, have certain similarities, yet each drug has subtle differences that make it unique.

Class I—Sodium Channel Blockers
Class I antiarrhythmic drugs have a membrane-stabilizing or anesthetic effect on the cells of the myocardium. Class I contains the largest number of drugs of the four antiarrhythmic drug classifications. Because their actions differ slightly, the drugs are subdivided into classes IA, IB, and IC.

TABLE 37.1 Types of Arrhythmias

ARRHYTHMIA	DESCRIPTION
Atrial flutter	Rapid contraction of the atria (up to 300 bpm) at a rate too rapid for the ventricles to pump efficiently.
Atrial fibrillation	Irregular and rapid atrial contraction, resulting in a quivering of the atria and causing an irregular and inefficient ventricular contraction.
Premature ventricular contractions	Beats originating in the ventricles instead of the sinoatrial node in the atria, causing the ventricles to contract before the atria and resulting in a decrease in the amount of blood pumped to the body.
Ventricular tachycardia	A rapid heartbeat with a rate of more than 100 bpm, usually originating in the ventricles.
Ventricular fibrillation	Rapid, disorganized contractions of the ventricles resulting in the inability of the heart to pump any blood to the body, which will result in death unless treated immediately.

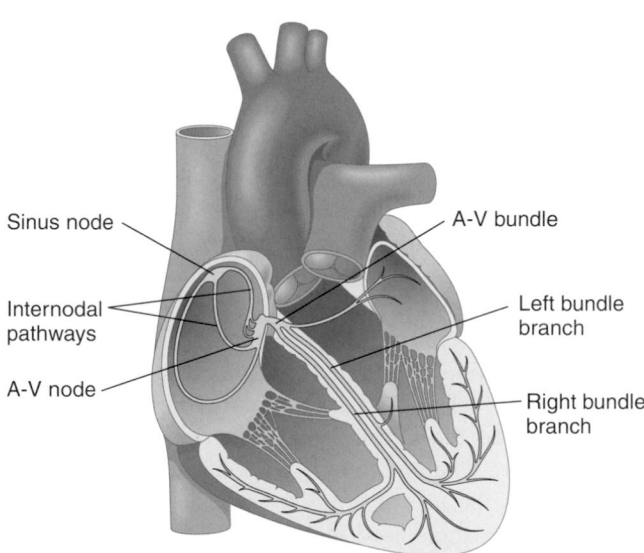

FIGURE 37.2 Electrical conduction of the heart.

Action Potential
All cells are electrically polarized, with the inside of the cell more negatively charged than the outside. The difference in the electrical charge is called the *resting membrane potential*. Nerve and muscle cells are excitable and can change the resting membrane potential in response to electrochemical stimuli. The *action potential* is an electrical impulse that passes from cell to cell in the myocardium, stimulating the fibers to shorten and causing muscular contraction (systole). An action potential generated in one part of the myocardium passes almost simultaneously through all the myocardial fibers, causing rapid contraction.

Refractory Period
Only one impulse can pass along a nerve fiber at any given time. After the passage of an impulse, there is a brief pause, or interval, before the next impulse can pass along the nerve fiber. This pause is called the *refractory period*, which is the period between the transmission of nerve impulses along a nerve fiber. Lengthening the refractory period decreases the number of impulses traveling along a nerve fiber within a given time.

Polarization
Nerve cells have positive ions on the outside and negative ions on the inside of the cell membrane when they are at rest. This is called polarization.

Depolarization
When a stimulus passes along the nerve, the positive ions move from outside to inside the cell and the negative ions move from inside to outside the cell. This movement of ions is called depolarization. Unless positive ions move into and negative ions move out of a nerve cell, a stimulus (or impulse) cannot pass along the nerve fiber.

Repolarization
Once the stimulus has passed along the nerve fiber, the positive and negative ions move back to their original place, that is, the positive ions on the outside and the negative ions on the inside of the nerve cell. This movement back to the original place is called *repolarization*.

Class IA Drugs
In general, class IA drugs act to:

- Prolong the action potential
- Produce moderate slowing of cardiac conduction.

For example, disopyramide (Norpace) decreases depolarization of myocardial fibers, prolongs the **refractory period**, and increases the action potential duration of cardiac cells (see Box 37.3).

Quinidine depresses myocardial excitability or the ability of the myocardium to respond to an electrical stimulus. By depressing the myocardium and its ability to respond to some, but not all, electrical stimuli, the pulse rate decreases and the heartbeat is corrected.

Class IB Drugs
Class IB drugs generally act to:

- Shorten the action potential duration
- Selectively depress cardiac conduction.

Lidocaine (Xylocaine) decreases diastolic depolarization, decreases automaticity of ventricular cells, and raises the threshold of the ventricular myocardium. **Threshold** is a term applied to any stimulus of the lowest intensity that will give rise to a response in a nerve fiber. A stimulus must be of a specific intensity (strength, amplitude) to pass along a given nerve fiber.

Some cardiac arrhythmias result from many stimuli present in the myocardium. Some of these are weak or of low intensity but are still able to excite myocardial tissue. Lidocaine raises the threshold of myocardial fibers, which in turn reduces the number of stimuli that will pass along these fibers and therefore decreases the pulse rate and corrects the arrhythmia.

Class IC Drugs
The general action of class IC drugs includes:

- Slight effect on **repolarization**
- Profound slowing of conduction.

Specifically, flecainide depresses fast sodium channels, decreases the height and rate of rise of action potentials, and slows conduction of all areas of the heart. Propafenone (Rythmol SR), which has a direct membrane-stabilizing effect on the myocardial membrane, prolongs the refractory period.

Class II—β-Adrenergic Blockers
The general action of drugs in class II is to indirectly block calcium channels and block catecholamine-caused arrhythmias. Acebutolol, esmolol, and propranolol (Inderal) act by blocking β-adrenergic receptors of the heart and kidney, reducing the influence of the sympathetic nervous system on these areas, decreasing the excitability of the heart and the release of renin (lowering heart rate and blood pressure). These drugs have membrane-stabilizing effects that contribute to their antiarrhythmic activity.

Class III—Potassium Channel Blockers
The general action of class III antiarrhythmic drugs is prolongation of repolarization. Amiodarone (Nexterone) appears to act directly on the cardiac cell membrane, prolonging the refractory period and repolarization and increasing the ventricular fibrillation threshold. Ibutilide acts by prolonging the action potential, producing a mild slowing of the sinus rate and AV conduction.

Class IV—Calcium Channel Blockers
In general, the class IV antiarrhythmic drugs act by:

- Depressing depolarization (phase 4)
- Lengthening phases 1 and 2 of repolarization.

Verapamil (Calan) is a calcium channel blocker. The calcium channel blocker inhibit the movement of calcium through channels across the myocardial cell membranes and vascular smooth muscle. Cardiac and vascular smooth muscles depend on the movement of calcium ions into the muscle cells through specific ion channels. When this movement is inhibited, the coronary and peripheral arteries dilate, thereby decreasing the force of cardiac contraction. This drug also reduces heart rate by slowing conduction through the SA and AV nodes. Additional information about the calcium channel blockers can be found in Chapter 34.

Class V—Other Agents
This is a category that was developed after the initial process of classification. Drugs such as digoxin, adenosine, and magnesium sulfate, which are used for very specific arrhythmias, are placed in this group because they do not fit easily into one of the other four classes.

USES
In general, the antiarrhythmic drugs are used to treat:

- Premature ventricular contractions (PVCs)
- Ventricular tachycardia
- Premature atrial contractions
- Paroxysmal atrial tachycardia
- Other atrial arrhythmias such as AF or atrial flutter
- Tachycardia when rapid but short-term control of ventricular rate is desirable.

Some of the antiarrhythmic drugs are used for other conditions. For example, propranolol is also used for clients with myocardial infarction. This drug has reduced the risk of death and repeated myocardial infarctions in those surviving the acute phase of a myocardial infarction. See the Summary Drug Table: Antiarrhythmic Drugs for more uses.

ADVERSE REACTIONS
Adverse reactions associated with the administration of specific antiarrhythmic drugs are given in the Summary Drug Table: Antiarrhythmic Drugs. General adverse reactions common to most antiarrhythmic drugs include the following:

Central Nervous System Reactions
- Lightheadedness
- Weakness
- Somnolence

Cardiovascular System Reactions
- Hypotension
- Arrhythmias
- Bradycardia

Other Reactions

- Urinary retention
- Local inflammation

All antiarrhythmic drugs may cause new arrhythmias or worsen existing arrhythmias, even though they are administered to resolve an existing arrhythmia. This phenomenon is called the proarrhythmic effect. This effect ranges from an increase in frequency of PVCs to the development of more severe ventricular tachycardia to ventricular fibrillation and the effect may lead to death. Proarrhythmic effects may occur at any time, but they occur more often when excessive dosages are given, when the preexisting arrhythmia is life-threatening, or when the drug is given IV.

 Lifespan Considerations

Gerontology

Older adults are at greater risk for adverse reactions such as additional arrhythmias or aggravation of existing arrhythmias, hypotension, and heart failure (HF). Careful monitoring is necessary for early identification and management of adverse reactions. Monitor the intake and output and report any signs of HF, such as an increase in weight, a decrease in urinary output, or shortness of breath. A dosage reduction may be indicated.

CONTRAINDICATIONS

The antiarrhythmic drugs are contraindicated in clients with known hypersensitivity to these drugs. They are contraindicated during pregnancy and lactation. The antiarrhythmic drug amiodarone is a pregnancy category D drug, indicating that fetal harm can occur when the agent is administered to a pregnant woman. It is used only if the potential benefits outweigh the potential hazards to the fetus. Antiarrhythmic drugs are contraindicated in clients with second- or third-degree AV block (if the client has no artificial pacemaker), severe HF, aortic stenosis, hypotension, and cardiogenic shock. Quinidine is contraindicated in clients with myasthenia gravis or systemic lupus erythematosus.

PRECAUTIONS

Antiarrhythmic drugs are used cautiously in clients with hepatic disease, electrolyte disturbances, HF (quinidine, flecainide, and disopyramide), and renal impairment.

Most antiarrhythmics are pregnancy category B or C drugs, indicating that safe use of these drugs during pregnancy or lactation, or in children, has not been established. Disopyramide is used cautiously in clients with myasthenia gravis, urinary retention, or glaucoma, as well as in men with prostate enlargement.

INTERACTIONS

When various antiarrhythmics are used with other medications, a host of different interactions may occur. Therefore refer to Table 37.2 where the specific antiarrhythmic drug and other agent interaction is described.

Owing to a specific enzyme reaction, grapefruit or its juice should not be taken if on the following drugs: amiodarone or any of the calcium channel blockers.

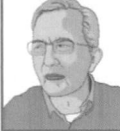 **PHARMACOLOGY IN PRACTICE**

ASSESSMENT

A nurse reviews the drug history of a client who has been prescribed disopyramide for the treatment of an arrhythmia. Which of the following drugs, if taken concurrently, can decrease the serum levels of disopyramide?

1. Erythromycin
2. Quinidine
3. Thioridazine
4. Rifampicin

TABLE 37.2 Interactions of Antiarrhythmics With Other Agents

INTERACTING DRUG	COMMON USES	EFFECT OF INTERACTION
Disopyramide		
Clarithromycin, erythromycin	Bacterial infections	Increased serum disopyramide levels
Fluoroquinolones	Infections	Risk of life-threatening arrhythmias
Quinidine	Cardiac problems	Increased serum levels of disopyramide
Rifampin	Antitubercular agent	Decreased disopyramide serum levels
Thioridazine, ziprasidone	Management of mental illness	Increased risk of life-threatening arrhythmias
Quinidine		
Cholinergic drugs	Treatment of glaucoma	Failure to terminate paroxysmal supraventricular tachycardia
Cimetidine	GI problems	Increased serum quinidine level
Hydantoins	Seizure control	Decreased therapeutic effect of quinidine
Nifedipine	Treatment of angina	Decreased action and serum level of quinidine
Cholinergic blocking drugs	GI problems	Additive vagolytic effect
Lidocaine		
β-Blockers	Hypertension and angina	Increased lidocaine levels
Cimetidine	GI problems	Decreased lidocaine clearance with possible toxicity
Flecainide		
Amiodarone	Cardiac problems	Increased serum flecainide levels
Cimetidine	GI problems	Increased serum flecainide levels
Disopyramide, verapamil	Cardiovascular problems	May increase negative inotropic properties; avoid using either of these drugs with flecainide
Propranolol and other β-blockers	Cardiovascular problems	Increased serum levels of propranolol and flecainide and additive negative inotropic effects
Local anesthetics	Anesthesia	Concurrent use (e.g., during pacemaker implantation, surgery, or dental use) may increase the risk of CNS side effects
Quinidine	Cardiac problems	Increased serum propafenone levels
SSRIs (antidepressants)	Relief of depression	Increased serum propafenone levels
Anticoagulants (e.g., warfarin)	Blood thinners	Increased prothrombin time and increased plasma warfarin levels
Digoxin	HF	Increased serum digoxin level
Theophylline	Management of asthma and COPD	Increased serum theophylline level

CNS, central nervous system; COPD, chronic obstructive pulmonary disease; GI, gastrointestinal; HF, heart failure; SSRIs, selective serotonin reuptake inhibitors.

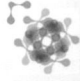

NURSING PROCESS: STEPS TO BUILD CLINICAL JUDGMENT
Client Receiving a Cardiotonic Drug

ASSESSMENT

Issues related to the medications used for both HF and arrhythmia have been identified in the previous chapters of this unit. Here we examine the needs of a client specifically being administered the cardiotonic, digoxin.

Preadministration Assessment

The cardiotonics are potentially toxic drugs; therefore clients are observed closely, especially during initial therapy.

Data gathering suggestions before the initial administration of the drug, digoxin, are listed in the following.
Objective data

- Vital signs (temperature, pulse both apical and radial, respirations, and blood pressure).
- Inspect physical appearance, noting skin color, temperature, and jugular vein distention

- Auscultate lungs, noting any unusual sounds during inspiration and expiration.
- Inspect sputum raised (if any), noting the appearance (e.g., frothy, pink tinged, clear, yellow).
- Palpate for pedal pulses and peripheral edema, noting rate and strength of pulses.
- Weigh the client.
- Laboratory tests—electrocardiogram, renal and hepatic function tests, complete blood count, and serum enzyme and electrolyte levels. Renal function is particularly important because diminished renal function could affect the prescribed dosage of digoxin.

Subjective data

- History of cardiac episodes, pain assessment if experiencing pain.
- Medical/family history.
- Drug therapy (list of all current drugs and supplements taken).

Ongoing Assessment

Before administering each dose of a cardiotonic take the apical pulse rate for 60 seconds (Fig. 37.3). Document the apical pulse rate in the designated area on the chart or the medication administration record. If the pulse rate is below 60 bpm in adults or greater than 100 bpm, withhold the drug and notify the primary health care provider, unless there is a written order giving different guidelines for withholding the drug.

 Lifespan Considerations

Pediatric

The drug is withheld and the primary health care provider is notified before administration of the drug if the apical pulse rate in a child is below 70 bpm, or below 90 bpm in an infant.

Weigh clients receiving a cardiotonic drug daily or as ordered. Intake and output are measured, especially if the client has edema or HF or is also receiving a diuretic.

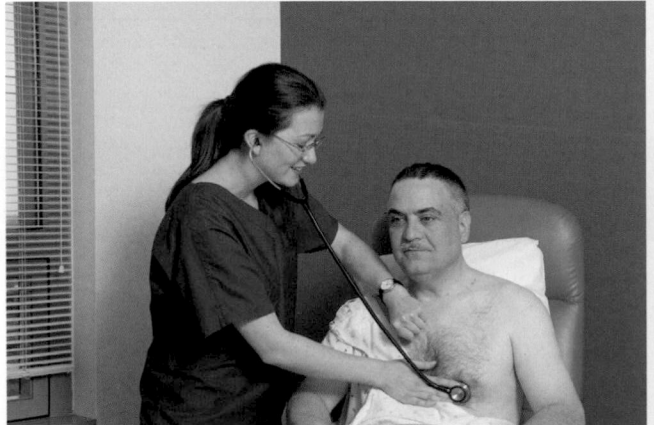

FIGURE 37.3 Nurse counts the apical pulse for 1 min before administering the cardiotonic.

Throughout therapy assess the client for peripheral edema and auscultate the lungs for crackles (formerly called *rales*). Serum electrolyte levels should be assessed periodically. Hypokalemia, hypomagnesemia, or hypercalcemia may increase the risk for toxicity. Any electrolyte imbalance is reported to the primary health care provider.

NURSING DIAGNOSES

Drug-specific nursing diagnoses include the following:

- **Malnutrition risk** related to anorexia, nausea, and vomiting.
- **Activity intolerance** related to weakness and drowsiness.
- **Injury risk** related to dizziness and lightheadedness.

Nursing diagnoses related to drug administration are discussed in Chapter 4.

PLANNING

The expected outcomes of the client depend on the specific reason for administering the drug but may include an optimal response to therapy, support of client needs related to the management of adverse reactions, and confidence in an understanding of the medication regimen.

IMPLEMENTATION

Promoting an Optimal Response to Therapy

Because other drugs are typically chosen to treat HF, it is the client who has been on this drug for a long time, often in a long-term care facility, who will be treated with digoxin. Great care must be taken when administering a cardiotonic drug because frail clients can become toxic before you notice an issue.

NURSING ALERT

Serum digoxin levels are monitored closely. Blood for serum level measurements should be drawn immediately before the next dose or 6–8 hr after the last dose regardless of the administration route. Therapeutic drug levels are between 0.8 and 2 ng/mL. Serum digoxin levels >2 ng/mL are considered toxic and are reported to the primary health care provider.

Periodic electrocardiograms, serum electrolytes, hepatic and renal function tests, and other laboratory studies also may be ordered. Diuretics (see Chapter 32) may be ordered for some clients receiving a cardiotonic drug. Diuretics, along with other conditions or factors, such as gastrointestinal (GI) suction, diarrhea, and old age, may produce low serum potassium levels (hypokalemia). The primary health care provider may order a potassium supplement to be given orally or IV.

NURSING ALERT

Hypokalemia makes the heart muscle more sensitive to digitalis, thereby increasing the possibility of developing digitalis toxicity. At frequent intervals closely observe clients who can become hypokalemic (diuretic therapy) for signs of digitalis toxicity.

Clients with hypomagnesemia (low serum magnesium levels) are at increased risk for digitalis toxicity. Individuals hospitalized in intensive care units with multiple alterations in nutrition, fluids, and medications are at greatest risk of hypomagnesemia. If low magnesium levels are detected, the primary health care provider may prescribe magnesium replacement therapy.

A cardiotonic can be given orally, IV, or intramuscularly (IM). When a cardiotonic drug is given IV, it is administered slowly (over at least 5 min), and the administration site is assessed for redness or infiltration. IM injection is not recommended for these drugs yet; they may be given through this route when needed urgently and IV access is not available. When giving a cardiotonic drug IM give the injection deep in the muscle and follow with massage to the site. No more than 2 mL should be injected IM.

Oral preparations can be given without regard to meals. Tablets can be crushed and mixed with food or fluids if the client has difficulty swallowing. Do not alternate between the dosage forms (i.e., tablets and capsules); these dosages are not the same. Owing to better absorption, the recommended dosage of the capsules is 80% of the dosage for tablets and elixir.

Monitoring and Managing Client Needs

Malnutrition Risk

If toxicity is suspected, then closely observe the client for adverse drug reactions such as anorexia, nausea, and vomiting. Carefully consider any client complaint or comment, document it on the client's record, and bring it to the attention of the primary health care provider. Other signs of digitalis toxicity include abdominal pain, visual disturbances (blurred, yellow, or green vision and white halos, borders around dark objects), and arrhythmias (any type).

If the nausea or anorexia is not a result of toxicity but an adverse reaction to the drug, then use nursing measures to help control the reactions. Offer frequent small meals rather than three large meals. Restricting fluids at meals and avoiding fluids 1 hr before and after meals helps control nausea. Helping the client to maintain good oral hygiene by brushing teeth or rinsing the mouth after ingesting food will also help with nausea.

Activity Intolerance

The client may experience weakness or drowsiness as adverse reactions associated with digoxin, which may lead to activity intolerance. The client is encouraged to increase daily activities gradually as tolerance increases and to plan adequate rest periods during the day.

Digitalis toxicity can occur even when normal doses are being administered or when the client has been receiving a maintenance dose. Many symptoms of toxicity are similar to the symptoms of the heart conditions for which the client is receiving the cardiotonic. The signs of digitalis toxicity are listed in Box 37.3. When digitalis toxicity develops, the primary health care provider may discontinue digitalis use until all signs of toxicity are gone. If severe bradycardia occurs,

> **BOX 37.3 Signs of Digitalis Toxicity**
>
> - Gastrointestinal—anorexia (usually the first sign), nausea, vomiting, diarrhea.
> - Muscular—weakness, lethargy.
> - Central nervous system—headache, drowsiness, visual disturbances (blurred vision, disturbance in yellow or green vision, halo effect around dark objects), confusion, disorientation, delirium.
> - Cardiac—changes in pulse rate or rhythm including electrocardiographic changes, such as bradycardia, tachycardia, and premature ventricular contractions.

atropine may be ordered. If digoxin has been given, the primary health care provider may order blood tests to determine serum drug levels. A digoxin serum level >2.0 ng/mL indicates toxicity.

Digoxin has a rapid onset and a short duration of action. Once the drug is withheld, the toxic effects of digoxin subside rapidly. Most often, digoxin toxicity can be treated successfully by simply withdrawing the drug.

 Lifespan Considerations

Gerontology

Older adults are particularly prone to digitalis toxicity. Some conditions such as dementia may have similar signs, such as confusion, as those of digitalis toxicity.

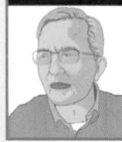 **PHARMACOLOGY IN PRACTICE**

MANAGING NEEDS

A client is being digitalized for HF. The primary health care provider assessing the client orders an analysis of serum electrolytes. Which of the following electrolyte changes indicates digoxin toxicity and needs to be reported? Select all that apply.
1. Hyponatremia
2. Hypokalemia
3. Hypomagnesemia
4. Hypocalcemia
5. Hypophosphatemia

Injury Risk

Hypotension and bradycardia caused by the cardiotonic or antiarrhythmic drugs may cause dizziness and lightheadedness, especially during early therapy. This places the client at greater risk of injury from falling. Postural hypotension may also occur during the first few weeks of therapy. Assist clients who are not on complete bed rest to ambulate until these symptoms subside. The client is advised to make position changes slowly.

Educating the Client and Family

In some instances, a cardiotonic drug may be prescribed for a prolonged period. If the primary health care provider wants the client to monitor the pulse rate daily during cardiotonic therapy, then show the client or a family member the correct technique for taking the pulse (see Client Teaching for Improved Outcomes: Monitoring Pulse Rate).

The primary health care provider may also want the client to omit the next dose of the drug and call them if the pulse rate falls below a certain level (usually 60 bpm in an adult, 70 bpm in a child, and 90 bpm in an infant). These instructions are emphasized at the time of client teaching.

Client Teaching for Improved Outcomes

Monitoring Pulse Rate

Monitoring a client's pulse rate is second nature when the client is in an acute care facility. However, when the client goes home with digoxin, they will need to monitor the pulse rate to prevent possible adverse reactions.

When you teach make sure your client understands the following:

✔ Have a watch with a second hand with you.
✔ Sit down and rest your nondominant arm on a table or chair armrest.
✔ Place the index and third fingers of your dominant hand just below the wrist bone on the thumb side of your nondominant arm.
✔ Feel lightly for a beating or pulsing sensation. This is your pulse.
✔ Count the number of beats for 30 seconds (if the pulse is regular) and multiply by 2. If the pulse is irregular count the number of beats for 60 seconds.
✔ Record the number of beats of your pulse and keep a log of your reading.
✔ If you notice the pulse is greater than 100 bpm or less than 60 bpm, then call your primary health care provider immediately.
✔ Should you plan to use a smartphone or watch, then be sure and talk to your primary health care provider regarding the type and functions they may want you to monitor.

As you develop a teaching plan include the following information:

• Do not discontinue use of this drug without first checking with the primary health care provider (unless instructed to do otherwise). Do not miss a dose or take an extra dose.
• Take this drug at the same time each day; a compartmentalized pill container may be helpful.

• Take your pulse before taking the drug, and withhold the drug and notify the primary health care provider if your pulse rate is less than 60 bpm or greater than 100 bpm.
• If you have a watch that records pulse, then try to look at it before take your medication—watch for patterns that you may need to notify your health care provider are happening.
• Avoid antacids and nonprescription cough, cold, allergy, antidiarrheal, and diet (weight-reducing) drugs unless their use has been approved by the primary health care provider. Some of these drugs interfere with the action of the cardiotonic drug or cause other potentially serious problems (see Interactions, earlier).
• Contact the primary health care provider if nausea, vomiting, diarrhea, unusual fatigue, weakness, vision change (such as blurred vision, changes in colors of objects, or halos around dark objects), or mental depression occurs.
• Carry medical identification describing the disease process and your medication regimen.
• Do not substitute tablets for capsules or vice versa.
• Follow the dietary recommendations (if any) made by the primary health care provider.
• When taking ivabradine use effective birth control and immediately notify your primary health care provider if you think you are pregnant.
• The primary health care provider will closely monitor therapy. Keep all appointments for primary health care provider visits or laboratory or diagnostic tests.

EVALUATION

• Therapeutic response is achieved, and the heart beats more efficiently.
• Adverse reactions are identified, reported to the primary health care provider, and managed successfully with appropriate nursing interventions:
  • Client maintains an adequate nutritional status.
  • Client carries out activities of daily living.
  • No evidence of injury is seen.
• Client and family express confidence and demonstrate an understanding of the drug regimen.

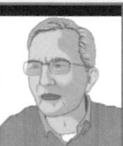

PHARMACOLOGY IN PRACTICE

USING CLINICAL REASONING

You asked Mr. Phillip to bring in his medications. Here is what he brought:

• seven bottles of various warfarin strengths,
• two bottles Zoloft 100 mg strength,
• Ambien,
• two bottles atenolol 50 mg strength,
• propranolol 60 mg strength.

He does not use a medication container because he "knows what to take out of each bottle." What action would you take next?

KEY POINTS

■ Heart failure, also known as congestive heart failure, is a condition in which the heart cannot pump enough blood to meet the tissue needs of the body. Left-sided failure (left ventricular dysfunction) leads to pulmonary symptoms such as dyspnea and moist cough. Right-sided failure (right ventricular dysfunction) can be seen with fluid backup in the body, such as distended neck veins, peripheral edema, and hepatic engorgement.

■ Cardiotonics increase the efficiency and improve the contraction of the heart muscle. Because of their toxic effects and use of other drugs such as ACE inhibitors or other hypertensive drugs, they are not used as frequently.

■ The heart has cardiac and nerve tissues; the nerves transmit an electrical impulse through the heart, which makes the muscles contract (a heartbeat). When there is an electrical conduction problem, it can affect the rate or the rhythm of the heartbeat. This irregularity is called a cardiac arrhythmia or dysrhythmia, which ranges from causing fatigue to being life-threatening.

■ Antiarrhythmic drugs include drugs that block impulses and are classified as class I—sodium channel blockers, class II—β-adrenergic blockers, class III—potassium channel blockers, and class IV—calcium channel blockers. Drugs not easily identified with other categories are in class V. Many of these drugs are also used for treating other cardiac conditions such as hypertension and heart failure.

■ Cardiac monitoring is important when therapy is started. Although the drugs are designed to correct an electrical conduction problem, they can also create new ones or extenuate existing problems—a proarrhythmic effect.

■ As with many of the drugs that affect the cardiovascular system, hypotension, lightheadedness, dizziness, and weakness are all adverse reactions that can lead to injury. When a cardiotonic is used, the pulse rate is monitored and the drug held if the client's heart rate is less than 60 bpm. Adverse reactions are typically GI in nature, and clients need to be monitored for toxicity to the drug, which can appear as GI distress, changes in vision, or muscle weakness.

SUMMARY DRUG TABLES
Cardiotonic Drugs

Generic Name	Trade Name	Uses	Adverse Reactions	Dosage Ranges
Cardiotonics				
digoxin *di-JOKS-in*	Lanoxin	Heart failure, atrial fibrillation	Headache, weakness, drowsiness, visual disturbances, nausea, vomiting, anorexia, arrhythmias	Loading dose:[a] 0.75–1.25 mg orally or 0.6–1 mg IV Maintenance: 0.125–0.25 mg/day orally Lanoxicaps: 0.1–0.3 mg/day orally
ivabradine *eye-VAB-ra-deen*	Corlanor	Low left ventricle ejection heart failure, stable angina if unable to take β-blocker	Bradycardia, increased blood pressure, visual brightness	5–7.5 mg twice daily orally
Miscellaneous Drugs				
milrinone *MIL-ri-none*		Short-term management of acute heart failure	Ventricular arrhythmias, hypotension, angina/chest pain, headaches, hypokalemia	Loading dose: 50 mcg/kg IV IV: Up to 1.13 mg/kg/day
valsartan/sacubitril *val-SAR-tan/sak-UE-bi-tril*	Entresto	Heart failure	Dizziness, cough, hyperkalemia	Titrated depending on ACEI dose; stop other drug 36 hr before switch

[a]Based on client lean body weight of 70 kg.

SUMMARY DRUG TABLES
Antiarrhythmic Drugs

Generic Name	Trade Name	Uses	Adverse Reactions	Dosage Ranges
Class I: Sodium Channel Blockers				
disopyramide *dye-soe-PEER-a-mide*	Norpace, Norpace CR	Life-threatening ventricular arrhythmias	Dry mouth, constipation, urinary hesitancy, blurred vision, nausea, fatigue, dizziness, headache, rash, hypotension, HF, proarrhythmic effect	Ventricular arrhythmias: dosage individualized, 400–800 mg/day orally in divided doses

Continued

SUMMARY DRUG TABLE (continued)
Antiarrhythmic Drugs

Generic Name	Trade Name	Uses	Adverse Reactions	Dosage Ranges
Class I: Sodium Channel Blockers (Continued)				
procainamide *pro-KANE-a-mide*		Ventricular arrhythmias	Hypotension, dizziness, urticaria, nausea, vomiting, arthralgia	IV titration not to exceed 1 g
quiNIDine *KWIN-i-deen*		Premature atrial and ventricular contractions, atrial tachycardia, chronic atrial fibrillation	Ringing in the ears, hearing loss, nausea, vomiting, dizziness	Administer test dose of one tablet orally or 200 mg IM to test for idiosyncratic reaction
lidocaine *LYE-doe-kane*	Xylocaine	Ventricular arrhythmias	Lightheadedness, nervousness, bradycardia, hypotension, drowsiness, apprehension, proarrhythmic effect	50–100 mg IV bolus; 1–4 mg/min IV infusion, 20–50 mg/kg/min; 300 mg IM
mexiletine *meks-IL-e-teen*		Life-threatening ventricular arrhythmias	Palpitations, nausea, vomiting, chest pain, heartburn, dizziness, lightheadedness, rash, agranulocytosis, proarrhythmic effect	Initial dose: 200 mg orally q8hr; maximum dosage, 1200 mg/day orally
flecainide *fle-KAY-nide*		Paroxysmal atrial fibrillation/flutter and supraventricular tachycardia	Dizziness, headache, faintness, unsteadiness, blurred vision, headache, nausea, dyspnea, HF, fatigue, palpitations, chest pain, proarrhythmic effect	Initial dose: 100 mg orally q12hr; maximum dosage, 390 mg/day
propafenone *pro-PAF-en-one*	Rythmol SR	Atrial fibrillation, ventricular arrhythmias, paroxysmal supraventricular tachycardia	Dizziness, nausea, vomiting, constipation, unusual taste, first-degree AV block, agranulocytosis, proarrhythmic effect	Initial dose: 150 mg orally q8hr; may be increased to 300 mg orally q8hr
Class II: Beta-Adrenergic Blockers				
acebutolol *a-se-BYOO-toe-lole*		Ventricular arrhythmias, hypertension	Hypotension, nausea, dizziness, bradycardia, vomiting, diarrhea, nervousness	Arrhythmias: 400–1200 mg/day orally in divided doses
esmolol *ES-moe-lol*	Brevibloc	Supraventricular tachycardia, noncompensatory tachycardia	Hypotension, weakness, lightheadedness, urinary retention	50–200 mcg/kg/min IV, loading dose may be as high as 500 mcg/kg over 1 min
propranolol *proe-PRAN-oh-lole*	Inderal	Cardiac arrhythmias, angina pectoris, hypertension, essential tremor, myocardial infarction, migraine headache, pheochromocytoma	Nausea, vomiting, bradycardia, dizziness, hypotension, hyperglycemia, diarrhea, bronchospasm, pulmonary edema	Cardiac arrhythmias: 10–30 mg orally TID or QID Life-threatening arrhythmias: 1–3 mg IV, may repeat once in 2 min Angina pectoris: 80–320 mg/day orally in 2–4 divided doses
Class III: Potassium Channel Blockers				
amiodarone *a-MEE-oh-da-rone*	Nexterone	Life-threatening ventricular arrhythmias	Malaise, fatigue, tremor, proarrhythmic effect, nausea, vomiting, constipation, ataxia, anorexia, bradycardia, photosensitivity	Loading dose: 800–1600 mg/day orally in divided doses Maintenance dose, 390 mg/day orally; up to 1000 mg/day over 24 hr IV
dofetilide *doe-FET-il-ide*	Tikosyn	Conversion of atrial fibrillation/flutter to normal sinus rhythm, maintenance of normal sinus rhythm	Headache, chest pain, dizziness, respiratory tract infection, dyspnea, nausea, flulike syndrome, insomnia, proarrhythmic effect	Dosage based on ECG response and creatinine clearance; range, 125–500 mg BID

Generic Name	Trade Name	Uses	Adverse Reactions	Dosage Ranges
dronedarone *droe-NE-da-rone*	Multaq	Paroxysmal atrial fibrillation, maintenance of normal sinus rhythm	Nausea, vomiting, diarrhea	400 mg orally BID
ibutilide *eye-BYOO-ti-lide*	Corvert	Atrial fibrillation/flutter	Headache, nausea, hypotension or hypertension, ventricular arrhythmias, proarrhythmic effect	Adults 60 kg and more: 1 mg infused over 10 min; may repeat in 10 min Adults under 60 kg: 0.1 mL/kg infused over 10 min; may repeat in 10 min
sotalol *SOE-ta-lole*	Betapace, Betapace AF	Treatment of life-threatening ventricular arrhythmias, reduction and delay of atrial fibrillation and flutter for ventricular arrhythmias (Betapace AF)	Drowsiness, difficulty sleeping, unusual tiredness or weakness, depression, decreased libido, bradycardia, HF, cold hands and feet, nausea, vomiting, nasal congestion, anxiety, life-threatening arrhythmias, proarrhythmic effect	Initially: 80 mg BID orally; may increase up to 239–320 mg/day (Betapace); up to 120 mg BID (Betapace AF)
Class IV: Calcium Channel Blockers				
dilTIAZem *dil-TYE-a-zem*	Cardizem, Cardizem CD, Tiazac	Hypertension, chronic stable angina, atrial fibrillation/flutter, paroxysmal superventricular tachycardia	Headache, dizziness, AV block, bradycardia, edema, dyspnea, rhinitis	Extended-release tablets/capsules: angina: 120–580 mg/day Exertional angina—immediate-release tablets: 30 mg QID Heart arrhythmias—injection: 0.25 mg/kg over 2 min, then titrated continuous infusion
verapamil *ver-AP-a-mill*	Calan, Covera HS, Verelan, Verelan PM	Supraventricular tachyarrhythmias, temporary control of rapid ventricular rate in atrial flutter/fibrillation, angina, unstable angina, hypertension	Constipation, dizziness, lightheadedness, headache, asthenia, nausea, vomiting, peripheral edema, hypotension, mental depression, agranulocytosis, proarrhythmic effect	Adults: oral—initial dose 80–120 mg TID; maintenance, 320–480 mg/day Hypertension: 239 mg/day orally; sustained release, in AM 80 mg TID; extended-release capsules, 100–300 mg orally at bedtime Parenteral: IV use only; initial dose 5–10 mg over 2 min; may repeat 10 mg 30 min later
Class V or Other Drugs				
adenosine *a-DEN-oh-seen*	Adenocard	Paroxysmal superventricular tachycardia	Headache, flushing, dyspnea, nausea, chest discomfort	3–12 mg IV bolus
digoxin *di-JOKS-in*	Lanoxin	HF, atrial fibrillation	Headache, weakness, drowsiness, visual disturbances, nausea, vomiting, anorexia, arrhythmias	Loading dose:[a] 0.75–1.25 mg orally or 0.6–1 mg IV Maintenance: 0.125–0.25 mg/day orally Lanoxicaps: 0.1–0.3 mg/day orally

[a]Based on client lean body weight of 70 kg.

CHAPTER REVIEW

Know Your Drugs

Clients sometimes know a medication by the brand (or trade) name and not the generic name. To recognize both names match the brand name with the generic name of the same medication.

Generic Name	Brand Name
1. lidocaine	A. Betapace
2. propranolol	B. Calan
3. sotalol	C. Inderal
4. verapamil	D. Xylocaine

Calculate Medication Dosages

1. Digoxin 0.5 mg orally via an enteral feeding tube is prescribed. The drug is available in a solution of 0.25 mg/mL. How many milliliters will the nurse prepare?
2. The primary health care provider prescribes verapamil 80 mg orally. The drug is available in 40-mg tablets. The nurse prepares _____.

Prepare for the NCLEX

RECALL THE FACTS

1. Which of the following serum digoxin levels in an adult would be most indicative that the client may be experiencing digoxin toxicity?
   1. 0.5 ng/mL
   2. 0.8 ng/mL
   3. 1.0 ng/mL
   4. 2.0 ng/mL
2. In which of the following situations would the nurse withhold a dose of digoxin and notify the primary health care provider?
   1. Pulse rate of 50 bpm
   2. Pulse rate of 87 bpm
   3. Pulse rate of 92 bpm
   4. Pulse rate of 64 bpm
3. An irregular, rapid atrial contraction resulting in quivering atria is best described as which of the following arrhythmias?
   1. Atrial fibrillation
   2. Premature ventricular contraction
   3. Ventricular tachycardia
   4. Ventricular fibrillation
4. Which of the following antiarrhythmic drugs are also used as antihypertensives?
   1. Sodium and calcium channel blockers
   2. β-Adrenergic and calcium channel blockers
   3. Potassium and sodium channel blockers
   4. β-Adrenergic and potassium channel blockers

5. Common adverse reactions of the antiarrhythmic drugs include _____.
   1. lightheadedness, hypotension, and weakness
   2. headache, hypertension, and lethargy
   3. weakness, lethargy, and hyperglycemia
   4. anorexia, gastrointestinal upset, and hypertension

ANALYZE THE FACTS

6. *The nurse suspects a client is experiencing digoxin toxicity. Which of the following symptoms would the client have reported to make the nurse suspicious of a toxic reaction?
   1. Insatiable hunger
   2. Constipation
   3. Halo in vision field
   4. Muscle cramping
7. Which of the following statements would the nurse include in a teaching plan for the client taking an antiarrhythmic drug on an outpatient basis?
   1. Take the drug without regard to meals.
   2. Limit fluid intake during the evening hours.
   3. Avoid drinking alcoholic beverages unless approved by the primary health care provider.
   4. Eat a diet high in potassium.
8. *Which of the following adverse reactions, if observed in a client prescribed propafenone, would indicate that the client may be developing agranulocytosis?
   1. Fever
   2. Ataxia
   3. Hyperactivity
   4. Dizziness

ALTERNATE-FORMAT QUESTIONS

9. Digoxin (Lanoxin) is prescribed for a client with heart failure. The primary health care provider prescribes digoxin (Lanoxin) 0.75 mg orally as the initial dose. Available are digoxin tablets of 0.5 and 0.25 mg. The nurse administers _____.
10. *The client's ventricular fibrillation has stabilized and the client is scheduled to see the nurse for medication review. The prescribed dose is amiodarone 400 mg daily. Look at the medication brought from home: how many tablets should the client be taking?

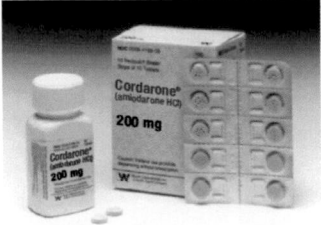

To check your answers, see Appendix F.

*Indicates the question is directly linked to the NCLEX-PN test plan in Appendix G.

WANT TO KNOW MORE? A wide variety of resources are available to enhance your learning and understanding of this chapter.

- Visit the**Point** for resources such as
  - NCLEX-Style Student Review Questions
  - Journal Articles
  - Dosage Calculations
  - Drug Monographs
  - Watch and Learn Videos
  - Concepts in Action Animations
- The *Study Guide to Accompany Introductory Clinical Pharmacology,* 12th edition, sold separately, will help you review and apply essential content.
- ✓*PrepU* is available to help students prepare for the NCLEX-PN examination.

UNIT 9
Drugs That Affect the Gastrointestinal System

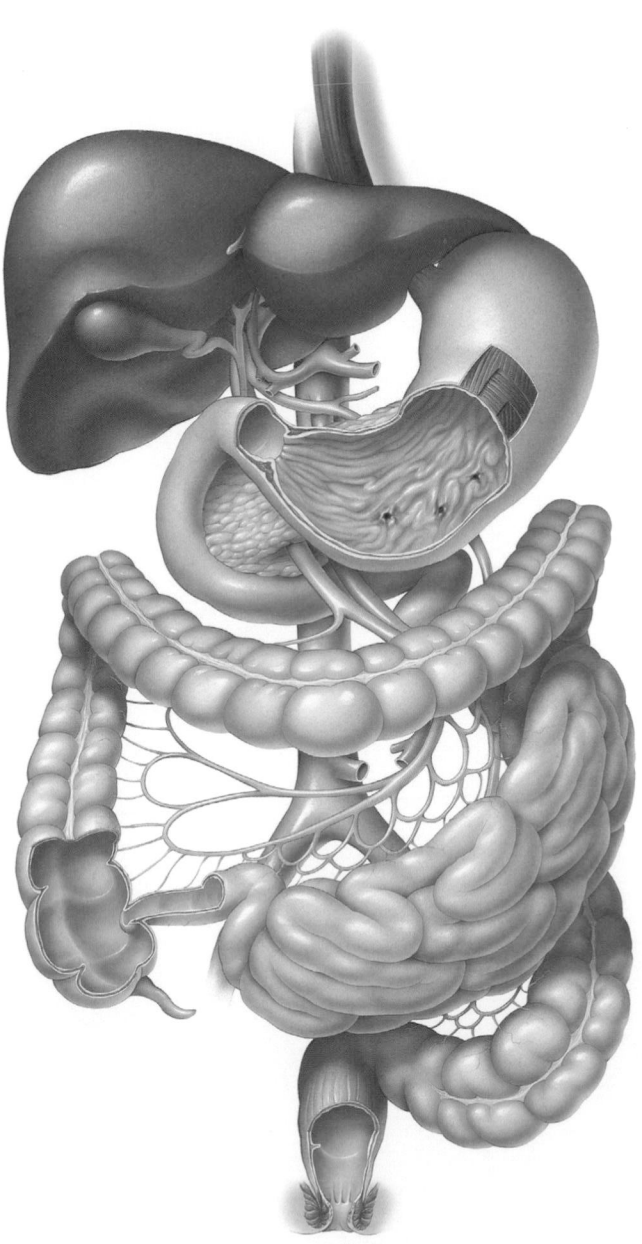

The gastrointestinal (GI) system is responsible for the ingestion and exchange of body nutrients. The process of digestion in the GI system begins with the breakdown of food and fluids in the mouth (oral cavity). In the stomach, foodstuffs are broken down by gastric acids and enzymes to prepare for absorption in the small intestine. After nutrients are absorbed in the small intestine, the large intestine is responsible for the reabsorption of water and the elimination of waste materials in the form of feces. As people age, the personal focus of health often centers on this body system. As aging occurs, individuals experience wear and tear on their teeth and the ability to produce saliva decreases; this changes the taste of foods. Also, as the body ages, motility and absorption in the GI system slow. Drugs are used to assist in the absorption of nutrients, either by altering the gastric acids for purposes of protection or by controlling the transit of food through the system by speeding up or slowing down the process.

Chapter 38 describes drugs used for protecting the structures of the upper GI system—mouth, esophagus, and stomach—from the effects of gastric acid. Drugs used to speed up or prevent emesis are also covered in this chapter.

Chronic illness, such as inflammatory bowel diseases, can affect how water and nutrients are absorbed. Drugs used to slow down or facilitate transit in the lower GI system— the small and large intestines—are covered in Chapter 39. The drugs used in the treatment of chronic GI diseases are also presented in Chapter 39.

An area of concern to you as the nurse caring for clients is the availability of nonprescription drugs for the GI system, thereby creating the potential for problems of misuse and overuse of the drugs, which may, in turn, disguise or delay diagnosis of more serious medical problems. This issue is addressed in Chapter 39 as well.

38

Upper Gastrointestinal System Drugs

Key Terms

chemoreceptor trigger zone (CTZ) group of nerve fibers located on the surface of the fourth ventricle of the brain that, when stimulated, results in vomiting

emetogenic causing vomiting

gastric stasis failure of the body to remove stomach contents normally

gastroesophageal reflux disease (GERD) reflux or backup of gastric contents into the esophagus

Helicobacter pylori stomach bacterium that causes peptic ulcer; also known as *H. pylori*

hydrochloric acid (HCl) stomach acid that aids in digestion

hyperphosphatemia elevated phosphorus levels in the body caused by chronic kidney disease

hypersecretory characterized by excessive secretion of a substance

nausea unpleasant and uncomfortable feeling in the stomach, sometimes followed by vomiting

vertigo feeling of a spinning or rotational motion; dizziness

vomiting spasmodic ejection of stomach contents through the mouth

Learning Objectives

On completion of this chapter, the student will:

1. Explain the general drug actions, uses, adverse reactions, contraindications, precautions, and interactions of drugs used to treat conditions of the upper gastrointestinal (GI) system.
2. Distinguish important preadministration and ongoing assessment activities the nurse should perform with the client receiving a drug used to treat conditions of the upper GI system.
3. List nursing diagnoses particular to a client receiving a drug used to treat conditions of the upper GI system.
4. Examine ways to promote an optimal response to therapy, how to manage adverse reactions, and important points to keep in mind when educating clients about the use of drugs to treat conditions of the upper GI system.

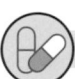 **Drug Classes**

Acid neutralizers
Acid reducers
- Histamine H_2 antagonists
- Proton pump inhibitors

GI stimulants
Antiemetics

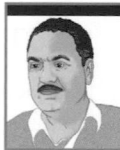 **PHARMACOLOGY IN PRACTICE**

Alfredo Garcia is being seen in the clinic for an upper respiratory infection. During the intake assessment, you find that his blood pressure is high and he complains of "heartburn." You ask him what helps relieve the heartburn. Mr. Garcia is attempting to use home remedies to decrease acid production in his stomach, and he tells you that he thinks he might have an ulcer, so he has been drinking cream and half-and-half to coat the ulcer. At one time, antiulcer diets included the use of dairy products with the intent of coating the mucosal lining of the stomach, protecting it from acid secretion. While reading this chapter, you will learn about the current method to treat peptic ulcers in the stomach.

The GI system is essentially a long tube in the body where ingested food and fluids are processed for absorption of the nutrients. The upper GI system consists of the mouth, esophagus, and stomach (Fig. 38.1). The mouth is responsible for breaking down food parts and mixing them with saliva to begin the digestion process. The tubular

493

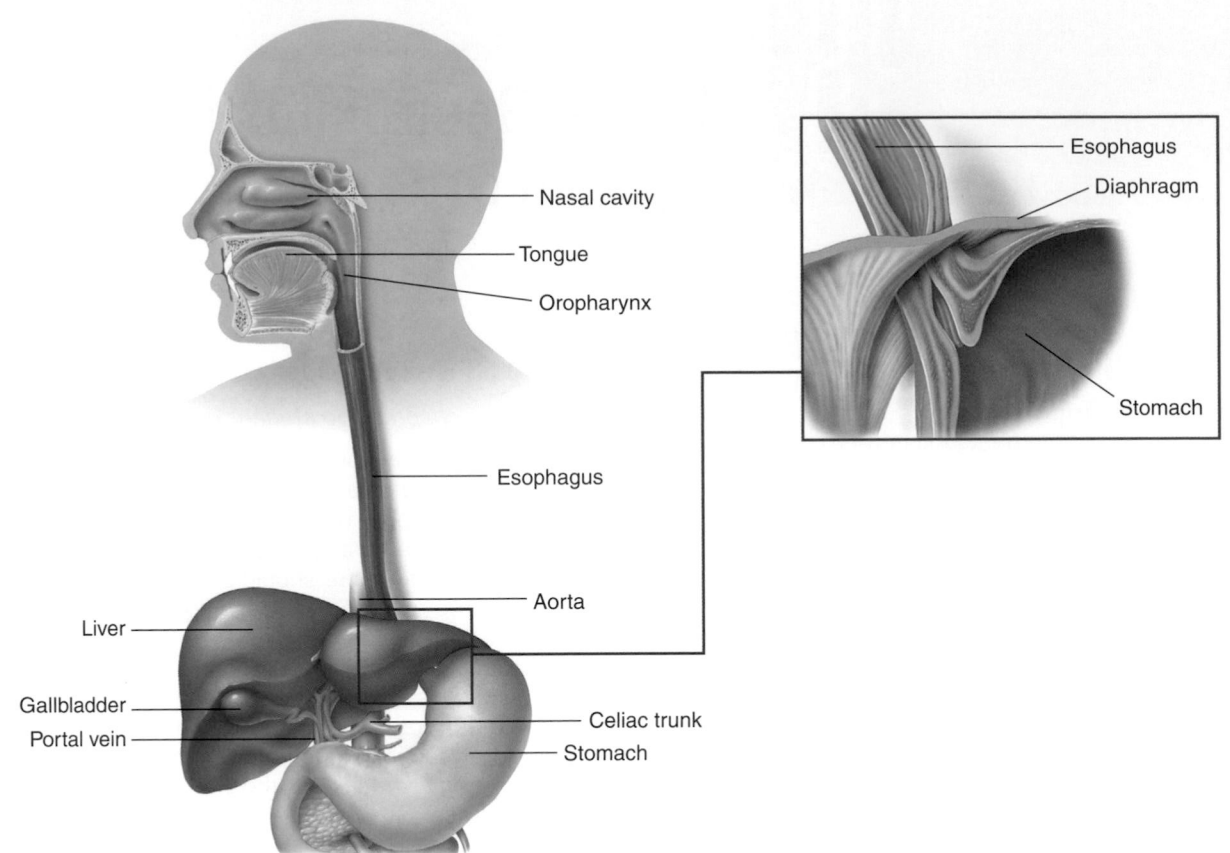

FIGURE 38.1 The upper GI system with esophagogastric junction featured.

esophagus connects the mouth to the stomach, where food is mixed with acids and enzymes to become a solution for absorption. Some of the cells of the stomach secrete **hydrochloric acid** (HCl), a substance that aids in the initial digestive process. Problems occur when acids or stomach contents reverse direction and come back up into the esophagus or stomach, which can create tissue damage and ulcers.

Drugs are presented in this chapter according to their function, whether they treat gastric acid production or prevent vomiting. Drugs that neutralize HCl and protect the mucosal lining are called *antacids*. Drugs that reduce the production and release of HCl include histamine type 2 receptor (H_2) antagonists, proton pump inhibitors, and miscellaneous acid-reducing agents. The proton pump inhibitors are particularly important in the treatment of *Helicobacter pylori* infection in clients with active duodenal ulcers. *H. pylori* is believed to cause a type of chronic gastritis and some peptic and duodenal ulcers as well (Olle, 2020). GI stimulants facilitate emptying of stomach contents into the small intestine and are used both as ulcer treatments and as antiemetics. Antiemetics are used to treat and prevent nausea and vomiting. Some of the more common drugs are listed in the Summary Drug Table: Upper Gastrointestinal System Drugs.

ACID NEUTRALIZERS: ANTACIDS

ACTIONS

Antacids ("against acids") are drugs that neutralize or reduce the acidity of stomach and duodenal contents by combining with HCl and increasing the pH of the stomach acid. Antacids do not "coat" the stomach lining, although they may increase the sphincter tone of the lower esophagus. Examples of antacids include aluminum (Amphojel), magaldrate (Riopan), and magnesium (milk of magnesia).

USES

Antacids are used in the treatment of hyperacidity caused by the following:

- Heartburn, acid indigestion, or sour stomach
- **Gastroesophageal reflux disease** (GERD; a reflux or backup of gastric contents into the esophagus)
- Peptic ulcer

Antacids may be used to treat conditions that are not associated with the GI system. For example, aluminum carbonate is a phosphate-binding agent and is used in treating **hyperphosphatemia** (often associated with chronic kidney disease) or as an adjunct to a low-phosphate diet to prevent formation of phosphate-based urinary stones. Calcium may be used in treating calcium deficiencies such as menopausal osteopenia/porosis. Magnesium may be used for treating magnesium deficiencies or magnesium depletion from malnutrition, restricted diet, or alcoholism.

ADVERSE REACTIONS

Antacids can have unpleasant reactions on the lower GI system producing either diarrhea or constipation. The magnesium- and sodium-containing antacids may have a laxative effect and may produce diarrhea. Aluminum- and calcium-containing products tend to produce constipation. Although the antacids have the potential for serious adverse reactions, they have a wide margin of safety, especially when used as prescribed. Adverse reactions of concern include:

- *Aluminum-containing antacids*—constipation, intestinal impaction, anorexia, weakness, tremors, and bone pain
- *Magnesium-containing antacids*—severe diarrhea, dehydration, and hypermagnesemia (nausea, vomiting, hypotension, decreased respirations)
- *Calcium-containing antacids*—rebound hyperacidity, metabolic alkalosis, hypercalcemia, vomiting, confusion, headache, renal calculi, and neurologic impairment
- *Sodium bicarbonate*—systemic alkalosis and rebound hyperacidity

CONTRAINDICATIONS AND PRECAUTIONS

The antacids are contraindicated in clients with severe abdominal pain of unknown cause and during lactation. Sodium-containing antacids are contraindicated in clients with cardiovascular problems, such as hypertension or heart failure, and those on sodium-restricted diets. Calcium-containing antacids are contraindicated in clients with renal calculi or hypercalcemia.

Aluminum-containing antacids are used cautiously in clients with gastric outlet obstruction or those with upper GI bleeding. Magnesium- and aluminum-containing antacids are used cautiously in clients with decreased kidney function. The calcium-containing antacids are used cautiously in clients with respiratory insufficiency, renal impairment, or cardiac disease. Antacids are classified as pregnancy category C drugs and should be used with caution during pregnancy.

INTERACTIONS

The following interactions may occur when an antacid is administered with another agent:

Interacting Drug	Common Use	Effect of Interaction
Digoxin, isoniazid, phenytoin, and chlorpromazine	Treatment of cardiac problems, infection, seizures, and nausea and vomiting, respectively	Decreased absorption of the interacting drugs results in a decreased effect of those drugs
Tetracycline	Anti-infective agent	Decreased effectiveness of anti-infective
Corticosteroids	Treatment of inflammation and respiratory problems	Decreased anti-inflammatory properties
Salicylates	Pain relief	Pain reliever is excreted more rapidly in the urine

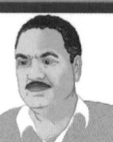

PHARMACOLOGY IN PRACTICE

DRUG RECOGNITION

A nurse has administered multiple doses of aluminum hydroxide gel to a client for the relief of stomach hyperacidity. What should the nurse begin to monitor for in this client after administration of a number of doses?
1. Complaints of headache
2. Constipation
3. Signs of electrolyte imbalance
4. Amount of fluid lost

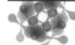 ACID-REDUCING AGENTS

Drugs that reduce the production of HCl include histamine H_2 antagonists, proton pump inhibitors, and miscellaneous drugs such as pepsin inhibitors, prostaglandins, and cholinergic blockers.

HISTAMINE H_2 ANTAGONISTS

ACTIONS

These drugs inhibit the action of histamine at H_2 receptor cells of the stomach, which then reduces the secretion of gastric acid. Because cholinergic blocking drugs typically block the action of histamine throughout the entire body, they are used less frequently. Histamine H_2 antagonists do not cause the generalized body effects of the cholinergic blockers, because they are selective only for the H_2 receptors in the stomach and not the general body H_2 receptors. When ulcers are present, the decrease in acid allows the ulcerated areas to heal. Examples of histamine H_2 antagonists include cimetidine or famotidine (Pepcid).

USES

These drugs are used prophylactically to treat stress-related ulcers and acute upper GI bleeding in critically ill clients. They are also used for the treatment of the following:

- Heartburn, acid indigestion, and sour stomach (frequently sold as over-the-counter remedies)
- GERD
- Gastric or duodenal ulcer
- Gastric **hypersecretory** conditions (excessive gastric secretion of HCl)

ADVERSE REACTIONS

Histamine H$_2$ antagonist adverse reactions are usually mild and transient as well as rare (affecting less than 2% of users) and include:

- Dizziness, somnolence, headache
- Confusion, hallucinations, diarrhea, and reversible impotence

CONTRAINDICATIONS AND PRECAUTIONS

The histamine H$_2$ antagonists are contraindicated in clients with a known hypersensitivity to the drugs. These drugs are used cautiously in clients with renal or hepatic impairment and in severely ill, older, or debilitated clients. Cimetidine is used cautiously in clients with diabetes. Histamine H$_2$ antagonists are pregnancy category B (cimetidine and famotidine) and C (nizatidine) drugs and should be used with caution during pregnancy and lactation.

LASA ALERT

The following drugs may sound alike; be sure to clarify when they are ordered:

Drug Name	Sounds Like
Axid	Ansaid
cimetidine	simethicone
famotidine	FLUoxetine, furosemide
nizatidine	tiZANidine

Drugs that look like a similar drug are noted in the Summary Drug Tables of each chapter.

PRACTICE CONSIDERATIONS

In 2020, the US Food and Drug Administration (FDA) requested all manufacturers of ranitidine to remove the product from the US market. A potential carcinogenic substance, N-nitrosodimethylamine was found in the drug product and noted to increase when stored at high room temperatures. The drug was removed from stores and pharmacies, and clients with the drug at home are asked to return the product to drug-take back locations near them (FDA, 2020).

INTERACTIONS

The following interactions may occur when a histamine H$_2$ antagonist is administered with another agent:

Interacting Drug	Common Use	Effect of Interaction
Antacids and metoclopramide	GI distress	Decreased absorption of the H$_2$ antagonists
Carmustine	Anticancer therapy	Decreased white blood cell count
Opioid analgesics	Pain relief	Increased risk of respiratory depression
Oral anticoagulants	Blood thinners	Increased risk of bleeding
Digoxin	Cardiac problems	May decrease serum digoxin levels

PROTON PUMP INHIBITORS

ACTIONS

Proton pump inhibitors are a group of drugs with antisecretory properties. These drugs suppress gastric acid secretion by inhibition of the hydrogen-potassium adenosine triphosphatase (ATPase) enzyme system of the gastric parietal cells. The ATPase enzyme system is also called the acid (proton) pump system. The proton pump inhibitors suppress gastric acid secretion by blocking the final step in the production of gastric acid by the gastric mucosa. Examples of proton pump inhibitors include esomeprazole (Nexium) and omeprazole (Prilosec).

USES

Proton pump inhibitors are used for treatment or symptomatic relief of various gastric disorders, including:

- Gastric and duodenal ulcers (specifically associated with *H. pylori* infections)
- GERD and erosive esophagitis
- Pathologic hypersecretory conditions
- Prevention of bleeding in high-risk clients using antiplatelet drugs

An important use of these drugs is combination therapy for the treatment of *H. pylori* infection in clients with duodenal ulcers. One treatment regimen used to treat infection with *H. pylori* is a triple-drug therapy, such as one of the proton pump inhibitors (e.g., omeprazole or lansoprazole) and two anti-infectives (e.g., amoxicillin and clarithromycin). Another triple-drug treatment regimen consists of bismuth plus two anti-infective drugs. Helidac, a triple-drug treatment regimen (bismuth, metronidazole, and tetracycline), may be given along with a histamine H$_2$ antagonist to treat disorders of the GI tract infected with *H. pylori*. Table 38.1 lists various drug combinations used in the treatment of *H. pylori* infection. Additional information concerning anti-infective agents is found in

TABLE 38.1 Agents Used to Eradicate *Helicobacter pylori* in Clients With Duodenal Ulcers

DRUG	RECOMMENDED USAGE	DOSAGE RANGE
Amoxicillin	In combination with lansoprazole and clarithromycin or lansoprazole alone	1 g BID for 14 days (triple therapy) or 1 g TID (double therapy)
Bismuth	In combination with other products	525 mg QID
Clarithromycin (Biaxin)	In combination with amoxicillin	500 mg TID
Lansoprazole (Prevacid)	In combination with clarithromycin or amoxicillin	30 mg BID for 14 days (triple therapy) or 30 mg TID for 14 days (double therapy)
Metronidazole (Flagyl)	In combination with other products	250 mg QID
Omeprazole (Prilosec)	In combination with clarithromycin	38 mg BID for 4 weeks and 20 mg/day for 15–28 days
Tetracycline	In combination with other products	500 mg QID
Combination Drug Packs	Brand Name	Dosing
Bismuth, metronidazole, tetracycline	Pylera, Helidac	Four times daily
Lansoprazole, amoxicillin, clarithromycin	*Formerly* Prevpac, now generic only	Twice daily
Omeprazole, amoxicillin, clarithromycin	Omeclamox—Pac	Twice daily
Omeprazole, amoxicillin, rifabutin	Talicia	Every 8 hours

Chapters 6 through 9. The Summary Drug Table: Upper Gastrointestinal System Drugs provides additional information on the proton pump inhibitor drugs used in treating *H. pylori* infection.

ADVERSE REACTIONS

The most common adverse reactions seen with the proton pump inhibitors include headache, nausea, diarrhea, and abdominal pain.

 Lifespan Considerations

Gerontology
When elderly clients are diagnosed with *C. diff* (*Clostridium difficile* diarrhea), the MAR should be checked for a proton pump inhibitor (PPI). Research shows a connection between long-term PPI administration and *C. difficile* infection in those aged 65+ years (Fisher, 2017).

CONTRAINDICATIONS AND PRECAUTIONS

PPIs are contraindicated in clients who are hypersensitive to any of the drugs. PPIs are used cautiously in older adults and in clients with hepatic impairment. Prolonged treatment may decrease the body's ability to absorb vitamin B_{12}, resulting in anemia. Omeprazole (pregnancy category C) and lansoprazole, rabeprazole, and pantoprazole (pregnancy category B) are contraindicated during pregnancy and lactation.

 Lifespan Considerations

Menopausal Women
An increase in fractures of the hip, wrist, and spine have been seen in those taking high doses of PPIs and undergoing treatment of osteoporosis with bisphosphonates.

LASA ALERT

The following drugs may sound alike; be sure to clarify when they are ordered:

Drug Name	*Sounds Like*
AcipHex	Acephen, Accupril, Aricept, pHisoHex
dexlansoprazole	aripiprazole, lansoprazole
Dexilant	DULoxetine
esomeprazole	ARIPiprazole, omeprazole
NexIUM	NexAVAR
omeprazole	ARIPiprazole, esomeprazole, fomepizole
pantoprazole	ARIPiprazole
Prevacid	Pravachol, Prevpac, PriLOSEC, Prinivil
PriLOSEC	Plendil, Prevacid, predniSONE, prilocaine, Prinivil, Pristiq, Proventil, PROzac
Protonix	Lotronex, Lovenox, protamine
RABEprazole	ARIPiprazole, donepezil, lansoprazole, omeprazole, raloxifene
Zegerid	Zestril

Drugs that look like a similar drug are noted in the Summary Drug Tables of each chapter.

INTERACTIONS

The following interactions may occur when a PPI is administered with another agent:

Interacting Drug	Common Use	Effect of Interaction
Sucralfate	Management of GI distress	Decreased absorption of the proton pump inhibitor
Ketoconazole and ampicillin	Anti-infective agent	Decreased absorption of the anti-infective
Oral anticoagulants	Blood thinners	Increased risk of bleeding
Digoxin	Cardiac problems	Increased absorption of digoxin
Benzodiazepines, phenytoin	Management of anxiety and seizure disorders	Risk for toxic level of antiseizure drugs
Clarithromycin (with omeprazole, specifically)	Anti-infective agent	Risk for an increase in plasma levels of both drugs
Bisphosphonates	Bone strengthening	Increased risk of fracture

MISCELLANEOUS ACID REDUCERS

Three other types of acid-reducing drugs that are less frequently used are the cholinergic blocking drugs (also called *anticholinergic* drugs), a pepsin inhibitor, and a prostaglandin drug. Cholinergic blocking drugs reduce gastric motility and decrease the amount of acid secreted by the stomach. These drugs have been largely replaced by histamine H_2 antagonists, which appear to be more effective and have fewer adverse effects. Examples of cholinergic blocking drugs used for GI disorders include propantheline and glycopyrrolate (Robinul). For information about specific cholinergic blocking drugs, see Chapter 26.

Sucralfate (Carafate) is known as a pepsin inhibitor or mucosal protective drug. The drug binds with protein molecules to form a viscous substance that buffers acid and protects the mucosal lining. Sucralfate is used in the short-term treatment of duodenal ulcers. It is the preferred drug in pregnant women who suffer from GERD symptoms and for treatment of stress ulcers. The most common adverse reaction is constipation. Drug interactions of sucralfate are similar to those of the PPIs.

A prostaglandin drug, misoprostol (Cytotec), has been used to reduce the risk of nonsteroidal anti-inflammatory drug (NSAID)–induced gastric ulcers in high-risk clients, such as older adults or the critically ill. Misoprostol both inhibits the production of gastric acid and has mucosal protective properties. Because this drug can cause abortion or birth defects, it is not recommended for use in ulcer reduction in women who are pregnant or may become pregnant or who are lactating. Adverse reactions include headache, nausea, diarrhea, and abdominal pain. The drug effects are decreased when it is taken with antacids.

GASTROINTESTINAL STIMULANT

ACTIONS

Metoclopramide (Reglan) is used to treat delayed gastric emptying and emesis—that is, it increases the motility of the upper GI tract without increasing the production of secretions. By sensitizing tissue to the effects of acetylcholine, the tone and amplitude of gastric contractions are increased, resulting in faster emptying of gastric contents into the small intestine. It also inhibits stimulation of the vomiting center in the brain.

USES

GI stimulants are used in the treatment of the following:

- GERD
- **Gastric stasis** (failure to move food normally out of the stomach) in diabetic clients, in clients with nausea and vomiting associated with cancer chemotherapy, and in clients in the immediate postoperative period

ADVERSE REACTIONS

Adverse reactions associated with metoclopramide are usually mild. Higher doses or prolonged administration may produce central nervous system (CNS) symptoms, such as restlessness, drowsiness, dizziness, extrapyramidal effects (tremor, involuntary movements of the limbs, muscle rigidity), facial grimacing, and depression.

CONTRAINDICATIONS AND PRECAUTIONS

The GI stimulant is contraindicated in clients with known hypersensitivity to the drug, GI obstruction, gastric perforation or hemorrhage, or pheochromocytoma. Clients with Parkinson disease or a seizure disorder who are taking drugs likely to cause extrapyramidal symptoms should not take these drugs.

This drug is used cautiously in clients with diabetes and cardiovascular disease. Metoclopramide is a pregnancy category B drug. The drug is secreted in breast milk and should be used with caution during pregnancy and lactation.

LASA ALERT

The following drugs may sound alike; be sure to clarify when they are ordered:

Drug Name	Sounds Like
metoclopramide	metOLazone, metoprolol, metroNIDAZOLE
Reglan	Megace, Regonol, Renagel, Regitine

Drugs that look like a similar drug are noted in the Summary Drug Tables of each chapter.

INTERACTIONS

The following interactions may occur when a GI stimulant is administered with another agent:

Interacting Drug	Common Use	Effect of Interaction
Cholinergic blocking drugs or opioid analgesics	Management of GI distress or pain relief	Decreased effectiveness of metoclopramide
Cimetidine	Management of GI distress	Decreased absorption of cimetidine
Digoxin	Management of cardiac problems	Decreased absorption of digoxin
Monoamine oxidase inhibitor antidepressants	Management of depression	Increased risk of hypertensive episode
Levodopa	Management of disease	Decreased metoclopramide and levodopa

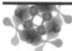 ANTIEMETICS

An antiemetic drug is used to treat or prevent **nausea** (unpleasant gastric sensation usually preceding vomiting) or **vomiting** (forceful expulsion of gastric contents through the mouth). The drugs discussed in this section are used to treat severe nausea and vomiting. Individuals may experience nausea owing to motion sickness or a condition called **vertigo** (a sensation of spinning or a rotation-type motion). Many of the drugs used to treat motion sickness can be purchased over the counter. Table 38.2 lists examples of drugs used in the treatment of motion sickness or vertigo.

ACTIONS

In addition to the stomach, the brain is involved in the sensation of nausea. The medulla has an area called the vomiting center. The process of vomiting happens when the area is stimulated directly by a nerve due to GI irritation, motion sickness, and vestibular neuritis (inflammation of the vestibular nerve). An adjacent area, the **chemoreceptor trigger zone** (CTZ), is a group of nerve fibers that sends signals to the vomiting center in the medulla when the metabolism is

TABLE 38.2 Motion Sickness Drugs

GENERIC NAME	TRADE NAME
dimenhydrinate	Dramamine
diphenhydramine	Benadryl
meclizine	Antivert
scopolamine	Transderm Scop (transdermal system)

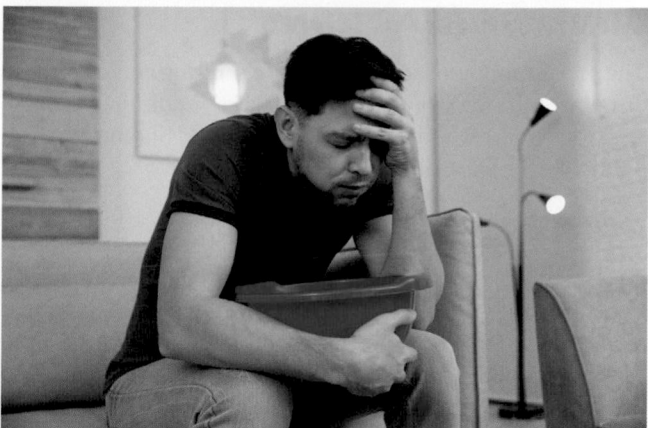

FIGURE 38.2 Antiemetic drugs work at the CTZ and peripherally at nerve endings to reduce nausea and vomiting.

unbalanced. When these nerves are stimulated by chemicals, such as drugs or toxic substances, impulses are sent to the vomiting center located in the medulla. Vomiting caused by drugs, radiation, and metabolic disorders often occurs because of stimulation of the CTZ. Antiemetics discussed here appear to act primarily by inhibiting the CTZ and the brain's primary neurotransmitters dopamine and acetylcholine.

The 5-hydroxytryptamine type 3 (5-HT3) receptor antagonists (such as ondansetron) target serotonin receptors both at the CTZ and peripherally at the nerve endings in the stomach. This action reduces the non-GI adverse effects that are often evident when nonspecific cholinergic blocking drugs are used (Fig. 38.2). Because of their localized action in the GI system, these drugs are being tested for use in irritable bowel syndrome as well.

USES

An antiemetic is used to treat nausea and vomiting, typically by preventive administration (prophylaxis):

- Before surgery to prevent vomiting during surgery
- Immediately after surgery when the client is recovering from anesthesia
- Before, during, and after administration of antineoplastic drugs that induce a high degree of nausea and vomiting
- During radiation therapy when the GI tract is in the treatment field
- During pregnancy for hyperemesis

Other causes of nausea and vomiting that may be treated with an antiemetic include bacterial and viral infections and adverse drug reactions. Some antiemetics also are used for motion sickness and vertigo. Dronabinol (Marinol) and nabilone are the only medically available cannabinoid (marijuana derivative) prescribed for antiemetic use. Approximately 35 states, Washington DC, and Guam allow marijuana use for medical purposes such as nausea. See Chapter 15 for a more in-depth discussion of marijuana use.

ADVERSE REACTIONS

The most common adverse reactions resulting from these drugs are varying degrees of drowsiness. Additional adverse reactions for each drug are listed in the Summary Drug Table: Upper Gastrointestinal System Drugs.

CONTRAINDICATIONS

Antiemetic drugs are contraindicated in clients with known hypersensitivity to these drugs or with severe CNS depression. The 5-HT3 receptor antagonists should not be used by clients with heart block or prolonged QT intervals. In general, these drugs are not recommended during pregnancy and lactation or for uncomplicated vomiting in young children. Prochlorperazine is contraindicated in clients with bone marrow depression, blood dyscrasia, Parkinson disease, or severe liver or cardiovascular disease.

PRECAUTIONS

Severe nausea and vomiting should not be treated with antiemetic drugs alone. The cause of the vomiting must be investigated. Antiemetic drugs may hamper the diagnosis of disorders such as brain tumor or injury, appendicitis, intestinal obstruction, and drug toxicity (e.g., digitalis toxicity). Delayed diagnosis of any of these disorders could have serious consequences for the client.

Cholinergic blocking antiemetics are used cautiously in clients with glaucoma or obstructive disease of the GI or genitourinary system, in those with renal or hepatic dysfunction, and in older men with possible prostatic hypertrophy. Promethazine is used cautiously in clients with hypertension, sleep apnea, or epilepsy. The 5-HT3 receptor antagonists should be used cautiously in clients with cardiac conduction problems or electrolyte imbalances.

5-HT3 receptor antagonists are pregnancy category B and used for hyperemesis. Perphenazine, prochlorperazine, promethazine, scopolamine, and chlorpromazine are pregnancy category C drugs. Other antiemetics are classified as pregnancy category B.

LASA ALERT

The following drugs may sound alike; be sure to clarify when they are ordered:

Drug Name	Sounds Like
Anzemet	Aldomet, Antivert, Avandamet
chlorproMAZINE	chlordiazePOXIDE, chlorproPAMIDE, clomiPRAMINE, prochlorperazine, promethazine
dolasetron	alosetron, granisetron, ondansetron, palonosetron
Tigan	Tiazac, Ticlid
trimethobenzamide	metoclopramide, trimethoprim

Drugs that look like a similar drug are noted in the Summary Drug Tables of each chapter.

INTERACTIONS

The following interactions may occur when an antiemetic is administered with another agent:

Interacting Drug	Common Use	Effect of Interaction
CNS depressants	Analgesia, sedation, or pain relief	Increased risk of sedation
Antihistamines	Management of allergy and respiratory distress	Increased adverse cholinergic blocking effects
Antacids	Management of gastric distress	Decreased absorption of antiemetic
Rifampin with 5-HT3 receptor antagonist	Tuberculosis/human immunodeficiency virus infection management	Decreased effectiveness of 5-HT3 receptor antagonist
Lithium with prochlorperazine	Management of bipolar disorder	Increased risk of extrapyramidal effects

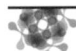 # EMETICS

Used for the opposite effect of an antiemetic drug, an *emetic* is a drug that *induces* vomiting. This is caused by local irritation of the stomach and by stimulation of the vomiting center in the medulla. Emetics are used to empty the stomach rapidly when an individual has accidently or intentionally ingested a poison or drug overdose. Not all poison ingestions or drug overdoses are treated with emetics. This is because more harm can occur from the vomiting of many substances. As a result, guidelines were established for the use of syrup of ipecac (see Client Teaching for Improved Outcomes: Using Emetics Properly).

 Herbal Considerations

Ginger, a pungent root, has been used medicinally for GI problems such as motion sickness, nausea, vomiting, and indigestion. In addition, it is recommended for the pain and inflammation of arthritis, and it may help lower cholesterol. The dosage of the dried form of ginger is 1 g (1000 mg) per day. Adverse reactions are rare, although heartburn has been reported by some individuals. Ginger should be used cautiously in clients with hypertension or gallstones and during pregnancy or lactation. As with any substance, a primary health care provider should be consulted before any ginger remedy is taken, although ginger has been consumed safely as a food by millions of individuals for centuries (DerMarderosian, 2003).

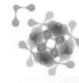

NURSING PROCESS: STEPS TO BUILDING CLINICAL JUDGMENT
Client Receiving a Drug for an Upper Gastrointestinal Condition

ASSESSMENT

Preadministration Assessment

Data gathering suggestions before the initial administration of an antiemetic or other upper GI drug include:
Objective data

- Vital signs (temperature, pulse, respirations, and blood pressure)
- Number of times emesis has occurred, approximate amount of fluid lost, content or blood
- Palpate for skin turgor
- Weight
- Laboratory tests—electrolyte panel if dehydration is suspected.

Subjective data

- Description of nausea, type and intensity of symptoms (e.g., pain, discomfort, nausea, vomiting)
- Remedies client has attempted before seeking treatment
- Medical history/drug therapy (list of all current drugs and supplements taken)

In the case of preventative administration of an antiemetic, explain the rationale for preventing an episode of nausea rather than waiting for symptoms to occur when the primary health care provider knows the drugs or treatments being given will cause this problem. Ask the client about any episodes of nausea or vomiting in anticipation of the therapy.

Ongoing Assessment

Monitor the client frequently for continued complaints of pain, sour taste, or the production of bloody or coffee-ground emesis. If vomiting is severe, observe the client for signs and symptoms of electrolyte imbalance and monitor the blood pressure, pulse, and respiratory rate every 2–4 hours or as ordered by the primary health care provider. Measure intake and output (urine, emesis) carefully until vomiting ceases and the client can take oral fluids in sufficient quantity.

Document in the client's record each time the client vomits, and notify the primary health care provider if there is blood in the emesis or if vomiting suddenly becomes more severe. If vomiting is severe, you may anticipate a nasogastric (NG) tube being inserted for suctioning to prevent aspiration of emesis (Fig. 38.3). You may need to measure the client's weight daily to weekly in clients with prolonged and repeated episodes of vomiting (e.g., those receiving chemotherapy for cancer). Assess the client at frequent intervals for the effectiveness of the drug in relieving symptoms (e.g., nausea, vomiting, or vertigo) and notify the primary health care provider if the drug fails to relieve or diminish symptoms.

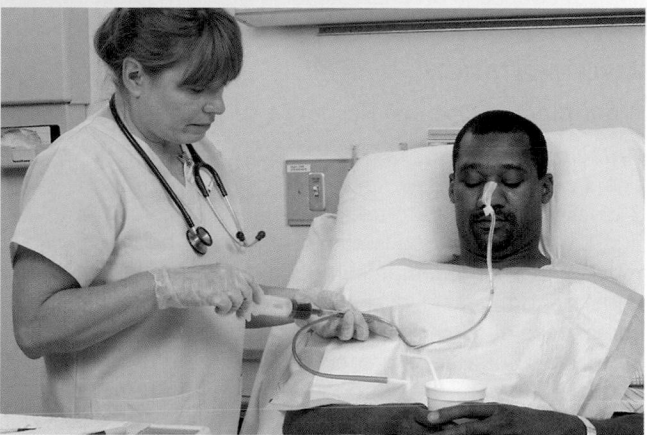

FIGURE 38.3 Placement of a nasogastric tube may be indicated with nausea and vomiting.

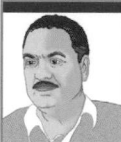

PHARMACOLOGY IN PRACTICE

ASSESSMENT

A nurse is caring for a client experiencing nausea and vomiting. The primary health care provider has prescribed antiemetic drug therapy for the client. Which of the following symptoms describe the possibility of dehydration? Select all that apply.

1. White streaks in stool
2. Decreased urinary output
3. Concentrated urine
4. Decreased respiratory rate
5. Dry mucous membranes

NURSING DIAGNOSES

Drug-specific nursing diagnoses include the following:

- **Risk for dehydration:** related to diarrhea, nausea, and vomiting
- **Malnutrition:** related to impaired ability to ingest and retain food and fluids, or offensive tastes and smells
- **Altered health maintenance:** related to inability to take oral form of medication
- **Injury risk:** related to adverse drug effects of drowsiness

Nursing diagnoses related to drug administration are discussed in Chapter 4.

PLANNING

The expected outcomes for the client depend on the reason the upper GI drug is administered but may include an optimal response to drug therapy, support of client needs related to the management of adverse reactions, and confidence in an understanding of the medication regimen.

IMPLEMENTATION

Promoting an Optimal Response to Therapy

Antacids

The antacid may be administered hourly for the first 2 weeks when used to treat acute peptic ulcer. After the first 2 weeks, the drug is administered 1–2 hours after meals and at bedtime. It is important for the client to understand that acid will be reduced, but with reduction comes less absorption of food and drugs from the stomach. Therefore, the antacids need to be taken later so that medicines have the opportunity to enter the circulation, before the acid is reduced. The primary health care provider may order that the antacid be left at the client's bedside for self-administration. Ensure that an adequate supply of water and cups for measuring the dose is available.

NURSING ALERT

Because of the possibility of an antacid interfering with the activity of other oral drugs, no oral drug should be administered within 1–2 hours of an antacid.

Non-oral Methods of Drug Administration

Clients taking acid-reducing drugs may not be able to take oral medications because of preparation for an operative procedure, postoperative nausea, or physical condition. Many of these drugs, other than antacids, come in forms for both intramuscular (IM) and intravenous (IV) administration. The IV route is typically preferred if the client has an existing IV line, because these drugs are irritating, and IM injections need to be given deep into the muscular tissue to minimize harm.

NURSING ALERT

When one of these drugs is given IV, monitor the rate of infusion at frequent intervals. Too rapid an infusion may induce cardiac arrhythmias.

Clients who are debilitated and require feeding from an NG tube are at risk for gastric ulcer development and may be prescribed acid-reducing drugs. Always check the medication label to see if the pill can be crushed or the capsule opened before doing so. These can be mixed with 40 mL of water or apple juice and administered through the NG tube. The tube is flushed with fluid afterward. Many of these drugs come in a liquid form as well as tablet or capsule. Request the liquid form when administration is in a tube to decrease the chance of a clogged NG tube due to improper flushing.

NURSING ALERT

Always use oral syringes to draw up drug solutions for enteral tube administration; this helps to avoid the accidental parenteral administration of an oral preparation.

Prevention of Nausea in Clients Undergoing Cancer Therapy

Different protocols for prechemotherapy nausea depend on the type of cancer treatment. Some cancer (antineoplastic) drugs rarely cause nausea, and others are highly **emetogenic**. Granisetron (Kytril), ondansetron (Zofran), and dolasetron (Anzemet) are examples of antiemetics used when cancer chemotherapy drugs are very likely to cause nausea and vomiting. These drugs are administered regardless of emesis history before the chemotherapy is given. The first dose is typically given IV during therapy, and then the client is asked to take it orally at home for a specified period. It is important to explain to the client that the drug prevents nausea and vomiting and to be sure to take the entire dose prescribed, even when the client feels fine at home. You may be asked to assist in the preadministration of antiemetics, yet the antineoplastics should always be given by a nurse trained in the administration of cancer chemotherapy.

Monitoring and Managing Client Needs

Risk for Dehydration

When antacids are given, keep a record of the client's bowel movements, because these drugs may cause constipation or diarrhea. If the client experiences diarrhea, accurately record fluid intake and output along with a description of the diarrhea stool. Uncontrolled diarrhea can lead to fluid loss and dehydration. Changing to a different antacid usually alleviates the problem. Diarrhea may be controlled by combining a magnesium antacid with an antacid containing aluminum or calcium.

Dehydration is a serious concern in the client experiencing nausea and vomiting. It is important to observe the client for signs of dehydration, which include poor skin turgor, dry mucous membranes, decrease in or absence of urinary output, concentrated urine, restlessness, irritability, increased respiratory rate, and confusion. Monitor the input and output (urine and emesis) and document findings every 8 hours. If the client is able to take and retain small amounts of oral fluids, offer sips of water at frequent intervals. In addition, it is important to observe the client for signs of electrolyte imbalance, particularly sodium and potassium deficit (see Chapter 54). If signs of dehydration or electrolyte imbalance are noted, contact the primary health care provider, because parenteral administration of fluids or fluids with electrolytes may be necessary.

 Chronic Care Considerations

Observations for fluid and electrolyte disturbances are particularly important in the older adult or chronically ill clients in whom severe dehydration may develop quickly. Immediately report symptoms of dehydration, such as dry mucous membranes, decreased urinary output, concentrated urine, restlessness, or confusion. Dehydration can lead to confusion and dizziness. Dizziness increases the risk for falls in the older adult. Assistance is needed for ambulatory activities. The environment is made safe by removing throw rugs, small pieces of furniture, and the like. Report any change in orientation to the primary health care provider.

Malnutrition

Nausea, vomiting, vertigo, and dizziness are disagreeable sensations. Provide the client with an emesis basin and check the client at frequent intervals. If vomiting occurs, empty the emesis basin and measure and document the volume in the client's record. Offer comfort measures such as giving the client a damp washcloth and a towel to wipe the hands and face as needed. It is also a good idea to give the client mouthwash or frequent oral rinses to remove the disagreeable taste that accompanies vomiting (Fig. 38.4).

Nausea may make the client lose their appetite and decrease nutritional intake. It is important to make the environment as pleasant as possible to enhance the client's appetite. Remove items with strong smells and odors. Change the client's bedding and clothing or gown as needed, because the odor of vomit may intensify the sensations of nausea and further decrease appetite. Ask visitors to refrain from wearing strong perfumes and colognes.

Altered Health Maintenance

When antacids are given, instruct the client to chew the tablets thoroughly before swallowing and then drink a full glass of water or milk. If the client expresses a dislike for the taste of the antacid or has difficulty chewing the tablet form, contact the primary health care provider. A flavored antacid may be ordered if the client finds the taste unpleasant. A liquid form may be ordered if the client has difficulty chewing a tablet. Liquid antacid preparations must be shaken thoroughly immediately before administration. Liquid antacids are followed by a small amount of water.

If the client cannot retain the oral form of the drug (other than the antacids), it may be given parenterally or as a rectal suppository (if the prescribed drug is available in these forms). If only the oral form has been ordered and the client cannot retain the drug, contact the primary health care provider regarding an order for a parenteral

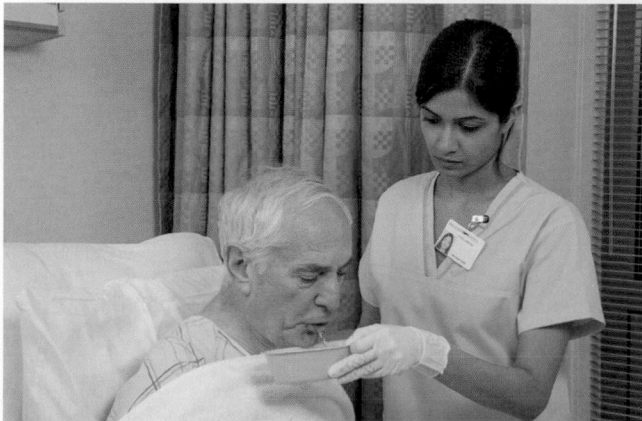

FIGURE 38.4 Provide comfort measures for the nauseated client.

or suppository form of this or another antiemetic drug. Should you send a client home with instructions to use a suppository, be sure to include disposable gloves or finger cots (medical supplies used to cover one or more fingers when a full glove is unnecessary) for administration.

When administering scopolamine for motion sickness, one transdermal system is applied behind the ear approximately 4 hours before the antiemetic effect is needed. Approximately 1 g of scopolamine is administered every 24 hours for 3 days. Advise the individual to discard any disk that becomes detached and to replace it with a fresh disk applied behind the opposite ear.

Injury Risk

Administration of these drugs may result in varying degrees of drowsiness. To prevent accidental falls and other injuries, assist the client who is allowed out of bed with ambulatory activities. If extreme drowsiness is noted, instruct the client to remain in bed and provide a call light for assistance.

! NURSING ALERT

Tardive dyskinesia (nonreversible, involuntary muscle spasms), which is typically associated with conventional antipsychotics, is known to occur with long-term use (12 weeks or more) of metoclopramide. Immediately report extrapyramidal symptoms to prevent tardive dyskinesia from occurring.

Educating the Client and Family

When a drug to treat the upper GI system is prescribed for outpatient use, and as you develop a teaching plan, include the following information:

- If drowsy, avoid driving or performing other hazardous tasks when taking these drugs.
- Do not use antacids indiscriminately. Check with a primary health care provider before using an antacid if other medical problems, such as a cardiac condition, exist (some antacids contain sodium).
- Do not increase the frequency of use or the dose if your symptoms become worse; instead, see the primary health care provider as soon as possible.
- Because antacids impair the absorption of some drugs, do not take other drugs within 2 hours before or after taking the antacid unless use of an antacid with a drug is recommended by the primary health care provider.
- If pain or discomfort remains the same or becomes worse, if the stools turn black, or if vomitus resembles coffee grounds, contact the primary health care provider as soon as possible.
- Magnesium-containing products may produce a *laxative* effect and may cause diarrhea; aluminum- or calcium-containing antacids may cause *constipation*.
- Taking too much antacid may cause the stomach to secrete excess stomach acid. Consult the primary health care provider or pharmacist about appropriate dose. Do not use the maximum dose for more than 2 weeks, except under the supervision of a primary health care provider.

- When taking PPIs, swallow the tablet whole at least 1 hour before eating. Do not chew, open, or crush.
- When taking metoclopramide, immediately report any of the following signs: difficulty speaking or swallowing; mask-like face; shuffling gait; rigidity; tremors; uncontrolled movements of the mouth, face, or extremities; and uncontrolled chewing or unusual movements of the tongue.

  🍷 Avoid the use of alcohol and other sedative-type drugs unless use has been approved by the primary health care provider.

- Take antiemetics for cancer chemotherapy as prescribed. Do not omit a dose. Consult the primary health care provider if you have forgotten a dose of the medication.
- When using rectal suppositories, remove foil wrapper and immediately insert the pointed end into the rectum without using force.

Client Teaching for Improved Outcomes

Using Emetics Properly

Before an emetic is given, it is extremely important to know the chemicals or substances that have been ingested, the time they were ingested, and what symptoms were noted before seeking medical treatment. This information will probably be obtained from a family member or friend, but the adult client may also contribute to the history. You should inform clients there are times when syrup of ipecac is contraindicated.

The FDA approved the following warnings for the labeling of syrup of ipecac:

✔ Do not use in persons who are not fully conscious.
✔ Do not use this product unless directed by a health care professional. Do not use if turpentine; corrosives, such as alkalis (lye) or strong acids; or petroleum distillates, such as kerosene, paint thinner, cleaning fluid, or furniture polish, have been ingested.

Manoguerra (2005) has expanded the contraindications for ipecac syrup to include situations in which:

✔ The client is comatose or has altered mental status, and the risk of aspiration of stomach contents is high.
✔ The client is having convulsions.
✔ The substance ingested is capable of causing altered mental status or convulsions.
✔ The substance ingested is a caustic or corrosive agent.
✔ The substance ingested is a low-viscosity petroleum distillate (e.g., gas or kerosene) with the potential for pulmonary aspiration and the development of chemical pneumonitis.
✔ The client has a medical condition that may be exacerbated by vomiting (e.g., severe hypertension, bradycardia, hemorrhagic diathesis).

Remember: The primary health care provider or nurse should also contact the local poison control center to obtain information regarding treatment.

- Motion sickness drugs should be taken about 1 hour before travel.
- Misoprostol: Because this drug may cause spontaneous abortion, women of childbearing age need to use a reliable contraceptive. If pregnancy is suspected, discontinue use of the drug and notify the primary health care provider. Report severe menstrual pain, bleeding, or spotting as well.

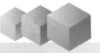

PHARMACOLOGY IN PRACTICE

SAFE DRUG ADMINISTRATION

An urgent care triage nurse receives a call about a client who has ingested a poison. What priority information should the nurse obtain from a family member or friend of the client before discussing with the PHCP on duty? Select all that apply.

1. Substances that have been ingested
2. Reason for ingesting the poison
3. Approximately when the substances were ingested
4. Client's mental status before taking the poison
5. Symptoms noted before seeking medical treatment

Concept Mastery Alert

Nurses should warn a client taking magnesium- and sodium-containing antacids about the potential of diarrhea, which is more common when magnesium products are taken.

EVALUATION

- Therapeutic effect is achieved and nausea or pain is controlled.
- Adverse reactions are identified, reported to the primary health care provider, and managed successfully through appropriate nursing interventions:
  - Fluid volume balance is maintained.
  - Client maintains an adequate nutritional status.
  - Client manages the therapeutic regimen effectively.
  - No evidence of injury is seen.
- Client or family expresses confidence and demonstrates an understanding of the drug regimen.

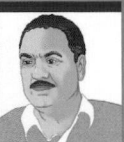

PHARMACOLOGY IN PRACTICE

USING CLINICAL REASONING

Alfredo Garcia was found to have GERD, not a peptic ulcer. During your client teaching, how would you explain to Mr. Garcia that using dairy products to coat the stomach lining is not helpful in reducing acid secretions? Instead, he is instructed to buy the antacid of his choice for the heartburn. He can't understand why he should coat his stomach with medicine instead of cream. Explain how antacids work.

KEY POINTS

■ The upper GI system includes the mouth, esophagus, and stomach. We take in food and fluids that are processed and absorbed for use by our cells. Hydrochloric acid is secreted in the stomach to help in the digestion process.

■ Problems occur when the digestive juices reverse and go into the esophagus or backflow into the stomach from the small intestine. Drugs discussed in this chapter focus on acid reduction or neutralization and increasing motility to move contents through the system. Antiemetics used to reduce or prevent nausea and vomiting are also discussed.

■ Antacids do not actually coat the stomach; instead, they neutralize the acid in the stomach. Because acid is needed for proper absorption, these drugs should not be taken within 2 hour of other drugs. Acid-reducing drugs such as the his-

tamine antagonists and PPIs reduce the gastric acid secretion. The decrease in acid aids in the healing process when an ulcer is present. Stimulants are used to promote GI motility, which, in turn, will reduce nausea. Antiemetics currently used inhibit neuronal transmission of sensation from the gut or the signal to vomit.

■ Common adverse reactions include headache, nausea, diarrhea, or abdominal pain. Metoclopramide, when used long term, can cause extrapyramidal effects, which can lead to the irreversible condition of tardive dyskinesia.

■ Multiple over-the-counter products exist to treat GI symptoms. Clients need confidence in understanding how to purchase and take these products because the majority of users do so without health care provider supervision.

SUMMARY DRUG TABLE
Upper Gastrointestinal System Drugs

Generic Name	Trade Name	Uses	Adverse Reactions	Dosage Ranges
Acid Neutralizers				
aluminum carbonate *a-LOO-mi-num*	Basaljel	Symptomatic relief of peptic ulcer and stomach hyperacidity, hyperphosphatemia	Constipation, bone softening, neurotoxicity	Two tablets or capsules (10 mL of regular oral suspension) as often as q2hr, up to 12 times daily
aluminum hydroxide	Alternagel, Amphojel, Gaviscon	Same as aluminum carbonate	Same as aluminum carbonate	500–1500 mg (5–30 mL in oral suspension) 3–6 times daily orally between meals and at bedtime
calcium carbonate *KAL-see-um*	Tums, Maalox, (multiple trade names)	Symptomatic relief of peptic ulcer and stomach hyperacidity, calcium deficiencies (osteopenia)	Acid rebound	0.5–1.5 g orally
magnesia (magnesium hydroxide) *mag-NEE-zhum*	Milk of Magnesia, Phillips MOM	Symptomatic relief of peptic ulcer and stomach hyperacidity, constipation	Diarrhea, bone loss in clients with chronic renal failure	Antacid: 622–1244 mg (5–15 mL in suspension) orally QID Laxative: 15–60 mL orally
magnesium oxide	Mag-Ox	Same as magnesia	Same as magnesia	140–800 mg/day orally
sodium bicarbonate *SOW-dee-um*	Bell/ans	Symptomatic relief of peptic ulcer and stomach hyperacidity	Electrolyte imbalance and metabolic alkalosis	0.3–2 g orally 1–4 times daily
Combined-Product Acid Neutralizer				
magaldrate (magnesium/ aluminate)	Iosopan, Mylanta, Riopan	Symptomatic relief of peptic ulcer and stomach hyperacidity	Constipation, diarrhea	5–10 mL orally between meals and at bedtime
famotidine/calcium carbonate/ magnesium hydroxide	Duo Fusion, Pepcid Complete	Symptomatic relief of peptic ulcer and stomach hyperacidity	See separate drugs	

Continued

SUMMARY DRUG TABLE (continued)
Upper Gastrointestinal System Drugs

Generic Name	Trade Name	Uses	Adverse Reactions	Dosage Ranges
Acid Reducers				
Histamine H₂ Antagonists				
cimetidine[a] *sye-MET-i-deen*	Tagamet (only in OTC form)	Gastric/duodenal ulcers, GERD, gastric hypersecretory conditions, GI bleeding, heartburn	Headache, somnolence, diarrhea	800–1600 mg/day orally; 300 mg q6hr IM or IV
famotidine[a] *fa-MOE-ti-deen*	Pepcid	Same as cimetidine	Same as cimetidine	20–40 mg orally; IV if unable to take orally
nizatidine[a] *ni-ZA-ti-deen*	Axid (only in OTC form)	Same as cimetidine	Same as cimetidine	150–300 mg/day orally in one dose or divided doses
Proton Pump Inhibitors				
dexlansoprazole *deks-lan-SOE-pra-zole*	Dexilant	Erosive esophagitis, reflux disease	Headache, nausea, diarrhea	30–60 mg/day orally
esomeprazole *es-oh-ME[a]pray-zole*	NexIUM	Erosive esophagitis, GERD, *H. pylori* eradication, NSAID-associated gastric ulcers	Headache, nausea, diarrhea	20–40 mg/day orally
lansoprazole[a] *lan-SOE-pra-zole*	Prevacid	Same as esomeprazole, hypersecretory conditions, cystic fibrosis (intestinal malabsorption)	Same as esomeprazole	15–30 mg/day orally
omeprazole[a] *oh-MEP-ra-zole*	Prilosec, (Zegerid—combined with sodium bicarbonate or magnesium)	Same as esomeprazole, hypersecretory conditions, heartburn, reduce risk of upper GI bleeding	Same as esomeprazole	20–60 mg/day orally
pantoprazole *pan-TOE-pra-zole*	Protonix	GERD, erosive esophagitis, and hypersecretory conditions	Same as esomeprazole	40 mg/day orally or IV Hypersecretion: 80 mg IV q12hr
RABEprazole *ra-BEP-ra-zole*	AcipHex	Same as esomeprazole	Same as esomeprazole	20 mg/day orally
Miscellaneous Acid Reducers				
sucralfate *soo-KRAL-fate*	Carafate	Short-term duodenal ulcer treatment	Constipation	1 g/day orally in divided doses
miSOPROStol *mye-soe-PROST-ole*	Cytotec	Prevention of gastric ulcers in clients taking NSAIDs	Headache, nausea, diarrhea, abdominal pain	100–200 mcg orally QID
GI Stimulant				
metoclopramide *met-oh-KLOE-pra-mide*	Reglan, Gimoti (nasal spray)	Diabetic gastroparesis, GERD, prevention of nausea and vomiting	Restlessness, dizziness, fatigue, extrapyramidal effects	10–15 mg orally; 10–20 mg IM, IV
Antiemetics				
5-HT₃ Receptor Antagonists				
dolasetron *dol-A-se-tron*	Anzemet	Prevention of chemotherapy-induced and postoperative nausea, vomiting	Headache, fatigue, fever, abdominal pain	100 mg orally or 1.8 mg/kg IV
granisetron[b] *gra-NI-se-tron*	Sustol (parenteral), Sancuso (transdermal)	Prevention of chemotherapy/radiation-induced nausea, vomiting	Headache, asthenia, diarrhea, constipation	10 mcg/kg IV; transdermal patch applied 2 days before to 5 days after chemotherapy treatment

Generic Name	Trade Name	Uses	Adverse Reactions	Dosage Ranges
ondansetron[b] *on-DAN-se-tron*	Zofran, Zuplenz	Prevention of chemotherapy-induced and postoperative nausea, vomiting, hyperemesis in pregnancy, bulimia, spinal analgesia–induced or gallbladder-induced pruritus	Headache, fatigue, drowsiness, sedation, constipation, hypoxia	8 mg orally BID or TID; 32 mg IV
palonosetron[b] *pal-oh-NOE-se-tron*	Aloxi	Prevention of chemotherapy-induced and postoperative nausea, vomiting	Headache, fatigue, fever, abdominal pain	0.25–0.5 mg in a single dose
netupitant/ palonosetron	Akynzeo	Chemotherapy-induced nausea, vomiting	Headache, fatigue, fever, abdominal pain	Dosed prior to chemotherapy
Antidopaminergics				
chlorproMAZINE *klor-PROE-ma-zeen*		Control of nausea and vomiting, intractable hiccoughs	Drowsiness, hypotension, dry mouth, nasal congestion	Nausea and vomiting: 10–25 mg orally q4–6hr; 50–100 mg rectal suppository q6–8hr; 25–50 mg IM q3–4hr Hiccoughs: 25–50 mg orally, IM, slow IV infusion
perphenazine *per-FEN-a-zeen*		Same as chlorpromazine	Same as chlorpromazine	8–16 mg/day orally in divided doses, 5–10 mg IM, IV q6hr
prochlorperazine *proe-klor-PER-a-zeen*		Control of nausea and vomiting	Same as chlorpromazine	Orally: 5–10 mg TID or QID IM, IV: 5–10 mg Rectal suppository: 25 mg BID Sustained release: 10–15 mg
promethazine *proe-METH-a-zeen*		Control of nausea and vomiting associated with anesthesia and surgery, motion sickness	Same as diphenhydramine (Benadryl)	Nausea and vomiting: 12.5–25 mg orally, IM, IV, rectally Motion sickness: 25 mg orally 1–2 hours before travel, repeat 8–12 hours
Miscellaneous Antiemetics				
aprepitant/ fosaprepitant[b] *ap-RE-pi-tant*	Emend	Prevention of chemotherapy-induced and postoperative nausea, vomiting	Headache, fatigue, stomatitis, constipation	125 mg 1 hour before chemotherapy and 80 mg daily for 3 days
dronabinol[b] *droe-NAB-i-nol*	Marinol, Syndros	Prevention of chemotherapy-induced nausea and vomiting, appetite stimulant for clients with human immunodeficiency virus infection	Drowsiness, somnolence, euphoria, dizziness, vomiting	5 mg/m² 1–3 hr before chemotherapy Appetite stimulant: 2.5 mg orally BID
nabilone[b] *NA-bi-lone*		Prevention of chemotherapy-induced nausea and vomiting	Drowsiness, vertigo, euphoria, dry mouth, psychohallucinations	1–2 mg BID up to 48 hours following chemotherapy dose
trimethobenzamide *trye-meth-oh-BEN-za-mide*	Tigan	Control of nausea and vomiting	Hypotension (IM use), Parkinson-like symptoms, blurred vision, drowsiness, dizziness	250 mg orally or 200 mg IM, rectal suppository TID or QID

These drugs are taken at least 30 min before meals and at bedtime.

[a]These drugs are sold over the counter in smaller doses than those listed for therapeutic interventions.

[b]These drugs are administered according to specific protocols; consult the order before administration.

CHAPTER REVIEW

Know Your Drugs

Clients sometimes know a medication by the brand (or trade) name and not the generic name. To help you recognize both names, match the brand name with the generic name of the same medication.

Generic Name	Brand Name
1. cimetidine	A. Nexium
2. esomeprazole	B. Pepcid
3. famotidine	C. Tagamet
4. ondansetron	D. Zofran

Calculate Medication Dosages

1. Esomeprazole 40 mg once daily is prescribed. The drug is available in 20-mg capsules. How many will the nurse administer? _____
2. Sucralfate 2 g twice daily is prescribed. The drug comes in an oral suspension sucralfate 1 g/10 mL. How many milliliters will the nurse administer in each dose? _____

Prepare for the NCLEX

RECALL THE FACTS

1. How would the nurse correctly administer an antacid to a client taking other oral medications?
   1. With the other drugs
   2. Thirty minutes before or after administration of other drugs
   3. Two hours before or after administration of other drugs
   4. In early morning and at bedtime
2. When a histamine H_2 antagonist drug is prescribed for the treatment of a peptic ulcer, the nurse monitors the client for which of the following adverse effects?
   1. Dry mouth, urinary retention
   2. Edema, tachycardia
   3. Constipation, anorexia
   4. Headache, somnolence
3. What is the most common adverse reaction the nurse would expect in a client receiving an antiemetic?
   1. Occipital headache
   2. Drowsiness
   3. Edema
   4. Nausea
4. When explaining how to use transdermal scopolamine, the nurse tells the client to apply the system to _____.
   1. a non-hairy region of the chest
   2. the upper back
   3. behind the ear
   4. the forearm

ANALYZE THE FACTS

5. *Select the most helpful resource for the nurse assisting the client to determine the best antacid to purchase.
   1. Scan magazines and newspaper ads.
   2. Discuss with the clinical pharmacist.
   3. Search the Internet for drug ads.
   4. Contact the drug company.
6. *Which of the following statements made by the client would be of concern to the nurse?
   1. "Take this pill if I feel nauseated."
   2. "I will take this antacid right before I eat."
   3. "I should avoid drinking alcoholic beverages for a while."
   4. "Eating a diet high in protein will help me feel better."
7. If a client is taking metoclopramide, which of the following behaviors indicates an irreversible condition that should be reported immediately to the primary health care provider?
   1. Muscle rigidity, dry mouth, insomnia
   2. Rhythmic, involuntary movements of the tongue, face, mouth, or jaw
   3. Muscle weakness, paralysis of the eyelids, diarrhea
   4. Dyspnea, somnolence, muscle spasms

ALTERNATE-FORMAT QUESTIONS

8. Match the antacid with the adverse reaction it causes:

1. Constipation	A. Milk of magnesia
2. Diarrhea	B. Amphojel
	C. Tums
	D. Bell/ans

9. Prochlorperazine 10 mg orally is prescribed. Use the drug label below to prepare the correct dosage. The nurse would administer _____.

NDC 00xx-0000-0x

PROCHLORPERAZINE SYRUP

5 mg/5 mL

℞ only.

10. The client is to receive 400 mg cimetidine (Tagamet) orally. Available for use is the cimetidine shown below. The nurse administers _____.

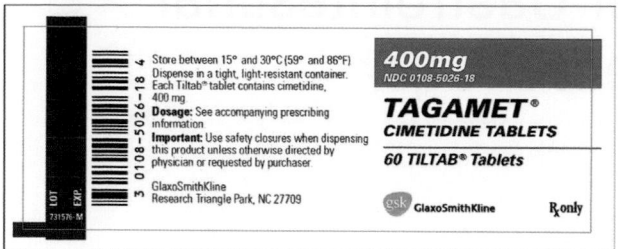

To check your answers, see Appendix F.

---

*Indicates the question is directly linked to the NCLEX-PN test plan in Appendix G.

WANT TO KNOW MORE? A wide variety of resources are available to enhance your learning and understanding of this chapter.

■ Visit thePoint for resources such as:
  • NCLEX-Style Student Review Questions
  • Journal Articles
  • Dosage Calculations
  • Drug Monographs
  • Watch and Learn Videos
  • Concepts in Action Animations
■ The *Study Guide to Accompany Introductory Clinical Pharmacology*, 12th edition, sold separately, will help you review and apply essential content.
■ ✓*PrepU* is available to help students prepare for the NCLEX-PN examination.

Lower Gastrointestinal System Drugs

Key Terms

antiflatulents   drugs that work against flatus (gas)

constipation   hardened fecal material that is difficult to pass

diarrhea   loose, watery stool

dyspepsia   fullness or epigastric discomfort

inflammatory bowel disease   inflammation of the bowel (e.g., Crohn disease and ulcerative colitis)

obstipation   watery stool leakage around a hard fecal impaction

Learning Objectives

On completion of this chapter, the student will:

1. Describe how inflammatory bowel disease alters function of the lower gastrointestinal (GI) system.
2. List the types of drugs prescribed or recommended for lower GI disorders.
3. Explain the uses, general drug actions, general adverse reactions, contraindications, precautions, and interactions associated with lower GI drugs.
4. Distinguish important preadministration and ongoing assessment activities the nurse should perform on the client taking a lower GI drug.
5. List nursing diagnoses particular to a client taking a lower GI drug.
6. Examine ways to promote an optimal response to therapy, how to manage common adverse reactions, and important points to keep in mind when educating clients about the use of lower GI drugs.

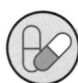 **Drug Classes**

Inflammatory Bowel Disease	Antidiarrheals
• Aminosalicylates	Antiflatulents
• Immunotherapy	Laxatives

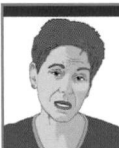 **PHARMACOLOGY IN PRACTICE**

Betty Peterson comes into the clinic and states, "Things just aren't right." During your assessment you learn she has become constipated after taking a cold preparation recently. After reading this chapter, determine why Betty has constipation and what should be recommended to help her.

The large intestine is responsible for the absorption of water and some of the nutrients from the food and fluids we eat. The speed of transit determines what will be absorbed. Transit of contents rapidly through the bowel is called **diarrhea**. When contents move sluggishly, more water is absorbed, and the fecal material gets harder, resulting in **constipation**. Transit can be triggered by many things. Illness, such as irritable bowel syndrome (IBS) or ulcerative colitis; bacterial infection; or drugs such as anti-infectives can make transit faster, resulting in diarrhea. Conditions such as Parkinson disease can slow the bowel, causing constipation. Treatment with opioid drugs and the after effects of abdominal surgery can also cause constipation.

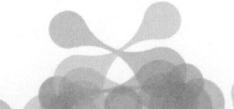

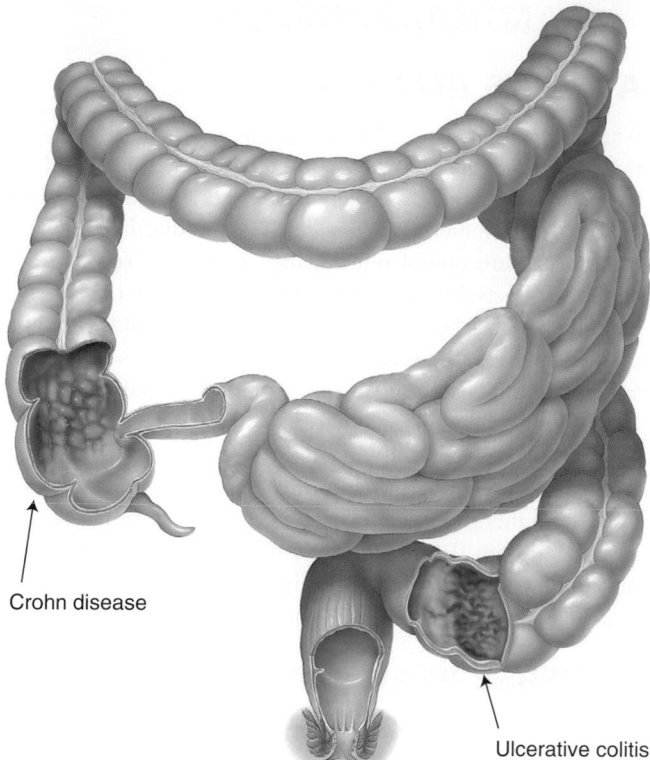

FIGURE 39.1 Examples of inflammatory bowel diseases. (Courtesy of Anatomical Chart Co.)

Crohn disease

Ulcerative colitis

Conditions that affect the function of the lower GI system can have a significant impact on activities of daily living; if proper absorption does not occur, people may not have the energy to engage in activities. One such condition that affects function is **inflammatory bowel disease** (IBD; Fig. 39.1). Another condition, IBS, also affects the lower GI system. The pain and bloating of a sluggish bowel or fear of stool incontinence may prevent people from socializing, again affecting daily life. The drugs described in this chapter affect the function of the bowel. Antidiarrheals and laxatives, as well as drugs to treat IBD and IBS, are presented. Some of the more common drugs are listed in the Summary Drug Table: Lower Gastrointestinal System Drugs.

INFLAMMATORY BOWEL DISEASE

According to the Crohn's and Colitis Foundation of America (2021), as many as 1.6 million Americans have IBD. The term IBD is used collectively for Crohn disease and ulcerative colitis, diseases that cause inflammation in the intestines. The cause of these diseases is unknown, but a number of genes have been identified that are associated with IBD. It is thought that genetic susceptibility and a virus or bacterial organism interacting with the body's immune system may be the cause (CCFA, 2021). Clinical manifestations of Crohn disease include abdominal pain and distention. As the disease progresses, other GI symptoms present, such as

anorexia, diarrhea, weight loss, dehydration, and nutritional deficiencies. Ulcerative colitis has a more abrupt onset; clients experience the sudden need to defecate, resulting in severe, blood- and mucus-filled diarrhea or no stool at all. Pain and fatigue accompany this disorder as well. No evidence has been found to support the theory that IBD is caused by tension, anxiety, or any other psychological factor or disorder (NIH, 2012). Drugs used to treat IBD include antibiotics, corticosteroids, biologic agents, and aminosalicylates. Aminosalicylates are described in this chapter; other drugs used in the treatment of IBD are included in their respective chapters.

AMINOSALICYLATES

ACTIONS AND USES

Aminosalicylates are aspirin-like compounds with anti-inflammatory action. You may also hear them called 5-aminosalicylate acid or 5-ASA medications. The drugs exert a topical anti-inflammatory effect in the bowel. The exact mechanism of action of these drugs is unknown. The aminosalicylates are used to treat Crohn disease and ulcerative colitis as well as other inflammatory diseases.

ADVERSE REACTIONS

Because these drugs are topical anti-inflammatory drugs, the most common adverse reactions happen in the GI system and include abdominal pain, nausea, and diarrhea. Other general adverse reactions include headache, dizziness, fever, and weakness.

CONTRAINDICATIONS AND PRECAUTIONS

Aminosalicylates are contraindicated in clients with a known hypersensitivity to the drugs or salicylate-containing drugs. In addition, these drugs are contraindicated in clients who have hypersensitivity to sulfonamides and sulfites or intestinal obstruction, and in children younger than 2 years. Aminosalicylates are pregnancy category B drugs (except olsalazine, which is in pregnancy category C); all are used with caution during pregnancy and lactation (safety has not been established).

LASA ALERT

The following drugs may sound alike; be sure to clarify when they are ordered:

Drug Name	*Sounds Like*
Colazal	Clozaril

Drugs that look like a similar drug are noted in the Summary Drug Tables of each chapter.

INTERACTIONS

The following interactions may occur when an aminosalicylate is administered with another agent:

Interacting Drug	Common Use	Effect of Interaction
Digoxin	Cardiac problems	Reduced absorption of digoxin
Methotrexate	Cancer and autoimmune conditions	Increased risk of immunosuppression
Oral hypoglycemic drugs	Diabetes mellitus management	Decreased blood glucose level
Warfarin	Blood thinner	Increased risk of bleeding

Immunomodulators and biologics are playing a greater role in the treatment of IBD. Although these drugs are not aminosalicylates, the biologic agents are being developed for a number of conditions that are caused by issues of immunity (see Unit 12). The immunomodulators include drugs such as infliximab (Remicade), which works to suppress the body's immune reactions. At one time reserved for those who did not respond to aminosalicylates or corticosteroids, immunotherapy is becoming more prevalent for both induction and remission of inflammatory bowel activity (Bhattacharya & Osterman, 2020).

PRACTICE CONSIDERATIONS

Alosetron is a 5-HT$_3$ receptor antagonist (like the antiemetics) used to treat IBS. It was temporarily pulled off market in the early 2000s because of an adverse reaction of significantly reducing blood supply to the colon (ischemic colitis). After changes were made, the US Food and Drug Administration (FDA) has approved the drug for administration without REMS oversite and guidelines restricting use to female clients only.

Clients should be alerted to call their health care provider if they have stomach pain, become constipated, or pass bloody stools. Be aware that Lotronex can be confused with Lovenox or Protonix.

 Herbal Considerations

Chamomile has several uses in traditional herbal therapy, including as a mild sedative and for treatment of digestive upsets, menstrual cramps, and stomach ulcers. It has been used topically for skin irritation and inflammation. Chamomile is on the FDA list of herbs generally recognized as safe. It is one of the most popular teas in Europe. When used as an infusion, it appears to produce an antispasmodic effect on the smooth muscle of the GI tract and to protect against the development of stomach ulcers. Although the herb is generally safe and nontoxic, the infusion is prepared from the pollen-filled flower heads and has resulted in mild symptoms of contact dermatitis to severe anaphylactic reactions in individuals hypersensitive to ragweed, asters, and chrysanthemums (DerMarderosian & Beutler, 2003).

 # ANTIDIARRHEALS

ACTIONS AND USES

Antidiarrheals are used in the treatment of diarrhea. Difenoxin (Motofen) and diphenoxylate (Lomotil) are chemically related to opioid drugs; therefore, they decrease intestinal peristalsis, which often is increased when the client has diarrhea. Because these drugs are opioid related, they may have sedative and euphoric effects, but no analgesic activity. A drug dependence potential exists; therefore, the drugs are combined with atropine (a cholinergic blocking drug), which causes dry mouth and other mild adverse effects. Abuse potential is reduced because of these unpleasant adverse effects.

Loperamide (Imodium) acts directly on the muscle wall of the bowel to slow motility and is not related to the opioids. It therefore is also used in treating chronic diarrhea associated with IBD. The drug crofelemer blocks the secretion of chloride, which causes high water volume loss in the diarrhea associated with HIV and AIDS.

ADVERSE REACTIONS

Gastrointestinal System Reactions
- Anorexia, nausea, vomiting, and constipation
- Abdominal discomfort, pain, and distention

OTHER SYSTEM REACTIONS

- Dizziness, drowsiness, and headache
- Sedation and euphoria
- Rash

CONTRAINDICATIONS AND PRECAUTIONS

These drugs are contraindicated in clients whose diarrhea is associated with organisms that can harm the intestinal mucosa (*Escherichia coli*, *Salmonella*, and *Shigella* spp.). Clients with pseudomembranous colitis, abdominal pain of unknown origin, and obstructive jaundice also should not take antidiarrheals. Antidiarrheal drugs are contraindicated in children younger than 2 years.

(!) NURSING ALERT

When taking over-the-counter (OTC) antidiarrheal drugs, if diarrhea persists for more than 2 days the client should discontinue use and seek treatment from the primary health care provider.

The antidiarrheal drugs are used cautiously in clients with severe hepatic impairment. Antidiarrheals are classified as pregnancy category C drugs and should be used cautiously during pregnancy and lactation. Loperamide is a pregnancy category B drug but is not recommended for use during pregnancy and lactation. Although crofelemer is labeled pregnancy category C, it has not been studied adequately for pregnancy, lactation, and pediatric use.

LASA ALERT

The following drugs may sound alike; be sure to clarify when they are ordered:

Drug Name	Sounds Like
Imodium	Indocin
Lomotil	LaMICtal, LamISIL, lamoTRIgine, Lanoxin, Lasix, loperamide
loperamide	furosemide, Lomotil

Drugs that look like a similar drug are noted in the Summary Drug Tables of each chapter.

INTERACTIONS

The following interactions may occur when an antidiarrheal drug is administered with another agent:

Interacting Drug	Common Use	Effects of Interaction
Antihistamines, opioids, sedatives, or hypnotics	Allergy treatment (antihistamines), sedation, or pain relief	Increased risk of central nervous system (CNS) depression
Antihistamines and general antidepressants	Allergy relief and depression management	Increased cholinergic blocking adverse reactions
Monoamine oxidase inhibitor (MAOI) antidepressants	Depression management	Increased risk of hypertensive crisis

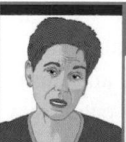 **PHARMACOLOGY IN PRACTICE**

ASSESSMENT
When assessing a client's use of OTC antidiarrheals, the client should be taught to seek treatment from a primary health care provider if diarrhea persists for how long?
1. 1 day
2. 12 hr
3. 2 days
4. 7 days

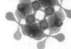 ## ANTIFLATULENTS

ACTIONS

Simethicone and charcoal are used as **antiflatulents** (drugs that reduce flatus or gas in the intestinal tract). These drugs do not absorb or remove gas; rather, they act to help the body release the gas by belching or flatus (passing gas). Simethicone has a defoaming action that disperses and prevents the formation of gas pockets in the intestine. Charcoal helps bind gas for expulsion.

USES

Antiflatulents are used to relieve painful symptoms of excess gas in the digestive tract that may be caused by the following:

- Postoperative gaseous distention and air swallowing
- **Dyspepsia** (fullness or epigastric discomfort)
- Peptic ulcer
- IBS or diverticulosis

In addition to its use for the relief of intestinal gas, charcoal may be used in the prevention of nonspecific pruritus associated with kidney dialysis treatment and as an antidote in poisoning. Simethicone is in some antacid products, such as Mylanta Liquid and Di-Gel Liquid.

ADVERSE REACTIONS

No adverse reactions have been reported with the use of antiflatulents.

CONTRAINDICATIONS AND PRECAUTIONS

Antiflatulents are contraindicated in clients with known hypersensitivity to any components of the drug. The pregnancy category of simethicone has not been determined; because it is not absorbed, it may be safe for use during pregnancy, although the primary health care provider should be consulted whenever any drug is to be taken. Charcoal is a pregnancy category C drug.

INTERACTIONS

There may be a decreased effectiveness of other drugs because of adsorption by charcoal, which can also adsorb other drugs in the GI tract. There are no known interactions with simethicone.

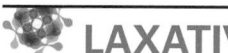 ## LAXATIVES

ACTIONS

There are various types of laxatives (see the Summary Drug Table: Lower Gastrointestinal System Drugs). The action of each laxative is somewhat different, yet they all produce the same result—relief of constipation. The manner of action of the various laxative groups is explained in Box 39.1.

USES

A laxative is most often prescribed for the short-term relief or prevention of constipation. Specific uses of laxatives include:

- *Stimulant, emollient, and saline laxatives*—evacuate the colon for rectal and bowel examinations
- *Stool softeners or mineral oil*—prevention of strain during defecation (after anorectal surgery or a myocardial infarction)
- *Psyllium and polycarbophil*—IBS and diverticular disease
- *Hyperosmotic (lactulose) agents*—reduction of blood ammonia levels in hepatic encephalopathy

when bulk-forming laxatives are administered without adequate fluid intake or in clients with intestinal stenosis.

 Chronic Care Considerations

The very young, the very old, and debilitated clients are at greatest risk for aspiration of mineral oil into the lungs when it is taken orally for constipation. Aspiration of mineral oil can lead to a lipid pneumonitis.

CONTRAINDICATIONS AND PRECAUTIONS

Laxatives are contraindicated in clients with known hypersensitivity and those with persistent abdominal pain, nausea, vomiting of unknown cause, or signs of acute appendicitis, fecal impaction, intestinal obstruction, or acute hepatitis. These drugs are used only as directed because excessive or prolonged use may cause physical dependence on them for normal bowel movements.

Magnesium is used cautiously in clients with any degree of renal impairment. Laxatives are used cautiously in clients with rectal bleeding, in pregnant women, and during lactation. The following laxatives are pregnancy category C drugs: cascara sagrada, docusate, glycerin, phenolphthalein, magnesium, and senna. These drugs are used during pregnancy only when the benefits clearly outweigh the risks to the fetus.

INTERACTIONS

- Mineral oil may impair the GI absorption of fat-soluble vitamins (A, D, E, and K).
- Laxatives may reduce absorption of other drugs present in the GI tract by combining with them chemically or hastening their passage through the intestinal tract.
- When surfactants are administered with mineral oil, they may increase mineral oil absorption.
- Milk, antacids, histamine H_2 antagonists, and proton pump inhibitors should not be administered 1–2 hr before bisacodyl tablets because the enteric coating may dissolve early (before reaching the intestinal tract), resulting in gastric lining irritation or dyspepsia and decreasing the laxative effect of the drug.

PRACTICE CONSIDERATIONS

Constipation due to opiate use is an adverse reaction that never develops tolerance. Methylnaltrexone (Relistor) acts by blocking opioid binding to receptors specifically in the GI tract, which reduces the decreased motility and transit delays that cause opiate-induced constipation.

ADVERSE REACTIONS

Constipation may occur as an adverse drug reaction. When the client has constipation as an adverse reaction to another drug, the primary health care provider may prescribe a stool softener or another laxative to prevent constipation during the drug therapy. Box 39.2 lists some of the drug classifications known to cause constipation.

Laxatives may cause diarrhea and a loss of water and electrolytes, abdominal pain or discomfort, nausea, vomiting, perianal irritation, fainting, bloating, flatulence, cramps, and weakness.

Prolonged use of a laxative can result in serious electrolyte imbalances, as well as the "laxative habit," that is, dependence on a laxative to have a bowel movement. Some of these products contain tartrazine (a yellow food dye), which may cause allergic-type reactions (including bronchial asthma) in susceptible individuals. Obstruction of the esophagus, stomach, small intestine, and colon has occurred

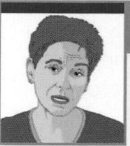

PHARMACOLOGY IN PRACTICE

SAFE DRUG ADMINISTRATION

A nurse is caring for a client taking a bulk laxative for the treatment of watery, loose stools. The overuse of the drug results in constipation in the client. What instruction should the nurse offer the client to avoid constipation?
1. Take commercial electrolytes.
2. Take the drug with food.
3. Drink an increased amount of fluid.
4. Avoid milk products.

inhibiting lipase, an enzyme that breaks down dietary fat. As a result, the fat eaten is indigestible and passes through the intestine without being absorbed. Although this drug is not a laxative, the action of the drug results in loose stools and increased flatus. Adverse reactions at the start of therapy may also include fecal urgency and incontinence with fat or oily stools. These typically diminish by the fourth week of therapy, yet can occur again when a meal high in fat (over 30%) is eaten. When taking a history of a client with diarrhea or increased flatus, be sure to review medications use for agents such as orlistat. This drug should not be used if the client has gallstones.

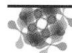

WEIGHT MANAGEMENT AGENTS

Orlistat (Xenical or Alli) is a drug used for obesity management (body mass index over 30). The drug works by

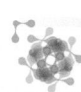

NURSING PROCESS—STEPS TO BUILDING CLINICAL JUDGMENT
Client Receiving a Drug for a Lower Gastrointestinal Condition

ASSESSMENT

Preadministration Assessment
Data gathering suggestions before the initial administration of a lower GI drug include:
Objective data

- Vital signs (temperature, pulse, respirations, and blood pressure)
- Auscultate for bowel sounds
- Palpate for abdomen, note guarding or discomfort
- Weigh the client
- Laboratory tests—electrolyte panel if severe diarrhea is evident.

Subjective data

- Description of type and intensity of symptoms (e.g., pain, discomfort, diarrhea or constipation, stool description)
- Remedies client has attempted before seeking treatment
- Medical history/drug therapy (list of all current drugs and supplements taken)

Note when a client describes their bowel patterns—loose stool may indicate diarrhea; however, hypoactive bowel sounds in severe cases of **obstipation** (liquid stool leaked around the fecal mass, presenting as loose stool) are evidence that the client is constipated, which would indicate very different drug therapy.

Ongoing Assessment
Assess the client receiving one of these drugs for relief of symptoms (e.g., diarrhea, pain, or constipation). Instruct the client regarding loose, frequent stools and diarrhea. The client may report multiple trips to the bathroom with formed stool as diarrhea. For the best treatment you need

to know the difference so you can report relief or continued symptoms to the primary health care provider. Monitoring vital signs if the client has severe diarrhea may help you to discover issues such as dehydration in addition to the bowel problem. Observe the client for adverse drug reactions associated with the specific GI drug being administered and report any adverse reactions to the primary health care provider before the next dose is due (Fig. 39.2).

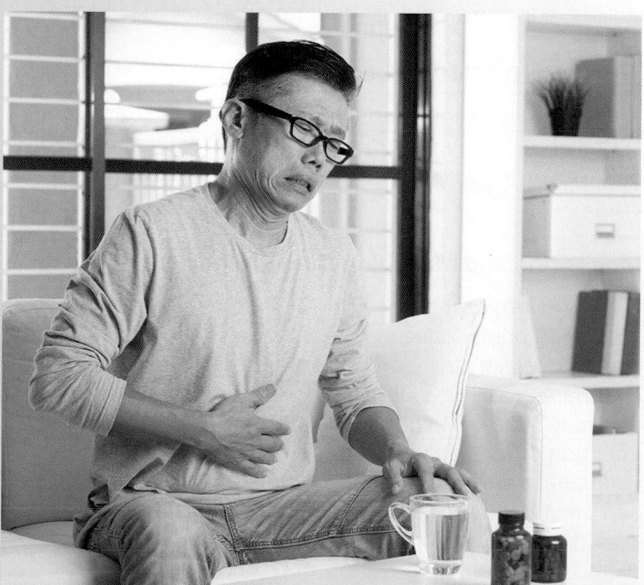

FIGURE 39.2 Disruption in bowel routine can have an impact on the activities of daily living for the client.

NURSING DIAGNOSES

A drug-specific nursing diagnosis is the following:

- **Risk for dehydration** related to diarrhea

Nursing diagnoses related to drug administration are discussed in Chapter 4.

PLANNING

The expected outcomes for the client depend on the reason for administration of the drug but may include an optimal response to drug therapy, support of client needs related to the management of adverse reactions, and confidence in an understanding of the medication regimen.

IMPLEMENTATION

Promoting an Optimal Response to Therapy

Ways in which you can help promote an optimal response to therapy when administering lower GI drugs follow.

Antidiarrheals

When diarrhea is severe, these drugs may be ordered to be given after each loose bowel movement. This may concern the client that the opposite will happen, that is, becoming constipated. Ask the client to describe or check each bowel movement before making a decision to administer the drug. Crofelemer is a drug taken twice daily orally. It is a delayed-release drug and should not be crushed or chewed.

Laxatives

Give bulk-producing or stool-softening laxatives with a full glass of water or juice. The administration of a bulk-producing laxative is followed by an additional full glass of water. Mineral oil preferably is given to the client with an empty stomach in the evening. Immediately before administration, thoroughly mix and stir laxatives that are in powder, flake, or granule form. If the laxative has an unpleasant or salty taste, explain this to the client. The taste of some of these preparations may be disguised by chilling, adding to juice, or pouring over cracked ice.

> **! NURSING ALERT**
>
> Because activated charcoal can absorb other drugs in the GI tract, when used as an antiflatulent it should not be taken 2 hr before or 1 hr after the administration of other drugs.

Monitoring and Managing Client Needs

Risk for Dehydration

Notify the primary health care provider if the client experiences an elevation in body temperature, severe abdominal pain, or abdominal rigidity or distention because this may indicate a complication of the disorder, such as infection or intestinal perforation. If diarrhea is severe, additional treatment measures, such as intravenous fluids and electrolyte replacement, may be necessary.

If diarrhea is chronic, encourage the client to drink extra fluids. Weak tea, water, bouillon, or a commercial electrolyte preparation may be used.

Monitor fluid intake and output closely. In some instances, the primary health care provider may prescribe an oral electrolyte supplement to replace electrolytes lost by frequent loose stools. Clients with fluid volume losses taking drugs that cause drowsiness or dizziness are at greater risk for injury. The client may require assistance with ambulatory activities. For perianal irritation caused by loose stools, instruct the client or caregiver to cleanse the area with mild soap and water after each bowel movement, dry the area with a soft cloth, and apply an emollient, such as petrolatum.

When a laxative is administered, document the bowel movement results on the client's chart. If excessive bowel movements or severe, prolonged diarrhea occurs, or if the laxative is ineffective, notify the primary health care provider. If a laxative is ordered for constipation, encourage a liberal fluid intake and an increase in foods high in fiber to prevent a repeat of this problem.

Educating the Client and Family

Because clients frequently begin use of OTC products for lower GI conditions before discussing with health care providers, develop teaching plans to include the following general points about these medications at any teaching session:

Antidiarrheals

- Do not exceed the recommended dosage.
- Observe caution when driving or performing other hazardous tasks because the drug may cause drowsiness.
  - 🍷 Avoid the use of alcohol or other CNS depressants (e.g., tranquilizers, sleeping pills) and other nonprescription drugs unless use has been approved by the primary health care provider.
- Notify the primary health care provider if diarrhea persists or becomes more severe.

Antiflatulents

- Take simethicone after each meal and at bedtime. Thoroughly chew tablets because complete particle dispersion enhances antiflatulent action.
- Notify the health care provider if symptoms are not relieved within several days.

Laxatives

- Avoid long-term use of these products unless use of the product has been recommended by the primary health care provider. Long-term use may result in the "laxative habit," which is dependence on a laxative to have a normal bowel movement. Constipation may also occur with overuse of these drugs. Laxatives are not to be used for weight loss. Read and follow the directions on the label.
- Do not use these products in the presence of abdominal pain, nausea, or vomiting.
- Notify the primary health care provider if constipation is not relieved or if rectal bleeding or other symptoms occur.
- To avoid constipation, drink plenty of fluids, get exercise, and eat foods high in bulk or roughage.
- Senna—may discolor urine: pink-red, red-violet, red-brown, yellow-brown, or black.

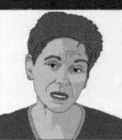

PHARMACOLOGY IN PRACTICE

MANAGING NEEDS

A nurse is caring for a radiation outpatient experiencing treatment-related diarrhea. Which of the following instructions should the nurse include in the teaching plan for this client? Select all that apply.
1. Get sufficient exercise.
2. If drowsy, observe caution when driving.
3. Avoid the use of alcohol.
4. Eat a variety of fruits and vegetables.
5. Avoid the use of nonprescription drugs.

EVALUATION

- Therapeutic drug effect is achieved, and bowel movements are appropriate for the client's normal routine.

- Adverse reactions are identified, reported to the primary health care provider, and managed successfully through appropriate nursing interventions:
  - Client maintains an adequate fluid volume.
- Client and family express confidence and demonstrate an understanding of the drug regimen.

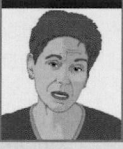

PHARMACOLOGY IN PRACTICE

USING CLINICAL REASONING

Betty shares the medications she is currently taking:

amitriptyline
acetaminophen
diphenhydramine cold preparation
ferrous sulfate
lisinopril/HCTZ

Based on this list of medications being taken, what type of laxative preparation would be best for Betty's constipation problem?

KEY POINTS

■ The lower GI system includes the small and large intestines. Other organs secrete into the system but are not mentioned in this chapter. Absorption of both nutrients and fluids occurs in the intestines, as does the exchange of waste products.

■ Drugs to reduce inflammation or an immune response are used for chronic conditions such as inflammatory bowel disease.

■ Drugs that slow down transit or speed up the process maybe used by clients at home or as part of an institutional treatment plan.

■ Adverse reactions include abdominal pain or perianal irritation associated with moving or slowing content transit in the bowel, or issues associated with fluid depletion such as dizziness, drowsiness, or headache.

■ Multiple OTC products exist to treat GI symptoms. Clients need confidence in understanding how to purchase and take these products because the majority of users do so without health care provider supervision.

SUMMARY DRUG TABLE
Lower Gastrointestinal System Drugs

Generic Name	Trade Name	Uses	Adverse Reactions	Dosage Ranges
Drugs Used to Treat Inflammatory Bowel Disease				
Aminosalicylates (5-ASA)				
balsalazide bal-SAL-a-zide	Colazal	Active ulcerative colitis	Headache, abdominal pain	2250 mg orally TID for 8 weeks
mesalamine me-SAL-a-meen	Asacol HD, Pentasa, Rowasa (rectal form)	Active ulcerative colitis, proctosigmoiditis or proctitis	Headache, abdominal pain, nausea	800–1000 mg orally TID or QID Suspension enema: 4 g daily
olsalazine ole-SAL-a-zeen	Dipentum	Maintenance of remission of ulcerative colitis	Diarrhea, abdominal pain and cramping	1 g/day orally in two divided doses
sulfaSALAzine sul-fa-SAL-a-zeen	Azulfidine	Ulcerative colitis, rheumatoid arthritis	Headache, nausea, anorexia, vomiting, gastric distress, reduced sperm count	Initial: 3–4 g/day orally in divided doses Maintenance: 2 g orally QID

Continued

SUMMARY DRUG TABLE (continued)
Lower Gastrointestinal System Drugs

Generic Name	Trade Name	Uses	Adverse Reactions	Dosage Ranges
Biologics for Bowel Disorders				
adalimumab a-da-LIM-yoo-mab	Humira	Crohn disease, ulcerative colitis	Irritation at injection site, increased risk of infections	160 mg subcut day 1, 80 mg in 2 weeks, 40 mg every 2 weeks
certolizumab cer-to-LIZ-u-mab	Cimzia	Crohn disease, rheumatoid arthritis	URI and urinary tract infection (UTI) symptoms	400 mg subcut every 2 weeks or monthly
golimumab goe-LIM-ue-mab	Simponi	Ulcerative colitis, arthritis—psoriatic, rheumatoid	URI symptoms, rhinitis, irritation at injection site, increased risk of infections	50 mg subcut weekly
infliximab in-FLIKS-e-mab	Remicade	Crohn disease, ulcerative colitis	Fever, chills, headache	5 mg/kg IV infusion at specified weekly intervals
natalizumab na-ta-LIZ-u-mab	Tysabri	Crohn disease, multiple sclerosis	Headache, muscle aches, diarrhea	300 mg IV every 4 weeks
tofacitinib toe-fa-SYE-ti-nib	Xeljanz	Ulcerative colitis, arthritis—psoriatic, rheumatoid	URI symptoms, rhinitis	5–11 mg orally, 1–2 times daily
ustekinumab you-stek-in-YOU-mab	Stelara	Crohn Disease, ulcerative colitis, plaque/arthritic psoriasis	Infection potential, URI	Based on weight, IV or subcut
vedolizumab ve-doe-LIZ-ue-mab	Entyvio	Crohn Disease, ulcerative colitis	Headache, URI, arthralgia	300 mg IV infusion every 8 weeks
Miscellaneous Drugs for Bowel Disorders				
alosetron a-LOE-se-tron	Lotronex	Second-line treatment of female irritable bowel syndrome (IBS) with severe diarrhea	Gastric distress, hemorrhoids, constipation	0.5–1 mg orally twice daily; Special permission must be obtained for therapy
alvimopan al-VI-moe-pan	Entereg	Accelerate upper/lower GI recovery following surgery	Indigestion, hypokalemia, fatigue	12 mg orally twice daily for no more than 15 doses
eluxadoline el-ux-AD-oh-leen	Viberzi	IBS with diarrhea	Constipation, nausea	75–100 mg orally twice daily
linaclotide lin-AK-loe-tide	Linzess	Chronic idiopathic constipation, IBS with constipation	Diarrhea	145–290 mcg orally daily
methylnaltrexone meth-il-nal-TREKS-one	Relistor	Opioid-induced constipation	Gastric distress, nausea, vomiting, diarrhea	450 mg orally, 12 mg subcut once daily
plecanatide ple-KAN-a-tide	Trulance	Chronic idiopathic constipation, IBS with constipation	Diarrhea	3 mg orally once daily
tenapanor ten-A-pa-nor	Ibsrela	IBS with diarrhea	Diarrhea	50 mg orally twice daily
Antidiarrheals				
Bismuth BIZ-muth	Bismatrol, Pepto-Bismol, Pink Bismuth	Nausea, diarrhea, abdominal cramps, *Helicobacter pylori* infection with duodenal ulcer	Same as difenoxin	Two tablets or 30 mL orally every 30 min to 1 hr, up to 8 doses in 24 hr
crofelemer kroe-FEL-e-mer	Mytesi	HIV/AIDS-related diarrhea	URI, bronchitis	125 mg orally twice daily
difenoxin with atropine dye-fen-OKS-in, A-troe-peen	Motofen	Symptomatic relief of acute diarrhea	Dry skin and mucous membranes, nausea, constipation, lightheadedness	Initial dose: two tablets orally, then one tablet after each loose stool (not to exceed eight tablets per day)

Generic Name	Trade Name	Uses	Adverse Reactions	Dosage Ranges
Antidiarrheals				
diphenoxylate with atropine *dye-fen-OKS-i-late*	Lomotil	Same as difenoxin	Same as difenoxin	5 mg orally QID
loperamide *loe-PER-a-mide*	Imodium,	Same as difenoxin	Same as difenoxin	Initial dose 4 mg orally; then 2 mg after each loose stool (not to exceed 16 mg/day)
tincture of opium	Paregoric	Severe diarrhea	Somnolence, constipation	0.6 mL orally QID
Antiflatulents				
Charcoal	CharcoCaps, Flatulex (combined with simethicone)	Intestinal gas, diarrhea, poisoning antidote	Vomiting, constipation, diarrhea, black stools	520 mg orally after meals (not to exceed 4–16 g/day)
simethicone *sye-METH-i-kone*	Gas-X, Mylicon, Maalox Anti-Gas, Mylanta Gas	Postoperative distention, dyspepsia, IBS, peptic ulcer	Bloating, constipation, diarrhea, heartburn	40–125 mg orally QID after meals and at bedtime
Laxatives				
Bulk-Producing Laxatives				
methylcellulose *meth-il-SEL-yoo-lose*	Citrucel, Unifiber	Relief of constipation, IBS, severe watery diarrhea	Diarrhea, nausea, vomiting, bloating, flatulence, cramping, perianal irritation, fainting	Follow directions given on the container
psyllium *SIL-i-yum*	Fiberall, Genfiber, Metamucil, Perdiem	Same as methylcellulose	Same as methylcellulose	Powder, granules, or wafers taken as directed on package
polycarbophil *pol-i-KAR-boe-fil*	Equalactin, FiberCon	Same as methylcellulose	Same as methylcellulose	1 g daily to QID or as needed (do not exceed 4 g in 24 hr)
Emollients				
mineral oil	Kondremul	Relief of constipation, fecal impaction	Perianal discomfort and itching due to anal seepage	15–45 mL orally at bedtime
Stool Softeners/Surfactants				
docusate (dioctyl; DDS) *DOK-yoo-sate*	Colace, Ex-Lax Stool Softener, Modane Soft, Surfak Liquigels	Relief of constipation, prevention of straining during bowel movement	Diarrhea, nausea, vomiting, bloating, flatulence, cramping, perianal irritation, fainting	Follow directions given on the container; comes in enema form
Hyperosmotic Agents				
glycerin *GLIS-er-in*	Colace Suppositories, Sani-Supp, Fleet Babylax	Relief of constipation	Same as docusate	Rectal suppository, use as directed
lactitol *LAK-ti-tol*	Pizensy	Chronic idiopathic constipation, hepatic encephalopathy	Same as docusate	10–20 g once daily
lactulose *LAK-tyoo-lose*	Constulose, Enulose, Generlac, Kristalose	Relief of constipation, hepatic encephalopathy	Same as docusate	Constipation: 15–30 mL/day orally Hepatic encephalopathy: 30–45 mL orally QID, may give enema form
lubiprostone *loo-bi-PROS-tone*	Amitiza	Chronic idiopathic constipation	Headache, nausea, diarrhea	24 mcg orally BID

Continued

SUMMARY DRUG TABLE (continued)
Lower Gastrointestinal System Drugs

Generic Name	Trade Name	Uses	Adverse Reactions	Dosage Ranges
Irritant or Stimulant Laxatives				
bisacodyl *bis-a-KOE-dil*	Dulcolax, Correctol	Relief of constipation	Diarrhea, nausea, vomiting, bloating, flatulence, cramping, perianal irritation	Tablets: 10–15 mg daily orally Rectal suppositories: 10 mg daily; comes in enema form
sennosides *SEN-na-sides*	Agoral, Senokot	Relief of constipation	Same as biscadoyl	Follow directions given on the container
Saline Laxatives				
magnesium preparations	Milk of Magnesia, Magnesium Citrate, Fleets (enema preparation)	Evacuate colon for endoscopy, relieve constipation	Same as docusate sodium	Follow directions given on the container
Bowel Evacuants				
polyethylene glycol (PEG) solution *pol-i-ETH-i-leen*	MiraLAX	Relieve constipation	Same as sodium docusate	Follow directions given on the container
polyethylene glycol-electrolyte solution (PEG-ES) *pol-ee-eth'-ih-leen*	Colyte, GoLYTELY, NuLYTELY, OCL	Evacuate colon for endoscopy, relieve constipation	Same as sodium docusate	4 L oral solution to be drunk in 3 hr
sodium picosulfate/ magnesium oxide/ citric acid	Clenpiq	Evacuate colon for endoscopy	Same as sodium docusate	Follow directions given on the container

CHAPTER REVIEW

Know Your Drugs

Clients sometimes know a medication by the brand (or trade) name and not the generic name. To help you recognize both names, match the brand name with the generic name of the same medication.

Generic Name	Brand Name
1. diphenoxylate	A. Colace
2. docusate	B. Lomotil
3. polyethylene glycol	C. Metamucil
4. psyllium	D. MiraLAX

Calculate Medication Dosages

1. Balsalazide (Colazal) 2250 mg orally TID is prescribed. If the drug comes in 750-mg capsules, the nurse administers _____ capsules with each dose.
2. Diphenoxylate (Lomotil) one tablet BID is prescribed. If the drug comes in 2.5-mg tablets, how much diphenoxylate will the client take in 24 hr?

Prepare for the NCLEX

RECALL THE FACTS

1. In which area of the GI tract is water primarily reabsorbed?
   1. Stomach
   2. Small intestine
   3. Large intestine (colon)
   4. Pancreas

2. Which of the following is the best description of the cause of Crohn disease?
   1. Somatic response to psychological stress
   2. Infection due to bacteria or parasites
   3. Inflammatory response in the colon
   4. Precancerous stage in the bowel

3. The client asks how stool softeners relieve constipation. Which of the following would be the best response by the nurse? Stool softeners relieve constipation by _____.
   1. stimulating the walls of the intestine
   2. promoting the retention of sodium in the fecal mass
   3. promoting water retention in the fecal mass
   4. lubricating the intestinal walls

4. The nurse administers antidiarrheal drugs _____.
   1. after each loose bowel movement
   2. hourly until diarrhea ceases
   3. with food
   4. three times a day

5. The pregnancy category for the antiflatulent drug simethicone is _____.
   1. pregnancy category A
   2. pregnancy category C
   3. pregnancy category X
   4. pregnancy category unknown

ANALYZE THE FACTS

6. When recording the administration of diphenoxylate for multiple loose stools:
   1. document the daily number of drugs given
   2. record all stools once each shift
   3. indicate all stools on the medication administration record (MAR) next to the drug
   4. document each dose on the MAR

7. Which of the following points should be included in a teaching plan for a client taking a laxative?
   1. They may be used for minor weight loss
   2. Drink more fluid and eat more high-fiber foods
   3. The abdominal pain is probably gas buildup
   4. Using daily promotes good bowel health

8. Why is atropine put in an antidiarrheal?
   1. To neutralize acid
   2. To kill bacteria in the bowel
   3. To reduce addictive property
   4. To promote bowel health

ALTERNATE-FORMAT QUESTIONS

9. Harmful drug interactions exist when aminosalicylates are taken with the following drugs. **Select all that apply.**
   1. Cardiotonics
   2. Beta-adrenergic blockers
   3. Oral hypoglycemics
   4. Anticoagulants

10. *A client is to drink 4 L of polyethylene glycol electrolyte solution (GoLYTELY) the night before an outpatient colonoscopy. If the directions state, "Drink 240 mL every 10 minutes," the nurse tells the client the solution must be completely drunk in _____ hours.

To check your answers, see Appendix F.

---

*Indicates the question is directly linked to the NCLEX-PN test plan in Appendix G.

WANT TO KNOW MORE? A wide variety of resources are available to enhance your learning and understanding of this chapter.
- Visit the**Point** for resources such as:
  - NCLEX-Style Student Review Questions
  - Journal Articles
  - Dosage Calculations
  - Drug Monographs
  - Watch and Learn Videos
  - Concepts in Action Animations
- The *Study Guide to Accompany Introductory Clinical Pharmacology*, 12th edition, sold separately, will help you review and apply essential content.
- ✓*PrepU* is available to help students prepare for the NCLEX-PN examination.

UNIT 10
Drugs That Affect the Endocrine System

The endocrine system consists of a group of glands situated throughout the body. The work of the endocrine system is to provide hormones (chemicals that assist in body functions) to various organs in the body. Hormones are produced and circulated through the blood to target receptors on certain cells in specific organs to assist in function. Glands that make up the endocrine system are (from head to toe) the pituitary, thyroid, pancreas, adrenal glands, and sex organs. In this unit, we will discuss them in a slightly different order.

The unit begins with a chapter about the pancreas and information on diabetes. The pancreas is part of the gastrointestinal (GI) system. This organ provides enzymes to assist in the digestion of food and provides the body with the hormone insulin to help cells use the glucose from food sources. Diabetes mellitus is a chronic condition characterized by problems with the body's production or use of insulin. According to recent studies, almost half of the adult population in the United States is either diabetic or prediabetic (Menke et al., 2015). About 30.3 million people or 9.4% of the adult population are considered diabetic (CDC, 2020). These statistics make the discussion of diabetes important and the first in this unit of drugs affecting the endocrine system. Chapter 40 discusses both insulin and the oral antidiabetic drugs used in treating diabetes mellitus.

Chapter 41 returns to the top of the head, where the pituitary gland sits at the base of the brain and helps with the function of many different organs in the body. Its hormones are secreted and sent to a variety of organs to promote and regulate growth and maturation, fluid and electrolyte balance, and metabolism. These hormones and the drugs that affect them are covered in Chapter 41. The adrenal glands are crucial in the secretion of corticosteroids, which are used to treat many conditions, these are also covered in the chapter.

An estimated 20 million Americans have some form of thyroid disease, and up to 60% of these people are unaware of their condition (ATA, 2019). Located in the lower anterior portion of the neck, the thyroid's purpose is to help control metabolism. In Chapter 42, you will learn about the function of the thyroid and its hormones as well as drugs used to supplement or reduce the function of the thyroid gland.

Last, hormones play a major role in the development of the reproductive system as people go through puberty. The ovaries in the female and the testes in the male produce hormones that aid in the development of secondary sexual characteristics such as hair, voice, and musculature. Reproduction is controlled by the secretion of hormones, too. Chapters 43 and 44 describe the function of these hormones and the drugs used to promote optimal reproductive health.

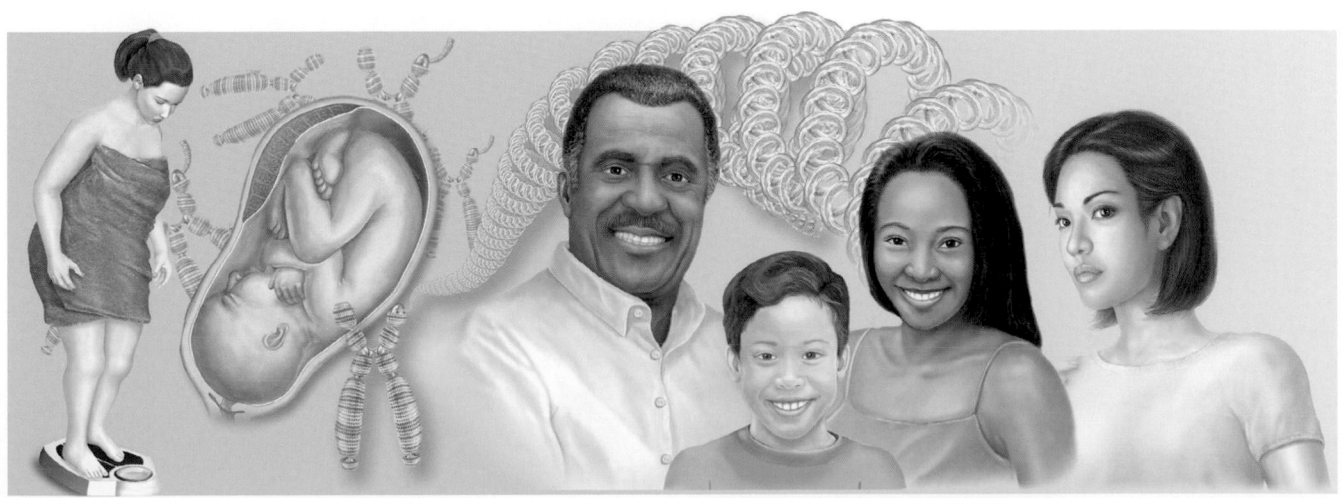

Courtesy of Anatomical Chart Co.

Antidiabetic Drugs

Key Terms

basal/bolus insulin dose the routine of taking a long-acting insulin to keep blood glucose levels stable during fasting periods and shorter-acting insulin to prevent rises in blood glucose after meals

diabetes mellitus disease in which insulin does not help glucose enter the cell

diabetic ketoacidosis (DKA) life-threatening deficiency of insulin resulting in severe hyperglycemia and excessively high levels of ketones in the blood

glucagon hormone secreted by the alpha cells of the pancreas that increase the concentration of glucose in the blood

glucometer device to monitor blood glucose level

glycosylated hemoglobin blood test that monitors average blood glucose level over a 3- to 4-month period

hyperglycemia high blood glucose (sugar) level

hypoglycemia low blood glucose (sugar) level

incretin hormones hormones that stimulate an increase of insulin from the beta cells of the pancreas; they slow gastric emptying and inhibit glucagon release

lipodystrophy atrophy of subcutaneous fat

polydipsia excessive thirst

polyphagia eating large amounts of food

polyuria increased urination

prediabetes a condition of a blood glucose higher than normal, yet not to diabetic level as evidence by an impaired glucose tolerance/fasting glucose, or metabolic syndrome

Learning Objectives

On completion of this chapter, the student will:

1. Describe the two types of diabetes mellitus.
2. Explain the types, uses, general drug actions, adverse reactions, contraindications, precautions, and interactions of the antidiabetic drugs.
3. Distinguish important preadministration and ongoing assessment activities the nurse should perform with the client taking an antidiabetic drug.
4. List nursing diagnoses particular to a client taking an antidiabetic drug.
5. Examine ways to promote an optimal response to therapy, how to manage common adverse reactions, and important points to keep in mind when educating clients about the use of antidiabetic drugs.

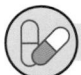 **Drug Classes**

Insulin products   Antidiabetic hypoglycemics

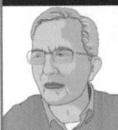 **PHARMACOLOGY IN PRACTICE**

When Mr. Phillip was seen for atrial fibrillation, it was discovered that he had not been seen by a health care provider in more than 5 years. The first priority was to stabilize his heart and coagulation status. He was then given an appointment to come to the clinic for a complete physical examination. During the clinic visit, Mr. Phillip was found to be in relatively good physical condition, yet his blood chemistries showed an elevation in his blood glucose level (153 mg/dL) and his HbA$_{1c}$ reading was 8%. When his wife was alive, he remembers she started fixing food in a different way because of the doctor's concerns about eating too much sugar. When you finish this chapter, you should better understand the meaning of these laboratory values and know what client interventions and instruction should follow.

Glucose is essential for cells to produce energy. A hormone produced by the pancreas, insulin is required for the proper use of glucose (carbohydrate) and for the proper metabolism of protein and fat in our bodies. These processes are accomplished by the release of small amounts of insulin into the bloodstream throughout the day in response to changes in blood glucose levels. In addition, insulin lowers blood glucose levels by inhibiting glucose production by the liver. Insulin also controls the storage and utilization of amino acids and fatty acids.

When insulin is not sufficiently produced to meet the demands of glucose in the blood, antidiabetic drugs help the body to stabilize and control blood glucose level. Some drugs help the body to control rising blood glucose, whereas others supplement insulin when it is not produced sufficiently by the body.

Diabetes mellitus (often referred to as simply *diabetes*) is a complicated, chronic disorder characterized either by insufficient insulin production by the beta (β) cells of the pancreas or by cellular resistance to insulin. Insulin insufficiency results in elevated blood glucose levels, or *hyperglycemia*. As a result of the disease, individuals with diabetes are at greater risk for a number of disorders, including myocardial infarction, cerebrovascular accident (stroke), blindness, kidney disease, vascular, and neurologic impairment in the extremities.

Insulin and antidiabetic drugs, along with diet and exercise, are the cornerstones of treatment for diabetes. They are used to prevent episodes of *hypoglycemia* and normalize carbohydrate metabolism.

There are two major types of diabetes mellitus:

- Type 1—formerly known as insulin-dependent diabetes mellitus or IDDM
- Type 2—formerly known as non–insulin-dependent diabetes mellitus or NIDDM

Another form of diabetes may occur with some pregnant women; this is termed gestational diabetes because it typically subsides when the child is born. Women who experience this condition are at a higher risk of developing type 2 diabetes later (Vann, 2009).

Lifespan Considerations

Pregnancy

Pregnancy makes diabetes more difficult to manage. Insulin requirements usually decrease in the first trimester, increase during the second and third trimesters, and decrease rapidly after delivery. The client with diabetes or a history of gestational diabetes must be encouraged to maintain good metabolic control before conception and throughout pregnancy.

Those with type 1 diabetes do not produce enough insulin and therefore must have insulin supplementation to survive (Fig. 40.1). Type 1 diabetes usually has a rapid onset, occurs before age 20 years, produces more severe symptoms swifter than type 2 diabetes, and is more difficult to control.

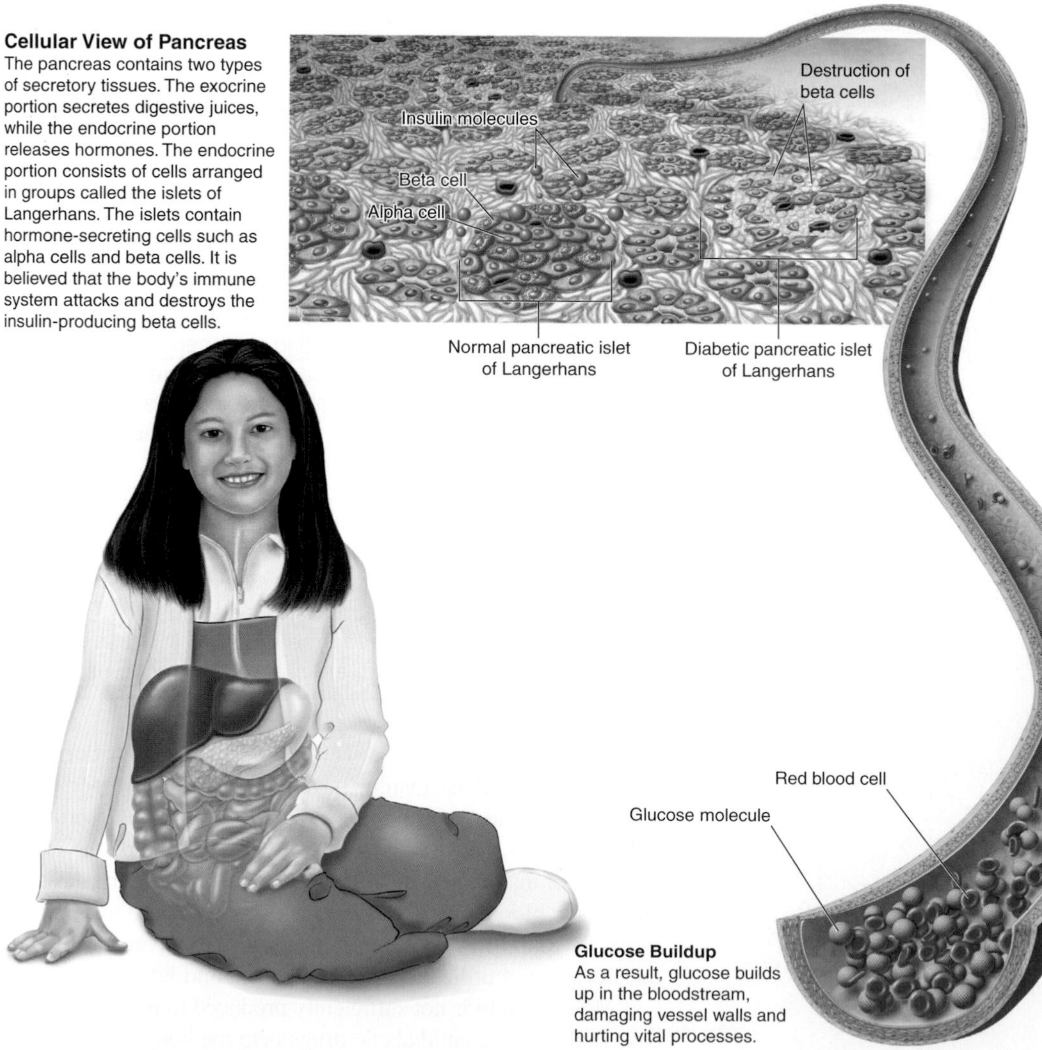

Cellular View of Pancreas
The pancreas contains two types of secretory tissues. The exocrine portion secretes digestive juices, while the endocrine portion releases hormones. The endocrine portion consists of cells arranged in groups called the islets of Langerhans. The islets contain hormone-secreting cells such as alpha cells and beta cells. It is believed that the body's immune system attacks and destroys the insulin-producing beta cells.

Insulin molecules

Beta cell

Alpha cell

Destruction of beta cells

Normal pancreatic islet of Langerhans

Diabetic pancreatic islet of Langerhans

Red blood cell

Glucose molecule

Glucose Buildup
As a result, glucose builds up in the bloodstream, damaging vessel walls and hurting vital processes.

FIGURE 40.1 Cellular view of type 1 diabetes. (Courtesy of Anatomical Chart Co.)

Major symptoms of types 1 and 2 diabetes include hyperglycemia, **polydipsia** (increased thirst), **polyphagia** (increased appetite), **polyuria** (increased urination), and weight loss. Control of type 1 diabetes is particularly difficult because of the lack of insulin production by the pancreas. Treatment requires a strict regimen that typically includes a carefully calculated diet, planned physical activity, home glucose testing several times a day, and daily supplement of insulin by injections or pump.

About 90%–95% of individuals with diabetes mellitus have type 2 diabetes. Those with type 2 diabetes are affected either by decreased production of insulin by the beta cells of the pancreas or by decreased sensitivity of the body cells to insulin, making the cells insulin resistant (Fig. 40.2).

What Causes Type 2 Diabetes?

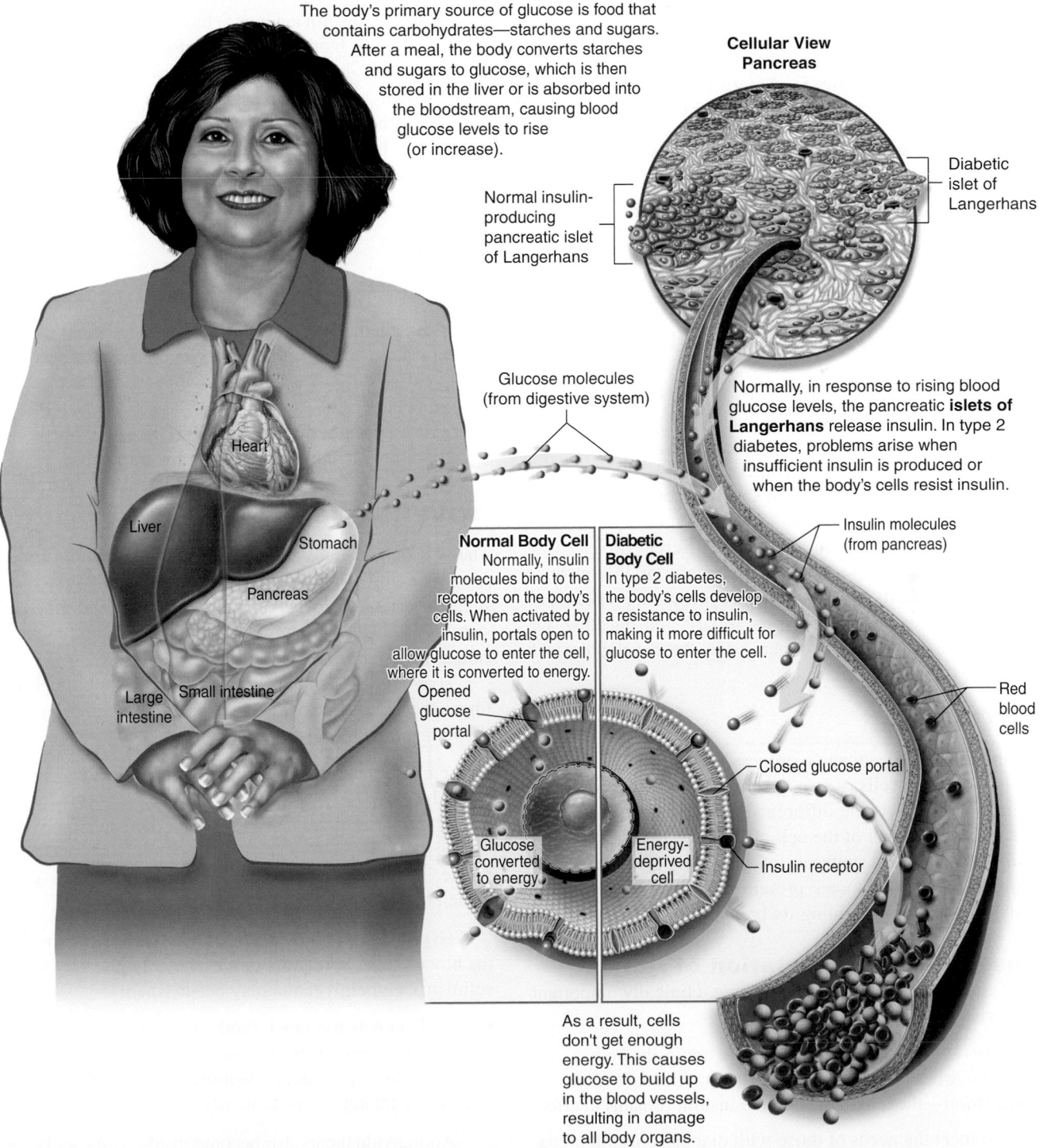

The body's primary source of glucose is food that contains carbohydrates—starches and sugars. After a meal, the body converts starches and sugars to glucose, which is then stored in the liver or is absorbed into the bloodstream, causing blood glucose levels to rise (or increase).

Cellular View Pancreas

Normal insulin-producing pancreatic islet of Langerhans

Diabetic islet of Langerhans

Glucose molecules (from digestive system)

Heart

Liver

Stomach

Pancreas

Large intestine   Small intestine

Normally, in response to rising blood glucose levels, the pancreatic **islets of Langerhans** release insulin. In type 2 diabetes, problems arise when insufficient insulin is produced or when the body's cells resist insulin.

Insulin molecules (from pancreas)

Normal Body Cell
Normally, insulin molecules bind to the receptors on the body's cells. When activated by insulin, portals open to allow glucose to enter the cell, where it is converted to energy.
Opened glucose portal

Glucose converted to energy

Diabetic Body Cell
In type 2 diabetes, the body's cells develop a resistance to insulin, making it more difficult for glucose to enter the cell.

Closed glucose portal

Energy-deprived cell

Insulin receptor

Red blood cells

As a result, cells don't get enough energy. This causes glucose to build up in the blood vessels, resulting in damage to all body organs.

FIGURE 40.2 Cellular view of type 2 diabetes. (Courtesy of Anatomical Chart Co.)

Although type 2 diabetes may occur at any age, the disorder occurs most often after age 40 years. The onset of type 2 diabetes is usually insidious. Symptoms begin to show less severely than type 1 diabetes. Risk factors for type 2 diabetes include:

- Obesity
- Older age
- Family history of diabetes
- History of gestational diabetes (diabetes that develops during pregnancy but disappears when pregnancy is over)
- Impaired glucose tolerance
- Minimal or no physical activity
- Race/ethnicity (African Americans, Hispanic/Latino Americans, Native Americans, and some Asian Americans)

In many individuals with type 2 diabetes, the disorder can be controlled with diet, exercise, and oral antidiabetic drugs. However, about 40% of those with type 2 diabetes respond poorly to the oral antidiabetic drugs and require insulin to control the disorder.

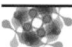 INSULIN PRODUCTS

Insulin is a hormone manufactured by the beta cells of the pancreas. Until the 1980s, animal-source insulins were used, yet sensitivity was a problem. In 1982, the first human insulin derived from a biosynthetic process (recombinant DNA or rDNA) was developed from bacterial sources and marketed as Humulin (Gebel, 2013). By manipulation of the amino acids in insulin, a slightly different product was made: insulin (Gebel, 2013). The benefit of insulin analogues is the ability to change the properties and make them faster acting such as with lispro, aspart, and glulisine. Or they can be made to act longer, as in the development of glargine.

ACTIONS

Insulin appears to activate a process that helps glucose molecules enter the cells of striated muscle and adipose tissue. Figure 40.2 depicts the difference between normal glucose metabolism and that of the cell affected by diabetes. Insulin also stimulates the synthesis of glycogen by the liver. In addition, insulin promotes protein synthesis and helps the body store fat by preventing its breakdown for energy.

Onset, Peak, and Duration of Action

Onset, peak, and duration are three clinically important properties of insulin:

- *Onset*—when insulin first begins to act in the body
- *Peak*—when the insulin is exerting maximum action
- *Duration*—the length of time the insulin remains in effect

To meet the needs of those with diabetes, insulin preparations are classified as rapid and short acting, intermediate acting, or long acting depending upon the onset, peak, and duration properties of the drug. Various insulin preparations have been developed to speed up or delay the onset and prolong the duration of action of the drug. Examples are the insulin analogues (lispro, aspart, and glulisine), which have an onset of 15 min. This is much less than regular insulin (30–60 min), making the insulin analogues better for pre-meal coverage or constant administration in an insulin pump (lispro and aspart are used for this purpose) (Dinsmoor, 2014).

Glargine (insulin analogue) has a slower and more even release into the bloodstream; therefore, it does not have a "peak action" compared with the traditional long-acting insulin such as NPH. Other analogue insulins are slow release, so their durations are very long, making them good choices for basal insulin administration. For more specifics concerning the onset, peak, and duration of various insulins see the Summary Drug Table: Insulin Preparations.

USES

Insulin products are used to:

- Replace the hormone insulin in type 1 diabetes
- Supplement insulin production in type 2 diabetes when uncontrolled by diet, exercise, weight reduction, or other antidiabetic agents
- Treat severe **diabetic ketoacidosis** (DKA) or diabetic coma
- Treat hypokalemia in combination with glucose

ADVERSE REACTIONS

The two major adverse reactions seen with insulin product administration are **hypoglycemia** (low blood glucose or sugar level) and **hyperglycemia** (elevated blood glucose or sugar level). The symptoms of hypoglycemia and hyperglycemia are listed in Table 40.1.

Hypoglycemia may occur when there is too much insulin in the bloodstream in relation to the available glucose (hyperinsulinism). Hypoglycemia may occur when:

- The client eats too little food or goes too long between meals.
- The client has drastically increased demands (activity or illness).
- The insulin given is incorrectly measured and is greater than that prescribed.

Hyperglycemia may occur if there is too little insulin in the bloodstream in relation to the available glucose (hypoinsulinism). Hyperglycemia may occur when:

- The client eats too much food.
- Too little or no insulin is given.
- The client experiences emotional stress, infection, surgery, pregnancy, or an acute illness.

An individual can also become insulin resistant because antibodies develop against insulin. These clients have impaired

TABLE 40.1 Hypoglycemia Versus Hyperglycemia

SYMPTOMS	HYPOGLYCEMIA (INSULIN REACTION)	HYPERGLYCEMIA (DIABETIC COMA, KETOACIDOSIS)
Onset	Sudden	Gradual (hours or days)
Blood glucose level	Less than 60 mg/dL	More than 200 mg/dL
Central nervous system	Fatigue, weakness, nervousness, agitation, confusion, headache, diplopia, convulsions, dizziness, unconsciousness	Drowsiness, dim vision
Respirations	Normal to rapid, shallow	Deep, rapid (air hunger)
Gastrointestinal	Hunger, nausea	Thirst, nausea, vomiting, abdominal pain, loss of appetite
Skin	Pale, moist, cool, diaphoretic	Dry, flushed, warm
Pulse	Normal or uncharacteristic	Rapid, weak
Miscellaneous	Numbness, tingling of the lips or tongue	Acetone breath, excessive urination

receptor function and become so unresponsive to insulin that the dose requirement may be in excess of 500 units/day, rather than the usual 40 to 60 units/day. A long-acting glargine (insulin analogue) marketed as Toujeo contains 300 units/mL. This high-potency insulin product in a concentrated form is used for clients requiring more than 200 units/day.

CONTRAINDICATIONS AND PRECAUTIONS

Specific insulin products are contraindicated when the client is hypoglycemic. Insulin is used cautiously in clients with renal or hepatic impairment and during pregnancy and lactation. The insulins are grouped in pregnancy category B, except for insulin glargine and insulin aspart, which are in pregnancy category C. Insulin appears to inhibit milk production in lactating women and could interfere with breastfeeding. Lactating women may require adjustment in insulin dose and diet.

LASA ALERT

The following drugs may sound alike; be sure to clarify when they are ordered:

Drug Name	*Sounds Like*
Apidra	Spiriva
HumuLIN N	HumuLIN R, HumaLOG, Humira
HumuLIN 70/30	HumaLOG Mix 75/25, HumuLIN R, NovoLIN 70/30, NovoLOG Mix 70/30
insulin glargine	insulin glulisine
Lantus	latanoprost, Latuda, Xalatan
Levemir	Lovenox
NovoLOG	HumaLOG, HumuLIN R, Nimbex, NovoLIN N, NovoLIN R, NovoLOG Mix 70/30
Tresiba	Tarceva, Toujeo, Tradjenta, Trulicity

Drugs that look like a similar drug are noted in the Summary Drug Tables of each chapter.

INTERACTIONS

When certain drugs are administered with insulin, a resultant decrease or increase in hypoglycemic effect can occur. Box 40.1 identifies selected drugs that decrease and increase the hypoglycemic effect of insulin.

Clients may not volunteer information regarding their use of complementary and alternative remedies. You should always inquire about use of herbal products. Although laboratory testing is not conclusive, medical reports indicate a possible interaction with eucalyptus products, causing decreased blood sugar.

ORAL ANTIDIABETIC DRUGS AND OTHER AGENTS

When type 2 diabetes is initially diagnosed, insulin is typically not the first-choice drug. Weight management by lifestyle, exercise, and diet changes is encouraged and blood work is monitored. The goal of these interventions is to reduce the risk of type 2 diabetes or a condition called prediabetes. **Prediabetes** is diagnosed when a client presents with impaired glucose tolerance/fasting glucose, or metabolic syndrome. A prediabetic client may be started on oral antidiabetic drugs to reduce the risk of developing type 2 diabetes. Oral antidiabetic drugs (also called hypoglycemics) are used to reduce glucose blood levels in clients with type 2 diabetes. *These drugs are not effective for treating type 1 diabetes.*

USES

A number of oral antidiabetic drugs are currently in use, and these are usually initiated using one drug (*monotherapy*) with others added as needed to control blood glucose levels. These drugs may also be used with insulin

BOX 40.1 Drugs That Alter Insulin Effectiveness

Selected Drugs That Decrease the Effect (More Insulin May Be Required)

acetazolamide	diltiazem	morphine
albuterol	diuretics	niacin
antipsychotics (atypical or second generation)	dobutamine	nicotine
	epinephrine	phenothiazines
asparaginase	estrogens	phenytoin
calcitonin	glucagon	progestogens
contraceptives, oral	human immunodeficiency virus (HIV) antivirals	protease inhibitors
corticosteroids		somatropin
cyclophosphamide	isoniazid	terbutaline
danazol	lithium	thyroid hormones

Drugs That Increase the Effect (Less Insulin May Be Required)

angiotensin-converting enzyme (ACE) inhibitors	clonidine	pentamidine
	disopyramide	pentoxifylline
alcohol	fluoxetine	pyridoxine
anabolic steroids	fibrates	salicylates
antidiabetic drugs, oral	lithium	somatostatin analogue
beta-blocking drugs	MAOIs	sulfonamides
calcium	mebendazole	tetracycline

in the management of some clients with type 2 diabetes. Figure 40.3 illustrates the American Association of Clinical Endocrinologists (AACE) treatment protocol for administration of antidiabetic drugs for type 2 diabetes.

The liver normally releases glucose by detecting the level of circulating insulin. When insulin levels are high, glucose is available in the blood, and the liver produces little or no glucose. When insulin levels are low, there is little circulating glucose, so the liver produces more glucose. In type 2 diabetes, the liver may not detect levels of glucose in the blood and, instead of regulating glucose production, releases glucose despite adequate blood glucose levels. In addition, injectable **incretin hormones** (increase insulin production, slow gastric emptying, and inhibit glucagon release) are used in combination therapy.

The following classes of antidiabetic drugs are listed by suggested use according to the 2020 AACE treatment protocol for administration.

BIGUANIDES

The drug class biguanides sensitizes the liver to circulating insulin levels, reduces intestinal glucose absorption, and reduces hepatic glucose production. Metformin, the only drug approved for use in the United States from the biguanide class, is the first choice drug used for initial type 2 diabetes or when a prediabetic client is started on antidiabetic drug therapy. This drug is usually started alone in what is called monotherapy. These drugs do not increase insulin levels or cause weight gain.

ADVERSE REACTIONS

Alone, metformin rarely causes hypoglycemia. However, clients receiving this drug in combination with insulin or other hypoglycemics (see other agents listed below) are at

greater risk for hypoglycemia. A reduction or titration in the dosage of one of the antidiabetic drugs may be required to prevent episodes of hypoglycemia when combination therapy is initiated.

Nausea, vomiting, diarrhea, and increased flatulence are adverse reactions of metformin. It is taken with food to minimize adverse gastrointestinal (GI) effects.

CONTRAINDICATIONS, PRECAUTIONS, AND INTERACTIONS

Metformin should not be used if the client has poor kidney function (FDA, 2016). Risk for problems such as lactic acidosis is greater when the kidneys are impaired (stages 3–5). There is a risk of acute kidney failure, which can lead to lactic acidosis, when contrast medium is used for radiologic studies. When contrast medium is used, metformin (or a product containing the drug) is stopped on the day of and 48 hr after the radiologic study. Metformin may lead to vitamin B_{12} malabsorption; clients should be monitored and supplements given as needed. The drug is also contraindicated in clients older than 80 years and during pregnancy (pregnancy category B) and lactation.

LASA ALERT

The following drugs may sound alike; be sure to clarify when they are ordered:

Drug Name	Sounds Like
MetFORMIN	metroNIDAZOLE

Drugs that look like a similar drug are noted in the Summary Drug Tables of each chapter.

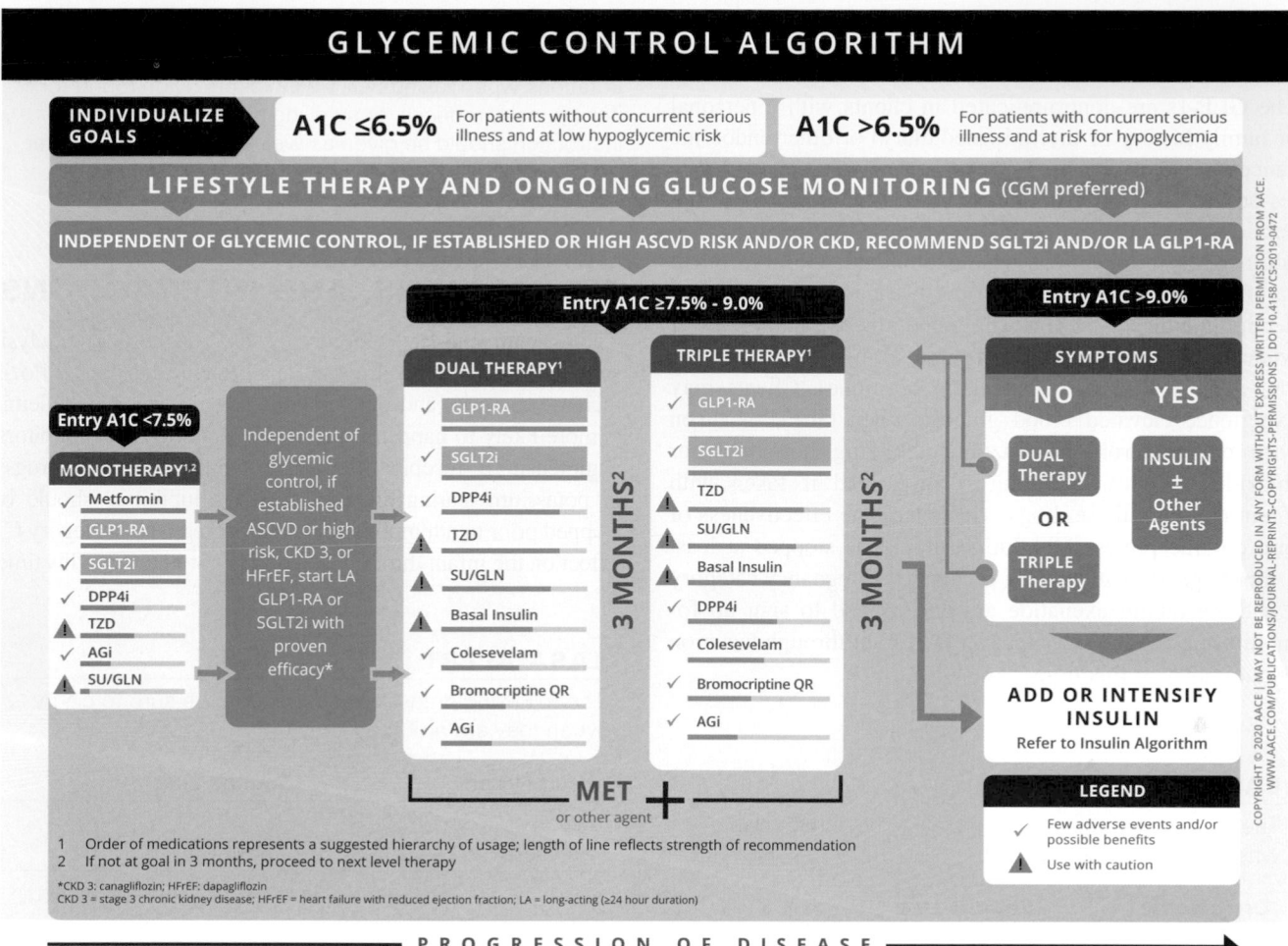

FIGURE 40.3 AACE/ACE comprehensive type 2 diabetes management algorithm. (Reprinted with permission from American Association of Clinical Endocrinologists © 2020 AACE. Garber, A. J., Handelsman, Y., Grunberger, G., et al. (2020). AACE/ACE comprehensive type 2 diabetes management algorithm 2020. *Endocrine Practice, 26*, 107–139.)

Metformin use is temporarily discontinued for surgical procedures. The drug therapy is restarted when the client's oral intake has been resumed and kidney function is normal. There is an increased risk of lactic acidosis when metformin is administered with the glucocorticoids.

> ⓘ **NURSING ALERT**
>
> Lactic acid is a normal muscle by-product of exercise when the cells do not get enough oxygen. Lactic acidosis happens when lactic acid builds up in the bloodstream faster than it can be removed. Symptoms include malaise (vague feeling of bodily discomfort), abdominal pain, rapid respirations, shortness of breath, and muscular pain. Cardiovascular collapse can occur if not recognized and treated.

GLUCAGON-LIKE PEPTIDE-1 AGONISTS

Incretin hormones are involved in the physiologic regulation of glucose balance. They increase insulin release and decrease glucagon levels in the circulation depending upon glucose levels. Glucagon-like peptide-1 (GLP-1) agonists are injectable drugs that mimic the incretin hormone, GLP-1. This hormone stimulates insulin release when a person eats; it also reduces glucagon and slows gastric emptying. Albiglutide, dulaglutide, exenatide, and semaglutide are used to treat type 2 diabetes. In addition to treating type 2 diabetes, liraglutide is used for chronic weight management of those with a body mass index greater than 27 who also have hypertension or dyslipidemia. Semaglutide is now available in an oral form, which should be taken in the morning at least 30 min before eating.

ADVERSE REACTIONS

Adverse reactions are typically GI in nature: diarrhea, nausea and vomiting, and heartburn. Clients taking exenatide or liraglutide may experience headaches, and all clients should monitor injection sites for local irritation.

CONTRAINDICATIONS, PRECAUTIONS, AND INTERACTIONS

The GLP-1s are contraindicated in clients with a personal or family history of thyroid (medullary) or other endocrine cancers. This drug should not be used to treat type 1 diabetes or DKA. GLP-1s should not be used with the dipeptidyl peptidase-4 (DPP-4) inhibitors because of the increased additive glycemic effect when combined. Observe client carefully for signs or symptoms of acute pancreatitis or declining kidney function. The blood glucose can fall lower when taken with the following drugs: androgens, insulins, and pegvisomant (a somatostatin hormone). Clients may experience elevated blood glucose when GLP-1 is taken with corticosteroids, danazol, luteinizing hormones, or thiazide diuretics. Bleeding is prolonged if taken with vitamin K, and these drugs will reduce the effectiveness of oral contraceptives. Albiglutide should be stopped at least 1 month prior to attempting pregnancy (pregnancy category C); those taking exenatide are encouraged to sign up for monitoring programs. Effect on the infant through lactation is not known at this time.

> **LASA ALERT**
>
> The following drugs may sound alike; be sure to clarify when they are ordered:
>
> | Drug Name | Sounds Like |
> | --- | --- |
> | Trulicity | Toujeo, Tradjenta, Tresiba |
>
> Drugs that look like a similar drug are noted in the Summary Drug Tables of each chapter.

SODIUM-GLUCOSE LINKED TRANSPORTER-2 INHIBITORS

Glucose is reabsorbed in the kidney by the sodium-glucose linked transporter-2 (SGLT-2). This process is decreased by the class of inhibiting drugs, SGLT-2 inhibitors. As a result the renal glucose threshold is lowered, allowing more glucose to leave the body via the urine. When this drug is administered, clients experience a drop in the HbA_{1c}, weight, and systolic blood pressure. There may also be a reduction in low-density lipoprotein.

ADVERSE REACTIONS

Yeast infections of the genital area can occur due to excretion of glucose in the urine. A rare, yet serious bacterial infection (necrotizing fasciitis) may result. Clients taking these drugs may experience hypotension and hyperkalemia.

> **NURSING ALERT**
>
> Clients should be taught to observe for early genital irritations when taking SGLT-2 inhibitors. Monitoring for itching, pain, redness, or swelling in the perineal area instruction should be given as well as noting a fever over 100.4 °F and general malaise or fatigue.

CONTRAINDICATIONS, PRECAUTIONS, AND INTERACTIONS

Clients with end-stage kidney disease or those on dialysis should not take these drugs. Canagliflozin and dapagliflozin increase diuresis, and dehydration may result. Hyperkalemia is more likely to happen if the client is taking ACE inhibitors, angiotensin II receptor blockers (both hypertension drugs), or potassium-sparing diuretics. SGLT-2 inhibitors should be stopped prior to attempting pregnancy (pregnancy category C). Effect on the infant through lactation is not known at this time.

> **LASA ALERT**
>
> The following drugs may sound alike; be sure to clarify when they are ordered:
>
> | Drug Name | Sounds Like |
> | --- | --- |
> | Farxiga | Fetzima |
> | Steglatro | Spravato |
>
> Drugs that look like a similar drug are noted in the Summary Drug Tables of each chapter.

DIPEPTIDYL PEPTIDASE-4 INHIBITORS

Dipeptidyl peptidase-4 inhibitors (also called gliptins) lower the blood glucose level of those with type 2 diabetes by enhancing the secretion of the incretin hormone produced by the body. This in turn reduces glucagon and lowers blood glucose levels.

ADVERSE REACTIONS

Headache and upper respiratory tract symptoms such as nasopharyngitis are the most frequent adverse reactions when taking this medication.

CONTRAINDICATIONS, PRECAUTIONS, AND INTERACTIONS

These drugs should not be used for DKA or if the client has type 1 diabetes. A gliptin should be used cautiously in clients with chronic kidney disease or in older adults. This drug has not been studied in pregnant women but is believed to be a category B drug from animal studies, and it should be used cautiously in lactating women.

THIAZOLIDINEDIONES

The thiazolidinediones (TZDs) improve insulin sensitivity in muscle and fat cells. These drugs also inhibit gluconeogenesis (formation of glucose from glycogen). As a result of reduced insulin resistance in the cell, the HbA_{1c} significantly lowers.

ADVERSE REACTIONS

Adverse reactions associated with the administration of TZDs include upper respiratory infections, sinusitis, headache, pharyngitis, myalgia, diarrhea, and back pain. Weight gain and hypoglycemia are more evident when used in combination therapy.

CONTRAINDICATIONS, PRECAUTIONS, AND INTERACTIONS

TZDs are contraindicated for clients with symptomatic heart failure. TZDs are not used to treat type 1 diabetes. Rosiglitazone specifically should not be used in combined therapy with insulin products. These drugs are used cautiously in clients with edema, cardiovascular disease, and liver or kidney disease. Monitor both sexes for bone fractures, especially of upper limbs after the first year of therapy. TZDs are pregnancy category C. Premenopausal women, who do not ovulate, may begin to ovulate again and effective barrier birth control is recommended because TZD can decrease the effectiveness of oral contraceptives.

ALPHA-GLUCOSIDASE INHIBITORS

The alpha-glucosidase (α-glucosidase) inhibitors, acarbose (Precose) and miglitol (Glyset), prevent the after-meal surge in blood glucose by delaying the digestion absorption of carbohydrates in the intestine.

ADVERSE REACTIONS

Increasing the dose of these drugs should be done slowly to reduce the GI adverse reactions of bloating, flatulence, and diarrhea. The use of these drugs in the United States is limited because of the unpleasant and not well-tolerated adverse GI reactions.

CONTRAINDICATIONS, PRECAUTIONS, AND INTERACTIONS

Alpha-glucosidase inhibitors are contraindicated in clients with preexisting GI problems, such as irritable bowel syndrome or Crohn disease. They should not be used for DKA or if the client has cirrhosis. Digestive enzymes may reduce the effect of miglitol. Acarbose and miglitol are used cautiously in clients with renal impairment. Considered pregnancy category B drugs, they have not been studied sufficiently to render safe to take while pregnant or when lactating.

AMYLINOMIMETIC

Amylin is a hormone produced by the pancreas along with insulin. This injectable drug mimics the endogenous amylin effects by delaying gastric emptying, decreasing glucagon release, and decreasing appetite. When used with insulin at meal times (endogenous or administered) it can reduce blood glucose (HbA_{1c} levels) and help reduce weight.

ADVERSE REACTIONS

Adverse reactions of amylin include nausea, vomiting, decreased appetite, abdominal pain, headache, pain or irritation at injection site, and hypoglycemia.

CONTRAINDICATIONS, PRECAUTIONS, AND INTERACTIONS

Do not use if problems with stomach emptying exist. This drug should not be used if client is taking a drug that slows GI motility, such as an alpha-glucosidase inhibitor. Pramlintide injection will delay the onset of action if taken at the same time as an oral antidiabetic medication. Considered pregnancy category C drugs, they have not been studied sufficiently to render safe to take while pregnant or when lactating.

 Chronic Care Considerations

Type 1 Diabetic
There is a greater risk of severe hypoglycemic reactions when pramlintide is given at the same time as insulin. These two drugs should be given as separate injections and not be mixed in the same syringe.

SULFONYLUREAS

Sulfonylureas appear to lower blood glucose by stimulating the beta cells of the pancreas to release insulin. This lowering is measured by a 1%–2% reduction in HbA_{1c}. Sulfonylureas are not effective if the beta cells of the pancreas cannot release a sufficient amount of insulin to meet the individual's needs. The most commonly used sulfonylureas are the second- and third-generation drugs, such as glimepiride, glipizide, and glyburide. The first-generation sulfonylureas (e.g., chlorpropamide, tolazamide, and tolbutamide) are rarely used today because they have a long duration of action and a higher incidence of adverse reactions and are more likely to react with other drugs.

ADVERSE REACTIONS

Adverse reactions associated with sulfonylureas include hypoglycemia, anorexia, nausea, vomiting, epigastric discomfort, weight gain, heartburn, and various vague neurologic symptoms, such as weakness and numbness of the extremities. Manipulating the dosing of these drugs can often reduce the unpleasant reactions.

CONTRAINDICATIONS, PRECAUTIONS, AND INTERACTIONS

The first-generation sulfonylureas (chlorpropamide, tolazamide, and tolbutamide) are contraindicated in clients with coronary artery disease or liver or renal dysfunction. Other sulfonylureas are used cautiously in clients with impaired liver function because liver dysfunction can prolong the drug's effect. In addition, sulfonylureas are used cautiously in clients with renal impairment and severe cardiovascular

disease. There is a risk for cross-sensitivity with sulfonylureas and sulfonamides (sulfa anti-infectives).

Sulfonylureas may have an increased hypoglycemic effect when administered with anticoagulants, clofibrate, fluconazole, histamine H_2 antagonists, methyldopa, monoamine oxidase inhibitors, nonsteroidal anti-inflammatory drugs, salicylates, sulfonamides, and tricyclic antidepressants. The hypoglycemic effect of sulfonylureas may be decreased when the agents are administered with beta blockers, calcium channel blockers, cholestyramine, corticosteroids, estrogens, hydantoins, isoniazid, oral contraceptives, phenothiazines, rifampin, thiazide diuretics, and thyroid agents.

LASA ALERT

The following drugs may sound alike; be sure to clarify when they are ordered:

Drug Name	Sounds Like
Amaryl	Altace, Amerge
chlorproPAMIDE	chlorproMAZINE
Diabinese	DiaBeta
glimepiride	glipizide, glyBURIDE
Glucotrol	Glucophage, glyBURIDE, GlycoTrol
TOLAZamide	terbutaline, TOLBUTamide, tolcapone

Drugs that look like a similar drug are noted in the Summary Drug Tables of each chapter.

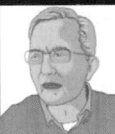 **PHARMACOLOGY IN PRACTICE**

SAFE DRUG ADMINISTRATION
A nurse is asked to check the medical history of a client who is to be administered glimepiride. Which of the following allergies would alert the nurse to a possible reaction when taking this drug?
1. Penicillin
2. Ragweed
3. Sulfa
4. Peanuts

MEGLITINIDES

Like the sulfonylureas, the meglitinides act to lower blood glucose levels by stimulating the release of insulin from the pancreas. This action depends on the ability of the beta cells in the pancreas to produce some insulin. However, the action of the meglitinides is more rapid than that of the sulfonylureas and their duration of action much shorter. Because of this, they must be taken three times a day.

The two meglitinides currently marketed in the United States include nateglinide (Starlix) and repaglinide.

ADVERSE REACTIONS

Adverse reactions associated with the administration of the meglitinides include upper respiratory tract infection, headache, rhinitis, bronchitis, headache, back pain, and hypoglycemia.

CONTRAINDICATIONS, PRECAUTIONS, AND INTERACTIONS

Drugs reducing the hypoglycemic effect of meglitinides include corticosteroids, carbamazepine, and rifampin. Debilitated, malnourished, or older clients are typically more susceptible to the hypoglycemic effects when taking these drugs. Considered pregnancy category C drugs, they have not been studied sufficiently to render safe to take while pregnant or when lactating.

LASA ALERT

The following drugs may sound alike; be sure to clarify when they are ordered:

Drug Name	*Sounds Like*
repaglinide	Rasagiline

Drugs that look like a similar drug are noted in the Summary Drug Tables of each chapter.

OTHER AGENTS

The bile acid sequestrant, colesevelam, is US Food and Drug Administration (FDA) approved as an adjunctive therapy to improve glycemic control in adults with type 2 diabetes. Bromocriptine, a dopamine agonist, acts on circadian neuronal activities and may help regulate the hypothalamus to normalize blood glucose in clients with insulin resistance.

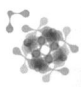

NURSING PROCESS—STEPS TO BUILDING CLINICAL JUDGMENT
Client Receiving Insulin and/or an Antidiabetic Drug

ASSESSMENT

Preadministration Assessment

Data gathering suggestions before antidiabetic drugs are administered include:
Objective data

- General client appearance, emphasis on skin (mucous membranes and extremities, with special attention given to any sores or cuts that appear to be infected or healing poorly, as well as any ulcerations or other skin or mucous membrane changes)
- Vital signs (temperature, pulse, respirations, and blood pressure)
- Weight, note gain or loss
- Laboratory results—HbA$_{1c}$, glucose tolerance/fasting levels, and lipid panel

Subjective data

- Current hyper/hypoglycemia symptoms experienced by client
- Dietary, activity history
- Family history of diabetes or other chronic health conditions

Typically, type 2 diabetes is not a sudden diagnosis. When blood glucose testing results fall into specific ranges a client is diagnosed as prediabetic or diabetic, see Table 40.2. Client laboratory tests are viewed over time and efforts at lifestyle modifications to lower blood glucose readings are encouraged.

Before antidiabetic medications are initiated, other laboratory testing may be done for baseline

TABLE 40.2 Blood Test Levels for Prediabetes and Diabetes Diagnosis

	HBA$_{1c}$ (%)	FASTING BLOOD GLUCOSE (MG/DL)	ORAL GLUCOSE TOLERANCE TEST (MG/DL)
Diabetes	6.5 or greater	126 or greater	200 or greater
Prediabetes	5.8–6.4	100–125	140–199
Normal	4–5.7	99 or lower	139 or lower

Adapted from ADA, 2012.

comparisons. For example, glomerular filtration rate to measure kidney function may be done before prescribing metformin.

If the client has diabetes and has been receiving insulin or an oral antidiabetic drug, include the type and dosage of drug used, dietary habits, and the frequency and methods used for glucose testing in the client's record.

Ongoing Assessment

The most important aspect of the ongoing assessment is tracking and treatment of high or low blood sugars (see Table 40.1). Frequent observation of the client for symptoms of hypoglycemia, particularly during initial therapy or after a change in dosage, is an important ongoing assessment. The client taking insulin products is particularly prone to hypoglycemic reactions at the time of peak insulin action (see the Summary Drug Table: Insulin Preparations) or when they have not eaten for some time or has skipped a meal. In acute care settings, frequent blood glucose monitoring is routinely done to help detect abnormalities of blood glucose.

Clients in the acute care setting are also monitored closely for hyperglycemia. Insulin needs increase in times of stress or illness. For a person without diabetes, blood glucose levels are considered within normal limits when the measure is 60–100 mg/dL. For a person with diabetes, the health care provider may have higher levels as the parameters for the client. When products such as insulin glargine (Lantus) are used, the insulin levels do not fluctuate as often.

When ready for discharge, newly diagnosed clients will need to be taught to use a glucometer for self-monitoring of blood glucose levels (see Client Teaching for Improved Outcomes: Obtaining a Blood Glucose Reading Using a Glucometer). Review monitoring with a teach-back demonstration of all clients to be sure they are correctly using equipment. The best way to monitor long-term glycemic control and response to treatment is with HbA_{1c} levels measured at 3-month intervals. If the first HbA_{1c} indicates that glycemic control during the last 3 months was inadequate, the dosages may be increased for better control.

Special populations may use continuous glucose monitoring (CGM). This method works best with those who have large swings in their blood sugars or gestational diabetes and if the client has an insulin pump. Using a small device that is inserted in the skin of the belly, CGM records blood sugar levels all day long at 1-, 5-, or 10-minute increments. The FDA has just approved devices so these can be viewed electronically by the health care provider or even by the client themselves with a smartphone. It is particularly helpful when blood sugar levels can get dangerously high or low.

NURSING DIAGNOSES

Drug-specific nursing diagnoses include the following:

- **Acute confusion** related to hypoglycemia effects on mentation
- **Hypovolemia/dehydration** related to fluid loss during DKA
- **Anxiety** related to uncertainty of diagnosis, testing own glucose levels, self-injection, dietary restrictions, other factors (specify)
- **Altered breathing pattern** related to hyperventilation in lactic acidosis with metformin use

Nursing diagnoses related to drug administration are discussed in Chapter 4.

PLANNING

The expected outcomes of the client may include an optimal response to therapy, support of client needs related to the management of adverse reactions, a reduction in anxiety, improved ability to cope with the diagnosis, and confidence in an understanding of the medication regimen.

IMPLEMENTATION

Nursing management of a client with diabetes requires diligent, skillful, and comprehensive nursing care.

Promoting an Optimal Response to Therapy

There are no fixed drug dosages in antidiabetic therapy. The drug regimen is individualized on the basis of the effectiveness and tolerance of the drug(s) used and the maximum recommended dose of the drug(s).

Blood Glucose Monitoring

Blood glucose levels are monitored often in the client with diabetes. The primary health care provider may order blood glucose levels to be tested before meals, after meals, and at bedtime. Less frequent monitoring may be performed if the client's glucose levels are well controlled. The **glucometer** is a device used by the client with diabetes or the nursing personnel to monitor

---

Client Teaching for Improved Outcomes

Obtaining a Blood Glucose Reading Using a Glucometer

When you teach, make sure your client understands the following:

- ✔ Before initial use, carefully read the manufacturer's instructions, because blood glucose monitoring devices vary greatly.
- ✔ Prepare the finger by cleansing the area with warm, soapy water. Rinse with warm water and dry well. (If the client cannot prepare the area, the caregiver should wear gloves to comply with Standard Precautions, the guidelines of the Centers for Disease Control and Prevention.)
- ✔ Remove a test strip and close the container to prevent damage to the remaining strips. Insert the strip into the meter if the instructions call for this before obtaining the blood sample.
- ✔ Using the lancet (needle) device, perform a finger stick *on the side* of a finger (not the tip), where there are fewer nerve endings and more capillaries.
- ✔ Gently massage the finger to produce a large, hanging drop of blood. Using this technique to obtain a blood sample will help prevent inaccurate readings. *Note:* Do not smear the blood or try to obtain an extra drop.
- ✔ Drop the blood sample on the test strip and read the number on the meter. *Note:* Some glucometers, especially institutional devices, may have slightly different procedures.
- ✔ Record the time and test results in the record-keeping method recommended by your primary health care provider.
- ✔ Clean and calibrate the device according to the manufacturer's recommendations to maintain accurate readings.

blood glucose levels. Nursing or laboratory personnel are responsible for obtaining blood glucose levels during hospitalization, but the client must be taught to monitor blood glucose levels after discharge from the acute care setting (see Client Teaching for Improved Outcomes: Obtaining a Blood Glucose Reading Using a Glucometer).

Urine testing was widely used to monitor glucose levels in the past, but this method has largely been replaced with blood glucose monitoring. Urine testing can play a role in identifying kidney involvement or ketone excretion in clients prone to ketoacidosis. If urine testing is done, it is usually recommended to use the second voided specimen (i.e., fresh urine collected 30 min after the initial voiding) to check glucose or acetone levels, rather than the first specimen obtained.

The **glycosylated hemoglobin** (HbA$_{1c}$) test is a blood test used to monitor the client's average blood glucose level throughout a 3- to 4-month period. When blood glucose levels are high, glucose molecules attach to hemoglobin in the red blood cell. The longer the hyperglycemia lasts, the more glucose binds to the red blood cell and the higher the glycosylated hemoglobin. This binding lasts for the life of the red blood cell (about 4 months). When the client's diabetes is well controlled with normal or near-normal blood glucose levels, the overall HbA$_{1c}$ level will not be greatly elevated. However, if blood glucose levels are consistently high, the HbA$_{1c}$ level will be elevated. The test result (expressed as a percentage) refers to the average amount of glucose that has been in the blood throughout the last 4 months. Results vary with the laboratory method used for analysis, but, in general, levels between 6.5% and 7% indicate good control of diabetes. Results of 10% or greater indicate poor blood glucose control for the last several months. The HbA$_{1c}$ is useful in evaluating the success of diabetes treatment, comparing new treatment regimens with past regimens, and individualizing treatment.

Insulin Product Administration

Sometimes the health care provider finds that the client achieves best control with one injection of insulin per day; sometimes the client requires two or more injections per day. In addition, two different types of insulin may be combined, such as a rapid-acting and a long-acting preparation. The number of insulin injections, dosage, times of administration, and type of insulin are determined by the health care provider after careful evaluation of the client's metabolic needs and response to therapy. The dosage prescribed for the client may require changes until the dosage is found that best meets the client's needs.

NURSING ALERT

Insulin requirements may change when the client experiences any form of stress and with any illness, particularly illnesses resulting in nausea and vomiting.

Insulin is ordered by the generic name (e.g., insulin aspart) or the trade (brand) name (e.g., NovoLog; see the Summary Drug Table: Insulin Preparations). One brand of insulin must never be substituted for another unless the substitution is approved by the primary health care provider, because some clients may be sensitive to changes in brands of insulin. In addition, it is important never to substitute one type of insulin for another. For example, do not use long-acting insulin instead of the prescribed short-acting insulin.

When administering insulin, care must be taken to use the correct insulin. Names and packaging are similar and can easily be confused. Carefully read all drug labels before preparing any insulin preparation. For example, Humalog (lispro) and Humulin R (regular human insulin) are easily confused because of the similar names.

Insulin cannot be administered orally, because it is a protein and readily destroyed in the GI tract. Insulin must be administered by the parenteral route, usually the subcutaneous (subcut) route. Aspiration for blood return does not need to be done when given subcut. Regular insulin is the only insulin preparation given intravenously (IV).

RAPID- AND SHORT-ACTING INSULIN PRODUCTS. Regular insulin is given 30–60 min before a meal to achieve optimal results.

Aspart is given immediately before a meal (within 5–10 min of beginning a meal). Lispro is given 15 min before a meal or immediately after a meal. Aspart and lispro make insulin product administration more convenient for many clients who find taking a drug 30–60 min before meals bothersome. In addition, lispro appears to lower the blood glucose level 1–2 hr after meals better than does regular human insulin, because it more closely mimics the body's natural insulin. It also lowers the risk of low blood glucose reactions from midnight to 6 a.m. in clients with type I diabetes.

INTERMEDIATE- AND LONG-ACTING INSULIN PRODUCTS. Many clients are maintained on a single dose of intermediate-acting insulin administered subcut in the morning. The longer-acting insulins are given before breakfast or at bedtime (depending on the primary health care provider's instructions).

Glargine is given subcut once daily at bedtime. This type of insulin product maintains a steady blood level and is used in treating adults and children with type 1 diabetes and in adults with type 2 diabetes who need long-acting insulin for the control of hyperglycemia.

Insulin products are available in concentrations of U100 and U300. You must read the label of the insulin bottle carefully for the name and the number of units per milliliter. The dose of insulin is measured in units. U100 insulin has 100 units in each milliliter; U300 has 300 units in each milliliter. Most people with diabetes use the U100 concentration. Clients who are resistant to insulin and require large insulin doses use the U300 concentration.

MIXING INSULINS. If the client is to receive regular insulin and NPH (isophane insulin suspension) insulin, clarify with the primary health care provider whether two separate injections are to be given or if the insulins may be mixed in the same syringe. If the two insulins are to be given in the same syringe, the short-acting insulin (regular or lispro) is drawn into the syringe first (Fig. 40.4). Even small amounts of intermediate- or long-acting insulin, if mixed with the short-acting insulin, can bind with the short-acting insulin and delay its onset.

> ⓘ **NURSING ALERT**
>
> Regular insulin is clear, whereas intermediate- and long-acting insulins are cloudy. The clear insulin should be drawn up first. When insulin lispro is mixed with a longer-acting insulin, the insulin lispro is drawn up first.

An unexpected response may be obtained when changing from mixed injections to separate injections or vice versa. If the client had been using insulin mixtures before admission, ask whether the insulins were given separately or together.

Several types of premixed insulins are available. These insulins combine regular insulin with the longer-acting NPH insulin. The mixtures are prescribed as ratios, such as 70/30, meaning 70% of NPH to 30% of regular insulin (the larger proportion long acting). Although these premixed insulins are helpful for clients who have difficulty drawing up their insulin or seeing the markings on the syringe, they prohibit individualizing the dosage. For clients who have difficulty controlling their diabetes, these premixed insulins may not be effective.

> ⓘ **NURSING ALERT**
>
> Do not mix or dilute glargine with any other insulin or solution, because glucose control will be lost and the insulin will not be effective.

PREPARING INSULIN FOR ADMINISTRATION. Always check the expiration date printed on the label of the insulin bottle before withdrawing the insulin. An insulin syringe that matches the concentration of insulin to be given is always used. For example, a syringe labeled as U100 is used only with insulin labeled U100. U300 insulin is given only by the subcut or intramuscular (IM) route. Never substitute a tuberculin syringe for an insulin syringe.

When insulin is in a suspension (this can be seen when looking at a vial that has been untouched for about 1 hr), gently rotate the vial between the palms of the hands and tilt it gently end to end immediately before withdrawing the insulin. This ensures even distribution of the suspended particles. Care is taken not to shake the insulin vigorously.

Carefully check the primary health care provider's order for the type and dosage of insulin immediately before withdrawing the insulin from the vial. All air bubbles must be eliminated from the syringe barrel and hub of the needle before withdrawing the syringe from the insulin vial.

> ⓘ **NURSING ALERT**
>
> Accuracy is of the utmost importance when measuring any insulin preparation because of the potential danger of administering an incorrect dosage. If possible, check and consult with another nurse for accuracy of the insulin dosage by comparing the insulin container, the syringe, and the primary health care provider's order before administration.

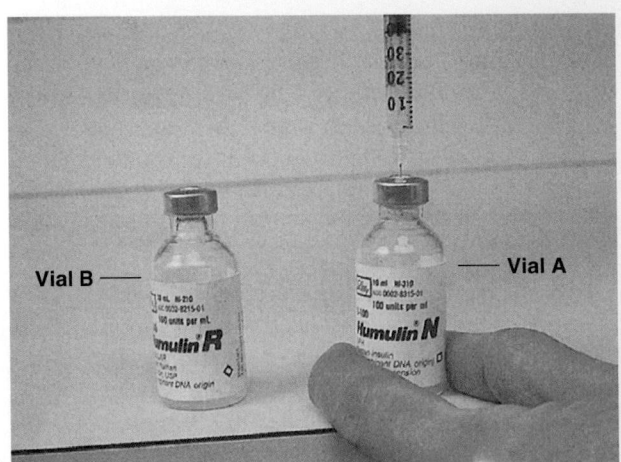
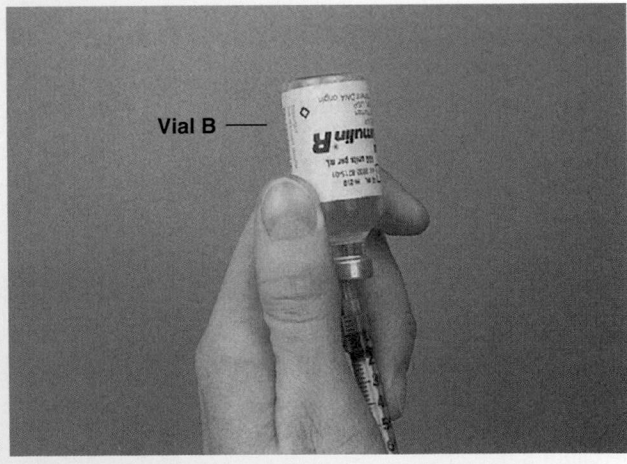

FIGURE 40.4 Drawing up two types of insulin into one syringe. **A.** After cleansing tops of both insulin vials, with the container upright, the nurse injects air into the Humulin N (intermediate-acting) insulin equal to the prescribed dosage of Humulin N. The nurse removes the needle without touching any fluid, then injects the amount of air equal to the prescribed dosage of the Humulin R (regular) insulin and withdraws the prescribed dosage of regular insulin into the syringe. **B.** After removing any air bubbles and determining what the total combined volume of the two insulins would measure, the nurse inverts the vial with the NPH (intermediate-acting) insulin and carefully withdraws the correct volume of medication. (*Note:* The nurse should have a second nurse independently check medication and dosage again before administering the insulin.)

ROTATING INJECTION SITES. Insulin may be injected into the arms, thighs, abdomen, or buttocks. Because absorption rates vary at the different sites, with the abdomen having the most rapid rate of absorption, followed by the upper arm, thigh, and buttocks, some health care providers recommend rotating the injection sites within one specific area, rather than rotating areas. For example, all available sites within the abdomen would be used before moving to the thigh.

Sites of insulin injection are rotated to prevent **lipodystrophy** (atrophy of subcut fat), a problem that can interfere with the absorption of insulin from the injection site. Lipodystrophy appears as a slight dimpling or pitting of the subcut fat.

With many tasks to learn in caring for diabetes, some manufactures provide numbered charts or templates to guide site rotation. Use these teaching tools as a method to instruct clients in self-management as well as providing care. Before each dose of insulin is given, check the client's record for the site of the previous injection and use the next site (according to the rotation plan) for injection. Ask the client to validate the site last used, too. If able, always ask the client if they prefer to self-inject, rather than assuming the person is too sick to do the task. After giving the injection, document the site used. Every time insulin is given, previous injection sites are inspected for inflammation, which may indicate a localized allergic reaction.

METHODS OF ADMINISTERING INSULIN. Several methods can be used to administer insulin: needle and syringe, pen, and by pump. Figure 40.5 illustrates these three methods of insulin administration. The most common method is the use of a needle and syringe. These items are both plentiful and inexpensive compared with other methods. Use of microfine needles has reduced the discomfort associated with an injection.

Another method is the pen injection system, which uses a cartridge that is prefilled with a specific type of insulin product (e.g., NPH insulin). This method is convenient for clients who self-administer their own insulin products. The pens are meant for single client use and should never be used with more than one client.

The desired units are selected by turning a dial and the locking ring. The dose is determined by the number of clicks heard. The needle portion is replaced between each injection. Although expensive, these are helpful for clients with trouble holding or seeing the syringe.

! NURSING ALERT

Insulin pens are client specific. They are designed for one client to use multiple times. A separate needle is used in these devices, yet can still be contaminated by the client's blood and should never be shared by more than one client.

Another method of insulin delivery is the insulin pump. This system attempts to mimic the body's normal pancreatic function, uses only rapid-acting insulin analogues, is battery powered, and requires insertion of a needle into subcut tissue. The needle is changed every 1–3 days. The amount of insulin injected can be adjusted according to blood glucose levels, which are monitored four to eight times per day.

DOSING. Individuals diagnosed with type 1 diabetes will always need to take insulin. The insulin dosage pattern that most closely follows normal insulin production is a multiple-dose plan sometimes called *intensive insulin therapy*. Dosing consists of **basal and bolus insulin**. A person eats food and it becomes glucose in the bloodstream; additionally, while asleep the liver also secretes glucose, which can increase glucose in the blood. The purpose of basal insulin is to keep blood glucose levels even when the person is fasting (such as being asleep) by helping the glucose get into cells so it can be burned for energy. In this regimen, a

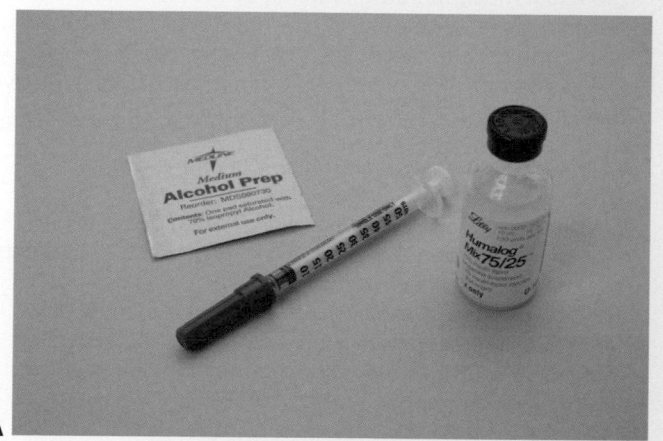
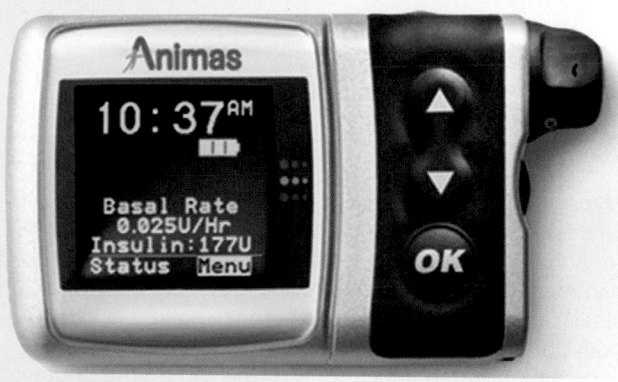
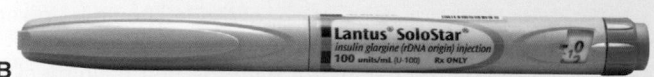

FIGURE 40.5 Insulin products can be administered using **(A)** a needle and syringe, **(B)** an insulin pen, or **(C)** an insulin pump. (From Carter, P. J. (2016). *Lippincott textbook for nursing assistants* (4th ed.). Wolters Kluwer.)

single dose of intermediate- or long-acting insulin is taken in the morning or at bedtime. Small doses (bolus) of rapid-acting insulin are taken before meals based on the client's blood glucose levels and HbA$_{1c}$. This allows for greater flexibility in the client's lifestyle, but it can also be an inconvenience to the client (e.g., the need always to carry supplies, the lack of privacy, inconvenient schedules).

Depending on the client's condition, an order for rapid- or short-acting insulin as a supplement to the drug regimen to "cover" any episodes of hyperglycemia may be used. For example, when client is hospitalized, blood glucose levels may be monitored every 6 hr or before meals and at bedtime, with regular (short-acting) insulin in a standardized protocol prescribed to cover any hyperglycemia detected. This coverage is sometimes referred to by the health care providers as a sliding scale, or insulin coverage. The supplemental insulin is administered based on blood glucose readings and the amount of insulin prescribed by the primary health care provider in the regular insulin coverage protocol. Even when a protocol is in use, you should immediately notify the primary health care provider if the blood glucose level is greater than 400 mg/dL.

Inhaled rapid-acting human insulin delivery is available and marketed as Afrezza. It is prescribed only under a Risk Evaluation and Mitigation Strategy (REMS) program. This is because of the risk of acute bronchospasm in client with chronic lung diseases such as asthma or chronic obstructive pulmonary disease. Inhaled insulin is also in the research process for use in clients with mild cognitive impairment and Alzheimer disease (Craft et al., 2012).

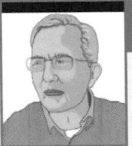

PHARMACOLOGY IN PRACTICE

DRUG RECOGNITION
A client with gestational diabetes is administered insulin with an insulin pump. Which of the insulin products will be used in the pump?
1. Lantus
2. Aspart
3. Regular
4. Glargine

Hypoglycemics
Oral and parenteral forms of hypoglycemics are available for administration. The incretin hormone preparations are parenteral and administered using a syringe pen. This is similar to insulin administration. These solutions should never be mixed with an insulin product. GLP-1 agonists should be injected subcut only at the same time of day on the same day each week.

Glycemic control is initially started with one drug. If blood glucose levels do not decrease, a second oral medication is added to the drug regimen. The choice of a second medication varies from client to client and is prescribed by the primary health care provider. Glucovance, which includes both glyburide and

metformin, is one example of the use of combination drugs for glycemic control. The combination drugs are useful for individuals who have other chronic conditions necessitating the administration of multiple pills, capsules, or tablets. Some chronically ill individuals may have well over 25–30 different drugs to take daily. Combination drugs in one form helps to lessen the burden of potentially missed medications by reducing the number of items being taken.

! NURSING ALERT
Exposure to stress, such as infection, fever, surgery, or trauma, may cause a loss of control of blood glucose levels in clients who have been stabilized with oral antidiabetic drugs. Should this occur, the primary health care provider may discontinue use of the oral drug and administer insulin product.

Oral antidiabetic drugs are given as a single daily dose or in divided doses. The following sections provide specific information for each group of oral antidiabetic drugs.

METFORMIN. The client is instructed to take metformin two or three times a day with meals. If the client has not experienced a response in 4 weeks using the maximum dose of metformin, the primary health care provider may add an oral sulfonylurea while continuing metformin at the maximum dose. Glucophage XR (metformin, extended release) is administered once daily with the evening meal, and should not be crushed or chewed.

SGLT-2. SGLT-2 medication should be taken at the same time each day. If a dose is missed, the drug should be taken as soon as this is recognized, but not two doses at once.

THIAZOLIDINEDIONES. Pioglitazone and rosiglitazone are given with or without meals. If the dose is missed at the usual meal, the drug is taken at the next meal. If the dose is missed on one day, it is not doubled the following day. If the drug is taken, the meal must not be delayed. Delay of a meal for as little as 30 min can cause hypoglycemia.

ALPHA-GLUCOSIDASE INHIBITORS. Acarbose and miglitol are given three times a day with the first bite of the meal, because food increases absorption. Some clients begin therapy with a lower dose once daily to minimize GI effects such as abdominal discomfort, flatulence, and diarrhea. The dose is then gradually increased to three times daily. Response to these drugs is monitored by periodic testing. Dosage adjustments are made at 4- to 16-week intervals based on blood glucose levels.

SULFONYLUREAS. Chlorpropamide, tolazamide, and tolbutamide are given with food to prevent GI upset. However, because food delays absorption, glipizide should be given 30 min before a meal. Glyburide and glimepiride are administered with breakfast or with the first main meal of the day.

MEGLITINIDES. Repaglinide can be taken immediately or up to 30 min before meals. Nateglinide is taken up to 30 min before meals.

Monitoring and Managing Client Needs

Acute Confusion

Mental confusion may be a sign that a client has low blood sugar. Close observation of the client with diabetes is important, especially when diabetes is newly diagnosed, the medication dosage changes, the client is pregnant, the client has a medical illness or surgery, or the client fails to adhere to the prescribed diet. Older, debilitated, or malnourished clients are also more likely to experience hypoglycemia. Episodes of hypoglycemia are corrected as soon as the symptoms are recognized. A client who has had this reaction before may be able to tell you that their blood sugar is low; check their blood sugar.

Methods of terminating a hypoglycemic reaction include the administration of one or more of the following rescue foods:

- 4 ounce of orange juice or other fruit juice
- Hard candy or one tablespoon of honey
- Commercial glucose products such as glucose gel or glucose tablets
- **Glucagon** by the subcut, IM, or IV routes
- Glucose 10% or 50% IV

Selection of any one or more of these methods for terminating a hypoglycemic reaction, as well as other procedures to be followed, such as drawing blood for glucose levels, depends on the written order of the primary health care provider or hospital policy. Never give oral fluids or substances (such as candy) to a client when the swallowing and gag reflexes are absent. Absence of these reflexes may result in aspiration of the oral fluid or substance into the lungs, which can result in extremely serious consequences and even death. If swallowing and gag reflexes are absent, or if the client is unconscious, glucose or glucagon is given by the parenteral route.

⚠ NURSING ALERT

When a hypoglycemic client is taking an alpha-glucosidase inhibitor (e.g., acarbose or miglitol), give the client an oral form of glucose, such as glucose tablets or dextrose, rather than juice, honey, or candy (sucrose). Absorption of sugar is blocked by acarbose or miglitol.

Glucagon is a hormone produced by the alpha (α) cells of the pancreas; it acts to increase blood glucose by stimulating the conversion of glycogen to glucose in the liver. A return of consciousness is observed within 5–20 min after parenteral administration of glucagon. Glucagon is effective in treating hypoglycemia only if glycogen is available from the liver.

Contact the primary health care provider when a hypoglycemic reaction occurs; note the substance and amount used to terminate the reaction, blood samples

drawn (if any), the length of time required for the symptoms of hypoglycemia to disappear, and the current status of the client. After termination of a hypoglycemic reaction, closely observe the client for additional hypoglycemic reactions. The length of time that close observation is required depends on the peak and duration of the insulin administered.

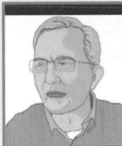

PHARMACOLOGY IN PRACTICE

MANAGING NEEDS

A client has been prescribed miglitol. The administration of miglitol causes hypoglycemia in the client. What is the nurse's priority intervention in such a situation?

1. Discuss the disease and methods of control with the client.
2. Administer insulin to the client.
3. Administer the client glucose tablets rather than sugar candy.
4. Obtain capillary blood specimens from the client.

Hypovolemia/Dehydration

Dehydration occurs with DKA. DKA is a potentially life-threatening deficiency of insulin (hypoinsulinism), resulting in severe hyperglycemia and requiring prompt diagnosis and treatment. Because insulin is unavailable to allow glucose to enter the cell, dangerously high levels of glucose build up in the blood (hyperglycemia). The body, needing energy, begins to break down fat for energy. As fats break down, the liver produces ketones. As more and more fat is used for energy, higher levels of ketones accumulate in the blood. Symptoms of hyperglycemia include elevated blood glucose levels (over 200 mg/mL); headache; increased thirst; epigastric pain; nausea; vomiting; hot, dry, flushed skin; restlessness; and diaphoresis (sweating). This increase in ketones disrupts the acid–base balance in the body, leading to DKA. DKA is treated with fluids, correction of acidosis and hypotension, and low doses of regular insulin.

Anxiety

The client with newly diagnosed diabetes may have difficulty accepting the diagnosis, and the complexity of the therapeutic regimen can seem overwhelming. The client with newly diagnosed diabetes often has many concerns regarding the diagnosis. For some, initially coping with diabetes and the methods required for controlling the disorder creates many problems. Some of the issues and concerns of these clients may include uncertainty regarding the ability to self-administer an injection, following a diet, weight control, complications associated with diabetes, and changes in eating times and habits.

An effective teaching program helps the client master the skills of self-care. Use principles of adult learning to start with small, obtainable goals. You may begin with blood sugar monitoring, then the skill of injection before discussing long-term complications. Success in small increments can help these clients gradually accept the diagnosis and begin to understand their feelings. In turn, this empowers the client and reduces uncertainty that leads to anxiety. The client in this situation gains confidence and then is able to talk about the disorder, express concerns, and ask questions.

Altered Breathing Pattern

When taking metformin, the client is at risk for lactic acidosis. Monitor the client for symptoms of lactic acidosis, which include unexplained hyperventilation, myalgia, malaise, GI symptoms, or unusual somnolence. If the client experiences these symptoms, contact the primary health care provider at once. Elevated blood lactate levels exceeding 5 mmol/L are associated with lactic acidosis and should be reported immediately. Once a client's diabetes is stabilized on metformin therapy, the adverse GI reactions that often occur at the beginning of such therapy are unlikely to be related to the drug therapy. A later occurrence of GI symptoms is more likely to be related to lactic acidosis or other serious disease.

Educating the Client and Family

Consistent adherence is a problem in some clients with diabetes, making client and family teaching vital to the proper management of diabetes. Clients may occasionally lapse in adhering to the prescribed diet, especially around holidays or other special occasions. This slip may not cause a problem if it is brief and not excessive and if the client immediately returns to the prescribed regimen. However, some clients frequently stray from the prescribed regimen, take extra insulin to cover dietary indiscretions, fast for several days before follow-up blood glucose determinations, and engage in other dangerous behaviors. Clients taking an oral antidiabetic drug may feel the disease is not serious *because* they are not taking insulin, or they may feel they lack control of the disease and express concern about the possibility of having to take insulin in the future. Although some clients can be convinced that failure to adhere to the prescribed therapeutic regimen is detrimental to their health, others continue to deviate from the prescribed regimen until serious complications develop. Every effort is made to stress the importance of adherence to the prescribed treatment during the initial teaching session and during follow-up office or clinic visits. Chronic illness workshops and support groups are helpful for some clients and family members to help them get back on track and stay motivated.

Include the following information in a teaching plan:

- *Identification*—wear identification, such as a MedicAlert bracelet, to inform medical personnel and others of the use of antidiabetic drugs or insulin to control the disease.
- *Diet*—importance of following the prescribed diet; calories allowed; food exchanges; planning daily menus; establishing meal schedules; selecting food from a restaurant menu; reading food labels; use of artificial sweeteners. Avoid alcohol, dieting, and commercial weight loss products not recommended by your health care team.
- *Blood glucose or urine testing*—the testing material recommended by the primary health care provider; a

review of the instructions included with the glucometer or the materials used for urine testing; the technique of collecting the specimen; interpreting test results; number of times a day or week the blood or urine is tested (as recommended by the primary health care provider); a record of test results.

- *Hypoglycemia/hyperglycemia*—signs and symptoms of hypoglycemia and hyperglycemia; food or fluid used to terminate a hypoglycemic reaction; importance of notifying the primary health care provider immediately if either reaction occurs.
- *Personal hygiene*—importance of good skin and foot care, personal cleanliness, frequent dental checkups, and routine eye examinations.
- *Exercise*—importance of following the primary health care provider's recommendations regarding physical activity. Do not engage in strenuous exercise programs unless use or participation has been approved by the primary health care provider.
- *When to notify the primary health care provider*—increase in blood glucose levels; urine positive for ketones; if pregnancy occurs; occurrence of antidiabetic or hyperglycemic episodes; occurrence of illness, infection, or diarrhea (insulin dosage may require adjustment); appearance of new problems (e.g., leg ulcers, numbness of the extremities, significant weight gain or loss).
- *Traveling*—importance of carrying an extra supply of oral medicines or insulin and a prescription for needles and syringes; always keep medications in the original container; storage of insulin when traveling; protecting needles and syringes from theft; airports typically have disposal containers for used equipment. It is important to discuss travel plans (especially foreign travel) with the primary health care provider.

Injectables

- *Insulin*—types; how dosage is expressed; calculating the insulin dosage; importance of using only the type, source, and brand name recommended by the primary health care provider; importance of not changing brands unless the health care provider approves; keeping a spare vial on hand; prescription for insulin purchase not required.
- *Storage of insulin*—insulin is kept at room temperature away from heat and direct sunlight if used within 1 month (and up to 3 months if refrigerated); vials not in use are stored in the refrigerator; prefilled insulin in glass or plastic syringes is stable for 1 week under refrigeration. Keep filled syringes in a vertical or oblique position with the needle pointing upward to avoid plugging the needle.
- *Needle and syringe*—purchase the same brand and needle size each time; parts of the syringe; reading the syringe scale.
- *Disposal of the needle and syringe*—puncture-proof containers specifically used for disposal may be obtained from pharmacies, clinics, or the primary health care provider. Clients are cautioned not to dispose in home

trash; rather, the filled container should be returned to where the container was purchased for disposal. Local hospitals will also take containers.

- Insulin needs may change in clients who become ill, especially with vomiting or fever, and during periods of stress or emotional disturbance. Contact the primary health care provider if these situations occur.

Oral Hypoglycemics

- Take the drug exactly as directed on the container (e.g., with food, 30 min before a meal).
- An antidiabetic drug is not oral insulin and cannot be substituted for insulin.
- Never stop taking this drug or increase or decrease the dose unless told to do so by the primary health care provider.
- Take the drug at the same time or times each day.
- Metformin—there is a risk of lactic acidosis when using this drug. Discontinue the drug therapy and notify the primary health care provider immediately if any of the following occur: respiratory distress, muscular aches, unusual somnolence, unexplained malaise, or nonspecific abdominal distress.
- SGLT2—sugar will be positive on a urine test. This makes you more at risk for a yeast infection (vaginal or penis) or urinary tract infection. Report signs or symptoms of infection immediately for treatment. Do not begin self-treatment until you have contacted the primary health care provider.
- Alogliptin—report severe and persistent abdominal pain, this may be acute pancreatitis.

EVALUATION

- Therapeutic drug effect is achieved and normal or near-normal blood glucose levels are maintained.
- Hypoglycemia and other adverse reactions are identified, reported to the primary health care provider, and managed successfully through appropriate nursing interventions:

  - Orientation and mentation remain intact.
  - Adequate fluid volume is maintained.
  - Anxiety is managed successfully.
  - An adequate breathing pattern is maintained.

- Client and family express confidence and demonstrate an understanding of the drug regimen.

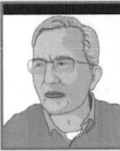

PHARMACOLOGY IN PRACTICE

USING CLINICAL REASONING

Mr. Phillip is sent home with a blood glucometer to check his own blood daily and is instructed to call the nurse after 1 week with the readings. The readings indicated that he most likely has type 2 diabetes. The primary health care provider prescribes glyburide. Mr. Phillip gets upset, telling you that when his wife was alive he did not take any medicines and was fine, so why is he so sick now? Discuss the instructions and information you would share with him.

KEY POINTS

■ Insulin is a hormone produced by the pancreas that regulates how glucose gets into cells and is used for energy. Protein and fat metabolism also require insulin.

■ Diabetes mellitus is a chronic condition where insufficient insulin is produced by the pancreatic beta cells (type 1) or in addition to less insulin produced the body cells become resistant to insulin (type 2). About 90%–95% of cases of diabetes are of the type 2 variety; many of these can be controlled with diet, exercise, and possibly the addition of an oral hypoglycemic drug.

■ Insulin is used to treat type 1 diabetes and may be used along with oral antidiabetic agents to treat type 2 diabetes. When insulin is given, the onset, peak, and duration of action are all properties that direct the administration schedule. Insulin is used to supplement the endogenous supply.

■ Oral hypoglycemics are not used to treat type 1 diabetes; oral agents stimulate the pancreas to release insulin or reduce the liver's tendency to release glucose into the circulating blood. Hormone injections may help stimulate the pancreas.

■ Self-management is an important concept in diabetic care and includes learning to monitor blood glucose, modify diet and exercise, control weight, and administer the drugs prescribed.

■ One of the primary tasks in diabetic management is monitoring for the adverse reactions or signs of hyperglycemia and hypoglycemia when a person assumes drug management for the disease. Adverse reactions associated with the oral hypoglycemic drugs are of the GI nature—nausea, metallic taste, cramping, and diarrhea.

SUMMARY DRUG TABLE
Insulin/Insulin Analogue Preparations

Types of Insulin	Trade Name	Activity		
		Onset	Peak	Duration
Short- and Rapid-Acting Insulins				
regular insulin (human)	HumuLIN R, Myxredlin, NovoLIN R	30–60 min	2–4 hr	5–8 hr
aspart (insulin analogue)[a]	Fiasp, NovoLOG	5–15 min	1–3 hr	3–5 hr
glulisine (insulin analogue)	Apidra	15–30 min	30–60 min	4 hr
lispro (insulin analogue)[a]	Admelog, HumaLOG, Lyumjev	5–10 min	30 min–1.5 hr	3–5 hr
Intermediate-Acting Insulins				
insulin isophane suspension (NPH)	HumuLIN N, NovoLIN N	1.5 hr	4–10 hr	14 hr
Long-Acting Insulins (All Insulin Analogues)				
insulin degludec	Tresiba	1 hr	9 hr	25 hr
insulin detemir	Levemir	3–4 hr	6–8 hr	24 hr
insulin glargine	Basaglar, Lantus, Semglee, Toujeo (300 U/mL)	1 hr	Steady, no peak	24 hr
Combined Insulins (Long/Short Acting)				
70% insulin aspart protamine/30% insulin aspart	NovoLOG 70/30	10–20 min	1–1.5 hr	18–24 hr
70% insulin analogue degludec/30% insulin analogue aspart	Ryzodeg 70/30	15 min	72 min	24 hr
70% isophane insulin suspension (NPH)/30% regular insulin	HumuLIN 70/30, NovoLIN 70/30	30–60 min	2–4 hr	18–24 hr
50% insulin lispro protamine/50% insulin lispro	HumaLOG Mix 50/50	15-30 min	1-5 hr	14–24 hr

[a]Used in insulin infusion pumps.

SUMMARY DRUG TABLE
Oral Antidiabetic Drugs (Hypoglycemics) and Other Agents

Generic Name	Trade Name	Uses	Adverse Reactions	Dosage Ranges
Biguanide				
metFORMIN *met-FOR-min*	Fortamet, Riomet	Prediabetes, type 2 diabetes monotherapy; combotherapy to improve glycemic control	Nausea, vomiting, flatulence, diarrhea	500–3000 mg/day orally; XR (extended release): 500–2000 mg/day
Glucagon-Like Peptide-1 (GLP-1) Agonists				
[a]**albiglutide** *al-bi-GLOO-tide*		Type 2 diabetes	Nausea, vomiting, diarrhea, injection site reaction	30 mg subcut, weekly
[a]**dulaglutide** *doo-la-GLOO-tide*	Trulicity	Type 2 diabetes	Same as albiglutide	1.5 mg subcut, weekly
[a]**exenatide** *ex-EN-a-tide*	Byetta (daily), Bydureon (weekly)	Type 2 diabetes	Same as albiglutide	5 mcg subcut, 1 hr after meal, twice daily; 2 mg subcut, weekly
[a]**liraglutide** *lir-a-GLOO-tide*	Victoza, Saxenda (obesity)	Type 2 diabetes, obesity	Headache, nausea, vomiting, diarrhea, constipation, local irritation at injection site	0.6–1.8 mg subcut daily
[a]**lixisenatide** *lix-i-SEN-a-tide*	Adlyxin	Type 2 diabetes		10–20 mcg subcut daily in morning
semaglutide *sem-a-GLOO-tide*	Ozempic, Rybelsus (oral)	Type 2 diabetes, Obesity	Decreased appetite, diarrhea	0.25–1 mg subcut weekly

Generic Name	Trade Name	Uses	Adverse Reactions	Dosage Ranges
Sodium-Glucose Linked Transporter-2 Inhibitors (SGLT-2is)				
canagliflozin *kan-a-gli-FLOE-zin*	Invokana	Type 2 diabetes	Genital/urinary yeast infections	100 mg orally daily
dapagliflozin *dap-a-gli-FLOE-zin*	Farxiga	Type 2 diabetes	Hypoglycemia, genital/urinary yeast infections	5 mg orally daily
empagliflozin *em-pa-gli-FLOE-zin*	Jardiance	Type 2 diabetes	Hypoglycemia, genital/urinary yeast infections	10 mg orally daily
ertugliflozin *er-too-gli-FLOE-zin*	Steglatro	Type 2 diabetes	Hypoglycemia, genital/urinary yeast infections	5–15 mg orally daily
Dipeptidyl Peptidase-4 Inhibitors (Gliptins)				
alogliptin *al-oh-GLIP-tin*	Nesina	Type 2 diabetes	Headache, nasopharyngitis	25 mg orally daily
linagliptin *lin-a-GLIP-tin*	Tradjenta	Type 2 diabetes	Nasopharyngitis	5 mg orally daily
SAXagliptin *sax-a-GLIP-tin*	Onglyza	Type 2 diabetes	Headache, upper respiratory infection, urinary tract infection	2.5–5 mg orally daily
SITagliptin *sit-ah-GLIP-tin*	Januvia	Type 2 diabetes	Headache, nasopharyngitis, upper respiratory infection	100 mg orally daily
Thiazolidinediones (TZD)				
pioglitazone *pye-oh-GLI-ta-zone*	Actos	Type 2 diabetes mono/combotherapy	Headache, back pain, respiratory symptoms	5–15 mg orally TID
rosiglitazone *roh-zsi-GLI-ta-zone*	Avandia	Type 2 diabetes mono/combotherapy	Headache, back pain, respiratory symptoms	4–8 mg/day orally
Alpha-Glucosidase Inhibitors (AGIs)				
acarbose *AY-car-bose*	Precose	Type 2 diabetes mono/combotherapy	Flatulence, bloating, diarrhea, abdominal pain	25–100 mg orally TID
miglitol *MIG-li-tol*	Glyset	Same as acarbose	Same as acarbose	25–100 mg orally TID
Amylinomimetic				
ᵃpramlintide *PRAM-lin-tide*	Symlin	Type 2 diabetes, type 1 adjunct	Headache, nausea, anorexia, injection site reaction	Type 2: 60–120 mcg subcut Type 1: 15–60 mcg subcut
Sulfonylureas				
Third Generation				
glimepiride *GLYE-me-pye-ride*	Amaryl	Type 2 diabetes mono/combotherapy	Nausea, weight gain, headache, epigastric discomfort, heartburn, hypoglycemia	1–4 mg/day orally
Second Generation				
glipiZIDE *GLIP-i-zide*	Glucotrol	Type 2 diabetes monotherapy	Same as glimepiride	5–40 mg/day orally
glyBURIDE *GLYE-byoor-ide*	DiaBeta, Glynase	Type 2 diabetes monotherapy	Same as glimepiride	1.25–20 mg/day orally
First Generation				
chlorproPAMIDE *klor-PROE-pa-mide*	Diabinese	Type 2 diabetes, diabetes insipidus	Same as glimepiride	100–250 mg/day orally
TOLAZamide *toll-AZ-a-mide*		Type 2 diabetes	Same as glimepiride	100–1000 mg/day orally
TOLBUTamide *toll-BYOO-ta-mide*		Type 2 diabetes	Same as glimepiride	0.25–3 g/day orally

Continued

SUMMARY DRUG TABLE (continued)
Oral Antidiabetic Drugs (Hypoglycemics) and Other Agents

Generic Name	Trade Name	Uses	Adverse Reactions	Dosage Ranges
Meglitinides				
nateglinide *na-te-GLYE-nide*	Starlix	Type 2 diabetes mono/ combotherapy	Upper respiratory tract infection, back pain, flu-like symptoms	60–120 mg orally TID before meals
repaglinide *re-PAG-li-nide*		Same as nateglinide	Hypoglycemia, upper respiratory tract infection, headache	0.5–4 mg orally before meals (maximum dose, 16 mg/day)
Other Agents				
bromocriptine *broe-moe-KRIP-teen*	Cycloset (approved for DM)	Parkinson disease, female endocrine imbalances, adjuvant in type 2 diabetes	Drowsiness, sedation, dizziness, faintness, epigastric distress, anorexia	10–40 mg/day orally
colesevelam *koh-le-SEV-e-lam*	WelChol	Hyperlipidemia, adjuvant in type 2 diabetes	Constipation, cramping, nausea	3–7 tablets/day orally
Glucose-Elevating Agents				
diazoxide *dye-az-OKS-ide*	Proglycem	Hypoglycemia caused by hyperinsulinism	Sodium and fluid retention, hyperglycemia, glycosuria, tachycardia, congestive heart failure	3–8 mg/kg/day orally in two or three equal doses q8–12hr
glucagon *GLOO-ka-gon*	Glucagon Emergency Kit, Baqsimi (intranasal)	Hypoglycemia	Nausea, vomiting, generalized allergic reactions	See instructions on the product

ªParenteral drug, comes in single patient injectable pen form.

SUMMARY DRUG TABLE
Oral Antidiabetic Combination Drugs

Antidiabetic Combination Drugs	
Generic Drugs	**Combination Drug Trade Name**
metformin/alogliptin	Kazano
metformin/canagliflozin	Invokamet
metformin/dapagliflozin	Xigduo XR
metformin/empagliflozin	Synjardy
metformin/empagliflozin/linagliptin	Trijardy XR
metformin/ertugliflozin	Segluromet
metformin/glyburide	NONE
metformin/glipizide	NONE
metformin/linagliptin	Jentadueto
metformin/pioglitazone	Actoplus
metformin/repaglinide	Prandimet
metformin/saxagliptin	Kombiglyze
metformin/saxagliptin/dapagliflozin	Qternmet XR
metformin/sitagliptin	Janumet
alogliptin/pioglitazone	Oseni
linagliptin/empagliflozin	Glyxambi
pioglitazone/glimepiride	Duetact
saxagliptin/dapagliflozin	Qtern
sitagliptin/ertugliflozin	Steglujan

CHAPTER REVIEW

Know Your Drugs

Clients sometimes know a medication by the brand (or trade) name and not the generic name. To help you recognize both names, match the brand name with the generic name of the same medication.

Generic Name	Brand Name
1. glyburide	A. DiaBeta
2. metformin	B. Fortamet
3. nateglinide	C. Januvia
4. sitagliptin	D. Starlix

Calculate Medication Dosages

1. A client is prescribed rosiglitazone (Avandia) 8 mg orally daily. Available are 2-mg tablets. The nurse would administer _____.

2. A client is prescribed 40 units NPH insulin mixed with 5 units of regular insulin. What is the total insulin dosage?

Prepare for the NCLEX

RECALL THE FACTS

1. Where is insulin produced in the body?
   1. Lining of the gut
   2. Pancreas
   3. Gallbladder
   4. Thyroid

2. Which of the following medications may be used for both type 1 and 2 diabetes?
   1. Regular insulin
   2. Januvia injection
   3. Metformin
   4. Chlorpropamide

3. Which of the following would the nurse mostly likely choose to treat a hypoglycemic reaction?
   1. Regular insulin
   2. NPH insulin
   3. Orange juice
   4. Crackers and soda

4. Which of the following would be the correct method of administering glargine an insulin analogue?
   1. Within 10 min of meals
   2. Immediately before meals
   3. Any time within 30 min before or 30 min after a meal
   4. At bedtime

5. Which of the following symptoms would alert the nurse to a possible hyperglycemic reaction?
   1. Fatigue, weakness, confusion
   2. Pale skin, elevated temperature
   3. Thirst, abdominal pain, nausea
   4. Rapid, shallow respirations, headache, nervousness

ANALYZE THE FACTS

6. A client with diabetes received a glycosylated hemoglobin test result of 9%. This indicates _____.
   1. the diabetes is well controlled
   2. poor blood glucose control
   3. the need for an increase in the insulin dosage
   4. the client is at increased risk for hypoglycemia

7. The mental health center is writing new admission protocols. Which client population should be routinely tested for elevated blood sugars?
   1. Obsessive–compulsive clients on antianxiety drugs
   2. Clinically depressed clients
   3. Schizophrenic clients on second-generation antipsychotics
   4. Older clients on haloperidol

ALTERNATE-FORMAT QUESTIONS

8. *List in order the following steps in drawing up two types of insulin.
   1. Remove air bubbles from syringe, and withdraw the Humulin N insulin prescribed.
   2. Remove the needle from the vial without getting fluid (insulin) on the needle.
   3. After cleansing both vials, inject air into the Humulin N insulin vial.
   4. Inject air into the regular insulin vial, and invert and withdraw the prescribed amount.

9. *A client is prescribed 40 units NPH insulin mixed with 5 units of regular insulin. What is the total insulin dosage? Describe how you would prepare the insulins.

10. A client is prescribed metformin (Glucophage) 1000 mg orally BID. The drug is available in 500-mg tablets. The nurse administers _____. What is the total daily dosage of metformin?

To check your answers, see Appendix F.

---

*Indicates the question is directly linked to the NCLEX-PN test plan in Appendix G.

WANT TO KNOW MORE? A wide variety of resources are available to enhance your learning and understanding of this chapter.
- Visit thePoint for resources such as:
  - NCLEX-Style Student Review Questions
  - Journal Articles
  - Dosage Calculations
  - Drug Monographs
  - Watch and Learn Videos
  - Concepts in Action Animations
- The *Study Guide to Accompany Introductory Clinical Pharmacology*, 12th edition, sold separately, will help you review and apply essential content.
- ✓PrepU is available to help students prepare for the NCLEX-PN examination.

41

Pituitary and Adrenocortical Hormones

Key Terms

adrenal insufficiency diminished adrenal gland production resulting in a deficiency in corticosteroids

anovulatory a menstrual cycle in which ovulation (release of egg) does not occur

cryptorchism failure of the testes to descend into the scrotum

cushingoid group of symptoms (including moon face, buffalo hump) caused by the disease due to the overproduction of endogenous glucocorticoids

diabetes insipidus disease caused by failure of the pituitary gland to secrete vasopressin or by surgical removal of the pituitary

feedback mechanism method used by glands to signal the need for or cessation of hormonal production

gonads glands responsible for sexual activity and characteristics

hirsutism excess growth of facial and body hair in women

hyperstimulation syndrome sudden ovarian enlargement caused by overstimulation

Learning Objectives

On completion of this chapter, the student will:

1. List the hormones produced by the pituitary gland and the adrenal cortex.
2. Explain general actions, uses, adverse reactions, contraindications, precautions, and interactions of the pituitary and adrenocortical hormones.
3. Distinguish important preadministration and ongoing assessment activities the nurse should perform with the client taking a pituitary or adrenocortical hormone.
4. List nursing diagnoses particular to a client taking a pituitary or adrenocortical hormone.
5. Examine ways to promote an optimal response to therapy, how to manage common adverse reactions, and important points to keep in mind when educating clients about the use of pituitary and adrenocortical hormones.

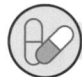 **Drug Classes**

Posterior pituitary hormones
• Vasopressin
Anterior pituitary hormones
• Gonadotropins

• Somatropin
• Adrenocorticotropic hormone
Glucocorticoids
Mineralocorticoids

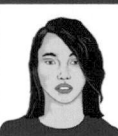 **PHARMACOLOGY IN PRACTICE**

Janna Wong is at the clinic for a sports physical. As you measure her height and weight, she tells you about a girl on the team who was sick and is now taking hormones and has grown 4 in. over the summer. Janna says that the coach favored this girl and let her use the bathroom whenever she felt like it. The classmate that Janna is describing had a pituitary tumor and needs to receive hormonal replacement for the rest of her life. Think about this situation as you read this chapter.

The pituitary gland is about the size of a green pea and lies deep within the cranial vault. The gland is not part of the brain; rather, it is suspended from the hypothalamus by the pituitary stalk and is protected by an indentation of the sphenoid bone called the *sella turcica*. The pituitary gland has two lobes:

• Anterior pituitary (adenohypophysis)
• Posterior pituitary (neurohypophysis)

The pituitary gland is often referred to as the "master gland" because it secretes many hormones that regulate numerous vital processes. The

548

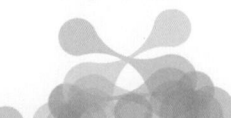

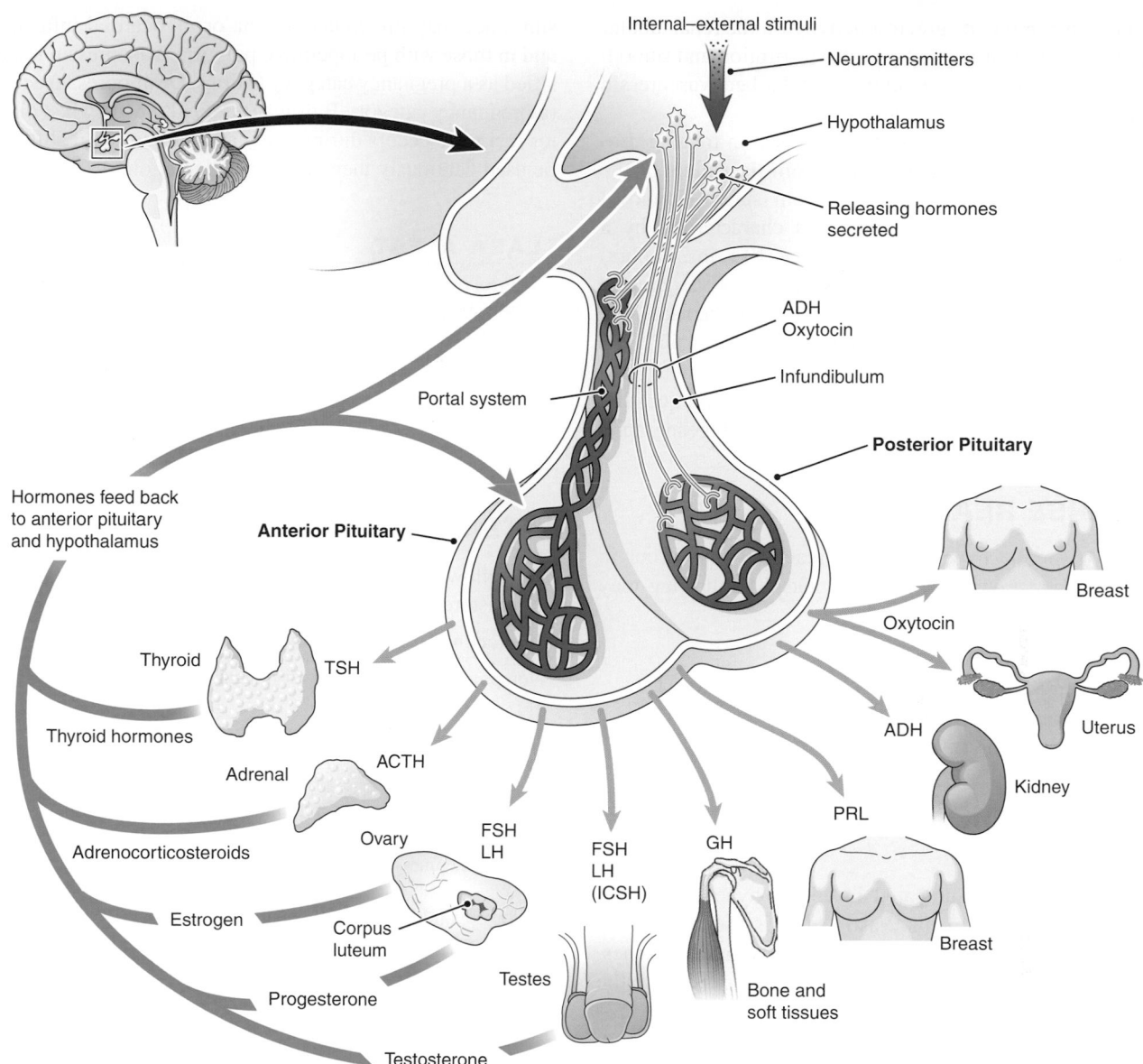

FIGURE 41.1 The pituitary gland and the hormones secreted by the anterior pituitary and the posterior pituitary. ADH, antidiuretic hormone; ACTH, adrenocorticotropic hormone; FSH, follicle-stimulating hormone; GH, growth hormone; ICSH, interstitial cell–stimulating hormone; LH, luteinizing hormone; PRL, prolactin; TSH, thyroid-stimulating hormone. (From Cohen, B. J., & Taylor, J. J. (2005). *Memmler's the human body in health and disease* (10th ed.). Lippincott Williams & Wilkins.)

pituitary regulates growth, metabolism, the reproductive cycle, electrolyte balance, and water retention or loss. The hormones secreted by the anterior and posterior pituitary and the organs influenced by these hormones are shown in Figure 41.1.

POSTERIOR PITUITARY HORMONES

The posterior pituitary gland produces two hormones: vasopressin (antidiuretic hormone [ADH]) and oxytocin (uterine stimulant). Vasopressin is discussed in this chapter and oxytocin is presented in Chapter 44.

VASOPRESSIN

ACTIONS AND USES

Vasopressin and its derivative, desmopressin (DDAVP), regulate the reabsorption of water by the kidneys. Vasopressin is secreted by the pituitary when body fluids must be conserved. This mechanism may be activated when, for example, an individual has severe vomiting and diarrhea with little or no fluid intake. When this and similar conditions are present, the posterior pituitary releases the hormone vasopressin, water in the kidney is reabsorbed into the blood (i.e., conserved), and the urine becomes concentrated.

Vasopressin exhibits its greatest activity on the renal tubular epithelium, where it promotes water resorption and smooth muscle contraction throughout the vascular bed. Vasopressin also has some vasopressor activity.

Vasopressin and its derivative are used in treating **diabetes insipidus**, a disease resulting from the failure of the pituitary to secrete vasopressin or from surgical removal of the pituitary. Diabetes insipidus is characterized by a marked increase in urination (as much as 10 L in 24 hours) and excessive thirst by inadequate secretion of vasopressin (ADH). Treatment with vasopressin therapy replaces the hormone in the body and restores normal urination and thirst. Vasopressin may also be used for preventing and treating postoperative abdominal distention and for dispelling gas interfering with abdominal roentgenography (radiographic studies).

ADVERSE REACTIONS

Local or systemic hypersensitivity reactions may occur in some clients receiving vasopressin, and the following may also be seen:

- Tremor, sweating, vertigo
- Nasal congestion
- Nausea, vomiting, abdominal cramps
- Water intoxication (overdosage, toxicity)

CONTRAINDICATIONS AND PRECAUTIONS

Vasopressin is contraindicated in clients hypersensitive to the drug or its components. Vasopressin is used cautiously in clients with a history of seizures, migraine headaches, asthma, heart failure (HF), or vascular disease (because the

substance may precipitate angina or myocardial infarction) and in those with perioperative polyuria. Vasopressin is classified as a pregnancy category C drug. Desmopressin acetate (a pregnancy category B drug) is typically used when diabetes insipidus occurs during pregnancy; however, it still must be used cautiously then and during lactation.

LASA ALERT

The following drugs may sound alike; be sure to clarify when they are ordered:

Drug Name	Sounds Like
desmopressin	vasopressin

Drugs that look like a similar drug are noted in the Summary Drug Tables of each chapter.

INTERACTIONS

The following interactions may occur when vasopressin is administered with another agent:

Interacting Drug	Common Use	Effect of Interaction
Norepinephrine	Neurostimulant	Decreased antidiuretic effect
Lithium	Management of psychological problems	Decreased antidiuretic effect
Oral anticoagulants	Blood thinners	Decreased antidiuretic effect
Carbamazepine	Anticonvulsant	Increased antidiuretic effect
Chlorpropamide	Antidiabetic (diabetes mellitus) agent	Increased antidiuretic effect

---

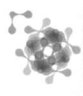

NURSING PROCESS: STEPS TO BUILDING CLINICAL JUDGMENT
Client Receiving Vasopressin

ASSESSMENT

Preadministration Assessment
Clients experiencing diabetes insipidus process large amounts of fluid in their bodies.

Data gathering suggestions before vasopressin is administered are listed in the following.
Objective data

- General client appearance, emphasis on signs of dehydration.
- Vital signs (temperature, pulse, respirations, and blood pressure).
- Weight.
- Measurement of intake and output over a specified period.

- Laboratory results—serum electrolytes, specifically sodium.
- Urinalysis, both sample and 24-hour specimen, fluid deprivation study.
- Magnetic resonance imaging of internal organs.

Subjective data

- Symptoms experienced by client regarding fluid intake/output.
- Family history of diabetes or other chronic health conditions.

If administering vasopressin to relieve abdominal distention, auscultate the abdomen and record the findings. Additionally measure and document the client's abdominal girth.

Ongoing Assessment

During the ongoing assessment of a hospitalized client monitor the blood pressure, pulse, and respiratory rate every 4 hours or as ordered by the primary health care provider. The client's fluid intake and output are strictly measured. The primary health care provider is notified if there are any significant changes in these vital signs because a dosage adjustment may be necessary.

The dosage of vasopressin or its derivatives may require periodic adjustments. After administration of the drug observe the client every 10–15 minutes for signs of an excessive dosage (e.g., blanching of the skin, abdominal cramps, and nausea). If these occur, reassure the client that recovery from these effects will occur in a few minutes.

NURSING DIAGNOSES

Drug-specific nursing diagnoses include the following:

- **Dehydration** related to inability to replenish fluid intake secondary to diabetes insipidus
- **Acute pain** related to abdominal distention

Nursing diagnoses related to drug administration are discussed in Chapter 4.

PLANNING

The expected outcomes for the client may include an optimal response to therapy, support of client needs related to the management of adverse reactions, and confidence in an understanding of the medication regimen.

IMPLEMENTATION

Promoting an Optimal Response to Therapy

Vasopressin may be given intramuscularly (IM) or sub-cutaneously (subcut) to an inpatient to treat diabetes insipidus. To prevent or relieve abdominal distention, the first dose is given 2 hours before radiographic examination and the second dose is given 30 minutes before the testing. An enema may be given before the first dose.

Desmopressin may be given orally, intranasally, subcut, or intravenously (IV). When the condition becomes chronic and the client learns to self-administer the drug, adjustments are made according to the client's response to therapy. Clients learn to regulate their dosage based on the frequency of urination and increase of thirst. A higher dose of the drug may be taken at night to reduce thirst and urination while sleeping.

Monitoring and Managing Client Needs

The adverse reactions associated with vasopressin, such as skin blanching, abdominal cramps, and nausea, may be decreased by administering the agent with one or two glasses of water. If these adverse reactions occur, inform the client that they are not serious and should subside within a few minutes.

NURSING ALERT

Excessive dosage is manifested as water intoxication (fluid overload). Symptoms of water intoxication include drowsiness, listlessness, confusion, and headache (which may precede convulsions and coma). If signs of excessive dosage occur, notify the primary health care provider before the next dose of the drug is due; a change in the dosage, the restriction of oral or IV fluids, and the administration of a diuretic may be necessary.

Dehydration

The symptoms of diabetes insipidus include the voiding of a large volume of urine at frequent intervals during the day and throughout the night. Accompanying this frequent urination is the need to drink large volumes of fluid because clients with diabetes insipidus are continually thirsty and need to be supplied with large amounts of drinking water. Take care to refill the water container at frequent intervals. This is especially important when the client has limited ambulatory activities. Until controlled by a drug, the symptoms of frequent urination and excessive thirst may cause a great deal of anxiety. Reassure the client that with the proper drug therapy, these symptoms will most likely be reduced or eliminated.

Fluid intake and output are accurately measured and the client is observed for signs of dehydration (dry mucous membranes, concentrated urine, poor skin turgor, flushing, dry skin, and confusion). This is especially important early in treatment and until such time as the optimum dosage is determined and symptoms have diminished. If the client's output greatly exceeds intake, contact the primary health care provider. In some instances, the primary health care provider may order specific gravity and volume measurements of each voiding or at hourly intervals. Document these results in the chart to aid the primary health care provider in adjusting the dosage to the client's needs.

 Chronic Care Considerations

Diabetes Insipidus

If a person with diabetes insipidus is unable to take routine medication, a fluid deficit can rapidly occur. Therefore, individuals with diabetes insipidus should wear a medical alert bracelet so that emergency personnel can be aware of this need for the medication and dosing can be continued if the clients are unable to take the drug themselves.

Acute Pain

If the client is receiving vasopressin for abdominal distention, explain the details of treating this problem and the necessity of monitoring drug effectiveness (e.g., auscultation of the abdomen for bowel sounds, insertion of a rectal tube, and measurement of the abdomen). If a rectal tube is ordered after administration of vasopressin for abdominal distention, the lubricated end of the tube is inserted past the anal sphincter and taped in place. The tube is left in place for 1 hour or as prescribed by the primary health care provider. Auscultate the abdomen every 15–30 minutes and measure abdominal girth hourly, or as ordered by the primary health care provider.

Educating the Client and Family

If desmopressin is to be used nasally, ensure that the client masters the technique of instillation. Provide illustrated client instructions with the drug and review them with the client. You should discuss the need to take the drug as directed by the primary health care provider. The client should change the dosage (i.e., the prescribed number or frequency of sprays) only after consulting with the primary health care provider.

Emphasize the importance of adhering to the prescribed treatment program to control symptoms. In addition to instruction on administration include the following in a client and family teaching plan:

- Wear medical identification naming the disease and the drug regimen.
- Carry a sport drink bottle to be sure to have liquids available at all times.

- Monitor the amount of fluids taken each day.
- Monitor the amount and frequency of urine for each 24-hour period, reporting changes to daily patterns to your nurse.
- Carry extra doses of the drug in case you do not make it home in time for your next dose.

🍷 Avoid the use of alcohol while taking these drugs.

- Rotate injection sites for parenteral administration.
- Contact the primary health care provider immediately if any of the following occurs: a significant increase or decrease in urine output, abdominal cramps, blanching of the skin, nausea, signs of inflammation or infection at the injection sites, confusion, headache, or drowsiness.

EVALUATION

- Therapeutic effect is achieved.
- Adverse reactions are identified, reported to the primary health care provider, and managed successfully through appropriate nursing interventions:
  - Fluid volume balance is maintained.
  - Acute pain is relieved.
- Client and family express confidence and demonstrate an understanding of the drug regimen.

ANTERIOR PITUITARY HORMONES

The hormones of the anterior pituitary include:

- thyroid-stimulating hormone (TSH)
- adrenocorticotropic hormone (ACTH)
- luteinizing hormone (LH)
- follicle-stimulating hormone (FSH)
- growth hormone (GH)
- prolactin (PRL)

The anterior pituitary hormone TSH is discussed in Chapter 42. The remaining hormones are covered in this chapter and can be classified as follows:

- ACTH is produced by the anterior pituitary and stimulates the adrenal cortex to secrete the corticosteroids in response to biologic stress.
- FSH and LH are called gonadotropins because they influence the gonads (the organs of reproduction).
- GH, also called somatropin, contributes to the growth of the body during childhood, especially the growth of muscles and bones.
- PRL, which is also secreted by the anterior pituitary, stimulates the production of breast milk in the postpartum client. Additional functions of PRL are not well understood. PRL is the only anterior pituitary hormone that is not used medically.

GONADOTROPINS: FOLLICLE-STIMULATING HORMONE AND LUTEINIZING HORMONE

The gonadotropins (FSH and LH) influence the secretion of sex hormones, the development of secondary sex characteristics, and the reproductive cycle in both men and women.

ACTION AND USES

These drugs are purified preparations of the gonadotropins (FSH and LH) extracted from the urine of postmenopausal women or produced by a recombinant form of DNA. Gonadotropins are used to induce ovulation and pregnancy in **anovulatory** women (women whose bodies fail to produce an ovum or fail to ovulate). These drugs are also used in assisted reproductive technology (ART) programs to stimulate multiple follicles for in vitro fertilization. Besides their use in treating female infertility, some of these drugs are used in men. Human chorionic gonadotropin (HCG) is extracted from human placentas. The actions of HCG are identical to those of the pituitary LH. This drug is also used in boys to treat prepubertal **cryptorchism** (failure of the testes to descend into the scrotum) and in men to treat selected cases of hypogonadotropic hypogonadism. Follistim AQ is used to induce sperm production (spermatogenesis). For additional information on the gonadotropins see the Summary Drug Table: Pituitary and Adrenocortical Hormones.

Clomiphene and the gonadotropin-releasing hormone antagonists are synthetic nonsteroidal compounds that bind to estrogen receptors, decreasing the amount of available estrogen receptors and causing the anterior pituitary to increase secretion of FSH and LH. These drugs are used to induce ovulation in anovulatory (nonovulating) women.

ADVERSE REACTIONS

Hormone-associated reactions
- Vasomotor flushes (which are like the hot flashes of menopause)
- Breast tenderness
- Abdominal discomfort, ovarian enlargement
- Hemoperitoneum (blood in the peritoneal cavity)

Generalized reactions
- Nausea, vomiting
- Headache, irritability, restlessness, fatigue
- Edema and irritation at the injection site

 Lifespan Considerations

Childbearing Women
Fetal effects have been demonstrated in animal studies when gonadotropins have been administered. Birth defects have been reported in human studies; therefore, gonadotropins should not be administered to women known to be pregnant.

CONTRAINDICATIONS, PRECAUTIONS, AND INTERACTIONS

These drugs are contraindicated in clients who are hypersensitive to the drug or any component of the drug. The gonadotropins are contraindicated in clients with high gonadotropin levels, thyroid dysfunction, adrenal dysfunction, liver disease, abnormal bleeding, ovarian cysts, or sex hormone–dependent tumors or in those with an organic intracranial lesion (pituitary tumor). Gonadotropins are contraindicated during pregnancy (pregnancy category X).

These drugs are used cautiously in clients with epilepsy, migraine headaches, asthma, or cardiac or renal dysfunction and during lactation. There are no known clinically significant interactions with the gonadotropins.

LASA ALERT
The following drugs may sound alike; be sure to clarify when they are ordered:

Drug Name	Sounds Like
elagolix	cetrorelix, degarelix, ganirelix
nafarelin	Anafranil, enalapril
Orilissa	orlistat

Drugs that look like a similar drug are noted in the Summary Drug Tables of each chapter.

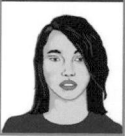 **PHARMACOLOGY IN PRACTICE**

SAFE DRUG ADMINISTRATION
A nurse is caring for a client who is taking ganirelix for ovulation induction. When are these injections given to the client?
1. When pregnancy is established to prevent miscarriage
2. Two weeks post partum
3. Before pregnancy to stimulate ovulation
4. If pregnancy attempts are unsuccessful in women with thyroid disease

---

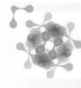 **NURSING PROCESS: STEPS TO BUILDING CLINICAL JUDGMENT**
Client Receiving a Gonadotropin

ASSESSMENT

Preadministration Assessment
These drugs are almost always administered on an outpatient basis and may be self-administered by the client.
 Data gathering suggestions before any of these drugs are administered include the following.
Objective data

- General client appearance.
- Vital signs (temperature, pulse, respirations, and blood pressure).
- Weight.
- Diagnostic testing for ovarian function and tubal patency.
- Pelvic examination may be performed by the primary health care provider to rule out ovarian enlargement, pregnancy, or uterine problems.

Subjective data
- Symptoms experienced by the client.
- Medical and family history.

Ongoing Assessment
At the time of each office or clinic visit ask the client about the occurrence of adverse reactions and document the client's vital signs and weight.

NURSING DIAGNOSES

Drug-specific nursing diagnoses include the following:

- **Acute pain** related to adverse reactions (ovarian enlargement, irritation at the injection site).
- **Anxiety** related to inability to conceive, treatment outcome, and other factors.

Nursing diagnoses related to drug administration are discussed in Chapter 4.

PLANNING

The expected outcomes of the client may include an optimal response to drug therapy, support of client needs related to the management of adverse reactions, reduction in anxiety, and confidence in an understanding of the medication regimen.

IMPLEMENTATION

Promoting an Optimal Response to Therapy

Gonadotropin injections are given in the primary health care provider's office or the clinic or they may be self-administered. These drugs must be administered IM or subcut because they are destroyed in the gastrointestinal (GI) tract; therefore, they cannot be taken orally. Injection sites are rotated and previous sites are checked for redness and irritation.

> **! NURSING ALERT**
>
> If the client complains of visual disturbances, the drug therapy is discontinued and the primary health care provider notified. An examination by an ophthalmologist is usually indicated.

Monitoring and Managing Client Needs

Acute Pain

Female clients taking these drugs are usually examined by the primary health care provider frequently to detect excessive ovarian stimulation, called **hyperstimulation syndrome** (sudden ovarian enlargement with ascites). The client may or may not report pain. This syndrome usually develops quickly, within 3–4 days.

> **! NURSING ALERT**
>
> The client is checked for signs of excessive ovarian enlargement (abdominal distention, pain, ascites [with serious cases]). The drug use is discontinued at the first sign of ovarian stimulation or enlargement. The client is usually admitted to the hospital for supportive measures.

Anxiety

Clients seeking treatment to become pregnant often experience a great deal of anxiety because of past failed attempts. In addition, when taking these drugs, the client faces the possibility of multiple births. The success rate of these drugs varies and depends on many factors. The primary health care provider usually discusses the value of this, as well as other approaches, with the client and her sexual partner. Allow the client time to talk about her concerns about the proposed treatment program.

Educating the Client and Family

Clients are instructed by the primary health care provider about the frequency of sexual intercourse. You can assess whether the client understands the directions given by the primary health care provider. When a gonadotropin is prescribed, you may instruct the client how to use the device to inject the hormone, to keep all primary health care provider appointments, and to report adverse reactions to the nurse or primary health care provider. Include the following information when a gonadotropin is prescribed.

Hormonal Ovarian Stimulants

- Before beginning therapy be aware of the possibility of multiple births and birth defects.
- It is a good idea to use a calendar to track the treatment schedule and ovulation.
- Report bloating, abdominal pain, flushing, breast tenderness, and pain at the injection site.

Nonhormonal Ovarian Stimulants

- Take the drug as prescribed (5 days) and do not stop taking the drug before the course of therapy is finished unless told to do so by the primary health care provider.
- Notify the primary health care provider if bloating, stomach or pelvic pain, jaundice, blurred vision, hot flashes, breast discomfort, headache, nausea, or vomiting occurs.
- Keep in mind that if ovulation does not occur after the first course of therapy, a second or third course may be used. If therapy does not succeed after three courses, the drug is considered unsuccessful and is use is discontinued.

EVALUATION

- Therapeutic effect is achieved.
- Adverse reactions are identified, reported to the primary health care provider, and managed successfully through appropriate nursing interventions:
  - Client is free of pain.
  - Anxiety is managed successfully.
- Client expresses confidence and demonstrates an understanding of the drug regimen.

🔬 GROWTH HORMONE

GH, also called *somatotropic hormone,* is secreted by the anterior pituitary. This hormone regulates the growth of the individual until approximately early adulthood or the time when the person no longer gains height.

ACTION AND USES

GH is available as the synthetic product somatropin. Somatropin is of recombinant DNA origin, and it is identical to human GH and produces skeletal growth in children. This drug is administered to children who have not grown because of a deficiency of pituitary GH; it must be used before closure of the child's bone epiphyses. Bone epiphyses are the ends of bones. They are separated from the main bone but joined to it by cartilage, which allows for growth or lengthening of the bone. GH is ineffective in clients with closed epiphyses because when the epiphyses close, growth (in length) can no longer occur.

GH is used in adults to supplement the lack of endogenous (naturally occurring) hormone. This may occur in conditions such as chronic renal failure or pituitary disease. The drug Serostim is also used in clients with human immunodeficiency virus infection to stop severe muscle wasting.

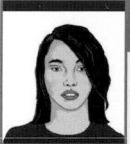

PHARMACOLOGY IN PRACTICE

PHYSIOLOGY

Which of the hormones is responsible for the growth of the body during childhood, especially the growth of muscles and bones?

1. Vasopressin
2. Somatotropin
3. Gonadotropin
4. ACTH

ADVERSE REACTIONS

Somatropin causes few adverse reactions when administered as directed. Antibodies to somatropin may develop in a small number of clients, resulting in a failure to experience response to therapy, namely, failure of the drug to produce

growth in the child. Some clients may experience hypothyroidism or insulin resistance. Swelling, joint pain, and muscle pain may also occur.

CONTRAINDICATIONS, PRECAUTIONS, AND INTERACTIONS

Somatropin is contraindicated in clients with known hypersensitivity to somatropin or sensitivity to benzyl alcohol and in those with epiphyseal closure or underlying cranial lesions (e.g., pituitary tumor). The drug is used cautiously in clients with thyroid disease or diabetes and during pregnancy (pregnancy category C) and lactation. Excessive amounts of glucocorticoids may decrease the response to somatropin.

LASA ALERT

The following drugs may sound alike; be sure to clarify when they are ordered:

Drug Name	Sounds Like
Humatrope	homatropine
octreotide	lanreotide, pasireotide
SandoSTATIN	SandIMMUNE, SandoSTATIN LAR, sargramostim, simvastatin
somatropin	homatropine, sumatriptan

Drugs that look like a similar drug are noted in the Summary Drug Tables of each chapter.

NURSING PROCESS: STEPS TO BUILDING CLINICAL JUDGMENT
Client Receiving Growth Hormone

ASSESSMENT

Preadministration Assessment

A thorough physical examination and laboratory and diagnostic tests are performed before a child is accepted into a GH program.

Data gathering suggestions before any of these drugs are administered include the following:

Objective data

- General client appearance
- Vital signs (temperature, pulse, respirations, and blood pressure)
- Height and weight measurements

Subjective data

- Medical and family history

Ongoing Assessment

Children may increase their growth rate from 3.5 to 4 cm/year before treatment to 8–10 cm/year during the first year of treatment. Each time the child visits the primary health care provider's office or clinic (usually every 3–6 months) measure and document the child's height and weight to evaluate the response to therapy. Bone age is monitored

periodically for growth and to detect epiphyseal closure, at which time therapy must stop.

NURSING DIAGNOSES

A key nursing diagnosis for clients receiving GH therapy is:

- **disturbed body image** related to changes in appearance, physical size, or failure to grow

Nursing diagnoses related to drug administration are discussed in Chapter 4.

PLANNING

The expected outcomes of the client may include an optimal response to drug therapy, support of client needs related to the management of adverse reactions, reduction in anxiety, and confidence in an understanding of the medication regimen.

IMPLEMENTATION

Promoting an Optimal Response to Therapy

GH is administered subcut. The vial containing the hormone is not shaken but swirled to mix. The solution is clear; do not administer it if it is cloudy. The weekly dosage is divided and given in three to seven doses throughout the week. The drug may (if possible) be given at bedtime to adhere most closely to the body's natural release of the hormone. Periodic testing of GH levels, glucose tolerance, and thyroid function may be done during treatment.

Monitoring and Managing Client Needs

Disturbed Body Image

Children requiring treatment are usually of short stature. The parents, and sometimes the children, may be concerned about the success or possible failure of treatment with GH. The child is provided with the opportunity to share fears, concerns, or anger. Acknowledge these feelings as normal and discuss any misconceptions the child or parents may have concerning treatment. Families may be surprised by the growth changes once treatment is started. Children may experience stretch marks or sizable changes in body structure and appearance. A child may become shy, reserved, or uncomfortable with their new body image. Time is allowed for the parents and children to ask questions not only before therapy is started but also during the months of treatment.

Educating the Client and Family

When the client is receiving GH, the primary health care provider discusses in detail the therapeutic regimen for increasing growth (height) with the child's parents or guardians. If the drug is to be given at bedtime and not in the outpatient clinic, instruct the parents on the proper injection technique. The parents are encouraged to keep all clinic or office visits with the child. You will want to explain that the child may experience sudden growth and increase in appetite and instruct the parents to report lack of growth, symptoms of diabetes (e.g., increased hunger, increased thirst, or frequent voiding), or symptoms of hypothyroidism (e.g., fatigue, dry skin, and intolerance to cold).

EVALUATION

- Therapeutic effect is achieved and the child grows in height.
- Adverse reactions are identified, reported to the primary health care provider, and managed successfully through appropriate nursing interventions:
  - Positive body image is maintained.
- Client and family express confidence and demonstrate an understanding of the drug regimen.

ADRENOCORTICAL HORMONES AND CORTICOTROPIN

This section discusses the hormones produced by the adrenal cortex or the adrenocortical hormones, which are the glucocorticoids and mineralocorticoids. These hormones are essential to life and influence many organs and structures of the body. The glucocorticoids and mineralocorticoids are collectively called *corticosteroids*.

Corticotropin (ACTH) is an anterior pituitary hormone that stimulates the adrenal cortex to produce and secrete adrenocortical hormones, primarily the glucocorticoids. Corticotropin is used for diagnostic testing of adrenocortical function.

The adrenal gland lies on the superior surface of each kidney. It is a double organ composed of an outer cortex and an inner medulla (Fig. 41.2). In response to ACTH secreted by the anterior pituitary, the adrenal cortex secretes several hormones (glucocorticoids, mineralocorticoids, and small amounts of sex hormones).

GLUCOCORTICOIDS

Glucocorticoids influence or regulate functions such as the immune response; glucose, fat, and protein metabolism; and the anti-inflammatory response. Table 41.1 describes the activity of glucocorticoids in the body.

ACTIONS

Glucocorticoids enter target cells and bind to receptors, initiating many complex reactions in the body. Some of the actions are considered undesirable, depending on the indication for which these drugs are used. Examples of the glucocorticoids include cortisone, hydrocortisone, prednisone, prednisolone, and triamcinolone. The Summary Drug Table: Pituitary and Adrenocortical Hormones provides information concerning these hormones.

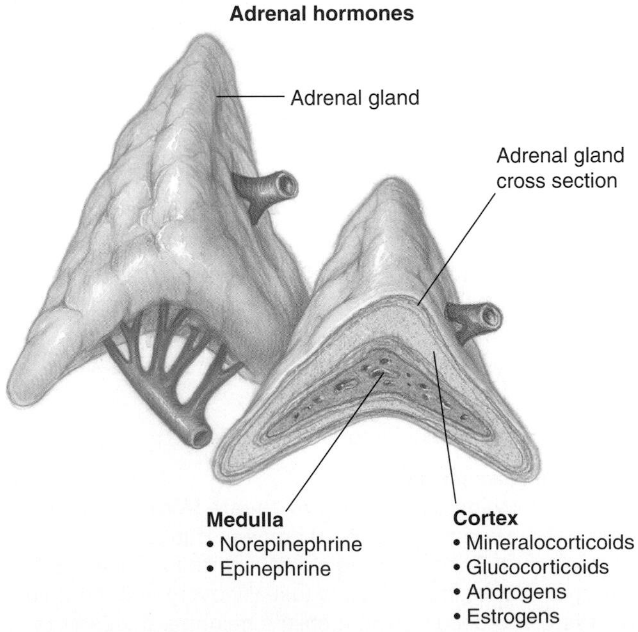

FIGURE 41.2 The adrenal gland hormones. (Courtesy of Anatomical Chart Co.)

TABLE 41.1 Activity of Glucocorticoids in the Body

FUNCTION WITHIN THE BODY	DESCRIPTION OF BODILY ACTIVITY
Anti-inflammatory	Stabilizes lysosomal membrane and prevents the release of proteolytic enzymes during the inflammatory process.
Regulation of blood pressure	Potentiates vasoconstrictor action of norepinephrine. Without glucocorticoids the vasoconstricting action is decreased and blood pressure decreases.
Metabolism of carbohydrates and protein	Facilitates the breakdown of protein in the muscle, leading to increased plasma amino acid levels. Increases activity of enzymes necessary for glucogenesis, producing hyperglycemia, which can aggravate diabetes, precipitate latent diabetes, and cause insulin resistance.
Metabolism of fat	A complex phenomenon that promotes the use of fat for energy (a positive effect) and permits fat stores to accumulate in the body, causing buffalo hump and moon-shaped or round face (a negative effect).
Interference with the immune response	Decreases the production of lymphocytes and eosinophils in the blood by causing atrophy of the thymus gland; blocks the release of cytokines, resulting in a decreased performance of T and B monocytes in the immune response. (This action, coupled with the anti-inflammatory action, makes the corticosteroids useful in delaying organ rejection in clients who underwent a transplant.)
Protection during stress	As a protective mechanism, the corticosteroids are released during periods of stress (e.g., injury or surgery). The release of epinephrine or norepinephrine by the adrenal medulla during stress has a synergistic effect along with the corticosteroids.
Central nervous system responses	Affects mood and possibly causes neuronal or brain excitability, causing euphoria, anxiety, depression, psychosis, and an increase in motor activity in some individuals.

USES

Glucocorticoids are used to treat the following:

- Adrenocortical insufficiency (replacement therapy)
- Allergic reactions
- Collagen diseases (e.g., systemic lupus erythematosus)
- Dermatologic conditions
- Rheumatic disorders
- Shock
- Multiple other conditions (Box 41.1)

BOX 41.1   Uses of Glucocorticoids

- **Endocrine disorders:** Primary or secondary adrenal cortical insufficiency, congenital adrenal hyperplasia, nonsuppurative thyroiditis, and hypercalcemia associated with cancer.
- **Rheumatic disorders:** Short-term management of acute ankylosing spondylitis, acute and subacute bursitis, acute nonspecific tenosynovitis, acute gouty arthritis, psoriatic arthritis, rheumatoid arthritis, posttraumatic osteoarthritis, synovitis of osteoarthritis, and epicondylitis.
- **Collagen diseases:** Systemic lupus erythematosus, acute rheumatic carditis, and systemic dermatomyositis.
- **Dermatologic disorders:** Pemphigus, bullous dermatitis herpetiformis, severe erythema multiforme (Stevens–Johnson syndrome), exfoliative dermatitis, mycosis fungoides, severe psoriasis, severe seborrheic dermatitis, angioedema, urticaria, and various skin disorders (e.g., lichen planus or keloids).
- **Allergic states:** Control of severe or incapacitating allergic conditions not controlled by other methods, bronchial asthma (including status asthmaticus), contact dermatitis, atopic dermatitis, serum sickness, and drug hypersensitivity reactions.
- **Ophthalmic diseases:** Severe acute and chronic allergic and inflammatory processes, keratitis, allergic corneal marginal ulcers, herpes zoster of the eye, iritis, iridocyclitis, chorioretinitis, diffuse posterior uveitis, optic neuritis, sympathetic ophthalmia, and anterior segment inflammation.
- **Respiratory diseases:** Seasonal allergic rhinitis, berylliosis, fulminating or disseminating pulmonary tuberculosis, and aspiration pneumonia.
- **Hematologic disorders:** Idiopathic or secondary thrombocytopenic purpura, hemolytic anemia, red blood cell anemia, and congenital hypoplastic anemia.
- **Neoplastic diseases:** Leukemia, lymphomas.
- **Edematous states:** Induction of diuresis or remission of proteinuria in nephrotic syndrome.
- **GI diseases:** During critical period of ulcerative colitis, regional enteritis, and intractable sprue.
- **Nervous system disorders:** Acute exacerbations of multiple sclerosis.

The anti-inflammatory activity of these hormones makes them valuable for suppressing inflammation and modifying the immune response.

ADVERSE REACTIONS

The adverse reactions that may result from the administration of glucocorticoids are given in Box 41.2. Long- or short-term high-dose therapy may also produce many of the signs and symptoms seen with Cushing syndrome, a disease caused by the overproduction of endogenous glucocorticoids. Some of the signs and symptoms of this Cushing-like (**cushingoid**) state include a buffalo hump (a hump on the back of the neck), moon face, oily skin and acne, osteoporosis, purple striae on the abdomen and hips, altered skin pigmentation, and weight gain. When a serious disease or disorder is treated, it is often necessary to allow these effects to occur because therapy with these drugs is absolutely necessary.

CONTRAINDICATIONS, PRECAUTIONS, AND INTERACTIONS

Glucocorticoids are contraindicated in clients with serious infections, such as tuberculosis and fungal and antibiotic-resistant infections. Glucocorticoids are administered with caution to clients with renal or hepatic disease, hypothyroidism, ulcerative colitis, diverticulitis, peptic ulcer disease, inflammatory bowel disease, hypertension, osteoporosis, convulsive disorders, or diabetes. Glucocorticoids are classified as pregnancy category C drugs and should be used with caution during pregnancy and lactation. Clients taking ACTH should avoid any vaccinations with live virus. The live virus vaccines can potentiate virus replication with ACTH, increase any adverse reaction to the vaccine, and decrease the client's antibody response to the vaccine.

Multiple drug interactions may occur with the glucocorticoids. Table 41.2 identifies selected clinically significant interactions.

MINERALOCORTICOIDS

ACTIONS AND USES

The natural mineralocorticoids consist of aldosterone and desoxycorticosterone and play an important role in conserving sodium and increasing potassium excretion. Because of these activities, mineralocorticoids are important in controlling salt and water balance. Aldosterone is the more potent of these two hormones. Deficiencies of mineralocorticoids result in a loss of sodium and water and a retention of potassium. Fludrocortisone is a drug that has both glucocorticoid and mineralocorticoid activity and is the only currently available mineralocorticoid drug. Fludrocortisone is used for replacement therapy for primary and secondary adrenocortical deficiency. Even

---

BOX 41.2 Adverse Reactions Associated With Glucocorticoids

- **Fluid and electrolyte disturbances:** Sodium and fluid retention, potassium loss, hypokalemic alkalosis, hypertension, hypocalcemia, hypotension, or shocklike reactions.
- **Musculoskeletal disturbances:** Muscle weakness, loss of muscle mass, tendon rupture, osteoporosis, aseptic necrosis of femoral and humeral heads, and spontaneous fractures.
- **Cardiovascular disturbances:** Thromboembolism or fat embolism; thrombophlebitis; necrotizing angiitis; syncopal episodes; cardiac arrhythmias; aggravation of hypertension; fatal cardiac arrhythmias with rapid, high-dose IV methylprednisolone administration; and HF in susceptible clients.
- **GI disturbances:** Pancreatitis, abdominal distention, ulcerative esophagitis, nausea, vomiting, increased appetite and weight gain, possible peptic ulcer or bowel perforation, and hemorrhage.
- **Dermatologic disturbances:** Impaired wound healing; thin, fragile skin; petechiae; ecchymoses; erythema; increased sweating; suppression of skin test reactions; subcut fat atrophy; purpura; striae; hirsutism; acneiform
- eruptions; urticaria; angioneurotic edema; and perineal itch.
- **Neurologic disturbances:** Convulsions, increased intracranial pressure with papilledema (usually after treatment is discontinued), vertigo, headache, neuritis or paresthesia, steroid psychosis, and insomnia.
- **Endocrine disturbances:** Amenorrhea, other menstrual irregularities, development of cushingoid state, suppression of growth in children, secondary adrenocortical and pituitary unresponsive (particularly in times of stress), decreased carbohydrate tolerance, manifestation of latent diabetes mellitus, and increased requirements for insulin or oral hypoglycemic agents (in diabetic clients).
- **Ophthalmic disturbances:** Posterior subcapsular cataracts, increased intraocular pressure, glaucoma, and exophthalmos.
- **Metabolic disturbances:** Negative nitrogen balance (caused by protein catabolism).
- **Other disturbances:** Anaphylactoid or hypersensitivity reactions, aggravation of existing infections, malaise, and increase or decrease in sperm motility and number.

TABLE 41.2 Selected Drug Interactions of Glucocorticoids

PRECIPITANT DRUG	OBJECT DRUG	DESCRIPTION
Cholestyramine	Hydrocortisone	Effects of hydrocortisone may be decreased.
Oral contraceptives	Corticosteroids	Effects of corticosteroid may be increased.
Estrogens	Corticosteroids	Effects of corticosteroid may be increased.
Hydantoins	Corticosteroids	Effects of corticosteroid may be decreased.
Ketoconazole	Corticosteroids	Effects of corticosteroid may be increased.
Rifampin	Corticosteroids	Effects of corticosteroid may be decreased.
Corticosteroids	Anticholinesterases	Anticholinesterase effects may be antagonized in myasthenia gravis.
Corticosteroids	Oral anticoagulants	Anticoagulant dose requirements may be reduced.
		Corticosteroids may decrease the anticoagulant action.
Corticosteroids	Digitalis glycosides	Coadministration may enhance the possibility of digitalis toxicity associated with hypokalemia.
Corticosteroids	Isoniazid	Isoniazid serum concentrations may be decreased.
Corticosteroids	Potassium-depleting diuretics	Hypokalemia may occur.
Corticosteroids	Salicylates	Corticosteroids will reduce serum salicylate levels and may decrease their effectiveness.
Corticosteroids	Theophyllines	Alterations in the pharmacologic activity of either agent may occur.

though this drug has both mineralocorticoid and glucocorticoid activity, it is used only for its mineralocorticoid effects.

ADVERSE REACTIONS

Adverse reactions may occur if the dosage is too high or prolonged or if withdrawal is too rapid. Administration of fludrocortisone may cause:

- Edema, hypertension, HF, enlargement of the heart
- Increased sweating, allergic skin rash
- Hypokalemia, muscular weakness, headache, hypersensitivity reactions

Because this drug has glucocorticoid and mineralocorticoid activity and is often given with glucocorticoids, adverse reactions of glucocorticoids must be closely monitored as well (see Box 41.2).

CONTRAINDICATIONS, PRECAUTIONS, AND INTERACTIONS

Fludrocortisone is contraindicated in clients with hypersensitivity to fludrocortisone and in those with systemic fungal infections. Fludrocortisone is used cautiously in clients with Addison disease or infection and during pregnancy (pregnancy category C) and lactation. Fludrocortisone decreases the effects of hydantoins and rifampin. There is a decrease in serum levels of salicylates when those agents are administered with fludrocortisone.

LASA ALERT

The following drugs may sound alike; be sure to clarify when they are ordered:

Drug Name	Sounds Like
cortisone	Cardizem, Cortizone
Cortef	Coreg, Lortab
Cortrosyn	colchicine, corticorelin, corticotropin, Cotazym
cosyntropin	corticorelin, corticotropin
Decadron	Percodan
dexAMETHasone	desoximetasone, dexMEDEtomidine, dextroamphetamine
hydrocortisone	hydrocodone, hydroxychloroquine, hydroCHLOROthiazide
Kenalog	Ketalar
methylPREDNISolone	medroxyPROGESTERone, methotrexate, methylTESTOSTERone, predniSONE
prednisoLONE	predniSONE
predniSONE	methylPREDNISolone, Pramosone, prazosin, prednisoLONE, PriLOSEC, primidone, promethazine
Solu-CORTEF	SOLU-Medrol

Drugs that look like a similar drug are noted in the Summary Drug Tables of each chapter.

NURSING PROCESS: STEPS TO BUILDING CLINICAL JUDGMENT
Client Receiving a Glucocorticoid or Mineralocorticoid

ASSESSMENT

Preadministration Assessment

Assessments depend on the client's condition and diagnosis.

Data gathering suggestions before vasopressin is administered are listed in the following:

Objective data

- General client appearance, emphasis on assessment of area involved
- Vital signs (temperature, pulse, respirations, and blood pressure)
- Weight
- Laboratory results—serum electrolytes and complete blood count
- Urinalysis
- Radiography of chest or upper GI tract

Subjective data

- Symptoms experienced by client
- Family history of other health conditions

Ongoing Assessment

Ongoing assessments of the client receiving a glucocorticoid, and the frequency of these assessments, depend largely on the disease being treated. Take and record vital signs every 4–8 hours if the client is not continuously monitored. Weigh the client daily to weekly, depending on the diagnosis and the primary health care provider's orders. More frequent assessment may be necessary if a glucocorticoid is used for emergency situations.

Assess for signs of adverse effects of the mineralocorticoid or glucocorticoid, particularly signs of electrolyte imbalance, such as hypocalcemia, hypokalemia, and hypernatremia (see Chapter 54). Be alert for changes in the client's mental status, especially if there is a history of depression or other psychiatric problems or if high doses of the drug are prescribed. Monitor for signs of an infection, which may be masked by glucocorticoid therapy. The blood of the client without diabetes is checked weekly for elevated glucose levels because glucocorticoids may aggravate latent diabetes. Those with diabetes must be checked more frequently.

When administering fludrocortisone check the client's blood pressure at frequent intervals. Hypotension may indicate insufficient dosage. Weigh the client daily and assess for edema, particularly swelling of the feet and hands. The lungs are auscultated for adventitious sounds (e.g., crackles).

NURSING DIAGNOSES

Drug-specific nursing diagnoses include the following:

- **Infection risk** related to immune suppression or impaired wound healing
- **Acute confusion** related to adverse drug reactions
- **Injury risk** related to muscle atrophy, osteoporosis, or spontaneous fractures

- **Acute pain** related to epigastric distress of gastric ulcer formation
- **Fluid overload** related to adverse reactions (sodium and water retention)
- **Disturbed body image** related to adverse reactions (cushingoid appearance)

Nursing diagnoses related to drug administration are discussed in Chapter 4.

PLANNING

The expected outcomes of the client include an optimal response to therapy, support of client needs related to the management of adverse reactions, and confidence in an understanding of the medication regimen.

IMPLEMENTATION

Promoting an Optimal Response to Therapy

Glucocorticoids may be administered orally, IM, subcut, IV, topically, or as an inhalant. The primary health care provider may also inject the drug into a joint (intra-articular), a lesion (intralesional), soft tissue, or bursa. The drug dosage is individualized and based on the severity of the condition and the client's response.

> ! **NURSING ALERT**
>
> Never omit a dose of a glucocorticoid. If the client cannot take the drug orally because of nausea or vomiting, contact the primary health care provider immediately because the drug needs to be ordered given by the parenteral route. Clients who can receive nothing by mouth for any reason must have the glucocorticoid given by the parenteral route.

Daily oral doses are usually given before 9 a.m. to minimize adrenal suppression and to coincide with normal adrenal function. However, alternate-day therapy may be prescribed for clients receiving long-term therapy. Fludrocortisone is given orally and is well tolerated in the GI tract.

 Lifespan Considerations

Gerontology

Corticosteroids are administered with caution in older adults because they are more likely to have preexisting conditions, such as heart failure (HF), hypertension, osteoporosis, and arthritis, which may be worsened by use of such agents. Monitor older adults for exacerbation of existing conditions during corticosteroid therapy. In addition, lower dosages may be needed because of the effects of aging, such as decreases in muscle mass, renal function, and plasma volume.

Alternate-Day Therapy

The alternate-day therapy approach to glucocorticoid administration is used in treating diseases and disorders requiring long-term therapy, especially arthritic disorders. This regimen involves giving twice the daily dose of the glucocorticoid every other day. The drug is given only once on the alternate day, before 9 a.m. The purpose of alternate-day administration is to provide the client requiring long-term glucocorticoid therapy with the beneficial effects of the drug while minimizing certain undesirable reactions (see Box 41.2).

Plasma levels of the endogenous adrenocortical hormones vary throughout the daytime and nighttime hours. They are normally higher between 2 and 8 a.m. and lower between 4 p.m. and midnight. When plasma levels are lower, the anterior pituitary releases ACTH, which in turn stimulates the adrenal cortex to manufacture and release glucocorticoids. When plasma levels are high, the pituitary gland does not release ACTH. The response of the pituitary to high or low plasma levels of glucocorticoids and the resulting release or nonrelease of ACTH is an example of the feedback mechanism, which may also be seen in other glands of the body, such as the thyroid gland.

The **feedback mechanism** (also called the *feedback control*) is the method by which the body maintains most hormones at relatively constant levels in the bloodstream. When the hormone concentration falls, the rate of production of that hormone increases. Likewise, when the hormone level becomes too high, the body decreases production of that hormone.

Administration of a short-acting glucocorticoid on alternate days and before 9 a.m., when glucocorticoid plasma levels are still relatively high, does not affect the release of ACTH later in the day yet gives the client the benefit of exogenous glucocorticoid therapy.

Client With Diabetes
Clients with diabetes who are receiving a glucocorticoid may require frequent adjustment of their insulin or oral antidiabetic drug dosage. Blood glucose levels may be monitored more frequently than when the client is at home. If the blood glucose levels increase or urine is positive for ketones, notify the primary health care provider. Some clients may have latent (hidden) diabetes. In these cases, the corticosteroid may precipitate hyperglycemia. Therefore, all clients, those with and those without diabetes, should have blood glucose levels checked frequently.

Adrenal Insufficiency
Administration of the glucocorticoids poses the threat of adrenal gland insufficiency (particularly if the alternate-day therapy is not prescribed). Administration of glucocorticoids several times a day and during a short time (as little as 5–10 days) results in shutting off the pituitary release of ACTH because there are always high levels of glucocorticoids in the plasma (caused by the body's own glucocorticoid production plus the administration of a glucocorticoid drug). Eventually, the pituitary atrophies and ceases to release ACTH. Without ACTH, the adrenals fail to manufacture and release (endogenous) glucocorticoids. When this happens, the client has acute adrenal insufficiency, which is

a life-threatening situation until corrected with the administration of an exogenous glucocorticoid.

Adrenal insufficiency is a critical deficiency of mineralocorticoids and glucocorticoids; the disorder requires immediate treatment. Symptoms of adrenal insufficiency include fever, myalgia, arthralgia, malaise, anorexia, nausea, orthostatic hypotension, dizziness, fainting, dyspnea, and hypoglycemia. Death due to circulatory collapse will result unless the condition is treated promptly. Situations producing stress (e.g., trauma, surgery, severe illness) may precipitate the need for an increase in dosage of corticosteroids until the crisis or stressful situation is resolved.

NURSING ALERT
Glucocorticoid therapy should never be discontinued suddenly. When administration of a glucocorticoid extends beyond 5 days and the drug therapy is to be discontinued, the dosage must be reduced gradually (tapered) over several days. In some instances, it may be necessary to taper the dose over 7–10 or more days. Tapering the dosage allows normal adrenal function to return gradually, thereby preventing adrenal insufficiency.

Monitoring and Managing Client Needs

Infection Risk
Report any slight rise in temperature, sore throat, or other signs of infection to the primary health care provider as soon as possible because decreased resistance to infection may occur during glucocorticoid therapy. Nursing personnel and visitors with any type of infection or recent exposure to an infectious disease should avoid client contact.

Acute Confusion
Glucocorticoid drugs can also cause disturbances in mental processing. Monitor and report any evidence of behavior change, such as depression, insomnia, euphoria, mood swings, or nervousness. If disturbances occur provide a quiet, nonthreatening environment and spend time actively listening as the client talks. It is important to encourage verbalization of fears and concerns. Anxiety usually decreases with understanding of the therapeutic regimen. Allow time for a thorough explanation of the drug regimen and answering of questions.

Injury Risk
Clients receiving long-term glucocorticoid therapy, especially those with limited activity, should be monitored for signs of compression fractures of the vertebrae and pathologic fractures of the long bones. If the client reports back or bone pain, contact the primary health care provider. Extra care is also necessary to prevent falls and other injuries when the client is confused or is allowed out of bed. If the client is weak, provide assistance to the client to the bathroom or when ambulating. Edematous extremities are handled with care to prevent skin tears and trauma.

Acute Pain
Peptic ulcer has been associated with glucocorticoid therapy. Encourage the client to report complaints of

epigastric burning or pain, bloody or coffee-ground emesis, or the passing of tarry stools. Giving oral corticosteroids with food or a full glass of water may minimize gastric irritation.

Fluid Overload

Fluid and electrolyte imbalances, particularly when it results in excess fluid volume in the tissues and circulation, are common with corticosteroid therapy. Scan the client for visible edema, keep an accurate fluid intake and output record, obtain daily weights, and restrict sodium if indicated by the primary health care provider. Edematous extremities are elevated and the client's position is changed frequently. Inform the primary health care provider if signs of electrolyte imbalance or glucocorticoid drug effects are noted. Dietary adjustments are made for the increased potassium loss and sodium retention, if necessary. Consultation with a dietitian may be indicated.

Disturbed Body Image

A body image disturbance may occur, especially if the client experiences cushingoid effects (e.g., buffalo hump, moon face), acne, or hirsutism. If continuation of drug therapy is necessary, explain the reason for the cushingoid appearance and emphasize the necessity of continuing the drug regimen. Assess the client's emotional state and help the client express feelings and concerns. Offer positive reinforcement, when possible. Instruct the client experiencing acne to keep the affected areas clean and in the use of over-the-counter acne drugs and water-based cosmetics or creams.

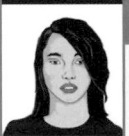

PHARMACOLOGY IN PRACTICE

MANAGING NEEDS

A client with acute shortness of breath is prescribed dexamethasone. Which of the following adverse reactions should the nurse monitor for in the client? Select all that apply.
1. Nasal congestion
2. Acneiform eruptions
3. Increased sweating
4. Perineal itch
5. Abdominal cramps

Educating the Client and Family

To support adherence provide the client and family with thorough instructions and educational materials about the drug regimen.

- These drugs may cause GI upset. To decrease GI effects take the oral drug with meals or snacks.
- Take antacids between meals to help prevent peptic ulcer.
- Carry client identification, such as a MedicAlert tag, so that drug therapy will be known to medical personnel during an emergency situation.
- Keep follow-up appointments to determine if a dosage adjustment is necessary.

Short-Term Glucocorticoid Therapy

- Take the drug exactly as directed in the prescription container. Do not increase, decrease, or omit a dose unless advised to do so by the primary health care provider.
- Take single daily doses before 9 a.m.
- Follow the instructions for tapering the dose because they are extremely important.
- If the problem does not improve, contact the primary health care provider.

Alternate-Day Oral Glucocorticoid Therapy

- Take this drug before 9 a.m. once every other day. Use a calendar or some other method to identify the days of each week to take the drug.
- Do not stop taking the drug unless advised to do so by the primary health care provider.
- If the problem becomes worse, especially on the days the drug is not taken, contact the primary health care provider.
- Most of the following teaching points may also apply to alternate-day therapy, especially when higher doses are used and therapy extends over many months.

Long-Term or High-Dose Glucocorticoid Therapy

- Do not omit this drug or increase or decrease the dosage except on the advice of the primary health care provider.
- Inform other primary health care providers, dentists, and all medical personnel of therapy with this drug. Wear medical identification or another form of identification to alert medical personnel of long-term therapy with a glucocorticoid.
- Do not take any nonprescription drug unless its use has been approved by the primary health care provider.
- If you go to get a vaccine ask if it is a "live virus." Do not receive the vaccine if it is a live preparation because of the risk for a lack of antibody response. (This does not include clients receiving corticosteroids as replacement therapy.)
- Whenever possible avoid exposure to infections. Contact the primary health care provider if minor cuts or abrasions fail to heal, persistent joint swelling or tenderness is noted, or fever, sore throat, upper respiratory infection, or other signs of infection occur.
- If the drug cannot be taken orally for any reason or if diarrhea occurs, contact the primary health care provider immediately. If you are unable to contact the primary health care provider before the next dose is due go to the nearest urgent care or hospital emergency department (preferably where the original treatment was started or where the primary health care provider is on the hospital staff) because the drug must be given by injection.
- Weigh yourself weekly. If significant weight gain or swelling of the extremities is noted contact the primary health care provider.
- Remember that dietary recommendations made by the primary health care provider are an important part of therapy and must be followed.
- Follow the primary health care provider's recommendations regarding periodic eye examinations and laboratory tests.

Intra-articular or Intralesional Administration
- Do not overuse the injected joint, even if the pain is gone.
- Follow the primary health care provider's instructions concerning rest and exercise.
- Commit to the prescribed exercise routines as instructed by the physical therapist.

Mineralocorticoid (Fludrocortisone) Therapy
- Take the drug as directed. Do not increase or decrease the dosage except as instructed to do so by the primary health care provider.
- Do not discontinue use of the drug abruptly.
- Inform the primary health care provider if the following adverse reactions occur: edema, muscle weakness, weight gain, anorexia, swelling of the extremities, dizziness, severe headache, or shortness of breath.

EVALUATION

- Therapeutic effect is achieved.
- Adverse reactions are identified, reported to the primary health care provider, and managed successfully through appropriate nursing interventions:

- No evidence of infection is seen.
- Orientation and mentation remain intact.
- No evidence of injury is seen.
- Client is free of pain.
- Fluid volume balance is maintained.
- Positive body image is maintained.
- Client expresses confidence and demonstrates an understanding of the drug regimen.

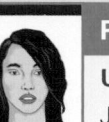

PHARMACOLOGY IN PRACTICE

USING CLINICAL REASONING

Janna's classmate was showing her the numerous medications she has to take on a daily basis. She wonders why her friend has to take two tablets of desmopressin during the day and three in the evening. Explain the reasoning for this schedule for the drug desmopressin.

KEY POINTS

■ The pituitary is a small gland suspended from the hypothalamus in the brain. The pituitary is called the "master gland" and controls many of the body processes. The gland has two lobes, the anterior and posterior pituitary.

■ The posterior pituitary secretes two hormones, oxytocin and vasopressin. Vasopressin regulates the reabsorption of fluid by the kidney. Diabetes insipidus occurs when vasopressin is not secreted properly. This results in unquenchable thirst and copious urination.

■ Clients taking vasopressin replacement can easily become dehydrated if they are unable to take the medication; therefore, a medical alert identification should always be worn.

■ The anterior pituitary secretes many hormones, including PRL, LH, FSH, TSH, ACTH, and GH. These all help in the regulation of growth, metabolism, reproduction, and stress.

■ Hormones to stimulate ovulation are given as an injection because the hormones are destroyed by GI fluids. Pain may be an indicator of hyperstimulation syndrome and the medication use is then stopped. Injection of GHs can lead to sudden growth spurts and leave the client with body image issues. ACTH influences the adrenal glands to secrete glucocorticoids; often this is triggered by biologic stress.

■ Corticosteroids influence metabolism, the immune response, and electrolyte and fluid balance. When replacement or supplementation is indicated, the drug use should be tapered off rather than stopped abruptly, as adrenal insufficiency can result.

SUMMARY DRUG TABLE
Pituitary and Adrenocortical Hormones

Generic Name	Trade Name	Uses	Adverse Reactions	Dosage Ranges
Posterior Pituitary Hormones				
desmopressin *des-moe-PRES-in*	DDAVP, Stimate	Diabetes insipidus, hemophilia A, von Willebrand disease, nocturnal enuresis	Headache, nausea, nasal congestion, abdominal cramps	Doses are individualized, administered orally, intranasally, or subcut
vasopressin *vay-soe-PRES-in*	Vasostrict	Shock from vasodilation shock, cadaver organ recovery, diabetes insipidus, prevention and treatment of postoperative abdominal distention, to dispel gas interfering with abdominal radiographic examination	Tremor, sweating, vertigo, nausea, vomiting, abdominal cramps, headache	Diabetes insipidus: 5–10 units IM, subcut q3–4hr, parenteral solution may be used intranasally

Continued

SUMMARY DRUG TABLE (continued)
Pituitary and Adrenocortical Hormones

Generic Name	Trade Name	Uses	Adverse Reactions	Dosage Ranges
Anterior Pituitary Hormones and Hormone Inhibitors				
Gonadotropins: Ovarian Stimulants				
choriogonadotropin alfa (recombinant) *kor-ee-ik-goe-NAD-oh-troe-pin*	Ovidrel	Ovulation induction, follicular maturation	Vasomotor flushes, breast tenderness, abdominal pain, ovarian overstimulation, nausea, vomiting	Injection following follicle stimulation drugs
chorionic gonadotropin (human) *kor-ee-ON-ik- goe-NAD-oh-troe-pin*	Novarel Pregnyl	Male pituitary deficiency, spermatogenesis, cryptorchidism, ovulation induction	Pain injection site, headache, fatigue, gynecomastia, precocious puberty	Weekly IM injections
follitropin alfa *foe-li-TRO-pin-AL-fa*	Gonal-F	Ovulation induction, spermatogenesis	Injection site pain, headache, acne, abdominal pain, nausea	Daily IM for ovulation, weekly for spermatogenesis
follitropin beta *foe-li-TRO-pin-BAY-ta*	Follistim AQ	Ovulation induction, spermatogenesis	Injection site pain, headache, acne, pelvic pain, nausea	Daily IM for ovulation, twice weekly for spermatogenesis
urofollitropin *yoor-oh-fol-li-TROE-pin*	Bravelle	Ovulation induction	Headache	Daily subcut
menotropin *men-oh-TROE-pin*	Menopur	Assisted reproductive technology	Abdominal pain, nausea, multiple gestations	Individualized dosing dependent on client outcome
Gonadotropin-Releasing Hormones/Synthetics				
elagolix *EL-a-GOE-lix*	Orilissa	Endometriosis	Hot flashes, night sweats, headache, decreased bone density	150–200 mg orally daily
nafarelin *naf-a-REL-in*	Synarel	Endometriosis, precocious puberty	Hot flashes, decreased libido, vaginal dryness, headache, emotional lability	400 mcg/day intranasally in two doses
Gonadotropin-Releasing Hormone Antagonists				
cetrorelix *set-roe-REL-iks*	Cetrotide	Infertility (controlled ovarian stimulation)	Ovarian overstimulation, nausea, vomiting	Dose individualized during cycle
degarelix *deg-a-REL-iks*	Firmagon	Advanced prostate cancer	Hot flashes, weight gain, injection site pain	80–240 mg subcut monthly
ganirelix *ga-ni-REL-iks*		Infertility (adjunct to control ovarian hyperstimulation)	Abdominal pain, fetal death, headache	250 mcg/day subcut during cycle
Nonsteroidal Ovarian Stimulant				
clomiPHENE *KLOE-mi-feen*		Ovulatory failure	Vasomotor flushes, breast tenderness, abdominal discomfort, ovarian enlargement, nausea, vomiting	50 mg/day orally for 5 days, may be repeated
Growth Hormone and Hormone Inhibitors				
somatropin *soe-ma-TROE-pin*	Genotropin, Humatrope, Norditropin, Omnitrope, Serostim	Growth failure caused by deficiency of pituitary GH in children, replacement of endogenous GH in adults	With injection: diarrhea, arthralgia / Long term: growth problems—bone, ear, edema	Doses are individualized, administered by subcut injection weekly
octreotide *ok-TREE-oh-tide*	SandoSTATIN	Reduction of GH in acromegaly and treatment of certain tumors, bleeding esophageal varices	Nausea, diarrhea, abdominal pain, sinus bradycardia, hypoglycemia, injection site pain	50 mcg subcut or IV BID or TID

Generic Name	Trade Name	Uses	Adverse Reactions	Dosage Ranges
ACTH				
corticotropic repository hormone (ACTH) *core-tih-koe-TROE-pik*		Diagnose adrenocortical function, nonsuppurative thyroiditis, hypercalcemia, multiple sclerosis	See Box 41.2	20 units IM, subcut QID
cosyntropin *koe-sin-TROE-pin*	Cortrosyn	Screening for adrenal insufficiency	Dizziness, nausea, vomiting	See package insert
Glucocorticoids				
betamethasone *bay-ta-METH-a-sone*	Celestone Soluspan	See Box 41.1	See Box 41.2	Individualize dosage; syrup or injectable, see package insert
budesonide *byoo-DES-oh-nide*	Entocort EC, Ortikos, Uceris	Crohn disease	See Box 41.2	9 mg QD in a.m. for 8 weeks
cortisone *KO-ti-sone*		See Box 41.1	See Box 41.2	25–300 mg/day orally
deflazacort *de-FLAZE-a-kort*	Emflaza	Duchenne muscular dystrophy	See Box 41.2	0.9 mg/kg orally daily
dexAMETHasone *deks-a-METH-a-sone*	Decadron, TaperDex	Cerebral edema, other conditions listed in Box 41.1	See Box 41.2	Individualize dosage based on the severity of the condition and response
hydrocortisone (cortisol) *hye-droe-KOR-ti-sone*	Cortef, Solu-CORTEF	See Box 41.1	See Box 41.2	Individualize dosage based on the severity of the condition and response
methylPREDNISolone *meth-il-pred-NIS-oh-lone*	Medrol, Depo-Medrol, Solu-Medrol	See Box 41.1	See Box 41.2	Individualize dosage based on the severity of the condition and response
prednisoLONE *pred-NIS-oh-lone*	Millipred	See Box 41.1	See Box 41.2	200 mg/day for 1 week, then 80 mg every other day
predniSONE *PRED-ni-sone*		See Box 41.1	See Box 41.2	Individualize dosage: initial dose usually between 5 and 60 mg/day orally
triamcinolone *trye-am-SIN-oh-lone*	Kenalog, Zilretta	See Box 41.1	See Box 41.2	Joint and soft tissue injection: 2–80 mg
Mineralocorticoids				
fludrocortisone *floo-droe-KOR-ti-sone*		Partial replacement therapy for Addison disease, salt-losing adrenogenital syndrome	See Box 41.2	0.1 mg three times a week to 0.2 mg/day orally
Miscellaneous Hormones and Hormone Inhibitors				
bromocriptine *broe-moe-KRIP-teen*	Parlodel	Hyperprolactinemia, acromegaly, (Parkinson disease, T2D)	Headache, dizziness, fatigue, nausea	5–7.5 mg/day orally
cabergoline *ca-BER-goe-leen*		Same as bromocriptine	Same as bromocriptine	1 mg twice weekly orally
osilodrostat *oh-SIL-oh-DROE-stat*	Isturisa	Cushing disease when surgical removal is not an option	Edema, acne, rash, nausea, vomiting, diarrhea, generalized aches, fatigue, runny nose	30 mg orally twice daily

CHAPTER REVIEW

Know Your Drugs

Clients sometimes know a medication by the brand (or trade) name and not the generic name. To recognize both names match the brand name with the generic name of the same medication.

Generic Name	Brand Name
1. betamethasone	A. Prelone
2. hydrocortisone	B. Medrol
3. methylprednisolone	C. Cortef
4. prednisolone	D. Celestone

Calculate Medication Dosages

1. Hydrocortisone 5 mg twice daily is prescribed. The drug is available in 2.5-mg tablets. The nurse prepares to administer _____.

2. Desmopressin 0.2 mg orally is prescribed. The drug is available in 0.1-mg tablets. The nurse administers _____.

Prepare for the NCLEX

RECALL THE FACTS

1. Where is the pituitary gland located?
   1. Inside the brain
   2. On top of the kidney
   3. Suspended from the hypothalamus
   4. Directly in front of the trachea

2. The pituitary gland secretes hormones. Which one is secreted by the posterior lobe?
   1. Growth hormone
   2. Luteinizing hormone
   3. Prolactin
   4. Vasopressin

3. Which of the following adverse reactions would the nurse expect with the administration of clomiphene?
   1. Edema
   2. Vasomotor flushes
   3. Sedation
   4. Hypertension

4. Which of the following signs would lead the nurse to suspect a cushingoid appearing adverse reaction in a client taking a corticosteroid?
   1. Moon face, hirsutism
   2. Kyphosis, periorbital edema
   3. Pallor of the skin, acne
   4. Exophthalmos

5. Adverse reactions to the administration of fludrocortisone include _____.
   1. hyperactivity, headache
   2. sedation, lethargy
   3. edema, hypertension
   4. dyspnea, confusion

ANALYZE THE FACTS

6. Which of the following assessments would be critical for the nurse to make when a child receiving GH comes to the primary health care provider's office?
   1. Blood pressure, pulse, and respiration
   2. Diet history
   3. Height and weight
   4. Measurement of abdominal girth

7. Which of the following statements, if made by the client, would indicate a possible adverse reaction to the administration of vasopressin?
   1. "I am unable to see well at night."
   2. "My stomach is cramping."
   3. "I have a sore throat."
   4. "I am hungry all the time."

8. *The client makes the following statement: "This is our last try to have a baby." Select the most appropriate nursing diagnosis.
   1. Body image disturbance
   2. Anxiety
   3. Acute confusion
   4. Dehydration

9. Harmful drug interactions exist when glucocorticoids are taken with selected drugs. Which drug increases the effect of the glucocorticoids when taken together?
   1. Cholestyramine
   2. Oral contraceptives
   3. Hydantoins
   4. Rifampin

ALTERNATE-FORMAT QUESTIONS

10. Match the lobe of the pituitary gland with the hormone it secretes.

1. Anterior	A. ACTH
2. Posterior	B. FSH
	C. Oxytocin
	D. TSH

To check your answers, see Appendix F.

---

*Indicates the question is directly linked to the NCLEX-PN test plan in Appendix G.

> **WANT TO KNOW MORE?** A wide variety of resources are available to enhance your learning and understanding of this chapter.
> - Visit **thePoint** for resources such as
>   - NCLEX-Style Student Review Questions
>   - Journal Articles
>   - Dosage Calculations
>   - Drug Monographs
>   - Watch and Learn Videos
>   - Concepts in Action Animations
> - The *Study Guide to Accompany Introductory Clinical Pharmacology*, 12th edition, sold separately, will help you review and apply essential content.
> - **✓PrepU** is available to help students prepare for the NCLEX-PN examination.

42

Thyroid and Antithyroid Drugs

Key Terms

euthyroid   normal thyroid function

goiter   enlargement of the thyroid gland causing a swelling in the front part of the neck, usually caused by hyperthyroidism

Graves disease   autoimmune disorder leading to overactivity of the thyroid gland

Hashimoto thyroiditis   autoimmune disease attacking the thyroid typically resulting in hypothyroid function

hyperthyroidism   overactive thyroid function

hypothyroidism   underactive thyroid function

thyrotoxicosis   severe hyperthyroidism characterized by high fever, extreme tachycardia, and altered mental status (also called *thyroid storm*)

Learning Objectives

On completion of this chapter, the student will:

1. Identify the hormones produced by the thyroid gland.
2. Explain the uses, general drug actions, adverse reactions, contraindications, precautions, and interactions of thyroid and antithyroid drugs.
3. Distinguish important preadministration and ongoing assessment activities the nurse should perform with the client taking a thyroid or antithyroid drug.
4. Examine ways to promote an optimal response to therapy, how to manage adverse reactions, and important points to keep in mind when educating clients about the use of thyroid and antithyroid drugs.

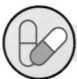 **Drug Classes**

Antithyroid drugs	Thyroid hormones

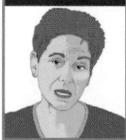

PHARMACOLOGY IN PRACTICE

Betty Peterson's neighbor will receive a dose of radioactive iodine for a hyperthyroid illness. Betty is concerned about bringing her daughter's new baby home, thinking that her neighbor may be radioactive after the procedure. Learn in this chapter how to respond to Betty's concerns.

The thyroid gland is located in the neck in front of the trachea (Fig. 42.1). This highly vascular gland manufactures and secretes two hormones: thyroxine (T_4) and triiodothyronine (T_3). These hormones help control the body metabolism. When the thyroid functions properly, this is known as a **euthyroid** (normal thyroid) state.

When the thyroid functions normally and the level of circulating thyroid hormone decreases, the anterior lobe of the pituitary secretes thyroid-stimulating hormone (TSH). TSH stimulates the cells of the thyroid to release stored thyroid hormones. This process is an example of the feedback mechanism described in Chapter 41.

When the thyroid does not work correctly, one of two conditions related to the hormone-producing activity of the thyroid gland may occur:

- **hyperthyroidism**—an increase in the amount of thyroid hormones manufactured and secreted
- **hypothyroidism**—a decrease in the amount of thyroid hormones manufactured and secreted

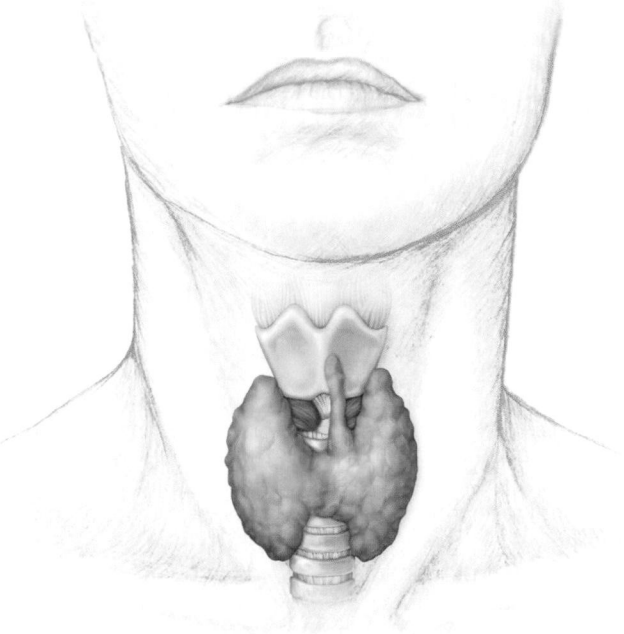

FIGURE 42.1 A normal thyroid gland. (Courtesy of Anatomical Chart Co.)

The symptoms of hypothyroidism and hyperthyroidism are described in Table 42.1.

HYPERTHYROIDISM

If the client has a condition such as **Graves disease** (auto-immune disorder), then the thyroid gland works harder to produce hormone and individuals may develop a **goiter** (enlarged thyroid gland). Hyperthyroidism can also be caused by inflammation and this condition is called **thyrotoxicosis**.

If hyperthyroidism, is caused by a condition, such as pregnancy and is correctable, it may be treated with one of the antithyroid drugs. If the condition is not correctable, then radioactive iodine is swallowed to destroy the thyroid so that it stops overproducing the hormones. In some cases, the thyroid may be removed surgically; however, it is a difficult procedure to remove the entire gland and that is why irradiation is the usual treatment.

HYPOTHYROIDISM

When the thyroid is surgically or radiologically removed, the client becomes *hypothyroid*, and without a functioning thyroid the individual must take thyroid supplements for the remainder of their life.

TABLE 42.1 Signs and Symptoms of Thyroid Dysfunction

BODILY SYSTEM OR FUNCTION	HYPOTHYROIDISM	HYPERTHYROIDISM
Metabolism	Decreased, with anorexia, intolerance to cold, low body temperature, weight gain despite anorexia	Increased, with increased appetite, intolerance to heat, elevated body temperature, weight loss despite increased appetite
Cardiovascular	Bradycardia, moderate hypotension	Tachycardia, moderate hypertension
Central nervous system	Lethargy, sleepiness	Nervousness, anxiety, insomnia, tremors, exophthalmos
Skin, skin structures	Pale, cool, dry skin; face appears puffy; coarse hair; nails thick and hard	Flushed, warm, moist skin; thinning hair; goiter
Ovarian function	Heavy menses, may be unable to conceive, loss of fetus possible	Irregular or scant menses
Testicular function	Low sperm count	

Figures Courtesy of Anatomical Chart Co.

Hypothyroidism can also be caused by a disease such as **Hashimoto thyroiditis**. An autoimmune disease, Hashimoto thyroiditis causes the thyroid to become inflamed. Rather than increasing hormone production, in this situation the inflammation keeps the gland from producing hormones. Thyroid hormones are again taken for supplement until the condition can be corrected.

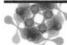 THYROID HORMONES

Thyroid hormones used as supplements include both the natural and synthetic hormones. The synthetic hormones are generally preferred because they are more uniform in potency than the natural hormones obtained from animals. Thyroid hormones are listed in the Summary Drug Table: Thyroid and Antithyroid Drugs.

ACTIONS

Thyroid hormones influence every organ and tissue of the body. These hormones increase the metabolic rate of tissues and result in increased heart and respiratory rate, raised body temperature, cardiac output, oxygen consumption, and the metabolism of fats, proteins, and carbohydrates. The exact mechanisms by which the thyroid hormones exert their influence on body organs and tissues are not well understood.

USES

Thyroid hormones are used in the treatment or prevention of *hypothyroidism* caused by the following:

- Subacute or chronic thyroiditis (Hashimoto disease or viral thyroiditis)
- Hormone supplement after hyperthyroid treatment
- Euthyroid goiter (enlargement of a normal thyroid gland)
- Thyroid nodules and multinodular goiter
- Some types of depression
- Thyroid cancer.

Levothyroxine (Synthroid) is the drug of choice for hypothyroidism because it is relatively inexpensive, requires once-a-day dosage, and has a more uniform potency than other thyroid hormone replacement drugs. Thyroid hormones also may be used as a diagnostic measure to differentiate suspected hyperthyroidism from euthyroidism.

> **NURSING ALERT**
>
> Thyroid hormones should not be used as a means of weight loss. When combined with other weight loss agents, life-threatening toxicity can occur.

ADVERSE REACTIONS

Treatment of hypothyroidism is based on individualized doses of the hormone. During initial therapy, the most common adverse reactions are signs of overdose and

hyperthyroidism as titration of the drug is being attempted (see Table 42.1). Adverse reactions other than symptoms of hyperthyroidism are rare.

CONTRAINDICATIONS AND PRECAUTIONS

These drugs are contraindicated in clients with known hypersensitivity to the drug, an uncorrected adrenal cortical insufficiency, or thyrotoxicosis. These drugs should not be used as a treatment for obesity or infertility. Thyroid hormone should not be used after a recent myocardial infarction. When hypothyroidism is a cause or a contributing factor to a myocardial infarction or heart disease, the physician may prescribe small doses of thyroid hormone.

These drugs are used cautiously in clients with cardiac disease and during lactation. Thyroid hormones are classified as pregnancy category A and their use should be continued by hypothyroid women during pregnancy.

LASA ALERT

The following drugs may sound alike; be sure to clarify when they are ordered:

Drug Name	*Sounds Like*
levothyroxine	lamoTRIgine, Lanoxin, levoFLOXacin, liothyronine
levoxyl	Lanoxin, Levaquin, Luvox
Liothyronine	levothyroxine
Synthroid	Symmetrel

Drugs that look like a similar drug are noted in the Summary Drug Tables of each chapter.

INTERACTIONS

The following interactions may occur with thyroid hormones:

Interacting Drug	Common Use	Effect of Interaction
Digoxin, β-blockers	Management of cardiac problems	Decreased effectiveness of cardiac drug
Oral antidiabetics and insulin	Treatment of diabetes	Increased risk of hyperglycemia
Oral anticoagulants	Blood thinners	Prolonged bleeding
Selective serotonin reuptake inhibitor antidepressants	Treatment of depression	Decreased effectiveness of thyroid drug
All other antidepressant drug categories	Treatment of depression	Increased effectiveness of thyroid drug
Decongestants	Treatment of nasal symptoms	Increased adverse reactions of thyroid drug

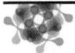 ANTITHYROID DRUGS

Antithyroid drugs or thyroid antagonists are used to treat *hyperthyroidism*. In addition to the antithyroid drugs, hyperthyroidism may be treated by the use of radioactive iodine (^{131}I) or by surgical removal of some or almost all of the thyroid gland (subtotal thyroidectomy).

ACTIONS

Antithyroid drugs inhibit the manufacture of thyroid hormones. They do not affect existing thyroid hormones circulating in the blood or stored in the thyroid gland. For this reason, therapeutic effects of the antithyroid drugs may not be observed for 3–4 weeks. Antithyroid drugs are listed in the Summary Drug Table: Thyroid and Antithyroid Drugs.

Radioactive iodine (^{131}I) is used because the thyroid has an affinity for iodine. The radioactive isotope accumulates in the cells of the thyroid gland, where destruction of thyroid cells occurs without damaging other cells throughout the body. Because the radioactive material is carried in iodine, it is important to assess the client's potential for iodine allergy (Greenfield, 2010).

PRACTICE CONSIDERATION

Providers continue to believe that shellfish allergy means an iodine hypersensitivity. As a result, contrast dyes and radioactive iodine might not be used when called for in health care. Researchers have found the allergen is the shellfish protein, not iodine, when a shellfish allergy is discovered (Schabelman & Witting, 2009).

Although using isotopes is preferable, it may not be recommended for all clients; therefore, a thyroidectomy may be necessary. Antithyroid drugs may be administered before surgery to return the client temporarily to a euthyroid state. When used for this reason, the vascularity of the thyroid gland is reduced typically using potassium iodide, and the tendency to bleed excessively during and immediately after surgery is decreased.

USES

Methimazole (Tapazole) and propylthiouracil (PTU) are used for the medical management of hyperthyroidism. Potassium iodide may be given orally with methimazole or PTU to prepare for thyroid surgery. Radioactive iodine (^{131}I)

is used for the treatment of hyperthyroidism and thyroid cancer. The drug is given orally either as a solution or in a gelatin capsule.

ADVERSE REACTIONS

Generalized System Reactions

- Hay fever, sore throat, skin rash, fever, headache
- Nausea, vomiting, paresthesias

Severe System Reactions

- Agranulocytosis (decrease in the number of white blood cells)
- Exfoliative dermatitis, granulocytopenia, hypoprothrombinemia
- Drug-induced hepatitis, acute pancreatitis

CONTRAINDICATIONS, PRECAUTIONS, AND INTERACTIONS

The antithyroid drugs are contraindicated in clients with hypersensitivity to the drug or any constituent of the drug. Mothers taking methimazole or PTU should not breastfeed their children. Radioactive iodine (pregnancy category X) is contraindicated during pregnancy and lactation.

Methimazole and PTU are used with extreme caution during pregnancy (pregnancy category D) because they can cause hypothyroidism in the fetus. However, if an antithyroid drug is necessary during pregnancy, PTU is the preferred drug because it does not cross the placenta. The potential for bleeding increases when these products are taken with oral anticoagulants.

LASA ALERT

The following drugs may sound alike; be sure to clarify when they are ordered:

Drug Name	Sounds Like
methIMAzole	methazolAMIDE, metOLazone

Drugs that look like a similar drug are noted in the Summary Drug Tables of each chapter.

PRACTICE CONSIDERATIONS

Currently methimazole is being reviewed for links with vasculitis and acute pancreatitis. The Canadian Health system has issued warnings, but at this writing the FDA has not (Agito & Manni, 2015; Hacking et al., 2019).

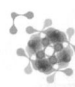

NURSING PROCESS: STEPS TO BUILD CLINICAL JUDGMENT
Client Receiving an Antithyroid Drug, Followed by Thyroid Hormone Supplement

ASSESSMENT

Often a client is diagnosed with hyperthyroidism, is treated and becomes hypothyroid, and subsequently requires supplementation. Nursing care described here covers the entire continuum of that care sequence.

Preadministration Assessment

Data gathering suggestions before a thyroid hormone or drug is administered include the following:

Objective Data

- General client appearance (see Table 44.1).
- Vital signs (temperature, pulse, respirations, and blood pressure).
- Weight, note gain or loss.
- Laboratory results—TSH, T_3, and T_4 levels, possibly serum thyroid antibody levels.

Subjective Data

- Current symptoms (see Table 44.1) experienced by client.
- Allergy history, particularly iodine or contrast dyes (which contain iodine).
- History of symptoms or other chronic health conditions.

Lifespan Considerations

Gerontology

Hypothyroidism may be confused with other conditions associated with aging, such as depression, cold intolerance, weight gain, confusion, or unsteady gait. These symptoms should be thoroughly evaluated before thyroid treatment is started.

Ongoing Assessment

During the ongoing assessment observe the client for adverse drug effects.

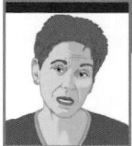

PHARMACOLOGY IN PRACTICE

ASSESSMENT

A nurse is assessing a client diagnosed with hypothyroidism. Which of the following symptoms would the nurse most likely document regarding the client during the preadministration assessment? Select all that apply.
1. Weight loss
2. Cold intolerance
3. Confusion
4. Sweating
5. Unsteady gait

Antithyroid Treatment

During the short-term therapy of radioactive treatment, adverse drug reactions are usually minimal. Long-term therapy is usually on an outpatient basis. Ask the client about relief of symptoms, as well as signs or symptoms indicating agranulocytosis, a possible adverse reaction

related to a decrease in blood cell numbers. Inquire about symptoms such as fatigue, fever, sore throat, easy bruising or bleeding, fever, cough, or any other signs of infection. Also monitor the client for signs of thyrotoxicosis (high fever, extreme tachycardia, diarrhea, vomiting, and altered mental status), which can occur in clients in whom hyperthyroidism increases rather than decreases during therapy. When these symptoms occur rapidly, it is termed as thyrotoxic crisis or thyroid storm.

Thyroid Supplement

The full effects of thyroid hormone replacement therapy may not be apparent for several weeks or more, but early effects may be apparent in as little as 48 hr. Signs of a therapeutic response include weight loss, mild diuresis, increased appetite, an increased pulse rate, and decreased puffiness of the face, hands, and feet. The client may also report an increased sense of well-being and increased mental activity.

! NURSING ALERT

Thyroid hormone replacement drugs are not equivalent to each other. Clients should not change brands or types of thyroid hormone without first checking with the primary health care provider. The primary health care provider needs to determine the equivalent dosages when changing medication brands.

NURSING DIAGNOSES

Drug-specific nursing diagnoses include the following:

- **Ineffective protection** related to urinary elimination of radioactive isotopes.
- **Altered health maintenance** related to consistent dosing or titrating doses.
- **Infection risk** related to adverse reactions.
- **Altered skin integrity risk** related to adverse reactions.

Nursing diagnoses related to drug administration are discussed in Chapter 4.

PLANNING

The expected outcomes of the client may include an optimal response to therapy, support of client needs related to the management of adverse reactions, and confidence in an understanding of the medication regimen.

IMPLEMENTATION

Promoting an Optimal Response to Therapy

Antithyroid Treatment

The client with hyperthyroidism may also have cardiac symptoms such as tachycardia or palpitations. Propranolol, an adrenergic blocking drug (see Chapter 24), may be prescribed by the primary health care provider as an adjunctive treatment for several weeks until the therapeutic effects of the antithyroid drug are obtained.

Prior home arrangements are made for isolated activities when the client with an enlarged thyroid gland is given radioactive iodine. The client stops taking antithyroid drugs about 3 days before the procedure. After midnight, no food or drink is taken; the client comes to the nuclear medicine department of a facility, swallows the preparation, and returns home. The effects of iodides are evident within 24 hr, with maximum effects attained after 10–15 days. If the client is hospitalized, radiation safety precautions identified by the hospital's department of nuclear medicine are followed.

Thyroid Supplement

Once a euthyroid state is achieved, the primary health care provider may begin a thyroid hormone supplement to prevent or treat hypothyroidism, which may develop slowly during long-term antithyroid drug therapy or after administration of [131]I. Thyroid hormones are administered once a day, early in the morning and preferably before breakfast. An empty stomach increases the absorption of the drug. Thyroid hormone replacement therapy in clients with diabetes may increase the intensity of the symptoms or the diabetes. Closely monitor the client with diabetes during thyroid hormone replacement therapy for signs of hyperglycemia (see Chapter 40) and notify the primary health care provider if this problem occurs.

 Lifespan Considerations

Gerontology

The older adult is at increased risk for adverse cardiovascular reactions when taking thyroid drugs. The initial dosage is smaller for an older adult, and increase in dosages, if they are necessary, is made in smaller increments during a period of about 8 weeks.

Carefully monitor clients with cardiovascular disease who take thyroid hormones. The development of chest pain or worsening of cardiovascular disease should be reported to the primary health care provider immediately because the client may require a reduction in the dosage of the thyroid hormone.

Monitoring and Managing Client Needs

Ineffective Protection

When the client returns home after taking the radioactive preparation, a place in the home where other individuals can be avoided should have been arranged. Avoiding contact with small children and pregnant women is especially important. Private toilet facilities should be provided and the client flushes twice each time. Eating utensils and laundry should be cleaned separately and the client should sleep alone. Instructions will be given as to how long the client should do activities by themselves and away from others; typically this lasts for 2–4 days.

Altered Health Maintenance

The client with hyperthyroidism may be concerned with the results of medical treatment and with the problem of taking the drug at regular intervals around the clock (usually every 8 hr—7 a.m., 3 p.m., and 11 p.m.). While some clients may be awake early in the morning and retire late

at night, others may experience difficulty with this 8-hour dosage schedule. Another concern may be a tendency to forget the first dose early in the morning, thus causing a problem with the two following doses.

If the client expresses a concern about the dosage schedule, suggest other options such as awaking at 6 a.m., taking the drug, and returning to bed. The drug absorbs better on an empty stomach, so this schedule would be ideal. Medication dispensers with alarms are available as well as simply posting a notice on a bathroom mirror to remind the individual that the first dose is due immediately after rising. After a week or more of therapy, most clients remember to take their morning dose on time.

For the client with hypothyroidism, once thyroid supplement is started, dosing is individualized to the needs of the client. If the dosage is inadequate, the client will continue to experience signs of hypothyroidism. If the dosage is excessive, the client will exhibit signs of hyperthyroidism. It is important to teach the client how to monitor reactions and document them well to provide information for correct dosing. This may be a frustrating process for the client, as the primary health care provider makes dose adjustments based on the client's hormone responses.

Infection Risk

Monitor the client throughout therapy for adverse drug reactions. Teach the client about signs of agranulocytosis. It is important that the client learn these signs because reduced white blood cells will put the client at greater risk of infections, particularly upper respiratory tract infections.

Altered Skin Integrity Risk

If the client experiences a rash while taking methimazole or PTU, soothing creams or lubricants may be applied, and soap is used sparingly, if at all, until the rash subsides. Drug dosing may need to be changed; report any indication of rash immediately.

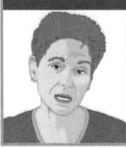 **PHARMACOLOGY IN PRACTICE**

SAFE DRUG ADMINISTRATION
When should the nurse advise a client to take levothyroxine (Synthroid)?
1. In the morning on an empty stomach
2. In the morning on a full stomach
3. In the evening on an empty stomach
4. In the evening on a full stomach

Educating the Client and Family

Thyroid hormones and antithyroid drugs are usually taken on an outpatient basis. Client instruction should include the importance of taking the drug exactly as directed and not stopping the drug use even though symptoms have improved. The drugs absorb better on an empty stomach, so meal timing should be taken into consideration. As you develop a teaching plan for the client include the following points.

Methimazole and Propylthiouracil

- Take these drugs at regular intervals around the clock (e.g., every 8 hr) unless directed otherwise by the primary health care provider.
- Do not take these drugs in larger doses or more frequently than as directed on the prescription container.
- Notify the primary health care provider promptly if any of the following occur: sore throat, fever, cough, easy bleeding or bruising, headache, or a general feeling of malaise.
- Record weight twice a week and notify the primary health care provider if there is any sudden weight gain or loss. (Note: The primary health care provider may also want the client to monitor pulse rate. If this is recommended, the client needs instruction in the proper technique and a recommendation to record the pulse rate and bring the record to the primary health care provider's office or clinic.)
- Avoid the use of nonprescription drugs unless the primary health care provider has approved the use of a specific drug.

Radioactive Iodine

- Follow the directions of the department of nuclear medicine regarding precautions to be taken.
- Keep in mind that tenderness and swelling of the neck, sore throat, and cough may occur in 2–3 days after the procedure.

Thyroid Hormone

- Replacement therapy is for life, with the exception of transient hypothyroidism seen in those with thyroiditis.
- Do not increase, decrease, or skip a dose unless advised to do so by the primary health care provider.
- Take this drug in the morning, preferably before breakfast, unless advised by the primary health care provider to take it at a different time of day.
- Notify the primary health care provider if any of the following occur: headache, nervousness, palpitations, diarrhea,

excessive sweating, heat intolerance, chest pain, increased pulse rate, or any unusual physical change or event.
- Do not change from one brand of the drug to another without consulting the primary health care provider.

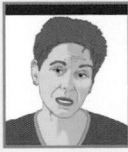

PHARMACOLOGY IN PRACTICE

ASSESSMENT

A client undergoing PTU drug therapy is discharged from the clinic facility. What instruction should the nurse include in the teaching plan? Select all that apply.
1. Take the drug at regular intervals.
2. Record weight twice a week.
3. Notify the primary health care provider when palpitations go away.
4. Avoid taking the drug in larger doses.

EVALUATION

- Therapeutic effect is achieved.
- Adverse reactions are identified, reported to the primary health care provider, and managed successfully through appropriate nursing interventions:
  - Client protects others effectively.
  - Client manages the therapeutic regimen effectively.
  - No evidence of infection is seen.
  - Skin remains intact.
- Client and family express confidence and demonstrate an understanding of the drug regimen.

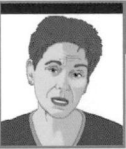

PHARMACOLOGY IN PRACTICE

USING CLINICAL REASONING

Does Betty have cause for concern about her neighbor being able to contaminate the baby? Discuss how you would present information to Betty to help deal with her fear.

KEY POINTS

■ The thyroid gland secretes the hormones thyroxine and triiodothyronine, which help control metabolism. This process is controlled by the pituitary gland when it secretes TSH.

■ Hashimoto thyroiditis is an example of a condition that causes hypothyroidism. When a person has hypothyroidism, the presenting problems include decreased metabolism, weight gain, low body temperature, lethargy, and pale, cool, dry skin, along with other symptoms. Graves disease is an example of a condition that causes hyperthyroidism. When a person has hyperthyroidism, the presenting problems include increased metabolism; weight loss; intolerance to heat; tachycardia; nervousness; anxiety; exophthalmos; flushed, warm skin; and possible goiter, along with other symptoms.

■ Hyperthyroid conditions are treated with antithyroid drugs or radioactive iodine to slow or completely eliminate function. Hypothyroidism is treated with thyroid hormone supplementation.

■ Common adverse reactions include the opposite action, such as symptoms of hyperthyroidism resulting from too much thyroid hormone replacement.

SUMMARY DRUG TABLE
Thyroid and Antithyroid Drugs

Generic Name	Trade Name	Uses	Adverse Reactions	Dosage Ranges
Thyroid Hormones				
levothyroxine (T₄) *lee-voe-thye-ROKS-een*	Euthyrox, Levoxyl, Synthroid,	Hypothyroidism, thyroid-stimulating hormone suppression, thyroid diagnostic testing	Palpitations, tachycardia, headache, nervousness, insomnia, diarrhea, vomiting, weight loss, fatigue, sweating, flushing	100–125 mcg/day orally
liothyronine (T₃) *lye-oh-THYE-roe-neen*	Cytomel	Same as levothyroxine	Same as levothyroxine	25–75 mcg/day orally
thyroid, desiccated	Armour	Same as levothyroxine	Same as levothyroxine	Maintenance: 60–120 mg/day orally
Antithyroid Preparations				
methIMAzole *meth-IM-a-zole*	Tapazole	Hyperthyroidism, thyrotoxicosis	Numbness, headache, loss of hair, skin rash, nausea, vomiting, agranulocytosis	5–40 mg/day orally, divided doses at 8-hour intervals
propylthiouracil (PTU) *proe-pil-thye-oh-YOOR-a-sil*		Same as methimazole	Same as methimazole	300–900 mg/day orally, divided doses at 8-hour intervals
Iodine Products				
radioactive iodide (¹³¹I) *eye'-oh-dyde*	Isotope	Eradicate hyperthyroidism, selected cases of thyroid cancer	Bone marrow depression, nausea, vomiting, tachycardia, itching, rash, hives	Measured by a radioactivity calibration system before administering orally 4–10 μCi Thyroid cancer: 50–150 μCi

CHAPTER REVIEW

Know Your Drugs

Clients sometimes know a medication by the brand (or trade) name and not the generic name. To recognize both names match the brand name with the generic name of the same medication.

Generic Name	Brand Name
1. levothyroxine	A. Armour
2. methimazole	B. PTU (common abbreviation)
3. propylthiouracil	C. Synthroid
4. thyroid, desiccated	D. Tapazole

Calculate Medication Dosages

1. Methimazole 40 mg is prescribed. The drug is available in 10-mg tablets. The client is taught to take _____.

2. Levothyroxine 0.2 mg orally is prescribed. Available are 0.1-mg tablets. The client is taught to take _____.

Prepare for the NCLEX

RECALL THE FACTS

1. What is the function of the thyroid gland?
   1. Secrete hormones produced in the pituitary gland
   2. Aid in digestion
   3. Control metabolism
   4. Facilitate breathing

2. Graves disease is an autoimmune disorder that causes which of the following symptoms?
   1. Tachycardia
   2. Low body temperature
   3. Thick, hard fingernails
   4. Low sperm count

3. Hypothyroidism is treated with which of the following interventions?
   1. Surgery
   2. Hormone replacement
   3. Radioactive iodine
   4. Tapazole

4. What condition is most likely to occur in a client taking a thyroid hormone?
   1. Heart failure
   2. Hyperthyroidism
   3. Hypothyroidism
   4. Euthyroidism
5. The nurse informs the client that therapy with a thyroid hormone may not initially produce a therapeutic response for _____.
   1. 24–48 days
   2. 1–3 days
   3. several weeks or more
   4. 8–12 months

ANALYZE THE FACTS

6. Which of the following symptoms best indicate a rare but serious adverse reaction is developing in a client receiving methimazole (Tapazole)?
   1. Fever, sore throat, bleeding from an injection site
   2. Cough, periorbital edema, constipation
   3. Constipation, anorexia, blurred vision
   4. Unsteady gait, blurred vision, insomnia
7. Which of the following statements made by a client would indicate to the nurse that the client is experiencing an adverse reaction to radioactive iodine?
   1. "I am sleepy most of the day."
   2. "I am unable to sleep at night."
   3. "My throat hurts when I swallow."
   4. "My body aches all over."
8. *Which of the following food allergies is of highest concern to the client about to take radioactive iodine?
   1. Peanut or other tree nuts
   2. Seafood
   3. Wheat products
   4. Lactose intolerance

ALTERNATE-FORMAT QUESTIONS

9. Which drugs are used to treat hypothyroidism? **Select all that apply.**
   1. T_4
   2. Synthroid
   3. Thyroid-stimulating hormone
   4. PTU
10. Which hormones are produced by the thyroid gland? **Select all that apply.**
    1. T_3
    2. T_4
    3. Thyroid-stimulating hormone
    4. Thyroxine

To check your answers, see Appendix F.

_____

*Indicates the question is directly linked to the NCLEX-PN test plan in Appendix G.

WANT TO KNOW MORE? A wide variety of resources are available to enhance your learning and understanding of this chapter.
- Visit forthePoint resources such as
  - NCLEX-Style Student Review Questions
  - Journal Articles
  - Dosage Calculations
  - Drug Monographs
  - Watch and Learn Videos
  - Concepts in Action Animations
- The *Study Guide to Accompany Introductory Clinical Pharmacology,* 12th edition, sold separately, will help you review and apply essential content.
- ✓*PrepU* is available to help students prepare for the NCLEX-PN examination.

43

Male and Female Hormones

Key Terms

anabolism tissue-building process

androgens male hormones, responsible for sexual maturity and characteristics

catabolism tissue-depleting process

endogenous pertaining to something that normally occurs or is produced within the organism

estrogen female hormones, responsible for sexual maturity and characteristics

gynecomastia male breast enlargement

menarche age of onset of first menstruation

progesterone female hormone produced by the corpus luteum that works in the uterus (along with estrogen) to prepare the uterus for possible conception

testosterone primary male sex hormone; acts to stimulate development of the male reproductive organs and secondary sex characteristics

virilization acquisition of male sexual characteristics by a woman

Learning Objectives

On completion of this chapter, the student will:

1. Explain the medical uses, actions, adverse reactions, contraindications, precautions, and interactions of the male and female hormones.
2. Distinguish important preadministration and ongoing assessment activities the nurse should perform with the client taking male or female hormones.
3. List nursing diagnoses particular to a client taking male or female hormones.
4. Examine ways to promote an optimal response to therapy, how to manage adverse reactions, and important points to keep in mind when educating the client about the use of male or female hormones.

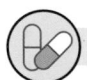 **Drug Classes**

Androgens	Estrogens	Progestins

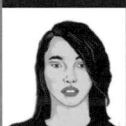 **PHARMACOLOGY IN PRACTICE**

Janna Wong is at the clinic for a sports physical examination. After the physical examination, Janna lingers in the examination room. You knock and ask if everything is okay. She asks you to come in and says she would like to get birth control. After reading the chapter, determine how you would respond to Janna's request.

Male and female hormones help us display gender. They play a vital role in the development and maintenance of secondary sex characteristics, and they are necessary for human reproduction. Although hormones are naturally produced by the body, administration of a male or female hormone may be indicated in the treatment of certain disorders, such as advanced-stage cancer, male hypogonadism, and male or female hormone deficiency. Hormones also are used as contraceptives and for treating the symptoms of menopause (Chapter 45).

A hormone use that is more overtly prevalent in our society today is hormone replacement both during and after gender reassignment for transgender individuals. Although it may seem simple enough to just add the opposite gender hormone, it is much more complex. Male and female hormones alone cannot change the effects of birth when puberty has started. Instead, the hormones of birth must be stopped, then hormone replacement will help to develop secondary sexual characteristics of the desired sex (Gromko, 2020). Other medications (e.g., spirolactone,

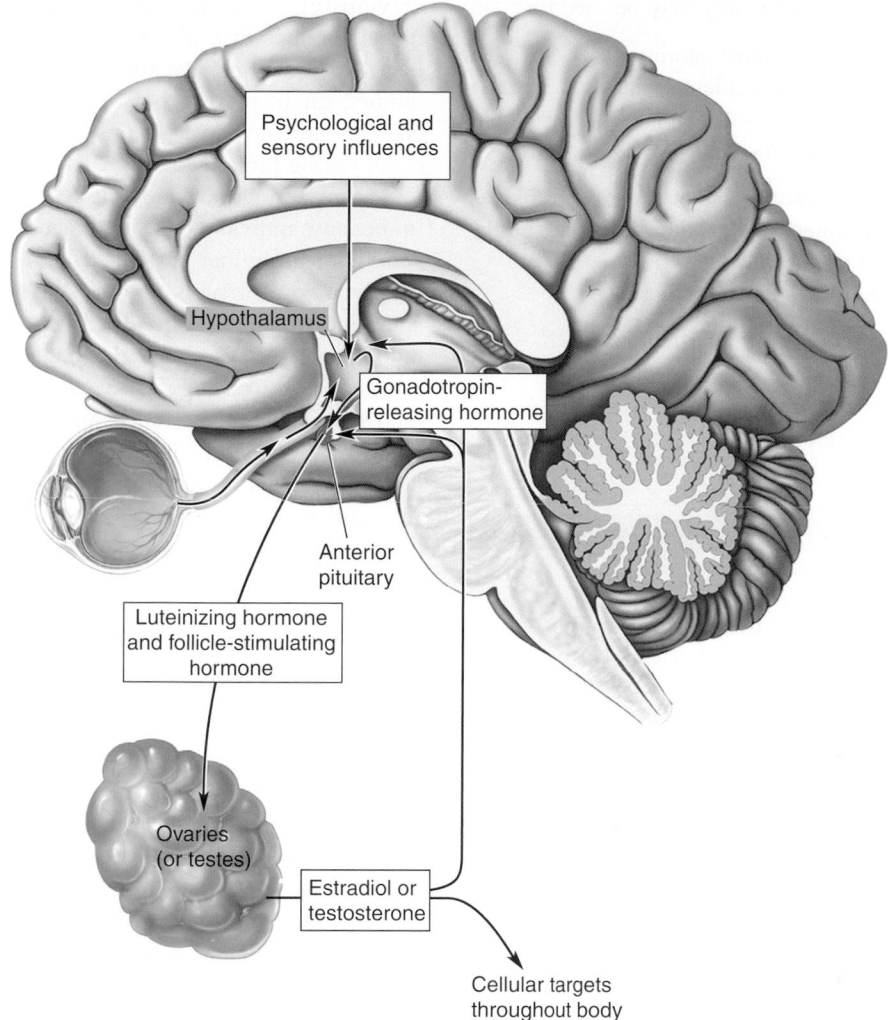

FIGURE 43.1 The sex hormone relationship of the pituitary and hypothalamus. (From Bear, M. F., Connors, B. W., & Parasido, M. A. (2001). *Neuroscience—Exploring the brain* (2nd ed.). Lippincott Williams & Wilkins.)

histrelin), growth hormones, and antihormone drugs in combination with counseling and surgical procedures are some of the strategies used to treat gender dysphoria.

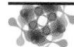 **MALE HORMONES**

Male hormones—**testosterone** and its derivatives—are collectively called androgens. **Androgen** secretion is influenced by the anterior pituitary gland. Small amounts of male and female hormones are also produced by the adrenal cortex (see Chapter 41). The anabolic steroids are closely related to the androgen testosterone and have both androgenic and anabolic (stimulate cellular growth and repair) activity. Androgen hormone inhibitors reduce the conversion of testosterone into a potent androgen (Fig. 43.1).

ACTIONS

Androgens

The male hormone testosterone and its derivatives cause the reproductive maturation in the adolescent boy. From puberty onward, androgens continue to aid in the development and

maintenance of secondary sex characteristics: facial hair, deep voice, body hair, body fat distribution, and muscle development. Testosterone also stimulates the growth in size of the sex organs (penis, testes, vas deferens, prostate) at the time of puberty. The androgens also promote tissue-building processes (**anabolism**) and reverse tissue-depleting processes (**catabolism**).

Anabolic Steroids

Anabolic steroids are synthetic drugs chemically related to androgens. Like the androgens, they promote tissue-building processes. Given in normal doses, they have a minimal effect on the accessory sex organs and secondary sex characteristics.

USES

Androgen therapy may be given as replacement therapy for the following:

- Testosterone deficiency
- Hypogonadism (failure of the testes to develop)
- Delayed puberty
- Development of testosterone deficiency after puberty

In the female client, androgen therapy may be used for:

- Postmenopausal, metastatic breast carcinoma
- Premenopausal, hormone-dependent metastatic breast carcinoma
- Transgender therapy female-to-male (FTM)

The transdermal testosterone system is used as replacement therapy when endogenous (produced by the body) testosterone is deficient or absent.

Anabolic steroid use includes the following:

- Management of anemia of renal insufficiency
- Control of metastatic breast cancer in women
- Promotion of weight gain in those with weight loss after surgery, trauma, or infections

 Lifespan Considerations

Young Athletes

The use of anabolic steroids to promote an increase in muscle mass and strength is a serious problem. Athletes ranging from high school to professionals have used anabolic steroids to gain strength and performance in sports. Routine testing for steroid use in areas such as professional sports and the Olympics, plus banning athletes found to be using drugs, has resulted in a decline of use in recent years. Yet, young athletes should continue to be taught proper training techniques and discouraged from use of anabolic steroids to boost performance.

ADVERSE REACTIONS

Androgens

In men, administration of androgen may result in breast enlargement (**gynecomastia**), testicular atrophy, and inhibition of testicular function, impotence, enlargement of the penis, nausea, vomiting, jaundice, headache, anxiety, male-pattern baldness, acne, and depression. Fluid and electrolyte imbalances, which include sodium, water, chloride, potassium, calcium, and phosphate retention, may also occur.

In women receiving an androgen preparation for breast carcinoma, the most common adverse reactions are amenorrhea, menstrual irregularities, and **virilization** (acquisition of male sexual characteristics by a woman). Virilization produces facial hair, a deepening of the voice, and enlargement of the clitoris. Male-pattern baldness and acne may also result.

Anabolic Steroids

Virilization in a woman is the most common reaction associated with anabolic steroids, especially when higher doses are used. Acne occurs frequently in all age groups and both sexes. Nausea, vomiting, diarrhea, fluid and electrolyte imbalances (the same as for the androgens, discussed

previously), testicular atrophy, jaundice, anorexia, and muscle cramps may also be seen. Blood-filled cysts of the liver and sometimes the spleen, malignant and benign liver tumors, an increased risk of atherosclerosis, and mental changes are the most serious adverse reactions that may occur during prolonged use.

Many serious adverse drug reactions are being reported in healthy individuals using anabolic steroids. There is some indication that prolonged high-dose use has resulted in psychological and possibly physical dependence and some individuals have required treatment in drug rehabilitation centers. Severe mental changes, such as uncontrolled rage (called "roid rage"), severe depression, and suicidal tendencies; malignant and benign liver tumors; aggressive behavior; increased risk of atherosclerosis; inability to concentrate; and personality changes are not uncommon. In addition, the incidence of the severe adverse reactions cited earlier appears to be increased in those using anabolic steroids for this purpose.

CONTRAINDICATIONS AND PRECAUTIONS

The male hormones are contraindicated in clients with known hypersensitivity to the drugs, liver disorders, or serious cardiac disease, and in men with prostate gland disorders (e.g., prostate carcinoma and prostate enlargement). These drugs are classified as pregnancy category X drugs and should not be administered during pregnancy and lactation. Anabolic steroids are contraindicated for use to enhance physical appearance or athletic performance. Anabolic steroids should be used cautiously in older men because of increased risk of prostate enlargement and prostate cancer.

LASA ALERT

The following drugs may sound alike; sure to clarify when they are ordered:

Drug Name	Sounds Like
methylTESTOSTERone	medroxyPROGESTERone, methylPREDNISolone

Drugs that look like a similar drug are noted in the Summary Drug Tables of each chapter.

INTERACTIONS

The following interactions may occur with the male hormones:

Interacting Drug	Common Use	Effect of Interaction
Oral anticoagulants	Blood thinners	Increased antidiuretic effect
Imipramine and androgen	Treatment of depression	Increased risk of paranoid behavior
Sulfonylureas and anabolic steroids	Diabetes	Increased risk of hypoglycemia

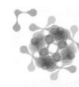

NURSING PROCESS: STEPS TO BUILDING CLINICAL JUDGMENT
Client Receiving a Male Hormone

ASSESSMENT

Preadministration Assessment

Assessment of the client receiving an androgen or anabolic steroid depends on the drug, the client, and the reason for administration.

Androgens

In most instances, androgens or anabolic steroids are administered to the man on an outpatient basis.

Data gathering suggestions before androgens/anabolic steroids are administered include:

Objective data

- General client appearance, emphasis on secondary sex characteristics
- Vital signs (temperature, pulse, respirations, and blood pressure)
- Weight
- Lab results—serum electrolytes, complete blood count, hepatic function, serum/urinary calcium levels

Subjective data

- Symptoms experienced by client
- Dietary history for women with advanced cancer, pain, and limits to range of motion for bone metastasis
- Emotional and social history for females seeking transgender therapy
- Family history of heart disease, deep vein thrombosis, or other chronic health conditions

Ongoing Assessment

The ongoing assessment depends on the reason the drug was prescribed and the condition of the client. Men receiving an androgen or anabolic steroid are questioned regarding the effectiveness of drug therapy.

Track the weight of the client with advanced breast carcinoma daily or as ordered by the primary health care provider. Contact the primary health care provider if there is a significant (5-lb) increase or decrease in weight. Check the lower extremities frequently for signs of edema.

Teach the client or caregiver to observe for adverse drug reactions, especially signs of fluid and electrolyte imbalance, jaundice (which may indicate hepatotoxicity), and virilization. The primary health care provider must be alerted to any signs of fluid and electrolyte imbalance or jaundice.

When the client is hospitalized, review vital signs every 4–8 hr, depending on the client's condition, and then evaluate the client's response to drug therapy based on original assessment findings. Possible responses include a decrease in pain, an increase in appetite, and a feeling of well-being.

 Chronic Care Considerations

Diabetes

When the androgens are administered to a client with diabetes, blood glucose levels should be measured frequently because glucose tolerance may be altered. Adjustments may need to be made in insulin dosage, oral antidiabetic drugs, or diet.

When anabolic steroids are used for weight gain, the client is weighed at intervals ranging from daily to weekly. A good dietary regimen is necessary to promote weight gain. Consult the dietitian if the client eats poorly.

NURSING DIAGNOSES

Drug-specific nursing diagnoses include the following:

- **Fluid overload** related to adverse reactions (sodium and water retention)
- **Altered body image perception** (in the female) related to adverse reactions (virilization)

Nursing diagnoses related to drug administration are discussed in Chapter 4.

PLANNING

The expected outcomes of the client may include an optimal response to therapy, support of client needs related to the management of adverse reactions, and confidence in an understanding of the medication regimen.

IMPLEMENTATION

Promoting an Optimal Response to Therapy

If the androgen is to be administered as a buccal tablet, show the client how to place the tablet and warn the client not to swallow the tablet but to allow it to dissolve in the mouth. Remind the client not to smoke or drink water until the tablet is dissolved. Oral and parenteral androgens are often taken or given by injection on an outpatient basis. When given by injection, the injection is administered deep intramuscularly (IM) into the gluteal muscle. Alternatively, a pellet dose is placed under the skin and repeated every 3–6 months. Oral testosterone is given with or before meals to decrease gastrointestinal (GI) upset.

Androderm is a transdermal system that is applied nightly to clean, dry skin on the abdomen, thigh, back, or upper arm. This system is not applied to the scrotum. Sites are rotated, with 7 days between applications to any specific site. The system is applied immediately after opening the pouch and removing the protective covering. If the client has not exhibited a therapeutic response after 8 weeks of therapy, another form of testosterone replacement therapy should be considered.

When the system is removed it should be folded in half on itself to prevent accidental dosing if touched.

Testosterone gel (AndroGel) is applied once daily (preferably in the morning) to clean, dry, intact skin of the shoulders and upper arms or abdomen. After the packet is opened, the contents are squeezed into the palm of the hand and immediately applied to the application sites. The application sites are allowed to dry before the client gets dressed. The gel is not applied to the genitals. Wear gloves if applying to another person; wash hands well with soap and water for self-applications.

ⓘ NURSING ALERT

Always instruct and remind clients about disposal procedures for androgen gels and transdermal patches. Virilization in children inadvertently exposed to testosterone products has occurred when products are not disposed properly. Provide written instructions in disposal, using gels on exposed skin, and hand hygiene after self-administration.

Axiron is a liquid preparation that is sprayed into the axillae daily. It is a fast-drying liquid being tested for ease of use.

The pellet method has gain popularity for clients who prefer not to deal with medications daily or become fearful of repeated injections (Gromko, 2020). A stab wound is made into the skin after a local anesthetic numbs the area and it is cleaned. Then a trocar is inserted and the pellets are placed under the skin, the trocar is removed and the wound is stitched or Steri-Strips are applied. It is a good idea to order more pellets than the amount needed because they are small and may inadvertently fall to the floor during handling.

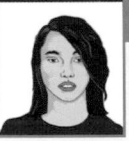

PHARMACOLOGY IN PRACTICE

DRUG RECOGNITION
The androgen testosterone is available in several dosage forms. In which of the following routes is testosterone not able to be given?

1. Intravenously
2. Topically
3. Orally
4. Subcutaneously

Monitoring and Managing Client Needs
Observe the client receiving an androgen or anabolic steroid for signs of adverse drug reactions.

Fluid Overload
Sodium and water retention may also occur with androgen or anabolic steroid administration, causing the client to become edematous. In addition, other electrolyte imbalances, such as hypercalcemia, may occur. Monitor the client for fluid and electrolyte disturbances.

Lifespan Considerations

Gerontology
Older adults with cardiac problems or kidney disease are at increased risk for sodium and water retention when taking androgens or anabolic steroids.

To monitor for fluid retention, make a daily comparison of the client's preadministration weight with current weights and make sure to note the appearance of puffy eyelids and dependent swelling of the hands or feet (if the client is ambulatory) or the sacral area (if the client is nonambulatory), and report any findings to the primary health care provider. Daily fluid intake and output should be used to calculate fluid balance, too.

Altered Body Image Perception
With long-term administration of a male hormone, the female client may experience mild to moderate masculine changes (virilization), namely, facial hair, a deepening of the voice, and enlargement of the clitoris. Male-pattern baldness, patchy hair loss, skin pigmentation, and acne may also result. Although these adverse effects are not life-threatening, they often are distressing and only add to the client's discomfort and anxiety. These problems may be easy to identify, but they are not always easy to solve. If hair loss occurs, suggest wearing head coverings such as hats, scarves, or a wig; mild skin pigmentation maybe covered with makeup; but severe and widespread pigmented areas and acne are often difficult to conceal. Each client is different, and the emotional responses to these outward changes may range from severe depression in a woman to a positive attitude and acceptance in a transgender man. Work with the client as an individual, first identifying the problems, and then helping the client, when possible, to deal with these changes.

Educating the Client and the Family
Explain the dosage regimen and possible adverse drug reactions to the client and family and develop a teaching plan to include the following points:

Androgens
- Notify the primary health care provider if any of the following occurs: nausea, vomiting, swelling of the legs, or jaundice. Women should report any signs of virilization to the primary health care provider.
- Oral tablets—take with food or a snack to avoid GI upset.
- Buccal tablets—place the tablet between the cheek and molars and allow it to dissolve in the mouth. Do not smoke or drink water until the tablet is dissolved.
- Testosterone transdermal system—apply according to the directions supplied with the product. Be sure the

skin is clean and dry and the placement area is free of hair. Do not store outside the pouch or use damaged systems. Discard systems in household trash in a safe manner to prevent ingestion/touching by children or pets.

Anabolic Steroids

- Anabolic steroids may cause nausea and GI upset. Take this drug with food or meals.
- Keep all primary health care provider or clinic visits because close monitoring of therapy is essential.
- Female clients: Notify the primary health care provider if signs of virilization occur.

EVALUATION

- Therapeutic response is achieved.
- Adverse reactions are identified, reported to the primary health care provider, and managed successfully with appropriate nursing interventions:
  - Adequate fluid volume is maintained.
  - Perceptions of body changes are managed successfully.
- Client and family express confidence and demonstrate an understanding of the drug regimen.

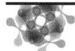 # FEMALE HORMONES

The two endogenous (produced by the body) female hormones are **estrogen** and **progesterone**. Like the androgens, their production is under the influence of the anterior pituitary gland. The endogenous estrogens are estradiol, estrone, and estriol. The most potent of these three estrogens is estradiol. Examples of estrogens used as drugs include estropipate and estradiol.

There are natural and synthetic progesterones, which are collectively called progestins. Examples of progestins used as drugs include medroxyprogesterone and norethindrone.

ACTIONS

Estrogens

Estrogens are secreted by the ovarian follicle and in smaller amounts by the adrenal cortex. Estrogens are important in the development and maintenance of the female reproductive system and the primary and secondary sex characteristics. At puberty, they promote growth and development of the vagina, uterus, fallopian tubes, and breasts. They also affect the release of pituitary gonadotropins (see Chapter 41).

Other actions of estrogen include fluid retention, protein anabolism, thinning of the cervical mucus, and inhibition or facilitation of ovulation. Estrogens contribute to the conservation of calcium and phosphorus, the growth of pubic and axillary hair, and pigmentation of the breast areolae and genitals. Estrogens also stimulate contraction of the fallopian tubes (which promotes movement of the ovum). They modify the physical and chemical properties of the cervical mucus and restore the endometrium after menstruation.

Progestins

Progesterone is secreted by the corpus luteum, placenta, and (in small amounts) adrenal cortex. Progesterone and its derivatives (the progestins) transform the proliferative endometrium into a secretory endometrium. Progestins are necessary for the development of the placenta and inhibit the secretion of pituitary gonadotropins, which in turn prevents maturation of the ovarian follicle and ovulation. The synthetic progestins are usually preferred for medical use because of the decreased effectiveness of progesterone when administered orally.

USES

Estrogens

Estrogen is most commonly used in combination with progesterones as a contraceptive agent (Table 43.1) or in postmenopausal women as estrogen replacement therapy (ERT) or in combination with progesterone as hormonal replacement therapy (HRT). In sexual reassignment, once male hormones are diminished, estrogen is used to enhance secondary sex characteristics in male-to-female (MTF) treatment. Replacement therapy and other uses of postmenopausal estrogen are discussed in Chapter 45.

Progestins

Progestins are used in the treatment of amenorrhea, endometriosis, and functional uterine bleeding. Progestins are also used as oral contraceptives, either alone or in combination with estrogen (see the Summary Drug Table: Male and Female Hormones; see also Table 43.1).

Contraceptive Hormones

Combination estrogens and progestins are used as oral contraceptives. There are four types of estrogen and progestin combination oral contraceptives: monophasic, biphasic, triphasic, and quad-phasic. Oral contraceptives have changed a great deal since their introduction in the 1960s. Today, lower hormone dosages provide reduced levels of hormones compared with the older formulations, while retaining the same degree of effectiveness (more than 99% when used as prescribed). The different formulations of hormones are described in Table 43.1.

Taking contraceptive hormones provides health benefits not related to contraception, such as regulating the menstrual cycle and decreasing menstrual blood loss, the incidence of iron-deficiency anemia, and dysmenorrhea. Health benefits

TABLE 43.1 Examples of Oral Contraceptives

TYPE OF COMBINATION	TRADE (GENERIC) NAMES
Monophasic Oral Contraceptives Constant dose of estrogen and progestin for entire 21-day cycle	Levora (estradiol and levonorgestrel) Gildagia (estradiol and norethindrone) Yaz (estradiol and drospirenone)
Biphasic Oral Contraceptives Progestin dose is changed at midcycle	Seasonique (estradiol and levonorgestrel)
Triphasic Oral Contraceptives Contains three different doses of progestin with gradual estrogen increase over the cycle	Enpresse (estradiol and levonorgestrel) Nortrel (estradiol and norethindrone) Velivet (estradiol and desogestrel)
Quad-phasic Oral Contraceptives Mimics the natural hormonal menstrual cycle, reduce side effects, but errors in dosing can be greater	Natazia (estradiol and dienogest)
Progestin-only Contraceptive (Minipill) Used when health condition warrants no estrogen (e.g., breastfeeding, DVT risk, heart disease, migraine headaches)	Camila (norethindrone)

DVT, deep vein thrombosis.

related to the inhibition of ovulation include a decrease in ovarian cysts and ectopic pregnancies. In addition, there is a decrease in fibrocystic breast disease, acute pelvic inflammatory disease, endometrial cancer, and ovarian cancer; improved maintenance of bone density; and a decrease in symptoms related to endometriosis in women taking contraceptive hormones. Newer combination contraceptives such as drospirenone and ethinyl estradiol combinations (YAZ) have been shown to help reduce moderate acne and maintain clear skin in women 15 years of age or older (who menstruate, want contraception, and have no response to topical antiacne medications).

ADVERSE REACTIONS: ESTROGENS

Administration of estrogens by any route may result in many adverse reactions, although the incidence and intensity of these reactions vary. Some of the adverse reactions seen with the administration of estrogens follow.

Central Nervous System Reactions
- Headache, migraine
- Dizziness, mental depression

Dermatologic Reactions
- Dermatitis, pruritus
- Chloasma (pigmentation of the skin) or melasma (discoloration of the skin), which may continue when use of the drug is discontinued

Gastrointestinal Reactions
- Nausea, vomiting
- Abdominal bloating and cramps

Genitourinary Reactions
- Breakthrough bleeding, withdrawal bleeding, spotting, change in menstrual flow
- Dysmenorrhea, premenstrual-like syndrome, amenorrhea
- Vaginal candidiasis, cervical erosion, vaginitis

Local Reactions
- Pain at injection site or sterile abscess with parenteral form of the drug
- Redness and irritation at the application site with transdermal system

Ophthalmic Reactions
- Steepening of corneal curvature
- Intolerance to contact lenses

MISCELLANEOUS REACTIONS
- Edema, rhinitis, changes in libido
- Breast pain, enlargement, and tenderness
- Reduced carbohydrate tolerance
- Venous thromboembolism, pulmonary embolism
- Weight gain or loss
- Generalized and skeletal pain

Warnings associated with the administration of estrogen include an increased risk of endometrial cancer, gallbladder disease, hypertension, hepatic adenoma (a benign tumor of the liver), cardiovascular disease, and thromboembolic disease, and hypercalcemia in those with breast cancer and bone metastases.

ADVERSE REACTIONS: PROGESTINS

Administration of progestins by any route may result in many adverse reactions, although the incidence and intensity of these reactions vary. Progestin administration may result in the following:

- Breakthrough bleeding, spotting, change in menstrual flow, amenorrhea
- Breast tenderness, edema, weight increase or decrease
- Acne, chloasma or melasma, insomnia, mental depression

In addition to the adverse reactions seen with progestins, the use of a levonorgestrel implant system may result in bruising after insertion, scar tissue formation at the site of insertion, and hyperpigmentation at the implant site. The use of medroxyprogesterone contraceptive injection may result in the same adverse reactions as those associated with administration of any progestin.

TABLE 43.2 Estrogen and Progestin: Excess and Deficiency

HORMONE[a]	SIGNS OF EXCESS	SIGNS OF DEFICIENCY
Estrogen	Nausea, bloating, cervical mucorrhea (increased cervical discharge), polyposis (numerous polyps), hypertension, migraine headache, breast fullness or tenderness, edema	Early or midcycle breakthrough bleeding, increased spotting, hypomenorrhea, melasma (discoloration of the skin)
Progestin	Increased appetite, weight gain, tiredness, fatigue, hypomenorrhea, acne, oily scalp, hair loss, hirsutism (excessive growth of hair), depression, monilial vaginitis, breast regression	Late breakthrough bleeding, amenorrhea, hypermenorrhea

[a]Hormonal balance is achieved by adjusting the estrogen/progestin dosage. Oral contraceptives have different amounts of progestin and estrogen, varying the estrogenic and progestational activity in each product.

ADVERSE REACTIONS: CONTRACEPTIVE HORMONES

When estrogen–progestin combinations are used as oral contraceptives, these drugs may exhibit adverse reactions that vary depending on their estrogen or progestin content, so the adverse reactions of each must be considered. Table 43.2 identifies the symptoms of estrogen and progestin excess or deficiency. The adverse effects are minimized by adjusting the estrogen–progestin balance or dosage.

CONTRAINDICATIONS AND PRECAUTIONS

Estrogen and progestin therapy is contraindicated in clients with known hypersensitivity to the drugs, breast cancer (except for metastatic disease), estrogen-dependent neoplasms, undiagnosed abnormal genital bleeding, and thromboembolic disorders. The progestins also are contraindicated in clients with cerebral hemorrhage or impaired liver function. Both the estrogens and progestins are classified as pregnancy category X drugs and are contraindicated during pregnancy.

Estrogens are used cautiously in clients with gallbladder disease, hypercalcemia (may lead to severe hypercalcemia in clients with breast cancer and bone metastasis), cardiovascular disease, and liver impairment. Cardiovascular complications are greater in women who smoke and use estrogen. Progestins are used cautiously in clients with a history of migraine headaches, epilepsy, asthma, and cardiac or renal impairment.

PRACTICE CONSIDERATIONS

The FDA has issued concerns about the increased risk of birth control pills containing drospirenone. Research indicates chances of developing a blood clot may be double that of other pills without drospirenone. Those most at risk are women with high blood pressure or cholesterol, diabetes, or are overweight. Women are encouraged to discuss their individual risk for blood clots with their primary health care provider before starting birth control pills with drospirenone (Casciotti et al., 2015).

The warnings associated with the use of oral contraceptives, notably the combined drug contraceptives, are the same as those for the estrogens and progestins and include cigarette smoking (especially those older than 35 years of age), which increases the risk of cardiovascular side effects, such as venous and arterial thromboembolism, myocardial infarction, and thrombotic and hemorrhagic stroke. Also reported with oral contraceptive use are hepatic adenomas and other tumors, visual disturbances, gallbladder disease, hypertension, and fetal abnormalities.

LASA ALERT

The following drugs may sound alike; be sure to clarify when they are ordered:

Drug Name	Sounds Like
Depo-Provera	DEPO-Medrol, depo-subQ provera 104
medroxyPROGES-TERone	HYDROXYprogesterone caproate, methylPREDNISolone, methylTESTOSTERone
Premarin	Primaxin, Provera, Remeron
Provera	Covera, Femara, Parlodel, Premarin, Proscar, PROzac

Drugs that look like a similar drug are noted in the Summary Drug Tables of each chapter.

INTERACTIONS

The following interactions may occur with female hormones:

Interacting Drug	Common Use	Effect of Interaction
Estrogens		
Oral anticoagulants	Blood thinners	Decreased anticoagulant effect
Tricyclic antidepressants	Treatment of depression	Increased effectiveness of antidepressant
Rifampin	Anti-infective	Increased risk of breakthrough bleeding
Hydantoins	Seizure control	Increased risk of breakthrough bleeding and pregnancy

Interacting Drug	Common Use	Effect of Interaction
Progestins		
Anticonvulsants or rifampin	Seizure control or anti-infective, respectively	Decreased effectiveness of progestin
Penicillins or tetracyclines	Anti-infective agents	Decreased effectiveness of oral contraceptives

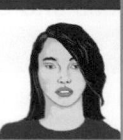

PHARMACOLOGY IN PRACTICE

INTERVENTION
A woman taking oral contraceptives has heard about health benefits associated with oral contraceptive use, apart from contraception, and is eager to know more about it. Which of the following risks are reduced with oral contraceptive use? Select all that apply.

1. Iron deficiency anemia
2. Ovarian cancer
3. Cervical erosion
4. Osteoporosis
5. Vaginal candidiasis

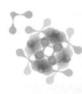

NURSING PROCESS: STEPS TO BUILDING CLINICAL JUDGMENT
Client Receiving a Female Hormone

ASSESSMENT

Preadministration Assessment
Data gathering suggestions before an estrogen or progestin are administered include:

Objective data

- General client appearance
- Vital signs (temperature, pulse, respirations and blood pressure)
- Weight
- Breast and pelvic examination with a Papanicolaou (Pap) test to rule out cervical cancer or human papillomavirus (HPV)
- Lab results – serum electrolytes, complete blood count, hepatic function

Subjective data

- Client health history, including menstrual history, menarche (age of onset of first menstruation), menstrual pattern, and changes in the menstrual pattern (including a menopause history when applicable)
- Vaccine history especially HPV
- Sexual history and reason for contraception
- Smoking history
- Emotional and social history for females seeking transgender therapy
- Family history of vascular disease, thrombophlebitis, or liver disease

Assess the understanding of safe sexual practices and understanding that hormonal contraceptives do not protect against sexually transmitted infections (STIs).

Ongoing Assessment
At the time of each office or clinic visit, the blood pressure, pulse, respiratory rate, and weight are checked. Ask the client about any adverse drug effects as well as the result of drug therapy. Weigh the client and report a steady weight gain or loss. A periodic (usually annual) physical examination is performed by the primary health care provider and may include a pelvic examination, breast examination, Pap test, and laboratory tests.

NURSING DIAGNOSES

Drug-specific nursing diagnoses include the following:

- **Altered Health Seeking Behavior** related to administration of medications routinely despite adverse reactions
- **Fluid Overload** related to sodium and water retention
- **Altered Tissue Perfusion** related to thromboembolic effects
- **Malnutrition Risk** related to weight gain or loss

Nursing diagnoses related to drug administration are discussed in Chapter 4.

PLANNING

The expected outcomes of the client may include an optimal response to therapy, support of client needs related to the management of adverse reactions, and confidence in an understanding of the medication regimen.

IMPLEMENTATION

Promoting an Optimal Response to Therapy

Estrogens
Estrogens may be administered orally, IM, intravenously (IV), transdermally, or intravaginally. Outpatient use as a contraceptive is typically self-administered by the oral route. The transdermal delivery route has been found to be safer, especially for women with elevated triglycerides, type 2 diabetes, hypertension, or migraine headaches, or those who smoke.

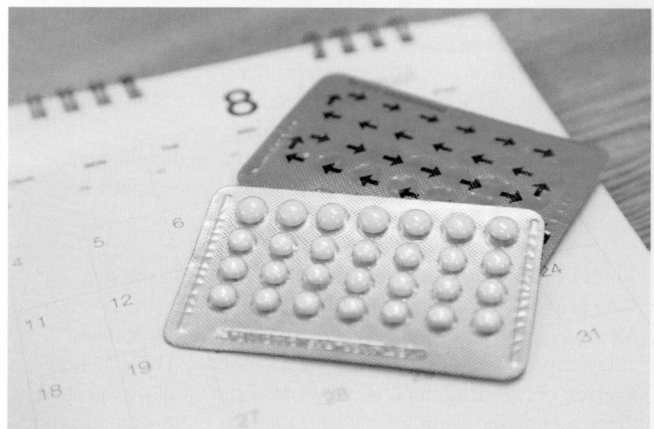

FIGURE 43.2 Oral contraceptives in a monthly (28 day) pack where 21 pills are active ingredients.

Contraceptive Hormones

Monophasic oral contraceptives are administered on a 21-day regimen, with the first tablet taken on the first Sunday after the menses begin or on the day the menses begin if the menses begin on Sunday. After the 21-day regimen, the next 7 days are skipped (or a benign pill is taken to maintain the daily habit, see Fig. 43.2), and then the cycle is begun again. With the biphasic oral contraceptives, the first phase is 10 days of a smaller dosage of progestin, and the second phase is a larger amount of progestin. The estrogen dosage remains constant for 21 days, followed by no estrogen for 7 days. Some regimens contain seven placebo tablets for easier management of the therapeutic regimen. With the triphasic oral contraceptives, the estrogen amount stays the same or may vary, and the progestin amount varies throughout the 21-day cycle. The quad-phasic oral contraceptives have an even greater progression of progestin through the month, bringing this

pill closest to a normal menstrual cycle. Progestin-only oral contraceptives are taken daily and continuously.

 Lifespan Considerations

Childbearing Age Women

When using oral contraceptives for dysmenorrhea or endometriosis, the practice of skipping 4–7 days per month is eliminated. As a result, oral contraceptive products are now produced (Seasonale, Seasonique), which maintain 84-day cycles. Many women without gynecologic issues prefer this extended cycle form of birth control because monthly menstrual periods are eliminated (Golobof, 2016).

Contraceptive Implant System

Levonorgestrel, a progestin, is available as an implant contraceptive system (Norplant system). Six capsules, each containing levonorgestrel, are implanted using local anesthesia in the subdermal (below the skin) tissues of the midportion of the upper arm. The capsules provide contraceptive protection for 5 years but may be removed at any time at the request of the client. See Box 43.1 for more information on ways to promote an optimal response when taking the contraceptive hormones.

Medroxyprogesterone Contraceptive Injection

Medroxyprogesterone (Depo-Provera), a synthetic progestin used in the treatment of abnormal uterine bleeding and secondary amenorrhea, is also used as a contraceptive. This drug is given IM every 3 months, and the initial dosage is given within the first 5 days of menstruation or within 5 days postpartum. When this drug is given IM, the solution must be shaken vigorously before use to ensure uniform suspension, and the drug is given deep IM into the gluteal or deltoid muscle.

BOX 43.1 Alternatives to Oral Contraceptive Hormones

Clients who choose to use contraceptive hormone preparations need to be fully informed of their benefits and drawbacks. You can be instrumental in educating clients about these drugs. Included here are contraceptive methods used by women in place of the traditional oral contraceptive pills.

Emergency Contraceptives (Aftera, EContra, React, Preventesa, Take Action, Plan B, My Way, Ella [ulipristal])
These preparations are used for emergency contraception after unprotected intercourse or known contraceptive failure. They prevent pregnancy; they do not work if the client is already pregnant.
- When using high-dose levonorgestrel (plan B), take one tablet within 72 hr after unprotected intercourse. Take the second dose of plan B 12 hr later.
- Ella can be taken within 5 days of unprotected intercourse
- This drug can be used any time during the menstrual cycle.
- If vomiting occurs within 1 hr after taking either dose, notify the primary health care provider.

- Emergency contraceptives are not effective in terminating an existing pregnancy.
- Emergency contraceptives should not be used as a routine form of contraception.

Etonogestrel/Ethinyl Estradiol Vaginal Ring (NuvaRing)
- The woman inserts the vaginal ring into the vagina, where it remains continuously for 3 weeks. It is removed for 1 week, during which bleeding usually occurs (usually 2–3 days after removal).
- Insert a new ring 1 week after the last ring was removed, on the same day of the week as it was inserted in the previous cycle. Do this even if bleeding is not finished.
- *Insertion:* Position for insertion by the woman may be standing with one leg up, squatting, or lying down. Compress the ring and insert into the vagina. (The exact position of the vaginal ring inside the vagina is not critical to its effectiveness.)
- The vaginal ring is removed after 3 weeks on the same day of the week as it was started. Removal is accomplished

BOX 43.1   Alternatives to Oral Contraceptive Hormones (continued)

by hooking the index finger under the forward rim or by grasping the rim between the thumb and index finger and pulling it out. Discard the used ring in the foil pouch in a waste receptacle out of the reach of children or pets. (Do not flush the ring down the toilet.)

- Consider the menstrual cycle, timing of ovulation, and possibility of pregnancy before beginning treatment.
- The vaginal ring may be accidentally expelled (e.g., when it was not inserted properly, during straining for defecation, while removing a tampon, or with severe constipation). If this occurs, rinse the vaginal ring with lukewarm water and reinsert promptly. (If the ring has been out of the vagina for more than 3 hr, contraceptive effectiveness may be reduced and an alternative contraceptive must be used for the next 7 days.)
- The most common adverse effects leading to discontinuation of contraceptive use involve device-related problems, such as foreign body sensations, coital problems, and device expulsion.
- Other adverse effects include vaginitis, headache, upper respiratory tract infection, leukorrhea, sinusitis, weight gain, and nausea.

Levonorgestrel/Etonogestrel Implants (Norplant System/Nexplanon)

This is a long-term (5-year, 3-year for Nexplanon) reversible contraceptive system, and an informed consent may be required in some institutions before implementing this procedure. The client needs to know that a surgical incision is required to insert six capsules and that removal also requires surgical intervention.

Levonorgestrel-Releasing Intrauterine System (Mirena, Skyla)

The capsules of the levonorgestrel-releasing intrauterine system (LRIS) are inserted during the first 7 days of the menstrual cycle or immediately after a first-trimester abortion. LRIS is an intrauterine contraception device for use for not more than 5 years. Before insertion, provide the client with the client package insert. Also, before insertion, a complete medical and social history, including that of the partner, is obtained to determine conditions that might influence the use of an intrauterine device (IUD). Several client teaching points follow:

- Irregular menstrual bleeding, spotting, prolonged episodes of bleeding, and amenorrhea may occur. These symptoms diminish with continued use. The client should check after each menstrual period to ensure that the thread attached to the LRIS still protrudes from the cervix. Caution her not to pull the thread.
- If pregnancy occurs with the LRIS in place, the LRIS should be removed. If the LRIS is not removed there is an increased risk of miscarriage/abortion, sepsis, premature labor, and premature delivery.
- The client should self-monitor for flu-like symptoms, fever, chills, cramping, pain, bleeding, vaginal discharge, or leakage of fluid.
- Reexamination and evaluation are done shortly after the first menses or within the first 3 months after insertion.

- Menstrual flow usually decreases after the first 3 to 6 months of LRIS use; therefore, an increase of menstrual flow may indicate expulsion of the device.
- Symptoms of partial or complete expulsion include pain and bleeding. However, the LRIS also can be expelled without any noticeable effects.

Medroxyprogesterone Contraceptive Injection (Depo-Provera)

Medroxyprogesterone is available as a long-term injectable contraceptive administered IM every 3 months. The injection is given only during the first 5 days after the onset of a normal menstrual period, within 5 days postpartum if the woman is not breastfeeding, or at 6 weeks postpartum. Client teaching points include the following:

- Bleeding irregularities may occur (i.e., irregular or unpredictable bleeding or spotting, or heavy continuous bleeding). Bleeding usually decreases to amenorrhea as treatment continues.
- Women tend to gain weight while using this form of contraception.
- The drug is not readministered if there is a sudden partial or complete loss of vision or if the client experiences ptosis, diplopia, depression, or migraine.

Norelgestromin/Ethinyl Estradiol Transdermal System (Ortho Evra, Xulane)

- The system is designed around a 28-day cycle, with a new patch applied each week for 3 weeks. Week 4 is patch free.
- Apply the new patch on the same day each week (note patch change day on the calendar).
- Discard used patch (only wear one patch at a time).
- Use no creams or lotions on area where patch is to be applied. Apply patch to clean, dry, intact, healthy skin on the buttock, abdomen, upper outer arm, or upper torso in a place where the patch will not be rubbed by clothing. Patch should not be placed on the breast or on areas that are red or irritated.
- *Beginning treatment:* First-day start (apply first patch on the first day of the menstrual cycle) or Sunday start (apply first patch on the first Sunday after the menstrual period begins).
- A backup contraceptive should be used for the first week of the *first* treatment cycle.
- If the patch partially or completely detaches for less than 24 hr, reapply to the same place or replace with a new patch immediately (no backup contraception needed).
- If the patch detaches for more than 24 hr, apply a new patch immediately (new patch change day). Backup contraception is needed for the first week (7 days) of the new cycle.
- If the patch change is forgotten, begin again immediately, making this day the new patch change day. (Backup contraception is needed for the first 7 days.)
- If breakthrough bleeding continues longer than a few cycles, a cause other than the patch should be considered. Do not stop patch if bleeding occurs.
- Bleeding should occur during the patch-free week. If no bleeding occurs, consider the possibility of pregnancy.
- If pregnancy is confirmed, discontinue treatment.

(Continued)

If the interval is greater than 14 weeks between the IM injections of medroxyprogesterone, be certain that the client is not pregnant before administering the next injection.

Monitoring and Managing Client Needs

Altered Health Seeking Behavior

The client prescribed female hormones usually takes them for several months or years. Throughout that time, the client must be monitored for adverse reactions. These drugs are self-administered at home. Clients may decide to regulate their own drug doses to alleviate adverse reactions; this can lead to ineffective dosing and more unwanted reactions such as pregnancy. Therefore, client education is an important avenue for detecting and managing adverse reactions.

With estrogens, it is important to monitor for breakthrough bleeding. If breakthrough bleeding occurs with either estrogen or progestin, the client notifies the primary health care provider. A dosage change may be necessary.

GI upsets such as nausea, vomiting, abdominal cramps, and bloating may also occur. Nausea usually decreases or subsides within 1–2 months of therapy. However, until then the discomfort may be decreased if the drug is taken with food. If nausea is continual, frequent small meals may help. If nausea and vomiting persist, an antiemetic may be prescribed. Bloating may be alleviated with light to moderate exercise or by limiting fluid intake with meals.

Carefully monitor the client with diabetes who is taking female hormones. The primary health care provider is notified if blood glucose levels are elevated or the urine is positive for ketone bodies, because a change in the dosage of insulin or the oral antidiabetic drug may be required. See Chapter 40 for the management of hypoglycemic and hyperglycemic episodes.

Fluid Overload

Sodium and water retention may occur during female hormone therapy. In addition to reporting any swelling of the hands, ankles, or feet to the primary health care provider, weigh the hospitalized client daily, keep an accurate record of the intake and output, encourage ambulation (if not on bed rest), and help the client to eat a diet low in sodium (if prescribed by the primary health care provider).

Altered Tissue Perfusion

Teach the client how to monitor for signs of thromboembolic effects, such as pain, swelling, and tenderness in the extremities, headache, chest pain, and blurred vision. These adverse effects are reported immediately to the primary health care provider. Clients with previous venous insufficiency, who are on bed rest for other medical reasons, taking combined drug contraceptives, or who smoke are at increased risk for thromboembolic effects. Encourage the client to elevate the lower extremities when sitting, if possible, and to exercise the lower extremities by walking.

There is an increased risk of postoperative thromboembolic complications in women taking oral contraceptives. If possible, use of the drug is discontinued at least 4 weeks before a surgical procedure associated with thromboembolism or during prolonged immobilization. Women must be counseled to use another form of contraception during this time period.

Malnutrition Risk

Alterations in nutrition can occur, resulting in significant weight gain or loss. Weight gain occurs more frequently than weight loss. Encourage a daily diet that includes adequate amounts of protein and carbohydrates and is low in fats. A variety of nutritious foods (fruits, vegetables, grains, cereals, meats, and poultry) should be included in the daily diet, with portion sizes decreased to meet individual needs. A dietitian may be consulted if necessary. An exercise program is helpful in both losing weight and maintaining weight loss.

Weight loss is often as difficult to manage as weight gain. When a client taking the female hormones has a decrease in appetite and loses weight, encourage the individual to increase protein, carbohydrates, and calories in the diet. Small feedings with several daily snacks are usually better tolerated in those with a loss of appetite than are three larger meals. Clients are encouraged to eat foods they like. Dietary supplements may be necessary if a significant weight loss occurs. A dietitian may be consulted if necessary. Weights are usually taken on a weekly, rather than daily, basis.

Educating the Client and Family

The instructions for starting oral contraceptive therapy vary with the product used. Each product has detailed client instruction sheets regarding starting oral contraceptive therapy. The instructions for missed doses also are included in the package insert and are reviewed with the client. Advise those taking oral contraceptives that skipping a dose could result in pregnancy. See Box 43.1 for more information to include in a teaching plan for a woman taking contraceptive hormones. Be sure the client is confident in understanding the directions provided for contraception.

In most instances, the primary health care provider performs periodic examinations, such as laboratory analyses, a pelvic examination, or a Pap test. The client is encouraged to keep all appointments for follow-up evaluation of therapy. Include the following points in your teaching plan:

Estrogens and Progestins

- Carefully read the client package insert available with the drug. If there are any questions about this information, discuss them with the primary health care provider.

- If GI upset occurs, take the drug with food.
- Notify the primary health care provider if any of the following occurs: pain in the legs or groin area; sharp chest pain or sudden shortness of breath; lumps in the breast; sudden severe headache; dizziness or fainting; vision or speech disturbances; weakness or numbness in the arms, face, or legs; severe abdominal pain; depression; or yellowing of the skin or eyes.
- If pregnancy is suspected or abnormal vaginal bleeding occurs, stop taking the drug and contact the primary health care provider immediately.
- Client with diabetes: Check the blood glucose daily, or more often. Contact the primary health care provider if the blood glucose is elevated. An elevated blood glucose level may require a change in diabetic therapy (insulin, oral antidiabetic drug) or diet; these changes must be made by the primary health care provider.

Oral Contraceptives
- A package insert is available with the drug. Read the information carefully. Begin the first dose as directed in the package insert or as directed by the primary health care provider. If there are any questions about this information, discuss them with the primary health care provider.
- To obtain a maximum effect, take this drug as prescribed and at intervals not exceeding once every 24 hr. An oral contraceptive is best taken with a routine daily behavior, such as with the evening meal or at bedtime. The effectiveness of this drug depends on following the prescribed dosage schedule. Failure to comply with the dosage schedule may result in a pregnancy.
- Use an additional method of birth control (as recommended by the primary health care provider) until after the first week in the next cycle.
- If 1 day's dose is missed, take the missed dose as soon as remembered or take two tablets the next day. If 2 days are missed, take two tablets for the next 2 days and continue on with the normal dosing schedule. However, another form of birth control must be used until the cycle is completed and a new cycle is begun. If 3 days in a row or more are missed, discontinue use of the drug and use another form of birth control until a new cycle can begin. Before restarting the dosage regimen, make sure a pregnancy did not result from the break in the dosage regimen.
- If there are any questions regarding what to do about a missed dose, discuss the procedure with the primary health care provider.
- Avoid smoking or excessive exposure to second-hand smoke while taking these drugs; cigarette smoking during estrogen therapy may increase the risk of cardiovascular effects.

- Report adverse reactions such as fluid retention or edema to the extremities; weight gain; pain, swelling, or tenderness in the legs; blurred vision; chest pain; yellowed skin or eyes; dark urine; or abnormal vaginal bleeding.
- Remember that while taking these drugs, clients need periodic examinations by the primary health care provider and laboratory tests.

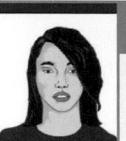

PHARMACOLOGY IN PRACTICE

SAFE DRUG ADMINISTRATION
A 30-year-old female client arrives at the health care center complaining of abnormal uterine bleeding. Diagnosis indicates endometrial hyperplasia and the client is prescribed Depo-Provera (medroxyprogesterone). Which of the following should the nurse keep in mind when administering this drug?

1. The drug is implanted in the subdermal tissue.
2. The drug is to be shaken vigorously before use.
3. First dose is given on the 10th day of a menstrual cycle.
4. The drug provides contraception for 5 years.

EVALUATION

- Therapeutic effect is achieved.
- Adverse reactions are identified, reported to the primary health care provider, and managed using appropriate nursing interventions.
  - Client manages the therapeutic regimen effectively.
  - Adequate fluid volume is maintained.
  - Tissue perfusion is maintained.
  - Client maintains an adequate nutritional status.
- Client expresses confidence and verbalizes the importance of adhering to the prescribed therapeutic regimen.

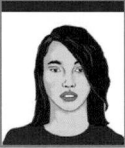

PHARMACOLOGY IN PRACTICE

USING CLINICAL REASONING
What are some assessment questions you will ask Janna about her request for birth control? Can she make this request without her mother's permission at age 16 in your community? How might you help Janna discuss the question of using birth control with her mother?

KEY POINTS

■ Secondary sex characteristics as well as human reproduction are directed by male and female hormones. Supplement of naturally occurring hormones is necessary for some conditions, in treating certain cancers, and when a deficiency occurs.

■ Testosterone and its derivatives are called androgens—or the male hormones—and are secreted by the anterior pituitary gland. These hormones promote reproductive maturation and the development of secondary sex characteristics (e.g., facial hair and deeper voice). They also promote tissue and muscle building. Anabolic steroids are synthetic drugs chemically similar to androgens.

■ Adverse reactions include gynecomastia, testicular atrophy, impotence, nausea, vomiting, and male-pattern baldness. When used to reduce female hormone production in women, menstrual issues and virilization are adverse reactions.

■ Estrogen and progesterone are the two hormones produced in the female body. Estrogen is secreted by the anterior pituitary gland and progesterone by the corpus luteum of the ovary. These hormones promote reproductive maturation and the development of secondary sex characteristics (e.g., breast development and pigmentation of areolae and genitals).

■ Estrogen is used for contraception and replacement therapy following menopause, and progestin is used for both contraception and menstrual issues.

■ Adverse reactions include headache, depressive mood, nausea, vomiting, skin discoloration, and menstrual irregularities.

SUMMARY DRUG TABLE
Male and Female Hormones

Generic Name	Trade Name	Uses	Adverse Reactions	Dosage Ranges
Androgens				
fluoxymesterone *floo-oks-i-MES-te-rone*		Males: hypogonadism, delayed puberty; Females: inoperable advanced breast cancer	Nausea, vomiting, acne, hair thinning, headache, libido changes, anxiety, mood changes, hematopoietic and electrolyte imbalances; Males: gynecomastia, testicular atrophy, erectile dysfunction; Females: amenorrhea, virilization	Males: 5–20 mg/day orally; Females: 10–40 mg/day orally
methylTESTOSTERone *meth-il-tes-TOS-te-rone*	Methitest	Same as fluoxymesterone	Same as fluoxymesterone	Males: 10–50 mg/day orally; Females: 50–200 mg/day orally
testosterone *tes-TOS-ter-one*	AndroGel, Androderm (patch), Testim, Vogelxo (Transdermal) Aveed, Delatestryl, Depo-Testosterone (injectable), Testopel (pellet insert), Axiron (axilla spray), Natesto (inhaled), Xyosted	Primary or hypogonadotropic hypogonadism, delayed puberty	Same as fluoxymesterone	Buccal: 30 mg BID; Gel: apply daily; Injectable: 50–400 mg every 2–4 weeks; Pellet: 150–450 mg subcut every 3–6 months; Transdermal: 6 mg/day, apply patch daily; Spray: 30–120 mg daily
Anabolic Steroids				
oxymetholone *oks-i-METH-oh-lone*	Anadrol-50	Anemia	Same as nandrolone	1–5 mg/kg/day orally
oxandrolone *oks-AN-droe-lone*		Bone pain, weight gain, protein catabolism	Acne, hair thinning, libido changes, anxiety, mood changes, edema, electrolyte imbalances; Males: gynecomastia, testicular atrophy, sexual dysfunction; Females: amenorrhea, virilization	2.5–20 mg/day orally in divided doses

Continued

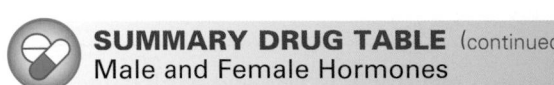

SUMMARY DRUG TABLE (continued)
Male and Female Hormones

Generic Name	Trade Name	Uses	Adverse Reactions	Dosage Ranges
Estrogens				
estrogens, conjugated *ES-troe-jenz*	Premarin	Oral: hypogonadism, primary ovarian failure. Parenteral: abnormal uterine bleeding from hormonal imbalance	Headache, dizziness, melasma, venous thromboembolism, nausea, vomiting, abdominal bloating and cramps, breakthrough bleeding/spotting, vaginal changes, rhinitis, changes in libido, breast enlargement and tenderness, weight changes, generalized pain	0.3–2.5 mg/day orally IM: 25 mg/injection
estrogens, esterified	Menest	Same as conjugated estrogens	Same as conjugated estrogens	0.3–1.25 mg/day orally
estradiol cypionate *es-tra-DYE-ole*	Depo-Estradiol	Female hypogonadism, male-to-female therapy (MTF)	Same as conjugated estrogens; pain at injection site	1–5 mg IM every 3–4 weeks
estradiol transdermal system	Alora, Climara, Divigel, Dotti, Estraderm, Menostar, Vivelle	Same as conjugated estrogens, MTF	Same as conjugated estrogens	Variable doses, applied to skin weekly
estradiol valerate *es-tra-DYE-ole*	Delestrogen	Female hypogonadism, Menopause symptoms, MTF, prostate cancer	Same as conjugated estrogens; pain at injection site	10–30 mg IM every 2–4 weeks
estropipate *ES-troe-pih-pate*		Female hypogonadism, Menopause symptoms	Same as conjugated estrogens	0.625–9 mg/day orally
Progestins				
progesterone *proe-JES-ter-one*	Crinone, Milprosa, Prometrium	Endometrial hyperplasia (oral), breast enhancement (MTF), amenorrhea, abnormal uterine bleeding (injection), infertility (gel)	Breakthrough bleeding, spotting, change in menstrual flow, amenorrhea, breast tenderness, weight gain or loss, melasma, insomnia	Orally: 200 mg for 12 days of cycle IM: 5–10 mg/day for 6–8 days Gel: 90 mg/day
medroxyPROGESTERone *me-DROKS-ee-proe-JES-te-rone*	Depo-Provera, Provera	Amenorrhea, abnormal uterine bleeding, endometrial hypoplasia	Same as progesterone	5–10 mg/day orally
norethindrone *nor-ETH-in-drone*	Aygestin	Amenorrhea, abnormal uterine bleeding, endometriosis	Same as hydroxyprogesterone caproate	2.5–10 mg/day for 5–10 days of cycle

CHAPTER REVIEW

Know Your Drugs

Clients sometimes know a medication by the brand (or trade) name and not the generic name. To help you recognize both names, match the brand name with the generic name of the same medication.

Generic Name	Brand Name
1. conjugated estrogen	A. Climara
2. medroxyprogesterone	B. Premarin
3. methyltestosterone	C. Provera
4. transdermal estradiol	D. Testred

Calculate Medication Dosages

1. Medroxyprogesterone 650 mg IM is prescribed. The drug is available in a solution of 400 mg/mL. The nurse administers _____.

2. Nandrolone 100 mg IM is prescribed. The drug is available in a solution of 100 mg/mL. The nurse administers _____.

Prepare for the NCLEX

RECALL THE FACTS

1. Which hormone is secreted by the posterior pituitary gland?
   1. Estrogen
   2. Oxytocin
   3. Progesterone
   4. Testosterone

2. The nurse monitors the client taking an anabolic steroid for adverse reactions, which is the most severe reaction?
   1. Anorexia
   2. Nausea and vomiting
   3. Severe mental changes
   4. Acne

3. The nurse must be aware that older men taking androgens are _____.
   1. prone to urinary problems
   2. at greater risk for hypertension
   3. at increased risk for confusion
   4. at increased risk for prostate cancer

4. When monitoring a client taking an oral contraceptive, the nurse would observe the client for signs of excess progestin. Which of the following reactions would indicate to the nurse that a client has an excess of progestin?
   1. Increased appetite, hair loss
   2. Virilization, constipation
   3. Nausea, early breakthrough bleeding
   4. Deepening of the voice, lightheadedness

5. When teaching the client taking an oral contraceptive for the first time, the nurse emphasizes the importance of taking _____.
   1. two tablets per day at the first sign of ovulation
   2. the drug at the same time each day
   3. the drug early in the morning before arising
   4. the drug each day for 20 days beginning on the first of the month

6. Which hormone when given to women can cause virilization?
   1. Androgen
   2. Estrogen
   3. Progesterone
   4. Thyroid

ANALYZE THE FACTS

7. A client calls the outpatient clinic and says that she missed 1 day's dose of her "birth control pills." Which of the following statements would be most appropriate for the nurse to make to the client?
   1. Do not take an additional tablet but resume the regular schedule today.
   2. Discontinue use of the drug and use another type of contraceptive until after your next menstrual period.
   3. Take two tablets today; then resume the regular daily schedule.
   4. Come into the office immediately for a pregnancy test.

8. The following statement indicates that the client understands the purpose of birth control pills:
   1. "These will protect me from STIs."
   2. "I must take one each time I have sex to prevent pregnancy."
   3. "If I miss a couple of days, I should use an additional birth control method."
   4. "I put the medicine in water and it works better."

ALTERNATE-FORMAT QUESTIONS

9. The drug YAZ is a combination of different medications. Which drugs are in this pill? **Select all that apply.**
   1. Estradiol
   2. Drospirenone
   3. Levonorgestrel
   4. Norethindrone

10. The anabolic steroids can cause which of the following unpleasant adverse reactions? **Select all that apply.**
    1. Gynecomastia
    2. Jaundice
    3. Testicular atrophy
    4. Virilization

To check your answers, see Appendix F.

WANT TO KNOW MORE? A wide variety of resources are available to enhance your learning and understanding of this chapter.

- Visit the**Point** for resources such as:
  - NCLEX-Style Student Review Questions
  - Journal Articles
  - Dosage Calculations
  - Drug Monographs
  - Watch and Learn Videos
  - Concepts in Action Animations
- The *Study Guide to Accompany Introductory Clinical Pharmacology*, 12th edition, sold separately, will help you review and apply essential content.
- ✓**PrepU** is available to help students prepare for the NCLEX-PN examination.

Uterine Drugs

Key Terms

albuminuria excessive protein in the urine

antepartum the time during pregnancy before childbirth

eclampsia a condition where seizures and possible coma happens in pregnancy after 20 weeks in a woman who has become hypertensive, with excess protein found in the urine

placenta previa during pregnancy the placenta implants in the lower part of the uterus, possibly over the cervix

preeclampsia a condition in pregnancy after 20 weeks in a woman when she becomes hypertensive, with excess protein found in the urine

tocolysis to prevent preterm labor

uterine atony marked relaxation of the uterine muscle

water intoxication fluid overload in the body when electrolytes are imbalanced

Learning Objectives

On completion of this chapter, the student will:

1. Explain the actions, uses, adverse reactions, contraindications, precautions, and interactions of drugs acting on the uterus.
2. Distinguish important preadministration and ongoing assessment activities the nurse should perform with the client taking an oxytocic or tocolytic drug.
3. List some nursing diagnoses particular to a client taking an oxytocic or tocolytic drug.
4. Examine ways to promote an optimal response to therapy, how to manage adverse reactions, and important points to keep in mind when educating clients about the use of an oxytocic or tocolytic drug.

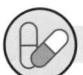 **Drug Classes**

Oxytocic drugs   Tocolytics

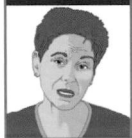 **PHARMACOLOGY IN PRACTICE**

Betty Peterson's daughter has been admitted to the obstetric unit and is being induced. This is her daughter's first child, and Betty is extremely anxious. After reading this chapter, think about the information that would be helpful to the family.

When developing a birth plan, if drugs are in it, the women typically chooses which pain medications to include. The use of medication for labor and the delivery of babies is not frequently included in the birth plans pregnant women develop with their providers. Yet, drug therapy can be beneficial for use in labor and delivery to promote the well-being of a woman and her fetus. Depending on the client's need, drugs may be used to stimulate, intensify, or inhibit uterine contractions. Two classes of drugs—oxytocics and tocolytics—and their effect on the uterus are presented in this chapter. The specific drugs acting on the uterus are listed in the Summary Drug Table: Uterine Drugs.

OXYTOCIC DRUGS

An oxytocic drug is one that stimulates the uterus. Oxytocic drugs are used in the **antepartum** (before birth of the neonate) setting to induce uterine contractions similar to those of normal labor. These drugs are

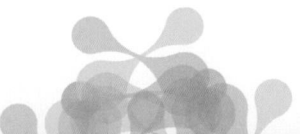

administered before vaginal delivery to initiate labor and after delivery to help contract the uterus.

ACTION AND USES

Oxytocin

Oxytocin is an endogenous hormone produced by the posterior pituitary gland (Fig. 44.1). This hormone has uterus-stimulating properties, acting on the smooth muscle of the uterus, especially when pregnant. As pregnancy progresses, the sensitivity of the uterus to oxytocin increases, reaching a peak, immediately before the birth of the infant. This sensitivity enables oxytocic drugs to exert their full therapeutic effect on the uterus and produce the desired results: stimulation of contractions. Oxytocin also has antidiuretic and vasopressor effects.

Oxytocin is administered intravenously (IV) for starting or improving labor contractions. Drugs may be used to induce an early vaginal delivery when there are fetal or maternal problems, such as a woman with diabetes and a large fetus, Rh problems, premature rupture of the membranes, uterine inertia, and **preeclampsia** (also called pregnancy-induced hypertension). Preeclampsia is a condition of pregnancy characterized by hypertension, headache, **albuminuria** (protein in the urine), and edema of the lower extremities occurring at, or near, term. The condition may progressively worsen until **eclampsia** (a serious condition occurring between the 20th week of pregnancy and the end of the first week postpartum and characterized by convulsive seizures and coma) occurs.

Oxytocin may also be used in managing inevitable or incomplete abortion. Additionally, when the birthing mother does not have parenteral access (an IV line), oxytocin can be given intramuscularly (IM) during the third stage of labor (period from the time the baby is born until the placenta is expelled) to produce uterine contractions and control postpartum bleeding and lessen hemorrhage potential (Barbieri, 2016).

Some women find that when taken intranasally, oxytocin may stimulate the milk ejection (milk letdown) reflex, and they can breastfeed more successfully. Although intranasal preparations are not commercially available, compounding pharmacies have made them for women. When the hormone prolactin (produced by the anterior pituitary) is low, another drug has been tried to increase milk supply, with variable success. Metoclopramide (Reglan) blocks the production of dopamine in the brain and increases prolactin levels with the intent of producing a greater milk supply (Bonyata, 2016).

Other Uterine Stimulants

Uterine stimulants increase the strength, duration, and frequency of uterine contractions and are used to decrease the incidence of postpartum hemorrhage (or uterine bleeding). Misoprostol used orally is becoming more popular for labor induction than oxytocin (Young, 2020). It has been found to be safer and easier to assist women during induction than oxytocin, dinoprostone, and vaginal misoprostol (Alfirevic, 2014). The issue remains that it is still considered an off-label use by the Food and Drug Administration (FDA).

Other drugs given after the delivery of the placenta and used to prevent postpartum and postabortal hemorrhage caused by **uterine atony** (marked relaxation of the uterine muscle) include methylergonovine and carboprost.

ADVERSE REACTIONS

Oxytocin

Administration of oxytocin may result in the following:
For the mother

- Nausea, vomiting, cardiac arrhythmias, anaphylactic reactions
- Uterine rupture, uterine hypertonicity

For the fetus

- Bradycardia

Oxytocin is similar to the hormone vasopressin and because of its antidiuretic effect, serious water intoxication (fluid overload, fluid volume excess) may occur, particularly when the drug is administered by continuous infusion and the client is receiving fluids by mouth.

Other Uterine Stimulants

Adverse reactions associated with other uterine stimulants include the following (to the mother):

- Nausea, vomiting, diarrhea
- Elevated blood pressure, temporary chest pain
- Dizziness, water intoxication, headache

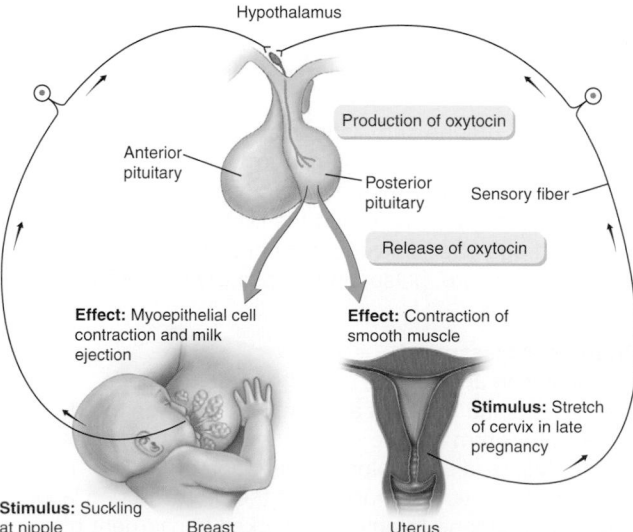

FIGURE 44.1 Regulation and effect of the hormone oxytocin. (From Premkumar, K. (2004). *The massage connection: Anatomy and physiology.* Lippincott Williams & Wilkins.)

Allergic reactions may also occur. In some instances, hypertension associated with seizure or headache may occur.

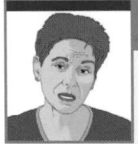

PHARMACOLOGY IN PRACTICE

SAFE DRUG ADMINISTRATION
Which of the following is an adverse effect caused by all uterine stimulants because of their antidiuretic effect?

1. Dehydration
2. Hypotension
3. Water intoxication
4. Polydipsia

CONTRAINDICATIONS, PRECAUTIONS, AND INTERACTIONS

Oxytocin is contraindicated in clients with known hypersensitivity to the drug, cephalopelvic disproportion, and unfavorable fetal position or presentation. It is also contraindicated in obstetric emergencies, situations of fetal distress when delivery is not imminent, severe preeclampsia, eclampsia, and hypertonic uterus, as well as during pregnancy when there is total placenta previa. It should not be used as an agent to induce labor when vaginal delivery is contraindicated. Oxytocin is not expected to be a risk to the fetus when administered as indicated. When oxytocin is administered with vasopressors, however, severe maternal hypertension may occur.

Misoprostol should not be prescribed where a spontaneous labor and vaginal delivery would be contraindicated, including women who have had a prior cesarean delivery or major uterine surgery. Precaution in using with clients who have cardiovascular or renal disease.

Methylergonovine and carboprost are not used before delivery of the fetus. They are contraindicated in those with known hypersensitivity to the drug or hypertension. These drugs are used cautiously in clients with heart disease, vascular disease with narrowed vessels, and renal or hepatic disease, and during lactation. When methylergonovine is administered concurrently with vasopressors or to clients who are heavy cigarette smokers, excessive vasoconstriction may occur.

LASA ALERT

The following drugs may sound alike; be sure to clarify when they are ordered:

Drug Name	Sounds Like
Cytotec	Cytoxan
Methergine	Brethine
MiSOPROStol	Metoprolol, miFEPRIStone
Prostin E2	Prostin VR (alprostadil)

Drugs that look like a similar drug are noted in the Summary Drug Tables of each chapter.

NURSING PROCESS: STEPS TO BUILDING CLINICAL JUDGMENT
Client Receiving an Oxytocic Drug

ASSESSMENT

Preadministration Assessment
Data gathering suggestions before oxytocic drugs are administered include:
Objective data

- General client appearance
- Vital signs (temperature, pulse, respirations, and blood pressure)
- Weight
- Fetal positioning and heart tones
- Uterine activity (strength, duration, and frequency of contractions)
- Support person present/available

Subjective data

- Symptoms of labor
- Obstetrical history (e.g., parity, gravidity, previous obstetric problems, type of labor, stillbirths, abortions, live-birth infant abnormalities),
- Review birth plan for induction circumstances
- General health history

When oxytocin is used, monitor uterine contractions as well as the fetus. Monitoring uterine contractions for strength and length of the contractions is done with an external monitor or by an internal uterine catheter with an electronic monitor. In addition to uterine contractions, the fetal heart rate (FHR) is also monitored. Note when internal monitoring is done, the mother is no longer able to ambulate.

The other uterine stimulants may be given orally, rectally, or IM during the postpartum period to reduce the possibility of postpartum hemorrhage and to prevent relaxation of the uterus. When the client is to receive any of these drugs after delivery, it is important to document the blood pressure, pulse, and respiratory rate before administration.

Ongoing Assessment
After injecting an oxytocic drug, both the mother's contractions and the FHR are continuously monitored. Three to four firm uterine contractions should occur every 10 min, followed by a palpable relaxation of the uterus. Be aware that hyperstimulation of the uterus during labor may lead to uterine tetany with marked impairment of the uteroplacental blood flow, uterine rupture, cervical rupture, amniotic fluid embolism, and trauma to the infant. Overstimulation of the uterus is dangerous to both the

fetus and the mother and may occur even when the drug is administered properly in a uterus that is hypersensitive to oxytocin.

NURSING ALERT

All clients receiving IV oxytocin must be under constant observation to identify complications. In addition, the health care provider attending the delivery should be immediately available at all times.

When monitoring uterine contractions, notify the health care provider attending the delivery immediately if any of the following occurs:

- A significant change in the FHR or rhythm
- A marked change in the frequency, rate, or rhythm of uterine contractions; uterine contractions lasting more than 60 seconds; or contractions occurring more frequently than every 2–3 min, or no palpable relaxation of the uterus
- A marked increase or decrease in the client's blood pressure or pulse or any significant change in the client's general condition (vital signs are typically obtained every 15–30 min in active labor)

If any of these conditions are noted, immediately discontinue the oxytocin infusion and run the primary IV line at the rate prescribed by the health care provider attending the delivery until the client is examined.

Report any signs of water intoxication or fluid overload (e.g., drowsiness, confusion, headache, listlessness, and wheezing, coughing, or rapid breathing) to the health care provider attending the delivery.

When the woman does not have parenteral access (IV line) oxytocin may be given IM after delivery of the placenta. After administering the drug, continue to take vital signs every 5–10 min. Palpate the client's uterine fundus for firmness and position. Immediately report any excess bleeding to the health care provider attending the delivery.

When administering methylergonovine IM after delivery, monitor vital signs every 4 hr and also, note the character and amount of vaginal bleeding. The client may report abdominal cramping with the administration of these drugs. If cramping is moderately severe to severe, contact the health care provider attending the delivery because it may be necessary to discontinue use of the drug.

NURSING ALERT

Although studies show rectal misoprostol does not achieve serum levels sufficient to stimulate uterine contractions, it is acceptable to use when parenteral drugs are not available to prevent postpartum hemorrhage (Barbieri, 2016).

NURSING DIAGNOSES

Drug-specific nursing diagnoses include the following:

- **Anxiety** related to fears associated with the process of labor and delivery
- **Injury Risk** (fetal) related to adverse drug effects of oxytocin on the fetus (fetal bradycardia)
- **Fluid Overload** related to administration of IV fluids and the antidiuretic effects associated with oxytocin
- **Acute Pain** related to adverse reactions (abdominal cramping, nausea, headache)

Nursing diagnoses related to drug administration are discussed in Chapter 4.

PLANNING

The expected client outcomes may include an optimal response to drug therapy (e.g., initiation of the normal labor process), adverse reactions (e.g., absence of a fluid volume excess with oxytocin administration) identified and reported to the health care provider attending the delivery, and confidence in an understanding of the medication regimen.

IMPLEMENTATION

Promoting an Optimal Response to Therapy

Misoprostol
Although misoprostol can be administered orally, vaginally, or rectally, most times it is given orally. The vaginal insert is not available in the United States, yet tablets inserted vaginally have been used. The medication is taken in the labor and delivery unit during a planned induction, when cervical ripening is indicated and birth is anticipated within 24 hr. Typically, IV access is started for fluids or later medication administration. Monitoring of the fetus and uterus should start within about 30 min and activity should begin within 30–60 min. A second dose may be given in 3–6 hr. If drug administration is switched to oxytocin, it should not be started until at least 4 hr after the last dose of misoprostol was given. Misoprostol tablets are administered rectally to induce or augment uterine contractions in the home setting when IV access is not viable.

Oxytocin
When oxytocin is prescribed, the drug typically comes in a premixed solution such as 20 units in 1000 mL of solution, and delivered as units/minute. By using premixed solutions, errors are prevented because all clients are using the same dilution in a solution. An infusion pump is used to control the infusion rate. Frequently, health care providers attending deliveries establish protocol guidelines for administering the oxytocin solution and for increasing or decreasing the flow rate or discontinuing the administration of oxytocin. The flow rate is usually increased every 20–30 min, but this may vary according to the client's response. The strength, frequency, and duration of contractions and the FHR are monitored closely.

Methylergonovine
Administer methylergonovine at the direction of the health care provider attending the delivery. Methylergonovine is usually given IM at the time of the delivery of the anterior shoulder or after the delivery of the placenta. The drug is not given routinely IV because it may produce sudden hypertension and stroke. If the drug is ordered IV,

administer it slowly over a period of 1 min or more with close monitoring of the client's blood pressure. Although you may try to explain the purpose of the drug, which is to improve the tone of the uterus and help the uterus to return to its (near) normal size, the excitement of a new baby may interfere with the mother's understanding. You may need to repeat this should she wonder about the uterine sensations.

Carboprost is administered IM, and its advantage is that it can be given to a hypertensive woman. Care should be taken that hyperstimulation of the uterus causing uterine tetany does not occur.

Monitoring and Managing Client Needs

Anxiety

When given to induce or stimulate contractions, oxytocin is administered in an IV infusion. The client receiving oxytocin may have concern over the use of the drug to produce contractions. This may be contrary to the birth plan of the mother. By explaining the purpose of the IV infusion and the expected results to the client, you can be supportive of her desires for a successful birth. Because the client receiving oxytocin must be closely supervised, use the time with the client to offer encouragement and reassurance to help reduce anxiety.

Injury Risk (Fetal)

When oxytocin is administered, some adverse reactions must be tolerated or treated symptomatically until therapy is discontinued. For example, if the client is nauseated, provide an emesis basin and perhaps a cool towel for the forehead. If vomiting occurs, provide rinsing solutions to freshen the mouth.

If contractions are frequent, prolonged, or excessive, the infusion is stopped to prevent fetal anoxia or trauma to the uterus. Excessive stimulation of the uterus can cause uterine hypertonicity and possible uterine rupture. To keep the fetus oxygenated, place the client on her left side and provide supplemental oxygen. The effects of the drug diminish rapidly, because oxytocin is a short-acting drug.

Fluid Overload

Track fluid intake and output; when oxytocin is administered IV, there is a danger of an excessive amount of systemic fluid retention (water intoxication) because of the antidiuretic effect of oxytocin. In some instances, hourly measurements of output are necessary. Observe the client for signs of fluid overload (see Chapter 54). If any of these signs or symptoms is noted, immediately discontinue the oxytocin infusion but let the primary IV line run at the rate ordered until the client is examined.

Acute Pain

When methylergonovine is administered for uterine atony and hemorrhage, abdominal cramping can occur and is usually an indication of drug effectiveness. The uterus is palpated in the lower abdomen as small, firm, and round. However, report persistent or severe cramping to the primary health care provider.

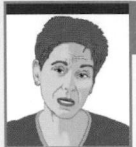

PHARMACOLOGY IN PRACTICE

MANAGING NEEDS

A client is receiving oxytocin to induce labor and is concerned about the use of the drug. Which of the following interventions should the nurse implement to help alleviate the client's anxiety? Select all that apply.

1. Explain the purpose of the IV infusion.
2. Do not inform the client of the expected outcome.
3. Administer an antianxiety drug to the client.
4. Offer encouragement and reassurance.
5. Spend time with the client.

Educating the Client and Family

The treatment regimen is explained to the client and family (when appropriate). Answer any questions the client may have regarding treatment and instruct the client to report any adverse reactions. Also inform the client and family about the therapeutic response during administration of the drug, and if nasal spray is to be used, teach the client the proper technique.

EVALUATION

- Therapeutic effect is achieved and normal labor is initiated.
- Adverse reactions are identified, reported to the primary health care provider, and managed successfully through appropriate nursing interventions:
  - Anxiety is managed successfully.
  - No evidence of injury is seen.
  - Fluid volume balance is maintained.
  - Client is free of pain.
- Client expresses confidence and demonstrates an understanding of the drug regimen.

TOCOLYTICS

Premature births make up 10% of all the births in the United States, with some states almost at 13% (March of Dimes, 2019). When a baby is born early all the organs may not be mature, especially the lungs. This is of concern because it can lead to significant problems and even death. In some developing countries, the rate of premature birth is as high as 18% (March of Dimes, 2019). In our country, minority groups also have more premature births with the highest rates seen in black and Native American populations (March of Dimes, 2019).

Preterm labor (PTL) is one of the leading causes of premature births. **Tocolysis** is a term meaning to prevent PTL. Therefore, tocolytic drugs are used to stop labor (Fig. 44.2). Although a number of studies have been done, the conclusions do not strongly support using drugs to stop PTL. Progesterone and rest are the first-line treatments. Tocolytics are indicated

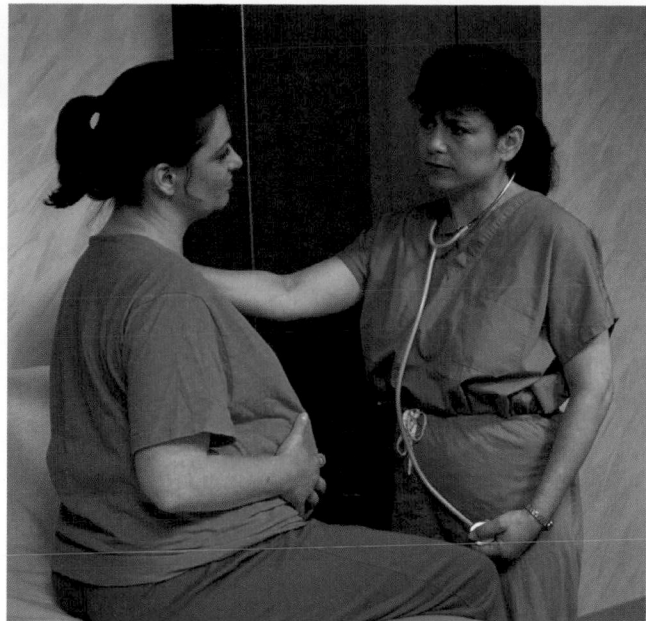

FIGURE 44.2 Tocolytic agents help stop contractions and gain time for fetal organ maturity.

when the rate of contractions is more than 6 per hour and produce cervical changes. Researchers do agree that gaining a few days for the fetus to stay in the uterus is beneficial for organ maturation (Valdes, 2012).

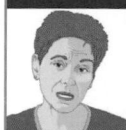

PHARMACOLOGY IN PRACTICE

PATHOPHYSIOLOGY

PTL can have severe consequences when an infant is born early. Tocolytic drugs are used to stop PTL to allow which body system in the fetus to gain maturity?

1. Heart
2. Lungs
3. Kidneys
4. Brain

ACTIONS AND USES

Tocolytics are generally used when contractions begin for a pregnancy between 24 and 33 weeks' gestation. Indomethacin and magnesium are the most commonly used tocolytics. Indomethacin is a nonsteroidal anti-inflammatory drug that blocks the production of substances called *prostaglandins* (see Chapter 14), which contribute to uterine contractions. Before the use of indomethacin, magnesium was the most commonly used drug to decrease uterine muscle contractions and is also used for seizure control with eclampsia. Magnesium is a calcium

antagonist that works to decrease the force of uterine contractions. Drugs, such as nifedipine, block the contractions of the smooth muscle of the uterus. This calcium channel blocker and the beta$_2$-adrenergic (β_2-adrenergic) drug (terbutaline) are used to delay the delivery process for 24–48 hr. This amount of time is often sufficient to allow the pregnant woman to be transferred to an acute care facility that deals with preterm deliveries or gives time to administer corticosteroids to the fetus in utero to enhance organ maturity.

ADVERSE REACTIONS

Adverse reactions include the following:
To the mother

- Fatigue, flushing, headache, dizziness, diplopia
- Nausea, vomiting, stomach upset, heartburn
- Prolonged vaginal bleeding
- Sweating, hypotension, depressed reflexes, and flaccid paralysis are other adverse reactions associated with IV administration. They are related to hypocalcemia induced by the therapy

To the fetus

- Increased heart rate
- Increased blood sugar

CONTRAINDICATIONS, PRECAUTIONS, AND INTERACTIONS

Magnesium and calcium channel blockers are contraindicated in clients with known hypersensitivity to these drugs, in clients with heart block or myocardial damage, and when the woman is within 2 hr of delivery. Terbutaline should not be used in women with heart disease, hyperthyroid, or poorly controlled diabetes. Magnesium is classified as a pregnancy category A drug, calcium channel blockers are pregnancy category C, and indomethacin is a pregnancy category B drug. Although these drugs are given for PTL, they still should be given cautiously during pregnancy.

! **NURSING ALERT**

Because of the risk of serious adverse reactions, the use of terbutaline for more than 48 hr or in the home setting is not advised. Terbutaline in oral form is not recommended for use as a tocolytic.

There is an increased effectiveness of central nervous system depressants (e.g., opioids, analgesics, and sedatives) when magnesium is administered. The effectiveness of neuromuscular blocking agents is enhanced as well. See Chapters 14 and 34, respectively, for drug interactions with indomethacin and calcium channel blockers.

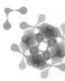

NURSING PROCESS: STEPS TO BUILDING CLINICAL JUDGMENT
Client Receiving a Tocolytic Agent

ASSESSMENT

Preadministration Assessment

Data gathering suggestions before oxytocic drugs are administered include:

Objective data

- General client appearance, respiratory assessment
- Neurological examination (mentation, cranial nerves, deep tendon reflexes—when using magnesium)
- Vital signs (temperature, pulse, respirations, and blood pressure)
- Weight
- Monitoring of uterine/fetal activity
- Results of vaginal fetal fibronectin test (protein)
- Complete blood count, creatinine level (when using magnesium)
- Liver function and amniotic fluid index (when using indomethacin)

Subjective data

- Symptoms of PTL, back pain, cramping, discharge, fluid from vagina
- Obstetrical history (e.g., PTL, preeclampsia)
- General health history, include risk factors—infections, cigarette smoking

Ongoing Assessment

During the ongoing assessment of a client receiving a tocolytic drug, nursing activities include the following at 15- to 30-min intervals:

- Obtaining blood pressure, pulse, and respiratory rate
- Monitoring FHR
- Checking the IV infusion rate
- Examining the area around the IV needle insertion site for signs of infiltration
- Monitoring uterine contractions (frequency, intensity, length)
- Measuring maternal intake and output
- Maternal reflexes (if using magnesium)

NURSING DIAGNOSES

Drug-specific nursing diagnoses include the following:

- **Anxiety** related to fears concerning PTL
- **Impaired Gas Exchange** related to pulmonary edema from drug therapy and IV fluids

  Nursing diagnoses related to drug administration are discussed in Chapter 4.

PLANNING

The expected outcomes of the client may include an optimal response to therapy, a reduction in anxiety, and confidence in an understanding of the treatment of PTL.

IMPLEMENTATION

Promoting an Optimal Response to Therapy

For IV administration, the solution is prepared according to the primary health care provider's instructions. An infusion pump is used to control the flow rate. The medication will be piggybacked to the primary line, allowing the client to maintain IV access should it become necessary to temporarily discontinue the drug infusion. In some cases, the primary health care provider may prescribe indomethacin for administration by the rectal or oral route throughout the treatment, rather than by the IV route.

Terbutaline can be given IV or subcutaneously. The drug is easy to administer using the upper arm site for subcutaneous injection. If the first 0.25 mg dose does not significantly decrease contractions, a second dose is given after 15–30 min. Other treatments are considered after an unsuccessful second dose. Some providers are attempting to deliver terbutaline via pump as a continuous subcutaneous infusion; unfortunately, the outcomes are yet to justify the expense of using this route (Kelbach, 2016).

In any case, the client is continuously monitored to recognize hypotension should it occur, at which time the client is placed in a left lateral position unless the primary health care provider orders a different position.

The primary health care provider is kept informed of the client's response to the drug, because a dosage change may be necessary. The primary health care provider establishes guidelines for the regulation of the IV infusion rate, as well as the blood pressure and pulse ranges that require stopping the IV infusion.

Monitoring and Managing Client Needs

During administration of the drug, monitor maternal and fetal vital signs every 15 min and uterine contractions frequently throughout the infusion.

Anxiety

The client in PTL may have many concerns about her pregnancy as well as the effectiveness of drug therapy. The woman is encouraged to verbalize any fears or concerns. Actively listen to the client's concerns and carefully and accurately answer any questions she may have concerning drug therapy. In addition, offer emotional support and encouragement while the drug is being administered. The presence of family members may decrease anxiety in the woman experiencing PTL; learn your institutional policy for the number of visitors that can be at the bedside.

Impaired Gas Exchange

If the mother's pulse rate increases to 140 bpm or there is persistent elevation of pulse rate, irregular pulse, or increase in respiratory rate of more than 20 respirations per minute, notify the primary health care provider. Assess the respiratory status for symptoms of pulmonary edema (e.g., dyspnea, tachycardia, increased respiratory rate, crackles, and frothy sputum). If these reactions occur, immediately notify the primary health care provider. Usually, the drug may be discontinued or the dosage decreased. After contractions cease, taper the dosage to the lowest effective dose by decreasing the drug infusion rate at regular intervals prescribed by the primary health care provider. The infusion continues for at least 12 hr after uterine contractions cease. Because treatment duration is brief, coach the client through mild adverse reactions. If adverse reactions are severe, use of the drug is discontinued or the dosage decreased.

Educating the Client and Family

Carefully and gently explain the treatment regimen to the client. Remember that anxiety about the condition of the fetus may hamper her ability to focus on your words. The primary health care provider usually discusses the expected outcome of treatment with the client and answers any questions regarding therapy. Although the client is monitored closely during therapy, the client is instructed to immediately use the call light if any of the following occurs: nausea, vomiting, palpitations, or shortness of breath.

EVALUATION

- Therapeutic drug effect is achieved and labor is stopped.
- Adverse reactions are identified, reported to the primary health care provider, and managed successfully through appropriate nursing interventions:
  - Anxiety is managed successfully.
  - Gas exchange is maintained.
- Client expresses confidence and demonstrates an understanding of the drug regimen.

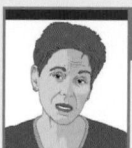

PHARMACOLOGY IN PRACTICE

USING CLINICAL REASONING

As the clinic nurse you know that Betty has some mental health issues and gets anxious about issues easily. What role might anxiety play in the birthing process? How can you explain induction while being supportive to Betty and her daughter?

KEY POINTS

■ Oxytocin is a hormone produced in the posterior pituitary gland. The hormone stimulates the smooth muscle of the uterus. In a pregnant woman, oxytocin stimulation causes uterine contractions. The hormone is used to start or induce labor in pregnant women and may be used to expel the placenta after the baby is delivered.

■ The oxytocin hormone also has antidiuretic and vasopressor effects. Adverse reactions to be aware of include water intoxication (holding water in the body because of the hormone) or high blood pressure. Use of the hormone is contra-indicated when the fetus is not in proper position or when placenta previa or other conditions exist as described.

■ If premature labor threatens a pregnancy, tocolytic drugs may be used to diminish contractions to allow for maturity of fetal organs before delivery. These drugs affect the mother in the opposite manner of the hormone oxytocin, reducing uterine contractions and possibly lowering the mother's blood pressure.

■ Both maternal and fetal vital signs should be monitored when these drugs are used.

SUMMARY DRUG TABLE
Uterine Drugs

Generic Name	Trade Name	Uses	Adverse Reactions	Dosage Ranges
Oxytocics				
carboprost *KAR-boe-prost*	Hemabate	Postpartum uterine hemorrhage, termination	Nausea, flushing	250 mcg IM may repeat in 15–90 min, not to exceed 2 mg total dose
methylergonovine *meth-il-er-goe-NOE-veen*	Methergine	Control of postpartum bleeding and hemorrhage, uterine atony	Dizziness, headache, nausea, vomiting, elevated blood pressure	0.2 mg IM, IV, orally after delivery of the placenta
mifepristone *mi-FE-pris-tone*	Mifeprex	Termination of pregnancy (adjunct to misoprostol)	Headache, nausea, cramping, diarrhea, vomiting	200 mg orally in single dose
miSOPROStol *mye-soe-PROST-ole*	Cytotec	Postpartum hemorrhage, cervical ripening	Headache, nausea, diarrhea, abdominal pain	600 mcg orally to induce, 100-mcg tablet rectally administered
oxytocin *oks-i-TOE-sin*	Pitocin	Antepartum: To initiate or improve uterine contractions Postpartum: Control of postpartum bleeding and hemorrhage	Nausea, vomiting, pelvic hematoma, postpartum bleeding, cardiac arrhythmias, anaphylactic reactions	Induction of labor: Individualize dose not to exceed 10 units/min Postpartum bleeding: IV infusion of 10–40 units in 1000-mL IV solution or 10 units IM after placenta delivery

Continued

SUMMARY DRUG TABLE (continued)
Uterine Drugs

Generic Name	Trade Name	Uses	Adverse Reactions	Dosage Ranges
Agents for Cervical Ripening				
dinoprostone *dye-noe-PROST-one*	Cervidil, Prepidil, Prostin E2	Prepare near/term cervix for labor induction	Uterine contraction, gastrointestinal (GI) effect	As directed on package insert
Tocolytics				
nifedipine *nye-FED-i-peen*	Procardia	Preterm labor	Headache, dizziness, weakness, edema, nausea, muscle cramps, cough, nasal congestion, wheezing	20 mg orally q3–8hr
indomethacin *in-doe-METH-a-sin*	Indocin	Preterm labor before 31 weeks' gestation	Headache, dizziness, nausea, vomiting, stomach upset or heartburn, prolonged vaginal bleeding	100 mg rectally, then 50 mg orally q6hr for a total of eight doses
magnesium *mag-NEE–zhum*		Preterm labor, seizure control	Fatigue, headaches, flushing, diplopia	4–6 g IV over 2 min, then infuse 1–4 g/hr
terbutaline *ter-BYOO-ta-leen*	Brethine	Preterm labor	Nervousness, restlessness, tremor, headache, anxiety, hypertension, palpitations, arrhythmias, hypokalemia, pulmonary edema	Subcut: 250 mcg; second dose in 15–30 min

CHAPTER REVIEW

Know Your Drugs

Clients sometimes know a medication by the brand (or trade) name and not the generic name. To help you recognize both names, match the brand name with the generic name of the same medication.

Generic Name	Brand Name
1. dinoprostone	A. Indocin
2. indomethacin	B. Pitocin
3. nifedipine	C. Prepidil
4. oxytocin	D. Procardia

Calculate Medication Dosages

1. Terbutaline 2.5 mg is prescribed. The drug is available in 5-mg/mL vial. The nurse administers _____.
2. Methylergonovine 0.2 mg IM is prescribed. The drug is available as 0.2 mg/mL. The nurse administers _____.

Prepare for the NCLEX

RECALL THE FACTS

1. The function of the hormone oxytocin is to stimulate
   1. Blood pressure
   2. Cardiac muscle
   3. Kidney processing
   4. Uterine smooth muscle

2. Which gland produces oxytocin?
   1. Adrenal
   2. Pituitary
   3. Thyroid
   4. Uterus

3. When oxytocin is administered over a prolonged time, which of the following adverse reactions would be most likely to occur?
   1. Hyperglycemia
   2. Renal impairment
   3. Increased intracranial pressure
   4. Water intoxication

4. What percentage of births in the United States is considered preterm?
   1. 10%
   2. 11%
   3. 45%
   4. 89%

5. Which nursing diagnosis would the nurse anticipate when administering either a uterine stimulant or tocolytic?
   1. Anxiety
   2. Impaired gas exchange
   3. Fluid overload
   4. Altered tissue perfusion

6. Magnesium is used as a tocolytic drug. What other condition is treated with this drug?
   1. Uterine atony
   2. Preeclampsia
   3. Placenta previa
   4. Eclampsia

ANALYZE THE FACTS

7. IV oxytocic and tocolytic drugs should be administered:
   1. As immediate push drugs in a syringe
   2. In a syringe pump into a heparin lock device
   3. Directly in a primary IV line
   4. Secondary or piggybacked into a primary line

8. When the client is receiving oxytocin, which of the following situations should the nurse immediately notify the health care provider attending the delivery?
   1. Uterine contractions occurring every 5–10 min
   2. Uterine contractions lasting more than 60 seconds or contractions occurring more frequently than every 2–3 min
   3. Client experiencing pain during a uterine contraction
   4. Client experiencing increased thirst

ALTERNATE-FORMAT QUESTIONS

9. *Oxytocin is prepared in a solution of 10 units in 1000 mL (0.01 units/1 mL). If the nurse is ordered to give 0.05 units of oxytocin per minute, how many milliliters would that be?

10. Name the drug and class of the nonobstetric drugs that have tocolytic properties.
    1. A drug and a class of drugs used for pain relief
    2. A drug and a class of drugs used for lowering blood pressure
    3. A drug and a class of drugs used for bronchial dilation

To check your answers, see Appendix F.

*Indicates the question is directly linked to the NCLEX-PN test plan in Appendix G.

WANT TO KNOW MORE? A wide variety of resources are available to enhance your learning and understanding of this chapter.

- Visit for thePoint resources such as:
  - NCLEX-Style Student Review Questions
  - Journal Articles
  - Dosage Calculations
  - Drug Monographs
  - Watch and Learn Videos
  - Concepts in Action Animations
- The *Study Guide to Accompany Introductory Clinical Pharmacology,* 12th edition, sold separately, will help you review and apply essential content.
- ✓*PrepU* is available to help students prepare for the NCLEX-PN examination.

UNIT 11
Drugs That Affect the Urinary System

The urinary system includes the kidneys, ureters, bladder, and urethra. This body system is responsible for the regulation and elimination of body fluids.

Each kidney contains about 1 million nephrons, which filter the blood to remove waste products. During this process, water and electrolytes are also selectively removed. It is an important body system to consider when discussing drug therapy, because it is one of the primary systems used to eliminate drugs from the body. If the system does not work properly, drugs continue to circulate in the body. This can lead to drug buildup, increased adverse reactions, or toxicity from the drug.

The focus of Chapter 45 is on issues that have an effect on both the urinary and reproductive systems as individuals age. The reproductive system (male and female reproductive organs) works in tandem with the urinary system. Although the reproductive system is not covered in detail in this unit, it plays a key role in the aging process. Issues arise as female hormones diminish and the reduction in estrogen affects many body systems. Because the uterus and vagina are interconnected structures, estrogen reduction also affects the function of the urinary system. In men, the urinary system is affected when there is enlargement of the prostate. This leads to concerns for both function and quality of relationships.

And why are aging urinary/reproductive systems of issue? It is because on January 1, 2011 (1–1–11), the first baby boomer turned 65 years of age. Furthermore, until 2031, it is estimated that 10,000 individuals will turn 65 on a *daily basis*, and as people age, their concerns about staying active and healthy increase. Keeping the urinary/reproductive organs in working order is a major part of that health concern.

The bladder is the storage area for urine before it is excreted from the body and is the focus of Chapter 46. The nature of the bladder and its contents make it susceptible to infection. In this chapter, discussion pertains to the drugs used specifically for treating urinary tract infections (UTIs) and the discomfort associated with those infections.

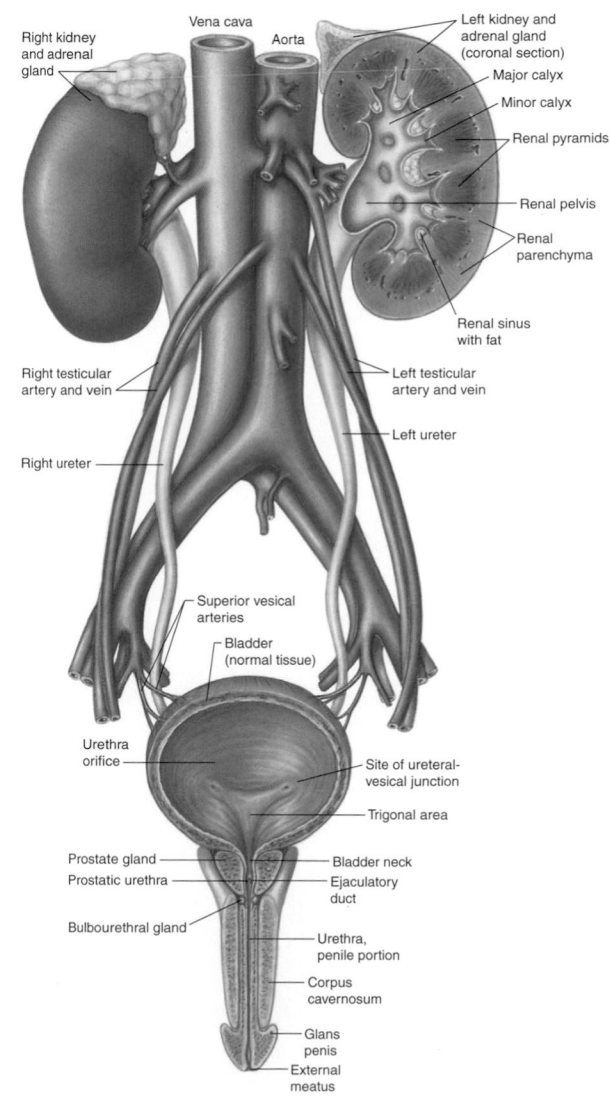

Kidneys and urinary tract

Menopause and Andropause Drugs

Key Terms

andropause   male menopause

dysuria   painful urination

menarche   age of onset of first menstruation

menopause   the cessation of menstruation; the end of monthly cycles, referring to the fertility cycle of women

neurogenic   impaired bladder function caused by a nervous system abnormality, typically an injury to the spinal cord

nocturia   voiding at night

overactive bladder (OAB)   sudden involuntary contraction of the muscular wall of the bladder

overactive bladder syndrome (OBS)   condition of urgency, frequency, and nocturia, with or without incontinence

priapism   prolonged, painful penile erection

stress incontinence   losing urine without meaning to during physical activity

urge incontinence   strong, sudden need to void because of bladder spasm or contraction

uroselective   antiadrenergic drug that is selective for alpha (α) receptors in the urinary system and not generalized

Learning Objectives

On completion of this chapter, the student will:

1. Describe changes occurring in the urinary and reproductive systems because of aging.
2. Explain the uses, general drug actions, adverse reactions, contraindications, precautions, and interactions of the drugs used to treat symptoms associated with menopause and andropause.
3. Distinguish important preadministration and ongoing assessment activities the nurse should perform with the client taking a drug for a change resulting from menopause or andropause.
4. List nursing diagnoses for a client taking a drug for a change resulting from menopause or andropause.
5. Examine ways to promote an optimal response to therapy, how to manage adverse reactions, and important points to keep in mind when educating clients about the use of drugs to treat a change resulting from menopause or andropause.

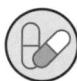 **Drug Classes**

Female hormones
- Estrogens
- Progestins

Selective Estrogen Receptor Modulators (SERMs).

Antispasmodics.

Benign prostatic hyperplasia (BPH) agents
- Alpha-adrenergic (α-adrenergic) blockers
- Androgen hormone inhibitors (AHIs)

Impotence agents.

Hormonal cancer agents.

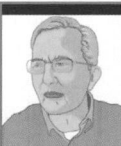

PHARMACOLOGY IN PRACTICE

Mr. Phillip, a 72-year-old widower who lives alone, was diagnosed with a urinary tract infection (UTI) 8 weeks ago. Having failed to come in for a follow-up urine sample 2 weeks after completing the course of drug therapy, he is at the clinic to see a primary health care provider because the UTI symptoms are now worse.

Aging reproductive system changes are closely related to changes in the urinary system for both men and women. Changes to a woman's reproductive system, the shared changes to the genitourinary system, and changes to the male are described in this chapter.

Menopause (the end of monthly cycles) makes changes for women very pronounced, because it is when fertility and menstrual bleeding stops. For men, the change is not as overt. Hormonal and urinary changes may be more subtle and are referred to as **andropause** (or a male form of menopause). Hormonal therapy for advanced cancer is also covered in this chapter because these drugs and treatments are often used in older individuals. The goal of drugs discussed in this chapter is to reduce symptoms related to the changes of aging reproductive and urinary tract systems.

MENOPAUSE

The female fertility cycle, which is under the influence of estrogen and progesterone, is described in Chapter 43. Estrogen is a hormone that thickens the lining of the uterus in preparation for egg implantation. Yet, these hormones serve the body in other ways, too. Estrogen helps the body process calcium to maintain bone structure, helps in keeping cholesterol levels in balance, and maintains vaginal health.

As women age, there is a complex change in estrogen and other hormones. Many of the physical changes throughout the body associated with loss of estrogen are illustrated in Figure 45.1. During menopause, estrogen and progesterone diminish and the menstrual cycle can become irregular until it stops altogether. With the onset of menopause, symptoms such as hot flashes, night sweats, vaginal dryness, painful intercourse, mood changes, and sleep problems may occur.

For many years, hormone replacement therapy (HRT) was prescribed for the treatment of menopausal symptoms and the reduction of risk for osteoporosis and heart disease. In 2002, an extensive study, the Women's Health Initiative, raised serious questions about replacement therapy benefits and risks. Many women became fearful and almost two-thirds of those using replacement therapy stopped (Shanahan, 2015).

Currently, when a woman begins to experience changes (perimenopausal), it is a good time to discuss options with her primary health care provider. Estrogen plus progestin, or what is now called HRT, may be suggested for the woman who still has her ovaries. Estrogen alone (estrogen replacement therapy [ERT]), is recommended when the woman no longer has ovaries (post complete hysterectomy). For women having moderate menopausal symptoms, replacement is recommended for no more than 5 years (Shanahan, 2015). The client should discuss the benefit of relief of symptoms (e.g., hot flashes) with negative impact on her body (e.g., blood pressure and lipid changes). Information about medications used to deal with aging and heart disease or bone changes of older women is discussed in Unit 8 and Chapter 29, respectively.

Aging specifically in the female genitourinary system includes fat atrophy and hormonal changes, which are responsible for the following:

- Vaginal walls become thinner, shorten, and lose some of their elasticity.
- The vagina produces less lubrication and at a slower rate during sexual arousal.
- The pH environment changes, making the vagina more susceptible to yeast infections.
- Pelvic floor muscles weaken and lead to stress incontinence.

Symptoms related to these changes can be reduced by replacing the lost hormones.

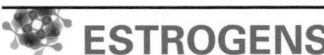 ESTROGENS

ACTIONS AND USES

In addition to contraception, estrogen is most commonly used in HRT (hormonal) or ERT in postmenopausal women. Changes to aging tissues can be lessened when estrogens are used for the following:

- Relief of moderate to severe vasomotor symptoms of menopause (flushing, sweating)
- Treatment of atrophic vaginitis
- Treatment of osteoporosis in women past menopause
- Palliative treatment of advanced prostatic carcinoma (in men)
- Selected cases of advanced breast carcinoma

The estradiol transdermal system is thought to be the most effective with the least adverse reactions. It is also used after removal of the ovaries in premenopausal women (female castration) and primary ovarian failure. Estrogen may also be given intramuscularly (IM) or intravenously (IV) to treat uterine bleeding caused by hormonal imbalance. When estrogen is used to treat menopausal symptoms in a woman with an intact uterus, concurrent use of progestin (HRT) is recommended to decrease the risk of endometrial cancer. After a hysterectomy, estrogen alone is prescribed because there is no fear of the effect on the endometrium when it has been removed.

ADVERSE REACTIONS

Administration of estrogens by any route may result in many adverse reactions, although the incidence and intensity of these reactions vary. Some of the adverse reactions seen with the administration of estrogens are as follows:

Central Nervous System Reactions
- Headache, migraine
- Dizziness, mental depression

Dermatologic Reactions
- Dermatitis, pruritus
- Chloasma (pigmentation of the skin) or melasma (discoloration of the skin), which may continue when use of the drug is discontinued

Changes Due to Menopause

Hair growth
- Thinning of scalp hair.
- Darkening or thickening of other body hair, such as facial hair.

Skin
- Loss of firmness, tension, and fluid.
- Decrease in melanocytes, which give skin pigment.
- Increased sensitivity to sun exposure.

Bone
- Becomes progressively more porous and brittle.
- Increased risk of osteoporosis.
- More subject to fractures.

Circulatory system
- Increased heart disease risk.
- Increased high–blood pressure risk.
- Increased high-cholesterol risk.

Breasts
- Less firm breasts. Glandular tissue is replaced with fat.

Reproductive system
- Few remaining follicles (egg cells) in ovaries.
- Reproductive organs decrease in size.
- Vaginal mucosa become thinner, less lubricated.
- Vaginal pH changes, increasing susceptibility to infection.
- Endometriosis disappears.

Urinary system
- Thinning of tissues in bladder and urethra.
- Increased risk of urinary tract infections.

Another health concern associated with menopause is weight gain.

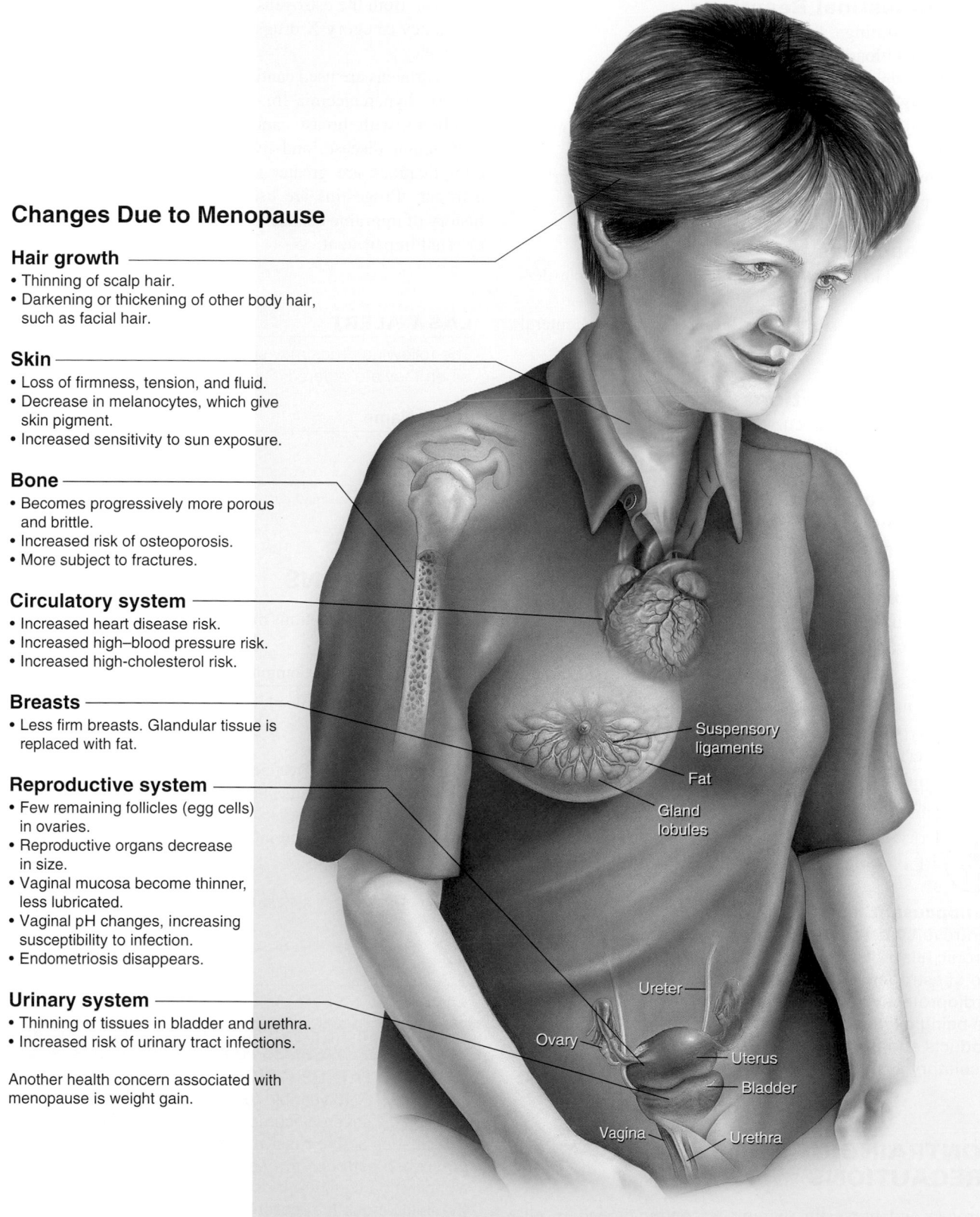

Suspensory ligaments

Fat

Gland lobules

Ureter

Ovary

Uterus

Bladder

Vagina

Urethra

FIGURE 45.1 Menopausal changes in the female body. (Asset provided by Anatomical Chart Co.)

Gastrointestinal Reactions

- Nausea, vomiting
- Abdominal bloating and cramps

Genitourinary Reactions

- Breakthrough bleeding, withdrawal bleeding, spotting, changes in menstrual flow
- Dysmenorrhea, premenstrual-like syndrome, amenorrhea
- Vaginal candidiasis, cervical erosion, vaginitis

Local Reactions

- Redness and irritation at the application site with transdermal system
- Pain at injection site or sterile abscess with parenteral form of the drug

Ophthalmic Reactions

- Steepening of corneal curvature
- Intolerance to contact lenses

Miscellaneous Reactions

- Edema, rhinitis, changes in libido
- Breast pain, enlargement, and tenderness
- Reduced carbohydrate tolerance
- Venous thromboembolism, pulmonary embolism
- Weight gain or loss
- Generalized and skeletal pain

Warnings associated with the administration of estrogen include an increased risk of endometrial cancer, gallbladder disease, hypertension, hepatic adenoma (a benign tumor of the liver), cardiovascular disease, and thromboembolic disease, and hypercalcemia in those with breast cancer and bone metastases.

 Lifespan Considerations

Menopausal Clients

Controversy persists over the increased risk for chronic heart disease and female cancers with the use of estrogen. Estrogen should not be used as a cardioprotective drug. Transdermal delivery systems are being explored to reduce the use of oral estradiol products and provide lower concentrations in the circulatory system.

CONTRAINDICATIONS AND PRECAUTIONS

Estrogen and progestin therapy is contraindicated in clients with known hypersensitivity to the drugs, breast cancer (except for metastatic disease), estrogen-dependent neoplasms, undiagnosed abnormal genital bleeding, and thromboembolic disorders. The progestins also are contraindicated in clients with cerebral hemorrhage or impaired liver function. Both the estrogens and progestins are classified as pregnancy category X drugs and are contraindicated during pregnancy.

Estrogens are used cautiously in clients with gallbladder disease, hypercalcemia (may lead to severe hypercalcemia in clients with breast cancer and bone metastasis), cardiovascular disease, and liver impairment. Cardiovascular complications are greater in women who smoke and use estrogen. Progestins are used cautiously in clients with a history of migraine headaches, epilepsy, asthma, and cardiac or renal impairment.

LASA ALERT

The following drugs may sound alike; be sure to clarify when they are ordered:

Drug Name	Sounds Like
Premarin	Primaxin, Provera, Remeron

Drugs that look like a similar drug are noted in the Summary Drug Tables of each chapter.

INTERACTIONS

The following interactions may occur with female hormones:

Interacting Drug	Common Use	Effect of Interaction
Oral anticoagulants	Blood thinners	Decreased anticoagulant effect
Tricyclic antidepressants	Treatment of depression	Increased effectiveness of antidepressant
Rifampin	Anti-infective	Increased risk of breakthrough bleeding
Hydantoins	Seizure control	Increased risk of breakthrough bleeding and pregnancy

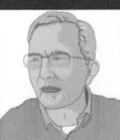 **PHARMACOLOGY IN PRACTICE**

PATHOPHYSIOLOGY

A 46-year-old female client complains of severe vasomotor symptoms of menopause (hot flushes and excessive sweating). The client is prescribed estrogen to treat menopausal symptoms along with a concurrent use of progestins. Which of the following is the reason for the concurrent use of progestins?
1. Reduce GI irritation caused by estrogen
2. Treat associated atrophic vaginitis
3. Reduce risk of endometrial carcinoma
4. Decrease risk of postmenopausal osteoporosis

Herbal Considerations

Black cohosh, an herb reported to be beneficial in managing symptoms of menopause, is generally regarded as safe when used as directed. Black cohosh is a member of the buttercup family. Black cohosh tea is not considered as effective as other forms. Boiling the root releases only a portion of the therapeutic constituents. The benefits of black cohosh (not to be confused with blue cohosh) include:

- Reduction in physical symptoms of menopause: hot flashes, night sweats, headaches, heart palpitations, dizziness, vaginal atrophy, and tinnitus (ringing in the ears).
- Decrease in psychological symptoms of menopause: insomnia, nervousness, irritability, and depression.
- Improvement in menstrual cycle regularity by balancing the hormones and reducing uterine spasms.

Adverse reactions are rare; the most common adverse reaction is nausea. Black cohosh is contraindicated during pregnancy. Toxic effects include dizziness, headache, nausea, impaired vision, and vomiting. This herb is nonhormonal and is an alternative for women with breast cancer. In addition to its popularity as an herb for women's hormonal balance, black cohosh has been used for muscular and arthritic pain, headache, and eyestrain (DerMarderosian & Beutler, 2003). Other herbs used to relieve menopausal symptoms include sage, dandelion, evening primrose oil, and calendula.

SELECTIVE ESTROGEN RECEPTOR MODULATORS

SERM drugs are proving to be a possible alternative to hormonal treatment for postmenopausal symptoms (Pinkerton & Thomas, 2014). SERM drugs act at estrogen receptor sites throughout the body. The first drug, clomiphene, is still used to stimulate ovulation. In attempts to create a new contraceptive, tamoxifen (a cancer agent), was discovered. Likewise, raloxifene developed unsuccessfully for breast cancer treatment, was found to prevent and treat postmenopausal osteoporosis (Maximov et al., 2013).

ACTIONS AND USES

Because of their selectiveness, these drugs may potentiate or block estrogen effects in different tissues. SERMs used in aging women include those for vaginal atrophy, osteoporosis prevention, and breast cancer treatment. Tamoxifen and toremifene are also used to treat breast cancer. Raloxifene works in the bone at the estrogen receptor, and decreases resorption and increases mineral density. Ospemifene is used to treat painful intercourse caused by vaginal atrophy.

ADVERSE REACTIONS

Common adverse reactions include hot flashes and vaginal discharge. Some women experience muscle spasms and excessive sweating. A greater risk of developing endometrial cancer may occur when using estrogen-based drugs together with a SERM.

Lifespan Considerations

Menopausal Women
There is an increased risk of deep vein thrombosis, stroke, and/or MI in women using SERM therapy. Discontinue immediately and seek medical assistance for any signs or symptoms of these disorders.

CONTRAINDICATIONS, PRECAUTIONS, AND INTERACTIONS

Ospemifene should not be used by women diagnosed with breast cancer or hepatic disease. It also should not be used with estrogens, estrogen antagonists, fluconazole, or rifampin. Raloxifene decreases the effectiveness of both warfarin and cholestyramine. Women taking raloxifene and having a procedure where prolonged bed rest is anticipated should discontinue the drug 72 hours prior to that procedure. These drugs are not to be used by pregnant women.

LASA ALERT

The following drugs may sound alike; be sure to clarify when they are ordered:

Drug Name	Sounds Like
Evista	AVINza, Eovist
raloxifene	ospemifene, toremifene

Drugs that look like a similar drug are noted in the Summary Drug Tables of each chapter.

Lifespan Considerations

Menopausal Cancer Survivors
Inadequate counseling for sexual dysfunction after cancer treatment is reported by almost 71% of female cancer survivors. One study using topical lidocaine compresses prior to sexual intercourse, found that 85% of the women resumed sexual relations. Coincidentally, none of the male partners reported penile numbness (Goetsch et al., 2015). This may be a good option for women who are not able to take hormonal drugs during menopause.

URINARY AGING

As a person's age increases, so do the number of urinary system disorders. All parts of the urinary system are affected by aging.

Changes in kidney size and blood flow to the kidney reduce renal function by almost 50% in older individuals. These changes decrease the filtration and the urine becomes more dilute. Diuretics (Chapter 32) are used to maintain function in the kidney as well as to reduce fluid in the body for hypertension control.

The urinary bladder diminishes in strength, flexibility, and capacity resulting in frequent urination, especially at night (**nocturia**). The urethra shortens and its lining becomes thinner, increasing susceptibility to infection. In addition to the effects of childbirth and loss of muscle tone in pelvic structures, the urinary sphincter becomes less flexible and is less able to close tightly, resulting in urine leakage (**stress incontinence**). This type of incontinence is typically treated with surgical or behavioral interventions.

Another continence issue can occur when the sensation of having to urinate is not as strong and may not be felt until the bladder is completely full. Then the need to void is sudden and urgent and there may be a loss of urine (**urge incontinence**). When bladder training exercises are not successful in relieving problems, urge incontinence can be treated with drugs called antispasmodics. **Overactive bladder syndrome** (or involuntary contractions of the detrusor or bladder muscle) also presents with urinary urgency. **Overactive bladder (OAB)** is estimated to affect more than 33 million individuals in the United States (AUA, 2020). This problem sometimes results from such disorders as cystitis or prostatitis or from abnormalities related to affected structures, such as the kidney or the urethra. Symptoms of an OAB include urinary urgency (a strong and sudden desire to urinate), frequent urination throughout the day and night, and urge incontinence. Another urinary issue in men involves an enlarged prostate, which can eventually interfere with urination. The enlarged prostate compresses the urethra, reducing the flow of urine from the bladder. This also makes men more susceptible to UTIs.

 # ANTISPASMODICS

ACTIONS AND USES

Antispasmodics are cholinergic blocking drugs that inhibit bladder contractions and delay the urge to void. These drugs counteract the smooth muscle spasm of the urinary tract by relaxing the detrusor and other muscles through action at the parasympathetic nerve receptors (see Chapter 26). Flavoxate is used primarily in men to relieve symptoms of dysuria (painful or difficult urination), urinary urgency, nocturia (excessive urination during the night), suprapubic pain and frequency, and urge incontinence. Mirabegron (Myrbetriq) is a beta$_3$-adrenergic (β_3-adrenergic) receptor agonist, which relaxes the smooth muscle as the bladder fills with urine. This action allows the bladder to hold a greater amount of urine. The other antispasmodic drugs are also used to treat bladder instability (i.e., urgency, frequency, leakage, incontinence, and painful or difficult urination) caused by a **neurogenic bladder** (impaired bladder function caused by a nervous system abnormality, typically an injury to the spinal cord).

ADVERSE REACTIONS

Adverse reactions to these drugs are similar to those with other cholinergic blocking drugs. They include the following:

- Dry mouth, drowsiness, constipation or diarrhea, decreased production of tears, decreased sweating, gastrointestinal (GI) disturbances, dim vision, and urinary hesitancy
- Nausea and vomiting, nervousness, vertigo, headache, rash, and mental confusion (particularly in older adults)

When reviewing adverse reactions with a client, it is important to know that before a drug is eliminated consider extended-release (ER) formulas. These drugs release less drug all at one time in the system, as a result, uncomfortable adverse reactions associated with cholinergic blockers are reduced. Clients should be told that antispasmodic drugs can discolor the urine (dark orange to brown) and stain undergarments that come in contact with the urine.

CONTRAINDICATIONS AND PRECAUTIONS

Antispasmodic drugs are contraindicated in those clients with known hypersensitivity to the drugs or with glaucoma. Other clients for whom antispasmodics are contraindicated are those with intestinal or gastric blockage, abdominal bleeding, myasthenia gravis, or urinary tract blockage.

These drugs should be used with caution in clients with GI infections, benign prostatic hypertrophy (BPH), urinary retention, hyperthyroidism, hepatic or renal disease, and hypertension. Antispasmodic drugs are classified as pregnancy category C drugs and are used only when the benefit to the woman outweighs the risk to the fetus.

LASA ALERT

The following drugs may sound alike; be sure to clarify when they are ordered:

Drug Name	Sounds Like
Detrol	Ditropan
Ditropan	Detrol, diazepam, Diprivan, dithranol
Enablex	Effexor XR
flavoxATE	fluvoxaMINE
oxybutynin	OxyCONTIN
tolterodine	fesoterodine, tolcapone
VESIcare	Vesanoid, Vessel Care

Drugs that look like a similar drug are noted in the Summary Drug Tables of each chapter.

INTERACTIONS

The following interactions may occur when an antispasmodic drug is administered with another agent:

Interacting Drug	Common Use	Effect of Interaction
Antibiotics/ antifungals	Fight infection	Decreased effectiveness of anti-infective drug
Meperidine, flurazepam, phenothiazines	Preoperative sedation	Increased effect of the antispasmodic
Tricyclic antidepressants	Management of depression	Increased effect of the antispasmodic
Haloperidol (Haldol)	Antianxiety/ antipsychotic agent	Decreased effectiveness of the antipsychotic drug
Digoxin	Management of cardiac problems	Increased serum levels of digoxin

ANDROPAUSE

Unlike women, men do not go through a major change in fertility like women as they experience menopause. Instead, changes occur gradually and are called andropause or the *male climacteric.* Aging changes in the male reproductive system occur primarily in the testes. Like the ovary, testicular tissue diminishes; what is different between the sexes is that the male sex hormone levels (of testosterone) remain relatively constant.

The change men often notice is prostate enlargement. The prostate gland is about the size of a walnut, it sits below the bladder, and wraps around the urethra. Scar tissue replaces prostate cells and causes the enlargement (Fig. 45.2). Fifty percent of men will experience BPH as they age. BPH may cause difficulty in urination, retention of urine, and incontinence. Prostate gland infections or inflammation (prostatitis) may also occur. The risk of prostate cancer is no greater in men with BPH. Although symptoms may be similar, prostate cancer is caused by a change in the prostate cells (see Chapter 50). Treatment for BPH is aimed at relieving symptoms and improving urinary flow.

⊘ NURSING ALERT

Early-stage prostate cancer may not have specific signs or symptoms. When men present with issues such as difficulty with urination, reduced flow, or blood in the urine, prostate cancer should always be ruled out before treatment for BPH is started.

DRUGS TO TREAT BPH

Treatment for BPH includes monitoring, medications, or invasive procedures. Drugs are used for mild to moderate symptoms of BPH (e.g., frequency, reduced flow, nocturia, and dysuria) and include androgen inhibitors and adrenergic blockers.

BENIGN PROSTATIC HYPERPLASIA

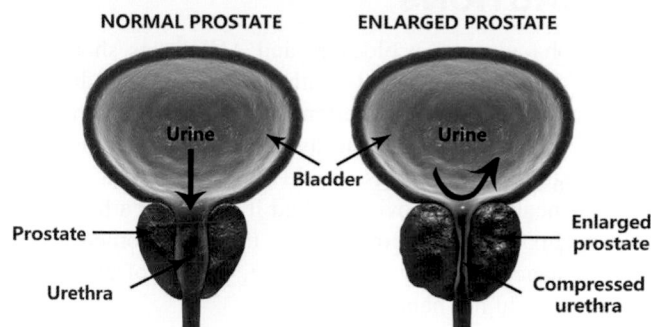

FIGURE 45.2 Enlarged prostate and narrowing of urethra result in reduced urinary flow.

ACTIONS AND USES

The most widely used drugs to treat BPH are the alpha-adrenergic (α-adrenergic) blockers. As discussed in Chapter 24, adrenergic blockers prevent the neurotransmission of norepinephrine. The drugs used for BPH are peripherally acting, alpha$_{1a}$-adrenergic (α$_{1a}$-adrenergic) blockers that exert their action primarily on the smooth muscle of the prostate and the bladder neck. By blocking norepinephrine, the muscles relax and this allows urine to flow from the bladder. Adrenergic blockers can be **uroselective**, meaning the alpha$_{1a}$-adrenergic blockers exert their action on the bladder with minimal action on the vascular system.

Androgen hormone inhibitors have been used for many years to deal with symptoms of BPH. The biggest drawback has been the adverse effects of erectile dysfunction (ED) and decreased libido. The AHIs prevent the conversion of testosterone into the androgen 5α-dihydrotestosterone (DHT). The growth of the prostate gland depends on DHT. The lowering of serum levels of DHT reduces the effect of this hormone on the prostate gland, resulting in a decrease in the size of the gland and the symptoms associated with prostatic gland enlargement.

The use of both types of drugs is proving successful based on the different sites of action of the drugs (Dhingra & Bhagwat, 2011). There is one drug on the market that combines an alpha$_{1a}$-adrenergic blocker with an AHI—Jalyn, a combination of dutasteride and tamsulosin.

ADVERSE REACTIONS

Adverse reactions usually are mild and do not require discontinuing use of the drug. Some of the adverse reactions seen with the administration of alpha-adrenergic blockers are as follows: weight gain, fatigue, dizziness, and transient orthostatic hypotension. Adverse reactions of the AHI drugs, when they occur, are related to the sexual drive and include impotence, decreased libido, and a decreased volume of ejaculation. Changes to breast tissue—pain or tenderness, nipple discharge, or enlargement—can occur while taking AHIs.

CONTRAINDICATIONS AND PRECAUTIONS

Both alpha-adrenergic blockers and AHI drugs should be used with caution in clients with hepatic or renal disease. Caution the client with hypertension when using both beta- and alpha (α)-blockers that hypotensive symptoms may be increased. These drugs should be discontinued and the primary health care provider called if angina or a heart-like pain occurs. Although not typically taken by women, AHIs are pregnancy category X. Therefore, women of childbearing age should not handle the drug.

PRACTICE CONSIDERATIONS

Dutasteride may pass in the blood; therefore, men should not donate blood while taking the drug and up to 6 months after discontinuing the drug. This is to prevent the possibility of a pregnant woman receiving the drug in a transfusion.

LASA ALERT

The following drugs may sound alike; be sure to clarify when they are ordered:

Drug Name	Sounds Like
Cardura	Cardene, Cordarone, Cordran, Coumadin, K-Dur, Ridaura
doxazosin	doxapram, doxepin, DOXOrubicin
finasteride	dutasteride, furosemide
Flomax	Flonase, Flovent, Foltx, Fosamax
Proscar	Prograf, ProSom, Provera, PROzac
Rapaflo	Rapamune
silodosin	sildenafil, sirolimus
tamsulosin	tacrolimus, tamoxifen, terazosin

Drugs that look like a similar drug are noted in the Summary Drug Tables of each chapter.

INTERACTIONS

The following interactions may occur when an alpha-adrenergic blocking drug is administered with another agent:

Interacting Drug	Common Use	Effect of Interaction
Antibiotics/ antifungals	Fight infection	Decreased effectiveness of anti-infective drug
Beta-blockers	Hypertension	Increased hypotension
Phosphodiesterase type 5 (PDE5) inhibitors	ED	Increased hypotension

Saw palmetto is used to relieve the symptoms of BPH (urinary frequency, decreased flow of urine, and nocturia). The herb is believed to reduce inflammation and the hormone DHT (responsible for prostate enlargement). Saw palmetto does not cause impotence, yet it can aggravate GI disorders such as peptic ulcer disease. Men report reduction in urinary symptoms in 1–3 months when 160 mg twice daily is taken. It is not recommended as a tea, because the active constituents are not water-soluble. It is usually recommended that the herb be taken for 6 months, followed by evaluation by a primary health care provider (Bent et al., 2006).

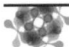 # DRUGS TO TREAT ED

In addition to slowed urination, BPH causes problems with ejaculation or the ability to have an erection. ED may be a concern for aging men. It is normal for erections to occur less frequently as men age. The ability to experience repeated ejaculation is reduced. However, ED is most often the result of a medical (90%) or psychological (10%) problem rather than simple aging. Medications (especially anti-hypertensive and antidepressants) can cause the inability to develop or maintain an erection. Disorders such as diabetes can also cause ED. ED that is caused by medications or illness is oftentimes successfully treated using drug therapy.

ACTIONS AND USES

Sexual stimulation causes a series of steps where chemicals are released and the smooth muscles of the penis (corpus cavernosum) become engorged with blood. ED results from a failure of the penis to become engorged, preventing sexual intercourse. PDE5 inhibitors are oral drugs that facilitate the enzyme that allows blood flow into the penis, resulting in an erection. Tadalafil (Cialis brand only) is also approved for daily use because it also relieves urinary difficulties resulting from an enlarged prostate.

Because the PDE5 inhibitors have vasodilating properties, both sildenafil (Revatio) and tadalafil (Adcirca) are used to treat pulmonary arterial hypertension (PAH) because they can relax smooth muscle in the pulmonary circulation and in return reduce pressure in the vessels. Different configurations of the drug are used, as is noted by the different brand name for the PAH agents compared to the names of the ED products. To better understand PAH, see Chapter 35.

ADVERSE REACTIONS, CONTRAINDICATIONS, AND PRECAUTIONS

The most common adverse reactions include headache, flushing, GI upset, nausea, and runny nose or congestion. Drugs for ED should not be taken by men who use nitrates (e.g., for anginal pain), because these drugs affect smooth muscle. Clients with preexisting cardiac problems, especially those using drugs to lower blood pressure, should discuss use with their primary health care provider before using the drug. Doses should be reduced in men with renal or hepatic impairment. Medical attention should be sought for erections sustained for more than 4 hours. Ocular problems may occur when using these drugs; again, the primary health care provider should be consulted before use.

LASA ALERT

The following drugs may sound alike; be sure to clarify when they are ordered:

Drug Name	Sounds Like
avanafil	sildenafil, tadalafil, vardenafil
Levitra	Kaletra, Lexiva
Revatio	ReVia, Revonto
sildenafil	Silodosin
Viagra	Allegra, Vaniqa

Drugs that look like a similar drug are noted in the Summary Drug Tables of each chapter.

INTERACTIONS

The following interactions may occur when a PDE5 inhibitor is administered with another agent:

Interacting Drug	Common Use	Effect of Interaction
Antiretrovirals	Viral infection	Increased effectiveness of ED drug
Antihypertensives	Reduce blood pressure	Increased effectiveness of antihypertensive

Both sildenafil and vardenafil work best when not taken immediately after food. There is no known food interaction with tadalafil or avanafil.

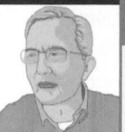

PHARMACOLOGY IN PRACTICE

MANAGING NEEDS

A nurse is caring for a male client who has been prescribed an ED medication. Which of the following is an adverse reaction of ED drugs?
1. Anginal pain
2. Gynecomastia
3. Headache
4. Frequent urination

HORMONES FOR CANCER TREATMENT

Hormones may be used in cancer therapy especially for advanced disease. Not to be confused with HRT used for aging conditions, anticancer hormones are used to block hormones or the actions which fuel cancer tumor growth.

Receptors for specific hormones needed for cell growth are found on the surface of some tumor cells. By stopping the production of a hormone, blocking hormone receptors, or substituting a drug for the actual hormone, cancer cells can be killed or their growth slowed. These drugs also appear to counteract the effect of male or female hormones in hormone-dependent tumors. Hormones are not used as curative drugs in cancer treatment; rather, they have an adjuvant, oftentimes, palliative role because of their ability to slow or reverse tumor growth.

Breast cancer is largely hormone-dependent. Almost 70% of all breast cancers are estrogen receptor-positive in postmenopausal women and 60% of the premenopausal breast cancers (ACS, 2020). Drugs used include aromatase inhibitors, progestins, and antiestrogens with the goal to decrease the amounts of estrogen and progestin feeding the tumor. Because these block hormones, reactions as noted with menopause may occur.

Gonadotropin-releasing hormone analogs, such as goserelin (Zoladex), appear to act by inhibiting the anterior pituitary secretion of gonadotropins, thus suppressing the release of pituitary gonadotropins. These drugs are used to treat breast, endometrial and prostate cancers.

Although slowing prostate tumor growth in early-stage disease may occur, over time the tumor cells become sensitized and antiandrogen drugs become less effective. One drug on the market, sipuleucel-T (Provenge), uses a man's own cells to sensitize the drug to target the prostate cancer cells. This requires taking white blood cells from the client, preparing the drug, then infusing the drug solution back into the client. For a listing of names, categories, and typical adverse reactions see the Summary Drug Table: Aging Urinary and Reproductive Drugs, Hormonal Therapy for Cancer.

LASA ALERT

The following drugs may sound alike; be sure to clarify when they are ordered:

Drug Name	Sounds Like
abiraterone	Apalutamide
anastrozole	anagrelide, letrozole
Arimidex	Aromasin
bicalutamide	apalutamide, enzalutamide, flutamide, nilutamide
degarelix	cetrorelix, ganirelix
estramustine	enzalutamide, exemestane
Femara	Famvir, femhrt, Provera
letrozole	Anastrozole
medroxyPROGESTERone	HYDROXYprogesterone caproate, methylPREDNISolone, methylTESTOSTERone
Provera	Covera, Femara, Parlodel, Premarin, Proscar, PROzac
tamoxifen	pentoxifylline, raloxifene, Tambocor, tamsulosin, temazepam, toremifene
toremifene	ospemifene, raloxifene
Zytiga	Jevtana, Xgeva, Xofigo, Xtandi, Zometa, Zydelig

Drugs that look like a similar drug are noted in the Summary Drug Tables of each chapter.

NURSING PROCESS—STEPS TO BUILDING CLINICAL JUDGMENT
Client Receiving an Aging Urinary or Reproductive Drug

ASSESSMENT

Preadministration Assessment

Many clients seeking treatment for urinary or reproductive issues related to aging will be seen as an outpatient or as a resident in a long-term care facility. For some providers it may be embarrassing to ask questions about urinary problems or sexual history. Because these are topics infrequently discussed, the provider should remember that it is also probably difficult for the client to bring these issues to the provider's attention.

Data gathering suggestions before the initial administration of a drug for aging urinary/reproductive issues include:

Objective data

- Description of OAB/incontinence issues
- Description of the urine—color, odor, concentration, or lack of clarity
- Use of protective pads/undergarments, number of changes per day
- Vital signs (temperature, pulse, respirations, and blood pressure)
- Dipstick testing for infection, blood or protein
- Residual urine measurement if indicated
- Renal and hepatic function tests, complete blood count, and urinalysis if client has impaired function in any of these body systems

Subjective data

- Sexual health history
- For women: Menstrual history, which includes the **menarche** (age of onset of first menstruation), menstrual pattern, and any changes in the menstrual pattern (including a menopause history when applicable)
- For men: Symptoms of BPH (frequency of voiding during the day and night and difficulty starting the urinary stream)
- Medical/treatment history, thrombophlebitis, smoking for HRT
- Allergy history, particularly a drug allergy

(see Fig. 45.3).

Ongoing Assessment

At the time of each office or clinic visit, the blood pressure, pulse, respiratory rate, and weight are checked. Ask the client about any adverse drug effects, as well as the result of drug therapy. For example, if the client is receiving estrogen for the symptoms of menopause, ask her to compare her original symptoms with the symptoms she is currently experiencing, if any. You may want to ask about any breakthrough bleeding or adverse reactions such as weight gain or leg pain (thromboembolism). When antispasmodics are prescribed, monitor the client for a reduction in the symptoms identified in the preadministration assessment, such as dysuria, urinary frequency, urgency, or nocturia. Ask about the relief of any pain associated with irritation of the lower genitourinary tract. For men being treated for BPH, inquire about

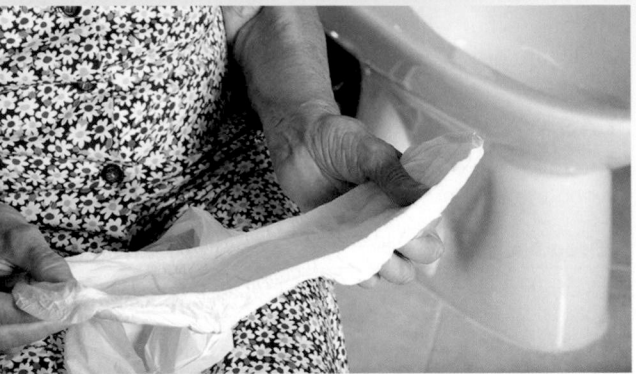

FIGURE 45.3 Clients may use pads or protective clothing for a considerable time period before seeking help. Supportive, active listening will help the client express feelings related to the loss of bodily functions.

changes in urinary flow patterns or if an ED medication has provided satisfactory results.

NURSING DIAGNOSES

Drug-specific nursing diagnoses include the following:

- **Knowledge deficiency** related to diagnosis, use of E(H)RT, or other factors
- **Impaired oral mucous membranes** related to dry mouth from anticholinergic
- **Injury risk** related to drowsiness, dizziness, or hypotension
- **Acute pain** related to priapism

Nursing diagnoses related to drug administration are discussed in Chapter 4.

PLANNING

The expected outcomes for the client may include an optimal response to drug therapy, support of client needs related to the management of adverse reactions, and confidence in an understanding of the medication regimen.

IMPLEMENTATION

Promoting an Optimal Response to Therapy

Estrogens maybe administered orally, IM, IV, transdermally, or intravaginally. Outpatient use as a hormone supplement is typically self-administered orally. The transdermal delivery route has been found to be safer, especially for women with elevated triglycerides, type 2 diabetes, hypertension, or migraine headaches, or those who smoke. When estrogens are given vaginally for atrophic vaginitis, the nurse gives the client instructions on proper use.

❗ NURSING ALERT

Women who are pregnant or may become pregnant should not handle crushed or broken finasteride (Propecia, Proscar) or dutasteride (Avodart) tablets or capsules. Absorption of the drug poses substantial risk for abnormal growth to a male fetus.

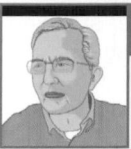

PHARMACOLOGY IN PRACTICE

SAFE DRUG ADMINISTRATION
Which of the following medications should not be touched by pregnant women?
1. Silodosin
2. Oxybutynin
3. Flavoxate
4. Dutasteride

Monitoring and Managing Client Needs

Knowledge Deficiency

The woman taking female hormones may have many concerns about therapy with these drugs. Some concerns may be based on inaccurate knowledge, such as incorrect facts about certain dangers associated with female hormones. Although there are dangers associated with long-term use of female hormones, these adverse reactions occur in a small number of clients. When the client is closely monitored by the primary health care provider, the dangers associated with long-term use are often minimized.

Some women may be anxious because of a fear of experiencing uterine cancer as the result of HRT. You may explain that taking progestin, which counteracts the negative effect of estrogen, can prevent estrogen-induced cancer of the uterus. Other women may fear the development of breast cancer or heart disease. Most research studies find that there is little risk for breast cancer developing and that the benefits of HRT often outweigh the risk of breast cancer. Studies questioned the effectiveness of HRT for postmenopausal women and the increased risk of cardiovascular disease. Newer studies demonstrate that lower doses orally or transdermally help reduce bone fractures in postmenopausal women. Encourage the client to ask questions about her therapy. Inaccurate information is clarified before starting therapy. Refer questions that cannot or should not be answered by a nurse to the primary health care provider.

The male client with advanced prostatic carcinoma also may have concerns about taking a female hormone. Assure the client that the dosage is carefully regulated and that feminizing effects, if they occur, will be dealt with by the provider.

Impaired Mucous Membranes

A common adverse reaction to antispasmodics (cholinergic blocking drugs) includes dry mouth. You may suggest that the client not only suck on hard candy, sugarless lozenges, or small pieces of ice but also perform frequent mouth care. Sometimes clients may think if they reduce fluid intake that will reduce urination and urinary issues. Be sure to instruct clients in ways to maintain fluid intake and that reducing fluids will actually make urinary problems worse. Tell clients that by increasing oral fluids this will minimize the chance of also becoming constipated. Should the client become constipated, again encourage fluids, a high-fiber diet, and fruits and vegetables with high water content, such as watermelon, strawberries, or spinach.

Injury Risk

Should a client be prescribed adrenergic blocking drugs for BPH, instruct the client on his chance of injury caused by a hypotensive reaction. A client may experience immediate lowering of his blood pressure, termed "first-dose orthostatic hypotension," when first starting these drugs. When starting the medication, the client may become dizzy during the first 60–90 minutes after taking the drug. Instruct the client to take the drug at bedtime or when less activity is anticipated. The important issue is to take the medication at about the same time each day. This reaction can also happen if the drug is stopped and started a week or more later.

Acute Pain

An uncommon but potentially serious adverse reaction of the ED drugs is **priapism** (an erection lasting more than 4–6 hours). This can be very painful and if not treated within a few hours, priapism can result in tissue damage and possible permanent impotence. Those more prone to priapism include clients with sickle cell anemia, multiple myeloma, leukemia, or an anatomic deformity of the penis. Because this can be an embarrassing adverse reaction, the client may be reluctant to seek medical attention. Acknowledge the discomfort of discussing this situation and provide instruction for self-management to empower the client.

The antidote for an erection lasting for more than 2 hours is pseudoephedrine (Sudafed) 120 mg orally, immediate-release tablets only. Men should be instructed to have this medication on hand while using drugs for ED and proper administration when priapism occurs. Health care providers should be contacted when an erection lasts for 3 hours or the pseudoephedrine does not work after 1 hour.

When a client with priapism seeks care, injection of alpha-adrenergic stimulants (e.g., phenylephrine or norepinephrine) may be helpful in treating priapism once the engorgement is drained. In some cases, surgical intervention may be required.

Educating the Client and Family

When educating the client and family about drugs to relieve symptoms of aging genitourinary and reproductive systems, remember that your client is typically older and may need repeated instruction to understand how to self-manage their issues and medications. The client and family should feel confident in understanding that the drug is to help reduce symptoms experienced that may be hard to discuss with others. As you develop a teaching plan be sure to include one or more of the following items of information:

Estrogens and Progestins

- Carefully read the client package insert available with the drug. If there are any questions about this information, discuss them with the primary health care provider.
- If GI upset occurs, take the drug with food.
- Notify the primary health care provider if any of the following occurs: pain in the legs or groin area; sharp chest pain or sudden shortness of breath; lumps in the breast; sudden severe headache; dizziness or fainting; vision or speech disturbances; weakness or numbness

in the arms, face, or legs; severe abdominal pain; depression; or yellowing of the skin or eyes.
- If pregnancy is suspected or abnormal vaginal bleeding occurs, stop taking the drug and contact the primary health care provider immediately.
- Client with diabetes: check the blood glucose daily, or more often. Contact the primary health care provider if the blood glucose is elevated. An elevated blood glucose level may require a change in diabetic therapy (insulin, oral antidiabetic drug) or diet; these changes must be made by the primary health care provider.

Estradiol Transdermal System
- Be sure to read the package insert carefully. Some systems are applied twice weekly; others are applied every 7 days.
- Apply the system immediately after opening the pouch, with the adhesive side down. Apply to clean, dry skin of the trunk, buttocks, abdomen, upper inner thigh, or upper arm. Do not apply to breasts, waistline, or a site exposed to sunlight. The area should not be oily or irritated. Be careful with heat sources such as an electric blanket that can increase the rate of absorption.
- Press the system firmly in place with the palm of the hand for about 10 seconds. The application site is rotated, with at least 1-week intervals between applications to a particular site.
- Avoid areas that may be exposed to rubbing or where clothing may rub the system off or loosen the edges.
- Remove the old system before applying a new system. Rotate application sites to prevent skin irritation.
- Follow the directions of the primary health care provider regarding application of the system (e.g., continuous, 3 weeks of use followed by 1 week off, changed weekly, or applied twice weekly).
- If the system falls off, reapply it or apply a new system. Continue the original treatment schedule. Dispose away from both children and pets.

Intravaginal Application
- Use the applicator correctly. Refer to the package insert for correct procedure. The applicator is marked with the correct dosage and accompanies the drug when purchased.
- Wash the applicator after each use in warm water with a mild soap and rinse well.
- Maintain a recumbent position for at least 30 minutes after instillation.
- Use a panty liner to protect clothing if necessary.
- Do not double the dosage if a dose is missed. Instead, skip the dose and resume treatment the next day.

Androgen Hormone Inhibitor
- Inform the primary health care provider immediately if sexual partner is or may become pregnant, because additional measures, such as discontinuing the drug or use of a condom, may be necessary.
- Women who are or may become pregnant should not handle this medication.

- Do not donate blood for at least 6 months after stopping medication because of potential effects on pregnant women who may receive the blood product.

Antiandrogens (Abiraterone)
- Abiraterone (Zytiga) is taken concurrently with prednisone; be sure ample supply of the steroid drug is dispensed.
- Women who are, or may become, pregnant should not handle this medication.

Gonadotropin-Releasing Hormones Analogs
- Provide postimplant care instructions including lifting limitations and bathing restrictions while healing

Antispasmodic Drugs
- Flavoxate: Take this drug three to four times daily as prescribed. This drug is used to treat symptoms; other drugs are given to treat the cause.
- Oxybutynin: Take this drug with or without food. Oxybutynin contains an outer coating that may not disintegrate and sometimes may be observed in the stool. This is not a cause for concern. If using the transdermal form (patch) of the drug, be sure to apply to a clean, dry area of the hip, abdomen, or buttocks. Remove the old patch and rotate sites of new application every 7 days.
- Antispasmodic drugs can cause heat prostration (fever and heat stroke caused by decreased sweating) in high temperatures. If you live in hot climates or will be exposed to high temperatures, take appropriate precautions.

EVALUATION
- Therapeutic effect is achieved and urinary or reproductive symptoms are relieved.
- Adverse reactions are identified, reported to the primary health care provider, and managed successfully through appropriate nursing interventions.
  - Knowledge level is enhanced.
  - Mucous membranes are moist and intact.
  - No injury is evident.
  - Client is free of pain.
- Client and family express confidence and demonstrate an understanding of the drug regimen.

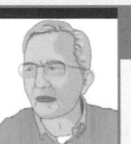

PHARMACOLOGY IN PRACTICE

USING CLINICAL REASONING

Mr. Phillip has returned to the clinic with continued UTI symptoms. The primary health care provider suspects that Mr. Phillip may have BPH and is reducing his own fluid intake to prevent himself from having to get up at night to urinate. Analyze the situation to determine what points you would stress in a teaching plan for this client.

KEY POINTS

■ During menopause, the hormone estrogen diminishes and the menstrual cycle can become irregular until it stops. This period is also called the female climacteric. Changes related to the cardiovascular, skeletal, urinary, and reproductive systems can cause uncomfortable symptoms. The hormone estrogen can be replaced, which helps to relieve flushing, sweating, and atrophy of vaginal and urinary tissues, and improves bones.

■ The number of urinary system disorders increases as people age. Renal function can be reduced to 50% and the urine becomes more dilute. Strength, flexibility, and the capacity of the bladder decrease. This can lead to pain, frequency, or incontinence. Antispasmodic agents reduce urinary smooth muscle spasms and improve urinary flow.

■ Urinary issues can also be a sign of prostate enlargement. BPH symptoms such as frequency, reduced flow, nocturia, and dysuria are treated with antiadrenergic or male hormone inhibitors. ED may result from use of certain medications or a medical condition such as diabetes or BPH. Medications used to treat ED are similar to others used to dilate circulatory vessels. Similar adverse reactions can present such as hypotension.

■ Advanced cancers of the reproductive systems in both men and women respond to hormonal manipulation. At this time these are used for palliative purposes and are not meant to cure the disease.

SUMMARY DRUG TABLE
Aging Urinary and Reproductive Drugs

Generic Name	Trade Name	Uses	Adverse Reactions	Dosage Ranges
Female Hormone: Estrogens				
estrogens, conjugated *ES-troe-jenz*	Premarin	Oral: vasomotor symptoms associated with menopause, atrophic vaginitis, osteoporosis, hypogonadism, primary ovarian failure, breast and prostate cancer palliation Parenteral: abnormal uterine bleeding from hormonal imbalance	Headache, dizziness, melasma, venous thromboembolism, nausea, vomiting, abdominal bloating and cramps, breakthrough bleeding/spotting, vaginal changes, rhinitis, changes in libido, breast enlargement and tenderness, weight changes, generalized pain	0.3–2.5 mg/day orally; IM: 25 mg/injection
estrogens, esterified	Menest	Same as conjugated estrogens	Same as conjugated estrogens	0.3–1.25 mg/day orally
estrogens, topical	Divigel, EstroGel (transdermal)	Vaginal atrophy and vasomotor symptoms associated with menopause	Rare: minor vaginal irritation or itching	Metered-dose for daily application
estrogens, vaginal	Estring, Femring, Ogen, and Premarin Vaginal Creams	Vaginal atrophy and vasomotor symptoms associated with menopause	Rare: minor vaginal irritation or itching	See package insert; used weekly or monthly
estradiol, oral *es-tra-DYE-ole*	Estrace	Vasomotor symptoms associated with menopause, osteoporosis prevention, hypoestrogenism palliative therapy for breast and prostate cancer	Same as conjugated estrogens	0.5–10 mg/day orally
estradiol cypionate	Depo-Estradiol	Moderate to severe vasomotor symptoms associated with menopause, female hypogonadism, male-to-female therapy (MTF)	Same as conjugated estrogens; pain at injection site	1–5 mg IM, every 3–4 weeks

Continued

SUMMARY DRUG TABLE (continued)
Aging Urinary and Reproductive Drugs

Generic Name	Trade Name	Uses	Adverse Reactions	Dosage Ranges
Female Hormone: Estrogens (continued)				
estradiol vaginal	Vagifem	Atrophic vaginitis	Same as conjugated estrogens	One tablet vaginally daily
estradiol transdermal system	Alora, Climara, Divigel, Dotti, Estraderm, Menostar, Vivelle	Same as conjugated estrogens, MTF therapy	Same as conjugated estrogens	Variable doses, applied to skin weekly
estropipate *ES-troe-pih-pate*	Ogen (cream), Ortho-Est (tablet)	Moderate to severe vasomotor symptoms associated with menopause, female hypogonadism, ovarian failure, osteoporosis	Same as conjugated estrogens	0.625–9 mg/day orally
synthetic conjugated estrogens, A		Moderate to severe vasomotor symptoms associated with menopause, vaginal atrophy	Same as conjugated estrogens	0.45 mg/day orally, then adjust according to symptoms
synthetic conjugated estrogens, B		Moderate to severe vasomotor symptoms associated with menopause	Same as conjugated estrogens	0.3 mg/day orally, then adjust according to symptoms
estrogens and progestins combined	Activella, Angeliq, Climara Pro, CombiPatch, Femhrt, Prempro, YAZ	Treatment of moderate to severe vasomotor symptoms associated with menopause, treatment of vulval and vaginal atrophy, osteoporosis	Adverse reactions of both hormones; same as synthetic conjugated estrogens and progesterone	Oral or transdermal, variable dosing, used daily or weekly. See package insert
Selective Estrogen Receptor Modulator				
ospemifene *os-PEM-i-feen*	Osphena	Dyspareunia, vaginal atrophy caused by menopause	Hot flashes, vaginal discharge	60 mg orally daily
raloxifene *ral-OKS-i-feen*	Evista	Treatment and prevention of postmenopausal osteoporosis	Leg cramps, dizziness, blood clots	60 mg orally daily
Estrogen/SERM Combination				
estrogen/bazedoxifene *ES-troe-jenz ba-ze-DOX-i-feen*	Duavee	Moderate to severe vasomotor symptoms associated with menopause *and osteoporosis prevention*	Same as conjugated estrogens	0.45/0.2 mg/day orally
Urinary Drugs (Antispasmodics)				
darifenacin *dar-i-FEN-a-sin*	Enablex	OAB w/urge incontinence, urgency/frequency	Dry mouth, constipation	7.5 mg/day orally
fesoterodine *fes-oh-TER-oh-deen*	Toviaz	OAB w/urge incontinence, urgency/frequency	Dry mouth	4–8 mg orally daily
flavoxATE *fla-VOKS-ate*		Male urinary symptoms caused by cystitis, prostatitis, and other urinary problems	Dry mouth, drowsiness, blurred vision, headache, urinary retention	100–200 mg orally TID or QID
mirabegron *mir-a-BEG-ron*	Myrbetriq	OAB w/urge incontinence, urgency/frequency	Constipation, diarrhea, dizziness, nausea	25 mg orally daily, titrate up to 50 mg/day
oxybutynin *oks-i-BYOO-ti-nin*	Ditropan XL	OAB w/urge incontinence, urgency/frequency, neurogenic bladder	Dry mouth, nausea, headache, drowsiness, constipation, urinary retention	5 mg orally, 2–3 times/day; 3.9 mg transdermal, use 3–4 days

Generic Name	Trade Name	Uses	Adverse Reactions	Dosage Ranges
solifenacin *sol-i-FEN-a-sin*	VESIcare	OAB w/urge incontinence, urgency/frequency	Dry mouth, constipation, blurred vision, dry eyes	5 mg/day orally
tolterodine *toll-TER-oh-deen*	Detrol, Detrol LA (long-acting, ER)	OAB w/urge incontinence, urgency/frequency	Dry mouth, constipation, headache, dizziness	2 mg orally TID; ER: 4 mg/day
⊘ **trospium** *TROSE-pee-um*		OAB w/urge incontinence, urgency/frequency	Dry mouth, constipation, headache	20 mg orally TID
Benign Prostatic Hypertrophy Drugs				
Antiadrenergic Drugs: Peripherally Acting				
alfuzosin *al-FYOO-zoe-sin*	Uroxatral	BPH	Headache, dizziness	10 mg orally daily
doxazosin *doks-AY-zoe-sin*	Cardura	Hypertension, BPH	Headache, dizziness, fatigue	Hypertension: 1–8 mg orally daily; BPH: 1–16 mg orally daily
silodosin *SI-lo-doe-sin*	Rapaflo	BPH, dislodge ureteral stones	Headache, dizziness, ejaculatory dysfunction, diarrhea, rhinitis	8 mg orally daily
tamsulosin *tam-SOO-loe-sin*	Flomax	BPH, dislodge ureteral stones	Headache, ejaculatory dysfunction, dizziness, rhinitis	0.4 mg orally daily
terazosin *ter-AY-zoe-sin*		Hypertension, BPH, dislodge ureteral stones	Dizziness, postural hypotension, headache, dyspnea, nasal congestion	Hypertension: 1–20 mg orally daily; BPH: 1–10 mg orally daily
Androgen Hormone Inhibitors				
dutasteride *doo-TAS-teer-ide*	Avodart	BPH	Impotence, decreased libido	0.5 mg/day orally
finasteride *fi-NAS-teer-ide*	Propecia, Proscar	Male-pattern baldness, BPH	Impotence, decreased libido, asthenia, dizziness, postural hypotension	1–5 mg/day orally
dutasteride/tamsulosin combination	Jalyn	BPH	See each separate drug	One capsule orally at the same time daily
Impotence Agents—Phosphodiesterase Type 5 (PD5E) Inhibitors				
avanafil *a-VAN-a-fil*	Stendra	ED	Headache, dyspepsia, nasal congestion, back pain	100–200 mg orally 30–60 minutes before sexual activity
sildenafil *sil-DEN-a-fil*	Viagra, Revatio	ED, PAH(Revatio only), altitude sickness	Headache, flushing, dyspepsia, nasal congestion	25–50 mg orally 30–60 minutes before sexual activity
tadalafil *tah-DA-la-fil*	Cialis, Adcirca, Alyq	ED, BPH, PAH(Adcirca, Alyq only)	Headache, dyspepsia, nasal congestion, back pain	5–20 mg orally, as needed for sexual activity / Up to 36 hours before sexual activity; maybe taken 5 mg daily for BPH/ED
vardenafil *var-DEN-a-fil*	Levitra, Staxyn	ED	Headache, flushing, dyspepsia, runny nose, back pain	5–20 mg orally 60 minutes before sexual activity 4 hours before sexual activity
Hormonal Therapy for Breast, Endometrial, and Prostate Cancer				
Gonadotropin-Releasing Hormone Antagonist				
degarelix *deg-a-REL-ix*	Firmagon	Advanced prostate cancer	Hot flashes, injection site pain, weight gain	80–240 mg subcut

Continued

SUMMARY DRUG TABLE (continued)
Aging Urinary and Reproductive Drugs

Generic Name	Trade Name	Uses	Adverse Reactions	Dosage Ranges
Gonadotropin-Releasing Hormone Analogs				
goserelin GOE-se-rel-in	Zoladex	Prostate and breast cancer, endometriosis, endometrial thinning	Headache, emotional lability, depression, sweating, acne, breast atrophy, sexual dysfunction, vaginitis, hot flashes, pain, edema	3.6-mg monthly implant, 10.8-mg q3mo implant
histrelin his-TREL-in	Vantas	Prostate cancer	Hot flashes, fatigue, implant site irritation	50–60 mcg/day delivered, for example, implant changed yearly
leuprolide loo-PROE-lide	Eligard, Lupron	Prostate cancer, endometriosis, precocious puberty, uterine leiomyomata	Hot flashes, edema, bone pain, electrocardiographic changes, hypertension	1 mg/day subcut, provided in monthly injection form and implant
triptorelin trip-toe-REL-in	Trelstar Mixject	Prostate cancer	Hot flashes, skeletal pain, headache, impotence	3.75 mg IM every 28 days
Antiandrogens				
abiraterone a-bir-A-ter-one	Yonsa, Zytiga	Prostate cancer	Hot flashes, nocturia, urinary frequency, peripheral edema, general pain, upper respiratory infection	1000 g/day with prednisone
apalutamide a-pa-LOO-ta-mide	Erleada	Prostate cancer	Hypertension, dizziness, fatigue, nausea, diarrhea, peripheral edema, skin rash, itching	240 mg/day orally
bicalutamide bye-ca-LOO-ta-mide	Casodex	Prostate cancer	Hot flashes, dizziness, constipation, nausea, diarrhea, nocturia, hematuria, peripheral edema, general pain, asthenia, infection	50 mg/day orally
darolutamide DAR-oh-LOO-ta-mide	Nubeqa	Prostate cancer	Fatigue, neutropenia, asthenia	600 mg twice daily orally
enzalutamide en-za-LOO-ta-mide	Xtandi	Prostate cancer	Hot flashes, numbness, headache, back pain, diarrhea	160 mg orally daily
flutamide FLOO-ta-mide		Prostate cancer	Hot flashes, loss of libido, impotence, diarrhea, nausea, vomiting, gynecomastia	250 mg/orally TID
nilutamide ni-LOO-ta-mide	Nilandron	Prostate cancer	Pain, headache, asthenia, flu-like symptoms, insomnia, nausea, constipation, testicular atrophy, dyspnea	300 mg/day for 1 month, then 150 mg/day orally
Estrogen				
estrogens, conjugated ES-troe-jenz	Premarin	Oral: prostate and breast cancer palliation	Headache, dizziness, melasma, venous thromboembolism, nausea, vomiting	0.3–2.5 mg/day orally; IM: 25 mg/injection
estradiol valerate es-tra-DYE-ole	Delestrogen	Prostate cancer, female hypogonadism, MTF therapy	Same as conjugated estrogens; pain at injection site	10–20 mg IM monthly

Generic Name	Trade Name	Uses	Adverse Reactions	Dosage Ranges
estramustine *es-tra-MUS-teen*	Emcyt	Prostate cancer	Breast tenderness and enlargement, nausea, diarrhea, edema	14 mg/kg/day orally in divided doses
Aromatase Inhibitors				
anastrozole *an-AS-troe-zole*	Arimidex	Breast cancer	Vasodilation, mood disturbances, nausea, hot flashes, pharyngitis, asthenia, pain	1 mg/day orally
exemestane *ex-e-MES-tane*	Aromasin	Breast cancer	Same as anastrozole	25 mg/day orally
letrozole *LET-roe-zole*	Femara	Breast cancer	Same as anastrozole	2.5 mg/day orally
Progestins				
medroxyPROGESTERone *me-DROKS-ee-proe-JES-te-rone*	Depo-Provera, Provera	Endometrial or renal cancer	Fatigue, nervousness, rash, pruritus, acne, edema	400–1000 mg/wk IM
megestrol *me-JES-trole*		Breast or endometrial cancer, appetite stimulant in human immunodeficiency virus (HIV) infection	Weight gain, nausea, vomiting, edema, breakthrough bleeding	40–320 mg/day orally in divided doses
Antiestrogen				
fulvestrant *fool-VES-trant*	Faslodex	Breast cancer	Nausea, vomiting, asthenia, pain, pharyngitis, headache	250 mg IM once monthly
Antiestrogens—SERM Class				
tamoxifen *ta-MOKS-i-fen*	Soltamox	Breast cancer, prophylactic therapy for women at high risk for breast cancer	Hot flashes, rashes, headaches, vaginal bleeding and discharge	20–40 mg/day orally
toremifene *tore-EM-i-feen*	Fareston	Breast cancer	Hot flashes, sweating, nausea, dizziness, edema, vaginal bleeding and discharge	60 mg/day orally

CHAPTER REVIEW

Know Your Drugs

Clients sometimes know a medication by the brand (or trade) name and not the generic name. To help you recognize both names, match the brand name with the generic name of the same medication.

Generic Name	Brand Name
1. avanafil	A. Ditropan XL
2. finasteride	B. Rapaflo
3. oxybutynin	C. Propecia
4. silodosin	D. Stendra

Calculate Medication Dosages

1. The primary health care provider prescribes fesoterodine 8 mg orally once a day for an OAB problem. The pharmacy dispenses the drug in 4-mg tablets. The nurse instructs the client to take _____.

2. The primary health care provider prescribes sildenafil 50 mg orally as needed for sexual relations. If the maximum dose is 100 mg in 24 hours, how many pills can the client take in 1 day?

Prepare for the NCLEX

RECALL THE FACTS

1. When a woman stops ovulating, this is referred to as _____.
   1. menarche
   2. andropause
   3. menopause
   4. HRT

2. Which of the following structures is in the upper urinary system?
   1. Bladder
   2. Prostate
   3. Urethra
   4. Kidney

3. What percentage of kidney function typically is reduced as people age?
   1. 10%
   2. 35%
   3. 50%
   4. 85%
4. The most common drugs used for BPH are _____.
   1. cholinergic blockers
   2. antiadrenergics
   3. hormones
   4. enzyme inhibitors
5. How many Americans suffer from an overactive bladder?
   1. 33 million
   2. billion
   3. 46,000
   4. 250,000
6. If a urinary drug has anticholinergic effects, the symptoms will be _____.
   1. slow heartbeat
   2. dry mouth
   3. wakefulness
   4. dry skin

ANALYZE THE FACTS

7. If the drug dutasteride is for BPH and used only for men, why is it rated pregnancy category X?
   1. To be sure it is not administered to women for menopausal symptoms.
   2. It can harm a male fetus if absorbed by a pregnant woman.
   3. To make it clear it is to be given to men only.
   4. All drugs are ranked no matter if only for men or not.

8. *A client calls regarding taking vardenafil. Which of the following statements would be of concern and should be reported immediately?
   1. "Nurse, my cheeks look like I'm having a hot flash."
   2. "My penis is still poking out now after 4 hours."
   3. "I can't take those pills because they give me a headache!"
   4. "My nose is suddenly stuffy, wonder if I have a cold."

ALTERNATE-FORMAT QUESTIONS

9. A client says they are stopping the antispasmodic drug because of dry mouth and constipation. What are some teaching tips the nurse can offer to reduce these adverse reactions? **Select all that apply.**
   1. Add more fiber to your diet.
   2. Limit fluid intake.
   3. Eat a piece of watermelon daily.
   4. Select meat cuts that are iron rich.
   5. Brush and floss your teeth regularly.
10. As the urinary bladder ages, which of the following cause nocturia? **Select all that apply.**
    1. Capacity increases.
    2. Flexibility is reduced.
    3. Prostate tissue obstructs flow.
    4. Bladder strength diminishes.

To check your answers, see Appendix F.

――――――――――

*Indicates the question is directly linked to the NCLEX-PN test plan in Appendix G.

WANT TO KNOW MORE? A wide variety of resources are available to enhance your learning and understanding of this chapter.
- Visit the Point for resources such as:
  - NCLEX-Style Student Review Questions
  - Journal Articles
  - Dosage Calculations
  - Drug Monographs
  - Watch and Learn Videos
  - Concepts in Action Animations
- The *Study Guide to Accompany Introductory Clinical Pharmacology,* 12th edition, sold separately, will help you review and apply essential content.
- ✓*PrepU* is available to help students prepare for the NCLEX-PN examination.

Urinary Tract Anti-Infectives and Other Urinary Drugs

Learning Objectives

On completion of this chapter, the student will:

1. Explain the uses, general drug actions, adverse reactions, contraindications, precautions, and interactions of the drugs used to treat infections and symptoms associated with urinary tract infections.
2. Distinguish important preadministration and ongoing assessment activities the nurse should perform with the client taking a drug for a urinary tract infection.
3. List nursing diagnoses particular to a client taking a drug for a urinary tract infection.
4. Examine ways to promote an optimal response to therapy, how to manage adverse reactions, and important points to keep in mind when educating clients about the use of drugs to treat urinary tract infections.

 Drug Classes

Urinary anti-infectives	Urinary analgesics

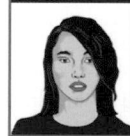

PHARMACOLOGY IN PRACTICE

Janna Wong is a 16-year-old high school gymnast. She is at the clinic for a routine physical examination. Vital signs show that Janna has a fever of 100.5 °F. She says she feels tired, yet is fidgety. When asked if she would like some water, Janna says no because she does not want to urinate until she gets home. Think about her remarks as you read this chapter.

This chapter discusses drugs used to treat urinary tract infections, which are frequently referred to as UTIs. A large number of health-related provider visits are related to UTI symptoms and treatment. About 10 million outpatient appointments and 3 million emergency department visits are due to complaints of UTI symptoms (Pinkerton et al., 2020). UTIs are also the most commonly treated infection in the long-term care setting (Abbo & Hooton, 2014). Typically, a course of anti-infectives is prescribed since the symptoms are uncomfortable.

One consequence of treating this vast number of UTIs is resistance to bacterial medications. Antibiotic resistance is a major factor when anti-infective drugs are frequently prescribed, especially in long duration (Abbo, 2014). Therefore, it is a difficult balancing of recognition and treatment versus too liberal guidelines for treatment of UTIs.

The drugs discussed in this chapter are primarily anti-infectives. They are used in the treatment of UTIs, and they have an effect on bacteria in the urinary tract. Although administered systemically, that is, by the oral or parenteral routes, they do not achieve significant levels in the bloodstream and are of no value in treating *systemic* infections. They are primarily excreted by the kidneys and exert their major antibacterial effects in the urine as it travels through the bladder.

Examples of the most common drugs used in treating UTIs include amoxicillin (broad-spectrum penicillins; see Chapter 7), trimethoprim (sulfonamides; see Chapter 6), and nitrofurantoin. Some drugs used in the treatment of UTIs, such as nitrofurantoin, do not belong to the antibiotic or sulfonamide groups of drugs. The anti-infective drugs known as fluoroquinolones (see Chapter 9) were initially approved for UTI treatment, but have become of greater use in systemic infection treatment. Combination drugs such as trimethoprim and sulfamethoxazole (Bactrim or Septra) are also used. The Summary Drug Table: Urinary Tract Anti-Infectives gives examples of the drugs used for UTIs.

Urinary analgesics are another drug category frequently used to treat UTIs and long-term interstitial cystitis, specifically to relieve the discomfort associated with these conditions.

URINARY ANTI-INFECTIVES

ACTIONS AND USES

Urinary tract infections are caused by pathogenic microorganisms of one or more structures of the urinary system (Fig. 46.1). Because the female urethra is considerably shorter than the male urethra, women are affected by UTIs much more frequently than men. The most common structure affected is the bladder. Clinical manifestations of a bladder UTI or bladder inflammation (**cystitis**) include urgency, frequency, pressure, burning pain on urination, and pain caused by spasm in the region of the bladder and the suprapubic area. With chronic UTIs, the urethra, prostate (**prostatitis**), and kidney (**pyelonephritis**) may also be affected.

Many of the anti-infective drugs used for treating UTIs are chosen because of the rapid excretion rate of the drugs rather than the way they act inside the body. As a result, these anti-infectives have a high concentration in the urine and appear to act by interfering with bacterial multiplication in the urine. Nitrofurantoin (Macrodantin) may be **bacteriostatic** (slows or retards the multiplication of bacteria) or **bactericidal** (destroys bacteria), depending on the concentration of the drug in the urine. See the specific anti-infective chapters for the manner in which other anti-infective drugs work.

Phenazopyridine is a dye that exerts a topical analgesic effect on the lining of the urinary tract. It does not have anti-infective activity. Phenazopyridine is available over the counter as a separate drug but is also included in some urinary tract anti-infective combination drugs.

ADVERSE REACTIONS

Adverse reactions are primarily gastrointestinal (GI) disturbances and include the following:

- Anorexia, nausea, vomiting, and diarrhea
- Abdominal pain or stomatitis

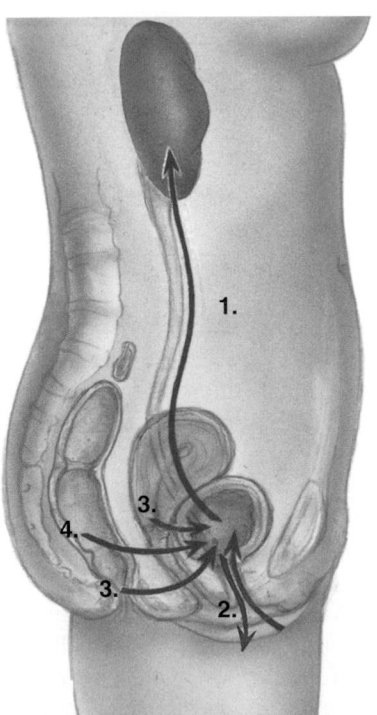
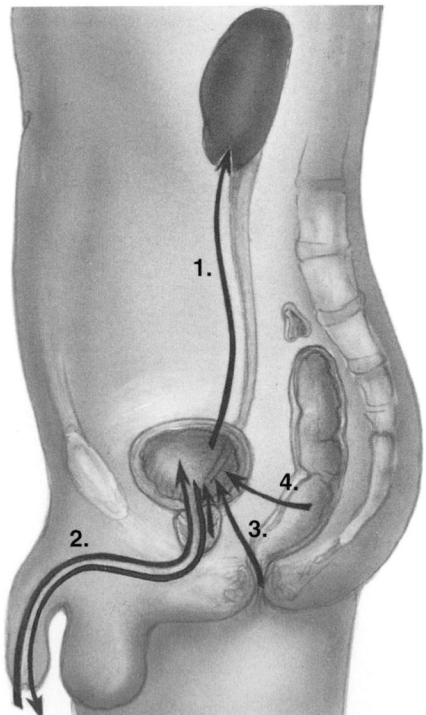

1. Ascending (reflux) from bladder to kidney

2. Ascending urethra to bladder; descending urethra from bladder

3. From rectum, cervix, and prostate to bladder

4. From bowel to bladder

FIGURE 46.1 Routes of infection in the urinary tract. (Asset provided by Anatomical Chart Co.)

Other generalized body system reactions include:

- Drowsiness, dizziness, headache, blurred vision, weakness, and peripheral neuropathy
- Rash, pruritus, photosensitivity reactions, and leg cramps

When these drugs are given in large doses, clients may experience burning on urination and bladder irritation; this should not be mistaken for a continued infection. Nitrofurantoin has been known to cause acute and chronic pulmonary reactions. Clients should be told that phenazopyridine will discolor the urine (dark orange to brown) and permanently stain undergarments that come in contact with the urine.

CONTRAINDICATIONS AND PRECAUTIONS

Anti-infectives are contraindicated in clients with a hypersensitivity to the drugs and during pregnancy (pregnancy category C) and lactation. One exception is nitrofurantoin, which is classified as a pregnancy category B drug and is used with caution during pregnancy.

The anti-infectives should be used cautiously in those with renal or hepatic impairment. Clients who are allergic to tartrazine (a food dye) should not take methenamine (Hiprex). This drug is used cautiously in clients with gout, because it may cause crystals to form in the urine. Nitrofurantoin is used cautiously in clients with cerebral arteriosclerosis, diabetes, or a glucose-6-phosphate dehydrogenase (G6PD) deficiency.

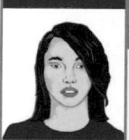

PHARMACOLOGY IN PRACTICE

SAFE DRUG ADMINISTRATION

A nurse receives an order to begin methenamine drug therapy. For which of the following client conditions is the use of this drug contraindicated? Select all that apply.
1. Cerebral arteriosclerosis
2. Asthma
3. Allergy to tartrazine
4. Chronic gout

LASA ALERT

The following drugs may sound alike; be sure to clarify when they are ordered:

Drug Name	Sounds Like
Amoxil	amoxapine
ampicillin	Aminophylline
Elmiron	Imuran
Hiprex	Mirapex
Macrobid	micro-K, Nitro-Bid
methenamine	mesalamine, methazolAMIDE, methionine
Monurol	Monopril
nitrofurantoin	Neurontin, nitroglycerin
pentosan	pentostatin
phenazopyridine	phenoxybenzamine
Pyridium	Dyrenium, Perdiem, pyridoxine, pyrithione

Drugs that look alike are noted in the Summary Drug Tables of each chapter.

INTERACTIONS
Anti-Infectives
The following interactions may occur when a specific urinary anti-infective is administered with another agent:

Interacting Drug	Common Use	Effect of Interaction
Sulfamethoxazole		
Oral anticoagulants	Blood thinner	Increased risk for bleeding
Nitrofurantoin		
Magnesium trisilicate or magaldrate	Relieve gastric upset	Decreased absorption of anti-infective
Anticholinergics	Relieve bladder spasm/ discomfort	Delay in gastric emptying, thereby increasing the absorption of nitrofurantoin
Fosfomycin (Monurol)		
Metoclopramide (Reglan)	Relieve gastric upset	Lowers plasma concentration and urinary tract excretion of fosfomycin

An increased urinary pH (alkaline urine) decreases the effectiveness of methenamine. Therefore, to avoid raising the urine pH when taking methenamine, the client should not use antacids containing sodium bicarbonate or sodium carbonate.

Herbal Considerations

Cranberry juice has long been recommended for use in treating and preventing UTIs. Clinical studies have confirmed that cranberry juice is beneficial to individuals with frequent UTIs. Cranberry juice inhibits bacteria from attaching to the walls of the urinary tract and prevents certain bacteria from forming dental plaque in the mouth. Cranberry juice is safe for use as a food and for urinary tract health. Cranberry juice and capsules have no contraindications, no known adverse reactions, and no drug interactions. The recommended dosage is 9–15 capsules a day (400–500 mg/day) or 4–8 ounce of juice daily (Brown, 2012).

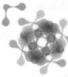

NURSING PROCESS: STEPS TO BUILDING CLINICAL JUDGMENT
Client Receiving a Urinary Tract Anti-Infective or Other Urinary Tract Drug

ASSESSMENT

Preadministration Assessment

Data gathering suggestions before the initial administration of a drug for urinary issues include:

Objective data

- Description of signs of infection, such as redness or distention of bladder
- Description of the urine—color, odor, concentration, or lack of clarity
- Vital signs (temperature, pulse, respirations, and blood pressure)
- Dipstick testing for infection, blood or protein
- Residual urine measurement if indicated
- Renal and hepatic function tests, complete blood count, and urinalysis if client has impaired function in any of these body systems

Subjective data

- Current symptoms of the infection (complaints of frequency, itching, pain)
- Confusion in the elderly
- Allergy history, particularly a drug allergy

Ongoing Assessment

Many UTIs are treated on an outpatient basis because hospitalization is seldom required. UTIs may affect the hospitalized client or nursing home resident especially with an indwelling urethral catheter, a disorder such as a stone in the urinary tract, or low fluid intake. The primary nursing interventions to prevent UTIs in the hospitalized client are good hand hygiene (handwashing) and frequent perineal care when an indwelling urinary catheter is in place.

When caring for a hospitalized client with a UTI, monitor the vital signs every 4 hours or as ordered by the primary health care provider (PHCP). Any significant rise in body temperature is reported to the PHCP, because intervention to reduce the fever or culture and sensitivity tests may need to be repeated.

If after several days the symptoms of the UTI do not improve or they become worse, contact the PHCP. Periodic urinalysis and urine culture and sensitivity tests may be ordered to monitor the effects of drug therapy.

NURSING DIAGNOSES

Drug-specific nursing diagnoses include the following:

- **Increased urinary frequency** related to discomfort of urinary tract infection
- **Altered breathing pattern** related to adverse reaction to drug

Nursing diagnoses related to drug administration are discussed in Chapter 4.

PLANNING

The expected outcomes for the client may include an optimal response to drug therapy, support of client needs related to the management of adverse reactions, and confidence in an understanding of the medication regimen.

IMPLEMENTATION

Promoting an Optimal Response to Therapy

To promote an optimal response to therapy, give urinary tract anti-infectives with food to prevent GI upset. Nitrofurantoin especially should be given with food, meals, or milk because this drug is particularly irritating to the stomach. Fosfomycin (Monurol) has special administration requirements; it comes in a 3-g, one-dose packet that must be dissolved in 90–120 mL of water (not hot water). Administer the drug immediately after dissolving it in water. The exception is pentosan which is administered after meals to prevent GI upset.

> **! NURSING ALERT**
>
> Instruct clients who are using phenazopyridine that it should not be taken for more than 2 days when used in combination with an antibacterial drug to treat a UTI. When used for more than 2 days, the drug may mask the symptoms of a more serious disorder.

Monitoring and Managing Client Needs

Observe the client for adverse drug reactions. If an adverse reaction occurs, contact the PHCP before the next dose of the drug is due. However, serious drug reactions, such as a pulmonary reaction, are reported immediately.

Increased Urinary Frequency

The client is encouraged to drink at least 2000 mL of fluid daily (if condition permits) to dilute urine and decrease pain on voiding. Drinking extra fluids aids in the physical removal of bacteria from the genitourinary tract and is an important part of UTI treatment (see Client Teaching for Improved Outcomes: Preventing and Treating UTIs). Offer fluids, preferably water, to the client at hourly intervals. Cranberry or prune juice is usually given rather than orange juice or other citrus or vegetable juices. Contact the PHCP if the client fails to drink extra fluids, if the urine output is low, or if the urine appears concentrated during daytime hours. The urine of those drinking 2000 mL or more daily appears dilute and light in color.

Older clients often have a decreased thirst sensation and must be encouraged to increase fluid intake. This is especially true if the individual is not able to obtain or reach the fluid container. Develop a schedule to offer fluids at regular intervals to older adult clients or those who seem unable to increase their fluid intake without supervision.

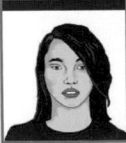

PHARMACOLOGY IN PRACTICE

MANAGING NEEDS

A nurse is caring for an older client receiving an anti-infective for the treatment of urinary problems. The client refuses to increase fluid intake, fearful of incontinence. What intervention should the nurse plan for the care of this client?

1. Increase the client's intake of fluids forcefully.
2. Stop administering the drug and call the PHCP.
3. Develop a schedule to offer the client fluids.
4. Administer the drug to the client with warm water.

Client Teaching for Improved Outcomes

Preventing and Treating UTIs

When you teach, make sure your client understands the following:

✔ How to accurately describe UTIs and their causes, and identifies what may be the cause.

✔ Able to review the drug therapy regimen, including prescribed drug, dose, and frequency of administration.

✔ Knows the importance of taking the entire drug even if the client feels better after a few doses.

✔ Describes ways to reduce UTIs, such as how to wipe front to back after going to the bathroom.

✔ Avoid tight clothing, prolonged wearing of pantyhose, tight pants, or wet bathing suits.

✔ Shower instead of bathing, rinsing well; avoid "overcleaning" and irritating the skin.

✔ Use tampons for menstrual periods instead of pads; make a habit of voiding every 4 hours and changing the tampon.

✔ After sexual contact, void and drink 2–8 ounce of water.

✔ Increase fluid intake, gauging the amount you drink to the color of your urine (it should be pale yellow during the day).

✔ Avoid eating foods or drinking liquids that irritate the bladder, such as coffee, tea, alcohol, artificial sweeteners, chocolate, and pepper.

✔ Vitamin C supplements and cranberry juice help maintain an acid environment in the bladder.

✔ Be sure to drink fluids and void regularly when cycling or horseback riding.

When administering these drugs, monitor the fluid intake and urinary output for volume and frequency. Measure and record the fluid intake and output every 8 hours, especially when the PHCP orders an increase in fluid intake or when a kidney infection is being treated. The PHCP may also order daily urinary pH levels when methenamine or nitrofurantoin is administered. These drugs work best in acid urine; failure of the urine to remain acidic may require administration of a urinary acidifier, such as ascorbic acid.

Altered Breathing Pattern

Pulmonary reactions have been reported with the use of nitrofurantoin and may occur within hours and up to 3 weeks after drug therapy is initiated. Signs and symptoms of an acute pulmonary reaction include dyspnea, chest pain, cough, fever, and chills. If these reactions occur, immediately notify the PHCP and withhold the next dose of the drug until the client is seen by a PHCP. In addition to the aforementioned signs and symptoms, a nonproductive cough or malaise may indicate a chronic pulmonary reaction, which may occur during prolonged therapy.

Educating the Client and Family

Educate regarding the importance for everyone to increase fluid intake to at least 2000 mL/day (unless contraindicated) to help remove bacteria from the genitourinary tract (see Client Teaching for Improving Outcomes: Preventing

---

and Treating UTIs). Be sure the client understands that phenazopyridine will cause a reddish-orange discoloration of the urine that stains clothing. In addition, the fluid that lubricates the eyes may change color, causing permanent discoloration of contact lenses. Reassure the client that this discoloration is normal and will subside when use of the drug is discontinued.

To ensure adherence to the prescribed drug regimen, educate about the importance of completing the full course of drug therapy even though symptoms have been relieved. A full course of therapy is necessary to ensure that all bacteria have been eliminated from the urinary tract. Include the following drug teaching points in a client and family teaching plan:

• Take the drug with food or meals (nitrofurantoin must be taken with food or milk). If GI upset occurs despite taking the drug with food, contact the PHCP.

• Take the drug at the prescribed intervals and complete the full course of therapy. Do not discontinue taking the drug even though the symptoms have disappeared, unless directed to do so by the PHCP.

• If drowsiness or dizziness occurs, avoid driving and performing tasks that require alertness.
🍷 Avoid alcoholic beverages and do not take any nonprescription drug unless its use has been approved by the PHCP.

• Notify the PHCP immediately if symptoms do not improve after 3 or 4 days.

• *Nitrofurantoin:* Take this drug with food or milk to improve absorption. Continue therapy for at least 1 week or for 3 days after the urine shows no signs of infection. Notify the PHCP immediately if any of the following occurs: fever, chills, cough, shortness of breath, chest pain, or difficulty breathing. Do not take the next dose of the drug until the PHCP has been contacted. The urine may appear brown during therapy with this drug; this is not abnormal.

• *Methenamine:* Avoid excessive intake of citrus products, milk, and milk products.

• *Fosfomycin* comes in dry form as a one-dose packet to be dissolved in 90–120 mL of water (not hot water). Drink immediately after mixing and take with food to prevent gastric upset.

• *Phenazopyridine:* This drug may cause a reddish-orange discoloration of the urine and tears and may stain fabrics or contact lenses. This is normal. Take the drug after meals. Do not take this drug for more than 2 days if you are also taking an antibiotic for the treatment of a UTI.

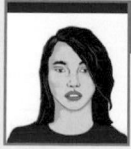

PHARMACOLOGY IN PRACTICE

TEACHING & LEARNING

The nurse advises clients taking phenazopyridine that their urine may become discolored and stain clothing. Which of the following colors might it become?
1. Orange
2. Blue
3. Purple
4. Green

EVALUATION

- Therapeutic effect is achieved and bladder symptoms are relieved.
- Adverse reactions are identified, reported to the PHCP, and managed successfully through appropriate nursing interventions.
  - Urinary elimination occurs without incident.
  - Adequate breathing pattern is maintained.
- Client and family express confidence and demonstrate an understanding of the drug regimen.

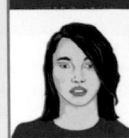

PHARMACOLOGY IN PRACTICE

USING CLINICAL REASONING

During your intake interview, you find that Janna drinks minimal amounts of water at school, waiting to get home to void instead of using the school facilities. Urinalysis shows cloudy, dark amber urine with white cells when you test it using a dipstick. In addition to antibiotic treatment, what are some important teaching points to review with Janna?

KEY POINTS

■ Urinary tract infections are caused by pathogenic microorganisms of one or more structures of the urinary tract. Because the female urethra is considerably shorter than the male urethra, women are affected by UTIs much more frequently than men. The most common structure affected is the bladder.

■ The anti-infectives used are the same as for other bacterial infections although taken orally they do not achieve significant levels in the bloodstream. The purpose of use is that they are rapidly excreted by the kidneys and exert their major antibacterial effects in the urine as it travels through the bladder.

■ Adverse reactions are GI such as nausea, diarrhea, and abdominal pain. If burning on urination occurs it should be determined if it is because of the medication or the infection.

SUMMARY DRUG TABLE
Urinary Tract Anti-Infectives

Generic Name	Trade Name	Uses	Adverse Reactions	Dosage Ranges
⊘ **amoxicillin** a-moks-i-SIL-in	Amoxil	Acute bacterial UTIs, other bacterial infections	Glossitis, stomatitis, gastritis, furry tongue, nausea, vomiting, diarrhea, rash, fever, pain at injection site, hypersensitivity reactions, hematopoietic changes	250–500 mg orally q8hr or 875 mg orally BID
fosfomycin fos-foe-MYE-sin	Monurol	Acute bacterial UTIs	Nausea, diarrhea, vaginitis, rhinitis, headache, back pain	3-g packet orally, provided in powder that must be mixed with fluid
methenamine meth-EN-a-meen	Hiprex	Chronic bacterial UTIs	Nausea, vomiting, abdominal cramps, bladder irritation	1 g orally BID
nitrofurantoin nye-troe-fyoor-AN-toyn	Macrobid, Macrodantin	Acute bacterial UTIs	Nausea, anorexia, peripheral neuropathy, headache, bacterial superinfection	50–100 mg orally QID
trimethoprim (TMP) trye-METH-oh-prim		Acute bacterial UTIs	Rash, pruritus, nausea, vomiting	200 mg/day orally
Urinary Anti-Infective Combinations				
trimethoprim and sulfamethoxazole (TMP-SMZ) trye-METH-oh-primsul-fa-meth-OKS-a-zoll	Bactrim	Acute bacterial UTIs, shigellosis, and acute otitis media	GI disturbances, allergic skin reactions, headache, anorexia, glossitis, hypersensitivity	160 mg TMP/800 SMZ orally q12hr; 8–10 mg/kg/day (based on TMP) IV in 2–4 divided doses
Other Urinary Drug (Analgesic)				
⊘ **pentosan** PEN-toe-san	Elmiron	Relief of pain associated with irritation of the bladder	Headache, diarrhea, stomach distress	100 mg orally TID
phenazopyridine fen-az-oh-PEER-i-deen	Pyridium	Relief of pain associated with irritation of the lower genitourinary tract	Headache, rash, pruritus, GI disturbances, red-orange discoloration of the urine, yellowish discoloration of the skin or sclera	200 mg orally TID

⊘ Take this drug at least 1 hour before or 2 hours after meals.

CHAPTER REVIEW

Know Your Drugs

Clients sometimes know a medication by the brand (or trade) name and not the generic name. To help you recognize both names, match the brand name with the generic name of the same medication.

Generic Name	Brand Name
1. trimethoprim/sulfamethoxazole	A. Amoxil
2. pentosan	B. Bactrim
3. nitrofurantoin	C. Macrodantin
4. amoxicillin	D. Elmiron

Calculate Medication Dosages

1. Amoxicillin 500 mg is prescribed. The drug is available in 250-mg tablets. The nurse administers _____.

2. Nitrofurantoin oral suspension 50 mg is prescribed. The oral suspension contains 25 mg/5 mL. The nurse administers _____.

Prepare for the NCLEX

RECALL THE FACTS

1. The nurse correctly administers nitrofurantoin (Macrodantin) _____.
   1. with food
   2. for no longer than 7 days
   3. without regard to food
   4. for no longer than 2 days
2. To avoid raising the pH of the urine when taking methenamine (Hiprex), the nurse advises the client to _____.
   1. use an antacid before taking the drug
   2. take an antacid immediately after taking the drug
   3. avoid antacids containing sodium bicarbonate or sodium carbonate
   4. avoid the use of antacids 1 hour before or 2 hours after taking the drug
3. What instruction would be most important to give a client prescribed fosfomycin (Monurol)?
   1. Drink one to two glasses of cranberry juice daily to promote healing of the urinary tract.
   2. You may take the drug without regard to meals.
   3. This drug comes in a one-dose packet that must be dissolved in 90 mL or more of fluids.
   4. This drug may cause mental confusion.

ANALYZE THE FACTS

4. *What statement(s) would be included in a teaching plan for a client prescribed phenazopyridine?
   1. There is a danger of heat prostration or heat stroke when taking phenazopyridine in a hot climate.
   2. This drug may turn the urine dark brown. This is an indication of a serious condition and should be reported immediately.
   3. This drug may cause photosensitivity. Take precautions when out in the sun by wearing sunscreen, a hat, and a long-sleeved shirt for protection.
   4. This drug may turn the urine reddish-orange. This is a normal occurrence that will disappear when use of the drug is discontinued.

ALTERNATE-FORMAT QUESTIONS

5. Match the inflammation to the organ affected.

1. Cystitis	A. Bladder
2. Prostatitis	B. Kidney
3. Pyelonephritis	C. Prostate
4. Urethritis	D. Urethra

To check your answers, see Appendix F.

---

*Indicates the question is directly linked to the NCLEX-PN test plan in Appendix G.

WANT TO KNOW MORE? A wide variety of resources are available to enhance your learning and understanding of this chapter.

- Visit thePoint for resources such as:
  - NCLEX-Style Student Review Questions
  - Journal Articles
  - Dosage Calculations
  - Drug Monographs
  - Watch and Learn Videos
  - Concepts in Action Animations
- The *Study Guide to Accompany Introductory Clinical Pharmacology*, 12th edition, sold separately, will help you review and apply essential content.
- ✔PrepU is available to help students prepare for the NCLEX-PN examination.

UNIT 12
Drugs That Affect the Immune System

The immune system is made up of a number of organs (thymus, tonsils/adenoids, spleen, portions of the gastrointestinal tract), the bone marrow, and a series of lymph vessels and nodes. Lymph flows through the entire body as a set of cells and fluid designed to recognize and respond to invasion. The function of the immune system is to protect our cells from invading substances, survey for intrusion, and maintain homeostasis. There are three levels of defense that the immune system uses to stop invasion and fight disease.

The first level of defense is a physical barrier. This barrier includes the skin surface and hairs, body secretions (such as tears and mucous), and the acid content in the stomach.

The second line of defense involves cells in the body that identify and attack an invasive threat and begin the inflammatory response. Sometimes called innate nonspecific immunity, it includes the phagocytes—natural killer cells, granulocytes, and macrophages.

The third line of defense differs from the second with the ability to create memory—learned specific or adaptive immunity. It is a slower response than the second-level response but can last much longer and targets specific microbes.

The term "immunotherapy" refers to the treatment of disease by inducing, enhancing, or suppressing an immune response (Stedman, 2020). The chapters in this unit describe the drugs used mainly on the second and third level (adaptive immunity) to support, modulate, or suppress the immune system in its efforts to recognize invasion of an outside pathogen or identifying the body's own cells growing out of control.

In this unit, we will discuss therapies designed to influence the immune system, reserving those that specifically treat cancer to Unit 13. In Chapter 47, vaccines (that stimulate us to make specific antibodies) are presented.

Chapter 48 focuses on the agents used to modulate or manipulate the immune system. Finally, Chapter 49 introduces drugs that are used to suppress an overactive immune system and are used for conditions such as rheumatoid arthritis or multiple sclerosis.

The COVID-19 pandemic has highlighted an area of concern for nurses and the significance of the immune system to many. Back in the early 1900s, communicable diseases and injuries were the primary illnesses health care providers treated. Communicable diseases, such as smallpox and polio have been almost completely eradicated by immunizing large populations of people at or near birth. We saw the transition as chronic illness took the forefront of healthcare time and resources. Immunology research also turned to modulating the immune system as part of care for chronic disorders. Yet, appearance of a virulent pathogen has healthcare again looking at acute illness. All areas of society have been impacted socially as well as economically by the coronavirus—SARs-CoV-2. COVID-19 has shown us the importance of vaccination for prevention and immunomodulation for treatment.

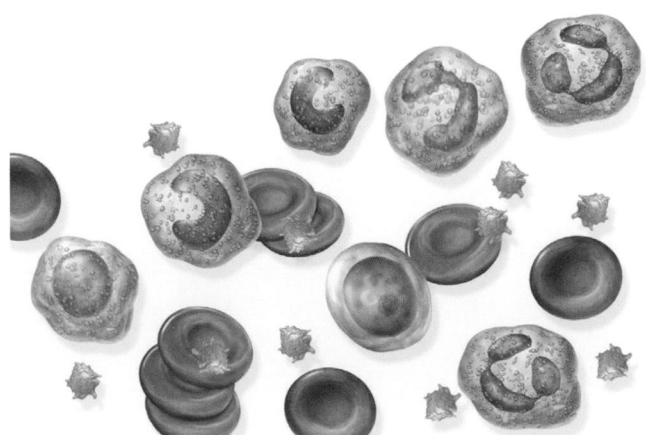

Vaccines

(continued)

Key Terms

active immunity type of immunity that occurs when the person is exposed to a disease and develops the disease and the body makes antibodies to provide future protection against the disease

adaptive immunity type of immunity that is pathogen specific and creates memory to the pathogen

antibody molecule with the ability to bind to a specific antigen

antigen substance that is capable of inducing a specific immune response

antigen–antibody response antibodies formed in response to exposure to a specific antigen

attenuate to weaken

booster immunogen injected after a specified interval; often after the primary immunization to stimulate and sustain the immune response

cell-mediated immunity immune reaction caused by white blood cells

globulins plasma proteins that are insoluble in water

humoral immunity antibody-mediated immune response of the body

immune globulins solution obtained from human or animal blood containing antibodies that have been formed by the body to specific antigens; administered to provide passive immunity to one or more infectious diseases

immunity resistance to infection

immunization the process in which a person is made immune or resistant to an infectious disease

innate immunity the part of the immune system that serves as the body's first line of defense

Learning Objectives

On completion of this chapter, the student will:

1. Discuss humoral immunity and cell-mediated immunity.
2. Compare and contrast the different types of immunity.
3. Explain the use of vaccines, toxoids, immune globulins, and antivenins to provide immunity against diseases.
4. Distinguish preadministration and ongoing assessments the nurse should perform, with the client receiving an immunologic agent.
5. Identify nursing diagnoses particular to a client receiving an immunologic agent.
6. Examine ways to promote an optimal response, management of common adverse reactions, special considerations, and important points to keep in mind when educating a client taking an immunologic agent.

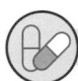

Drug Classes

Active immunity agents
- Vaccines, bacterial and viral
- Toxoids

Passive immunity agents
- Immune globulins
- Antivenins

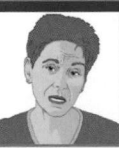

PHARMACOLOGY IN PRACTICE

Betty Peterson's niece, Rebecca, has been staying with Betty since Rebecca was laid off from her job. Rebecca has a young infant son, 4-month-old Jimmy. Rebecca received health insurance from her previous employer, but now that she is unemployed, she is taking her baby to the local health clinic. She is embarrassed because she misplaced the immunization information and cannot remember if he is due for any immunizations or which ones come next. Determine where he is in the immunization schedules assuming he is up to date with these.

mmunity refers to the ability of the body to identify and resist microorganisms that are potentially harmful. This ability enables the body to fight or prevent infectious disease and inhibit tissue and organ damage. Illustrated in Figure 47.1 are the branches of innate and adaptive immunity. This chapter discusses components that influence adaptive immunity; specifically vaccines that help the body to boost this process of gaining immunity.

The immune system is not confined to any one part of the body. Immune stem cells, formed in the bone marrow, may remain in the bone marrow until maturation, or they may migrate to different body sites

Cells of the immune system

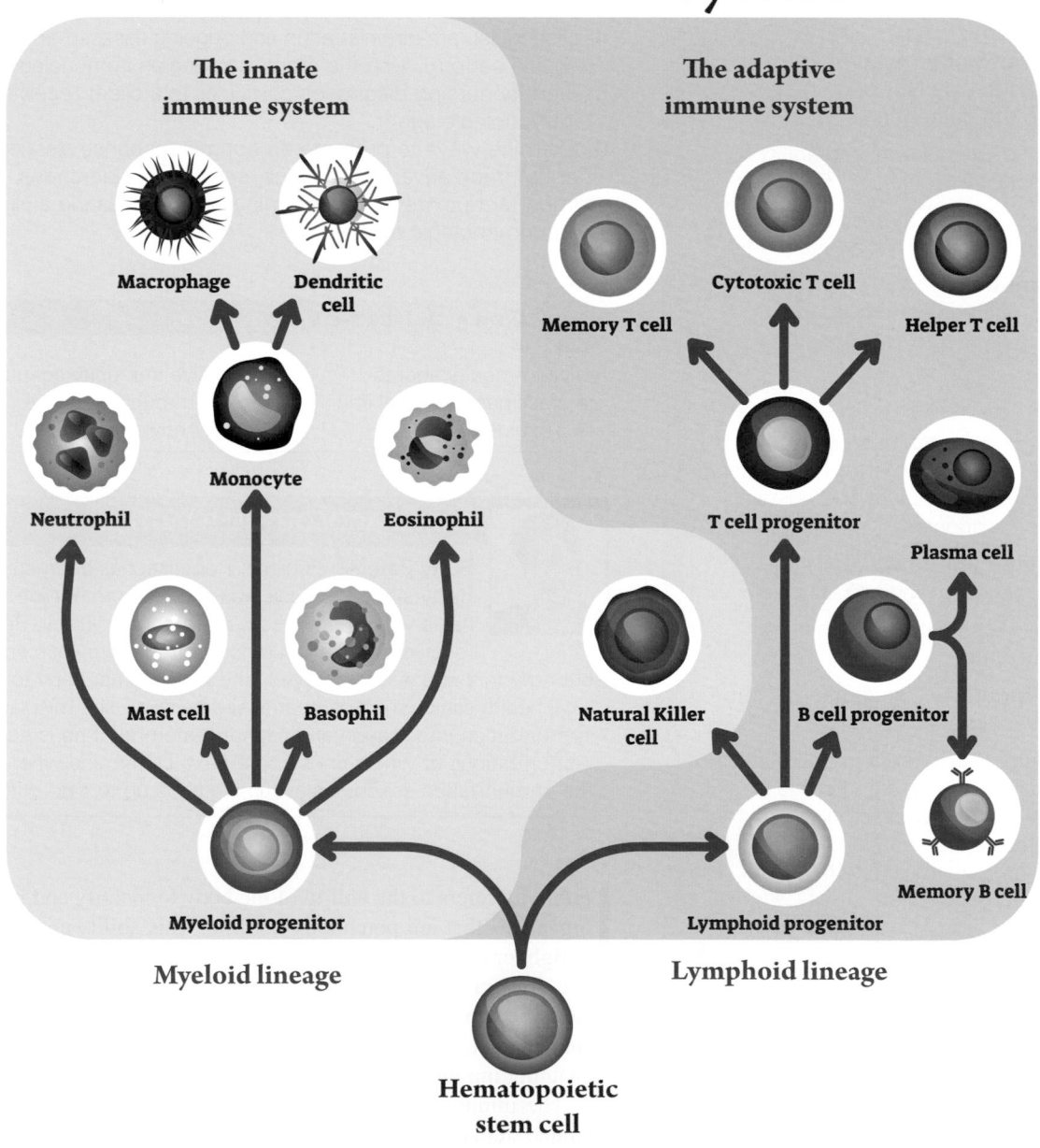

FIGURE 47.1 Innate and adaptive immune systems.

where they mature. After maturation, most immune cells circulate in the body and exert specific effects. The adaptive immunity has two distinct, but overlapping, mechanisms with which to fight invading organisms:

- Cell-mediated defenses (cell-mediated immunity)
- Antibody-mediated defenses (humoral immunity)

CELL-MEDIATED IMMUNITY (T CELLS)

Cell-mediated immunity (CMI) results from the activity of many leukocyte actions. This type of immunity is dependent upon the actions of the *T lymphocytes,* which are responsible for a delayed type of immune response. The T lymphocytes defend against viral infections, fungal infections, and some bacterial infections as described in the following:

- The T lymphocyte becomes sensitized by its first contact with a specific **antigen** (substance that elicits a specific immune response).
- Subsequent exposure to an antigen stimulates multiple reactions aimed at destroying or inactivating the offending antigen.
- T lymphocytes and macrophages (large cells that surround, engulf, and digest microorganisms and cellular debris) work together in CMI to destroy the antigen.
- T lymphocytes attack the antigens directly, rather than produce antibodies (as is done in humoral immunity). Cellular reactions may also occur without macrophages.

If CMI is reduced, as in the case of acquired immunodeficiency syndrome (AIDS), the body is unable to protect itself against many viral, bacterial, and fungal infections.

HUMORAL IMMUNITY (B CELLS)

Humoral immunity protects the body against bacterial and viral infections. Special lymphocytes (white blood cells), called *B lymphocytes,* produce circulating antibodies to act against a foreign substance. This type of immunity is based on the **antigen–antibody response**. An **antigen** is a substance, usually a protein, that stimulates the body to produce antibodies. An **antibody** is a globulin (protein) produced by the B lymphocytes as a defense against an antigen.

Specific antibodies are formed for specific antigens; for example, chickenpox antibodies are formed when the person is exposed to the chickenpox (varicella) virus (the antigen). Once manufactured, antibodies circulate in the bloodstream, sometimes only for a short time, but in other cases, for the lifetime of the person. When an antigen enters the body, specific antibodies neutralize the invading antigen; this condition is called **immunity**. Thus the individual with specific circulating antibodies is immune (or has immunity) to a specific antigen. Immunity is the resistance that an individual has against diseases.

CMI and humoral immunity are interdependent; CMI influences the function of the T lymphocytes and humoral immunity influences the function of the B lymphocytes.

ACTIVE AND PASSIVE IMMUNITY

Active and passive immunity involve the use of agents that stimulate antibody formation (active immunity) or the injection of ready-made antibodies found in the serum of immune individuals or animals (passive immunity). Figure 47.2 demonstrates a visual depiction of this process.

Active Immunity

When a person is exposed to certain infectious microorganisms (the source of antigens), the body actively builds an immunity (forms antibodies) to the invading pathogen. This is called **active immunity**. There are two types of active immunity: (1) naturally acquired active immunity and (2) artificially acquired active immunity. The Summary Drug Table: Immunization Agents identifies agents that produce active immunity.

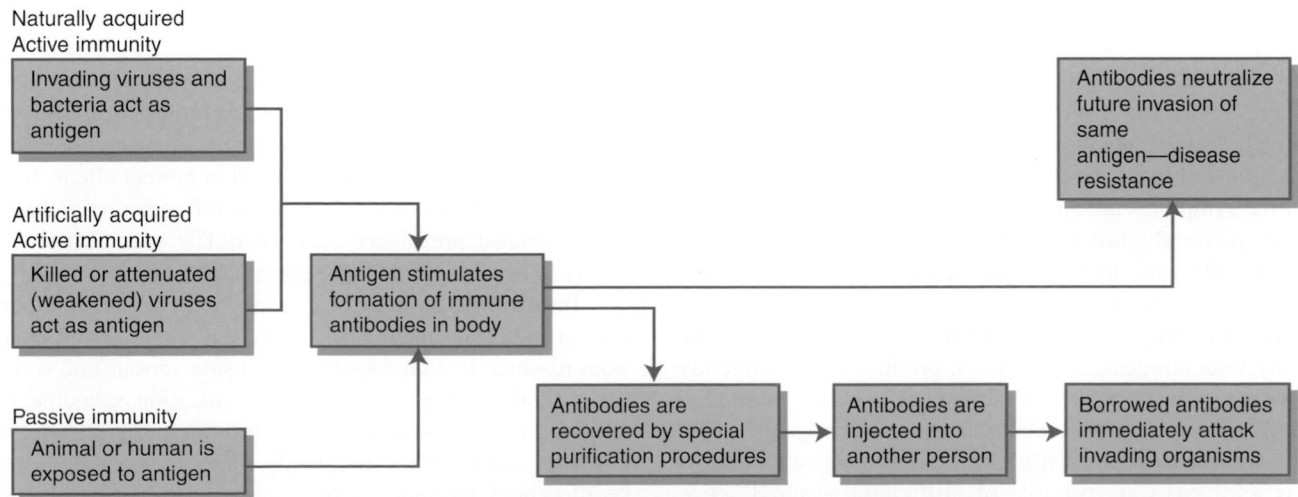

FIGURE 47.2 Active and passive immunity.

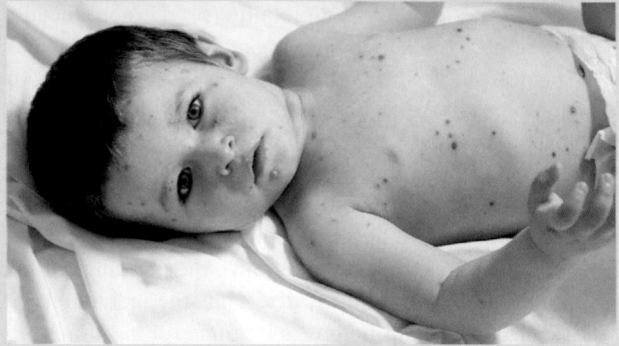

Naturally acquired active immunity is exemplified by an individual who is exposed to chickenpox (varicella virus) for the first time and who has no immunity to the disease. The body immediately begins to manufacture antibodies against the varicella virus. However, the production of a sufficient quantity of antibodies takes time and the individual gets the disease. At the time of exposure and while the individual still has chickenpox, the body continues to manufacture antibodies. These antibodies circulate in the individual's bloodstream for life. In the future, any exposure to the varicella virus results in the antibodies mobilizing to destroy the invading antigen.

Naturally Acquired Active Immunity

Naturally acquired active immunity occurs when the person is exposed to and experiences a disease and the body manufactures antibodies to provide future immunity to the disease. This is called *active immunity* because the antibodies are produced by the person who had *active* disease, such as a child who is sick with the chickenpox. Thus, having the disease produces immunity. Box 47.1 describes an example of naturally acquired active immunity.

Artificially Acquired Active Immunity

Artificially acquired active immunity occurs when an individual is given a killed or weakened viral antigen, which stimulates the formation of antibodies against the antigen. The antigen does not cause the disease, but the individual still manufactures specific antibodies against the disease. When a **vaccine** containing an **attenuated** (weakened) antigen is given, the individual may experience a few minor symptoms of the disease or even a mild form of the disease, but the symptoms are almost always milder than the disease itself and usually last for a short time.

The decision to use an attenuated rather than a killed virus as a vaccine to provide immunity is based on research in the laboratory to see what form is effective on the virus. Many viral antigens, when killed, produce a poor antibody response, whereas when the antigen is merely weakened, a good antibody response occurs. Immunization against a specific disease provides artificially acquired active immunity. Box 47.2 gives an example of artificially acquired active immunity.

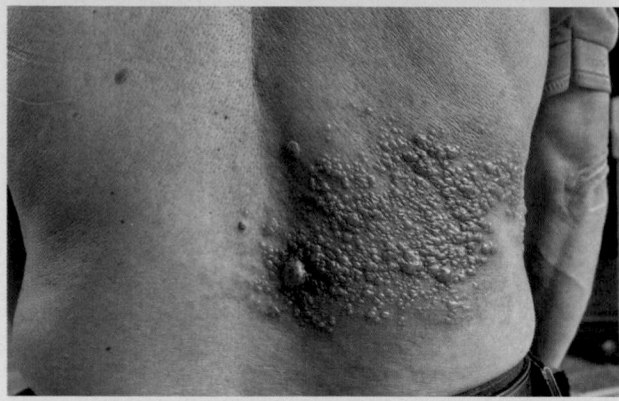

Although chickenpox may seem like a minor illness, later in life, it can cause herpes zoster (shingles), a painful condition. Once infected, the virus remains dormant in the nervous system. An example of the use of an attenuated virus is the administration of the varicella virus vaccine to an individual who has *not* had chickenpox (or to boost the immunity of a person who did have the disease) to prevent them from getting shingles. The varicella (chickenpox) vaccine contains the live, attenuated varicella virus. The individual receiving the vaccine develops a mild or modified chickenpox infection, which then produces immunity against the varicella virus. The varicella vaccine protects the recipient for several years or, in some individuals, for life.

Artificially acquired immunity against some diseases may require periodic **booster** injections to keep an adequate antibody level (or antibody titer) circulating in the blood. A booster injection is the administration of an additional dose of the vaccine to boost the production of antibodies to a level that will maintain the desired immunity. The booster is given months or years after the initial vaccine and may be needed because the life of some antibodies is short. An example of a killed virus used for immunization booster is the yearly influenza vaccine. These vaccines protect those who receive the vaccine for about 3–6 months. This is why they are given yearly. When given yearly, the configuration of the vaccine can be different so as to protect from the predominant strains of the virus for that specific year. For example, the influenza vaccine is designed to protect clients from three to four different viral strains of influenza predicted to be of greatest prevalence each year. The vaccine changes yearly to accommodate those specific strains.

Immunization is a form of artificial active immunity and an important method of controlling some of the infectious diseases that are capable of causing serious and sometimes fatal consequences. The immunization schedule for children, teenagers, and adults is provided in Appendix C. Changes can be made frequently to these schedules. It is best to check the most current immunization schedules for this and other age groups and late-start schedules, all of which can be obtained from the Centers for Disease Control and Prevention (CDC) website at http://www.cdc.gov/vaccines/. Currently, many infectious diseases may be prevented by vaccines (artificial active immunity). Examples of some of these diseases can be found in Box 47.3.

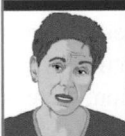

Passive Immunity

Passive immunity occurs when **immune globulins** or antivenins are administered. This type of immunity provides the individual with ready-made antibodies from another human or an animal (see Fig. 47.2). Passive immunity provides immediate immunity to the invading antigen but lasts for only a short time. Box 47.4 provides an example of passive immunity.

VACCINES AND TOXOIDS

Some immunologic agents capitalize on the body's natural defenses by stimulating the immune response, thereby creating protection against a specific disease within the body. Other immunologic agents supply ready-made antibodies to provide passive immunity. Examples of immunologic agents include vaccines, toxoids, and immune globulins.

ACTIONS AND USES

Antibody-producing tissues cannot distinguish between an antigen that is capable of causing disease (a live antigen), an attenuated antigen, or a killed antigen. Because of this phenomenon, vaccines, which contain either an attenuated or a killed antigen, have been developed to create immunity to certain diseases. The live antigens are either killed or weakened during the manufacturing process. The weakened or killed antigens contained in the vaccine do not have sufficient strength to cause disease. Although it is a rare occurrence, vaccination with any vaccine may not result in a protective antibody response in all individuals given the vaccine.

A toxin is a poisonous substance produced by a bacterium (such as *Clostridium tetani,* the bacterium that causes tetanus). A toxin is capable of stimulating the body to produce antitoxins, which are substances that act in the same manner as antibodies. Toxins are powerful substances and, like other antigens, they can be attenuated. A toxin that is attenuated (or weakened) but still capable of stimulating the formation of antitoxins is called a toxoid.

Both vaccines and toxoids are administered to stimulate the body's immune response to specific antigens or toxins. These agents must be administered before exposure to the disease-causing organism. The initiation of the immune response, in turn, produces resistance to a specific infectious disease. The immunity produced in this manner is active immunity.

Vaccines and toxoids are used for the following:

- Routine immunization of infants and children
- Immunization of adults against tetanus
- Immunization of adults at high risk for certain diseases (e.g., pneumococcal and influenza vaccines)
- Immunization of children or adults at risk for exposure to a particular disease (e.g., hepatitis A for those going to endemic areas)
- Immunization of prepubertal girls or nonpregnant women of childbearing age against rubella.

Gerontology

As individuals age, so does their immune system. Fewer antibodies are produced compared with a younger person, even after vaccinated. Fluzone High-Dose is an influenza vaccine with four times the amount of antigen than a normal vaccine dose. The greater amount of antigen is designed to boost the immune system higher and is recommended for clients over the age of 65 years. You may hear both clients and providers refer to this as the *Super Flu Vaccine*.

ADVERSE REACTIONS

Adverse reactions from the administration of vaccines or toxoids are usually mild. Chills, fever, muscular aches and pains, rash, and lethargy may be present. Pain and tenderness at the injection site may also occur. Although rare, a hypersensitivity reaction may occur. Some people concerned with egg allergies have refused vaccination. For these individuals, many of the routine vaccines, such as the yearly influenza vaccine, have an alternative preparation that is not made with eggs. The Summary Drug Table: Immunization Agents provides a listing of the typical adverse reactions.

CONTRAINDICATIONS AND PRECAUTIONS

Immunologic agents are contraindicated in clients with known hypersensitivity to the agent or any component of it. Allergy to eggs is a concern with some vaccines. It is recommended to see a primary health care provider familiar with egg allergies for vaccination if an allergy is suspected. Some people with "hive-only" reactions are able to tolerate vaccines without a problem (ACIP, 2012). The measles, mumps, rubella, and varicella vaccines are contraindicated in clients who have had an allergic reaction to gelatin, neomycin, or a previous dose of one of the vaccines. The measles, mumps, rubella, and varicella vaccines are contraindicated during pregnancy, especially during the first trimester, because of the danger of birth defects. Women are instructed to avoid becoming pregnant at least 3 months after receiving these vaccines. Vaccines and toxoids are contraindicated during acute febrile illnesses, leukemia, lymphoma, immunosuppressive illness or drug therapy, and nonlocalized cancer. Always ask about allergy history before preparing a vaccine for administration. See Box 47.5 for additional information on the contraindications to immunologic agents.

Owing to the possible reoccurrence of herpes zoster, adults with a history of shingles should receive a dose of the recombinant zoster vaccine (RZV). The Advisory Committee for Immunization Practices states

---

BOX 47.5   Contraindications to Immunization

- Moderate or severe illness, with or without fever.
- Anaphylactoid reactions (e.g., hives, swelling of the mouth and throat, difficulty breathing [dyspnea], hypotension, and shock).
- Known allergy to vaccine or vaccine constituents, particularly gelatin, eggs, or neomycin.
- Individuals with an immunologic deficiency should not receive a vaccine (virus is transmissible to the immunocompromised individual).
- Immunizations are postponed during the administration of steroids, radiation therapy, and antineoplastic (anticancer) drug therapy.
- Viral vaccines against measles, rubella, and mumps should not be given to pregnant women.
- Clients who experience severe systemic or neurologic reactions after a previous dose of the vaccine should not be given any additional doses.

---

that RZV may be used in adults aged 50 years or older, regardless of prior receipt of live zoster vaccine (ZVL), and does not require screening for a history of chickenpox (varicella). Clients with the acute stage of herpes zoster should delay vaccination until symptoms subside.

INTERACTIONS

Vaccinations containing live organisms are not administered within 3 months of immune globulin administration because antibodies in the globulin preparation may interfere with the immune response to the vaccination. Corticosteroids, antineoplastic drugs, and radiation therapy depress the immune system to such a degree that insufficient numbers of antibodies are produced to prevent the disease. When the salicylates are administered with the varicella vaccination, there is an increased risk of Reye syndrome developing (Box 47.6).

IMMUNE GLOBULINS AND ANTIVENINS

ACTIONS AND USES

Globulins are proteins present in blood serum or plasma that contains antibodies. *Immune globulins* are solutions obtained from human or animal blood containing antibodies that have been formed by the body to specific antigens. Because they contain ready-made antibodies, they are given for passive immunity against a disease. The immune globulins are administered to provide passive immunization to one or more infectious diseases. Those receiving immune globulins receive antibodies only to the diseases to which the donor blood is immune. The onset of protection is rapid but of short duration (1–3 months).

BOX 47.6   Covid-19 and the Pandemic of 2020

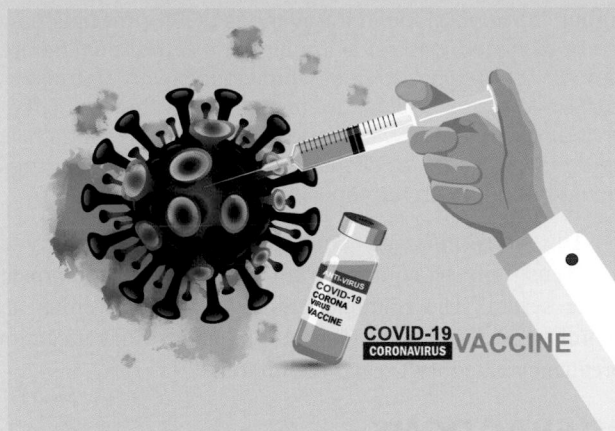

2020 was a trying year of infection, isolation, exhaustion, and for some extreme loneliness. This was also the year the public learned more about immunity, messenger RNA (mRNA), and vaccinations than in any other time in the 21st century.

The COVID-19 vaccines are currently the only mRNA vaccines licensed in the United States. However, researchers have been studying how to make mRNA vaccines for decades (Joseph, 2020). The vaccines take advantage of the process that cells use to make proteins. In comparison, most vaccines use weakened or inactivated components of the microorganism to stimulate the body's immune response to create antibodies. These vaccines use mRNA to trigger an immune response and build immunity to SARS-CoV-2, the virus that causes COVID-19 (CDC, 2021).

The use of cellular components, like mRNA, was developed decades ago to kill bacterial cells. As explained in Chapter 8, antibacterial agents are administered that interfere with the protein (*synthesis*) in the bacterial cell, which in turn kills the bacterial cell. As explained in Unit 2, new cells are made when

DNA strands unravel and messages are made with strands of mRNA, telling the cell how to build amino acids. The message is translated by ribosomes to make the string of amino acids that becomes a protein. As in the case of antibacterial drugs, they interfere with the process of protein synthesis, and the amino acids do not link together to make the protein and eventually the cell dies.

In contrast, the vaccine itself is a strand of mRNA in an injectable form. The message when injected as the vaccine is the "how to" instructions to make the unique protein spikes of the SARS-CoV-2 virus. As a result, the body's immune system is triggered to respond to the spiked protein (not the entire virus) and produce antibodies to fight off the assumed infection. This works because the virus has to use the Corona Spike to attach to a normal cell; as a result the vaccine has produced antibodies and activates our T cells to recognize and respond to the spike before it can attach. Lastly, the injected mRNA is broken down in the cell by enzymes and leaves the cell like other cellular waste products (CDC, 2021).

People are tentative about a vaccine that came about so quickly. The mumps vaccine was considered the vaccine with the most rapid development (4 years) cycle before the pandemic (Solis-Moreira, 2020). Although it seems like only a year at most, researchers have been studying the use of mRNA in pharmacology and immunity for a number of years. The earliest stages of clinical trials using mRNA vaccines have been carried out for other viruses, including influenza, Zika, rabies, and cytomegalovirus (Joseph, 2020).

By increasing funding, allowing development and clinical testing to move in tandem rather than sequentially, and emergency use of the vaccine granted, we are able to provide the ability to vaccinate worldwide at record speed (Solis-Moreira, 2020). As a result, we may see more vaccines developed and produced in a more rapid manner.

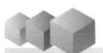 *Concept Mastery Alert*

Immune globulin or antivenin administration produces passive immunity for the client.

Antivenins are used for passive, transient protection from the toxic effects of bites by spiders (black widow and similar spiders) and snakes (rattlesnake, copperhead and cottonmouth, and coral). The most effective response is obtained when the drug is administered within 4 hr after exposure.

ADVERSE REACTIONS

Adverse reactions to immune globulins are rare. However, local tenderness and pain at the injection site may occur. The most common adverse reactions include urticaria, angioedema, erythema, malaise, nausea, diarrhea, headache, chills, and fever. Adverse reactions, if they occur, may last for several hours. Systemic reactions are extremely rare, with the exception of immune globulins given to prevent posttransplant rejection. These immune globulins are made from equine (horse) or rabbit serum and can produce anaphylactic reactions. They should be administered only under the direction of a physician specializing in transplantation medicine.

The antivenins may cause various reactions, with hypersensitivity being the most severe. Some antivenins are prepared from equine serum, and if a client is sensitive to equine serum, serious reactions or death may result. The immediate reactions usually occur within 30 min after administration of the antivenin. Symptoms include apprehension; flushing; itching; urticaria; edema of the face, tongue, and throat; cough; dyspnea; vomiting;

cyanosis; and collapse. Other adverse reactions are included in the Summary Drug Table: Immunization Agents.

CONTRAINDICATIONS AND PRECAUTIONS

Immunologic agents are used with extreme caution in individuals with a history of allergies. Sensitivity testing may be performed in individuals with a history of allergies. Because of the potential harm to a fetus, no adequate studies have been conducted in pregnant women, and it is also not known whether these agents are excreted in breast milk. Thus the immunologic agents (pregnancy category C) are used with caution in pregnant women and during lactation.

The immune globulins are contraindicated in clients with a history of allergic reactions after administration of human immunoglobulin preparations and in individuals with isolated immunoglobulin A (IgA) deficiency (individuals could have an anaphylactic reaction to subsequent administration of blood products that contain IgA).

 Chronic Care Considerations

Human immune globulin intravenous (IGIV) products have been associated with renal impairment, acute renal failure, osmotic nephrosis, and death. Individuals with a predisposition to acute renal failure (e.g., those with preexisting renal disease), those with diabetes mellitus, individuals older than 65 years, or clients receiving nephrotoxic drugs should not be given human IGIV products.

The antivenins are contraindicated in clients with hypersensitivity to equine serum or any other component of the serum. The immune globulins and antivenins are administered cautiously during pregnancy and lactation (pregnancy category C) and in children.

INTERACTIONS

Antibodies in the immune globulin preparations may interfere with the immune response to live virus vaccines, particularly measles, but including others such as mumps and rubella. It is recommended that the live virus vaccines be administered 14–30 days before or 6–12 weeks after the administration of immune globulins. No known interactions have been reported with antivenins.

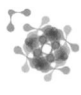 **NURSING PROCESS: STEPS TO BUILDING CLINICAL JUDGMENT**
Client Receiving a Vaccine

ASSESSMENT

Preadministration Assessment
Data gathering suggestions before vaccine administered include the following:
Objective data

- General client appearance.
- Vital signs (temperature, pulse, respirations, and blood pressure).

Subjective data

- Previous vaccine history.
- Basic medical history, e.g., cancer, leukemia, lymphoma, immunosuppressive drug therapy.
- Allergy history.

Some vaccines contain antibodies obtained from animals, whereas other vaccines may contain proteins or preservatives to which an individual may be allergic. A highly allergic person may have an allergic reaction that could be serious and even fatal. If the client has an allergy history, the primary health care provider may decide to perform skin tests for allergy to one or more of the components or proteins in the vaccine. You should also scan the record or ask the client about any conditions that contraindicate the administration of the agent.

Ongoing Assessment
The client is usually not hospitalized after administration of an immunologic agent (with the exception of transplant recipients). However, the client may be asked to stay in the clinic or office for observation for about 30 min after the injection to observe for any signs of hypersensitivity (e.g., laryngeal edema, hives, pruritus, angioneurotic edema, and severe dyspnea; see Chapter 1 for additional information). Emergency resuscitation equipment is kept available to be used in the event of a severe hypersensitivity reaction.

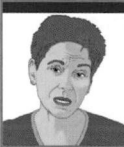 **PHARMACOLOGY IN PRACTICE**

SAFE DRUG ADMINISTRATION
A client is advised to stay in the clinic for observation for about 30 min after administering an immunologic agent. Which of the following signs should a nurse assess for to identify a hypersensitivity reaction? Select all that apply.

1. Pruritus
2. Laryngeal edema
3. Dyspnea
4. Renal failure
5. Convulsions

NURSING DIAGNOSES

Drug-specific nursing diagnoses include the following:

- **Acute pain** related to adverse reactions (pain and discomfort at the injection site, muscular aches and pain).
- **Altered health seeking behavior** related to the timing of immunization schedule.

Nursing diagnoses related to drug administration are discussed in Chapter 4.

PLANNING

The expected outcomes of the client may include an optimal response to the immunologic agent, support of client needs related to the management of common adverse drug effects, and confidence in an understanding of and adherence to the prescribed immunization schedule.

IMPLEMENTATION

Promoting an Optimal Response to Therapy

! NURSING ALERT

Most vaccine preparations require refrigeration. Always have a backup plan for storage of the vaccine should the health care facility lose power. Temperature fluctuations can harm the vaccines.

If a vaccine is not in a liquid form and must be reconstituted, then read the directions enclosed with the vaccine for reconstitution. It is important to follow the enclosed directions carefully to ensure proper action of the vaccine. Package inserts also contain information regarding dosage, adverse reactions, method of administration, and administration sites (when appropriate), as well as, when needed, recommended booster schedules.

Multiple Vaccines at One Visit

Forty years ago, children received five vaccines (about eight injections) by the age of 2 years. At the turn of the century that number became 11 vaccines given in 20 injections by age 2 years (Offit, 2002). Currently, by 6 years of age a child will receive 14 vaccines in almost 50 doses (NVIC, 2016). This amounts to receiving up to seven injections during a single office visit (Fig. 47.3).

Many manufacturers are preparing combination products to reduce the number of injections during the vaccination process. Examples include the measles, mumps, and rubella (MMR) vaccine; the diphtheria, tetanus, and pertussis (DTaP) vaccine; and the *Haemophilus* b (TriHIBit) vaccine. Even with these combination injections, infants and small children will continue to take multiple injections, which may cause distress for both children and parents. This distress can lead to delay in recommended vaccinations. Taddio (2015) describes a number of interventions nurses can use to reduce this distress, which include the following:

- Do not aspirate intramuscular (IM) vaccines.
- Give the most painful injection last.
- Use a pacifier during the procedure, if less than 2 years old (be sure all orals are given before).

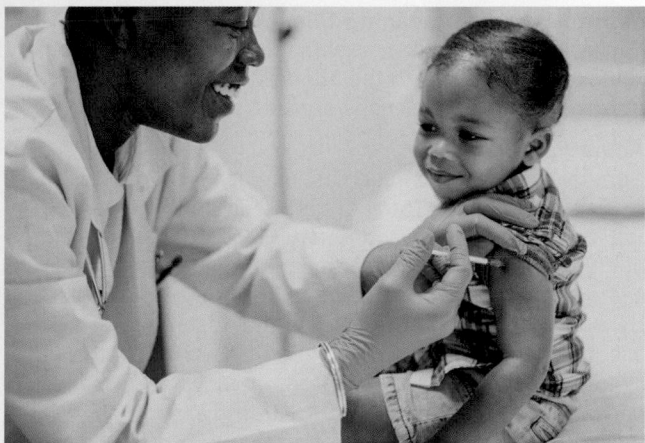

FIGURE 47.3 Swift and diligent actions on the part of the nurse during pediatric immunization will reduce parental anxiety; thus, promoting a successful outcome will help in maintaining adherence to vaccination schedules.

- Parent should be present and should hold the child; if the child is older than 3 years have them sit upright.
- Use a topical anesthetic (needs to be applied by parent before visit).

Delaying Immunization

On occasion, it may be necessary to postpone the regular immunization schedule, particularly for children. This is of special concern to parents. The decision to delay immunization because of illness or for other reasons must be discussed with the primary health care provider. However, the decision to administer or delay vaccination because of febrile illness (illness causing an elevated temperature) depends on the severity of the symptoms and the specific disorder. In general, all vaccines can be administered to those with minor illnesses, such as a cold, and to those with a low-grade fever. However, moderate or severe illness is a temporary contraindication. In instances of moderate or severe illness, vaccination is done as soon as the acute phase of the illness is over. Box 47.5 lists general contraindications to immunizations. Specific contraindications and precautions may be found in the package insert that comes with the drug or at the website of the Immunization Action Coalition (www.immunize.org).

Documentation of Immunization

State agencies, drug companies, and immunization organizations all provide standardized forms for parents or caregivers to document immunization history. In addition to your facility documentation provide or record in the document the following information presented by the parent or caregiver:

- Date of vaccination.
- Route and site, vaccine type, manufacturer.
- Lot number and expiration date.
- Name, address, and title of the individual administering the vaccine.
- Be sure to write down when to return if a booster is indicated.

Monitoring and Managing Client Needs

Minor adverse reactions, such as fever, rashes, and aching joints, are possible with the administration of a vaccine. In most cases, these reactions subside within 48 hr.

Acute Pain

General interventions, such as increasing the fluids in the diet, allowing for adequate rest, and keeping the atmosphere quiet and nonstimulating, may be beneficial. The primary health care provider may prescribe acetaminophen, every 4 hr, to control these reactions. Using the dominant arm helps in the absorption of the injection. Also, during the injection, aspiration of the syringe contents is not indicated for vaccines. Schedule pediatric clients when staffing patterns allow for more than one nurse to assist so that two nurses can inject opposite limbs simultaneously. Topical numbing preparations are available, yet they often require parents to apply the agent before coming to the clinic. This can add stress for the parent by adding one more item to do in preparing for the visit, especially if they have minimal help at home. If local irritation at the injection site occurs, it can be treated with warm or cool compresses, depending on the client's preference. A lump may be palpated at the injection site after a DTaP vaccination or other immunization. This is not abnormal and resolves itself within several days to weeks.

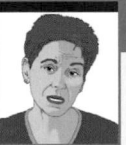

PHARMACOLOGY IN PRACTICE

MANAGING NEEDS

A child complains of pain at the injection site following the administration of the measles vaccine. Which of the following interventions should a nurse instruct the parent to implement for pain management following vaccine administration? Select all that apply.

1. Administer acetaminophen
2. Massage the injection site
3. Decrease fluid intake
4. Encourage adequate rest
5. Apply heat

Altered Health Seeking Behavior

Parents may seek your advice and counsel about vaccinations, especially regarding their fears of harm vs. protection to their child. This is your opportunity to advocate and educate the public about the advantages of immunization. Parents are encouraged to have infants and young children immunized as suggested by the Advisory Committee on Immunization Practices. These schedules are updated and published yearly; an example is provided in Appendix C. The CDC Immunization website offers downloadable personalized plans for the technology-minded parent. When the parents do not bring in a form or booklet to record the immunization, you should provide the parents with a copy of the record of immunizations. This is especially helpful if multiple providers will be involved in the immunization schedule.

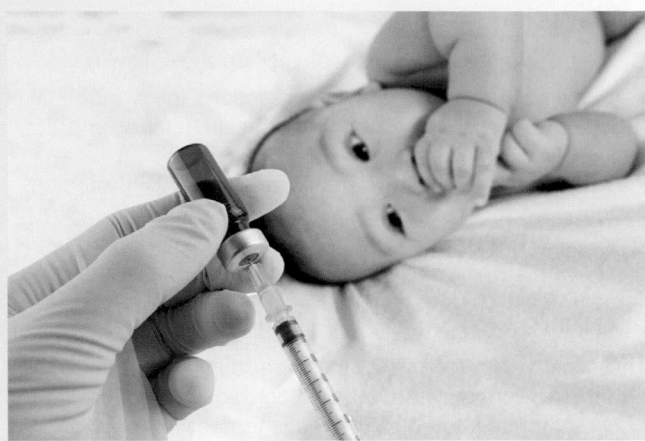

FIGURE 47.4 By maintaining adherence to immunization schedules, children enjoy healthy lives free of debilitating communicable diseases.

Because evidence of immunization is required by schools (even at the college level), the record provided to parents by the provider is even more important. Records can be downloaded regarding both information about immunizations and copies of blank record-keeping sheets from the CDC website or the Immunization Action Coalition. This helps empower the parent(s) caring for the child, making adherence to the routine immunization schedule likely (Fig. 47.4).

ⓘ NURSING ALERT

In most cases, the risk of serious adverse reactions from an immunization is much smaller than the risk of contracting the disease for which the immunizing agent is given.

Vaccine Reaction and Fear

Parents are sometimes concerned about serious adverse reactions that can harm a child following an immunization. Much of this fear stems from the widely publicized results of a study published in 1998 by Andrew Wakefield, a physician, making a correlation between autism and the MMR vaccine. This was also during the time when social media was developing, and his findings were circulated worldwide by celebrities as well as aired on television almost daily. This study was found to be fraudulent and Wakefield lost his license to practice medicine. Yet, individuals remain fearful of the adverse reactions of immunizations. Although the number of these incidents is small, a risk factor still remains when some vaccines are given.

Well-meaning parents want their children to be protected, yet they are fearful of stories they have heard about vaccines, many of which are given for diseases they have never seen. It is important for the parents to understand the risk associated with not receiving immunization against infectious diseases. The risk may be higher than and just as serious as the risk associated with the use of vaccines. Keep in mind that when a large segment of the population is immunized, the few not immunized are less likely to be exposed to and be infected with the disease-producing microorganism—they benefit from what is termed *herd immunity* (Quarles et al., 2002). However, when large numbers of the population are not immunized, there is a great increase in the chances of exposure to the infectious disease and a significant increase in the probability that the individual will experience the disease.

Educating the Client and Family

When an adult or child is receiving a vaccine for immunization explain to the client or a family member the possible reactions that may occur, such as soreness at the injection site or fever.

Advise those traveling to a foreign country to consult their primary health care provider or the CDC website well in advance of their departure date for information about the immunizations that will be needed. Some clinics specialize in overseas travel, as immunizations should be given well in advance of departure and it may take several weeks to produce adequate immunity.

Encourage the parents or guardians to become educated and advocate for their child's safety. Refer to the Immunization Action Coalition for information on both for and against immunization and learn the adverse reactions or serious adverse events that may occur after administration of a vaccine. Build trust and confidence in the parent or caregiver to discuss concerns that may make it necessary to report the event to the Vaccine Adverse Event Reporting System (VAERS) (Box 47.7).

The following list summarizes the information to be included when educating the parents of a child receiving a vaccine:

- Discuss briefly the risks of contracting vaccine-preventable diseases and the benefits of immunization.
- Instruct the parents to bring immunization records to all visits.
- Provide the date of return for the next vaccination with reminder mail or telephone messages.
- Discuss common adverse reactions (e.g., fever, soreness at the injection site) and methods to reduce these reactions (e.g., acetaminophen, warm compresses).
- Instruct the parents to report any unusual or severe adverse reactions after the administration of a vaccine.

BOX 47.7 Vaccine Adverse Event Reporting System

VAERS is a national vaccine safety surveillance program cosponsored by the CDC and the U.S. Food and Drug Administration (FDA). VAERS collects and analyzes information from reports of adverse reactions after immunization. Anyone can report to VAERS. Reports are sent in by vaccine manufacturers, health care providers, and vaccine recipients and their parents or guardians. Any clinically significant adverse event that occurs after the administration of any vaccine should be reported. Individuals are encouraged to provide the information on the form even if the individual is uncertain whether the event was related to the immunization. A copy of the form can be obtained by calling 1-800-822-7967 or by submitting the information through the Internet at http://www.vaers.hhs.gov/.

EVALUATION

- Therapeutic effect is achieved, and the disease for which immunization is given does not present itself.
- Adverse reactions are identified, reported to the primary health care provider, and managed successfully with appropriate nursing interventions:
  - Acute injection pain is managed successfully.
  - Client or parents/guardians adhere to the immunization schedule.
- Client and family express confidence and demonstrate an understanding of the drug regimen.

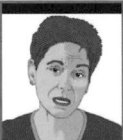

PHARMACOLOGY IN PRACTICE

USING CLINICAL REASONING

Jimmy Peterson, aged 4 months, has a slight cold with a runny nose when he comes for his regular well-baby checkup. His mother tells you that because Jimmy is sick, she does not think he needs his immunization at this time. She says that she will bring him in next month for the shot. Looking over his records, you see that the family has no insurance at this time and has to pay out of pocket for all visits and vaccinations. Analyze the situation to determine the best response to Jimmy's mother. Discuss any assessments that you think would be important to make before giving your response.

KEY POINTS

■ Immunity is the body's ability to identify and resist potentially harmful microorganisms. There are two types of immunity: cell mediated and antibody mediated.

■ CMI involves the T lymphocytes. When exposed to an antigen, the T cells become sensitized and subsequent exposures stimulate a reaction to destroy the offending antigen.

■ Antibody-mediated immunity involves the B lymphocytes and is referred to as humoral immunity. When exposed to an antigen, the B cells produce antibodies as a defense against the offending antigen.

■ The active and passive immunity of vaccinations focus on the antibody-mediated immunity. Since the advent of immunization, many childhood diseases have become almost non-existent (such as polio) and adults can be protected from conditions that can make them severely ill (such as the flu or shingles).

■ Adverse reactions typically are minor, yet sensational stories have made some parents or caregivers fearful of the dangers of immunization in comparison with the affliction itself.

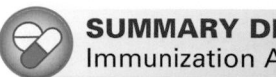

SUMMARY DRUG TABLE
Immunization Agents

Generic Drug	Trade Name	Uses	Adverse Reactions	Dosage Ranges
Agents for Active Immunity				
Vaccines, Bacterial (Routine Immunization)				
***Haemophilus influenzae* type b conjugate** *he-MOF-fi-lus in-floo-EN-zah*	ActHIB, Hiberix, PedvaxHIB	Routine immunization of children	Rare; minor local reactions such as local tenderness, pain at injection site, anorexia, fever, myalgia	0.5 mL IM, see immunization schedule
meningococcal *me-NIN-joe-kok-al*	Menactra, MenQuadfi, Menveo	Routine immunization of adolescents	Same as *H. influenzae* vaccine	0.5 mL subcut only
meningococcal B *me-NIN-joe-kok-al*	Bexsero, Trumenba	Routine immunization of ages 10–25 years	Same as *H. influenzae* vaccine	0.5 mL subcut only
pneumococcal (PCV or PPV) *noo-moe-KOK-al*	Pneumovax 23	Routine immunization of children, PPV is recommended for certain high-risk groups who cannot take PCV	Same as *H. influenzae* vaccine	0.5 mL subcut or IM, see immunization schedule
Vaccines, Bacterial (Special Populations)				
anthrax *AN-thraks*	BioThrax	Anthrax prevention pre-/postexposure	Injection site tenderness, redness, burning	0.5 mL IM day 0, day 1, and 6 months
BCG *Bee-see-jee*		Prevention of pulmonary TB in negative, high-risk populations (health care workers, infants and children in high-TB areas)	Same as *H. influenzae* vaccine	0.2–0.3 mL percutaneous, repeat in 2–3 months
pneumococcal 13-valent conjugate	Prevnar 13	Active immunization against *Streptococcus pneumoniae* for infants and toddlers, prevention of otitis media	Rare; minor local reactions such as local tenderness, pain at injection site, decreased appetite, irritability, drowsiness, fever	0.5 mL IM
typhoid *TYE-foyd*	Typhim Vi, Vivotif	Immunization against typhoid	Same as *H. influenzae* vaccine	Oral: total of four capsules 1 week before exposure Parenteral: adults and children 2 years and older, one dose of 0.5 mL IM
Vaccines, Viral (Routine Immunization)				
measles (rubeola), mumps, rubella, and varicella[a] *MEE-zels, mumpz, roo-BEL-a*	MMR II (live), ProQuad (attenuated)	Routine immunization of children	Mild fever, rash, cough, rhinitis	0.5 mL subcut
hepatitis A, inactivated *hep-a-TYE-tis A*	Havrix, Vaqta	Routine immunization of children	Same as measles vaccine	Administered IM; dosage varies with product; see package insert for specific dosages
hepatitis B, recombinant *hep-a-TYE-tis B*	Engerix-B, Recombivax HB	Routine immunization of children	Minor local reactions such as local tenderness, pain at injection site, anorexia, fever, myalgia	Three to four doses of 0.5–2 mL IM

Generic Name	Trade Name	Uses	Adverse Reactions	Dosage Ranges
human papillomavirus (HPV) *YU-man pap-ih-LO-ma VYE-rus*	Cervarix (female), Gardasil (male/female)	Prevention of diseases caused by HPV, genital warts, and certain cancers	Minor local reactions, such as local tenderness, pain at injection site	Three doses of 0.5 mL IM; initial, 2 months, 6 months
influenza A *in-floo-EN-za*	Afluria, FluMist, Fluarix, FluLaval, Fluvirin, Fluzone, Fluzone High Dose (over 65 years)	Active immunization against the specific influenza virus strains contained in the formulation ages 6 months and beyond	Same as measles vaccine	One dose 0.5 mL IM Nasal: one to two doses (FluMist only, may not be used each flu season)
poliovirus, inactivated (IPV) *POE-lee-oh-VYE-rus*	IPOL	Routine immunization of children	Rare; malaise, nausea, diarrhea, fever	0.5 mL IM or subcut; see immunization schedule
varicella *var-i-SEL-a*	Varivax	Routine immunization of children	Minor local reactions, such as local tenderness, pain at injection site, rash, fever, cough, irritability	0.5 mL subcut; see immunization schedule
zoster, recombinant (RZV) *ZOS-ter*	Shingrix	Prevention of shingles in people older than 50 years	Transient pain, erythema, swelling or itching at the injection site	Single dose subcut
Vaccines, Pandemic (Routine Immunization-Emergency Authorization)				
COVID-19 vaccine (mRNA) *CO-vide*	Moderna Covid-19, Pfizer-BioNTech Covid	Prevention of Coronavirus infection caused by SARS-CoV-2 (18 years or older)	Pain, swelling at injection site, muscle pain, chills, headache, fatigue, nausea	0.3–0.5 mL IM two doses given 3–4 weeks apart
COVID-19 adenovirus vector	Janssen Covid-19 (J&J), Sylvant	Prevention of Coronavirus infection caused by SARS-CoV-2 (18 years or older)	Pain, swelling at injection site, muscle pain, chills, headache, fatigue, nausea	0.5 mL IM, single dose; do not premedicate with analgesic/antihistamine
Vaccines, Viral (Special Populations)				
avian influenza (H5N1) *ay'-vee-an in-floo-en'-zah*	Seqirus, Audenz	Active immunization against avian influenza in adults (18–64 years)	Headache, malaise, nausea	Two 1-mL IM doses given 1 month apart
ebola Zaire vaccine *e-BO-luh-za-IR*	Ervebo	Active immunization against Zaire ebolavirus in adults	Pain, redness, swelling at injection site, chills	1-mL IM single dose
rotavirus *ROE-ta-vye-rus*	Rotarix, RotaTeq	Prevention of gastroenteritis caused by rotavirus serotypes contained in the vaccines	Fever, decreased appetite, abdominal cramping, irritability, decreased activity	Three 2.5-mL doses given orally
rabies vaccine *RAY-beez*	Imovax, RabAvert	Prevention of rabies in people with greater risk (e.g., veterinarians, animal handlers, forest rangers); postexposure prophylaxis: bite by an animal suspected of carrying rabies	Transient pain, erythema, swelling or itching at the injection site, headache, nausea, abdominal pain, muscle aches, dizziness	Preexposure prophylaxis: 1 mL IM, see package insert for dosing Postexposure: give vaccine IM after initial immune globulin injection
Toxoids (Routine Immunization)				
diphtheria and tetanus toxoids and acellular pertussis (DtaP) *dif-thair'-ee-ah, tet-ah-nuss tok'-soyds, ay-sell'-yoo-lar per-tuss'-uss*	Daptacel, Infanrix	Active immunization against diphtheria, tetanus, and pertussis	Headache, dizziness, rash, itching, nausea, fever	0.5 mL IM; see immunization schedule

Continued

SUMMARY DRUG TABLE (continued)
Immunization Agents

Generic Name	Trade Name	Uses	Adverse Reactions	Dosage Ranges
Combination Products (Viral/Bacterial Vaccine or Toxoid Together)				
hepatitis A and B combination	Twinrix	Twinrix for those older than 18 years traveling to endemic areas	See individual vaccines	See package insert for specific dosing
Agents for Passive Immunity				
Immune Globulins				
botulism immune globulin (BIG-IV) *BOT-yoo-lism*	BabyBIG	Treatment of infant botulism	Headache, chills, fever	IV administration only; see dosing schedule
cytomegalovirus immune globulin (CMV-IGIV) *sye-toe-meg-a-low-VYE-russ*	CytoGam	Prevention of CMV infection after organ transplant	Injection site: tenderness, pain, muscle stiffness Systemic: headache, chills, fever	See dosing schedule, varies weeks out from transplant
hepatitis B immune globulin (HBIG) *hep-a-TYE-tis*	HepaGam B, Nabi-HB	Prevention of hepatitis B after exposure to the disease (use if not previously immunized)	Same as CMV-IGIV	0.06 mL/kg (3–5 mL) IM
immune globulin (gamma globulin; IgG)	GamaSTAN	Prevention of disease after exposure (use if not previously immunized); hepatitis A, measles (rubeola), varicella, rubella, immunoglobulin deficiency	Same as CMV-IGIV	See dosing schedule, varies for disease
immune globulin intravenous (IGIV)	Octagam, Gammagard, Polygam S/D	Immunodeficiency syndrome, ITP, chronic lymphocytic leukemia, bone marrow transplant, pediatric human immunodeficiency virus infection	Headache, chills, fever	IV administration only; see dosing schedule, varies for disease
lymphocyte immune globulin[b] *lim'-foe-syte*	Atgam	Treatment of rejection after organ transplant, aplastic anemia	Chills, fever, arthralgia	After skin test dose, IV administration only; see dosing schedule, varies for disease
antithymocyte globulin[b]	Thymoglobulin	Treatment of acute rejection after kidney transplant, aplastic anemia	Chills, fever, arthralgia	IV administration only; see dosing schedule
rabies immune globulin (RIG) *RAY-beez*	HyperRAB, Imogam	Prevention of rabies after exposure to the disease (use if not previously immunized)	Same as CMV-IGIV	See dosing schedule
Rh immune globulin (IGIM)	Rhophylac, RhoGAM	Prevention of Rh hemolytic disease after birth	Same as CMV-IGIV	300 mcg (one vial) IM within 72 hr of delivery
Rh immune globulin (IGIV)	WinRho SDF	Suppression of Rh isoimmunization after termination of pregnancy; ITP	Headache, chills, fever	IV administration only; see dosing schedule
Rh immune globulin microdose (IG-microdose)	MICRhoGAM	Suppression of Rh isoimmunization after termination of pregnancy before 12 weeks' gestation	Same as CMV-IGIV	50 mcg (one vial) IM

Generic Name	Trade Name	Uses	Adverse Reactions	Dosage Ranges
respiratory syncytial virus immune globulin (RSV-IGIV) *sin-sish'-al vye'-russ*	RespiGam	Respiratory syncytial virus	Headache, chills, fever	IV administration only; see dosing schedule
tetanus immune globulin (TIG) *tet'-ah-nuss*	HyperTet	Tetanus prophylaxis after injury in clients whose immunization is incomplete or uncertain	Same as CMV-IGIV	250 units IM
varicella-zoster immune globulin (VZIG) *var-ih-sell'-ah zoss'-ter*	Varizig	Prevention of varicella in compromised clients after exposure to the disease (use if not previously immunized)	Same as CMV-IGIV	IM administration only; see dosing schedule
Antivenins				
Crotalidae polyvalent immune Fab *kroe-tal'-ih-day pol-ee-vay'-lent*	CroFab	For treatment of mild to moderate North American rattlesnake bites	Urticaria, rash	See package insert for mixing and administration
antivenin (*Micrurus fulvius*) *an-tee-venn'-in*		Passive transient protection for toxic effects of venoms of coral snake in the United States	Urticaria, rash	See package insert for mixing and administration

[a]The trivalent MMR vaccine is the preferred immunizing agent for most children and adults.
[b]Must be prescribed and administered by specialized physicians.

CHAPTER REVIEW

Know Your Drugs

Clients sometimes know a medication by the brand (or trade) name and not the generic name. To recognize both names, match the brand name with the generic name of the same medication.

Generic Name	Brand Name
1. Chickenpox (varicella)	A. Gardasil
2. HPV vaccine	B. RhoGam
3. Rh+ (immune globulin)	C. Varivax
4. Shingles (varicella-zoster)	D. Shingrix

Calculate Medication Dosages

1. FluLaval (influenza vaccine) is supplied in 5-mL vials. If each injection is 0.5 mL, how many vials will need to be ordered to inoculate 60 people?

Prepare for the NCLEX

RECALL THE FACTS

1. Humoral immunity involves which type of white blood cells?
   1. Macrophages
   2. Basophils
   3. B lymphocytes
   4. T lymphocytes

2. What type of immunity involves injecting ready-made antibodies?
   1. Artificially acquired active immunity
   2. Naturally acquired active immunity
   3. Passive immunity
   4. Cell-mediated immunity

3. When discussing the possibility of adverse reactions after receiving a vaccine, the nurse tells the parents of a young child that _____.
   1. adverse reactions may be severe and the child should be monitored closely for 24 hr
   2. adverse reactions are usually mild
   3. the child will likely experience a hypersensitivity reaction
   4. the most common adverse reaction is a severe headache

4. Which of the following statements made by the client would alert the nurse to a possibility of an allergy to the measles vaccine? "My child is allergic to _____."
   1. gelatin
   2. peanut butter
   3. sugar
   4. corn

5. What type of immunity does an antivenin produce?
   1. Artificially acquired active immunity
   2. Naturally acquired active immunity
   3. Passive immunity
   4. Cell-mediated immunity
6. What type of immunity is produced by the recombinant hepatitis B vaccine?
   1. Artificially acquired active immunity
   2. Naturally acquired active immunity
   3. Passive immunity
   4. Cell-mediated immunity

ANALYZE THE FACTS

7. *The nurse is monitoring a client receiving an intravenous (IV) infusion of respiratory syncytial virus immune globulin (RSV-IGIV). Which of the following symptoms may indicate an early allergic reaction?
   1. Chills
   2. Itching
   3. Soreness at infusion site
   4. Diarrhea

ALTERNATE-FORMAT QUESTIONS

8. Which of the following diseases does the MMR vaccine provide protection against? **Select all that apply.**
   1. Human papillomavirus (HPV) infection
   2. Measles
   3. Chickenpox
   4. Mumps
   5. Rubella

9. Which of the following provides protection against pertussis? **Select all that apply.**
   1. DTaP
   2. DTTd
   3. TriHiBit
   4. Pediarix
   5. Comvax

To check your answers, see Appendix F.

---

*Indicates the question is directly linked to the NCLEX-PN test plan in Appendix G.

WANT TO KNOW MORE? A wide variety of resources are available to enhance your learning and understanding of this chapter.

- Visit **thePoint** for resources such as:
  - NCLEX-Style Student Review Questions
  - Journal Articles
  - Dosage Calculations
  - Drug Monographs
  - Watch and Learn Videos
  - Concepts in Action Animations
- The *Study Guide to Accompany Introductory Clinical Pharmacology,* 12th edition, sold separately, will help you review and apply essential content.
- ✓**PrepU** is available to help students prepare for the NCLEX-PN (Practice Nurse) examination.

Immunostimulants and Immunomodulators

Key Terms

cytokines proteins, which aid cells, signal the immune response and stimulate cells to move to the site of inflammation

erythrocytes red blood cells (RBCs); one of several formed elements in the blood

erythropoiesis process of making RBCs

folinic acid rescue *in chemotherapy,* the technique of administering leucovorin after a large dose of methotrexate, thereby allowing normal cells to survive; also called *leucovorin rescue*

hematopoiesis undifferentiated stem cells are stimulated to become specific blood cells

intrinsic factor substance produced by the cells in the stomach and necessary for the absorption of vitamin B_{12}

iron deficiency anemia condition resulting when the body does not have enough iron to meet its need for iron

leukocytes white blood cells (WBCs)

macrocytic anemia anemia resulting from abnormal formation (enlargement) of erythrocytes

malaise a generalized feeling of discomfort and illness

megakaryocytes precursor cell to the platelets

megaloblastic anemia anemia characterized by large, abnormal, immature erythrocytes circulating in the blood; results from folic acid deficiency

thrombopoiesis formation of platelets (thrombocytes)

Learning Objectives

On completion of this chapter, the student will:

1. Describe how immunity related cells communicate to each other in the body.
2. Explain how interferons are used to treat multiple sclerosis.
3. Describe the function of the different types of blood cells.
4. List the drugs used in the treatment of anemia and bleeding and the prevention of infection.
5. Explain the actions, uses, general adverse reactions, contraindications, precautions, and interactions of the agents used in the treatment of anemia and bleeding and the prevention of infection.
6. Distinguish important preadministration and ongoing assessment activities the nurse should perform on a client receiving an agent used in the treatment of anemia and bleeding and the prevention of infection.
7. Identify nursing diagnoses particular to a client receiving an agent used in the treatment of anemia and bleeding and the prevention of infection.
8. Examine ways to promote an optimal response to therapy and important points to keep in mind when educating clients about the use of an agent used in the treatment of anemia and bleeding and the prevention of infection.

 Drug Classes

Interferons and interleukins
Immunostimulants for bleeding and infection
Hematopoietic factors for anemia

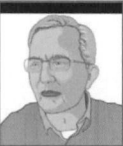

PHARMACOLOGY IN PRACTICE

Mr. Phillip, aged 72 years, has chronic kidney disease. He had a friend who was on dialysis about 5 years ago and complained of being tired all the time. They gave him "shots" to perk him up but instead he had a heart attack. Mr. Phillip is concerned about his kidney disease progressing and having to start dialysis and wonders if the same thing could happen to him.

mmunomodulators, as the name implies, are drugs that modify the actions of the immune system. These drugs work to mimic some of our natural bodily processes carried out by cytokines. **Cytokines** (see Fig. 48.1) are a broad group of proteins involved in cell-to-cell communication. They work to respond to disease and convey messages to

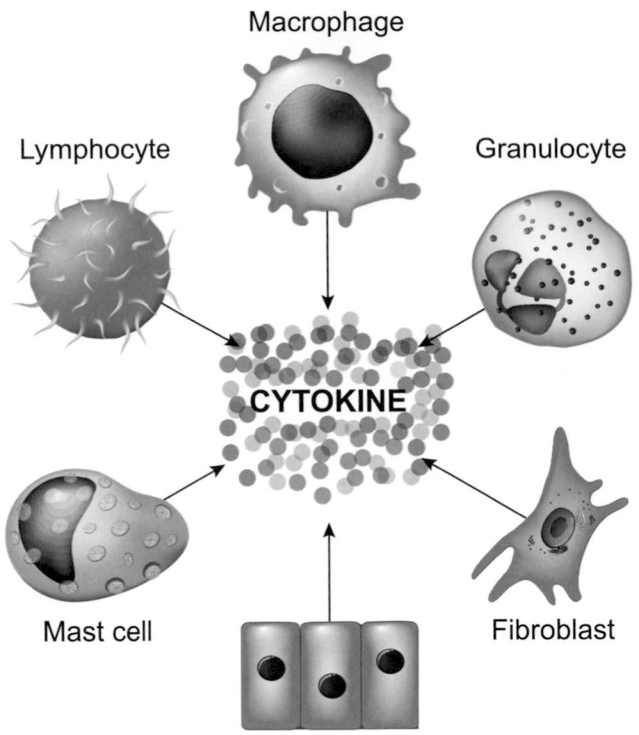

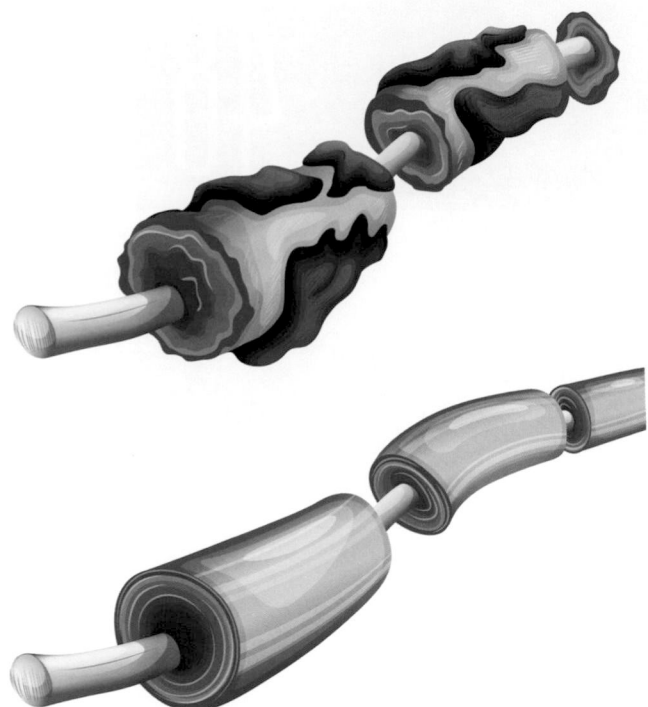

FIGURE 48.2 Nerve myelin deterioration in multiple sclerosis.

FIGURE 48.1 Cytokine communication in the body; this chapter focuses on communicating with the lymphocyte.

modulate the immune system. In addition to the cytokines that communicate in the immune system, drugs to support the hematopoietic system are included in this chapter. Two types of cytokines are discussed in this chapter: interferons and colony-stimulating factors (CSFs). A third type, interleukins, is covered in Chapter 51 in Unit 13.

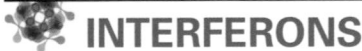

INTERFERONS

Interferons are cytokine antiviral agents that get their name from the ability to "interfere" with viral replication inside the cell. The cytokines that target white blood cells (WBCs, leukocytes) are called interleukins. Multiple sclerosis (MS) is one of the conditions in which interferons are used.

MULTIPLE SCLEROSIS

A progressive disease of the central nervous system, MS involves destruction of the myelin sheath that protects nerve fibers (see Fig. 48.2). When the sheath erodes, nerve impulses are altered and can result in impairment of sensation, movement, or vision (Britannica, 2021).

For many years, systemic treatment with corticosteroids was the primary treatment of MS. In 1993, interferon beta-1b (Betaseron) was the first interferon approved by the FDA for MS treatment. Interferon beta-1b is thought to enhance T-cell activity and in a series of steps reduces

inflammation in the central nervous system. In 1996, interferon beta-1a (Avonex) was approved. Now there are a number of interferons as well as other immunomodulators to treat MS on the market. Interferons continue to be widely used for relapsing MS (Filipi & Jack, 2020).

ACTIONS AND USES

Interferons are naturally occurring proteins produced within cells in response to a viral microorganism entering a cell (Olsen, 2018). The ability to manufacture interferons using recombinant DNA has increased their use as medications. They enhance the immune system's ability to protect the body without overtly attacking the foreign substance (bacteria, virus, cancer, etc). Interferons act in the following ways:

- Prevent viruses from replicating inside of host cells.
- Stimulate specific receptors on other healthy cells to prevent viral invasion.
- Inhibit tumors, stimulate T cells, and enhance the inflammatory response.
- Stimulate phagocytes to be more aggressive.
- Act as anti-infective to some bacterial and parasitic infections.

Interferons are identified as alfa, beta, gamma, and peginterferons. These drugs are used to treat a select group of cancers, MS, skin issues, and both hepatitis B and C.

ADVERSE REACTIONS

Because the interferons activate the immune response, a cluster of symptoms similar to fighting influenza occur. These are referred to as "flu-like symptoms" because they mimic the bodily response to fight the flu. Flu-like symptoms generally include:

- Chills
- Cough
- Fever
- Headache
- **Malaise** (generalized discomfort)

These adverse reactions are typically treated with acetaminophen and antihistamines.

PRACTICE CONSIDERATIONS

Patti et al. (2020) found that drug administration during evening hours reduced flu-like symptoms compared with those clients who injected themselves in the morning.

Other symptoms may include nausea, muscle aches, fatigue, sore throat, reduced appetite, or diarrhea. Skin rashes, injection pain and inflammation, edema in the extremities, and antibody development can occur.

Given parenterally, injection sites are rotated to reduce site reactions. Switching to a drug with less frequent dosing (three times/week to weekly drug) may help reduce injection site irritation and increase client compliance with the dosing schedule.

! NURSING ALERT

Given frequently by intramuscular (IM) or subcutaneous (subcut) injection; site reactions are common and include tenderness, redness, and warmth.

CONTRAINDICATIONS AND PRECAUTIONS

Interferons are contraindicated in clients with known hypersensitivity to the drug or any component of the drug. Neuropsychiatric symptoms including depression, confusion, and manic behavior have been noted in clients both with and without a psychiatric history. Asymptomatic elevation in liver enzyme levels has occurred; therefore, clients should be cautioned regarding alcohol intake while using the drug. Caution is used when administering to clients with cardiac or liver disease, a history of seizure disorder, and thyroid problems. A reduction in WBC count makes clients susceptible to infection.

Immunomodulators are not started during pregnancy, unless the woman is at high risk of MS activity. When on interferons, they are stopped when pregnancy is confirmed. Interferon has been found in breast milk (Hale, 2012).

 Chronic Care Considerations

Clients on interferon therapy should not be inoculated with live-attenuated vaccines (e.g., oral polio).

LASA ALERT

The following drugs may sound alike; be sure to clarify when they are ordered:

Drug Name	Sounds Like
Alferon	Alkeran
Avonex	Avelox
PEG-Intron	Intron A, Pegasys

Drugs that look alike are noted in the Summary Drug Tables of each chapter.

INTERACTIONS

The following interactions may occur when an interferon is administered with another agent:

Interacting Drug	Common Use	Effect of Interaction
Cladribine	Chemotherapy	Increased lymphopenia, adverse interferon reactions
Zidovudine	HIV antiretroviral	Increased adverse reactions of zidovudine

---

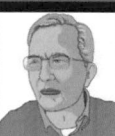 **PHARMACOLOGY IN PRACTICE**

PATHOPHYSIOLOGY

Interferons bolster the immune system by which of the following methods?

1. Direct attack on bacteria and viruses
2. As an antifungal agent
3. Stimulate healthy cells as viral protection
4. Stimulate B cells and the inflammatory response

STIMULATION OF THE HEMATOPOIETIC SYSTEM

Colony-stimulating factors are a group of immunostimulants used in cancer treatment and chronic renal failure to support the hematopoietic system. Many of the treatments used to fight cancer also kill fast growing cells of the hematopoietic system. The hematopoietic system is composed of fluids and particles that are known as *blood*. Blood is a complex fluid that circulates continuously through the heart and blood vessels and to the outermost cells of our body tissues. Three distinct cells circulate in the blood:

- Red blood cells (RBCs, **erythrocytes**) that supply our cells with oxygen from the lungs to the tissues
- WBCs (**leukocytes**) that protect our bodies from dangerous microorganisms
- Platelets (**megakaryocytes**) that control the bleeding from microscopic to major tears in our tissues

Chronic diseases such as chronic kidney disease or medical treatments such as chemotherapy can cause a hematologic failure. When this happens, inadequate numbers of cells are produced. As a result, the body can no longer meet the demands for oxygen transportation, blood coagulation, or prevention of invasion of microorganisms. Anemia, bleeding, and infection can result.

The goal for treating these hematologic problems is to stimulate the body to make more of the specific blood cells. This process is called **hematopoiesis**. During this process, undifferentiated stem cells in the bone marrow are signaled to multiply and differentiate into erythrocytes, leukocytes, or megakaryocytes (Fig. 48.3). Hematopoietic drugs help enhance this process and are used to treat anemia, bleeding, and infection.

COLONY-STIMULATING FACTORS—NEUTROPHILS

There are a number of different WBCs that protect the body from microbial invasion and infection. The WBC known as the neutrophil is one of the major cells in the line of defense against infection. *Neutropenia* is the term for the condition that results when the neutrophil level in the blood is low. Infection is likely to occur when a client is neutropenic. Neutrophils have an extremely short lifespan (6–8 hours), meaning that they rapidly grow and divide. Because of its rapid growth cycle, the neutrophil is a prime target for destruction by the cancer chemotherapy drugs, as well as the cancer cells themselves. Chemotherapy-induced neutropenia is a major reason that cancer treatments may be delayed or canceled. When this happens, the client is at a greater risk for continued growth of the cancer or illness from the treatment. CSFs are drugs used to stimulate the growth and production of WBCs to help fight off infection.

ACTIONS AND USES

CSFs are glycoproteins (cellular protein with attached sugar) that act on the hematopoietic cells to stimulate proliferation, differentiation, and maturation of WBCs. CSFs are used

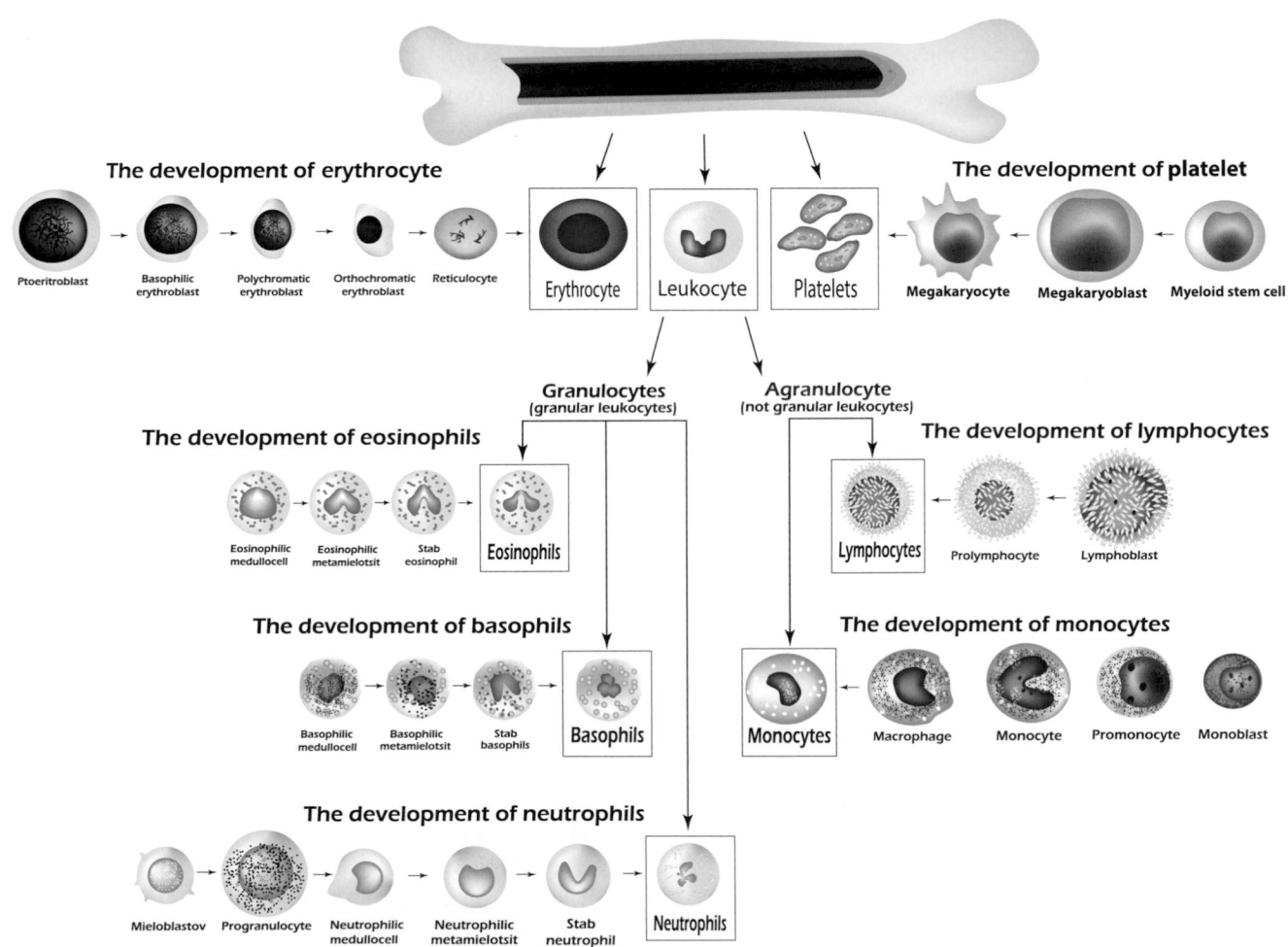

FIGURE 48.3 Hematopoiesis. (Photo by Timonina/Shutterstock)

to treat or prevent infection (by minimizing neutropenia) associated with the following:

- Chemotherapy-induced neutropenia during solid tumor cancer treatment
- Neutropenia during bone marrow transplant (BMT)
- Production of stem cells for harvest before BMT
- Neutropenia in those susceptible to symptomatic chronic infection

Injections of the CSF filgrastim are started at least 24 hours after the completion of a cycle of chemotherapy. The absolute neutrophil count (ANC) is monitored and therapy is continued until an ANC of at least 10,000/mm^3 is achieved. It is not recommended to use the drug for longer than 2 weeks, and treatment is discontinued at least 1 day before the next chemotherapy cycle is to begin. Special instruction is needed in cases of BMT or stem cell harvest.

Pegfilgrastim is similar to filgrastim but is given as a single dose between chemotherapy cycles. Sargramostim is used following BMT, following induction chemotherapy used with leukemia, and to stimulate stem cells for harvest.

ADVERSE REACTIONS

General System Reactions
- Bone pain
- Hypertension
- Nausea and vomiting
- Alopecia
- Hypersensitivity or allergic reactions

See the Summary Drug Table: Immunostimulants and Immunomodulator Drugs for more information on these drugs.

CONTRAINDICATIONS, PRECAUTIONS, AND INTERACTIONS

CSFs are contraindicated in clients with known hypersensitivity to the drug or any component of the drug. Filgrastim is used cautiously in clients with hypothyroid disease. The CSFs are pregnancy category C drugs, and caution is used when the client is breastfeeding. Pegfilgrastim can cause a sickle cell crisis in those with the disease. CSFs can cause hypersensitive reactions and should be treated with antihistamines, steroids, and bronchodilators to maintain their use. These drugs can stimulate cancer cell growth in cancer types that are stimulated by growth factors. An even higher increase in neutrophil count can occur when these drugs are taken with lithium, a drug used for the manic phase of mood disorders.

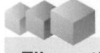 *Concept Mastery Alert*

Filgrastim (Neupogen) should be used with caution in clients with hypothyroidism.

COLONY-STIMULATING FACTORS—PLATELET DEVELOPMENT

Platelets are important to normal blood clotting. They are formed from megakaryocytes in the blood. The megakaryocyte is a large blood cell that can divide into many platelets. A low platelet count is a condition called *thrombocytopenia.* Decreased platelet production can also be caused by anemia. Sometimes the body does not make enough platelets because of unknown causes; this is termed idiopathic (or immune) thrombocytopenic purpura or ITP.

ACTIONS AND USES

A group of drugs called thrombopoietin receptor agonist stimulate megakaryocyte production (**thrombopoiesis**), resulting in more platelets. These drugs are used to prevent severe thrombocytopenia and reduce the need for multiple platelet transfusions.

Medication is started when platelet counts drop to less than 50,000/mm^3 in ITP and when clients with liver-disease-induced thrombocytopenia will have an invasive procedure with bleeding risk. Platelet counts are monitored and therapy is continued until a count of at least 50,000/mm^3 is achieved. It is not recommended for normalizing platelet counts.

Eltrombopag is used additionally for clients with aplastic anemia and those with chronic hepatitis C.

ADVERSE REACTIONS

General System Reactions
- Headache
- Fatigue
- Muscle aches
- Fever
- Allergic reactions

Cardiovascular System Reactions
- Peripheral edema
- Palpitations
- Atrial fibrillation
- Emboli resulting in stroke and pulmonary edema
- Capillary leak syndrome

Eltrombopag can be toxic to the liver. Liver function studies are done before starting the drug and every 2 weeks while on drug therapy. See the Summary Drug Table: Immunostimulants and Immunomodulator Drugs for more information on these drugs.

CONTRAINDICATIONS, PRECAUTIONS, AND INTERACTIONS

Thrombopoietin drugs are contraindicated in clients with known hypersensitivity to the drug or any component of the drug. These drugs are used cautiously in clients with renal failure and those with liver failure. Clients should be monitored for cataract (eye) formation. It is a pregnancy category C drug, so women should use effective contraception and lactating clients should stop breastfeeding.

Discontinuing either eltrombopag or romiplostim may result in platelet counts lower than the original diagnosed counts.

LASA ALERT

The following drugs may sound alike; be sure to clarify when they are ordered:

Drug Name	Sounds Like
Avatrombopag	eltrombopag, lusutrombopag
romiPLOStim	romiDEPsin

Drugs that look alike are noted in the Summary Drug Tables of each chapter.

COLONY-STIMULATING FACTORS—RED BLOOD CELL DEVELOPMENT

ANEMIA

Anemia is a condition caused by an insufficient amount of hemoglobin delivering oxygen to the tissues. Causes of anemia include a decrease in the number of RBCs, a decrease in the amount of hemoglobin in RBCs, or both. There are various types and causes of anemia. For example, anemia can result from blood loss, excessive destruction of RBCs, inadequate production of RBCs, and deficits in various nutrients, as in **iron deficiency anemia**. Figure 48.4 illustrates some of the changes in RBCs based on different anemias and sickle cell disease for comparison with a normal RBC. Once the type and cause have been identified, the primary health care provider selects a method of treatment.

The anemias discussed in this chapter include anemia in clients with chronic illness such as renal disease or caused by treatment, iron deficiency anemia, pernicious anemia, and anemia resulting from a folic acid deficiency. Table 48.1 defines these anemias.

Anemia may occur in clients with chronic illness as a result of disease treatment. Cancer and chronic kidney disease are two diseases that produce disease- or treatment-related anemia. Erythropoiesis-stimulating agents (ESAs) are glycoproteins that stimulate and regulate the production of erythrocytes. Chronic kidney disease reduces the kidney's ability to produce erythropoietin (EPO), which stimulates the production of RBCs. Cancer treatment reduces the bone marrow's ability to produce RBCs. Two examples of drugs used to treat anemia associated with chronic illness are epoetin alfa (Epogen) and darbepoetin alfa (Aranesp).

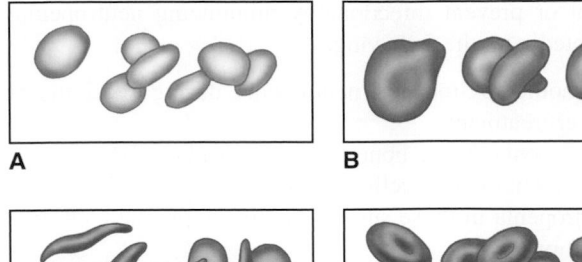
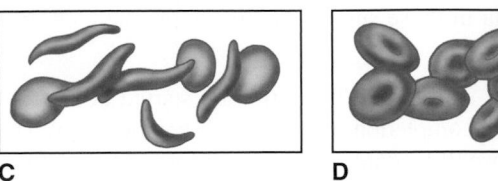

FIGURE 48.4 Changes in red blood cells compared to a normal cell. **A.** Iron deficiency anemia. **B.** Megaloblastic or folic acid deficiency anemia. **C.** Sickle cell disease. **D.** Normal red blood cell.

ACTIONS AND USES

ESAs are drugs that, like natural EPO, stimulate **erythropoiesis**, the process of making RBCs. ESAs are used to treat anemia associated with the following:

- Chronic kidney disease
- Chemotherapy for cancer treatment
- Zidovudine (AZT) therapy for human immunodeficiency virus (HIV) infection
- Postsurgical blood replacement in place of allogeneic (from others) transfusions

Darbepoetin alfa and methoxy polyethylene–epoetin β are erythropoiesis-stimulating proteins used to treat anemia associated with chronic kidney disease in clients receiving dialysis, as well as in clients who are not receiving dialysis. These drugs elevate or maintain RBC levels and decrease the need for transfusions.

TABLE 48.1 Anemias

TYPE OF ANEMIA	DESCRIPTION
Iron deficiency	Anemia characterized by an inadequate amount of iron in the body to produce hemoglobin
Anemia in chronic kidney disease	Anemia resulting from a reduced production of erythropoietin, a hormone secreted by the kidney that stimulates the production of RBCs
Pernicious anemia	Anemia resulting from lack of secretion by the gastric mucosa of the intrinsic factor essential to the formation of RBCs and the absorption of vitamin B_{12}
Folic acid deficiency	Anemia occurring because of a dietary lack of folic acid, a component necessary in the formation of RBCs

ADVERSE REACTIONS

Epoetin alfa (an EPO), darbepoetin alfa, and methoxy poly-ethylene are usually well tolerated when used to maintain a hemoglobin level no higher than 12 g/dL. The most common adverse reactions include:

- Hypertension
- Headache
- Nausea, vomiting, diarrhea
- Rashes
- Fatigue
- Arthralgia and skin reaction at the injection site

See the Summary Drug Table: Immunostimulants and Immunomodulator Drugs for more information on these drugs.

CONTRAINDICATIONS AND PRECAUTIONS

Epoetin alfa is contraindicated in clients with uncontrolled hypertension, those needing an emergency transfusion, and those with a hypersensitivity to human albumin. Darbepoetin alfa (Aranesp) is contraindicated in clients with uncontrolled hypertension or in those allergic to the drug. Polycythemia (an overload of RBCs in the circulation) can occur if the hemoglobin is not carefully monitored and the dosage is too high. This can result in increased mortality, serious cardio or thromboembolic events in any client, and possible tumor progression in cancer clients.

Epoetin alfa and darbepoetin alfa are used with caution in clients with hypertension, heart disease, congestive heart failure, or a history of seizures. Both these drugs are pregnancy category C drugs and are used cautiously during pregnancy and lactation.

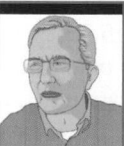

PHARMACOLOGY IN PRACTICE

SAFE DRUG ADMINISTRATION
A client is prescribed epoetin alfa for the treatment of anemia associated with chronic renal failure. With which of the following hemoglobin counts is epoetin alfa contraindicated?

1. 2 g/dL
2. 6 g/dL
3. 11 g/dL
4. 17 g/dL

DRUGS USED IN TREATING SPECIFIC ANEMIAS

IRON DEFICIENCY

The following drugs are not used in immunotherapy, yet when the body does not have enough iron to supply its own needs, the resulting condition is not unlike the anemia mentioned earlier. This is typically called *iron deficiency anemia*. Iron is the component in hemoglobin that picks up oxygen from the lungs and carries it to the body tissues. Iron deficiency anemia is a very common type of anemia. Approximately 50% of pregnant women and 20% of all women experience anemia. Decreased iron stores result from a decrease in RBCs; causes include heavy menstrual bleeding and poor absorption or lack of iron in the diet.

ACTIONS AND USES

Iron preparations act by elevating the serum iron concentration, which replenishes hemoglobin and depleted iron stores. Oral iron supplements are typically used. Iron is best absorbed on an empty stomach. Supplemental iron is needed during pregnancy and lactation because normal dietary intake rarely supplies the required amount.

Parenteral iron is used when the client cannot take oral drugs or when the client experiences gastrointestinal (GI) intolerance to oral iron administration. Other iron preparations, both oral and parenteral, used in treating iron deficiency anemia can be found in the Summary Drug Table: Immunostimulants and Immunomodulator Drugs.

ADVERSE REACTIONS

GI Reactions
- GI irritation
- Nausea, vomiting
- Constipation, diarrhea
- Darker (black) stools

Generalized System Reactions
- Headache
- Backache
- Allergic reactions

When given parenterally, additional adverse reactions include soreness, inflammation, and sterile abscesses at the IM injection site. When iron is administered by the IM route, a brownish discoloration of the skin may occur. Intravenous (IV) administration may result in phlebitis at the injection site.

CONTRAINDICATIONS AND PRECAUTIONS

Iron supplements are contraindicated in clients with known hypersensitivity to the drug or any component of the drug. Iron compounds are contraindicated in clients with hemochromatosis or hemolytic anemia. Iron compounds are used cautiously in clients with hypersensitivity to aspirin because these clients may have a hypersensitivity to the tartrazine or sulfite content of some iron compounds.

The parenteral form of iron can cause anaphylactic-type reactions and should be used only when oral supplement is contraindicated.

INTERACTIONS

The following interactions may occur when an iron preparation is administered with another agent:

Interacting Drug	Common Use	Effect of Interaction
Antibiotics	Fight infection	Decreased gastrointestinal absorption of the antibiotic
Levothyroxine	Treatment of hypothyroidism	Decreased absorption of levothyroxine
Levodopa, methyldopa	Treatment of Parkinson disease	Decreased effect of antiparkinsonian medication
Ascorbic acid (vitamin C)	Vitamin supplement	Increased absorption of iron

FOLIC ACID DEFICIENCY

Folic acid (folate) is required for the manufacture of RBCs in the bone marrow. Folic acid is found in leafy green vegetables, fish, meat, poultry, and whole grains. A deficiency of folic acid results in megaloblastic anemia. **Megaloblastic anemia** is characterized by the presence of large, abnormal, immature erythrocytes circulating in the blood.

ACTIONS AND USES

Folic acid is used in treating megaloblastic anemias that are caused by a deficiency of folic acid. Although neural tube defects are not related to anemia, studies indicate there is a decreased risk for embryonic neural tube defects if folic acid is taken before conception and during early pregnancy. Neural tube defects occur during early pregnancy, when the embryonic folds forming the spinal cord and brain join together. Defects of this type include anencephaly (congenital absence of brain and spinal cord), spina bifida (defect of the spinal cord), and meningocele (a saclike protrusion of the meninges in the spinal cord or skull). The U.S. Public Health Service recommends the use of folic acid for all women of childbearing age to decrease the incidence of neural tube defects. Dosages during pregnancy and lactation are as great as 0.8 mg/day.

Oral supplements are the first choice for megaloblastic anemia and folic acid deficiency treatment. If a client is unable to take oral medications, leucovorin may be used. This drug is a derivative (an active reduced form) of folic acid. Leucovorin is more commonly used to diminish the hematologic effects of methotrexate, a drug used in treating certain types of cancer (see Chapter 50). Leucovorin "rescues" normal cells from the destruction caused by methotrexate and allows them to survive. This technique of administering leucovorin after a large dose of methotrexate is called folinic acid rescue or *leucovorin rescue.*

ADVERSE REACTIONS

Few adverse reactions are associated with the administration of folic acid. Rarely, parenteral administration may result in allergic hypersensitivity.

CONTRAINDICATIONS AND PRECAUTIONS

Folic acid and leucovorin are contraindicated for treating pernicious anemia or for other anemias in which vitamin B_{12} is deficient. Folic acid is a pregnancy category A drug and is generally considered safe for use during pregnancy. Pregnant women are more likely to experience folate deficiency because folic acid requirements increase during pregnancy. Pregnant women with a folate deficiency are at increased risk for complications of pregnancy and fetal abnormalities. The recommended dietary allowance (RDA) of folate during pregnancy is 0.4 mg/day and during lactation, 0.26–0.28 mg/day. Although the potential for fetal harm appears remote, the drug should be used cautiously and only within the RDA guidelines.

INTERACTIONS

Signs of folate deficiency may occur when sulfasalazine is administered concurrently. An increase in seizure activity may occur when folic acid is administered with the hydantoins (antiseizure drugs).

VITAMIN B_{12} DEFICIENCY

Vitamin B_{12} is essential to growth, cell reproduction, the manufacture of myelin (which surrounds some nerve fibers), and blood cell manufacture. The **intrinsic factor**, which is produced by cells in the stomach, is necessary for the absorption of vitamin B_{12} in the intestine. A deficiency of the intrinsic factor results in abnormal formation of erythrocytes because of the body's failure to absorb vitamin B_{12}, a necessary component for blood cell formation. The resulting anemia is called **macrocytic anemia**.

ACTIONS AND USES

Vitamin B_{12} (cyanocobalamin) is used to treat clients with a vitamin B_{12} deficiency; this condition is seen in those who have:

- A strict vegetarian (vegan) lifestyle
- Total gastrectomy or subtotal gastric resection (in which the cells producing the intrinsic factor are totally or partially removed)
- Intestinal diseases such as ulcerative colitis or sprue
- Gastric carcinoma
- Congenital decrease in the number of gastric cells that secrete intrinsic factor

Vitamin B_{12} is also used to perform the Schilling test, which is used to diagnose pernicious anemia.

! NURSING ALERT

Pernicious anemia must be diagnosed and treated as soon as possible because vitamin B_{12} deficiency that is allowed to progress for more than 3 months may result in degenerative lesions of the spinal cord.

A deficiency of vitamin B_{12} caused by a low dietary intake is rare because the vitamin is found in meats, milk, eggs, and cheese. The body is also able to store this vitamin. A deficiency, for any reason, will not occur for 5–6 years from birth. Clients should be assessed for a history of vegan diet or gastric bypass surgery.

ADVERSE REACTIONS

Mild diarrhea and itching have been reported with the administration of vitamin B_{12}. Other adverse reactions that may be seen include a marked increase in RBC production, acne, peripheral vascular thrombosis, congestive heart failure, and pulmonary edema.

CONTRAINDICATIONS, PRECAUTIONS, AND INTERACTIONS

Vitamin B_{12} is contraindicated in clients who are allergic to cyanocobalamin. Vitamin B_{12} is a pregnancy category A drug if administered orally and a pregnancy category C drug if given parenterally. Vitamin B_{12} is administered cautiously during pregnancy and in clients with pulmonary disease and those with anemia. Alcohol, neomycin, and colchicine may decrease the absorption of oral vitamin B_{12}.

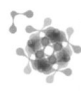

NURSING PROCESS: STEPS TO BUILD CLINICAL JUDGMENT
Client Receiving an Immunomodulating Drug Used in the Treatment of Anemia, Bleeding, or Infection

ASSESSMENT

Preadministration Assessment
Data gathering suggestions before the initial administration of an immunomodulating/anemia drug include the following:
Objective data

- Vital signs (temperature, pulse, respirations, and blood pressure).
- General appearance.
- Specific signs for anemia (listlessness, shortness of breath, pallor), bleeding (bruising, blood oozing from gums, or infection [fever]).
- Inspect general physical appearance, noting skin color, temperature, and any lesions, differences bilaterally.
- Laboratory tests—baseline blood counts and organ function.
- Weight, if certain drugs need for dose calculation.

Subjective data

- Description of type and intensity of symptoms (e.g., pain, discomfort, fatigue)
- Reported ability to carry out activities of daily living
- History of bowel issues and habits
- History of other current nonmalignant disease or disorder, such as autoimmune or diabetes, that may or may not be related to the malignant disease
- History of travel to areas of infectious diseases or having had an infectious disease

Ongoing Assessment
During the ongoing assessment, if the vital signs such as heart or respiration rate increase, this can indicate low RBCs; these should be frequently monitored especially if the client is moderately to acutely ill. Additionally, ask the client about adverse reactions and report any occurrence of adverse reactions to the primary health care provider before the next dose is due. Immediately report severe adverse reactions.

Monitor the client for relief of the symptoms (fatigue, shortness of breath, sore tongue, headache, pallor). Some clients may note a relief of symptoms after a few days of therapy. Periodic laboratory tests are necessary to monitor the results of therapy. Check for signs of bleeding and infection during the first few days of therapy with the CSF, as an increase in blood cells may take a few days once therapy is started.

When the client is receiving oral iron supplements inform the client that the color of the stool will become darker or black. If diarrhea or constipation occurs contact the primary health care provider.

If parenteral iron dextran is administered inform client that soreness at the injection site may occur. Teach the client to check injection sites daily for signs of inflammation, swelling, or abscess formation.

NURSING DIAGNOSES

Drug-specific nursing diagnoses include the following:

- **Fatigue** related to dilutional anemia caused by fluid retention.
- **Malnutrition** related to lack of iron, folic acid, and others (specify) in the diet.
- **Constipation** related to adverse reaction to iron therapy.

Nursing diagnoses related to drug administration are discussed in Chapter 4.

PLANNING

The expected outcomes for the client may include an optimal response to therapy, supporting the client needs related to the management of adverse reactions, and confidence in an understanding of and compliance with the prescribed treatment regimen.

IMPLEMENTATION

Promoting an Optimal Response to Therapy

Thrombopoietin Receptor Agonists
Taken orally, they should be at least 2 hours before or 4 hours after meals high in calcium (dairy products, calcium-fortified juices, or calcium-rich vegetables), antacids, or supplements. Oral syringes used with suspension products should not be reused. Missed doses should be taken as soon as discovered, but never more than one dose per day.

Epoetin Alfa
When epoetin alfa is administered to a client with hypertension monitor the blood pressure closely. Report any rise of 20 mm Hg or more in the systolic or diastolic pressure to the primary health care provider. The hematocrit is usually measured before each dose during therapy with epoetin alfa.

The drug is given three times weekly IV or subcut; if the client is receiving dialysis, the drug is administered into the venous access line. The drug is mixed gently during preparation for administration. Shaking may denature the glycoprotein. The vial is used for only one dose; any remaining or unused portion is discarded.

> **NURSING ALERT**
> The target hemoglobin level is no more than 11 g/dL. Myocardial infarction and stroke are more likely to occur when the hemoglobin level rises higher. Additionally, report any increase in the hematocrit of 4 points within any 2-week period because an exacerbation of hypertension is associated with an excessive rise of hematocrit. Withholding the drug use lowers the blood levels.

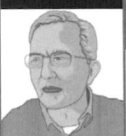

PHARMACOLOGY IN PRACTICE

MANAGING NEEDS
A nurse administers the CSF, filgrastim, following chemotherapy. During the ongoing assessment, which of the following data points would make the nurse call the primary health care provider with the intent to discontinue the daily injections?

1. Complaints of sore throat
2. Hemoglobin laboratory value of 12 g/dL
3. Neutrophil count of 30,000/mm³
4. Petechiae on the torso

Iron
Iron supplements are preferably given between meals with water, but many people cannot tolerate this and may need to take them with food. Milk and antacids may interfere with absorption of iron and should not be taken at the same time as iron supplements. If the client is receiving other drugs, then check with the clinical pharmacist regarding the simultaneous administration of iron salts with other drugs.

Parenteral iron can be given by the IM or IV route. IV route is preferred for clients on hemodialysis and to increase stores during surgical procedures when blood loss is anticipated (Ionescu et al., 2020). Before iron dextran is administered, a test dose (0.5 mL iron dextran) may be administered IV at a gradual rate over a period of 30 seconds or more. Newer preparations of iron (iron sucrose, ferric gluconate) make severe reaction less prevalent (Auerbach & Macdougall, 2014)

> **NURSING ALERT**
> Parenteral administration of iron dextran has resulted in fatal anaphylactic-type reactions. Instruct client to report immediately any of the following adverse reactions: dyspnea, urticaria, rashes, itching, and fever.

After the test dose, the prescribed dose of iron is administered IM. The drug is given into the muscle mass of the buttocks' upper outer quadrant (never into an arm or other area) using the Z-track method (see Chapter 2) to prevent leakage into the subcut tissue. A large-bore needle is required. If the client is standing, then have the client place weight on the leg not receiving the injection.

Vitamin B$_{12}$
Clients with vitamin B$_{12}$ anemia are treated with vitamin B$_{12}$ IM administered weekly. The parenteral route is used because the vitamin is ineffective orally, owing to the absence of the intrinsic factor in the stomach, which is necessary for utilization of vitamin B$_{12}$. After stabilization, maintenance (usually monthly) injections may be necessary for life. Vitamin B$_{12}$ is available in an intranasal form for those who are on maintenance therapy.

Monitoring and Managing Client Needs

Fatigue
During administration of the CSF drugs, the client may experience fluid retention. With the increase in fluid volume, this makes the ratio of cells to fluid in the blood less, which results in dilutional anemia. The client may experience fatigue because of this anemia. The client may need an explanation of this situation and to be given permission to feel tired. Teach the client and family energy-saving skills to help maintain the same level of activities of daily living.

Malnutrition
A balanced diet is recommended with an emphasis on foods that are high in iron (e.g., lean red meats, cereals, dried beans, and leafy green vegetables), folic acid

(e.g., green leafy vegetables, liver, and yeast), or vitamin B_{12} (e.g., beef, pork, eggs, milk, and milk products). Use the clinical dietitian or nutritionist to help the client make appropriate food selections when:

- the client is vegetarian or vegan and needs iron-rich foods.
- the client's appetite is poor or inadequate and needs increase in calories/proteins.
- specific anemia can be corrected with dietary interventions.
- the drug therapy has dietary restrictions/ contraindications.

Small portions of food may be more appealing than large or moderate portions. Provide a pleasant atmosphere and allow ample time for eating. If the client is unable to eat well, note this on the client's chart and bring the problem to the attention of the primary health care provider.

Constipation

Constipation may be a problem when a client is taking oral iron preparations. Instruct the client to increase fluid intake to 10–12 glasses of water daily (if the condition permits), eat a diet high in fiber, and increase activity. An active lifestyle and regular exercise (if condition permits) help decrease the constipating effects of iron. If constipation persists, the primary health care provider may prescribe a stool softener.

Educating the Client and Family

Explain the medical regimen thoroughly to the client and family and emphasize the importance of following the prescribed treatment regimen. Include the following points in a client and family teaching plan.

Hematopoietic Factors

- Keep all appointments with the primary health care provider. The drug is administered up to three times per week (by the subcut or IV route or through a dialysis access line). Periodic blood tests are performed to determine the effects of the drug and to determine dosage.
- Strict compliance with the antihypertensive drug regimen is important in clients with known hypertension during epoetin alfa therapy.
- The following adverse reactions may occur: dizziness, headache, fatigue, joint pain, nausea, vomiting, or diarrhea. Report any of these reactions.
- Clients might have heard about problems with the drug Leukine. The product was withdrawn temporarily because of reports of adverse reactions including syncope (fainting). This was correlated with a change in the formulation of the drug, which included edetate disodium (EDTA). This formula has been taken off the market and Leukine is now considered safe.

- If the client or caregiver is administering the injections at home, use puncture-resistant containers for disposal and return full containers to the proper agency for disposal.

Iron

- Take this drug with water on an empty stomach. If GI upset occurs, take the drug with food or meals.
- Do not take antacids, tetracyclines, penicillamine, or fluoroquinolones at the same time or 2 hours before or after taking iron without first checking with the primary health care provider.
- This drug may cause a darkening of the stools, constipation, or diarrhea. If constipation or diarrhea becomes severe contact the primary health care provider.
- Mix the liquid iron preparation with water or juice and drink through a straw to prevent staining the teeth.
- Avoid the indiscriminate use of advertised iron products. If a true iron deficiency occurs, the cause must be determined and therapy should be under the care of a health care provider.
- Have periodic blood tests during therapy to determine the therapeutic response.

Folic Acid

- Avoid the use of multivitamin preparations unless they have been approved by the primary health care provider.
- Follow the diet recommended by the primary health care provider because diet and drug are necessary to correct anemia associated with folic acid deficiency.

Leucovorin

- Megaloblastic anemia—adhere to the diet prescribed by the primary health care provider. If the purchase of foods high in protein (which can be expensive) becomes a problem, discuss this with the primary health care provider.

Vitamin B_{12}

- Nutritional deficiency of vitamin B_{12}—eat a balanced diet that includes seafood, eggs, meats, and dairy products.
- Pernicious anemia—lifetime therapy is necessary. Eat a balanced diet that includes seafood, eggs, meats, and dairy products. Avoid contact with infections, and report any signs of infection to the primary health care provider immediately because an increase in dosage may be necessary.
- Adhere to the treatment regimen and keep all appointments with the clinic or primary health care provider. The drug is given at periodic intervals (usually monthly for life). In some instances, parenteral or intranasal self-administration or parenteral administration by a family member is allowed (instruction in administration is necessary).

EVALUATION

- Therapeutic effect of the drug is achieved.
- Adverse reactions are identified, reported to the primary health care provider, and managed successfully with appropriate nursing interventions:
  - Client reports fatigue is manageable.
  - Client maintains an adequate nutritional status.
  - Client reports adequate bowel movements.
- Client and family express confidence and demonstrate an understanding of the drug regimen.

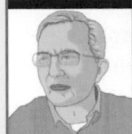

PHARMACOLOGY IN PRACTICE

USING CLINICAL REASONING

You learn that Mr. Phillip's wife was given CSFs during her breast cancer treatment. How could you explain the differences and similarities between these medications?

KEY POINTS

■ Immunomodulating agents are used to stimulate or suppress the immune system to treat a variety of diseases.

■ Chronic diseases such as kidney failure or treatments such as chemotherapy can reduce the number of cells in the circulation, causing fatigue, bleeding, or infection. CSFs are one type of immunostimulant that can boost the number of cells.

■ The hematopoietic system is composed of fluid and three types of cells. RBCs supply the body with oxygen, WBCs protect the body from microorganisms, and platelets control bleeding.

■ These drugs are fragile and must be mixed before administration. They are given subcut or IV. Adverse reactions include flu-like symptoms. A dramatic reduction in cells of the specific type stimulated will occur when the injections are stopped.

■ Anemia is a condition caused by reduced amounts of hemoglobin resulting in less oxygen to be delivered to the tissues. Anemia occurs because of chronic illnesses or specific deficiencies such as iron deficiency.

SUMMARY DRUG TABLE
Immunostimulants and Immunomodulator Drugs

Generic Name	Trade Name	Uses	Adverse Reactions	Dosage Ranges
Interferons				
interferon alfa-2b In-ter-FEER-on	Intron A	Chronic hepatitis B, Kaposi sarcoma, lymphoma, melanoma, hairy cell leukemia, genital warts	Flu-like symptoms (fever, headache, muscle ache), fatigue, nausea	Dependent on condition being treated, given subcut or IM
interferon alfa-n3 In-ter-FEER-on	Alferon N	Genital warts	Flu-like symptoms, nausea	250,000–2.5 million units injected into the base of wart twice a week
interferon beta-1a In-ter-FEER-on	Avonex, Rebif	Multiple sclerosis, relapsing	Flu-like symptoms, fatigue, nausea, UTI, injection site reaction	22–44 mcg IM weekly (Avonex), subcut three times weekly (Rebif)
interferon beta-1b In-ter-FEER-on	Betaseron, Extavia	Multiple sclerosis, relapsing	Flu-like symptoms, fatigue, skin rash, nausea, abdominal pain, urine urgency, injection site reaction	0.0625 mg titrated subcut to 0.25 mg every other day
interferon gamma-1b In-ter-FEER-on	Actimmune	Chronic granulomatous (immunodeficiency), severe osteopetrosis (overly dense bones)	Flu-like symptoms, fatigue, nausea, diarrhea, injection site reaction	50 mcg/m^2 subcut three times weekly

Generic Name	Trade Name	Uses	Adverse Reactions	Dosage Ranges
peginterferon alfa-2a *Peg-in-ter-FEER-on*	Pegasys	Chronic hepatitis B & C	Flu-like symptoms, fatigue, insomnia, alopecia, nausea, abdominal pain, cough, injection site reaction	180 mcg weekly subcut for 48 weeks
peginterferon alfa-2b *Peg-in-ter-FEER-on*	PegIntron	Chronic hepatitis C	Flu-like symptoms, fatigue, insomnia, alopecia, nausea, anorexia, abdominal pain, injection site reaction	6 mcg/kg/week subcut for 8 weeks, then 3 mcg/kg/week for up to 5 years
peginterferon beta-1a *Peg-in-ter-FEER-on*	Plegridy	Multiple sclerosis, relapsing	Flu-like symptoms, fatigue, insomnia, alopecia, nausea, abdominal pain, cough, injection site reaction	125 mcg, given subcut every other week
Interleukin				
aldesleukin *al-des-LOO-kin*	Proleukin	Metastatic melanoma and renal cell carcinoma	Flu-like symptoms, hypotension, rash, nausea, vomiting, diarrhea, dyspnea	Dependent on condition being treated, given IV in units per kilogram
Colony-Stimulating Factors				
Hematopoietic Factors for Infection				
filgrastim *fil-GRA-stim*	Neupogen, Nivestym, Granix, Zarxio	Treat or prevent severe neutropenia	Bone pain, nausea, vomiting, diarrhea, alopecia	5–10 mcg/kg subcut or IV daily
pegfilgrastim *peg-fil-GRA-stim*	Neulasta, Fulphila, Nyvepria, Udenyca, Ziextenzo	Treat or prevent severe neutropenia	Bone pain, nausea, vomiting, diarrhea, alopecia	Single 6-mg subcut injection per cycle
sargramostim *sar-GRAM-oh-stim*	Leukine	Treat or prevent severe neutropenia following BMT, induction chemotherapy	Headache, bone pain, nausea, vomiting, diarrhea, alopecia, skin rash	250 mcg/m² IV daily
Hematopoietic Factors for Bleeding				
avatrombopag *a-va-TROM-boe-PAG*	Doptelet	Severe chronic thrombocytopenia (ITP)	Headache, fatigue, fever	40 mg daily orally
eltrombopag *el-TROM-boe-pag*	Promacta	Severe chronic thrombocytopenia (ITP)	Nausea, excessive menstrual bleeding	Max. dose 75 mg/day orally
lusutrombopag *Loo-soo-TROM-boe-pag*	Mulpleta	Thrombocytopenia associated with chronic liver disease	Headache	3 mg daily orally for 1 week
romiPLOStim *roe-mi-PLOE-stim*	Nplate	Treatment of severe chronic thrombocytopenia (ITP)	Muscle pain, dizziness, insomnia	1 mcg/kg subcut weekly
Adjuvant Agents				
plerixafor *pler-IX-a-fore*	Mozobil	Use with G-CSF to mobilize hematopoietic stem cells for collection and autologous transplant	Headache, dizziness, fatigue, joint pain, nausea, vomiting, diarrhea	Injected approximately 11 hours before stem cell collection

Continued

SUMMARY DRUG TABLE (continued)
Immunostimulants and Immunomodulator Drugs

Generic Name	Trade Name	Uses	Adverse Reactions	Dosage Ranges
Hematopoietic Factors for Anemia				
darbepoetin alfa *dar-be-POE-e-tin*	Aranesp	Anemia associated with CKD and nonmyeloid cancers	Hypertension, hypotension, headache, diarrhea, vomiting, nausea, myalgia, arthralgia, cardiac arrhythmias, cardiac arrest	Titrated to hemoglobin (Hb) level
epoetin alfa (erythropoietin [EPO]) *e-POE-e-tin*	Epogen, Procrit, Retacrit	Anemias associated with CKD, zidovudine therapy in HIV-infected clients, clients with cancer receiving myelosuppressive chemotherapy, clients undergoing elective nonvascular surgery	Hypertension, headache, nausea, vomiting, fatigue, skin reaction at injection site	Titrated to Hb level
luspatercept *lus-PAT-er-sept*	Reblozyl	Anemias associated with thalassemia, myelodysplastic syndromes	Hypertension, nausea, abdominal pain, diarrhea, headache, dizziness, fatigue, muscle aches, cough	1.25–1.75 mg/kg dependent on Hb level
methoxy polyethylene (glycol-epoetin beta) *meth-OX-ee pl-i-ETH-i-leen*	Mircera	Anemia associated with CKD	Hypertension, hypotension, headache, diarrhea, vomiting, nausea	Titrated to Hb level
Adjuvant Agents				
ferrous *FER-us*	Feostat, Fergon, Feosol, Fer-In-Sol	Prevention and treatment of iron deficiency anemia	GI irritation, nausea, vomiting, constipation, diarrhea, allergic reactions	Daily requirements: males, 10 mg/day orally; females, 18 mg/day orally; during pregnancy and lactation: 30–60 mg/day orally Replacement in deficiency states: 90–300 mg/day (6 mg/kg/day) orally for 6–10 months
folic acid *FOE-lik* *AS-id*	Folvite	Megaloblastic anemia caused by deficiency of folic acid	Allergic sensitization	Up to 1 mg/day orally, IM, IV, subcut
iron dextran *EYE-ern DEKS-tran*	Dexferrum, INFeD	Iron deficiency anemia (only when oral form is contraindicated)	Anaphylactoid reactions, soreness and inflammation at injection site, chest pain, arthralgia, backache, convulsions, pruritus, abdominal pain, nausea, vomiting, dyspnea	Dosage (IV, IM) based on body weight and grams percentage (g/dL) of Hb
iron sucrose *EYE-ern SOO-krose*	Venofer	Iron deficiency anemia in kidney disease, via dialysis machine	Hypotension, cramps, leg cramps, nausea, headache, vomiting, diarrhea, dizziness	100 mg elemental iron by slow IV infusion or during dialysis session

Generic Name	Trade Name	Uses	Adverse Reactions	Dosage Ranges
leucovorin *loo-koe-VOR-in*		Treatment of megaloblastic anemia; leucovorin rescue after high-dose methotrexate therapy	Allergic sensitization, urticaria, anaphylaxis	See cancer therapy
sodium ferric gluconate complex	Ferrlecit	Iron deficiency	Flushing, hypotension, syncope, tachycardia, dizziness, pruritus, dyspnea, conjunctivitis, hyperkalemia	125 mg of elemental iron IV over at least 10 minutes
vitamin B$_{12}$ (cyanocobalamin) *sye-an-oh-koe-BAL-ah-min*		Vitamin B$_{12}$ deficiencies, GI pathology; Schilling test	Mild diarrhea, itching, edema, anaphylaxis	Schilling test: 100–1000 mcg/day for 2 weeks, then 100–1000 mcg IM every month

CHAPTER REVIEW

Know Your Drugs

Clients sometimes know a medication by the brand (or trade) name and not the generic name. To recognize both names match the brand name with the generic name of the same medication.

Generic Name	Brand Name
1. epoetin alfa	A. Neulasta
2. filgrastim	B. Plegridy
3. pegfilgrastim	C. Neupogen
4. peginterferon beta-1a	D. Procrit

Calculate Medication Dosages

1. The primary health care provider prescribes 25 mg iron dextran IM. The drug is available in a vial with 50 mg/mL. The nurse administers _____.
2. Folvite (folic acid) 1 mg subcut is prescribed. The drug is available in a vial with 5 mg/mL. The nurse administers _____.

Prepare for the NCLEX

RECALL THE FACTS

1. An erythrocyte is commonly known as a _____.
   1. WBC
   2. basophil
   3. RBC
   4. platelet
2. Which of the following drugs is approved to treat ITP?
   1. Folic acid
   2. Filgrastim
   3. Leucovorin
   4. RomiPLOStim

3. Which is the most common type of anemia?
   1. Iron deficiency anemia
   2. Folic acid anemia
   3. Pernicious anemia
   4. Megaloblastic anemia
4. Which of the following substances would decrease the absorption of oral iron?
   1. Antacids
   2. Levothyroxine
   3. Ascorbic acid
   4. Vitamin B$_{12}$
5. Filgrastim is contraindicated in which of the following conditions?
   1. Hypothyroidism
   2. Hyperthyroidism
   3. Pernicious anemia
   4. Pregnancy

ANALYZE THE FACTS

6. *When monitoring a client taking epoetin alfa, which of the following laboratory results should be reported immediately to the health care provider?
   1. Any increase in hematocrit of 4 points within a 2-week period
   2. Any increase in hematocrit of 2 points within a 2-week period
   3. A daily change in the hematocrit of 1 point or more
   4. A stabilization in the hematocrit in any 2-day period

7. When teaching a client about the use of vitamin B_{12}, the nurse would include which of the following statements?
   1. Take the oral form of vitamin B_{12} daily at bedtime on an empty stomach.
   2. Take the oral form of vitamin B_{12} when you begin to feel weak or experience a headache.
   3. You will require vitamin B_{12} injections monthly for life.
   4. You will require vitamin B_{12} injections every 2 weeks until remission occurs.

8. A vegan client has been diagnosed with iron deficiency. Which of the following foods would be recommended?
   1. Lean red meats
   2. Dried beans
   3. Egg yolks
   4. Pork

ALTERNATE-FORMAT QUESTIONS

9. A client with limited health literacy is prescribed oral iron tablets for anemia following blood loss during a surgical procedure. The iron is available in 10-mg tablets. The primary health care provider has ordered 30 mg on the first day, followed by 10 mg on days 2–5. The nurse shows the client how many tablets to be taken on the first day? _____
   How many on the last day of therapy? _____

10. Match the CSF with the sign or symptom it is used to treat:

1. Filgrastim	A. Fatigue
2. Eltrombopag	B. Bleeding
3. Darbepoetin	C. Infection

To check your answers, see Appendix F.

_____

*Indicates the question is directly linked to the NCLEX-PN test plan in Appendix G.

WANT TO KNOW MORE? A wide variety of resources are available to enhance your learning and understanding of this chapter.
- Visit thePoint for resources such as
  - NCLEX-Style Student Review Questions
  - Journal Articles
  - Dosage Calculations
  - Drug Monographs
  - Watch and Learn Videos
  - Concepts in Action Animations
- The *Study Guide to Accompany Introductory Clinical Pharmacology,* 12th edition, sold separately, will help you review and apply essential content.
- ✔*PrepU* is available to help students prepare for the NCLEX-PN examination.

Immune Blockers

Key Terms

antibody molecule with the ability to bind to a specific antigen

autoimmune a response where antibodies are formed against one's own body

cell-mediated immunity immune reaction caused by white blood cells

humoral immunity antibody-mediated immune response of the body

hypersensitive reaction undesirable reaction produced by a normal immune system

passive immunity type of immunity occurring from the administration of ready-made antibodies from another individual or animal, with no memory or antibody development to protect against later infection

Learning Objectives

On completion of this chapter, the student will:

1. List the classes of immune blockers used in the immuno-suppressive treatment of diseases.
2. Explain the uses, general drug actions, general adverse reactions, contraindications, precautions, and interactions of the immune blocker drugs.
3. Distinguish important preadministration and ongoing assessment activities the nurse should perform with the client receiving immune blocker drugs.
4. List nursing diagnoses particular to a client receiving immunotherapy drugs.
5. Examine ways to promote an optimal response to therapy, how to manage common adverse reactions, and important points to keep in mind when educating clients about the use of an immune blocker drug.

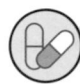 **Drug Classes**

Immunosuppressants
Monoclonal antibodies

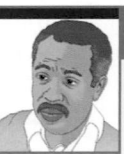 **PHARMACOLOGY IN PRACTICE**

Clients may learn about a specific drug from direct advertising. While his hip is healing, Mr. Park has been rather bored in the rehabilitation wing of the long-term care center. As a result, he has been watching a great deal of daytime television. During evening medication pass, he asks why his physician has not considered using Humira or Enbrel because he is diagnosed with arthritis. Think about how to respond as you learn about immunotherapy and suppression of the immune system.

Cell-mediated immunity involves the lymphatic system and the T lymphocytes (T cells). T cells circulate in the bloodstream and lymphatics, ever prepared to protect the body. The various kinds of T cells include the following:

- Helper T cells—coordinate the immune response and increase B-lymphocyte antibody production.
- Cytotoxic T cells—recognize specific antigens, then attack and kill the cell.

- Suppressor T cells—suppress the immune response once the threat is gone.
- Memory T lymphocytes—recognize previous contact with antigens and activate an immune response.

Other immune cells include the following:

- Natural killer cells—which attack cells directly by altering the cell membrane and causing cell lysis (destruction).
- Dendritic cells—the key initiators of the immune process, and they present the antigen to the T cells.

A defect in the T-cell system can lead to self-attack on one's own tissues resulting in **autoimmune** conditions such as rheumatoid arthritis and the insulin resistance of type 1 diabetes (Pullen, 2014).

Humoral immunity involves antibody creation. **Antibodies** are the proteins produced by the immune system in response to foreign antigens. They are Y-shaped molecules binding to antigens on a pathogenic cell, acting as a flag to the immune system to attack and destroy the cell. When the antibodies mistakenly identify one's own tissue as foreign, the immune system attacks the normal cells, and this is the underlying cause of autoimmune conditions such as systemic lupus erythematosus (SLE) and multiple sclerosis (MS) (Ogbru & Davis, 2021) (see Fig. 49.1).

IMMUNOSUPPRESSANT DRUGS

An immunosuppressive drug is an agent that reduces the strength of the body's own immune system. As noted earlier, autoimmune diseases, such as SLE and MS, cause the immune system to attack the body's own tissue. Immunosuppressant drugs are used to treat these diseases to weaken the immune system, thus suppressing the self-attack reaction. This helps reduce the impact of the autoimmune disease on the body.

AUTOIMMUNE DISEASE

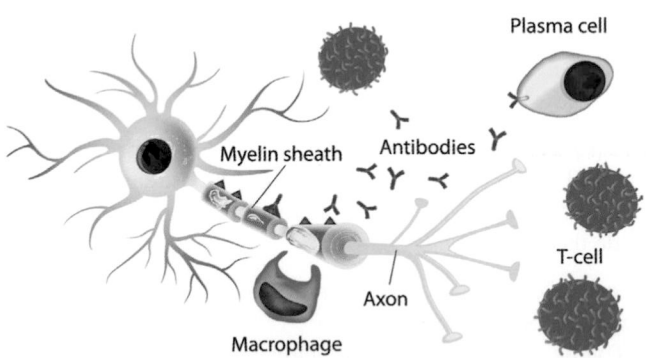

FIGURE 49.1 Autoimmune disease example of multiple sclerosis and the self-attack on nerve cells.

Drugs used to suppress immunity include the following:

- Corticosteroids (prednisone)—prevent production of cytokines and interleukins (ILs) so lymphocytes do not respond (see Chapter 41).
- Calcineurin inhibitors (tacrolimus or cyclosporine)—bind with calcineurin (protein that activates T cells) and prevent secretion of IL-2.
- mechanistic target Of rapamycin (mTOR) inhibitors (sirolimus)—prevent cell cycle completion of the lymphocyte cells.
- IMDH (inosine monophosphate dehydrogenase) inhibitors (azathioprine or mycophenolate)—antimetabolite, which inhibits enzymes and impairs B- and T-cell production.
- Biologics (etanercept)—lysis of lymphocytes.
- Monoclonal antibodies (mAbs, basiliximab)—prevent activation of T lymphocytes.

ACTION AND USES

In the situation of an autoimmune disease, the immune system, which defends the body against disease, malfunctions and attacks the body's own tissue as if it was a foreign tissue. Immunosuppressant drugs suppress this abnormal reaction by weakening the immune system.
Actions of an immunosuppressive drug include:

- inhibiting the inflammatory response.
- inhibiting the activation of T cells.
- reducing antibody formation.

Immunosuppressant drugs are used to treat autoimmune diseases and reduce organ rejection in transplant clients. Autoimmune disorders likely to be treated with immunosuppressive drugs include conditions such as psoriasis, MS, Crohn disease (gastrointestinal system), ulcerative colitis, and rheumatoid arthritis.

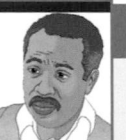

PHARMACOLOGY IN PRACTICE

PATHOPHYSIOLOGY
Immunosuppressants are used to dampen the cellular response of which cell line?
1. Erythrocytes
2. Lymphocytes
3. Megakaryocytes
4. Plasma cells

Organ Transplant

When an individual's organs begin to fail or are traumatically damaged, an organ transplant may be considered. In this situation, an organ (e.g., kidney) is taken from one body and placed in another. An organ transplant can be thought of as a client receiving a foreign object (the new organ), despite methods used to match the tissues between the two individuals.

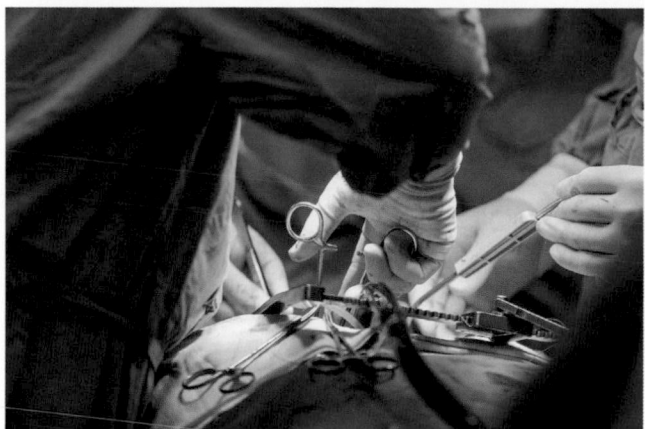

FIGURE 49.2 Reducing the chance of organ rejection is an important use of immunosuppressive drugs.

The new organ is as much a threat as a foreign microorganism like a virus or bacterial cell. The body's immune system recognizes a new organ as being a foreign object and in turn attacks the new organ, thus causing severe damage and leading to the body rejecting the organ. Immunosuppressant drugs are used in transplant clients to intentionally suppress the production and activity of immune cells; as a result, they do not recognize and attack the new organ. When used in this way, immunosuppressants are typically referred to as antirejection drugs and must be taken long term as ongoing protection to the new organ (Fig. 49.2).

ADVERSE REACTIONS

Because these drugs interfere with the immune system, common adverse reactions include headache, chills, and fever. Clients taking biologics may also feel nauseated or experience GI distress. Other adverse reactions experienced are itching, dizziness, and myalgias. Calcineurin inhibitors may cause gum hyperplasia, hair growth, or tremors.

CONTRAINDICATIONS, PRECAUTIONS, AND INTERACTIONS

Vaccination with live virus (such as the chickenpox or measles, mumps, and rubella [MMR] vaccines) should not be given if the client is on an immunosuppressant agent. Because these agents decrease immunity, there is an increased risk of infection. Therefore, clients should be routinely monitored for neutropenia and infectious diseases. Clients with HIV+ should not take alefacept (used for plaque psoriasis).

Calcineurin inhibitors are nephrotoxic in high doses and the BUN should be monitored frequently. Cardiac arrhythmias are more likely to occur if taking calcineurin inhibitors with antiarrhythmic medications. Severe reduction in red cells, white cells, and platelets is seen when those taking IMDH inhibitors are also taking angiotensin-converting enzyme inhibitor (ACEI) for hypertension. Many of the immunosuppressant agents interact with grapefruit

juice and other citrus; consult a clinical nutritionist for client instruction on dietary restrictions.

LASA ALERT

The following drugs may sound alike; so be sure to clarify when they are ordered:

Drug Name	Sounds Like
basiliximab	Bezlotoxumab
CycloSPORINE	cyclophosphamide, Cyklokapron, cycloSERINE
Prograf	Gengraf, PROzac
SandIMMUNE	SandoSTATIN
tacrolimus	everolimus, pimecrolimus, sirolimus, temsirolimus

Drugs that look like a similar drug are noted in the Summary Drug Tables of each chapter.

 ## MONOCLONAL ANTIBODIES

ACTIONS AND USES

Monoclonal antibodies (mAbs) are a **passive** type of immunity, therefore requiring multiple doses to provide ongoing protection. mAbs target specific antigens on the surface of a cell to reduce the immune response. Multiple diseases are treated with mAbs:

- Reducing inflammation and promoting clinical remission in clients with ulcerative colitis (Basson, 2019), skin conditions, and rheumatoid arthritis
- Targeting the allergy cascade in clients with severe asthma (Stephenson, 2017)
- Neutralizing key immune elements that attack the nervous system in clients with MS (Voge & Alvarez, 2019)
- Preventing migraine attacks
- Preventing new vessel formation in the eyes of clients with wet macular degeneration
- As an adjunct in fighting viral diseases, e.g., HIV and COVID-19

There are a number of mAbs on the market, and due to the manner in which mAbs are named, they can be confused with each other easily. Box 49.1 discusses the methodology used in naming the drugs, and this can be helpful in drug recognition.

ADVERSE REACTIONS

Central Nervous System Reactions
- Headache
- Dizziness

GI System Reactions
- Nausea
- Abdominal pain

BOX 49.1 | Naming of Monoclonal Antibodies

When looking at a list of mAb names, to the untrained eye, it appears to be an odd assortment of letters. Thus, making the recognition of mAb names and understanding the uses daunting. Yet the arrangement of those letters is very specific and designed to help in the understanding of mAb naming and function.

Let us use the example of a drug made to treat arthritis: *adalimumab* (Humira).

Monoclonal terminology is built from the back of the word forward. Starting with the end of the word, or suffix, *-mab* indicates it is a monoclonal antibody.

The next one or two letters indicate the type of tissue used to make the mAb. It can be pure tissue or a chimeric combination of tissue types.

- o, indicates from mouse tissue
- u, indicates from human tissue
- xi, combination of human and mouse tissues
- zu, combination of mouse and human, but the majority is human

-u-mab, this drug is made from human tissue.

The next section of the word indicates the target tissue. It may be one, two, or three letters. Over time, some of the letters have changed. The determination of the letters dealing more with the ability to say the word than the meaning.

- ba(c) = bacterial
- ci(r) = cardiovascular
- fu(ng) = fungal
- ki(n) = interleukin
- li(m) = immune system
- ne(ur) = neural
- os = bone
- tox(a) = toxin
- t(u)a = tumor
- vi(r) = viral

-lim-u-mab now means a monoclonal antibody, originating from human tissue, to target the immune system.

Lastly, the beginning of the word, or prefix, is what is given to the drug by the manufacturer. Hopefully, the letters chosen make the word flow and easy to say.

Ada-lim-u-mab, a monoclonal antibody, originating from human tissue, to target the immune system. It is a drug developed to treat arthritis and immune skin disorders. (Dyson, 2016)

Immune System Reactions

- Infection, skin eruptions
- Upper respiratory infection (URI) with cough
- Antibody development

Infusion Reactions

Many mAbs are administered intravenously (IV) or by subcutaneous injection. During IV infusion a **hypersensitive reaction** may occur. This is due to the sensitivity of the client to the tissue of origin of the mAb. Mouse and human tissues are used to make the drugs. When mAbs are composed of more mouse tissue than human tissue, a hypersensitive reaction is more likely to be experienced. Also, infusion-related reactions are more likely to occur during the first infusion than in subsequent treatments. Table 49.1 lists the adverse reactions potentially seen in an infusion reaction.

> **! NURSING ALERT**
>
> Although infusion reactions occur in about 3%–4% of those receiving mAbs, they are more likely to happen when they are derived from mouse tissue (Fig. 49.3). The key to knowing this is in the suffix of the drug name. Drugs ending in *-momab* are derived from mice and have the highest risk for hypersensitive reaction (Wujcik, 2018).

CONTRAINDICATIONS AND PRECAUTIONS

mAbs should not be used if a person has an active, severe infection. Live vaccine should not be given directly before, during, or immediately after mAb use. Viral infections, such as hepatitis B may be reactivated during therapy, and antiviral treatment should be initiated. Monitor for adverse reactions in

TABLE 49.1 Components of Infusion Reactions

BODY SYSTEM	ADVERSE REACTIONS
Generalized	Fever, chills, rigors, sweating, warm feeling
Cardiovascular	Chest pain, palpitations, hypo-/hypertension, tachy-/bradycardia, arrhythmia, edema, ischemia, infarction, cardiac arrest
CNS	Throbbing headache, dizziness, confusion, LOC
Integumentary	Rash, pruritis, urticaria, erythema, tearing, angioedema
GI	Nausea, vomiting, metallic taste, diarrhea, abdominal cramps/bloating
GU	Incontinence, uterine cramping, renal impairment
Multiple sclerosis	Arthralgias, myalgia, fatigue, tumor pain, hypotonia
Respiratory	Cough, dyspnea, nasal congestion, rhinitis, sneezing, hoarseness, tachypnea, wheezing, tightness, bronchospasm, laryngeal edema, stridor, cyanosis, acute respiratory distress syndrome

Vogel, W. (2010). Infusion reactions: diagnosis, assessment, and management. *Clinical Journal of Oncology Nursing, 14*(2), E10-E21. https://doi.org/10.1188/10.CJON.E10-E21.

clients with cardiac and renal impairment (hypertension and proteinuria). Observe for GI distress, change in bowel habits, and progress to colitis and possible bowel perforation. mAbs can cross the placenta and cause fetal harm; therefore, women are cautioned to use effective birth control and should not use the drug when pregnant. Lactation is discouraged during and 6 months after ending mAb treatment.

Therapeutic monoclonal antibody types nomenclature.

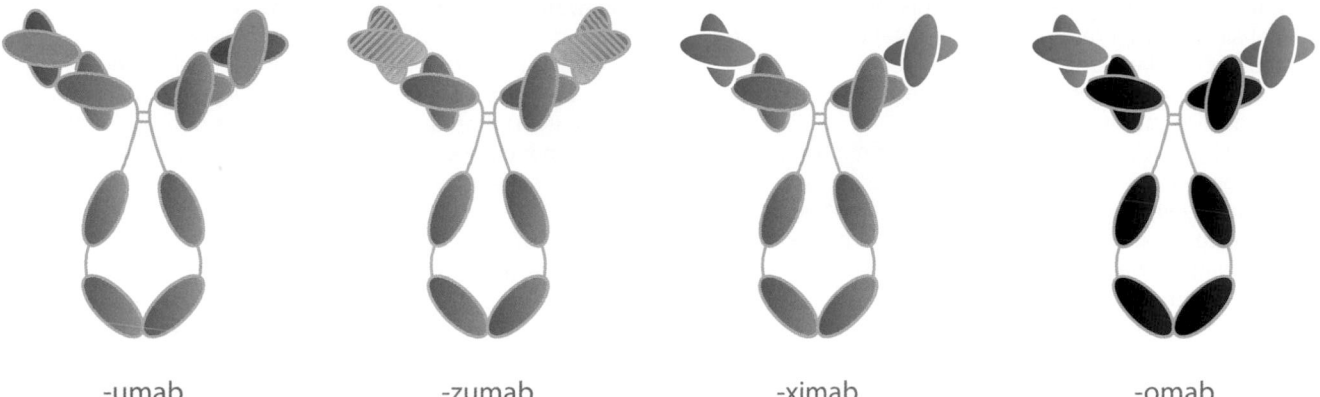

-umab   -zumab   -ximab   -omab

FIGURE 49.3 The different colors help illustrate how distinct mouse tissue is from human and chimeric tissues. (Photo by Visuta/ Shutterstock)

LASA ALERT

The following trade drugs may sound alike, so be sure to clarify when they are ordered:

Drug Name	Sounds Like
Rituxan	Remicade
Synagis	Synalgos-DC, Synflorix, Synvisc

Drugs that look alike are noted in the Summary Drug Tables of each chapter.

INTERACTIONS

The following interactions may occur when an mAb is administered with another agent:

Interacting Drug	Common Use	Effect of Interaction
Clozapine, promazine	Management of psychiatric problems	Increased risk for CNS toxicity
Roflumilast	Treatment of respiratory problems	Increased risk for immunosuppression
Vaccines (BCG, Covid-19, rabies)	Prevent viral disease	Decreased development of immunity to specified pathogen

BIOSIMILARS

By this chapter in the text, you are familiar with generic and trade names for drugs. Because mAbs and vaccines are biological products, the distinction between their equivalents is termed differently—biologic (reference) products and biosimilars. Biologics are produced using technology and living tissue from a type of cell (plant, animal, or microorganism). Because it is living tissue, each batch of product can be slightly different. This would be similar to saying each batch of a trade drug may be different.

Again, the difference is the ingredients used to make the medication; i.e., whether it is chemically synthesized to be exactly the same (trade drug) or if living tissue is used (biologic product). Because patents on many of these biologic products (or reference products) are beginning to expire, this is where biosimilars are seen. Much like trade drugs versus generic drugs, a biosimilar is like the original biologic, only some of the inactive portions may be different. The first drug to have a biosimilar created was infliximab (Remicade) in 2017.

To solve the issue of telling biologics from biosimilars, the FDA recommends that biosimilars have an additional suffix of four randomly generated letters included in the name, infliximab-dyyb (Inflectra). Since then, more biosimilars for this biologic are on the market, they include infliximab-axxq (Avsola) and infliximab-abda (Renflexis). See the Summary Drug Tables in chapters including biologics for more biosimilar names and products.

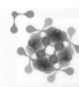

NURSING PROCESS: STEPS TO BUILD CLINICAL JUDGMENT
Client Receiving a Monoclonal Antibody Drug

ASSESSMENT

Preadministration Assessment

A client may be treated as an outpatient in the ambulatory setting or as an inpatient in a hospital. Where administration occurs is dependent upon the extent of the disease, comorbidity, or the complexity of this or other therapies. Data gathering suggestions before the initial administration of an immunotherapy drug include the following:

Objective data

- Note the type and location of the disease.
- Vital signs (temperature, pulse, respirations, and blood pressure) and weight.
- Inspect general physical appearance, noting skin lesions for baseline integumentary status.
- Neurological and psychosocial assessment to monitor for reactions.
- Laboratory and radiologic tests—electrocardiography (ECG), complete blood count (CBC), lipid profile, diabetes screening, and baseline organ function (e.g., liver and thyroid) and autoimmune status.
- Pregnancy testing if female.

Subjective data

- Client's knowledge or understanding of the proposed immunotherapy regimen.
- Previous or concurrent treatments (if any) and toleration of those treatments.
- History of other current diseases or disorder, such as diabetes, malignant disease.
- History of travel to areas where infectious diseases are prevalent.
- History of having had an infectious disease.
- Other factors, such as the client's age, financial problems that may be associated with a long-term illness, family cooperation and interest in client care, and the adequacy of health insurance coverage (which may be of great concern to the client).

Ongoing Assessment

As part of the ongoing assessment expect that the client will experience flu-like symptoms with administration as part of response to treatment. A generalized inflammatory response may occur; therefore, the nurse must anticipate appropriate interventions. If the inflammation worsens despite interventions, steroids may be ordered in an effort to minimize symptoms. Those with preexisting lung cancer should be monitored closely for inflammatory reactions in the respiratory system. Clients should be monitored for opportunistic infections due to the reduction of cells in the immune system and may need to be put on antifungal or antibacterial drugs.

NURSING DIAGNOSES

Drug-specific nursing diagnoses include the following:

- **Impaired comfort: flu-like symptoms** related to stimulation of the immune system.
- **Altered skin integrity** related to integumentary response to the generalized inflammatory process.

Nursing diagnoses related to drug administration are discussed in Chapter 4.

PLANNING

The expected outcomes for the client depend on the reason for administration but may include an optimal response to therapy, meeting client needs related to the management of adverse reactions, and confidence in an understanding of the medication regimen.

IMPLEMENTATION

Promoting an Optimal Response to Therapy

Nurses who are certified in immunotherapy drug administration administer these drugs, but any nurse may be involved in monitoring clients for adverse reactions (see Chapter 51). Immunotherapy drugs are potentially toxic drugs that can cause a variety of effects during and after their administration.

Monoclonal Antibodies

mAbs are usually given parenterally, by the IV route, or some are subcutaneously injected. When infused over time, carefully monitor and observe client for a hypersensitive reaction. To reduce reactions, the drug should be administered slowly. When a reaction does occur stop the infusion and administer IV steroids and/or diphenhydramine. Instruction to the client and family should include that the reactions decrease with ongoing therapy.

Hypersensitive infusion reactions can be somewhat lessened by premedication. Reassure the client that the medications administered before the immunotherapy will help ease the adverse reactions. Often, a combination of acetaminophen and diphenhydramine (with or without a steroid) are given 30 minutes before the infusion. Warm blankets should be provided for client comfort. If clients react a second time, often the treatment is discontinued and another treatment medication or option is considered.

For those self-administering the drug subcutaneously be sure the client or caregiver feels confident in the technique before this becomes a routine procedure carried out at home. Follow-up on knowledge of storage of drug, technique, potential site reactions, and disposal is important.

ⓘ NURSING ALERT

Clients with relapsing MS may be prescribed glatiramer (Copaxone) for self-administration. It comes in a 20 mg/mL formula used daily or 40 mg/mL taken three times weekly. These products are not interchangeable, and the 40 mg formula cannot be used for daily dosing.

For mAbs taken orally, there are no special precautions for handling, yet it is important to take it at the same time each day to support effectiveness. Food may exacerbate the skin rash of erlotinib if taken with food.

Typically, doses are not titrated to adverse reactions, clients will get the full dose, it will be held, or it will be completely discontinued.

Monitoring and Managing Client Needs

Impaired Comfort

Flu-like symptoms, as illustrated in Figure 49.4, can be an array of items including appetite loss, chills, fatigue, fever, headache and body ache, or gastric upset (nausea or diarrhea). For gastric upset, cold and salty foods are

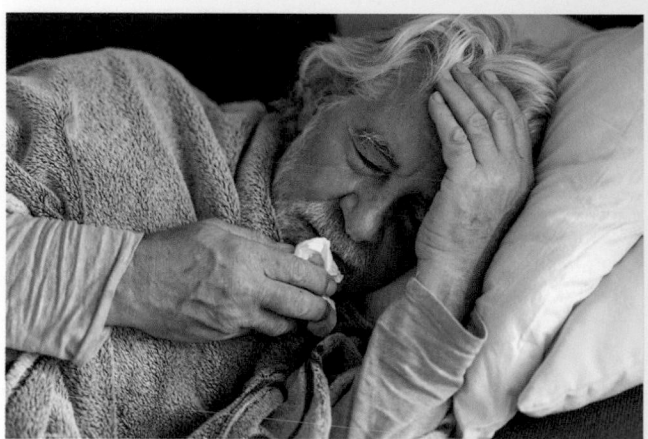

FIGURE 49.4 Flu-like symptoms present as a feeling of malaise and discomfort.

preferred over spicy, sweet, or greasy foods. Provide warm blankets and warm fluids to drink during infusion.

Encourage clients to balance activity with rest periods to reduce fatigue. Although it may sound counterintuitive, exercise helps reduce fatigue; encourage clients to take small walks or participate in activities such as yoga (Puksic et al., 2021).

Altered Skin Integrity
One aspect of the inflammatory reaction to mAb administration is seen as skin inflammation. It is not like a typical reaction to an external irritant, instead it is due to the inflammatory response from within. Do not use acne-type products on the rash (Houlihan et al., 2005). Typically, it presents anywhere on the body that is above the waist during the first week of treatment. Clients should avoid sunlight and use sunscreen even on cloudy days. Instruct the client to avoid rubbing the area and to wear clothing that is not rough or irritating. Using mild soaps and sensitive skin moisturizers can diminish itching. If pustules form instruct the client not to puncture them and monitor for bacterial infection. Harsh soaps and perfumed lotions are avoided.

Potential Medical Complication: Infusion Reactions
Clients should be taught before the drug is given when an infusion reaction is anticipated and may be uncomfortable. The risk of reaction is greater during the first few sessions of treatment. Reactions tend to be more pronounced when the mAb is produced from mouse tissue or a combination of tissues (Dyson, 2016).

> ## ! NURSING ALERT
> The risk of an infusion reaction can be predicted by examining the suffix of the drug being infused:
>
> - –momab (highest risk of infusion reaction)
> - –ximab
> - –zumab
> - –mumab (lowest risk of infusion reaction)

PHARMACOLOGY IN PRACTICE

INTERVENTIONS
A client in the outpatient infusion clinic complains of feeling nauseated and chilly during mAb infusion. Which of the following interventions should the nurse perform to provide comfort? Select all that apply.
1. Reduce the infusion rate.
2. Select a carbonated beverage/ice from the client supplies.
3. Tell the client to avoid sun on clear and cloudy days.
4. Obtain a new blanket from the warmer and soda crackers.

Educating the Client and Family
The health care provider usually discusses the proposed treatment and possible adverse drug reactions with the client and family members. As the nurse, you will briefly review these explanations immediately before administration of any immunotherapy drug.

Clients may receive immunotherapy orally, subcutaneously, or IV, and this could occur in hospitals, in ambulatory centers, or at home. For those receiving immunotherapy drugs orally at home, a client and family teaching plan is based on the drug prescribed, the health care provider's explanation of the drug therapy regimen and instructions for taking the drug, and the needs of the individual. The importance of taking the drug at the same time each day to maintain a consistent body level is emphasized. A calendar or automated medication box indicating the doses to take and dates the drug is to be taken is often helpful for the client. Discuss ways to ensure dosing even if the client does not feel well, such as help from a family member. Special precautions typically do not need to occur in the home other than keeping medications out of reach of children and animals.

Include the following points in a client and family teaching plan when oral/subcut therapy is prescribed:

- Take the drug only as directed on the prescription container.
- Familiarize yourself with the brand or trade name and the generic name to avoid confusion. If you live with another person at home ask that person to help you verify the correct drug and dose of the drug before you take it.
- When self-administering injectables inspect contents for flakes or cloudy fluid—if present do not use.
- Refrigerate in original carton and take out 15–30 minutes before injecting and allow to warm to room temperature; do not put medication in hot water or the microwave.

- Dispose of sharps appropriately in marked containers.
- Never increase, decrease, or omit a dose unless advised to do so by the health care provider. Set up reminders such as a calendar, cellphone alarm, or computer alert if dosing routinely becomes an issue.
- If any problems (adverse reactions) occur, no matter how minor, contact the health care provider immediately.
- All recommendations given by the health care provider, such as increasing the fluid intake or eating or avoiding certain foods, are important.
- The effectiveness or action of the drug could be altered if these directions are ignored. Other recommendations, such as checking the mouth for sores, taking your temperature, or taking care with skin products, are given to identify or minimize some of the effects these drugs have on the body.
- Keep all appointments for immunotherapy. These drugs must be given at certain intervals to be effective.
- Do not take any nonprescription drugs unless the use of a specific drug has been approved by the health care provider.
- Avoid drinking alcoholic beverages unless the health care provider has approved their use.
- Always inform other physicians, dentists, and medical personnel of therapy with this drug.
- Keep all appointments for the laboratory tests ordered by the health care provider. If you are unable to keep a laboratory appointment, then notify the health care provider immediately.

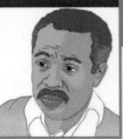

PHARMACOLOGY IN PRACTICE

MANAGING NEEDS

In your client teaching session, you are asked the best method to warm adalimumab for self-injection. Your best reply is _____.

1. In the microwave
2. Rolling the pen between your palms
3. On the counter, safely away from children
4. Running hot tap water on the pen

EVALUATION

- Therapeutic response is achieved and there is reduced evidence of disease.
- Adverse reactions are identified, reported to the primary health care provider, and managed successfully with appropriate nursing interventions:
  - Client reports comfort, with minimal fever or chills.
  - Skin is intact and irritation is reduced.
- Client and family express confidence and demonstrate understanding of the drug regimen.

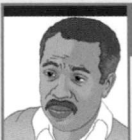

PHARMACOLOGY IN PRACTICE

USING CLINICAL REASONING

Using your concept map of Mr. Park review the medical conditions you have displayed on your map. What can you tell him about the immunotherapy drugs and why they are not used for his condition?

KEY POINTS

- The immune system can be overactivated in autoimmune diseases; antibodies mistake one's own tissues as foreign and self-attack the tissues

- Immunosuppressive drugs are used to weaken an overactive immune system or to diminish the immune response in an organ/tissue transplant.

- Monoclonal antibodies are a passive type of immunity and require multiple doses for ongoing protection.

- Given parenterally, immunotherapies are susceptible to hypersensitive reactions due to the tissues they are made from, i.e., mouse tissue.

- Flu-like reactions are due to the immune-generated response.

 SUMMARY DRUG TABLE
Drugs Used to Treat Autoimmune Diseases and Prevent Organ Rejection

Generic Name	Trade Name	Uses	Adverse Reactions	Dosage Ranges
Immune Suppressant Drugs				
Anti-Organ Rejection Agents				
antithymocyte globulin *an-te-THY-moe-site*	Thymoglobulin	Acute renal, heart, liver transplant rejection, chronic GVHD	GI distress, increased risk of infections	Administer IV infusion by weight
basiliximab *ba-si-LIK-si-mab*	Simulect	Acute renal rejection prophylaxis	GI distress, hypertension, increased risk of infections	20 mg IV infusion
belatacept *bel-AT-a-sept*	Nulojix	Acute renal, liver transplant rejection	GI distress, hypertension, increased risk of infections	Administer IV infusion by weight

Generic Name	Trade Name	Uses	Adverse Reactions	Dosage Ranges
cycloSPORINE *SYE-kloe-spor-een*	SandIMMUNE	Acute renal, heart, liver transplant rejection	GI distress, hypertension, increased risk of infections	Administer IV infusion by weight
mycophenolate *mye-koe-FEN-oh-late*	Cellcept	Acute organ rejection prophylaxis	GI distress, hypertension, increased risk of infections	1–1.5 g IV twice daily
sirolimus *sir-OH-li-mus*	Rapamune	Acute renal rejection prophylaxis, lymphangi-oleiomyomatosis	GI distress, edema, hypertension, increased risk of infections	40 mg orally daily
tacrolimus *ta-KROE-li-mus*	Astagraf XL, Envarsus XR, Prograf	Acute organ rejection prophylaxis, GVHD	GI distress, edema, hypertension, increased risk of infections	Administer IV infusion by weight

Disease-Specific Monoclonal Antibodies and Inhibitors

Asthma

benralizumab *ben-ra-LIZ-ue-mab*	Fasenra	Adjunct for severe asthma	Headache, pharyngitis, antibody development	30 mg subcut every 4 weeks for three doses, then every 8 weeks
dupilumab *doo-PIL-ue-mab*	Dupixent	Adjunct for severe asthma	Eye irritation, injection site irritation, antibody development	100 mg subcut every 2 weeks
mepolizumab *me-poe-LIZ-ue-mab*	Nucala	Adjunct for severe asthma	Headache, injection site irritation, antibody development	100 mg subcut once a month
omalizumab *oh-mah-lye-ZOO-mab*	Xolair	Moderate to severe persistent asthma	Injection site reaction, anaphylaxis	150–375 mg subcut every 2–4 weeks
reslizumab *res-LIZ-ue-mab*	Cinqair	Adjunct for severe asthma	Increased creatine, antibody development	3 mg/kg IV every 4 weeks

Migraine Headaches

eptinezumab *EP-ti-NEZ-ue-mab*	Vyepti	Migraine prophylaxis	Nasopharyngitis	100 mg IV infusion, given four times yearly
erenumab *e-REN-ue-mab*	Aimovig	Migraine prophylaxis	Constipation, injection site reaction, antibody dev.	70 or 140 mg subcut monthly
fremanezumab *free-ma-NEZ-ue-mab*	Ajovy	Migraine prophylaxis	Injection site reaction, antibody dev.	225 mg subcut monthly or 675 mg every 3 months
galcanezumab *GAL-ka-NEZ-ue-mab*	Emgality	Cluster and migraine prophylaxis	Injection site reaction, antibody dev.	Cluster: 300 mg subcut at onset; Migraine: 120 mg subcut monthly

Multiple Sclerosis

alemtuzumab *ay-lem-TU-zoo-mab*	Lemtrada	MS/leukemia	Rash, headache, fever	12 mg IV over 3 days, then yearly
dimethyl fumarate *dye-meth-il Fue-ma-rate*	Tecfidera	MS,– relapsing	Infection potential, flushing, abdominal pain, nausea, diarrhea	120 mg orally BID for 7 days, 240 mg BID maintenance
diroximel fumarate *dye-ROX-i-mel FUE-ma-rate*	Vumerity	MS, relapsing	Infection potential, flushing, abdominal pain, nausea, diarrhea	231 mg orally BID for 7 days, 462 mg BID maintenance
fingolimod *fin-GOL-i-mod*	Gilenya	MS, relapsing	Headache, URI symptoms, nausea, abdominal pain, diarrhea	0.5 mg orally daily

Continued

SUMMARY DRUG TABLE (continued)
Drugs Used to Treat Autoimmune Diseases and Prevent Organ Rejection

Generic Name	Trade Name	Uses	Adverse Reactions	Dosage Ranges
Disease-Specific Monoclonal Antibodies and Inhibitors (Continued)				
glatiramer gla-TIR-a-mer	Copaxone, Glatopa	MS, relapsing	Rash, sweating, flushing, nausea, reaction at injection site	20 mg daily or 40 mg three times weekly subcut
monomethyl fumarate MON-oh-METH-il FUE-ma-rate	Bafiertam	MS, relapsing	Infection potential, flushing, abdominal pain, nausea, diarrhea	95 mg orally BID for 7 days, 190 mg BID maintenance
natalizumab na-ta-LIZ-u-mab	Tysabri	MS, relapsing; Crohn disease	Headache, depression, fatigue, rash, nausea, muscle pain, URI, infusion reaction	300 mg IV infusion every 4 weeks
ocrelizumab ok-re-LIZ-ue-mab	Ocrevus	MS, relapsing	Infection potential, URI, infusion reaction	300 mg IV infusion initial dosing, 600 mg IV every 6 months
ofatumumab oh-fa-TOOM-yoo-mab	Kesimpta	MS/leukemia	Headache, URI symptoms	20 mg subcut weekly
ozanimod oh-ZAN-i-mod	Zeposia	MS, relapsing	Headache, URI symptoms	0.23–1 mg orally daily
siponimod si-PON-i-mod	Mayzent	MS, relapsing	Headache, hypertension	0.22–2 mg orally daily
teriflunomide ter-i-FLOO-noh-mide	Aubagio	MS, relapsing	Headache, alopecia, nausea, diarrhea	7–14 mg orally daily
Rheumatoid Arthritis				
abatacept ab-a-TA-sept	Orencia	Arthritis—juvenile idiopathic, psoriatic, rheumatoid	Headache, nasal congestion, URI symptoms, nausea	500–750 mg IV every 4 weeks
adalimumab a-da-LIM-yoo-mab	Humira	RA; other autoimmune disorders (e.g., Crohn disease)	Irritation at injection site, increased risk of infections	40 mg subcut every other week
anakinra an-a-KIN-ra	Kineret	RA, COVID-19, NOMID	Headache, irritation at injection site, pancytopenia	100 mg subcut daily
baricitinib bar-i-SYE-ti-nib	Olumiant	RA, when refractory to (TNF) therapies	URI symptoms, rhinitis	2 mg orally daily
certolizumab cer-to-LIZ-u-mab	Cimzia	RA, Crohn disease	URI and UTI symptoms	400 mg subcut every 2 weeks or monthly
etanercept et-a-NER-sept	Enbrel	Arthritis—juvenile idiopathic, psoriatic, rheumatoid	Headache, rhinitis, irritation at injection site, increased risk of infections	25 mg subcut twice weekly or 50 mg subcut weekly
golimumab goe-LIM-ue-mab	Simponi	Arthritis—psoriatic, rheumatoid, ulcerative colitis	URI symptoms, rhinitis, irritation at injection site, increased risk of infections	50 mg subcut weekly
inFLIXimab in-FLIKS-e-mab	Remicade	RA in combination with methotrexate, Crohn disease, ulcerative colitis	Fever, chills, headache	3–10 mg/kg IV infusion at specified weekly intervals
riTUXimab ri-TUK-si-mab	Rituxan, Ruxience (rituximab-pvvr), Truxima (rituximab-abbs)	Leukemia, lymphoma, inflammatory diseases, RA	Fever, chills, headache, URI symptoms	1 g IV every 2 weeks, 4 times per year
sarilumab sar-IL-ue-mab	Kevzara	RA	Increase liver enzyme levels, skin reactions	200 mg subcut every 2 weeks

Generic Name	Trade Name	Uses	Adverse Reactions	Dosage Ranges
tocilizumab *toe-si-LIZ-oo-mab*	Actemra	Arthritis—juvenile idiopathic, psoriatic, rheumatoid	Headache, nasal congestion, URI symptoms, increased blood pressure, elevated alanine aminotransferase level (liver function)	4 mg/kg IV every 4 weeks
tofacitinib *toe-fa-SYE-ti-nib*	Xeljanz	RA, ulcerative colitis, PA	URI symptoms, rhinitis	5–11 mg orally, one to two times daily
upadacitinib *ue-PAD-a-SYE-ti-nib*	Rinvoq	RA	URI symptoms, rhinitis	15 mg orally once daily
Psoriasis				
apremilast *a-PRE-mi-last*	Otezla	Psoriasis, PA, oral ulcers of Behcet disease	Nasopharyngitis, nausea, diarrhea, weight loss	10–20 mg daily or twice daily
brodalumab *broe-DAL-ue-mab*	Siliq	Plaque psoriasis	Nasopharyngitis	210 mg subcut, weekly, to biweekly for 16 weeks
guselkumab *gue-sel-KOO-mab*	Tremfya	Plaque psoriasis, PA	Infection potential, URI	100 mg subcut every 8 weeks
ixekizumab *ix-ee-KIZ-ue-mab*	Taltz	Plaque psoriasis, PA, ankylosing spondylitis	Infection potential, URI, injection site reaction	80–160 mg subcut every 4 weeks
risankizumab-rzaa *RIS-an-KIZ-ue-mab*	Skyrizi	Plaque psoriasis	Infection potential, URI	75–150 mg subcut every 12 weeks
secudinumab *sek-ue-KIN-ue_mab*	Cosentyx	Plaque psoriasis, PA, ankylosing spondylitis	Infection potential, URI	150–300 mg subcut every 4 weeks
tildrakizumab *til-dra-KIZ-ue-mab*	Ilumya	Plaque psoriasis	Infection potential, URI	100 mg subcut every 12 weeks
ustekinumab *you-stek-in-YOU-mab*	Stelara	Plaque psoriasis, PA, Crohn disease, ulcerative colitis	Infection potential, URI	Based on weight, IV or subcut
vedolizumab *ve-doe-LIZ-ue-mab*	Entyvio	Crohn disease, ulcerative colitis	Headache, URI, arthralgia	300 mg IV infusion every 8 weeks
VEGFR Antagonists—Eye Preparations for Macular Degeneration				
aflibercept *a-FLIB-er-sept*	Eylea	Macular degeneration, diabetic macular edema/retinopathy		Intravitreal injection monthly/bimonthly
brolucizumab *BROE-lue-SIZ-ue-mab*	Beovu	Macular degeneration—wet		Intravitreal injection monthly for 3 months
pegaptanib *peg-AP-ta-nib*	Macugen	Macular degeneration—wet		Intravitreal injection every 6 weeks
ranibizumab *ra-ni-BIZ-oo-mab*	Lucentis	Macular degeneration, diabetic macular edema/retinopathy		Intravitreal injection monthly
Adjuncts Used to Treat HIV Infection With Antiretrovirals				
ibalizumab *Eye-ba-LIZ-ue-mab*	Trogarzo	Drug-resistant HIV	Dizziness, nausea, rash, neutropenia, increased bilirubin	2000 mg IV loading dose, then 800 mg every 2 weeks for maintenance

CHAPTER REVIEW

Know Your Drugs

Clients sometimes know a medication by the brand (or trade) name and not the generic name. To recognize both names match the brand name with the generic name of the same medication.

Generic Name	Brand Name
1. mycophenolate	A. Skyrizi
2. etanercept	B. Cellcept
3. risankizumab-rzaa	C. Enbrel
4. tofacitinib	D. Xeljanz

Calculate Medication Dosages

1. Tofacitinib is infused every 4 weeks at 4 mg/kg. If the teen weighs 38 kg, what should the dose of tofacitinib be in this infusion? _____

Prepare for the NCLEX

RECALL THE FACTS

1. Which immune blockers are considered biologic products?
   1. Calcineurin inhibitors
   2. Monoclonal antibodies
   3. Corticosteroids
   4. IMDH inhibitors
2. Which of the following elements involves humoral immunity?
   1. Dendritic cells
   2. Suppressor T cells
   3. Antibodies
   4. Platelets
3. Immune blockers do all the following functions, except _____?
   1. inhibit the activation of T cells
   2. reduce antibody formation
   3. inhibit the inflammatory response
   4. reduce febrile episodes
4. A client will be starting reslizumab for asthma. They fearfully ask about infusion reactions. Your best response is _____.
   1. "Your drug is mouse free."
   2. "What have you heard about infusion reactions?"
   3. "Don't worry we can treat it if it happens"
   4. "Why are you worried, skin reactions are far worse."
5. During the preadministration assessment, the nurse is alerted by the following client statement.
   1. "We recently traveled to Canada."
   2. "I had my gallbladder removed 3 years ago."
   3. "My friend had a positive TB test."
   4. "My pregnant daughter just moved into our house."

6. *Flu-like symptoms include the following?
   1. Appetite increase, fatigue, nausea
   2. Fatigue, chills, body aches
   3. Fever, skin flushing, nausea
   4. Diarrhea, tachycardia, fatigue

ANALYZE THE FACTS

7. Which monoclonal antibody would you predict is greater for a hypersensitive reaction?
   1. certolizumab
   2. erenumab
   3. basiliximab
   4. dupilumab
8. Volunteers are making infusion comfort kits for the ambulatory clinic. Which item would be inappropriate?
   1. Sour hard candies
   2. Fleece quilts
   3. Coupon for local fast food
   4. Stretch elastic band

ALTERNATE-FORMAT QUESTIONS

9. The infusion room nurse suspects the client is reacting to the mAb infusion. Arrange the following actions as they should happen next:
   1. Call the provider
   2. Stop the infusion
   3. Replace blanket with a fresh one from the warmer
   4. Administer standing order steroids/antihistamine
10. The label in the IV piggyback reads tofacitinib 172 mg/100 mL. Is this an appropriate dose for a child weighing 76 pounds?

To check your answers, see Appendix F.

---

*Indicates the question is directly linked to the NCLEX-PN test plan in Appendix G.

> **WANT TO KNOW MORE?** A wide variety of resources are available to enhance your learning and understanding of this chapter.
> - Visit thePoint for resources such as
>   - NCLEX-Style Student Review Questions
>   - Journal Articles
>   - Dosage Calculations
>   - Drug Monographs
>   - Watch and Learn Videos
>   - Concepts in Action Animations
> - The *Study Guide to Accompany Introductory Clinical Pharmacology*, 12th edition, sold separately, will help you review and apply essential content.
> - ✓**PrepU** is available to help students prepare for the NCLEX-PN examination.

UNIT 13
Drugs That Fight Cancer

ancer is still dreaded in our culture. It is not one disease; rather, it is cells of any body part gone haywire. At one time, a diagnosis of cancer was akin to a death sentence. With the advent of numerous drugs, known as chemotherapy, cancer is now viewed as a chronic illness in which people may be diagnosed and treated, then monitored for the remainder of their lives and treated again should cancer cells reemerge. The information provided in this unit is about antineoplastic drugs and meant to inform you about these medications—not to prepare you to administer them. Most hospitals and clinics require that nurses receive specialized training and standardized educational preparation before they are permitted to administer antineoplastic drugs. The Oncology Nursing Society has developed guidelines and educational tools for credentialing nurses for certification in administering chemotherapy.

Many of the treatments today are limited only by the destruction to the good cells in the body. The information in Chapter 50 is based on the need of all nurses to be able to assess and treat clients undergoing chemotherapy, whether they present with adverse reactions in the primary health care provider's clinic setting, the hospital emergency department, or being treated in the acute care setting for other illnesses or injuries.

With the advent of immunotherapy agents, all nurses will see more cancer clients being treated in the community rather than sequestered in large, urban medical centers during the course of treatment. Coupled with information gained from Unit 12, Chapter 51 will increase the understanding of how immunotherapy agents are used to treat cancers by helping our own cells recognize and respond to cancer cells just as if they were foreign microorganisms.

Because these medications (immunotherapy) target the immune system and not the cancer cells themselves, these drugs are often given in tandem with traditional chemotherapy. The difference between conventional chemotherapy and the newer targeted immunotherapies can be

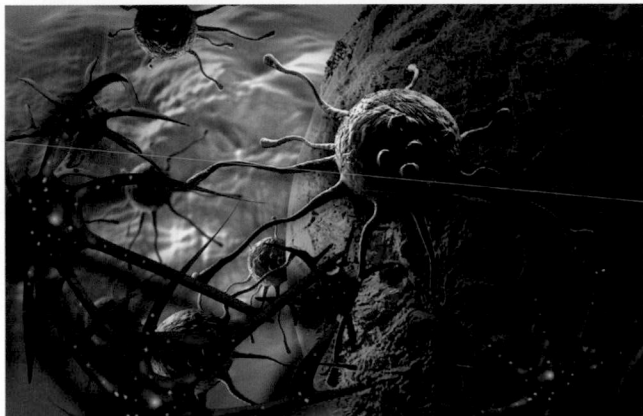

Jovan Vitanovski/Shutterstock.

described by the analogy of a car speeding out of control on the road.

> … A cancer cell is like a runaway car on the highway, where the gas pedal is stuck (the oncogenes are turned on). These cells are accelerating and continuously dividing. The brakes on the car (tumor suppressor genes) aren't working either. When conventional chemotherapy is used, it is like standing on the side of the highway, pointing a shotgun at the car and shooting it to make it stop. In this case there would be lots of collateral damage, to the road, other cars and innocent bystanders—likewise, many healthy cells are damaged in the form of adverse reactions to the traditional chemotherapy drugs. Targeted therapy is like putting a mechanic in the car to fix the gas pedal, and make the car stop. The effort is focused; less damage is done to structures around the cancer cell.
>
> (Ganguly, 2015)

With these drugs many more people may live longer, improved quality lives.

Drugs That Fight Cancer

Traditional Chemotherapy

Key Terms

alopecia abnormal loss of hair; baldness

anemia decrease in the number of red blood cells and hemoglobin value below normal

anorexia loss of appetite

antineoplastic drug used to treat neoplasia (cancer)

bone marrow suppression decreased production of all blood cells; also called *myelosuppression*

cell cycle nonspecific pertaining to a drug used in cancer treatment, effective in any phase of cell division

cell cycle specific pertaining to a drug used in cancer treatment, affecting a specific phase of cell division

chemotherapy drug therapy with a chemical, often used when referring to treatment with an antineoplastic drug

extravasation escape of fluid from a blood vessel into surrounding tissue

leukopenia decrease in the number of leukocytes (white blood cells)

metastasis spread of cancer outside the original organ or tissue

myelosuppression see bone marrow suppression

neoplasm a group of cells that undergo an abnormal growth pattern

neutropenia abnormally small number of neutrophils (infection-fighting type of white blood cell)

oncogenes a gene, which can make a cell become cancerous with specific circumstances

oral mucositis inflammation of the oral mucous membranes

palliation therapy designed to treat symptoms, not to produce a cure

stomatitis inflammation of a cavity opening, such as the oral cavity

thrombocytopenia decreased number of platelets in the blood

tumor suppressor genes a gene, which protects a cell from becoming cancerous

vesicant caustic drug substance

Learning Objectives

On completion of this chapter, the student will:

1. List the types of drugs used in the treatment of neoplastic diseases.
2. Explain the uses, general drug actions, general adverse reactions, contraindications, precautions, and interactions of the traditional chemotherapy drugs.
3. Distinguish important preadministration and ongoing assessment activities the nurse should perform with the client taking traditional chemotherapy drugs.
4. List nursing diagnoses particular to a client taking traditional chemotherapy drugs.
5. Examine ways to promote an optimal response to therapy, how to manage common adverse reactions, and important points to keep in mind when educating clients about the use of traditional chemotherapy drug.

 Drug Classes

Cell cycle–specific agents   Cell cycle–nonspecific agents

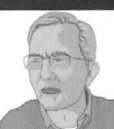 **PHARMACOLOGY IN PRACTICE**

Clients and families undergoing treatment for a malignant disease need special consideration, understanding, and emotional support. On occasion, these needs are unrecognized by members of the health care profession. Mr. Phillip comes to the clinic for a routine blood pressure check. As he sits at your desk he becomes tearful, telling you his wife fought breast cancer only to die in a car accident. As you read about the drugs used, think about your reaction to his grief situation.

D rugs, in addition to surgery and radiation, are tools used in the treatment of malignant diseases (i.e., cancer). The term **chemotherapy** is often used to refer to the drugs used to treat cancer. Another term seen is **antineoplastic**, meaning agents used to kill neoplasms or cancerous cells. Currently, there is a large number of drugs used and many biologic agents designed to target and kill cancer cells. This chapter discusses the traditional chemotherapy drugs used in the treatment of cancer—those which kill both cancerous and fast-growing tissues. The text in this chapter is designed to introduce you to the concepts of chemotherapy, in a manner which will help you in teaching your clients about the therapies.

Therapy typically has the goal of curing the client of their cancer. This is dependent many times on the stage or the advancement of the tumor cell growth. Although these drugs may not always lead to a complete cure of cancer, they often slow the rate of tumor growth and delay **metastasis** (spreading of cancer to other sites). These drugs can be used for cure, control, or **palliation** (comfort care, the relief of symptoms at the end of life).

THE CELL CYCLE

All cells grow in a specific pattern of growth called the *cell cycle* (Fig. 50.1). During the cell cycle, different components of a cell are synthesized, and the cell divides into two new cells.

The five phases of cell growth are:

1. G_1—RNA (ribonucleic acid) and proteins are built
2. S—DNA (deoxyribonucleic acid) is made from the components of the G_1 phase
3. G_2—RNA and protein synthesis preparing for cell division
4. M—mitotic cell division (the cell has doubled its contents and splits into two separate cells)
5. G_0—the dormant or resting phase

When the cell goes into a resting phase, the cell starts performing its usual function in the body (e.g., a white blood cell might "Go" to work fighting infection) or it prepares to start the cycle of cell division again. Some cells, such as blood cells, rapidly reproduce in a matter of hours. Other cells, such as nerve cells, complete their cell division and

then go into the resting phase for years. Some cells tend to stay in the resting phase but quickly divide if the tissue is injured. Liver cells are a good example of this behavior; they do not replicate unless there is damage to the liver. An important key point to remember is that the cells do not all go through the cycle at the same time.

Conventional antineoplastic drugs (or traditional chemotherapy) are designed to attack a cell during one or many of the phases of cell division. Drugs are categorized as **cell cycle specific** (meaning they target the cell in one of the phases of cell division) or as **cell cycle nonspecific** (they can target the cell at any phase of the cycle). Because the cancerous cells do not all reproduce at the same time, multiple chemotherapy drugs are given together to increase the chance that all cells will be affected by at least one of the drugs. Many subcategories of traditional chemotherapy drugs are available to treat malignancies. The traditional chemotherapy drugs covered in this chapter include the cell cycle–nonspecific and cell cycle–specific drugs.

The strategy of traditional chemotherapy is to affect cells that rapidly divide and reproduce. Malignant **neoplasms** or cancerous tumors usually consist of rapidly growing (abnormal) cells. Cancer cells have no biologic feedback controls to stop their growth or proliferation. Cancer cells are more sensitive to traditional chemotherapy drugs when the cells are in the process of growing and dividing. Chemotherapy is administered at the time the cell population is dividing as part of a strategy to optimize cell death. Using this approach, the faster the cancer grows, the faster it will die.

Because the drugs are given systemically (i.e., they circulate through the entire body), other rapidly growing cells are usually affected by these drugs. Rapidly growing normal cells in our bodies include: the lining of the oral cavity and gastrointestinal (GI) tract, cells of the gonads, bone marrow, hair follicles, and lymph tissue. Thus, traditional chemotherapy drugs affect these normal fast-growing tissues as well as malignant cells, causing unpleasant adverse reactions.

Chemotherapy is typically administered in a series of cycles to allow for recovery of normal cells and to destroy more malignant cells (Fig. 50.2). This timing of drug administration is based on the *fractional cell kill hypothesis*. For example, a group of drugs are selected and this drug regimen is intended to kill about 90% of the cancer cells during the first course of treatment. This means 10% of the cancer cells still remain in the body and continue to grow. Then the second course of chemotherapy is given, according to this theory, the chemotherapy targets the remaining cancer cells and reduces those cells by another 90%. Each cycle of treatment with the traditional chemotherapy drugs kills some, but by no means all, of the cancer cells. Theoretically, when only a few cells remain, the body's own immune system will be triggered and destroy what is left. By understanding the cell kill hypothesis and the cell cycle, one can appreciate the rationale for using repeated doses of chemotherapy with different traditional chemotherapy drugs. Various drugs that target cancer cells at various phases of the cell cycle are administered to kill as

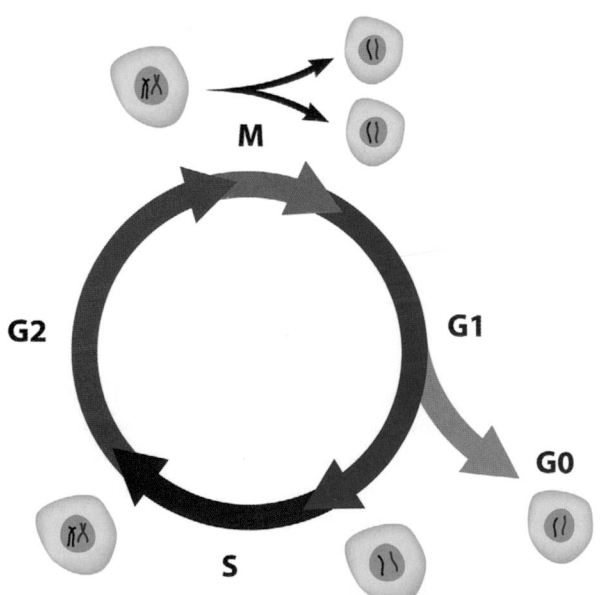

FIGURE 50.1 The cell cycle. G_1, RNA and protein synthesis; S, DNA synthesis; G_2, RNA and protein synthesis; M, mitotic cell division; G_0, cell resting phase, during which the cell either differentiates to perform its function or dies.

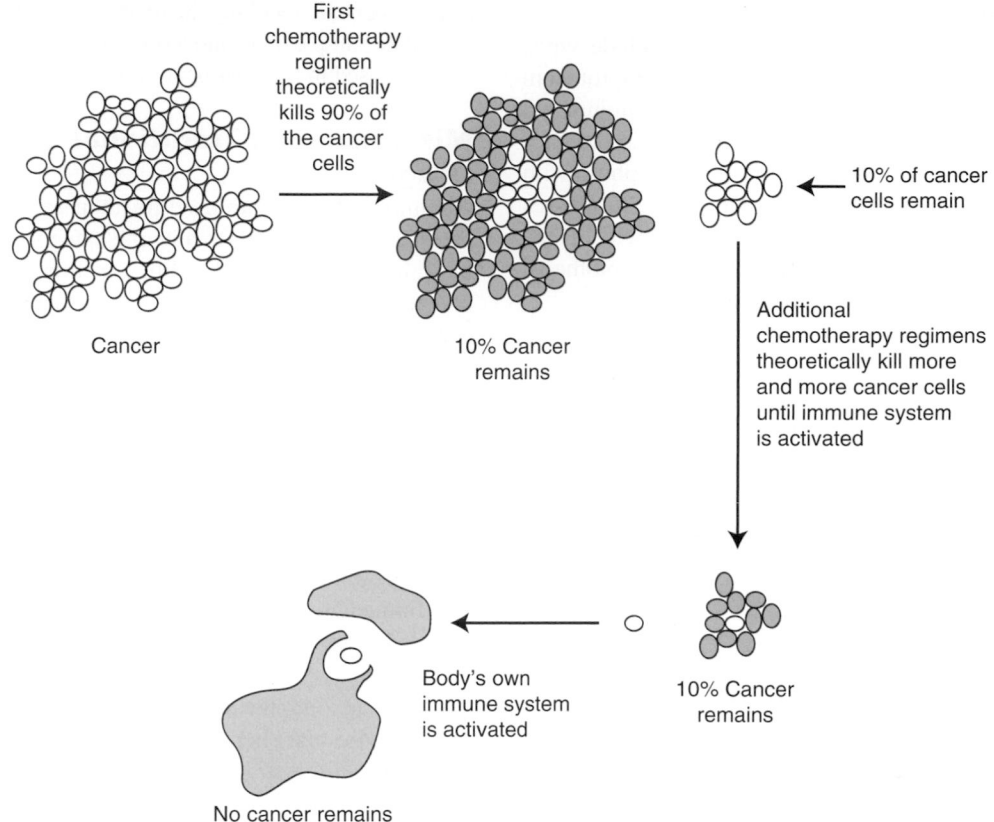

FIGURE 50.2 The fractional cell kill hypothesis: rationale for repeated chemotherapy regimens.

many cells as possible. Repeated courses of chemotherapy are used to kill an even greater proportion of the malignant cells until, theoretically, no cells are left.

 Herbal Considerations

Green tea and black teas come from the same plant. The difference is in the processing. Green tea is simply dried tea leaves, whereas black tea is fermented, giving it the dark color, stronger flavor, and the lowest amount of tannins and polyphenols. The beneficial effects of green tea lie in the polyphenols, or flavonoids, which have antioxidant properties. Antioxidants are thought to play a major role in preventing disease (e.g., colon cancer) and reducing the effects of aging. Green tea polyphenols are powerful antioxidants. The polyphenols are thought to act by inhibiting the reactions of free radicals in the body that are believed to play a role in aging. The benefits of green tea include an overall sense of well-being, cancer prevention, dental health, and maintenance of heart and liver health. Green tea taken as directed is safe and well-tolerated. Because green tea contains caffeine, nervousness, restlessness, insomnia, and GI upset may occur. Green tea should be avoided during pregnancy because of its caffeine content. Clients with hypertension, cardiac conditions, anxiety, insomnia, diabetes, and ulcers should use green tea with caution (DerMarderosian & Beutler, 2003).

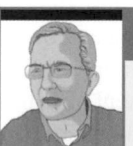

PHARMACOLOGY IN PRACTICE

PHYSIOLOGY

A nurse is caring for a client who is prescribed vinblastine. The nurse explains to the client that vinblastine is a cell cycle–specific drug. Which of the following is a characteristic of a cell cycle–specific drug?
1. Targets the cells at any phase of the cycle
2. Targets only the cells that are malignant
3. Targets the cells in various stages of cell division
4. Targets the cells in one of the phases of cell division

 CELL CYCLE–SPECIFIC DRUGS

ACTIONS AND USES

Cell cycle–specific drugs act on the cell in one specific phase of the process of cell division, affecting both malignant and normal cells. A combination of these drugs, all acting at different phases of cell division, is typically used to treat leukemias, lymphomas, and a variety of solid tumors. The site of action of each drug depends on the drug subcategory. See the Summary Drug Table: Traditional Chemotherapy Drugs for more information.

Plant Alkaloids

Drugs that are derived from plant alkaloids include vinca alkaloids, taxanes, podophyllotoxins, and camptothecin analog drugs. The vinca alkaloids interfere with amino acid production in the S phase and formation of microtubules in the M phase. Taxanes also interfere in the M phase with microtubules. Cells are stopped during the S and G_2 phases by the podophyllotoxins and thus are unable to divide. DNA synthesis during the S phase is inhibited by camptothecin analog drugs such as topotecan (Hycamtin).

Antimetabolites

Antimetabolite drugs are substances that incorporate themselves into the cellular components during the S phase of cell division. This interferes with the synthesis of RNA and DNA, making it impossible for the cancerous cell to divide into two daughter cells. These drugs are used for many of the leukemias, lymphomas, and solid tumors as well as autoimmune diseases. Methotrexate is an example of antimetabolite drugs.

CELL CYCLE–NONSPECIFIC DRUGS

ACTIONS AND USES

Cell cycle–nonspecific drugs interfere with the process of cell division of malignant and normal cells. Because they do not exert action specifically on one portion of the cell cycle, they are called *nonspecific* drugs. These drugs are used to cure, control, or provide palliation in the treatment of leukemias, lymphomas, and many different solid tumors, and are also used in the treatment of certain autoimmune diseases.

Alkylating Agents

Alkylating agents make the cell a more alkaline environment, which in turn damages the cell. Malignant cells appear to be more susceptible to the effects of alkylating drugs than normal cells. A number of subcategories are included in this group of cell cycle–nonspecific drugs. Nitrogen mustard derivatives, ethyleneimines, and platinum-based drugs all break or interfere with the crosslinks in the DNA structure. The alkyl sulfonate drug busulfan interferes with DNA of granulocytes and is used primarily for leukemias. The hydrazine group interferes with multiple phases in the synthesis of RNA, DNA, and protein. Nitrosoureas are unique in that they can cross the blood–brain barrier, and therefore are used in treating brain tumors.

Antineoplastic Antibiotics

Antineoplastic antibiotics, unlike their anti-infective antibiotic relatives, do not fight infection. Rather, their action is similar to alkylating drugs. Antineoplastic antibiotics appear to interfere with DNA and RNA synthesis, thereby delaying or inhibiting cell division and blocking the reproductive ability of malignant cells. An example of an antineoplastic antibiotic is doxorubicin, which is used in the treatment of many solid tumors.

Miscellaneous Traditional Chemotherapy Drugs

A number of drugs are used for their antineoplastic actions but they do not belong to any one category. The mechanism of action of many of the drugs in this unrelated group is not entirely clear. Examples of miscellaneous traditional chemotherapies are provided in the Summary Drug Table: Traditional Chemotherapy Drugs.

ADVERSE REACTIONS

Adverse reactions to traditional chemotherapy drugs can be viewed in three different time frames: immediate (during the actual administration), during therapy cycles, and long term (many years later, during survivorship).

Immediate adverse reactions occur as a result of administration. These include nausea and vomiting from highly emetic drugs or the potential of intravenous (IV) **extravasation** (leakage into the surrounding tissues) of irritating solutions. Traditional chemotherapy drugs are potentially toxic, and their administration is often associated with serious adverse reactions. At times, some of these adverse effects are allowed because the only alternative is to stop treatment of cancer. A treatment plan is developed that will prevent, lessen, or treat most or all of the symptoms of a specific adverse reaction. An example of prevention is giving an antiemetic before administering a traditional chemotherapy drug known to cause severe nausea and vomiting. Box 50.1 provides a list of those drugs most likely to cause nausea and vomiting.

An example of a treatment for an adverse reaction is the administration of an antiemetic and IV fluids with electrolytes when severe vomiting is anticipated. When the drugs

---

BOX 50.1	Emetic Potential of Traditional Chemotherapy Drugs

The following drugs have a 60% or greater (levels 4 and 5) chance of causing nausea and vomiting when administered to clients.

Alkylating Agents	**Antibiotics**
carboplatin	dactinomycin
carmustine	daunorubicin
cisplatin	doxorubicin
cyclophosphamide	mitoxantrone.
dacarbazine	
ifosfamide	**Antimetabolites**
lomustine	cytarabine
mechlorethamine	methotrexate.
melphalan	
procarbazine	**Plant Alkaloid**
streptozocin.	irinotecan.

listed in Box 50.1 are given, antiemetic protocols should always be followed to reduce adverse reactions. Some drugs, such as platinum-based agents, may damage certain organs during administration. Again, prechemotherapy protocols for IV fluid administration are initiated to prevent adverse reactions.

Some of these reactions are dose-dependent; that is, their occurrence is more common or their intensity is more severe when multiple doses (or cycles) are used. Because the traditional chemotherapy drugs affect cancer cells and rapidly proliferating normal cells (i.e., cells in the bone marrow, GI tract, reproductive tract, and hair follicles), adverse reactions occur as the result of action on these cells.

Adverse reactions common to many of the traditional chemotherapy drugs include **bone marrow suppression** (anemia, leukopenia, thrombocytopenia), **stomatitis** (inflammation of lining tissues), diarrhea, and hair loss. The most common reactions are **leukopenia** (reduced white blood cells) and **thrombocytopenia** (reduced platelets), which may cause cycles of chemotherapy to be delayed until blood cell counts can be raised. Some drugs, especially the alkaloids, affect the nervous system. These adverse reactions can range from a peripheral tingling sensation to *hand and foot syndrome* (tiny capillary leaks in extremities, causing symptoms from skin color changes to numbness).

Because the drugs used to treat cancer are effective, many people are living with the disease either cured or in remission. Some of the adverse reactions to traditional chemotherapy drugs can have long-lasting effects. These include damage to the gonads, causing fertility problems, and to other specific organ systems, leading to cardiac, pulmonary, or neurologic problems. In addition, secondary cancers like leukemia can be caused by the original cancer treatment. These problems are listed in the Summary Drug Table: Traditional Chemotherapy Drugs. Appropriate references should be consulted when administering these drugs, because there are a variety of uses and dose ranges and, in some instances, many adverse reactions.

PHARMACOLOGY IN PRACTICE

ASSESSMENT

The purpose of antineoplastic drugs is to affect cells that rapidly divide and reproduce. However, the adverse effects produced by traditional chemotherapy drugs are the result of their systemic use, which exposes nonmalignant cells in the body that are rapidly dividing and reproducing. Which of the following is **not** an example of a rapidly dividing and reproducing cell in the body?
1. Nerve cell
2. Bone marrow
3. Hair follicle
4. Oral mucosal cell

CONTRAINDICATIONS AND PRECAUTIONS

The information discussed in this section is general, and the contraindications, precautions, and interactions for each traditional chemotherapy drug vary. The chemotherapy nurse should consult appropriate sources before administering any traditional chemotherapy drug.

Traditional chemotherapy drugs are contraindicated in clients with leukopenia, thrombocytopenia, **anemia** (reduced red blood cells), serious infections, serious renal disease, or known hypersensitivity to the drug, and during pregnancy (see Box 50.2 for pregnancy classifications of selected traditional chemotherapy drugs) or lactation.

Traditional chemotherapy drugs are used cautiously in clients with renal or hepatic impairment, active infection, or other debilitating illnesses, or in those who have recently completed treatment with other traditional chemotherapy drugs or radiation therapy.

INTERACTIONS

A number of traditional chemotherapy drugs are harmful to normal cells as well as cancer cells. Cytoprotective agents are drugs used with the traditional chemotherapy drug to protect the normal cells or organs of the body. In this way, enough of the chemotherapeutic drug can be given to eradicate the cancer without irreversible harm to the client. Cytoprotective agents used with traditional chemotherapy drugs are listed in Box 50.3.

BOX 50.2	Pregnancy Classification for Selected Traditional Chemotherapy Drugs	
Pregnancy Category C		
asparaginase	mitotane	streptozocin
dacarbazine	pegaspargase	
Pregnancy Category D		
altretamine	docetaxel	mitoxantrone
azacitidine	doxorubicin	nelarabine
bleomycin	epirubicin	oxaliplatin
busulfan	eribulin	paclitaxel
cabazitaxel	etoposide	pemetrexed
capecitabine	fludarabine	pentostatin
carboplatin	fluorouracil	procarbazine
carmustine	gemcitabine	temozolomide
chlorambucil	hydroxyurea	thioguanine
cisplatin	idarubicin	thiotepa
cladribine	ifosfamide	topotecan
clofarabine	irinotecan	vinblastine
cyclophosphamide	ixabepilone	vincristine
cytarabine	lomustine	vinorelbine
dactinomycin	mechlorethamine	
daunorubicin	melphalan	
decitabine	mercaptopurine	
Pregnancy Category X		
methotrexate		
thalidomide		

BOX 50.3 Cytoprotective Agents

The following drugs function to protect cells or counteract adverse reactions resulting from therapeutic doses of the antineoplastic drugs.

- allopurinol, rasburicase (Elitek): Counteract the increase in uric acid and subsequent hyperuricemia resulting from the metabolic waste buildup from rapid tumor lysis (cell destruction)
- amifostine (Ethyol): Binds with metabolites of cisplatin to protect the kidneys from nephrotoxic effects, reduces xerostomia
- dexrazoxane (Zinecard): Cardioprotective agent used with doxorubicin
- famotidine (Pepcid): Used as premed with paclitaxel protocols to reduce hypersensitivity to the chemotherapy drug
- leucovorin (Wellcovorin), glucarpidase (Voraxaze): Provide folic acid to cells after methotrexate administration
- levoleucovorin (Fusilev): Counteracts with folic acid antagonists, used as rescue for high-dose methotrexate
- mesna (Mesnex): Binds with metabolites of ifosfamide to protect the bladder from hemorrhagic cystitis
- palifermin (Kepivance): Helps epithelial cells in the oral cavity recover after severe mucositis

The following table lists selected interactions of the plant alkaloids, antimetabolites, alkylating drugs, antibiotics, and miscellaneous antineoplastic drugs. Typically, additive bone marrow depressive effects occur when any category of traditional chemotherapy drug is administered with another chemotherapy drug or radiation therapy. Appropriate sources should be consulted by the chemotherapy nurse for a more complete listing of interactions before any antineoplastic drug is administered.

Interacting Drug	Common Use	Effect of Interaction
Plant Alkaloids		
Digoxin	Cardiac problems	Decrease serum level of digoxin
Phenytoin	Seizure disorders	Increased risk of seizures
Oral anticoagulants	Blood thinners	Prolonged bleeding
Antimetabolites		
Digoxin	Cardiac problems	Decrease serum level of digoxin
Phenytoin	Seizure disorders	Decreased need for antiseizure medication
Nonsteroidal anti-inflammatory drugs (NSAIDs)	Pain relief	Methotrexate toxicity
Alkylating Drugs		
Aminoglycosides	Anti-infective agents	Increased risk of nephrotoxicity and ototoxicity
Loop diuretics	Heart problems and edema	Increased risk of ototoxicity

Interacting Drug	Common Use	Effect of Interaction
Phenytoin	Seizure disorder	Increased risk of seizure
Antineoplastic Antibiotics		
Digoxin	Cardiac problems	Decrease serum level of digoxin
Miscellaneous Antineoplastic Drugs		
Insulin and oral antidiabetic	Diabetes management	Increased risk of hyperglycemia
Oral anticoagulants	Blood thinners	Prolonged bleeding
Antidepressants, antihistamines, opiates, or sedatives	Depression, allergy, pain relief, or sedation, respectively	Increased risk of central nervous system depression

LASA ALERT

Cell Cycle Specific Drugs

The following drugs may sound alike; be sure to clarify when they are ordered:

Drug Name	Sounds Like
azaCITIDine	azaTHIOprine, decitabine
cabazitaxel	DOCEtaxel, PACLitaxel
capecitabine	cabozantinib, capmatinib
cladribine	clevidipine, clofarabine, cytarabine, fludarabine, nelarabine
cytarabine	daunorubicin
Dacogen	DACTINomycin
eriBULin	epiRUBicin, erlotinib
etoposide	Teniposide
fludarabine	cladribine, floxuridine, flucytosine, fluorouracil, Flumadine
fluorouracil	floxuridine, flucytosine
Folotyn	Focalin
gemcitabine	gemtuzumab
Hycamtin	Mycamine
Jevtana	Xgeva, Xofigo, Xtandi, Zometa, Zytiga
methotrexate	mercaptopurine, methylPREDNISolone sodium succinate, metOLazone, metroNIDAZOLE, mitoXANTRONE, MXT Patch, PRALAtrexate
nelarabine	Clofarabine
PACLitaxel	cabazitaxel, DOCEtaxel, PARoxetine, Paxil
PEMEtrexed	methotrexate, pembrolizumab, PRALAtrexate, raltitrexed
pentostatin	pentamidine, pentosan
Taxol	Abraxane, Paxil, Taxotere
Taxotere	Abraxane, Taxol
thioguanine	Thiotepa
Trexall	Paxil
trifluridine	trifluoperazine
topotecan	Irinotecan
VinCRIStine	vinBLAStine, vinorelbine
Xeloda	Xenical, Xpovio

Drugs that look like a similar drug are noted in the Summary Drug Tables of each chapter.

LASA ALERT

Cell Cycle Non-Specific Drugs

The following drugs may sound alike; be sure to clarify when they are ordered:

Drug Name	Sounds Like
Adriamycin	Achromycin, Aredia, Idamycin
Alkeran	Alferon, Leukeran, Myleran
asparaginase	calaspargase pegol, pegaspargase
bendamustine	brentuximab, carmustine, lomustine
bleomycin	Cleocin
CARBOplatin	CISplatin, oxaliplatin
carmustine	bendamustine, lomustine
chlorambucil	Chloromycetin
cyclophosphamide	cycloSPORINE, ifosfamide
dacarbazine	dactinomycin, procarbazine
DACTINomycin	dacarbazine, Dacogen, DAPTOmycin, DAUNOrubicin
DAUNOrubicin	DACTINomycin, DOXOrubicin, epiRUBicin, IDArubicin, valrubicin
DOXOrubicin	DACTINomycin, DAUNOrubicin, doxapram, doxazosin, epiRUBicin, IDArubicin, valrubicin
Emcyt	Eryc
Erwinaze	Asparlas, Elaprase, Elspar, Oncaspar
estramustine	enzalutamide, exemestane.
ifosfamide	cyclophosphamide, fostamatinib
Leukeran	Alkeran, leucovorin, Leukine, Myleran
Matulane	Mitotane
melphalan	Mephyton, Myleran

Drug Name	Sounds Like
mitoMYcin	mitotane, mitoXANTRONE
mitoXANTRONE	methotrexate, mitoMYcin, mitotane, MTX Patch, Mutamycin
Paraplatin	Platinol
streptozocin	streptomycin
Temodar	Tambocor
temozolomide	temsirolimus
thiotepa	Thioguanine
valrubicin	DAUNOrubicin, DOXOrubicin, epirubicin, IDArubicin
Valstar	Varubi, valsartan

Drugs that look like a similar drug are noted in the Summary Drug Tables of each chapter.

 Herbal Considerations

The shiitake mushroom, an edible variety of mushroom, is associated with general health maintenance but not with any severe adverse reactions. Mild side effects, such as skin rashes and GI upset, have been reported. Lentinan, a derivative of the shiitake mushroom, is proving to be valuable in boosting the body's immune system and may prolong the survival time of clients with cancer by supporting immunity. In Japan, lentinan is commonly used to treat cancer. Additional possible benefits of this herb include lowering cholesterol levels by increasing the rate at which cholesterol is excreted from the body. Under no circumstances should shiitake or lentinan be used for cancer or any serious illness without consulting a primary health care provider (DerMarderosian & Beutler, 2003).

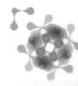 **NURSING PROCESS: STEPS TO BUILDING CLINICAL JUDGMENT**
Client Receiving a Traditional Chemotherapy Drug

ASSESSMENT

Preadministration Assessment

The extent of the preadministration assessment depends on the type of cancer and the client's general physical condition.

Data gathering suggestions before the initial administration of an antineoplastic drug include:

Objective data

- Note type and location of neoplastic lesion
- Stage of the disease, for example, early, metastatic, or terminal
- Vital signs (temperature, pulse, respirations, and blood pressure) and weight
- Inspect general physical appearance, noting skin color, temperature, and pain, differences bilaterally
- Laboratory and radiologic tests—to identify cancer or measure whether this dose of chemotherapy will need to be modified

Subjective data

- Client's knowledge or understanding of the proposed chemotherapy regimen
- Anxiety or fears the client may have regarding chemotherapy treatments or outcome
- Previous or concurrent treatments (if any), such as surgery, radiation therapy, other traditional chemotherapy drugs
- Other current nonmalignant disease or disorder, such as congestive heart failure or peptic ulcer, that may or may not be related to the malignant disease
- Other factors, such as the client's age, financial problems that may be associated with a long-term illness, family cooperation and interest in client care, and the adequacy of health insurance coverage (which may be of great concern to the client)

Accurate weight is important because the dosages of some antineoplastic drugs may be based on body surface measurements and are stated as a specific amount of drug per square meter (m^2) of the body surface. Additionally, the administration route of chemotherapy is routinely monitored; examples include assessment of vessel integrity for IV access or patency of venous access devices.

Some traditional chemotherapy drugs require treatment measures before administration. An example of preadministration treatment is hydration of the client with 1–2 L of IV fluid infused before administration of cisplatin or administration of an antiemetic before the administration of irinotecan (Camptosar). These measures are ordered by the oncology health care provider and, in some instances, may vary slightly from the manufacturer's recommendations.

Ongoing Assessment

The client who is acutely ill with many physical problems requires different ongoing assessment activities than does one who is ambulating and able to participate in the activities of daily living. Once the client's general condition is assessed and needs identified, develop a care plan to meet those needs. Clients receiving chemotherapy can be at different stages of their disease; therefore, you should individualize the nursing care of each client based on the client's needs, and not just on the type of drug administered.

In general, after the administration of a traditional chemotherapy drug, base your ongoing assessment on the following factors:

- Client's general condition
- Client's individual response to the drug
- Adverse reactions that may occur
- Guidelines established by the oncology health care provider or clinic
- Results of periodic laboratory tests and radiographic scans

Different types of laboratory tests may be used to monitor the client's response to therapy. Some of these tests, such as a complete blood count, may be used to determine the response of the bone marrow to the chemotherapy drug. Other tests, such as kidney function tests, may be used to detect nephrotoxicity, an adverse reaction that sometimes occurs with the administration of some of these drugs. Abnormal laboratory test results may also require a change in the nursing care plan. For example, a significant drop in the neutrophil count may require a delay in treatment, administration of colony-stimulating factors (see Chapter 48), and client teaching about ways to recognize and prevent infection and sepsis.

Review the results of all laboratory tests at the time they are reported. The oncology health care provider is notified of the results before the administration of successive doses of a chemotherapy drug. If these tests indicate a severe depressant effect on the bone marrow or other test abnormalities, the oncology health care provider may reduce the next drug dose or temporarily stop chemotherapy to allow the affected body systems to recover.

NURSING DIAGNOSES

The nursing diagnoses for the client with cancer are usually extensive and are based on many factors, such as the client's physical and emotional condition, the adverse reactions resulting from antineoplastic drug therapy, and the stage of the disease. Drug-specific nursing diagnoses include the following:

- **Malnutrition** related to anorexia, nausea, vomiting, and stomatitis
- **Fatigue** related to anemia and myelosuppression
- **Injury risk** related to thrombocytopenia and myelosuppression
- **Infection risk** related to neutropenia, leukopenia, and myelosuppression
- **Altered body image perception** related to adverse reactions of antineoplastic drugs (e.g., alopecia, weight loss)
- **Anxiety** related to diagnosis, necessary treatment measures, the occurrence of adverse reactions, other factors
- **Altered tissue integrity** related to adverse reactions of the antineoplastic drugs (radiation recall and extravasation)

Nursing diagnoses related to drug administration are discussed in Chapter 4.

PLANNING

The expected outcomes of the client may include an optimal response to therapy, support of client needs related to the management of adverse reactions, and confidence in an understanding of the prescribed treatment modalities.

IMPLEMENTATION

Promoting an Optimal Response to Therapy

Care of the client receiving an antineoplastic drug depends on factors such as the drug or combination of drugs given, the dosage of the drugs, the route of administration, the client's physical response to therapy, the response of the tumor to chemotherapy, and the type and severity of adverse reactions. Some drugs may be administered by various routes, depending on the cancer being treated. For example, thiotepa may be administered by the IV route for breast cancer, intravesicular route for superficial bladder cancer, intrapleural route for malignant pleural effusions, and intraperitoneal route for ovarian cancer. As the methods of administration have changed, so has the location for administration. Once given as long IV infusions over days or a week in the hospital, many of the traditional chemotherapy drugs are still given IV but as push or small-volume infusions, and they are delivered in an outpatient setting by highly skilled nurses.

Guidelines Established by the Setting for Care

In these settings (hospital, outpatient chemotherapy clinics, or office), policies are established to provide nursing personnel with specific guidelines for the assessment and care of clients receiving a single or combination chemotherapeutic drug regimen. During chemotherapy, the oncology health care provider may write orders for certain nursing procedures, such as measuring fluid intake and output, monitoring the vital signs at specific intervals, and increasing the fluid intake to a certain amount. Even when orders are written, you should increase the frequency of certain assessments, such as monitoring vital signs, if the client's condition changes. Some settings have written guidelines for nursing management when the client is receiving a specific chemotherapy drug. Incorporate these guidelines into the nursing care plan with nursing observations and assessments geared to the individual. At any time you may add further assessments to the nursing care plan when the client's condition changes.

If treatment is given in a setting where guidelines are not provided, it is important for you to review the drugs being given before their administration. These drugs should not be prescribed by a generalist health care provider; rather, antineoplastic drugs should be prescribed only by a provider trained specifically in the care of oncology clients. The clinical pharmacist consults appropriate references to obtain information regarding the preparation and administration of a particular drug, the average dose ranges, all the known adverse reactions, and the warnings and precautions given by the manufacturer.

Protection of the Provider

Those involved in the administration of antineoplastic drugs are at risk for many adverse reactions from accidental absorption of the drugs. Because so many of the drugs are given in the outpatient setting, personnel in clinics and offices are at high risk for exposure. It is important to follow the directions of the manufacturer regarding the type of solution to be used for preparation, dilution, or administration. The Occupational Safety and Health Administration (OSHA) guidelines state that antineoplastic drug preparation is to be performed in a biologic safety cabinet in a designated area. This is to prevent accidental inhalation and exposure to the person preparing the drugs. In addition, nurses need to be protected during administration and cleanup from accidental ingestion, inhalation, or absorption of the drugs (Menonna-Quinn et al., 2019). Table 50.1 outlines the protective items that should be available to staff working with antineoplastic drugs.

TABLE 50.1 Personal Protective Equipment for Safe Handling of Antineoplastic Drugs

ROUTE OF POTENTIAL EXPOSURE	SAFETY EQUIPMENT
Skin	Gowns—single-use, lint-free, disposable gowns with solid front and tight cuffs and made of impermeable or minimally permeable fabric (to the agents in use)
	Gloves (double gloving preferred)—powder-free; made of latex, nitrile, or neoprene; labeled and tested for use with chemotherapeutic drugs
Ingestion	Safety goggles with face shield—to protect face and eyes from possible splashes
Inhalation	National Institute for Occupational Safety and Health (NIOSH)-approved respirator—when inhalation is anticipated or a spill must be cleaned up

Based upon Polovich, M., (Ed.). (2011). Safe handling of hazardous drugs (2nd ed.). ONS publisher.

NURSING ALERT

Nurses who are pregnant, breastfeeding, or attempting to conceive should notify their employers regarding their condition and exposure to antineoplastic drugs. As a result, employers should provide alternate duty that does not include preparation, administration, or handling of hazardous drugs (ONS position statement, 2016).

Oral Administration

A number of antineoplastic drugs are administered orally. The oral route is convenient and noninvasive. Most oral drugs are well absorbed when the GI tract is functioning normally. Traditional chemotherapy drugs such as capecitabine (Xeloda) or temozolomide (Temodar) are given orally. Most oral drugs are administered by the client in a home setting. Many of the targeted agents come in oral form and should be taken with at least 8 ounce of fluid. Grapefruit juice should not be suggested because of its interaction with many targeted agents. The section on Educating the Client and Family provides information to include in a teaching plan.

Parenteral Administration

Although some of these drugs are given orally, others are given by the parenteral route. Traditional chemotherapy drugs may be administered subcutaneously (subcut), intramuscularly (IM), and IV. When giving these drugs IM, inject into the large muscles using the Z-track method (see Chapter 2) because administration can cause stinging or burning. When the subcut method of administration is used, the injection should contain no more than 1 mL, and injections are given in the usual subcut injection sites (see Chapter 2). If the injections are given frequently, the sites should be rotated and charted appropriately.

IV administration may be accomplished using a vascular access device, an Angiocath, or a butterfly needle. These devices have become common methods of drug delivery and, depending on the client's individual treatment regimen, may be inserted before therapy. Selection of the device depends on the type of therapy the client is to receive, the condition of the veins, and how long the treatment regimen is to be continued. Special directions for administration, stated by either the oncology health care provider or manufacturer, are also important. For example, cisplatin cannot be prepared or administered with needles or IV administration sets containing aluminum, because aluminum reacts with cisplatin, causing formation of a precipitate and loss of potency.

Nurses who are certified in chemotherapy drug administration administer these drugs, but any nurse may be involved in monitoring clients receiving traditional chemotherapy drugs. Traditional chemotherapy drugs are potentially toxic drugs that can cause a variety of effects during and after their administration. Box 50.4 summarizes important points to keep in mind when administering an antineoplastic drug.

Monitoring and Managing Client Needs

Not all clients have the same response to a specific antineoplastic drug. For example, an antineoplastic drug may cause vomiting, but the amount of fluid and electrolytes lost through vomiting may vary from client to client. One client may require additional sips of water once nausea and vomiting have subsided, whereas another may require IV fluid and electrolyte replacement. Nursing management is focused not only on what may or what did happen but also on the effects produced by a particular adverse reaction.

Malnutrition

Clients may not eat because they are tired or not hungry. **Anorexia** (loss of appetite resulting in the inability to eat) is a common occurrence with traditional chemotherapy drugs. This may be because of nausea, taste alterations, or sores in the GI system. Nausea and vomiting are common adverse reactions to some of the highly emetic antineoplastic drugs. To minimize this adverse reaction, the oncology health care provider may order an antiemetic, such as ondansetron (Zofran), to be given before treatment and continued for a few days after administration of the chemotherapy. Because this is an expensive drug, other protocols may include different (and less expensive) antiemetics. Some of these have adverse effects, such as a sedative action, which might add to the client's lack of desire to eat. In the example of the client who is vomiting, it is important to track accurately all fluid intake. To prevent handling of contaminated waste, use the client's weight instead of measuring urine or emesis to assess for fluid loss and observe the client for signs of dehydration and electrolyte imbalances. These measurements and observations aid the oncology health care provider in determining if fluid replacement is necessary.

Assess the nutritional status of the client before and during treatment. To stimulate appetite, provide small, frequent meals to coincide with the client's tolerance for food. Greasy or fatty foods and unpleasant sights, smells, and tastes are avoided. Cold foods, dry foods, and salty foods may be better tolerated. It is a good idea to provide diversional activities, such as music, television, and books. Relaxation, visualization, guided imagery, hypnosis, and other nonpharmacologic measures have been helpful to some clients.

It is not uncommon for the client to report alterations in the sense of taste during the course of chemotherapy. Some drugs give protein foods such as beef a bitter, metallic taste. Small, frequent meals (five to six meals daily) are usually better tolerated than are three large meals. Breakfast is often the best-tolerated meal of the day. Stress the importance of eating meals high in nutritive value, particularly protein (e.g., eggs, milk products, tuna, beans, peas, and lentils). Some clients prefer to have available high-protein finger foods such as cheese or peanut butter and crackers. Nutritional supplements may also be prescribed. Monitor the client's body weight weekly (or more often if necessary) and report any weight loss. If the client continues to lose weight, a feeding tube or total parenteral nutrition (TPN) may be used to supplement nutritional needs. Although this is not ideal, the client who is malnourished and weak may benefit from this intervention.

Because the cells in the mouth grow rapidly, they are particularly sensitive to the effects of the traditional chemotherapy drugs. Stomatitis or **oral mucositis** (inflammation of the oral mucous membranes) may appear 5–7 days after chemotherapy is started and continue up to 10 days after therapy. This adverse reaction is particularly uncomfortable because irritation of the oral mucous membranes affects the nutritional aspects of care. The client must avoid any foods or products that are irritating to the mouth, such as alcoholic beverages, spices, alcohol-based mouthwash, or toothpaste. Instruct caregivers to provide soft or liquid food high in nutritive value. The oral cavity is inspected for increased irritation. Teach the client to report any white patches on the tongue (possible *candidiasis* fungal infection), throat, or gums; any burning sensation; and bleeding from the mouth or gums. Mouth care is encouraged and should be performed every 4 hours, including a rinse with normal saline solution. Lemon/glycerin swabs are avoided because they tend to irritate the oral mucosa and complicate stomatitis. The oncology health care provider may order a topical viscous anesthetic, such as lidocaine viscous, to decrease discomfort.

Fatigue, Injury Risk, and Infection Risk

Many antineoplastic drugs interfere with the bone marrow's ability to make new cells. This interference is called *bone marrow suppression* or **myelosuppression** and is a potentially dangerous adverse reaction. Bone marrow suppression is manifested by abnormal laboratory test results and clinical evidence of leukopenia, thrombocytopenia, or anemia. For example, there is a decrease in the white blood cells or leukocytes (*leukopenia*), a decrease in the thrombocytes (*thrombocytopenia*), and a decrease in the red blood cells, resulting in anemia.

Anemia occurs as the result of a decreased production of red blood cells in the bone marrow and is characterized by fatigue, dizziness, shortness of breath, and palpitations. Teach the client to prioritize activities to conserve energy. Permission may need to be given to the active client to slow down and even take daytime naps. In some cases, the administration of blood transfusions may be necessary to correct the anemia.

Clients with **neutropenia** (reduction in the neutrophil type of white blood cells) have a decreased resistance to infection and must be monitored closely for any signs of infection. Combined therapy, such as chemotherapy and radiation together, can have an additive effect on the reduction of blood cells.

! NURSING ALERT

Because of the severity of leukopenia when taking temozolomide (Temodar) in conjunction with radiation to the brain, clients should be started on prophylactic therapy to prevent Pneumocystis pneumonia (PCP).

Clients are instructed to stay away from crowds or ill individuals while receiving myelosuppressive drugs. Sepsis, without the typical signs of infection, can affect clients because they lack neutrophils. The oncology health care provider may prescribe colony-stimulating factor injections to promote the production of blood cells between the chemotherapy cycles. Low-blood counts are one of the primary reasons a chemotherapy treatment may be delayed.

! NURSING ALERT

Report immediately any of the following signs of infection to the health care provider: temperature of 100.4 °F (38 °C) or higher, cough, sore throat, chills, frequent urination, or a white blood cell count of less than 2500/mm³.

Thrombocytopenia is characterized by a decrease in the platelet count (less than 100,000/mm³). Teach clients to monitor for bleeding tendencies and take precautions to prevent bleeding. Injections and multiple blood draws are avoided but, if necessary, then apply pressure to the injection site for 3–5 min to prevent bleeding into the tissue and the formation of a hematoma. Instruct the client to avoid the use of disposable razors, nail trimmers, dental floss, firm toothbrushes, or any sharp objects. The client is taught to refrain from contact and highly physical activities at this time. The client is monitored closely for easy bruising, skin lesions, and bleeding from any orifice (opening) of the body.

! NURSING ALERT

Teach the client to report to you or to the health care provider immediately any of the following: bleeding gums, easy bruising, petechiae (pinpoint hemorrhages), increased menstrual bleeding, tarry stools, bloody urine, or coffee-ground emesis.

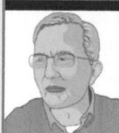

PHARMACOLOGY IN PRACTICE

MANAGING NEEDS
A client being treated with traditional chemotherapy is at a high risk for myelosuppression. Which of the following must the nurse consider with regard to injections and blood draws when the client is thrombocytopenic?
1. Use the same site for all withdrawals and injections
2. Apply pressure to the injection site for 3–5 min
3. Use straight razors when shaving
4. Keep the client's nails short

Altered Body Image Perception
Adverse reactions seen with the administration of these drugs may range from very mild to life-threatening. Some of these reactions, such as the loss of hair (**alopecia**), may have little effect on the physical status of the client but certainly may have a serious effect on the client's mental health. Because the practice of nursing is concerned with the whole client, such physically altering reactions that can have a profound effect on the client must be considered when planning nursing management.

Some drugs cause severe hair loss, whereas others cause gradual thinning. Examples of drugs commonly associated with severe hair loss are doxorubicin and vinblastine. If hair loss is associated with the traditional chemotherapy drug being given, inform the client that hair loss may occur. This problem may occur 10–21 days after the first treatment cycle. Hair loss is usually temporary, and hair will grow again when the drug therapy is completed. Forewarn the client that hair loss may occur suddenly and in large amounts (see Fig. 50.3). Hair will be lost not only from the head but also from the entire body. Although it is not life-threatening, alopecia can have an impact on temperature regulation, self-esteem, and body image, serving as a reminder that the individual is undergoing treatment for cancer.

Depending on the client, you may need to assist in making plans for the purchase of a wig or cap to disguise the hair loss until the hair grows back. Be aware that this

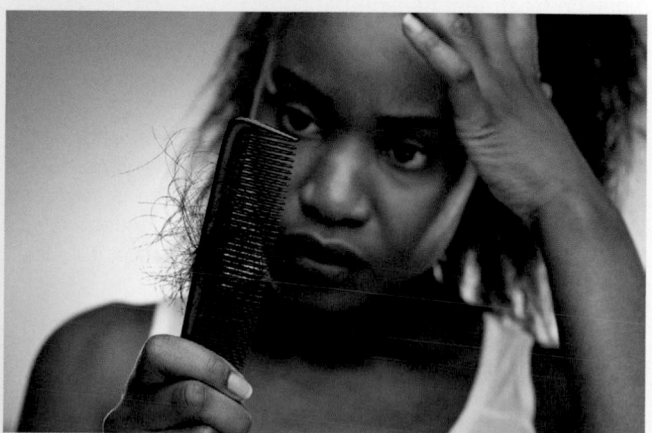

FIGURE 50.3 Hair loss can be sudden and surprise the client even when explained earlier by the nurse.

might be as great a problem to a male client as it is to a female client. The client is reminded about the importance of a head covering because of the large amount of body heat that can be lost with the hair gone.

Anxiety

The word *cancer* still evokes dread in people. Clients and family members are usually devastated by the diagnosis of cancer. Clients have to absorb much information and make quick, critical decisions about treatment. This can be especially demanding on both family and providers if English is not their first language. Obtaining information in the preferred language and interpreter services for provider interactions is both time-consuming and exhausting for the client and family members. The emphasis on the safety requirements of chemotherapy administration adds to the demands and fears placed on clients. The emotional impact of the disease may be forgotten or put aside by members of the health care team as they plan and institute therapy to control the disease. Because cancer treatment happens over time, you have the opportunity to offer consistent and empathetic emotional support to the client and family members. This support can help reduce some of the fear and anxiety experienced by the client and family during treatment.

Altered Tissue Integrity

Because the skin cells are rapidly growing cells, the integument is at risk for breakdown during antineoplastic drug therapy. As tender, new skin tissue grows it may be red, warm, and sometimes painful. This condition of the skin is called erythema. Care should be taken by clients to avoid the sun; to wear loose, protective clothing; and to watch areas of skinfolds for breakdown. Some traditional chemotherapy drugs have the ability to sensitize skin that has previously been irradiated. Be sure to instruct the client about this adverse reaction, because it can be both surprising and painful.

🛈 NURSING ALERT

Radiation recall is a skin reaction in which an area that was previously irradiated becomes reddened when a client is administered certain specific chemotherapy drugs. This is well-differentiated from a reaction exclusive to the drugs because of the defined outline of the previous radiation treatment field on the body.

Some traditional chemotherapy drugs are **vesicants** (i.e., they cause tissue necrosis if they infiltrate or extravasate out of the blood vessel and into the soft tissue). If **extravasation** occurs, underlying tissue is damaged. The damage can be severe, causing physical deformity or loss of vascularity or tendon function. If the damage is severe, skin grafting may be necessary to preserve function. Examples of vesicant drugs are daunorubicin, doxorubicin, and vinblastine.

🛈 NURSING ALERT

Clients at a greater risk for extravasation are those unable to communicate to the nurse about the pain of tissue injury, older adults, debilitated clients, or confused clients, and any client with fragile veins.

When the client is receiving a vesicant, ensure that extravasation protocol orders are signed and that an extravasation kit is on the unit before vesicant drugs are administered. The IV site is continuously monitored and checks for blood return are made frequently during IV push procedures (every 1–2 mL). If a vesicant is prescribed as an infusion, it is given only through a central line and checked every 1–2 hr. Keep the extravasation kit containing all materials necessary to manage an extravasation available, along with the extravasation policy and procedure guidelines.

Extravasation may occur without warning, or minor signs may be detected by an alert nurse. The earlier the extravasation is detected, the less likely soft-tissue damage will occur. Signs of extravasation include:

- Swelling (most common)
- Stinging, burning, or pain at the injection site (not always present)
- Redness
- Lack of blood return (if this is the only symptom, the IV line should be reevaluated; a lack of blood return alone is not always indicative of extravasation, and extravasation can occur even if a blood return is present)

If extravasation is suspected, the infusion is stopped immediately, antidotal procedures initiated, and the extravasation reported to the oncology health care provider.

Educating the Client and Family

The oncology health care provider usually discusses the proposed treatment and possible adverse drug reactions with the client and family members. As the nurse, you will briefly review these explanations immediately before administration of any antineoplastic drug.

Some traditional chemotherapy drugs are taken orally at home. The areas included in a client and family teaching plan for this type of treatment regimen are based on the drug prescribed, the oncology health care provider's explanation of the chemotherapy regimen and instructions for taking the drug, and the needs of the individual. To prevent unintended absorption, some pills or tablets should not be handled by others when administering the drugs. Family members are taught how to take out the medication from its container without touching the drug. Because the drugs are eliminated in body wastes, teach the client to double flush toilets and if able use a bathroom secluded from other family members when the drug is active in the body. Hospitals, clinics, or primary health care providers give printed instructions in the preferred language to the client. After the client has read them you will want to spend time with the client or family members to allow them to ask questions.

In some instances, a drug to prevent nausea may be prescribed to be taken at home before administration of the antineoplastic drugs in the outpatient setting. To obtain the best possible effects, stress to the client that the drug must be taken at the time specified by the oncology health care provider. It is important for the client to comply with the treatment regimen to maximize therapeutic effect. Most clients adhere to traditional chemotherapy; however, some of the drugs have modified schedules, such as when given in conjunction with radiation therapy with certain weeks on therapy and others off therapy, and these administration schedules can become confusing. Stress the importance of maintaining the dosing schedule exactly as prescribed. A calendar or automated medication box indicating the doses to take and dates the drug is to be taken is often helpful for the client. The client is instructed to bring the treatment calendar to each appointment, and they are questioned about any omitted or delayed doses. Nurses in the clinic, home health nurses, or caregivers are taught to fill the medication boxes. In general, one course of therapy is prescribed at a time to avoid inadvertent overdosing that could be life-threatening.

Include the following points in a client and family teaching plan when oral therapy is prescribed:

- Take the drug only as directed on the prescription container. Unless otherwise indicated, take the drug on an empty stomach with water to enhance absorption. However, the client should follow specific directions, such as "take on an empty stomach" or "take at the same time each day"; they are extremely important.
- Familiarize yourself with the brand or trade name and the generic name to avoid confusion. If you live with another person at home, ask that person to help you verify the correct drug and dose of the drug before you take it.
- Never increase, decrease, or omit a dose unless advised to do so by the oncology health care provider. Set up reminders such as a calendar, cellphone alarm, or computer alert if dosing routinely becomes an issue.
- If any problems (adverse reactions) occur, no matter how minor, contact the oncology health care provider immediately.
- All recommendations given by the oncology health care provider, such as increasing the fluid intake or eating or avoiding certain foods, are important.
- Some drugs leave the body relatively unchanged; therefore, to prevent contamination men should avoid using urinals and sit to urinate for at least 48 hours following the last dose of the drug. Toilets should be double flushed with the lid down to prevent spray in the bathroom.
- The effectiveness or action of the drug could be altered if these directions are ignored. Other recommendations, such as checking the mouth for sores, rinsing the mouth thoroughly after eating or drinking, or drinking extra fluids, are given to identify or minimize some of the effects these drugs have on the body. It is important to follow these recommendations.
- Keep all appointments for chemotherapy. These drugs must be given at certain intervals to be effective.
- Do not take any nonprescription drug unless the use of a specific drug has been approved by the oncology health care provider.
- Avoid drinking alcoholic beverages unless the oncology health care provider has approved their use.
- Always inform other physicians, dentists, and medical personnel of therapy with this drug.
- Keep all appointments for the laboratory tests ordered by the oncology health care provider. If you are unable to keep a laboratory appointment, notify the oncology health care provider immediately.

EVALUATION

- Therapeutic effect is achieved.
- Adverse reactions are identified, reported to the primary health care provider, and managed successfully using nursing interventions.
  - Client maintains an adequate nutritional status.
  - Client reports fatigue is managed appropriately.
  - No evidence of injury is seen.
  - No evidence of infection is seen.
  - Perceptions of body changes are managed successfully.
  - Anxiety is managed successfully.
  - Skin remains intact.
- Client and family express confidence and demonstrate an understanding of the drug regimen.

PHARMACOLOGY IN PRACTICE

USING CLINICAL REASONING

Some people do not think about survivorship when discussing cancer. Mr. Phillip's wife survived breast cancer, yet he still feels grief after losing her. Review Chapters 20 and 21 regarding the medications used to help him deal with his feelings. What other strategies would you now consider?

KEY POINTS

■ A neoplasm is a group of cells that do not maturate, but grow out of control. Traditional chemotherapy drugs are used to retard this process by interfering with specific portions of the cell cycle or disturbing the process.

■ Although chemotherapy literally means drug therapy, it is typically associated with anticancer drugs used in the cure, control, or palliation of the disease.

■ Because traditional chemotherapy drugs enter the body systemically, the same mechanism of action used to kill or retard cancerous cells can also harm other fast-growing cells in the body such as GI, blood component, skin, and other lining cells. Caution should be taken during administration with many of the drugs because of their ability to irritate tissues.

■ Adverse reactions to the platelets and red and white blood cells result in fatigue, bleeding, and infection. Nausea, vomiting, and diarrhea results from destruction of GI lining cells. Skin issues are the most common adverse reaction of targeted therapies. Peripheral nerve damage can result in numbness, tingling, or lack of sensation.

SUMMARY DRUG TABLE
Traditional Chemotherapy Drugs

Generic Name	Trade Name	Uses	Adverse Reactions
Cell Cycle–Specific Agents			
Plant Alkaloids			
VINCA ALKALOIDS			
vinBLAStine *vin-BLAS-teen*		Leukemia/lymphomas: Hodgkin disease, other lymphomas Solid tumors: testicular, breast, Kaposi sarcoma (KS) Nonmalignant: mycosis fungoides	Immediate: extravasation potential During therapy cycles: alopecia, anemia, leukopenia, paresthesias, nausea, vomiting, constipation Long term: fertility problems
vinCRIStine *vin-KRIS-teen*	Marqibo	Leukemia/lymphomas: acute leukemia, other lymphomas Solid tumors: rhabdomyosarcoma, bladder, breast, KS Nonmalignant: idiopathic thrombocytopenic purpura	Immediate: extravasation potential During therapy cycles: alopecia, anemia, leukopenia, paresthesias, nausea, vomiting, stomatitis, constipation Long term: renal, adrenal, fertility problems
vinorelbine *vi-NOR-el-been*	Navelbine	Solid tumors: non–small-cell lung cancer (NSCLC) Unlabeled use: other solid tumors, KS	Immediate: extravasation potential During therapy cycles: leukopenia, paresthesias, nausea, constipation, alopecia, radiation recall
Taxanes			
cabazitaxel *ca-baz-i-TAKS-el*	Jevtana	Solid tumors: prostate	Immediate: hypersensitivity reaction During therapy cycles: nausea, fever, anemia, leukopenia, vomiting, diarrhea, constipation, stomatitis, hematuria
DOCEtaxel *doe-se-TAKS-el*	Taxotere	Solid tumors: breast, NSCLC, prostate Unlabeled use: other solid tumors	Immediate: extravasation potential During therapy cycles: nausea, peripheral neuropathy, alopecia, cutaneous changes, fever, anemia, leukopenia, vomiting, diarrhea, stomatitis, fluid retention Long term: fertility problems
PACLitaxel *pac-li-TAKS-el*	Abraxane	Solid tumors: ovary, breast, NSCLC, KS Unlabeled use: other solid tumors	Immediate: cardiac changes, hypotension, extravasation potential During therapy cycles: nausea, vomiting, peripheral neuropathy, alopecia, fever, anemia, leukopenia, diarrhea, stomatitis Long term: fertility problems
Podophyllotoxins			
etoposide *e-toe-POE-side*	Etopophos, Toposar	Solid tumors: testicular, small-cell lung cancer (SCLC) Unlabeled use: other solid tumors, leukemias, and lymphomas	During therapy cycles: anemia, leukopenia, thrombocytopenia, alopecia, nausea, vomiting
teniposide *ten-i-POE-side*		Leukemia/lymphomas: acute lymphocytic leukemia (ALL)	Immediate: extravasation potential During therapy cycles: anemia, leukopenia, thrombocytopenia, alopecia, nausea, vomiting
Camptothecin Analogs			
irinotecan *eye-rye-no-TEE-kan*	Camptosar, Onivyde	Solid tumors: metastatic colon or rectal	Immediate: nausea, vomiting, diarrhea, inflammation potential (IV site) During therapy cycles: diarrhea, anemia, leukopenia, thrombocytopenia, asthenia, alopecia
topotecan *toe-poe-TEE-kan*	Hycamtin	Solid tumors: metastatic ovarian, SCLC	During therapy cycles: anemia, leukopenia, thrombocytopenia, alopecia, nausea, vomiting, diarrhea, constipation

Generic Name	Trade Name	Uses	Adverse Reactions
Antimetabolites			
azaCITIDine *ay-za-SYE-ti-deen*	Onureg, Vidaza	Myelodysplastic syndrome Unlabeled use: other leukemias and lymphomas	During therapy cycles: anemia, leukopenia, thrombocytopenia, nausea, vomiting
capecitabine *ka-pe-SITE-a-been*	Xeloda	Solid tumors: breast, colon	During therapy cycles: anemia, leukopenia, thrombocytopenia, diarrhea, hand and foot syndrome
cladribine *KLA-dri-been*		Leukemia/lymphomas: hairy cell leukemia Unlabeled use: other leukemias and lymphomas	During therapy cycles: anemia, leukopenia, thrombocytopenia, fever, nausea, rash
clofarabine *klo-FARE-a-been*	Clolar	Leukemia/lymphomas: ALL	During therapy cycles: anemia, leukopenia, thrombocytopenia, hyperuricemia
cytarabine (ara-C) *sye-TARE-a-been*	Cytosar-U	Leukemia/lymphomas: ALL, acute myelocytic leukemia (AML)	Immediate: nausea, vomiting During therapy cycles: anemia, leukopenia, thrombocytopenia
decitabine *de-SYE-ta-been*	Dacogen	Myelodysplastic syndrome Unlabeled use: other leukemias and lymphomas	During therapy cycles: anemia, leukopenia, thrombocytopenia, nausea, vomiting
floxuridine *floks-YOOR-i-deen*		Palliative treatment for solid tumors: colon	During therapy cycles: anemia, leukopenia, thrombocytopenia, nausea, vomiting
fludarabine *floo-DARE-a-been*		Leukemia/lymphomas: chronic lymphocytic leukemia (CLL) Unlabeled use: other leukemias and lymphomas	During therapy cycles: anemia, leukopenia, thrombocytopenia
fluorouracil (5-FU) *flure-oh-YOOR-a-sil*		Palliative treatment for solid tumors: breast, stomach, pancreas, colon, rectum	During therapy cycles: anemia, leukopenia, thrombocytopenia, nausea, vomiting, stomatitis, diarrhea, alopecia
gemcitabine *jem-SITE-a-been*	Infugem	Solid tumors: pancreatic, NSCLC	During therapy cycles: anemia, leukopenia, thrombocytopenia, fever, rash, nausea, vomiting, diarrhea, proteinuria
mercaptopurine (6-MP) *mer-kap-toe-PURE-een*	Purixan	Leukemia/lymphomas: ALL, AML Unlabeled use: inflammatory bowel disease	During therapy cycles: anemia, leukopenia, thrombocytopenia, hyperuricemia
methotrexate *meth-oh-TREKS-ate*	Trexall, Xatmep	Leukemia/lymphomas; ALL, non-Hodgkin lymphoma Solid tumors: breast, head/neck, choriocarcinomas, osteosarcomas Nonmalignant: mycosis fungoides, severe psoriasis, rheumatoid arthritis Unlabeled use: multiple sclerosis, inflammatory bowel disease	Immediate: nausea, vomiting (high dose) During therapy cycles: anemia, leukopenia, thrombocytopenia, stomatitis, diarrhea, renal damage Long term: hepatotoxicity
nelarabine *nel-AY-re-been*	Arranon	Leukemia/lymphomas: T-cell acute lymphoblastic leukemia and T-cell lymphoblastic lymphoma	During therapy cycles: fatigue, neurologic toxicity
PEMEtrexed *pem-e-TREKS-ed*	Alimta	Solid tumors: NSCLC, malignant pleural mesothelioma	During therapy cycles: anemia, leukopenia, thrombocytopenia, skin rashes
pentostatin *pen-toe-STAT-in*	Nipent	Leukemia/lymphomas: hairy cell leukemia Unlabeled use: other leukemias and lymphomas	During therapy cycles: anemia, leukopenia, thrombocytopenia, rash, itching, nausea, vomiting, diarrhea
PRALAtrexate *pral-a-TREX-ate*	Folotyn	T-cell lymphoma	During therapy cycles: anemia, leukopenia, thrombocytopenia, mucositis
trifluridine/tipiracil *trye-FLURE-i-deen*	Lonsurf	Metastatic colorectal tumors	During therapy cycles: anemia, leukopenia, thrombocytopenia, nausea, vomiting, diarrhea
thioguanine *thye-oh-GWAH-neen*	Tabloid	Acute leukemias Unlabeled use: severe psoriasis, inflammatory bowel disease	During therapy cycles: anemia, leukopenia, thrombocytopenia, hyperuricemia

Continued

SUMMARY DRUG TABLE (continued)
Traditional Chemotherapy Drugs

Generic Name	Trade Name	Uses	Adverse Reactions
Miscellaneous Agents			
eriBULin er-i-BUE-lin	Halaven	Solid tumors: advanced breast, liposarcoma	During therapy cycles: fatigue, peripheral neuropathy, neutropenia, nausea, diarrhea
ixabepilone ix-ab-EP-i-lone	Ixempra	Solid tumors: advanced breast	During therapy cycles: fatigue, peripheral neuropathy, neutropenia, alopecia, nausea, diarrhea
Cell Cycle–Nonspecific Agents			
Alkylating Drugs			
NITROGEN MUSTARD DERIVATIVES			
chlorambucil klor-AM-byoo-sil	Leukeran	Leukemia/lymphomas: CLL, lymphomas, Hodgkin disease	During therapy cycles: anemia, leukopenia, thrombocytopenia. Long term: fertility problems
cyclophosphamide sye-kloe-FOS-fa-mide		Leukemia/lymphomas: ALL, AML, CLL, advanced lymphomas, Hodgkin disease. Solid tumors: breast, ovary, neuroblastoma, retinoblastoma. Nonmalignant: mycosis fungoides, nephrotic syndrome (children), rheumatoid arthritis, systemic lupus erythematosus, multiple sclerosis	Immediate: nausea, vomiting. During therapy cycles: leukopenia, hemorrhagic cystitis, thrombocytopenia. Long term: fertility problems, secondary cancers
ifosfamide eye-FOSS-fa-mide	Ifex	Leukemia/lymphomas: unlabeled use (except AML). Solid tumors: testicular. Unlabeled use: lung, breast, ovary, gastric, pancreatic	Immediate: nausea, vomiting. During therapy cycles: leukopenia, thrombocytopenia, hemorrhagic cystitis, alopecia, somnolence, confusion
mechlorethamine me-klor-ETH-a-meen		Palliative treatment for CLL, chronic myelocytic leukemia (CML), advanced lymphomas, Hodgkin disease. Solid tumors: lung, metastatic disease, mycosis fungoides	Immediate: nausea, vomiting, extravasation potential, lymphocytopenia. During therapy cycles: anemia, leukopenia, thrombocytopenia, hyperuremia, diarrhea. Long term: fertility problems, secondary cancers
melphalan MEL-fa-lan	Alkeran, Evomela	Palliative/ hematopoietic stem cell transplant (HSCT) treatment for multiple myeloma. Solid tumors: ovary. Unlabeled use: testicular, breast, bone marrow transplantation	Immediate: nausea, vomiting. During therapy cycles: leukopenia, thrombocytopenia, diarrhea, alopecia. Long term: fertility problems, secondary cancers
Ethyleneimines			
altretamine (hexamethyl-melamine) al-TRET-a-meen		Palliative treatment for solid tumors: ovary	During therapy cycles: anemia, leukopenia, thrombocytopenia, nausea, vomiting, peripheral neuropathy, dizziness
bendamustine ben-da-MUS-teen	Belrapzo, Bendeka, Treanda	Leukemia/lymphomas: CLL, non-Hodgkin lymphoma	During therapy cycles: anemia, leukopenia, thrombocytopenia, nausea, vomiting, diarrhea
thiotepa thye-oh-TEP-a		Adjunct in stem cell transplant for CNS tumor, graft rejection	During therapy cycles: anemia, leukopenia, thrombocytopenia, alopecia. Long term: fertility problems
Alkyl Sulfonate			
busulfan byoo-SUL-fan	Busulfex, Myleran	Palliative/stem cell transplant treatment for CML	Immediate: induce seizures. During therapy cycles: anemia, leukopenia, thrombocytopenia, hyperuremia, graft-versus-host disease. Long term: fertility problems

Generic Name	Trade Name	Uses	Adverse Reactions
Hydrazines			
dacarbazine *da-KAR-ba-zeen*	DTIC	Leukemia/lymphomas: Hodgkin disease Solid tumors: melanoma Unlabeled use: pheochromocytoma, KS	Immediate: nausea, vomiting During therapy cycles: anemia, leukopenia, thrombocytopenia
procarbazine *proe-KAR-ba-zeen*	Matulane	Leukemia/lymphomas: Hodgkin disease Unlabeled use: other lymphomas, brain, SCLC, melanoma	Immediate: nausea, vomiting During therapy cycles: anemia, leukopenia, thrombocytopenia, peripheral neuropathy, alopecia
temozolomide *te-moe-ZOE-loe-mide*	Temodar	Solid tumors: glioblastoma, astrocytoma Unlabeled use: melanoma	During therapy cycles: leukopenia, thrombocytopenia, headache, nausea, vomiting, alopecia
Nitrosoureas			
carmustine (BCNU) *car-MUS-teen*	BiCNU, Gliadel (implant)	Palliative treatment for Hodgkin disease, multiple myeloma, various brain tumors Unlabeled use: T-cell lymphoma, melanoma	Immediate: nausea, vomiting During therapy cycles: leukopenia, thrombocytopenia Long term: pulmonary fibrosis
lomustine (CCNU) *loe-MUS-teen*	Gleostine	Leukemia/lymphomas: secondary treatment for Hodgkin disease Solid tumors: brain	Immediate: nausea, vomiting During therapy cycles: leukopenia, thrombocytopenia, alopecia, stomatitis Long term: pulmonary fibrosis, fertility problems
streptozocin *strep-toe-ZOE-sin*	Zanosar	Solid tumors: pancreatic	Immediate: nausea, vomiting During therapy cycles: azotemia, proteinuria, stomatitis
Platinum-Based Drugs			
CARBOplatin *KAR-boe-pla-tin*	Paraplatin	Solid tumors: ovarian Unlabeled use: lung, head and neck, testicular	During therapy cycles: anemia, leukopenia, thrombocytopenia
CISplatin *SIS-pla-tin*		Solid tumors: ovarian, testicular, bladder	Immediate: nausea, vomiting, renal damage During therapy cycles: anemia, leukopenia, thrombocytopenia tinnitus, hyperuricemia
oxaliplatin *ox-AL-i-pla-tin*		Solid tumors: colon, rectal	During therapy cycles: leukopenia, thrombocytopenia, peripheral neuropathy
Antibiotics			
bleomycin *blee-oh-MYE-sin*		Palliative treatment for lymphomas, pleural effusion Solid tumors: testicular, various types Unlabeled use: mycosis fungoides, KS	During therapy cycles: anemia, leukopenia, thrombocytopenia, vomiting, alopecia, skin erythema, cutaneous changes Long term: pneumonitis, pulmonary fibrosis
dactinomycin *dak-ti-noe-MYE-sin*	Cosmegen	Solid tumors: various sarcomas, Wilms tumor, gestational neoplasia, testicular	Immediate: nausea, vomiting, extravasation potential During therapy cycles: anemia, leukopenia, thrombocytopenia, alopecia, skin erythema Long term: fertility problems
DAUNOrubicin *daw-noe-ROO-bi-sin*		Leukemia/lymphomas: ALL, AML Solid tumors: KS	Immediate: nausea, vomiting, extravasation potential During therapy cycles: anemia, leukopenia, thrombocytopenia, alopecia, stomatitis, hyperuricemia, urine discoloration Long term: cardiotoxicity
DOXOrubicin *doks-oh-ROO-bi-sin*	Adriamycin, Doxil	Leukemia/lymphomas; ALL, AML, and various lymphomas Solid tumors: Wilms tumor, neuroblastoma, KS, various sarcomas, breast, lung, ovary, bladder, thyroid, gastric	Immediate: nausea, vomiting, extravasation potential During therapy cycles: anemia, leukopenia, thrombocytopenia, alopecia, cutaneous changes, stomatitis, hyperuricemia, urine discoloration, radiation recall, hand and foot syndrome Long term: cardiotoxicity

Continued

SUMMARY DRUG TABLE (continued)
Traditional Chemotherapy Drugs

Generic Name	Trade Name	Uses	Adverse Reactions
epiRUBicin *ep-i-ROO-bi-sin*	Ellence	Solid tumors: breast Unlabeled use: advanced esophageal	Immediate: extravasation potential During therapy cycles: anemia, leukopenia, thrombocytopenia, nausea, vomiting, alopecia, stomatitis, diarrhea, urine discoloration, radiation recall Long term: cardiotoxicity, fertility problems
idarubicin *eye-da-ROO-bi-sin*	Idamycin	Leukemia/lymphomas: AML	Immediate: extravasation potential During therapy cycles: anemia, leukopenia, thrombocytopenia, alopecia, nausea, vomiting, stomatitis, diarrhea, hyperuricemia, urine discoloration Long term: cardiotoxicity
mitoMYcin *MYE-toe-MYE-sin*	Jelmyto, Mutamycin	Solid tumors: stomach, pancreas	Immediate: extravasation potential During therapy cycles: anemia, leukopenia, thrombocytopenia, hyperuricemia
mitoXANTRONE *mye-toe-ZAN-trone*		Leukemia/lymphomas: acute nonlymphocytic leukemia Solid tumors: advanced prostate Nonmalignant: multiple sclerosis	Immediate: nausea, vomiting, extravasation potential During therapy cycles: leukopenia, nausea, alopecia Long term: cardiotoxicity, AML
valrubicin *val-ROO-bi-sin*	Valstar	Solid tumor: urinary bladder	During therapy cycles: urinary urge, frequency, pain, bleeding
Miscellaneous Agents			
DNA INHIBITOR			
hydroxyurea *hye-droks-ee-yoor-EE-a*	Droxia, Hydrea, Siklos	Solid tumors: melanoma, sickle cell anemia Unlabeled use: thrombocythemia, human immunodeficiency virus infection, psoriasis	During therapy cycles: anemia, leukopenia, thrombocytopenia, radiation recall
ADRENOCORTICAL INHIBITOR			
mitotane *MYE-toe-tane*	Lysodren	Solid tumors: adrenal cortex Unlabeled use: Cushing disease	During therapy cycles: nausea, vomiting, diarrhea
ENZYMES			
asparaginase *a-SPEAR-a-ji-nase*	Erwinaze	Leukemia/lymphomas: ALL	During therapy cycles: anemia, leukopenia, thrombocytopenia, hyperuricemia, rash, urticaria, acute anaphylaxis
calaspargase pegol *kal-AS-par-jase*	Asparlas	Leukemia/lymphomas: ALL	Same as asparaginase
pegaspargase *peg-AS-par-jase*	Oncaspar	Leukemia/lymphomas: ALL	Same as asparaginase
ANTIMICROTUBULE AGENTS			
estramustine (estradiol/ nitrogen mustard) *es-tra-MUS-teen*	Emcyt	Palliative treatment for solid tumors (e.g., prostate)	Immediate: nausea, diarrhea During therapy cycles: breast tenderness, thrombophlebitis, fluid retention Long term: gynecomastia, impotence
RETINOIDS			
alitretinoin *a-li-TRET-i-noyn*	Panretin	Kaposi sarcoma	Topical application
tretinoin *TRET-i-noyn*		Leukemia/lymphomas: acute promyelocytic leukemia	During therapy cycles: headache, fever, weakness, fatigue, edema, retinoic acid-acute promyelocytic leukemia (RA-APL) syndrome (acute anaphylactic reaction)
bexarotene *beks-AIR-oh-teen*	Targretin	Leukemia/lymphomas: cutaneous T-cell lymphoma	During therapy cycles: elevated blood lipids, rash, leukopenia, dry skin

CHAPTER REVIEW

Know Your Drugs

Clients sometimes know a medication by the brand (or trade) name and not the generic name. To help you recognize both names, match the brand name with the generic name of the same **medication**.

Generic Name	Brand Name
1. docetaxel	A. Arranon
2. ifosfamide	B. Taxotere
3. nelarabine	C. Ifex
4. temozolomide	D. Temodar

Calculate Medication Dosages

1. Chlorambucil dosage is calculated based on the client's body weight. The client weighs 64 kg. The prescribed dosage of chlorambucil is 0.2 mg/kg of body weight per day. What is the correct daily dosage for this client?
2. A client weighing 54 kg is to receive bleomycin 0.25 units/kg of body weight. What is the correct dosage of bleomycin?

Prepare for the NCLEX

RECALL THE FACTS

1. Cancerous cells grow when _____.
   1. the pH is too acid
   2. G_0 phase of the cell cycle is skipped
   3. too much wear and tear on the cells happens
   4. neutrophils are too low
2. During which phase of the cell cycle does a cell split into two daughter cells?
   1. G_1
   2. S
   3. G_2
   4. M
3. Which of the following findings would be most indicative to the nurse that the client has thrombocytopenia?
   1. Nausea
   2. Blurred vision
   3. Headaches
   4. Easy bruising
4. Which of the following adverse reactions to the antineoplastic drugs is most likely to affect the client's body image?
   1. Hematuria
   2. Alopecia
   3. Nausea
   4. Diarrhea
5. When assessing the client for leukopenia, the nurse _____.
   1. checks the client every 8 hr for hematuria
   2. monitors the client for fever, sore throat, and chills
   3. checks female clients for increased menstrual bleeding
   4. reports a white blood cell count of 5000/mm³

6. Which of the following interventions would be most helpful for a client with stomatitis?
   1. Mouth care should be provided at least once daily.
   2. Swab the mouth with lemon glycerin swabs every 4 hr.
   3. Provide frequent mouth care with normal saline.
   4. Use a hard bristle toothbrush to cleanse the mouth and teeth of debris.
7. *Which of the drugs listed is most likely to cause nausea or vomiting?
   1. Temozolomide
   2. Cetuximab
   3. Cisplatin
   4. Vincristine

ANALYZE THE FACTS

8. Which of the following is the most common symptom of extravasation?
   1. Swelling around the injection site
   2. Redness along the vein and around the injection site
   3. Pain at the injection site
   4. Tenderness along the path of the vein
9. A family member calls the nurse to report that the client is losing handfuls of hair. The nurse instructs the family member to:
   1. take the client to the emergency department.
   2. have the client scrub the head hard to get it all off.
   3. reassure the family member this is normal, and to support the client.
   4. rush to the store and purchase a wig or turban.

ALTERNATE-FORMAT QUESTIONS

10. *In what way might the nurse accidently be exposed to chemotherapy? **Select all that apply.**
    1. Direct skin contact
    2. Ingestion
    3. Inhalation
    4. Needle stick

To check your answers, see Appendix F.

_____

*Indicates the question is directly linked to the NCLEX-PN test plan in Appendix G.

WANT TO KNOW MORE? A wide variety of resources are available to enhance your learning and understanding of this chapter.
- Visit **thePoint** for resources such as:
  - NCLEX-Style Student Review Questions
  - Journal Articles
  - Dosage Calculations
  - Drug Monographs
  - Watch and Learn Videos
  - Concepts in Action Animations
- The *Study Guide to Accompany Introductory Clinical Pharmacology*, 12th edition, sold separately, will help you review and apply essential content.
- ✓**PrepU** is available to help students prepare for the NCLEX-PN examination.

Immune Modulating Therapies

Key Terms

adaptive immunity type of immunity that is pathogen specific and body creates immunologic memory to protect against pathogens

allogeneic from different sources than oneself

antigens unique proteins on the surface of cells

angiogenesis ability to grow blood vessels

autologous using one's own tissue

capillary leak syndrome massive leakage of plasma from blood vessels into surrounding tissues

chimeric combination of tissues used to make a monoclonal antibody

cytokines proteins, which aid cells, signal the immune response, and stimulate cells to move to the site of inflammation

cytokine storm immune system releases excessive cytokines resulting in an exaggerated immune response

cytotoxic poisonous to living cells

passive immunity type of immunity occurring from the administration of ready-made antibodies from another individual or animal, no memory or antibody development to protect against later infection

tumor lysis syndrome When large amounts of tumor cells are killed (lysed) releasing the cellular debris into the circulation, it can be life threatening if not treated

Learning Objectives

On completion of this chapter, the student will:

1. List the classes of immunotherapy used in the treatment of neoplastic diseases.
2. Explain the uses, general drug actions, general adverse reactions, contraindications, precautions, and interactions of the immunotherapy drugs.
3. Distinguish important preadministration and ongoing assessment activities the nurse should perform with the client receiving immunotherapy drugs.
4. List nursing diagnoses particular to a client receiving immunotherapy drugs.
5. Examine ways to promote an optimal response to therapy, how to manage common adverse reactions, and important points to keep in mind when educating clients about the use of an immunotherapy drug.

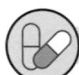 **Drug Classes**

Cytokines	Vaccines
Monoclonal antibodies	Adoptive cell therapy
Checkpoint inhibitors	

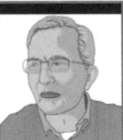 **PHARMACOLOGY IN PRACTICE**

As Mr. Phillip talks about his wife, he reminisces about going to the clinic with her for treatments. He says she was treated in the early summer and begins to chuckle. You ask what is funny and he tells you that she would put on a layer of sun screen then take her winter parka to wear during treatments. Learn about the immunotherapy drugs used to treat cancers and think about why she did this behavior.

Immunotherapy is a common pharmacologic intervention used in cancer care, or oncology. Immunotherapy as part of oncology care is used to treat cancers, restore or enhance the immune system's natural ability to fight the disease by:

- Stopping or slowing the growth of cancer cells.
- Preventing cancer from spreading in the body.
- Recognize cancer cells as foreign bodies and eliminate them.

(ASCO, 2020)

The immune system normally protects from foreign bodies or abnormal cells. It reads the proteins (**antigens**) on a cell's surface and identifies the cell as something abnormal. When antigens are detected, various components of the immune system are mobilized and the abnormal cell is destroyed. Unfortunately, cancers can evade these checkpoints and signals, resulting in continual cancer cell growth, the ability to grow their own blood vessels (**angiogenesis**), invade other tissues, and continue to evade the immune system. The goal of immunotherapy is to boost the immune response or enable the immune system to recognize and fight the cancers.

AGENTS THAT SUPPORT PASSIVE IMMUNITY

Tumor-associated antigens (TAAs) are not found on normal cells. TAAs can be on the surface of tumor cells or within the cell. The types of immunotherapy targeting the TAAs are monoclonal antibodies (mAbs), cytokines, and cancer vaccines. These various drugs enhance the immune cells' ability to recognize the TAA as foreign resulting in the body initiating the immune response, gain immunity to the cancer cells, and kill the cancer cells. Over 500 TAAs have been identified for cancers specifically (Olsen, 2018) (Fig. 51.1). Because of this ability to target just cancer cells, immunotherapy does not target and impact normal cells like traditional chemotherapy. Because the normal cells are not targeted, the adverse reactions people associate with chemotherapy do not occur as they do with traditional cancer drugs.

Monoclonal antibodies and cytokines work by **passive immunity**. These drugs target foreign objects but do not remember the invader. Therefore, these therapies must be repeated for ongoing protection.

CYTOKINES

Cytokines are proteins of the immune system involved in cell communication. In this chapter the cytokines, interferons and interleukins, are discussed.

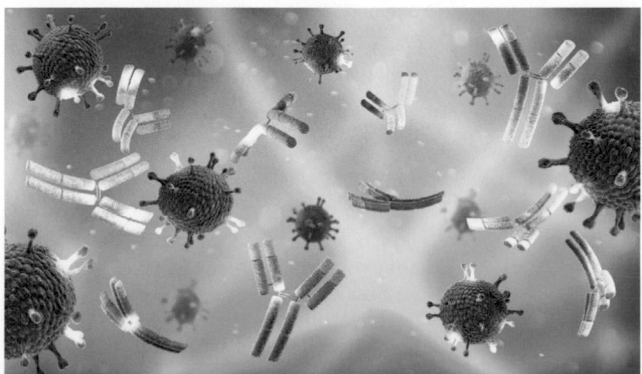

FIGURE 51.1 Monoclonal antibodies are attracted to the TAA on the cancer cell surfaces.

ACTIONS AND USES

Interferons are antiviral agents that have **cytotoxic** properties; interferon-alfa and -gamma are used in cancer treatment. The cytokines that activate killer cells are called interleukins.

Cytokines are used to:

- Enhance cytotoxic activities.
- Send signals to inhibit or promote cell death.
- Regulate antibody production and function of B/T cells.
- Interact with antigen presenting cells and NK cells.

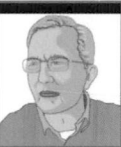

PHARMACOLOGY IN PRACTICE

PHYSIOLOGY

A nurse is caring for a client who is prescribed a monoclonal antibody. The nurse explains to the client that the drug supports passive immunity. Which of the following best describes the passive immunity of the mAb?
1. It creates memory like a cancer vaccine.
2. Signals are sent to white blood cells to attack.
3. Targets organelles inside the cell.
4. The function is much like the protection of our skin.

ADVERSE REACTIONS

Cytokines create an immune response, similar to having influenza and thus the symptoms experienced are referred to as "flu-like" symptoms. These symptoms include:

- Chills
- Cough
- Fever
- Headache
- Malaise

Other symptoms may include nausea, muscle aches, fatigue, sore throat, reduced appetite, or diarrhea. Skin rashes, injection pain and inflammation, edema in the extremities, and antibody development can occur. **Capillary leak syndrome** can occur due to increased vascular permeability. As a result of greater permeability, fluid leaks out of the circulation and into surrounding tissues, causing edema and dangerously low blood flow, which in turn can damage organs. **Cytokine storm** may also occur where the body is flooded with cytokines and again can lead to tissue damage or death if untreated.

CONTRAINDICATIONS, PRECAUTIONS, AND INTERACTIONS

Interferons are contraindicated in clients with known hypersensitivity to the drug or any component of the drug. A serious reaction of interferons may include neuropsychiatric symptoms, including depression, confusion, and manic behavior, which have been noted in clients both with and without a psychiatric history. Asymptomatic elevation in liver enzymes has occurred; therefore, clients should be cautioned regarding alcohol intake while using the drug. Caution is used when administering to clients with cardiac or liver disease, history of seizure disorder, and thyroid problems. A reduction in white blood cells makes clients susceptible to infection.

Immunomodulators are not started during pregnancy. When the client is on cytokines, they are stopped when pregnancy is confirmed. Cytokines have been found in breast milk (Hale, 2012); therefore, lactation is discouraged.

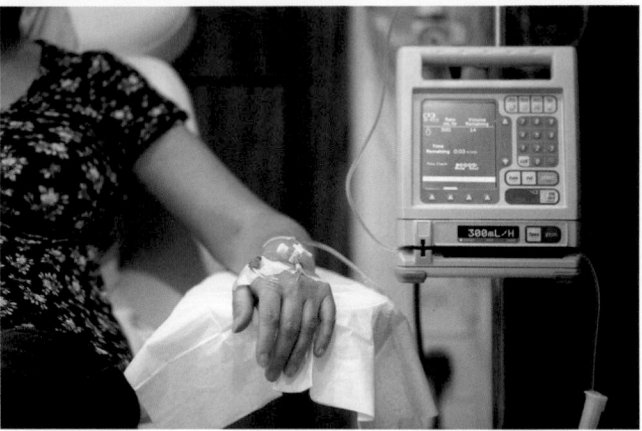

FIGURE 51.2 Frequently both immunotherapy and traditional chemotherapy are used as part of the treatment plan. (Photo by Brian A Jackson/Shutterstock)

ADVERSE REACTIONS

These drugs tend to have less adverse reactions than traditional chemotherapy because they do not interfere with healthy cells. Integumentary adverse reactions can range from rash to Stevens–Johnson syndrome.

Infusion reactions may appear as a hypersensitive reaction; this is due to the sensitivity of the client to the tissue of origin of the mAb. mAbs composed of more human tissue than nonhuman are less likely to have a reaction than those mAbs with more mouse tissue. Fatal infusion-related reactions are more likely to occur during the first infusion than in subsequent treatments. Table 51.1 lists the adverse reactions potentially seen in an infusion reaction.

LASA ALERT

The following drugs may sound alike; be sure to clarify when they are ordered:

Drug Name	Sounds Like
Alferon	Alkeran
Avonex	Avelox
PEG-Intron	Intron A, Pegasys

Drugs that look alike are noted in the Summary Drug Tables of each chapter.

INTERACTIONS

The following interactions may occur when an interferon is administered with another agent:

Interacting Drug	Common Use	Effect of Interaction
Cladribine	Chemotherapy	Increased lymphopenia, adverse interferon reactions
Zidovudine	HIV antiretroviral	Increased adverse reactions of zidovudine

MONOCLONAL ANTIBODIES

ACTIONS AND USES

Monoclonal antibodies (mAbs) target specific antigens on the surface of a tumor cell. Uses include:

- Flag cancer cells for destruction
- Block tumor growth and angiogenesis
- Deliver other agents to a tumor site

mAbs are typically used in combination with traditional chemotherapy (see Fig. 51.2) and/or radiation to improve therapy results (Olsen, 2018). Three of the most familiar agents include rituximab, trastuzumab, and bevacizumab.

TABLE 51.1 Components of Infusion Reactions

BODY SYSTEM	ADVERSE REACTION
Generalized	Fever, chills, rigors, sweating, warm feeling
Cardiovascular	Chest pain, palpitations, hypo/hypertension, tachy/bradycardia, arrhythmia, edema, ischemia, infarction, cardiac arrest
CNS	Throbbing headache, dizziness, confusion, loss of consciousness
Integumentary	Rash, pruritus, urticaria, erythema, tearing, angioedema
GI	Nausea, vomiting, metallic taste, diarrhea, abdominal cramps/bloating
GU	Incontinence, uterine cramping, renal impairment
Multiple sclerosis	Arthralgias, myalgia, fatigue, tumor pain, hypotonia
Respiratory	Cough, dyspnea, nasal congestion, rhinitis, sneezing, hoarseness, tachypnea, wheezing, tightness, bronchospasm, laryngeal edema, stridor, cyanosis, acute respiratory distress syndrome

Vogel, W. (2010). Infusion reactions: diagnosis, assessment, and management. *Clinical Journal of Oncology Nursing, 14*(2), E10-E21. https://doi.org/10.1188/10.CJON.E10-E21.

CONTRAINDICATIONS AND PRECAUTIONS

Monoclonal antibodies should not be used if a person has an active, severe infection. Live vaccine should not be given directly before, during, or immediately after mAbs. Viral infections, such as hepatitis B may be reactivated during therapy, and antiviral treatment should be initiated. Clients being treated for non-Hodgkin lymphoma with high tumor burden (volume) should prophylactically be treated for the possibility of **tumor lysis syndrome** (hyperkalemia, hypocalcemia, hyperuricemia, and hyperphosphatemia). Monitor for adverse reactions in clients with cardiac and renal impairment. mAbs can cross the placenta and cause fetal harm; therefore, women are cautioned to use effective birth control and should not use the drug when pregnant. Lactation is discouraged during and 6 months after ending mAbs treatment.

Owing to the manner in which monoclonal antibodies are named, they can be confused with each other easily. Be mindful to check the name carefully. Box 51.1 discusses the methodology used in naming the drugs; this can be helpful in drug recognition.

LASA ALERT

The following trade drugs may sound alike; be sure to clarify when they are ordered:

Drug Name	Sounds Like
Polivy	Poteligeo
Portrazza	Arzerra
Rituxan	Remicade

Drugs that look alike are noted in the Summary Drug Tables of each chapter.

INTERACTIONS

The following interactions may occur when a monoclonal antibody is administered with another agent:

Interacting Drug	Common Use	Effect of Interaction
Clozapine, promazine	Management of psychiatric problems	Increased risk for central nervous system (CNS) toxicity
roflumilast	Treatment of respiratory problems	Increased risk for immunosuppression
Vaccines (BCG, Covid-19, Rabies)	Prevent viral disease	Decreased risk for immunity to specified pathogen

CHECKPOINT AND OTHER INHIBITORS

The immune system has a set of checkpoints much like the traffic lights on a road. This system of signals prevents the immune system from becoming overstimulated. Some cancers have learned to evade this system so that the cancerous cell is not detected and basically gets the "green light" to continue unchecked growth (NCI, 2016).

ACTIONS AND USES

Checkpoint inhibitors are a subclass of monoclonal antibodies; Box 51.2 explains the naming of inhibitor drugs

---

BOX 51.1 Naming of Monoclonal Antibodies

When looking at a list of monoclonal antibody names, to the untrained eye, it appears to be an odd assortment of letters. Yet the arrangement of those letters is very specific and designed to help in the understanding of mAbs naming and function.

Let us use the example of a drug made to treat leukemia: riTUXimab (Rituxan).

This is a drug that can be confused with other drugs, therefore part of the name **TUX** is capitalized to heighten awareness, it does not impact the function of the drug.

Monoclonal terminology is built from the back of the word forward. Starting with the end of the word, or suffix, -*mab* indicates it is a monoclonal antibody.

The next one or two letters indicates the type of tissue used to make the mAb. It can be pure tissue or a **chimeric**, combination of tissue types.

- o, indicates from mouse tissue
- u, indicates from human tissue
- xi, combination human and mouse tissue
- zu, combination mouse and human, but the majority is human

-*xi-mab*, this drug is made from a combination of mouse and human tissue.

We know that drugs made from mouse tissue are more likely to cause a hypersensitive reaction, this portion of the word alerts us to that potential issue.

The next section of the word indicates the target tissue. It may be 1, 2, or 3 letters. Over time some of the letters have changed. The determination of the letters dealing more with the ability to say the word than the meaning.

- ba(c) = bacterial
- ci(r) = cardiovascular
- fu(ng) = fungal
- ki(n) = interleukin
- li(m) = immune system
- ne(ur) = neural
- os = bone
- tox(a) = toxin
- t(u)a = tumor
- vi(r) = viral

-*tu-xi-mab*, now means a monoclonal antibody, originating from chimeric tissue, targeting tumor tissue.

Lastly, the beginning of the word, or prefix, is what is given to the drug by the manufacturer. Hopefully the letters chosen make the word flow and easy to say.

Ri-tu-xi-mab, a monoclonal antibody, originating from chimeric tissue, to target tumor tissue, it is a drug developed to treat leukemia.

(Dyson, 2016)

BOX 51.2 Naming of Inhibitors

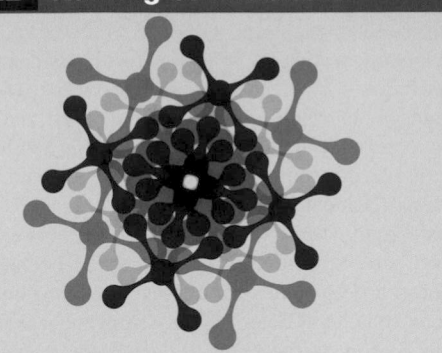

Inhibitor drug names are as confusing as the names of monoclonal antibodies. Yet, when examined, the names are created in a similar fashion (see Box 51.1), making the purpose of drug therapy understandable.

Unlike monoclonal antibodies, small molecule inhibitor drugs target processes within cells to inhibit cancer growth.

Monoclonal antibodies are given the suffix – *mab,* and *-ib* is the suffix to the small molecule inhibitors.

Inhibitors do not indicate the derived tissue type, yet they do indicate the type of inhibitor.

- *-anib* indicates angiogenesis inhibitors
- *-ciclib* indicates cyclin-dependent kinase inhibitors
- *-rafenib* indicates rapidly accelerated fibrosarcoma kinase inhibitors
- *-tinib* indicates tyrosine kinase inhibitors
- *-zomib* indicates proteasome inhibitors
(Scott, 2016)

compared with other monoclonal antibodies. Checkpoint inhibitors work inside cells interfering with specific cellular activity that caused the malignant change. There are a number of inhibiting agents; some block the action of certain enzymes, proteins, or other molecules involved in the growth and spread of cancer cells (Knoop, 2015). Depending upon the cancer cell type, the target can differ; examples include:

- Mutated protein in melanoma is *checked* by the drug vemurafenib (Zelboraf).
- In some leukemia cells two different genes can fuse together and become the *checkpoint* for imatinib (Gleevec).

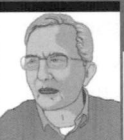

PHARMACOLOGY IN PRACTICE

DRUG RECOGNITION
Which of the following drugs is most likely a checkpoint inhibitor?

1. pertuzumab
2. tagraxofusp
3. erlotinib
4. alemtuzumab

ADVERSE REACTIONS AND PRECAUTIONS

Adverse reactions are typically inflammatory related and called *immune-related adverse events* (irAEs). They can start as generalized feelings of malaise and progress to life-threatening issues if not addressed quickly when identified (Rubin, 2015).

Integumentary System Reactions
Common adverse reactions of skin, nails, and hair include the following:

- Skin problems (rash, dry skin, nail changes, hair depigmentation)
- Photosensitivity

Gastrointestinal System Reactions
Diarrhea progressing to colitis, hepatitis, and elevated liver enzymes are common adverse reactions. For clients receiving sunitinib for gastrointestinal (GI) tumors, there is a rare but serious risk of bowel perforation (Kim, 2014).

Other Reactions
- Thyroid inflammation
- Pulmonary symptoms
- Neurological changes (hand and foot syndrome)
- Inflammatory arthritis
- Acute pancreatitis
- Inflammatory endocrine issues

Not all adverse reactions indicate a problem. Sometimes the reaction is a signal that the drug is working to kill the tumor cell. For example, clients treated with erlotinib or gefitinib have better outcomes (cancer improves) when the client develops an acne-like rash during therapy (Petrelli, 2012). Likewise, if a client experiences increased blood pressure when treated with bevacizumab, they tend to have a better outcome, too (Cai, 2013).

PRECAUTIONS

Caution is used in clients taking antidiabetic medications; they may experience more severe drops in blood sugar and should be more closely monitored. Monitor for increased bleeding if an anticoagulant is being taken. Studies in humans have not been adequately conducted to determine safety of checkpoint inhibitors while pregnant or lactating. Many of these agents may interfere with oral contraceptives; therefore, birth control should be discussed before therapy. Males may experience reduced sperm production. Clients taking vismodegib and sonidegib (used with metastatic basal cell cancers) should not give blood for at least a year following treatment because of the long half-life of these agents (Knoop, 2015).

Checkpoint inhibitors are less frequently prescribed for treatment of pediatric cancers, as children may experience greater immunosuppression.

INTERACTIONS

The following interactions may occur when checkpoint inhibitors are administered with another agent:

Interacting Drug	Common Use	Effect of Interaction
Antidiabetic	Treat diabetes	Increased blood sugar levels
Clozapine, promazine	Management of psychiatric problems	Increased risk for CNS toxicity
Antihypertensives	Treat high blood pressure	Increased risk of hypotension

AGENTS THAT SUPPORT ACTIVE IMMUNITY

A key concept in the success of immunotherapy is **adaptive immunity**. This is defined as the body's ability to actively recognize the antigen as the invader and present it to B or T lymphocytes. Subsequently, the body produces memory cells, which remember the antigen and prevent the same illness from affecting the individual more than once.

There are few of these therapies available, yet many are in the research process.

CANCER VACCINES

The function of vaccines is to trigger an immune response against a specific foreign body or pathogen. Although we may think of tumor tissue as an invader, it is not foreign tissue (King, 2004). Therefore, cancer vaccines are designed to make the tumor recognizable as "foreign" tissue. They develop antibodies and are capable of memory to fight ongoing disease.

Cancer vaccines differ from the ones discussed in Unit 12 in that most are being designed for treatment not prevention.

ACTIONS AND USES

Made to identify the molecular targets or genes that are different (tumor) from normal cells, an adaptive immune response gives the immune system memory to the abnormal cells. Uses include:

- Delay or stop cancer cell growth
- Cause tumor shrinkage
- Prevent cancer
- Eliminate cancer cells not killed by other methods

Currently, one treatment cancer vaccine is on the market, sipuleucel-T, used in the treatment of metastatic prostate cancer. Many more are in the research phase of development. See Chapter 47 for more information on preventative cancer vaccines, including the HPV vaccine.

ADVERSE REACTIONS, CONTRAINDICATIONS, AND PRECAUTIONS

Treatment cancer vaccines involve making the drug from the client's own tumor cells (**autologous**) or using many different cancer cells to induce a response (**allogeneic**). Clients are observed during and after infusion for reaction. Anaphylactic reactions may occur as an acute infusion reaction. Clients with cardiac or pulmonary conditions should be closely monitored during infusion.

Other adverse reactions include nausea, vomiting, fatigue, headache, and muscle and joint pain.

Because the drug is used to treat prostate cancer, it should not be given to women.

INTERACTIONS

The following interactions may occur when a cancer vaccine is administered with another agent:

Interacting Drug	Common Use	Effect of Interaction
Immunosuppressants	Reduce inflammatory response	Reduced vaccine effectiveness

ADOPTIVE CELL THERAPY

Adoptive cell therapy is a type of adaptive immunity using T cells because they have the ability to learn to tell cancer cells from healthy ones and have the memory to do so for years after treatment. Two types of therapy are being used currently, Chimeric Antigen Receptor T-Cell Transfer (CAR-T) therapy and Oncolytic viral therapy.

CAR-T involves the collection of T cells from a client's own blood, engineering them to recognize specific antigens on the cancer cell surface, and then infusing the cells back into the same client (Lamprecht, 2019). Infusions present with a high risk of cytokine release syndrome (CRS), or cytokine storm. The greater the amount of diseased tumor in the client at the time of reinfusion of cells, the more likely the client is to have a CRS reaction. Extremely high fever is typically the first indication a reaction is progressing.

Oncolytic viral therapy genetically modifies a virus to infect and destroy cancer cells. One drug has been produced to treat metastatic melanoma—talimogen laherparepvec. Because the drug is a virus, there are strict precautions that must be followed to protect the provider and others coming in contact with the drug.

NURSING PROCESS—STEPS TO BUILDING CLINICAL JUDGMENT
Client Receiving an Immune-Modulating Drug for Cancer

ASSESSMENT

Preadministration Assessment
A client may be treated as an outpatient in the ambulatory setting or as an inpatient in a hospital. Administration environment is dependent upon the extent of disease, comorbidity, or the complexity of this or other therapies. Data gathering suggestions before the initial administration of a cancer immunotherapy drug include:

Objective data
- Note type and location of neoplastic lesion
- Stage of the disease, for example, early, metastatic, or terminal
- Vital signs (temperature, pulse, respirations, and blood pressure) and weight
- Inspect general physical appearance, noting skin lesions for baseline integumentary status
- Neurological and psychosocial assessment to monitor for reactions
- Laboratory and radiologic tests—ECG, CBC, lipid profile, diabetes screening, and baseline organ function (e.g., liver and thyroid) and autoimmune status
- Pregnancy testing if female

Subjective data
- Client's knowledge or understanding of the proposed immunotherapy regimen
- History of bowel issues and habits
- Previous or concurrent treatments (if any), such as surgery, radiation therapy, or traditional chemotherapy drugs
- History of other current nonmalignant disease or disorder, such as autoimmune or diabetes, that may or may not be related to the malignant disease
- History of travel to areas of infectious diseases or having had an infectious disease
- Other factors, such as the client's age, financial problems that may be associated with a long-term illness, family cooperation and interest in client care, and the adequacy of health insurance coverage (which may be of great concern to the client)

Ongoing Assessment
As part of the ongoing assessment, anticipate that the client will experience the flu-like symptoms with administration as part of response to treatment. A generalized inflammatory response may occur, which is initially supported with nursing interventions. Should the inflammation advance, steroids may be added to treat the adverse reaction. Monitor respiratory status especially in clients being treated for lung cancer. Clients should be monitored for opportunistic infections owing to the reduction of cells in the immune system and may need to be put on antifungal or antibacterial drugs. A delayed clinical response can occur, *pseudo-progression*, where the tumor may appear to continue to grow up until about the 16th week after treatment was started. Clients need to be made aware of this happening, and one should assure them that the fear of lack of tumor response despite treatment is a normal feeling at this time (Rubin, 2015).

NURSING DIAGNOSES

Drug-specific nursing diagnoses include the following:
- **Impaired comfort: flu-like symptoms** related to stimulation of the immune system
- **Diarrhea** related to generalized inflammatory response in the bowel
- **Altered skin integrity** related to integumentary response to the generalized inflammatory process

Nursing diagnoses related to drug administration are discussed in Chapter 4.

PLANNING

The expected outcomes for the client depend on the reason for administration but may include an optimal response to therapy, meeting client needs related to the management of adverse reactions, and confidence in an understanding of the medication regimen.

IMPLEMENTATION

Promoting an Optimal Response to Therapy
Nurses who are certified in immunotherapy administer these drugs, but any nurse may be involved in monitoring clients for adverse reactions, see Chapter 50. Immunotherapy drugs are potentially toxic drugs that can cause a variety of effects during and after their administration.

Monoclonal Antibodies

mAbs are usually given parenterally—by the IV route, or some are subcutaneously injected. When infused over time, carefully monitor and observe client for a hypersensitive reaction. To reduce reactions the drug should be administered slowly and the client premedicated with acetaminophen and an antihistamine. Hypersensitive reactions become less likely with multiple treatments over time.

For those self-administering the drug, be sure the client or caregiver feels confident in technique before this becomes a routine procedure carried out at home. Follow-up on knowledge of storage of drug, technique, potential site reactions, and disposal is important.

For mAbs taken orally there are no special precautions for handling, yet it is important to take it at the same time daily to support effectiveness. Food may exacerbate the skin rash of erlotinib if taken with a meal.

Typically, doses are not titrated to adverse reactions, clients will get the full dose, it will be held or completely discontinued.

Monitoring and Managing Client Needs

Impaired Comfort

Flu-like symptoms can be an array of items including appetite loss, chills, fatigue, fever, head and body aches, or gastric upset (nausea, or diarrhea, see below). An example being an interleukin infusion, clients may experience chills and rigors within 30 minutes of starting the infusion. If warm blankets are not sufficient, IV meperidine may be given and premedication with acetaminophen and indomethacin planned for the next dose (Mavroukakis, 2001).

Encourage clients to balance activity with rest periods to reduce fatigue. Although it may sound counterintuitive to clients, exercise helps reduce fatigue; encourage clients to take small walks or participate in yoga (Puksic, 2021). For gastric upset, cold and salty foods are preferred over spicy, sweet, or greasy foods.

Diarrhea

Diarrhea may be a GI adverse reaction to immunotherapy, typically the inhibitors (Brahmer, 2018). It is due to the inflammatory response and is seen more frequently with GI or hormone-producing tumors (see Fig. 51.3). Because it can progress quickly from loose stools to colitis, clients and caregivers are taught to immediately inform the health care provider of bowel habit changes—abdominal pain, nausea, cramping, and bloody, mucous, or tarry stools. When the client is an inpatient, inspect stools for blood or mucus. Stool should be sent to rule out *C. difficile* (*C. diff*) or other pathogens. Viral screening, abdominal radiological tests, and endoscopy may be used to diagnose cause and guide treatment.

Instruct clients to avoid foods like caffeine, alcohol, and high roughage. Encourage foods with bulk such as pectin-containing fruits (apples), oatmeal, bananas, white rice, and cooked vegetables. Be sure the client drinks fluid to replace the loss from diarrhea. It is also important to maintain an accurate weight and intake and output record to help determine fluid balance.

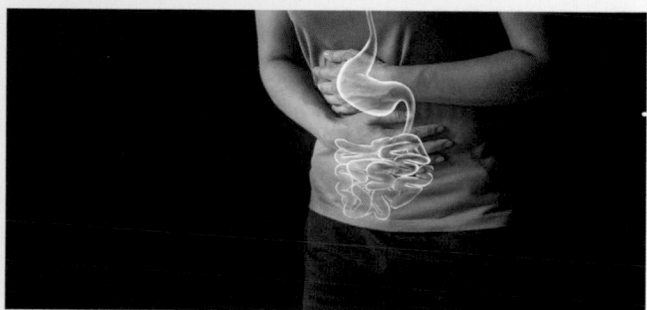

FIGURE 51.3 Diarrhea can progress quickly to colitis if interventions are not started quickly.

Because the immune system is affected by immunotherapy, observe the client for other signs and symptoms of a bacterial or fungal superinfection, such as vaginal or anal itching, sores in the mouth, diarrhea, fever, chills, and sore throat. It is important to report any new signs and symptoms occurring during therapy to the primary health care provider.

Altered Skin Integrity

Skin rash is an inflammatory reaction not a skin eruption like acne. Typically, it presents on the body, above the waist during the first week of treatment. Clients should avoid sunlight and use sunscreen even on cloudy days. Instruct the client to avoid rubbing the area and to wear clothing that is not rough or irritating. Using mild soaps and sensitive skin moisturizers can diminish itching. If pustules form, monitor for bacterial infection. Avoid the use of harsh soaps and perfumed lotions. Do not use acne products on the rash (Houlihan, 2005).

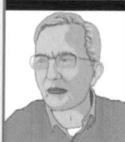

PHARMACOLOGY IN PRACTICE

MANAGING NEEDS

A client at the infusion center is ready for discharge after completing the first immunotherapy treatment. Which of the following instructions should the nurse give to the client? Select all that apply.

1. Use sunscreen, even on cloudy days.
2. Diarrhea is expected, you don't need to call just eat bulk foods.
3. If you feel tired don't go out and exercise.
4. If you experience chills call so we can premedicate you next time.

Potential Medical Complication: Infusion Reactions

Clients should be taught before the drug is given that an infusion reaction is anticipated and may be uncomfortable. Reactions tend to be more pronounced when the mAb is produced from mouse tissue or a combination of tissues (Dyson, 2016). Warm blankets should be provided for client comfort. Reassure the client that the medications administered before the immunotherapy will help to ease the adverse reactions. Instruction should include that the reactions decrease with ongoing therapy.

NURSING ALERT

The risk of an infusion reaction can be predicted by examining the suffix of the drug being infused:

- –momab (highest risk of infusion reaction)
- –ximab
- –zumab
- –mumab (lowest risk of infusion reaction)

Educating the Client and Family

The oncology health care provider usually discusses the proposed treatment and possible adverse drug reactions with the client and family members. As the nurse, you will briefly review these explanations immediately before administration of any immunotherapy drug.

Some immunotherapy drugs are taken orally at home. The areas included in a client and family teaching plan for this type of treatment regimen are based on the drug prescribed, the oncology health care provider's explanation of the drug therapy regimen and instructions for taking the drug, and the needs of the individual. The importance of taking the drug at the same time each day to maintain a consistent body level is emphasized. A calendar or automated medication box indicating the doses to take and dates the drug is to be taken is often helpful for the client. Discuss ways to ensure dosing even if the client does not feel well, such as help from a family member. Special precautions typically do not need to occur in the home, unless the client is participating in cancer vaccine therapy, then special instructions are given by the provider.

Include the following points in a client and family teaching plan when oral therapy is prescribed:

- Take the drug only as directed on the prescription container.
- Familiarize yourself with the brand or trade name and the generic name to avoid confusion. If you live with another person at home, ask that person to help you verify the correct drug and dose of the drug before you take it.
- Never increase, decrease, or omit a dose unless advised to do so by the oncology health care provider. Set up reminders such as a calendar, cellphone alarm, or computer alert if dosing routinely becomes an issue.
- If any problems (adverse reactions) occur, no matter how minor, contact the oncology health care provider immediately.

- All recommendations given by the oncology health care provider, such as increasing the fluid intake or eating or avoiding certain foods, are important.
- The effectiveness or action of the drug could be altered if these directions are ignored. Other recommendations, such as checking the mouth for sores, taking your temperature, or taking care with skin products, are given to identify or minimize some of the effects these drugs have on the body. It is important to follow these recommendations.
- Keep all appointments for immunotherapy. These drugs must be given at certain intervals to be effective.
- Do not take any nonprescription drug unless the use of a specific drug has been approved by the oncology health care provider.
  - Avoid drinking alcoholic beverages unless the oncology health care provider has approved their use.
- Always inform other physicians, dentists, and medical personnel of therapy with this drug.
- Keep all appointments for the laboratory tests ordered by the oncology health care provider. If you are unable to keep a laboratory appointment, notify the oncology health care provider immediately.

EVALUATION

- Therapeutic response is achieved and there is reduced evidence of disease.
- Adverse reactions are identified, reported to the primary health care provider, and managed successfully with appropriate nursing interventions:
  - Client reports comfort, with minimal fever or chills.
  - Client does not experience diarrhea.
  - Skin is intact and irritation is reduced.
- Client and family express confidence and demonstrate understanding of the drug regimen.

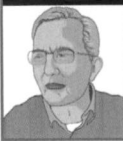

PHARMACOLOGY IN PRACTICE

USING CLINICAL REASONING

Mr. Phillip's wife received a drug called Herceptin. From the information you have learned about immunology determine what type of adverse reaction she had and her likelihood of experiencing reactions due to the immunology component of her treatments.

KEY POINTS

■ Immunotherapy treats cancer cells directly, restores or enhances the immune system's natural ability to fight cancerous cells.

■ Tumor-associated antigens on the surface of tumor cells are the targets of monoclonal antibodies, cytokines, and cancer vaccines. The immunotherapy drugs see the TAAs as being different and make the immune system think the cancer cell is foreign, resulting in the body initiating the immune response against the cancer cells.

■ Immunotherapies have less adverse reactions systemically than traditional chemotherapy since they focus on certain cells. Reactions of inflammation and hypersensitivity in the immune system are more predominant.

■ Although the reactions are not generalized to many body tissues, they can be of an emergent nature and need to be attended to even when a slight issue is noticed.

SUMMARY DRUG TABLE
Drugs Used to Treat Cancer (Immune Modulators)

Generic Name	Trade Name	Uses	Adverse Reactions
Passive Immunity			
Cytokines			
Interferons			
interferon Alfa-2b *In-ter-FEER-on*	Intron A	Lymphoma, melanoma, hairy cell leukemia, chronic hepatitis B, Kaposi sarcoma, genital warts	Flu-like symptoms, fatigue, insomnia, alopecia, nausea, abdominal pain, cough, injection site reaction
Interleukin			
aldesleukin *al-des-LOO-kin*	Proleukin	Metastatic melanoma and renal cell carcinoma	Flu-like symptoms, hypotension, rash, nausea, vomiting, diarrhea, dyspnea
tagraxofusp *tag-RAX-oh-fusp*	Elzonris	Leukemia/lymphoma	Same reaction for all drugs in this category
Monoclonal Antibodies			
ado-trastuzumab emtansine *a-do-tras-TU-xoo-mab* *em-TAN-seen*	Kadcyla	Solid tumors: HER2-positive breast	Flu-like symptoms, insomnia, skin rash, itching, nausea, diarrhea, nasopharyngitis, epistaxis, muscle aches, reduced lymphocytes, infusion reaction
alemtuzumab *ay-lem-TU-zoo-mab*	Lemtrada	Leukemia, multiple sclerosis	Same reaction for all drugs in this category
belantamab mafodotin- blmf *bel-AN-ta-mab mA-foe-DOE-tin*	Blenrep	Multiple myeloma	
bevacizumab *be-vuh-SIZ-uh-mab*	Avastin, Mvasi, Zirabev	Solid tumors: cervical, colon, brain	
blinatumomab *blin-a-TOOM-oh-mab*	Blincyto	Leukemia	
brentuximab vedotin *bren-TUX-i-mab* *ve-DOE-tin*	Adcetris	Lymphomas	
daratumumab *dar-a-TOOM-ue-mab*	Darzalex Darzalex Faspro (w/ hyaluronidase)	Multiple myeloma	
dinutuximab *din-ue-TUX-i-mab*	Unituxin	Solid tumors: neuroblastoma	
elotuzumab *el-oh-TOOZ-ue-mab*	Empliciti	Multiple myeloma	
enfortumab vedotin *en-FORT-ue-mab* *ve-DOE-tin*	Padcev	Solid tumors: bladder/urinary	
fam-trastuzumab detuxtecan-nxki *fam-tras-TU-zoo-mab* *de-RUX-the-can*	Enhertu	Solid tumors: HER2-positive breast	
gemtuzumab ozogamicin *gem-TOO-zoo-mab* *oh-zog-a-MY-sin*	Mylotarg	Leukemia	
ibritumomab tiuxetan *ib-ri-TYOO-mo-mab* *tye-TUX-e-tan*	Zevlin Y-90	Non-Hodgkin lymphoma	
intotuzumab ozogamincin *in-oh-TOOZ-ue-mab* *oh-zog-a-MY-sin*	Besponsa	Leukemia	

Continued

SUMMARY DRUG TABLE (continued)
Drugs Used to Treat Cancer (Immune Modulators)

Generic Name	Trade Name	Uses	Adverse Reactions
isatuximab *EYE-sa-TUX-i-mab*	Sarclisa	Multiple myeloma	
moxetumomab *mox-e-TOOM-oh-mab*	Lumoxiti	Hairy cell leukemia	
necitumumab *ne-si-TOOM-oo-mab*	Portrazza	Solid tumors: lung	
obinutuzumab *oh-bi-nue-TOOZ-ue-mab*	Gazyva	Leukemia/lymphoma	
ofatumumab *oh-fa-TOOM-yoo-mab*	Arzerra, Kesimpta	Leukemia/multiple sclerosis	
olaratumab *oh-lar-AT-ue-mab*	Lartruvo	Solid tumors: sarcoma	
pertuzumab *per-TU-zoo-mab*	Perjeta	Solid tumors: HER-positive breast	
polatuzumab vedotin *POL-a-TOOZ-ue-mab ve-DOE-tin*	Polivy	Lymphoma	
ramucirumab *ra-mue-SIR-ue-mab*	Cyramza	Solid tumors: colon, GI, liver, lung	
sacituzumab govitecan *SAK-i-TOOZ-ue-mab* *GOE-vi-TEE-kan*	Trodelvy	Solid tumors: triple-negative breast	
riTUXimab *ri-TUK-si-mab*	Rituxan, Ruxience (rituximab-pvvr), Truxima (rituximab-abbs), Rituxan Hycela (w/ hyaluronidase)	Leukemia, lymphoma, inflammatory diseases, rheumatoid arthritis	
tafasitamab *TA-fa-SIT-a-mab*	Monjuvi	Lymphoma	
trastuzumab *tras-TU-zoo-mab*	Herceptin, Herzuma (trastuzumab-pkrb), Ogivri (trastuzumab-dkst), Ontruzant (trastuzumab-dttb), Trazimera (trastuzumab-qyyp)	Solid tumors: breast, gastric	
Checkpoint and Other Inhibitors			
Checkpoint Inhibitors			
atezolizumab *a-te-zoe-LIZ-ue-mab*	Tecentriq	Solid tumors: breast, liver, melanoma, lung, bladder	Flu-like symptoms, peripheral edema, skin rash, itching, nausea, diarrhea, cough, arthralgia, reduced lymphocytes
avelumab *a-VEL-ue-mab*	Bavencio	Solid tumors: renal, urinary, Merkel	Same reaction for all drugs in this category
cemiplimab-rwlc *SEM-ip-LI-mab*	Libtayo	Squamous cell—local advanced, mets	
durvalumab *dur-VAL-ue-mab*	Imfinzi	Solid tumors: lung, bladder	
ipilimumab *ip-i-LIM-u-mab*	Vervoy	Solid tumors: lung, melanoma	
nivolumab *nye-VOL-ue-mab*	Opdivo	Solid tumors: colon, esophageal, head and neck, liver, lung, lymphoma, melanoma, renal, urothelial	
pembrolizumab *pem-broe-LIZ-ue-mab*	Keytruda	Lung, cervical, endometrial, squamous cell, lymphoma	
B-cell Lymphoma-2 Inhibitor			

Generic Name	Trade Name	Uses	Adverse Reactions
venetoclax *ven-ET-oh-klax*	Venclexta	Leukemia/lymphoma	Flu-like symptoms, peripheral edema, skin rash, itching, nausea, diarrhea, cough, arthralgia, reduced lymphocytes
EGFR Inhibitors			
afatinib *a-FA-ti-nib*	Gilortif	Solid tumors: lung	Nausea, diarrhea, rash, vision problems, hypomagnesia
cetuximab *se-TUK-see-mab*	Erbitux	Solid tumors: colon, head and neck	Same reaction for all drugs in this category
erlotinib *er-LOE-ti-nib*	Tarceva	Solid tumors: lung, pancreas	
gefitinib *ge-FI-ti-nib*	Iressa	Solid tumors: lung	
lapatinib *la-PA-ti-nib*	Tykerb	Solid tumors: breast	
panitumumab *pan-i-TOOM-yoo-mab*	Vectibix	Solid tumors: colon	
Hedgehog Pathway Inhibitors			
glasdegib *glas-DEG-ib*	Daurismo	leukemia	Fatigue, alopecia, nausea, vomiting, diarrhea, muscle pain and spasm
sonidegib *soe-ni-DEG-ib*	Odomzo	Solid tumors: locally advanced basal cell	Same reaction for all drugs in this category
vismodegib *vis-moe-DEG-ib*	Erivedge	Solid tumors: locally advanced basal cell	
Histone Deacetylase Inhibitors			
belinostat *be-LIN-oh-stat*	Beleodaq	Lymphoma	Fatigue, headache, fever, chills, rash, nausea, constipation, diarrhea
panobinostat *pan-oh-BIN-oh-stat*	Farydak	Multiple myeloma	Same reaction for all drugs in this category
romiDEPsin *roe-mi-DEP-sin*	Istodax	Lymphoma	
vorinostat *vor-IN-oh-stat*	Zolina	lymphoma	
IDH Inhibitors			
ivosidenib *EYE-voe-SID-e-nib*	Tibsovo	Leukemia	Fatigue, headache, fever, rash, peripheral edema, neuropathy, cough, nausea, constipation, diarrhea, arthralgia
enasidenib *en-a-SID-a-nib*	Idhifa	Leukemia	
Kinase Inhibitors			
abemaciclib *a-bem-a-SYE-klib*	Verzenio	Solid tumors: breast	Fatigue, headache, alopecia, peripheral edema, cough, nausea, diarrhea, arthralgia
alpelisib *AL-pe-LIS-ib*	Piqray	Solid tumors: breast	Same reaction for all drugs in this category
binimetinib *bin-i-ME-ti-nib*	Mektovi	Solid tumors: melanoma, colon	
capmatinib *kap-MA-ti-nib*	Tabrecta	Solid tumors: lung	
cobimetinib *koe-bi-ME-ti-nib*	Cotellic	Solid tumors: melanoma	

Continued

SUMMARY DRUG TABLE (continued)
Drugs Used to Treat Cancer (Immune Modulators)

Generic Name	Trade Name	Uses	Adverse Reactions
copanlisib koe-pan-LIS-ib	Aliqopa	Lymphoma	
dabrafenib da-BRAF-e-nib	Tafinlar	Solid tumors: melanoma, lung, thyroid	
dacomitinib DAK-oh-MI-ti-nib	Vizimpro	Solid tumors: lung	
duvelisib DOO-ve-LIS-ib	Copiktra	Leukemia/lymphoma	
encorafenib en-koe-RAF-e-nib	Braftovi	Solid tumors: melanoma, colon	
everolimus e-ver-OH-li-mus	Afinitor, Zortress (transplant only)	Solid tumors: breast, renal, neuroendocrine Renal/liver transplantation	
fedratinib fed-RA-ti-nib	Inrebic	Myelodysplastic/proliferative disorders	
gilteritinib GIL-te-RI-ti-nib	Xospata	Leukemia	
idelalisib eye-del-a-LIS-ib	Zydelig	Leukemia/lymphoma	
midostaurin mye-doe-STAW-rin	Rydapt	Leukemia	
palbociclib pal-boe-SYE-klib	Ibrance	Solid tumors: breast	
pralsetinib pral-se-TIN-ib	Gavreto	Solid tumors: lung	
ribociclib rye-boe-SYE-klib	Kisquali	Solid tumors: breast	
ruxolitinib rux-oh-LI-ti-nib	Jakafi	Myelodysplastic/proliferative disorders	
selpercatinib SEL-per-KA-tih-nib	Retevmo	Solid tumors: lung, thyroid	
selumetinib SEL-ue-ME-ti-nib	Koselugo	Neurofibromatosis	
trametinib tra-ME-ti-nib	Mekinist	Solid tumors: melanoma, lung, thyroid	
temsirolimus tem-sir-OH-li-mus	Torisel	Solid tumors: renal	
vemurafenib vem-ue-RAF-e-nib	Zelboraf	Solid tumors: melanoma, lung	
Anti-VEGF			
regorafenib re-goe-RAF-e-nib	Stivarga	Solid tumors: colon, liver, other GI cancers	Fatigue, headache, rash, hypertension, epistaxis
SORAfenib sor-AF-e-nib	NexAVAR	Solid tumors: renal, liver, thyroid	
Tyrosine Kinase/EGFR Inhibitors			
acalabrutinib a-KAL-a-broo-ti-nib	Calquence	Leukemia/lymphoma	Fatigue, nausea, vomiting, diarrhea, constipation, vision problems
alectinib al-EK-ti-nib	Alecensa	Solid tumors: lung	Same reaction for all drugs in this category
avapritinib A-vaPRI-ti-nib	Ayvakit	Solid tumors: GI	
axitinib ax-I-ti-nib	Inlyta	Solid tumors: renal, thyroid	

Generic Name	Trade Name	Uses	Adverse Reactions
bosutinib boe-SUE-ti-nib	Bosulif	Leukemia	
brigatinib bri-GA-ti-nib	Alunbrig	Solid tumors: lung	
cabozantinib ka-boe-Zan-ti-nib	Cabometyx, Cometriq	Solid tumors: liver, renal, thyroid	
ceritinib se-RI-ti-nib	Zykadia	Solid tumors: lung	
crizotinib kriz-OH-ti-nib	Xalkori	Solid tumors: lung	
dasatinib da-SA-ti-nib	Sprycel	Leukemia	
entrectinib en-TREK-ti-nib	Rozlytrek	Solid tumors: lung, various others	
erdafitinib er-da-FI-ti-nib	Balversa	Solid tumors: bladder, urinary	
ibrutinib eye-BROO-ti-nib	Imbruvica	Leukemia/myelodysplastic/ proliferative disorders	
imatinib eye-MAT-eh-nib	Gleevec	Leukemia/myelodysplastic/ proliferative disorders	
larotrectinib LAR-oh-TREK-ti-nib	Vitrakvi	Solid tumors: various	
lenvatinib len-VA-ti-nib	Lenvima	Solid tumors: endometrial, liver, renal, thyroid	
lorlatinib lor-LA-ti-nib	Lorbrena	Solid tumors: lung	
neratinib ne-RA-ti-nib	Nerlynx	Solid tumors: breast	
nilotinib nye-LOE-ti-nib	Tasigna	Leukemia	
osimertinib oh-si-mer-ti-nib	Tagrisso	Solid tumors: lung	
PAZOPanib paz-OH-pa-nib	Votrient	Solid tumors: renal, sarcoma, thyroid	
pemigatinib PEM-i-GA-ti-nib	Pemazyre	Solid tumors: bile duct	
PONATinib Poe-NA-ti-nib	Iclusig	Leukemia	
ripretinib rip-RE-ti-nib	Qinlock	Solid tumors: gastrointestinal stromal tumor (GIST)	
SUNItinib Su-NIT-e-nib	Sutent	Solid tumors: GIST, pancreas, renal, sarcoma, thyroid	
tucatinib too-KA-ti-nib	Tukysa	Solid tumors: breast	
vandetanib van-DET-a-nib	Caprelsa	Solid tumors: thyroid	
zanubrutinib ZAN-ue-BROO-ti-nib	Brukinsa	Lymphoma	
Nuclear Export Inhibitor			
selinexor SEL-i-NEX-or	Xpovio	Lymphoma/multiple myeloma	Fatigue, mental changes, peripheral edema, decreased appetite, nausea, vomiting, diarrhea, muscle pain

Continued

SUMMARY DRUG TABLE (continued)
Drugs Used to Treat Cancer (Immune Modulators)

Generic Name	Trade Name	Uses	Adverse Reactions
PARP Enzyme Inhibitors			
niraparib nye-RAP-a-rib	Zejula	Solid tumors: female genitourinary (GU)	Fatigue, headache, decreased appetite, taste changes, nausea, vomiting, diarrhea, muscle pain
olaparib oh-LAP-a-rib	Lynparza	Solid tumors: breast, ovarian, pancreas, prostate	
rucaparib roo-KAP-a-rib	Rubraca	Solid tumors: ovarian, prostate	
talazoparib tal-a-ZOE-pa-rib	Talzenna	Solid tumors: breast	
Proteasome Inhibitors			
bortezomib bore-TEZ-oh-mib	Velcade	Lymphoma/multiple myeloma	Fatigue, headache, neuropathy, rash, hypertension, diarrhea, nausea, pancytopenia
carfilzomib kar-FILZ-oh-mib	Kyprolis	Multiple myeloma	
ixazomib ix-AZ-oh-mib	Ninlaro	Multiple myeloma	
Protein Synthesis Inhibitors			
omacetaxine oh-ma-se-TAX-een	Synribo	Leukemia	Fatigue, headache, rash, hypertension, epistaxis
ziv-aflibercept ziv-a-FLIB-er-sept	Zaltrap	Solid tumors: colon	
Immunomodulators—Angiogenesis Inhibitors			
lenalidomide le-na-LID-oh-mide	Revlimid	Lymphoma reoccurrence, multiple myeloma	Fatigue, headache, dizziness, rash, edema, epistaxis
thalidomide tha-LI-doe-mide	Thalomid	Leprosum multiple myeloma	Lenalidomide, pomalidomide, and thalidomide are administered under strict supervision in special programs because of the severe birth defects that occur if taken while pregnant
pomalidomide poe-ma-LID-oh-mide	Pomalyst	Multiple myeloma, Kaposi sarcoma	
Active Immunity			
Vaccines			
sipuleucel-T si-pu-LOO-sel-tee	Provenge	Prostate cancer	Fever, chills, headache, flu-like symptoms
human papillomavirus (HPV) YU-man pap-ih-LO-ma VYE-rus	Cervarix (female), Gardasil (male/female)	Prevention of GU cancers, other conditions caused by HPV virus	Injection site reaction
Adoptive Cell Therapy			
axicabtagene ciloleucel ax-i-CAB-ta-jeen sye-LO-loo-sel	Yescarta	Lymphoma	Fatigue, fever, headache, tachycardia, hypotension, decreased appetite, nausea, diarrhea, cytokine release syndrome
brexucabtagene autoleucel BREX-ue-CAB-ta-jeen AW-toe-LOO-sel	Tecartus	Lymphoma	
tisagenlecleucel tis-a-jen-lek-LOO-sel	Kymriah	Leukemia/lymphoma	

CHAPTER REVIEW

Know Your Drugs

Clients sometimes know a medication by the brand (or trade) name and not the generic name. To help you recognize both names, match the brand name with the generic name of the same medication.

Generic Name	Brand Name
1. trastuzumab	A. Kisquali
2. pembrolizumab	B. Herceptin
3. ribociclib	C. Rituxan
4. rituximab	D. Keytruda

Calculate Medication Dosages

1. The cancer vaccine infusion reads 500 mL infused over 60 minutes. How long should a 125 mL IV bag be infused for?

Prepare for the NCLEX

RECALL THE FACTS

1. Which of the following agents involve active immunity?
   1. Cytokines
   2. Cancer vaccines
   3. Monoclonal antibodies
   4. Colony stimulating factors
2. The function of cytokines are to _____.
   1. Communicate in the immune system
   2. To invade cells and contaminate cytoplasm
   3. Interfere with the cell cycle
   4. Dampen the immune response
3. The term chimeric means _____.
   1. Massive plasma leakage into tissues
   2. Combining tissue groups to make a product
   3. Ability to make own blood vessels
   4. Poisonous to living cells
4. Adverse reactions typical of immunotherapy include _____.
   1. Capillary leak syndrome
   2. Flu-like symptoms
   3. Cytokine storm
   4. Tumor lysis syndrome
5. What would differentiate a more serious adverse reaction from the flu-like symptoms following drug administration?
   1. Appetite decreases, fatigue, nausea
   2. Fatigue, chills, body aches
   3. Fever, headache, nausea
   4. Malaise, multiple loose stools, chills

ANALYZE THE FACTS

6. The nurse is alerted by the following statement made by a client starting checkpoint inhibitor medications.
   1. "We recently traveled to Iowa."
   2. "I have always had a loose stool issue."
   3. "My great-grant parent had TB."
   4. "My pregnant daughter just moved into our house."

7. A client will be starting blinatumomab for leukemia. They fearfully ask about infusion reactions. Your best response is _____.
   1. "Your drug is mouse free."
   2. "What have you heard about infusion reactions?"
   3. "Don't worry we can treat it if it happens."
   4. "Why are you worried, skin reactions are far worse."
8. The infusion room nurse suspects the client is showing signs of capillary leak syndrome; which finding indicates this could be happening?
   1. Client is wearing a winter coat in the summer.
   2. Remarks on swollen feet, which they never had.
   3. Complains of ringing in the ears.
   4. Nausea feels like they are swaying on a boat.
9. Volunteers are making take home kits for the infusion clinic. Which item would be most appropriate?
   1. Paper tape and cotton dressings
   2. Flyers about local trail hikes
   3. Samples of sunscreen
   4. Sweet hard candies

ALTERNATE-FORMAT QUESTIONS

10. A client undergoing inhibitor therapy is having multiple stools, what should the nursing interventions be for this client? **Select all that apply.**
    1. Modify diet to remove caffeine and roughage.
    2. Send sample to laboratory to rule out pathogen.
    3. Start fluid restrictions.
    4. Begin accurate intake and output measures.

To check your answers, see Appendix F.

WANT TO KNOW MORE? A wide variety of resources are available to enhance your learning and understanding of this chapter.
- Visit thePoint for resources such as:
  - NCLEX-Style Student Review Questions
  - Journal Articles
  - Dosage Calculations
  - Drug Monographs
  - Watch and Learn Videos
  - Concepts in Action Animations
- The *Study Guide to Accompany Introductory Clinical Pharmacology,* 12th edition, sold separately, will help you review and apply essential content.
- √PrepU is available to help students prepare for the NCLEX-PN examination.

UNIT 14
Drugs That Affect Other Body Systems

This unit covers a variety of drugs affecting body systems not covered earlier in the text. Chapters in this unit include topical drugs used to treat skin disorders, otic (ear) and ophthalmic (eye) preparations, and fluids and electrolytes. Chapter 52 discusses topical drugs used in the treatment of skin disorders. The skin forms a barrier between the outside environment and the structures located beneath the skin. The *epidermis* is the outermost layer of the skin. Immediately below the epidermis is the *dermis*, which contains small capillaries that supply nourishment to the dermis and epidermis, sebaceous (oil-secreting) glands, sweat glands, nerve fibers, and hair follicles. Because of the skin's proximity to the outside environment, it is subject to various types of injury and trauma, as well as to changes in the skin itself. Topical drugs discussed include those used for infections, irritation, or to remove debris when cleaning.

Chapter 53 discusses drugs used to treat disorders of the eye and ear. Otic drugs may be used to treat infection and inflammation of the ear or to soften and remove cerumen (wax). Ophthalmic drugs are used for diagnostic and therapeutic purposes. As a diagnostic tool, ophthalmic drugs are used to anesthetize the eye, dilate the pupil, and stain the cornea to identify anomalies. Therapeutic purposes include the treatment of infection, allergy, and eye disorders such as glaucoma or macular degeneration.

The composition of body fluids remains relatively constant despite the many demands placed on the body each day. On occasion, these demands cannot be met, and electrolytes and fluids must be given intravenously (IV) in an attempt to restore equilibrium. In the many facilities where nurses work, the role you play in IV therapy differs.

No matter where you practice nursing, it is important to understand the basic concepts of fluid and electrolyte balance. The solutions used in managing body fluids discussed in Chapter 54 include intravenous fluid and electrolyte replacement, blood products, and total parenteral nutrition. Electrolytes are charged particles (ions) that are essential for normal cell function and are involved in various metabolic activities. The primary electrolytes discussed include potassium, calcium, magnesium, and sodium. Calculation of parenteral fluids and the conversion of IV fluids to other forms of pain medications are also included.

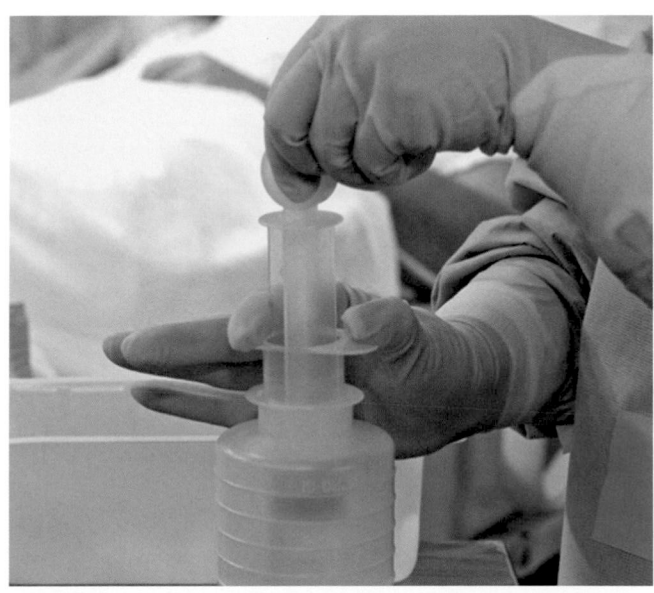

Drugs That Affect Other Body Systems

Skin Disorder Topical Drugs

Key Terms

bactericidal drug or agent that destroys or kills bacteria

bacteriostatic drug or agent that slows or retards the multiplication of bacteria

germicide agent that kills bacteria

keratolytic agent that removes excessive growth of the epidermis (top layer of skin)

necrotic pertaining to death of tissue

onychomycosis finger or toenail fungal infection

proteolysis enzymatic action that helps remove dead soft tissues by reducing proteins to simpler substances

purulent exudate fluid discharge of pus and white cells

superinfection overgrowth of bacterial or fungal microorganisms not affected by the antibiotic being administered

tinea corporis superficial fungal infection, commonly called *ringworm*

tinea cruris superficial fungal infection of the groin region, commonly called *jock itch*

tinea pedis superficial fungal infection of the foot, commonly called *athlete's foot*

tinea versicolor fungal infection that concentrates on the trunk of the body occurring in adolescents and young adults

Learning Objectives

On completion of this chapter, the student will:

1. List the types of drugs used in the treatment of skin disorders.
2. Explain the general drug actions, uses, and reactions to and any contraindications, precautions, and interactions associated with drugs used in treating skin disorders.
3. Distinguish important preadministration and ongoing assessment activities the nurse should perform on clients receiving a drug used to treat skin disorders.
4. List nursing diagnoses particular to a client using a drug to treat a skin disorder.
5. Examine ways to promote an optimal response to therapy and important points to keep in mind when educating the client about a skin disorder.

 Drug Classes

Retinoids	Topical immunomodulators
Antibiotic topicals	Antipsoriatic topicals
Antifungal topicals	Enzymes and keratolytics
Antiviral topicals	Local anesthetics
Antiseptics and germicides	
Corticosteroids	

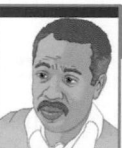

PHARMACOLOGY IN PRACTICE

The medication nurse in the long-term care facility caring for Mr. Park asks you about his shingles outbreak. Her cousin has cold sores and uses an acyclovir ointment when they first appear. She questions why Mr. Park was not prescribed a topical drug to ease the pain and irritation from the shingles lesions. Would not the same help Mr. Park? As you read about topical preparations, consider her question.

Typically, the most visible issue clients experience are conditions of the skin. Some of the most common include: acne, dermatitis, psoriasis, rosacea, and hair loss. These can be treated both topically or systemically; previous units have introduced you to drugs for systemic use of these and other conditions. In this chapter topical preparations are discussed. The drug classes are listed above in their respective categories. Drugs are categorized according to class, not ailment. For example, drugs used to treat acne may be in the retinoid category or antibiotic, antiseptic, or anti-inflammatory. This format will help you identify common side effects of topical drugs no matter the condition of use. See the Summary Drug Table: Topical Drugs for a listing of topical drugs and additional information.

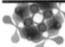 # RETINOIDS

Retinoids have become the first-line treatment of facial acne and many other skin problems. These drugs are used both systemically and topically. Issues of fetal defects make the oral products unsuitable for pregnant women. Below are the indications of topical use of Retinoids.

ACTIONS AND USES

Retinoids are chemically related to Vitamin A and regulate epithelial cell growth. Stimulation of new blood vessels in the skin helps bring nutrients to the skin. Topically, retinoids prevent dead skin cells from clogging tissue pores. These compounds are used to treat:

• Acne vulgaris
• Kaposi sarcoma
• Wrinkling

ADVERSE REACTIONS

Local irritation such as erythema, dryness, stinging or burning sensation, itching may occur, especially in the first 2–4 weeks of treatment. These reactions can become worse with the use of medicates, abrasive soaps or cleansers. Local reactions lessen with continued use over time. Sensitivity to weather extremes (hot or cold) may happen.

CONTRAINDICATIONS, PRECAUTIONS, AND INTERACTIONS

Those with a hypersensitivity to the drug or any components of it should not use retinoids. Preparations should not be used on damaged skin (cuts, sunburn, eczema). Hypersensitive reactions include facial edema, and should be stopped immediately. People should avoid sun or sun lamps while using and should not be used by pregnant women. There are no known drug interactions due to their limited use on the skin.

 Lifespan Considerations

Women and adolescents.
Females of childbearing age (including teenagers) prescribed retinoids must have a negative pregnancy test result before use and birth control is recommended while on the medication.

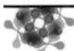 # TOPICAL ANTI-INFECTIVES

Localized skin infections may require the use of a topical anti-infective. The topical anti-infectives include antibiotic, antifungal, and antiviral drugs.

ACTIONS AND USES

Topical Antibiotic Drugs
Topical antibiotics exert a direct local effect on specific microorganisms and may be **bactericidal** (i.e., lethal to bacteria) or **bacteriostatic** (i.e., inhibit bacterial growth). Bacitracin, an antibacterial drug, inhibits cell wall synthesis and is an example of an antibiotic used in topical form.

These drugs are used to:

• Treat primary and secondary skin infections
• Prevent infection in minor cuts, wounds, scrapes, and minor burns
• Treat acne vulgaris

Topical Antifungal Drugs
Superficial mycotic (or fungal) infections occur on the surface of, or just below, the skin or nails. Surface fungal infections include athlete's foot (**tinea pedis**), jock itch (**tinea cruris**), ringworm (**tinea corporis**), and nail fungus (**onychomycosis**). In hot and humid climates a generalized fungal infection (**tinea versicolor**) is bothersome. Antifungal drugs exert a local effect by inhibiting growth of fungi. Antifungal drugs are used for treating:

• Athlete's foot, jock itch, ringworm
• Cutaneous candidiasis
• Other superficial fungal infections of the skin

Topical Antiviral Drugs
Acyclovir and penciclovir are topical forms of antiviral drugs used to treat oral herpes simplex virus (HSV). These drugs are used to inhibit viral activity:

• During initial episodes of HSV (prodrome phase)
• Directly on lesions to speed up recovery

Docosanol is a cream sold over the counter (OTC) and speeds healing as well.

ADVERSE REACTIONS

Adverse reactions to topical anti-infectives are usually mild. Occasionally, the client may experience a rash, itching, urticaria (hives), dermatitis, irritation, or redness, which may indicate a hypersensitivity (allergic) reaction to the drug. Prolonged use of topical antibiotic preparations may result in a superficial **superinfection** (an overgrowth of bacterial or fungal microorganisms not affected by the anti-infective being administered).

CONTRAINDICATIONS, PRECAUTIONS, AND INTERACTIONS

These drugs are contraindicated in clients with known hypersensitivity to the drugs or any components of the drug.

The topical antibiotics are pregnancy category C drugs and are used cautiously during pregnancy and lactation. Acyclovir and penciclovir are pregnancy category B drugs and are used cautiously during pregnancy and lactation.

The pregnancy categories of the antifungals are unknown except for econazole, which is in pregnancy category C, and ciclopirox, which is in pregnancy category B; both are used with caution during pregnancy and lactation. There are no significant interactions for the topical anti-infectives.

PRACTICE CONSIDERATIONS

Gentian violet is a bluish-violet dye with antiseptic properties. It is sometimes used to mark surgical areas and frequently used in veterinary practices. Some people feel it is a more homeopathic alternative for topical treatments of yeast and fungal infections than topical drugs. Studies conducted in Canada concluded in 2019 that there is a cancer risk to use and have banned the substance there and in other UK-associated countries (HC, 2019).

TOPICAL ANTISEPTICS AND GERMICIDES

An antiseptic is a drug that stops, slows, or prevents the growth of microorganisms. A **germicide** is a drug that kills bacteria.

ACTIONS

The exact mechanism of action of topical antiseptics and germicides is not well understood. These drugs affect a variety of microorganisms. Some of these drugs have a short duration of action, whereas others have a long duration of action. The action of these drugs may depend on the strength used and the time the drug is in contact with the skin or mucous membrane.

USES

Topical antiseptics and germicides are used for the following:

- To reduce the number of bacteria on skin surfaces
- As a surgical scrub and preoperative skin cleanser
- For performing hand hygiene before and after caring for clients
- In the home to cleanse the skin
- On minor cuts and abrasions to prevent infection

ADVERSE REACTIONS

Topical antiseptics and germicides provoke few adverse reactions. Occasionally, an individual may be allergic to the drug, and a skin rash or itching may occur. If an allergic reaction is noted, use of the topical drug is discontinued.

CONTRAINDICATIONS, PRECAUTIONS, AND INTERACTIONS

These drugs are contraindicated in clients with known hypersensitivity to the individual drug or any component of the preparation. There are no significant precautions or interactions when the drugs are used as directed.

TOPICAL CORTICOSTEROIDS

Topical corticosteroids vary in potency, depending on the concentration (percentage) of the drug, the vehicle (lotion, cream, aerosol spray) in which the drug is suspended, and the area (open or denuded skin, unbroken skin, thickness of the skin over the treated area) to which the drug is applied.

ACTIONS AND USES

Topical corticosteroids exert localized anti-inflammatory activity. When applied to inflamed skin, they reduce itching, redness, and swelling. These drugs are used in treating skin disorders such as:

- Psoriasis
- Dermatitis
- Rashes
- Eczema
- Insect bites
- First- and second-degree burns, including sunburn

Crisaborole is a topical medication used in the treatment of eczema that is not steroidal based. It is a phosphodiesterase 4 (PDE-4) inhibitor. PDE4 is an enzyme which regulates inflammation. Crisaborole blocks the production of the enzyme and reduces the inflammation associated with skin outbreak but does not have the risks of a steroid.

ADVERSE REACTIONS

Localized reactions may include burning, itching, irritation, redness, dryness of the skin, allergic contact dermatitis, and secondary infection. These reactions are more likely to occur if occlusive dressings are used. If liberally applied, some systemic absorption may occur. This is less likely when used as prescribed. Systemic reactions include hypothalamic–pituitary–adrenal axis suppression, Cushing syndrome, hyperglycemia, and glycosuria.

CONTRAINDICATIONS,

 Lifespan Considerations

Pediatric.
Because infants and children have a high ratio of skin surface area to body mass, they are at greater risk than adults for systemic adverse effects when treated with topical medication.

PRECAUTIONS, AND INTERACTIONS

Topical corticosteroids are contraindicated in clients with known hypersensitivity to the drug or any component of the drug; as monotherapy for bacterial skin infections; for use on the face, groin, or axilla (only the high-potency corticosteroids); and for ophthalmic use (may cause steroid-induced glaucoma or cataracts). The topical corticosteroids are not used as sole therapy in widespread plaque psoriasis. The topical corticosteroids are pregnancy category C drugs and are used cautiously during pregnancy and lactation. There are no significant interactions when these drugs are administered as directed.

Herbal Consideration

Aloe vera is used to prevent infection and promote healing of minor burns (e.g., sunburn) and wounds. When used externally, aloe helps to repair skin tissue and reduce inflammation. Aloe gel is naturally thick when taken from the leaf but quickly becomes watery because of the action of enzymes in the plant. Commercially available preparations have additive thickeners to make the aloe appear like the fresh gel. The agent can be applied directly from the fresh leaf by cutting the leaf in half lengthwise and gently rubbing the inner gel directly onto the skin. Commercially prepared products are applied externally as needed. Rare reports of allergy have been reported with the external use of aloe (DerMarderosian, 2003).

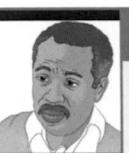

PHARMACOLOGY IN PRACTICE

PHYSIOLOGY

A client is seen at the urgent care facility with inflamed skin resulting from severe insect bites. The primary health care provider has prescribed topical corticosteroid therapy. The nurse caring for this client should know which of the following is the action of a topical corticosteroid?

1. Reduces itching, redness, and swelling
2. Reduces the number of bacteria on the skin
3. Prevents infection in the bite wounds
4. Cleanses the skin thoroughly

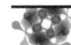 TOPICAL IMMUNOMODULATORS

ACTION AND USES

Immunomodulators reduce inflammation by stopping the production of cytokines. This is different than how steroids reduce inflammation. Additionally, immunomodulators are not systemically absorbed nor act on the collagen in the skin; therefore, they can be used in delicate areas such as the face and neck. The topical preparations are used to treat on a short-term basis:

- flare-ups of atopic eczema
- actinic keratosis (sun or aging spots)
- genital or perianal warts
- some skin cancers

ADVERSE REACTIONS

Reactions are localized to the skin tissues. Burning, itching, and skin redness are the primary local adverse reactions. Clients may develop photosensitivity of the skin and should

stay out of direct sunlight, even when not using the product. Some individuals may experience flu-like symptoms.

CONTRAINDICATIONS, PRECAUTIONS, AND INTERACTIONS

Because of the risk of greater immunosuppression and susceptibility to infection, immunocompromised clients should not use topical immunomodulators. Long-term use is contraindicated because of risk of skin malignancy. Caution is taken when pregnant or lactating since these drugs in topical form have not been studied in these populations of women. Tacrolimus should not be taken by clients allergic to the macrolide antibiotics (erythromycin, clarithromycin, or azithromycin).

Although not an immunomodulator, fluorouracil (an anticancer agent) is used to treat actinic keratosis topically. This agent causes redness and crusting of the skin. The cream should be handled like other chemotherapy agents and disposed of properly (see Chapter 50). Do not allow children, pets, or pregnant women to handle the agent or touch the cream when on the skin.

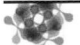 TOPICAL ANTIPSORIATICS

ACTION AND USES

Topical antipsoriatic drugs are drugs used to treat psoriasis (a chronic skin disease manifested by bright red patches covered with silvery scales or plaques) by helping to remove the plaques associated with the disorder.

ADVERSE REACTIONS

These drugs may cause burning, itching, and skin irritation. Anthralin may cause skin irritation, as well as temporary discoloration of the hair and fingernails.

CONTRAINDICATIONS, PRECAUTIONS, AND INTERACTIONS

Topical antipsoriatics are contraindicated in clients with known hypersensitivity to the drugs. Anthralin and calcipotriene, pregnancy category C drugs, are used cautiously during pregnancy and lactation.

TOPICAL ENZYMES

ACTIONS AND USES

A topical enzyme is used to help remove **necrotic** (dead) tissue from:

- Chronic dermal ulcers
- Severely burned areas

These enzymes aid in the removal of dead soft tissues by hastening the reduction of proteins into simpler substances. The process is called **proteolysis** or a proteolytic action. The components of certain types of wounds, namely, necrotic tissues and **purulent exudates** (pus-containing fluid), prevent proper wound healing. Removal of this type of debris by application of a topical enzyme aids in healing. Examples of conditions that may respond to application of a topical enzyme include second- and third-degree burns, pressure ulcers, and ulcers caused by peripheral vascular disease. An example of a topical enzyme is collagenase.

ADVERSE REACTIONS

The application of collagenase may cause mild, transient pain and possibly numbness and dermatitis. There is a low incidence of adverse reactions to collagenase.

CONTRAINDICATIONS, PRECAUTIONS, AND INTERACTIONS

Topical enzyme preparations are contraindicated in clients with known hypersensitivity to the drugs, in wounds in contact with major body cavities or where nerves are exposed, and in fungating neoplastic ulcers. These drugs are pregnancy category B drugs and are used cautiously during pregnancy and lactation. Enzymatic activity may be impaired by certain detergents and heavy metal ions, such as mercury and silver, which are used in some antiseptics. The optimal pH for collagenase is 6–8. Higher or lower pH conditions decrease the enzyme's activity.

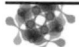 **KERATOLYTICS**

ACTIONS AND USES

A **keratolytic** is a drug that removes excess growth of the epidermis (top layer of skin) in disorders such as warts. These drugs are used to remove:

- Warts
- Calluses
- Corns
- Seborrheic keratoses (benign, variously colored skin growths arising from oil glands of the skin)

Examples of keratolytics include salicylic acid and masoprocol. Some strengths of salicylic acid are available as nonprescription products for the removal of warts on the hands and feet.

ADVERSE REACTIONS

These drugs are usually well tolerated. Occasionally a transient burning sensation, rash, dry skin, scaling, or flu-like syndrome may occur.

CONTRAINDICATIONS, PRECAUTIONS, AND INTERACTIONS

Keratolytics are contraindicated in clients with known hypersensitivity to the drugs and for use on moles, birthmarks, or warts with hair growing from them, on genital or facial warts, on warts on mucous membranes, or on infected skin. Prolonged use of the keratolytics in infants and in clients with diabetes or impaired circulation is contraindicated. Salicylic acid may cause salicylate toxicity with prolonged use. These drugs are pregnancy category C drugs and are used cautiously during pregnancy and lactation.

TOPICAL LOCAL ANESTHETICS

A topical anesthetic may be applied to the skin or mucous membranes.

ACTIONS AND USES

Topical anesthetics temporarily inhibit the conduction of impulses from sensory nerve fibers. These drugs may be used to relieve itching and pain caused by skin conditions, such as minor burns, fungal infections, insect bites, rashes, sunburn, and plant poisoning (e.g., poison ivy). Some are applied to mucous membranes as local anesthetics.

ADVERSE REACTIONS

Occasionally, local irritation, dermatitis, rash, burning, stinging, and tenderness may be noted.

CONTRAINDICATIONS, PRECAUTIONS, AND INTERACTIONS

These drugs are contraindicated in those with a known hypersensitivity to any component of the preparation. Topical anesthetics are used cautiously in clients receiving class I antiarrhythmic drugs such as tocainide and mexiletine, because the toxic effects are additive and potentially synergistic.

LASA ALERT

The following drugs may sound alike; be sure to clarify when they are ordered:

Drug Name	Sounds Like
bacitracin	Bactrim, Bactroban
benzoyl peroxide	benzyl alcohol
Cleocin	bleomycin, Clinoril, Cubicin, Lincocin
clindamycin	clarithromycin, Claritin, vancomycin
Cordran	Cardura, codeine, Cordarone
desoximetasone	Dexamethasone
erythromycin	azithromycin, clarithromycin
fluocinonide	flunisolide, fluocinolone
hydrocortisone	hydrocodone, hydroxychloroquine, hydrochlorothiazide
Kenalog	Ketalar
Lotrimin	Lotrisone
Nizoral	Nasarel, Neoral, Nitrol
Tretinoin	ISOtretinoin, Tenormin, triamcinolone, trientine

Drugs that look alike are noted in the Summary Drug Tables of each chapter.

NURSING PROCESS—STEPS TO BUILDING CLINICAL JUDGMENT
Client Receiving a Topical Drug for a Skin Disorder

ASSESSMENT

Preadministration Assessment

Data gathering suggestions before the initial administration of a topical drug include:

Objective Data

- Description of the skin lesions, such as rough, itchy patches; cracks between the toes; and sore and reddened areas
- Measure and document the areas of involvement, including the size, color, and appearance
- Vital signs (temperature, pulse, respirations, and blood pressure)
- Infection culture results
- Retinoids—result of pregnancy test (within 2 weeks) if female

A specific description is important so that changes indicating worsening or improvement of the lesions can be readily identified. Some agencies may provide a figure on which the lesions can be drawn, indicating the shape and distribution of the involved areas. Other agencies may document the appearance of the lesions using photography.

Figure 52.1 illustrates common types of lesions found on the skin.

Subjective Data

- Client's description of infection, including pain, burning, or itching
- Onset and duration of symptoms
- Allergy history, especially a history of drug allergies
- Remedies attempted before seeking care

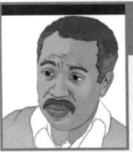

PHARMACOLOGY IN PRACTICE

ASSESSMENT

Which of the following herbal products might a client have used before being seen in the clinic to prevent infection and promote healing of minor burns and wounds?

1. Lemon balm
2. Aloe vera
3. Gentian Violet
4. Ginger

Ongoing Assessment

At the time of each application, inspect the affected area for changes (e.g., signs of improvement or worsening of the infection) and for adverse reactions, such as redness or rash. Contact the primary health care provider, and do not apply the drug if these or other changes are noted or if the client reports new problems, such as itching, pain, or soreness at the site. You may be responsible for checking the treatment sites 1 day or more after application and should inform the primary health care provider of any signs of extreme redness or infection at the application site.

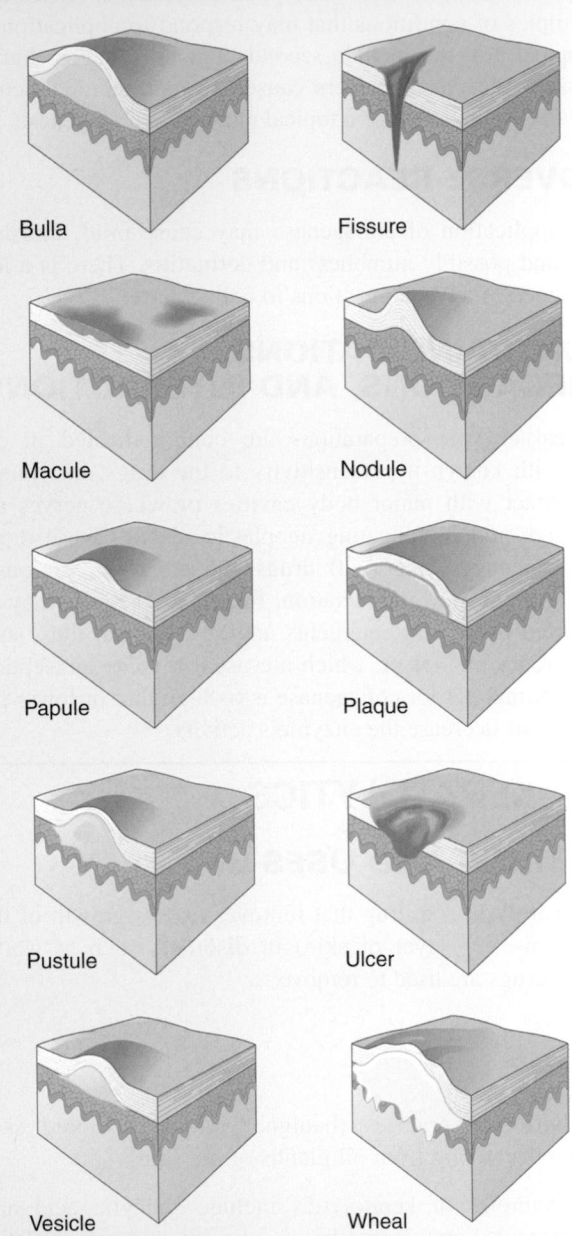

FIGURE 52.1 Types of skin lesions. (From Cohen, B. J. (2003). *Medical terminology* (4th ed.). Lippincott Williams & Wilkins.)

NURSING DIAGNOSES

Drug-specific nursing diagnoses include the following:

- **Altered skin integrity** related to the inflammatory process (increased sensitivity to the drug)
- **Acute pain** related to skin condition or increased sensitivity to drug therapy
- **Infection risk** related to entry of pathogens into affected areas
- **Altered body image perception** related to changes in skin and mucous membranes

Nursing diagnoses related to drug administration are discussed in Chapter 4.

PLANNING

The expected outcomes of the client may include an optimal response to drug therapy, support of client needs related to management of adverse drug reactions, and confidence in an understanding of the application or the reason for use of a topical drug.

IMPLEMENTATION

Promoting an Optimal Response to Therapy

Clients with wound-healing issues using these drugs may be institutionalized in acute rehab care or long-term care facilities. Oftentimes, devices to promote wound healing will be utilized and the application of the drug and device carried out by a nurse in these facilities. When the client is at home, frequently the nurse's involvement will be instructing the client or caregiver in the methods used to apply topical drugs.

Topical Anti-Infectives

Before each application, the area is cleansed with soap and warm water unless the primary health care provider orders a different method. The anti-infective is applied as prescribed (e.g., thin layer or applied liberally) and the area is either covered or left exposed as prescribed.

! NURSING ALERT

Care must be exercised when applying anti-infectives or any topical drug near or around the eyes. Damage to the corneal surface by the topical agent may impact vision.

Topical Antifungal Infection Preparations

When these drugs are applied topically to the skin, the area is inspected at the time of each application for localized skin reactions. When these drugs are administered vaginally, ask the client about any discomfort or other sensations experienced after insertion of the antifungal preparation. Note improvement or deterioration of lesions of the skin, mucous membranes, or vaginal secretions in the client record. It is important to evaluate and chart the client's response to therapy, too.

Topical Antiseptics and Germicides

Antiseptics and germicides are instilled or applied as directed by the primary health care provider or by the label on the product. Topical antiseptics and germicides are not a substitute for clean or aseptic techniques. Occlusive dressings are not to be used after application of these products unless a dressing is specifically ordered by the primary health care provider. Iodine permanently stains clothing and temporarily stains the skin. Care should be taken to remove or protect the client's personal clothing when applying iodine solution or tincture.

Antiseptic and germicidal drugs kept at the client's bedside must be clearly labeled with the name of the product, the strength, and, when applicable, the date of preparation of the solution. Be sure to replace hard-to-read or soiled, stained labels as needed. These solutions are not kept at the bedside of any client who is confused or disoriented, because the solution may be mistaken for water or another beverage.

Topical Corticosteroids

Before drug application, the area is washed with soap and warm water unless the primary health care provider directs otherwise. Topical corticosteroids are usually ordered to be applied sparingly. The primary health care provider also may order the area of application to be covered or left exposed to the air. Some corticosteroids are applied with an occlusive dressing. The drug is applied while the skin is still moist after washing with soap and water and a dressing is applied if ordered by the primary health care provider.

 Lifespan Considerations

Pediatric.

Do not use tight-fitting diapers or pants on a child treated in the diaper area. These types of clothing may work like an occlusive dressing and cause more of the drug to be absorbed into the child's body, resulting in a greater risk for adverse reactions.

Topical Enzymes

Certain types of wounds may require special preparations before applying the topical enzyme. The area is cleansed or prepared and the topical enzyme is applied as directed by the primary health care provider. Often a wound suction device may be applied to promote healing.

Topical Antipsoriatics

Care is exercised so that the product is applied only to the psoriatic lesions and not to surrounding skin. Instruct the client or caregiver to bring signs of excessive irritation to the attention of the primary health care provider.

 Lifespan Considerations

Gerontology.

Adults older than 65 years have more skin-related adverse reactions to calcipotriene (antipsoriatic). Use calcipotriene cautiously in older adults.

Topical Anesthetics

The anesthetic is applied as directed by the primary health care provider. Before the first application, cleanse and dry the area. For subsequent applications, all previous residue of the anesthetic should be removed.

When a topical gel, such as lidocaine viscous, is used for oral anesthesia, instruct the client not to eat food for 1 hour after use, because local anesthesia of the mouth or throat may impair swallowing and increase the possibility of aspiration.

Monitoring and Managing Client Needs

Most topical drugs cause few adverse reactions and, if they occur, discontinuing use of the drug maybe all that is necessary to relieve the symptoms.

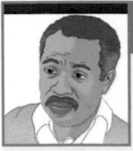

PHARMACOLOGY IN PRACTICE

ADVERSE REACTIONS
A nurse is caring for a client being treated for psoriasis with the topical drug, anthralin. Which of the following adverse reactions should the nurse observe for when a client is using anthralin?

1. Hypothalamic–pituitary–adrenal axis suppression
2. Cushing syndrome
3. Hyperglycemia and glycosuria
4. Temporary discoloration of the fingernails

Altered Skin Integrity

Dry skin increases the risk of skin breakdown from scratching. Advise the client to keep nails short, use warm water with mild soap for cleaning the skin, and rinse and dry the skin thoroughly.

Acute Pain

Occasionally, increased skin sensitivity occurs, causing greater redness, discomfort, and itching. Use cool, wet compresses for rashes or a bath to relieve the itching. Keeping the environment cool may also make the client more comfortable.

Infection Risk

Bath oils, creams, and lotions may be used, if necessary, as long as the primary health care provider is consulted before use. Dry, flaky skin is subject to breakdown and infection. Instruct the client or caregiver to observe the skin for signs of infection (e.g., redness, heat, pus, and elevated temperature and pulse) and immediately report any sign of infection.

Altered Body Image Perception

Some infections such as superficial and deep fungal infections respond slowly to therapy. The lesions caused by the fungal infections may cause the client to feel negatively about the body or a body part. They may be hesitant to go out in public during treatment, embarrassed by the infection when visible to others, see Figure 52.2. In addition, many clients experience anxiety and depression over the fact that therapy must continue for a prolonged period and that results are slow to appear. Depending on the method of treatment, clients may be faced with many problems during therapy and therefore, need time to talk about problems as they arise. Examples of these problems may be the cost of treatment, institutionalization (when required), the failure of treatment adequately to control the infection, and loss of income. It is important to develop a therapeutic nurse–client relationship that conveys an attitude of caring and fosters a sense of trust. Listen to the client's concerns and assist them in accepting the situation as temporary. Encourage the client to verbalize any feelings or anxiety about the effect of the disorder on body image. Explain the disorder and the treatment regimen in terms the client can understand and discuss the need at times for long-term treatment to eradicate the infection. Help the client and the family to understand that therapy must be

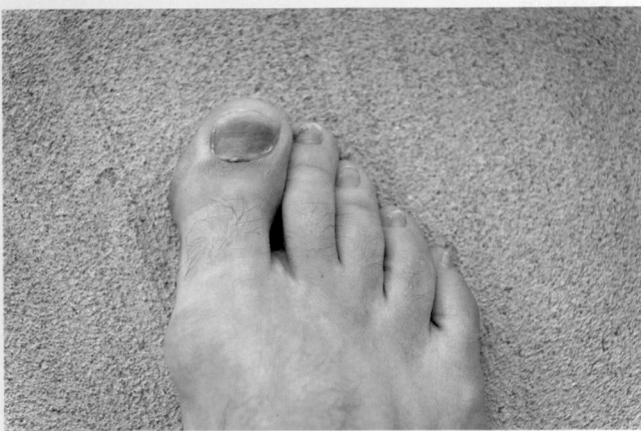

FIGURE 52.2 Clients may hesitate to go out in public places where others may see the infected body part. Nursing support to express feelings is important to keep clients active.

continued until the infection is under control. In some cases, therapy may take weeks or months.

Educating the Client and Family
If the primary health care provider has prescribed or recommended the use of a topical drug, note that most of the adverse effects that occur with topical drugs are a result of applying the drug improperly. Typically, if applied correctly, the drug usually is not systemically absorbed. However, sometimes clients think that if a little is good, then "more is better." Applying more than the amount necessary increases the client's risk for systemic absorption (see Client Teaching for Improved Outcomes: Application of Topical Drugs).

Client Teaching for Improved Outcomes

Application of Topical Drugs
Often, clients are required to apply topical drugs in the home setting. To ensure that the client applies the topical drug properly, *when you teach, make sure your client understands the following:*

✔ Gather all necessary supplies and wash hands before starting.
✔ Wash the area first to remove any debris and old drug.
✔ Pat the area dry with a clean cloth.
✔ Open the container (or tube) and place the lid or cap upside down on the counter or surface.
✔ Use a tongue blade, gloved finger (either with a nonsterile gloved hand or finger cot), cotton swab, or gauze pad to remove the drug, and then apply it to the skin.
✔ Wipe the drug onto the affected area using long smooth strokes in the direction of hair growth.
✔ Apply a thin layer of drug to the area (more is not better).
✔ Use a new tongue blade, applicator, or clean gloved finger to remove additional drug from the container (if necessary).
✔ Apply a clean, dry dressing (if appropriate) over the area.
✔ Wrap items for disposal and perform hand hygiene before engaging in other activities.

General Teaching Points

Wash the hands thoroughly before and after applying the product.

If the enclosed directions state that the product will stain clothing, be sure clothing is moved away from the treated area. If the product stains the skin, wear disposable gloves when applying the drug.

Follow the directions on the label or use as directed by the primary health care provider. Read any enclosed directions for use of the product carefully.

Prepare the area to be treated as recommended by the primary health care provider or as described in the directions supplied with the product.

Do not apply to areas other than those specified by the primary health care provider. Apply the drug as directed (e.g., thin layer or apply liberally).

Follow the directions of the primary health care provider regarding covering the treated area or leaving it exposed to air. The effectiveness of certain drugs depends on keeping the area covered or leaving it open.

Keep the product away from the eyes (unless use in or around the eye has been recommended or prescribed). Do not rub or put the fingers near the eyes unless the hands have been thoroughly washed and all remnants of the drug removed from the fingers. If the product is accidently spilled, sprayed, or splashed in the eye, wash the eye immediately with copious amounts of running water. Contact the primary health care provider immediately if burning, pain, redness, discomfort, or blurred vision persists for more than a few minutes.

The drug may cause momentary stinging or burning when applied.

Many of these preparations require consistent, long-term application for positive results. Incorporate application into daily hygiene routines such as after brushing teeth in the morning.

Discontinue use of the drug and contact the primary health care provider if rash, burning, itching, redness, pain, or other skin problems occur.

Retinoids

Females taking the drug—negative pregnancy test (within the last 2 weeks) and a form of birth control in use if sexually active, or possible activity

Anti-Infectives

Gentamicin may cause photosensitivity. Take measures to protect the skin from ultraviolet rays (e.g., wear protective clothing and use a sunscreen when out in the sun).

Topical clindamycin can be absorbed in sufficient amounts to cause systemic effects. If severe diarrhea, stomach cramps, or bloody stools occur, contact the primary health care provider immediately.

Antifungals

Clean the involved area and apply the ointment or cream to the skin as directed by the primary health care provider.

Do not increase or decrease the amount used or the number of times the ointment or cream should be applied, unless directed to do so by the primary health care provider.

During treatment for a ringworm infection, keep towels and facecloths for bathing separate from those of other family members to avoid the spread of the infection. It is important to keep the affected area clean and dry.

Antivirals

When applying ointment, use a finger cot (a medical supply used to cover one or more fingers when a full glove is unnecessary) or glove to prevent autoinoculation of other body sites.

This product will not prevent transmission of infection to others.

Transient burning, itching, and rash may occur.

Topical Corticosteroids

Apply ointments, creams, or gels sparingly in a light film; rub in gently.

Use only as directed. Do not use bandages, dressings, cosmetics, or other skin products over the treated area unless so directed by the primary health care provider.

Immunomodulators

Protect skin from sun exposure, even when not using the topical agent. Avoid tanning beds.

Use only on skin eruptions and a few weeks' duration, these are not meant for long-term treatment.

Enzyme Preparations

If, for any reason, it becomes necessary to inactivate collagenase, this can be accomplished by washing the area with povidone–iodine.

EVALUATION

- Therapeutic drug response is achieved.
- Adverse reactions are identified, reported to the primary health care provider, and managed successfully with appropriate nursing interventions:
  - Skin remains intact.
  - Client is free of pain.
  - No evidence of infection is seen.
  - Perceptions of body changes are managed successfully.
- Client or family member expresses confidence and demonstrates an understanding of the use and application of the prescribed or recommended drug.

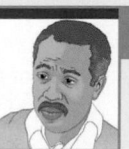

PHARMACOLOGY IN PRACTICE

USING CLINICAL REASONING

You point out to the medication nurse that Mr. Park is taking acyclovir orally. How would you explain the use of this medication in a systemic form rather than a topical form like the cousin's use for HSV?

KEY POINTS

■ A variety of topical drugs exist for many purposes. Retinoids used for acne. Anti-infectives treat bacterial, fungal, and viral infections of the skin. Antiseptic or germicidal solutions help to clean or kill bacteria on the skin or in wounds. Topical corticosteroids and immunomodulators when used reduce the itching, redness, and swelling associated with inflammation.

■ When used as directed, adverse reactions are minor, consisting of mild irritation or discomfort. Some products make the skin more sensitive to sunlight, and the client will need to wear protective clothing or use sunscreen when these products are used.

■ Agents used to treat plaques or wounds can be used alone or in conjunction with wound-healing systems.

■ Important nursing measures include thorough documentation of the site to be treated and instruction of appropriate use of drugs for the skin.

SUMMARY DRUG TABLE
Topical Drugs

Generic Name	Trade Name	Uses	Adverse Reactions	Dosage Ranges
Retinoids				
adapalene *a-DAP-a-leen*	Differin	Acne vulgaris, rosacea	Mild and transient pruritus, burning, stinging, erythema	Apply at bedtime
alitretinoin *a-li-TRET-i-noyn*	Panretin	Kaposi sarcoma skin lesions	Pruritus, burning, stinging, erythema	Apply twice daily to affected area
tazarotene *taz-AR-oh-teen*	Arazlo, Fabior, Tazorac	Acne vulgaris, psoriasis	Pruritus, burning, stinging, erythema, desquamation	Apply daily to affected area
tretinoin *TRET-i-noyn*	Altreno, Renova, Retin-A	Acne vulgaris, wrinkle remover (Renova)	Erythema, stinging, hypopigmentation	Apply at bedtime
trifarotene *trye-FAR-oh-teen*	Aklief	Acne vulgaris	Erythema, pruritus	Apply at bedtime
Antibiotic Drugs				
azelaic acid *a-zeh-LAY-ik*	Azelex, Finacea	Acne vulgaris, rosacea	Mild and transient pruritus, burning, stinging, erythema	Apply BID
bacitracin *basi-TRAY-sin*		Relief of skin infections, to help prevent infections in minor cuts and burns	Rare; occasionally redness, burning, pruritus, stinging	Apply daily or TID
benzoyl peroxide *BEN-zoe-il peer-OKS-ide*	Various brand names	Mild to moderate acne vulgaris and oily skin	Excessive drying, stinging, peeling, erythema, possible edema, allergic dermatitis	Apply daily or BID
clindamycin *klin-da-MYE-sin*	Cleocin T, ClindaMax, Clindets, Clindagel	Acne vulgaris, bacterial vaginitis	Dryness, erythema, burning, itching, peeling, oily skin, diarrhea, bloody diarrhea, abdominal pain, colitis	Apply a thin film daily (Clindagel) or BID to affected area
erythromycin *er-ith-roe-MYE-sin*	Erygel	Adjuvant for Acne vulgaris	Dryness, erythema, burning, itching, peeling	Apply daily or BID
gentamicin *jen-ta-MYE-sin*		Relief of primary and secondary skin infections	Mild and transient pruritus, burning, stinging, erythema, photosensitivity	Apply TID or QID to affected area
mafenide *MA-fe-nide*	Sulfamylon	Second- and third-degree burns	Pain or burning sensation, rash, itching, facial edema	Apply to burned area 1–2 times/day

Generic Name	Trade Name	Uses	Adverse Reactions	Dosage Ranges
metroNIDAZOLE *met-roe-NYE-da-zole*	MetroGel, MetroLotion, Noritate	Rosacea, bacterial vaginitis	Watery (tearing) eyes, redness, mild dryness, burning, skin irritation, nausea, tingling/numbness of extremities	Apply a thin film daily or BID to affected areas
mupirocin *myoo-PEER-oh-sin*		Impetigo infections caused by *Staphylococcus aureus* and *Streptococcus pyogenes,* used on facial burns Nasal: eradication of methicillin-resistant *S. aureus* (MRSA) as part of an infection control program to reduce the risk of institutional outbreaks of MRSA	Ointment: burning, stinging, pain, itching, rash, nausea, erythema, dry skin Cream: headache, rash, nausea, abdominal pain, burning at application site, dermatitis Nasal: headache, rhinitis, respiratory disorders (e.g., pharyngitis), taste perversion, burning, stinging, cough	Ointment: apply TID for 3–5 days Cream: apply TID for 10 days Nasal: divide the single-use tube between nostrils and apply BID for 5 days
ozenoxacin *oz-en-OX-a-sin*	Xepi	Impetigo caused by *Staphylococcus* or *Streptococcus*	Dermatitis rash	Apply a thin film daily or BID to affected areas
retapamulin *re-te-PAM-ue-lin*	Altabax	Impetigo caused by *Staphylococcus* or *Streptococcus*	Headache, pruritus	Apply a thin film daily or BID to affected areas
silver sulfadiazine *SIL-ver sul-fa-DYE-a-zeen*	Silvadene, Thermazene, SSD (cream)	Second- and third-degree burns	Leukopenia, skin necrosis, skin discoloration, burning sensation	Apply to burned area 1–2 times/day
sulfacetamide *sul fa SEE ta mide*	Klaron, Ovace	Acne vulgaris, facial bacterial infections		Apply BID
Antifungal Drugs				
butenafine *byoo-TEN-a-feen*	Mentax, Lotrimin Ultra	Dermatologic infections, tinea versicolor, tinea corporis (ringworm), tinea cruris (jock itch)	Burning, stinging, itching, worsening of the condition, contact dermatitis, erythema, irritation	Apply daily or BID for 2–4 weeks
ciclopirox *sye-kloe-PEER-oks*	Ciclodan, Loprox, Penlac	Loprox, cream and suspension: tinea pedis (athlete's foot), tinea cruris, tinea corporis, cutaneous candidiasis Gel: interdigital tinea pedis and tinea corporis, seborrheic dermatitis of the scalp Penlac: mild to moderate onychomycosis of fingernails and toenails	Cream: pruritus at the application site, worsening of clinical signs and symptoms, burning Loprox gel: burning sensation on application, contact dermatitis, pruritus, dry skin, acne, rash, alopecia, eye pain, facial edema Loprox shampoo: increased itching, burning, erythema, rash, headache Penlac: periungual erythema, irritation, ingrown toenail, burning of the skin	Apply to affected areas daily or BID Shampoo: see directions Penlac: apply daily preferably at bedtime or 8 hours before washing

Continued

SUMMARY DRUG TABLE (continued)
Topical Drugs

Generic Name	Trade Name	Uses	Adverse Reactions	Dosage Ranges
Antifungal Drugs (continued)				
clotrimazole *kloe-TRIM-a-zole*	Cruex, Lotrimin AF, Desenex	Tinea pedis, tinea cruris, and other skin infections caused by ringworm	Burning, itching, erythema, peeling, edema, general skin irritation	Apply thin layer to affected areas BID for 2–4 weeks
econazole *e-KONE-a-zole*	Ecoza	Tinea pedis, tinea cruris, tinea corporis, tinea versicolor, cutaneous candidiasis	Local burning, itching, stinging, erythema, pruritic rash	Apply to affected areas daily or BID
efinaconazole *ef'-in-a-KON-a-zole*	Jublia	Onychomycosis caused by *Trichophyton*	Local pain, irritation or rash	Apply once daily to affected area for 48 weeks
gentian violet *JEN-shun VYE-oh-let*		External treatment of abrasions, minor cuts, surface injuries, superficial fungal infections of the skin	Local irritation or sensitivity reactions	Apply locally BID Do not bandage
ketoconazole *kee-toe-KOE-na-zole*	Nizoral	Cream: tinea cruris, tinea corporis, tinea versicolor Shampoo: reduction of scaling caused by dandruff	Cream: severe itching, pruritus, stinging Shampoo: increase in hair loss, abnormal hair texture, scalp pustules, mild dryness of the skin, itching, oiliness/dryness of the hair	Cream: apply daily to affected areas for 2–6 weeks Shampoo: twice a week for 4 weeks with at least 3 days between each shampoo
luliconazole *loo-li-KON-a-zole*	Luzu	Tinea pedis, tinea cruris, tinea corporis	Local irritation, burning, cellulitis	Thinly cover affected area daily for 10 days
miconazole *mi-KON-a-zole*	Tetterine, Micatin, Monistat-Derm, Fungoid Tincture	Tinea pedis, tinea cruris, tinea corporis, cutaneous candidiasis	Local irritation, burning, maceration, allergic contact dermatitis	Cover affected areas BID
naftifine *NAF-ti-feen*	Naftin	Topical treatment of tinea pedis, tinea cruris, tinea corporis	Burning, stinging, erythema, itching, local irritation, rash, tenderness	Apply BID for 4 weeks
nystatin *nye-STAT-in*		Mycotic infections caused by *Candida albicans* and other *Candida* species	Virtually nontoxic and nonsensitizing; well tolerated by all age groups, even with prolonged administration; if irritation occurs, discontinue use	Apply BID or TID until healing is complete
oxiconazole *oks-i-KON-a-zole*	Oxistat	Tinea pedis, tinea cruris, tinea corporis	Pruritus, burning, stinging, irritation, contact dermatitis, scaling, tingling	Apply daily or BID for 1 months
sertaconazole *ser-ta-KON-na-zole*	Ertaczo	Tinea pedis	Pruritus, burning, stinging, irritation, contact dermatitis, scaling, tingling	Apply daily or BID for 1 months
sulconazole *sul-KON-a-zole*	Exelderm	Same as oxiconazole	Pruritus, burning, stinging, irritation	Apply daily or BID for 3–6 weeks
terbinafine *TER-bin-a-feen*	Lamisil AT	Same as oxiconazole	Same as oxiconazole	Apply BID until infection clears (1–4 weeks)
tolnaftate *tole-NAF-tate*	Tinactin	Same as oxiconazole	Same as oxiconazole	Apply BID for 2–3 weeks (4–6 weeks may be needed)

Generic Name	Trade Name	Uses	Adverse Reactions	Dosage Ranges
tavaborole *ta-va-BOR-ole*	Kerydin	Onychomycosis caused by *Trichophyton*	Local pain, irritation or rash	Apply once daily to affected area for 48 weeks
Topical Antivirals				
acyclovir *ay-SYE-kloe-veer*	Zovirax	HSV infections, varicella-zoster	Ointment: mild pain with transient burning/stinging Cream: pruritus, rash, vulvitis, edema or pain at application site	Ointment: apply to all lesions q3hr 6 times daily for 7 days Cream: apply 5 times daily for 4 days
docosanol *doe-KOE-san-ole*	Abreva	HSV-1 and -2 (cold sores)	Headache, skin irritation	Apply to lesions 5 times daily
penciclovir *pen-SYE-kloe-veer*	Denavir	HSV-1 and -2 (cold sores)	Headache, taste perversion	Apply q2hr for 4 days during waking hours
Antiseptics and Germicides				
chlorhexidine *klor-HEKS-i-deen*	BactoShield 2, Betasept, Exidine-2 Scrub, Hibiclens	Surgical scrub, skin cleanser, preoperative skin preparation, skin wound cleanser, preoperative showering and bathing	Irritation, dermatitis, photosensitivity (rare), deafness, mild sensitivity reactions	Varies, depending on administration
oxychlorosene *oks-i-KLOR-oh-seen*		Antiseptic for wound infections, remove necrotic tissue, counteract odors, UTI bladder irrigation	Pain, irritation if used in eye or bladder	Varies, depending on administration
povidone–iodine *POE-vi-done*	Acu-Dyne, Aerodine, Betadine	Microbicidal against bacteria, fungi, viruses, spores, protozoa, yeasts	Dermatitis, irritation, burning, sensitivity reactions	Varies, depending on administration
sodium hypochlorite *SOW-dee-um hye-poe-KLOR-ite*		Antiseptic against bacteria, fungi, viruses, spores, protozoa, yeasts; deodorizing properties	Chemical reaction or burn	Varies, depending on administration
triclosan *TRY-kloe-san*		Skin cleanser and degermer	None significant	Apply 5 mL on hands or face and rub thoroughly for 30 seconds, rinse thoroughly, pat dry
Corticosteroids, Topical				
alclometasone *al-kloe-MET-a-sone*		Treatment of various allergic/immunologic skin problems	Allergic contact dermatitis, burning, dryness, edema, irritation	Apply 1–6 times daily according to directions
amcinonide *am-SIN-oh-nide*		Same as alclometasone	Same as alclometasone	Apply 1–6 times daily according to directions
betamethasone *bay-ta-METH-a-sone*	Diprolene, Diprosone, Luxiq, Sernivo	Same as alclometasone	Same as alclometasone	Apply 1–4 times daily according to directions
desoximetasone *des-oks-i-MET-a-sone*	Topicort	Same as alclometasone	Same as alclometasone	Apply 1–4 times daily according to directions
diflorasone *dye-FLOR-a-sone*	Psorcon	Same as alclometasone	Same as alclometasone	Apply 1–4 times daily according to directions
fluocinolone *floo-oh-SIN-oh-lone*	Capex, Synalar	Same as alclometasone	Same as alclometasone	Apply 1–4 times daily according to directions
fluocinonide *floo-oh-SIN-oh-nide*	Vanos	Same as alclometasone	Same as alclometasone	Apply 1–4 times daily according to directions

Continued

SUMMARY DRUG TABLE (continued)
Topical Drugs

Generic Name	Trade Name	Uses	Adverse Reactions	Dosage Ranges
Corticosteroids, Topical (continued)				
flurandrenolide *flure-an-DREN-oh-lide*	Cordran, Nolix	Same as alclometasone	Same as alclometasone	Apply 1–4 times daily according to directions
hydrocortisone *hye-droe-KOR-ti-sone*	Bactine, Cort-Dome, Hytone, Locoid, Pandel	Same as alclometasone	Same as alclometasone	Apply 1–4 times daily according to directions
triamcinolone *trye-am-SIN-oh-lone*	Kenalog, Trianex, Triaderm	Same as alclometasone	Same as alclometasone	Apply 1–4 times daily according to directions
Topical Immunomodulators				
imiquimod *i-mi-KWI-mod*	Aldara, Zyclara	Keratitis, external genitalia and perianal warts	Local skin irritation, itching, excoriation, flaking	Apply externally 3 times weekly
ingenol mebutate *IN-je-nol MEB-u-tate*	Picato	Keratitis	Local skin irritation, itching, excoriation, flaking	Apply daily for 3 days
pimecrolimus *pim-e-KROE-li-mus*	Elidel	Atopic dermatitis	Local skin irritation, burning, itching, excoriation, flaking	Apply twice daily until symptoms are gone
tacrolimus *ta-KROE-li-mus*		Atopic dermatitis	Local skin irritation, itching, excoriation, flaking	Apply twice daily until symptoms are gone
Antipsoriatic Drugs				
anthralin *AN-thra-lin*	Drithocreme, Zithranol	Psoriasis	Few; transient irritation of normal skin or uninvolved skin	Apply daily
calcipotriene *kal-si-POE-try-een*	Dovonex, Sorilux	Psoriasis	Burning, itching, skin irritation, erythema, dry skin, peeling, rash, worsening of psoriasis, dermatitis, hyperpigmentation	Apply BID
selenium sulfide *se-LEE-nee-um*	Exsel, Head and Shoulders Intensive Treatment Dandruff Shampoo, Selsun Blue	Treatment of dandruff, seborrheic dermatitis of the scalp, and tinea versicolor	Skin irritation, greater than normal hair loss, hair discoloration, oiliness or dryness of hair	Massage 5–10 mL into wet scalp and allow to remain on scalp for 2–3 minutes, rinse
Enzyme Preparations				
collagenase *KOL-la-je-nase*	Santyl	For débriding chronic dermal ulcers and severely burned areas	Well tolerated and nonirritating; transient burning sensation may occur	Apply daily according to directions
Keratolytic Drugs				
masoprocol *mah-soe'-proe-koll*	Actinex	Actinic keratoses	Erythema, flaking, dryness, itching, edema, burning, soreness, bleeding, crusting, skin roughness	Apply BID
salicylic acid *sal-i-SIL-ik AS-id*	DuoFilm, Dr. Scholl's Wart Remover, Fostex, Fung-O, Mosco, Panscol	Aids in the removal of excessive keratin in hyperkeratotic skin disorders, including warts, psoriasis, calluses, and corns	Local irritation	Apply as directed in individual product labeling
Local Anesthetics				
benzocaine *BEN-zoe-kane*	Lanacane	Topical anesthesia in local skin disorders	Rare; hypersensitivity, local burning, stinging, tenderness, sloughing	Apply to affected area

Generic Name	Trade Name	Uses	Adverse Reactions	Dosage Ranges
Local Anesthetics (continued)				
dibucaine *DYE-byoo-kane*	Nupercainal	Topical anesthesia in local skin disorders, local anesthesia of accessible mucous membranes	Same as benzocaine	Topical: apply to affected area as needed Mucous membranes: dosage varies and depends on the area to be anesthetized
lidocaine *LYE-doe-kane*	DentiPatch, ELA-Max, Lidocaine Viscous, Xylocaine	Same as dibucaine	Same as benzocaine	Topical: apply to affected area as needed Mucous membranes: dosage varies and depends on the area to be anesthetized
butamben picrate *byoo'-tam-ben*		Topical anesthesia	Rare; local burning, stinging, tenderness	Apply to affected area
Misc. Agents				
minoxidil *mi-NOKS-i-dil*	Rogaine	Alopecia	Edema, blood pressure changes	Apply to scalp ½ capful twice daily
crisaborole *kris-a-BOR-ole*	Eucrisa	Atopic dermatitis— noncorticosteroid	Hypersensitivity, itching at site of application	Apply to affected area twice daily

CHAPTER REVIEW

Know Your Drugs

Clients sometimes know a medication by the brand (or trade) name and not the generic name. To help you recognize both names, match the brand name with the generic name of the same medication.

Generic Name	Brand Name
1. acyclovir	A. Desenex
2. chlorhexidine	B. Hibiclens
3. clotrimazole	C. Eucrisa
4. crisaborole	D. Zovirax

Prepare for the NCLEX

RECALL THE FACTS

1. Which is the outermost layer of skin tissue?
   1. Dermis
   2. Epidermis
   3. Subcutaneous
   4. Tendon
2. What reaction could occur with prolonged use of the topical antibiotics?
   1. Water intoxication
   2. Superficial superinfection
   3. Outbreak of eczema
   4. Cellulitis
3. Which of the following drugs has a proteolytic action?
   1. Amcinonide
   2. Collagenase
   3. Bacitracin
   4. Ciclopirox

4. A keratolytic agent would be safe to use on which of the following skin conditions?
   1. Moles
   2. Birthmarks
   3. Facial warts
   4. Calluses
5. What type of action do the corticosteroids have when used topically?
   1. Bactericidal activity
   2. Anti-inflammatory activity
   3. Antifungal activity
   4. Antiviral activity
6. What reaction could happen when a topical drug is covered with a heating pad?
   1. Increased drug absorption
   2. Slower wound healing
   3. Decreased drug absorption
   4. Bruising of surrounding area

ANALYZE THE FACTS

7. *The nurse is about to débride and cleanse an ulcerated wound. How should the nurse determine if pain medication is needed before starting the procedure?
   1. Wait for the client to ask for medication
   2. Check facial grimace when removing dressing
   3. Use the 0–10 scale for pain assessment
   4. Review medication administration record for past medication

8. *The nurse is gathering supplies to change the dressing of a client's central line (IV). Which of the following drugs is best suited to be used as a topical antiseptic?
   1. Amphotericin B
   2. Benzocaine
   3. Iodine
   4. Povidone–iodine

ALTERNATE-FORMAT QUESTIONS

9. Name the type of skin lesion illustrated below.

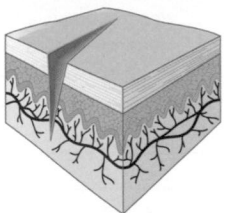

10. Dakin solution is ordered for home irrigation of a wound. The primary health care provider orders a 3:1 solution (water:Dakin) to be mixed with distilled water. How much water should be added to 10 mL of the Dakin solution?

To check your answers, see Appendix F.

WANT TO KNOW MORE? A wide variety of resources are available to enhance your learning and understanding of this chapter.
- Visit the**Point** for resources such as:
  - NCLEX-Style Student Review Questions
  - Journal Articles
  - Dosage Calculations
  - Drug Monographs
  - Watch and Learn Video
  - Concepts in Action Animations
- The *Study Guide to Accompany Introductory Clinical Pharmacology*, 12th edition, sold separately, will help you review and apply essential content.
- ✓*PrepU* is available to help students prepare for the NCLEX-PN examination.

Otic and Ophthalmic Preparations

Key Terms

cerumen ear wax

cycloplegia paralysis of the ciliary muscle, resulting in an inability to focus the eye

intraocular pressure (IOP) pressure within the eye

miosis constriction of the pupil of the eye

mydriasis dilation of the pupil

ophthalmic pertaining to the eye

otic pertaining to the ear, means *auditory* in Latin

otitis media infection of the middle ear

punctal occlusion procedure used when instilling eye drops to keep medication bathing eye and not immediately entering tear duct

superinfection overgrowth of bacterial or fungal microorganisms not affected by the antibiotic being administered

Learning Objectives

On completion of this chapter, the student will:

1. Explain the general actions, uses, adverse reactions, contraindications, precautions, and interactions of otic and ophthalmic preparations.
2. Distinguish important preadministration and ongoing assessment activities the nurse should perform on a client receiving otic and ophthalmic preparations.
3. List nursing diagnoses particular to a client taking an otic or ophthalmic preparation.
4. Examine ways to promote an optimal response to therapy, how to administer the preparations, and important points to keep in mind when educating clients about the use of otic or ophthalmic preparations.

 Drug Classes

Otic preparations	Ophthalmic preparations

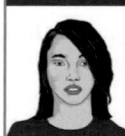 **PHARMACOLOGY IN PRACTICE**

Janna Wong, a 16-year-old high school student, recently switched from eyeglasses to contact lenses. She is experiencing minor eye irritation. In this chapter, you learn how to teach Janna the correct way to use her eye drops.

This chapter provides information on drugs that are topically applied to the ears and eyes. Because the ears and eyes help us to interpret our environment, any disease or injury that has the potential for partial or total loss of function of these organs should be treated.

OTIC PREPARATIONS

The term "**otic**" means *auditory* in Latin. It is important to remember the connection between the words "otic" and "ear," because harm can be done when these preparations are swallowed or administered into the eye.

Disorders of the ear are categorized according to the part of the ear affected: the outer, the middle, or the inner ear (Fig. 53.1). The disorders of the outer and middle ear are discussed in this chapter. **Otitis media**, by far the most common disorder of the middle ear, it is an accumulation of fluid in the middle ear accompanied by symptoms of intense local or systemic infection. The most common causes are viruses and bacteria.

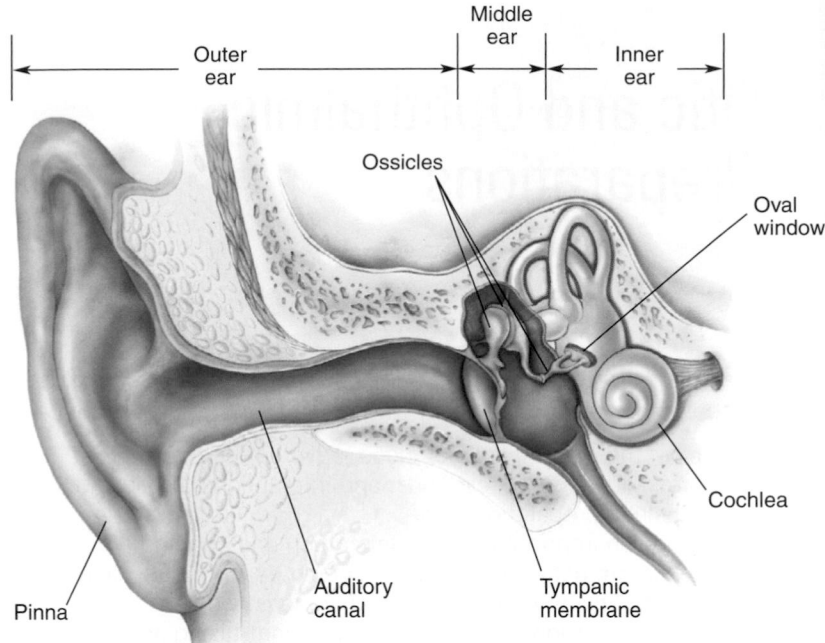

Symptoms include pain in the ear, drainage of fluid from the ear canal, and hearing loss. Other symptoms that may be present if the disorder becomes systemic include fever, irritability, headache, and anorexia.

ACTIONS

Otic preparations can be divided into three categories: (1) antibiotics, (2) corticosteroids, and (3) miscellaneous preparations. The miscellaneous preparations usually contain one or more of the following ingredients:

- Benzocaine—a local anesthetic used to temporarily relieve pain
- Phenylephrine—a vasoconstrictor decongestant
- Hydrocortisone/desonide—corticosteroid for anti-inflammatory and antipruritic effects
- Glycerin—an emollient and a solvent
- Antipyrine—an analgesic
- Acetic acid, boric acid, benzalkonium, aluminum (Burow Solution), benzethonium—provide antifungal or antibacterial action
- Carbamide peroxide/triethanolamine—aids in removing **cerumen** (yellowish or brownish ear wax) by softening and breaking up the wax

Examples of otic preparations are given in the Summary Drug Table: Selected Otic Preparations.

USES

Otic preparations are instilled in the external auditory canal and may be used to:

- Treat infection and inflammation
- Relieve pain
- Aid in the removal of cerumen

When the client has an inner ear infection, systemic antibiotic therapy is indicated.

ADVERSE REACTIONS

When otic drugs are applied topically, the amount of drug that enters the systemic circulation usually is not sufficient to produce adverse reactions. Local adverse reactions that may occur include:

- Ear irritation
- Itching
- Burning

Prolonged use of otic preparations containing an antibiotic, such as ciprofloxacin, may result in a **superinfection** (an overgrowth of bacterial or fungal microorganisms not affected by the antibiotic being administered).

LASA ALERT	
The following drugs may sound alike; be sure to clarify when they are ordered:	
Drug Name	*Sounds Like*
Cetraxal	cefTRIAXone
ciprofloxacin	Cephalexin
fluocinolone	fluocinonide
Drugs that look alike are noted in the Summary Drug Tables of each chapter.	

CONTRAINDICATIONS, PRECAUTIONS, AND INTERACTIONS

Otic drugs are contraindicated in clients with a known hypersensitivity to the drugs. The otic drugs are used with caution during pregnancy and lactation. The pregnancy category of most of these drugs is unknown when they are used as otic drugs. Drugs to remove cerumen are not used if ear drainage, discharge, pain, or irritation is present; if the eardrum is perforated; or after ear surgery. Otic drugs are available in dropper bottles and can be dangerous if ingested. Therefore, store these drugs safely out of the reach of children and pets.

If an allergy is suspected, the drug is not administered. No significant interactions have been reported with the use of otic preparations.

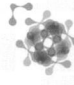

NURSING PROCESS: STEPS TO BUILDING CLINICAL JUDGMENT
Client Receiving an Otic Preparation

ASSESSMENT

Preadministration Assessment
When a client is seen in the clinic setting, here are the data gathering suggestions before administering an otic drug which include:
Objective data

- Examining the outer structures of the ear (i.e., the earlobe and the skin around the ear)
- Observe for the presence of any drainage or visible wax

Subjective data

- Complaints of ear pain, tinnitus, or changes in hearing
- Medication history, specifically looking at drugs taken systemically that may cause ototoxicity

Before prescribing an otic preparation, the primary health care provider examines the ear's external and internal structures. Perforated eardrums may be a contraindication to some of the otic preparations. Check with the primary health care provider before administering an otic preparation to a client with a perforated eardrum.

Ongoing Assessment
Assess the client's response to therapy. For example, a decrease in pain or inflammation should occur. Examine and palpate the outer ear and ear canal for any local redness or irritation that may indicate sensitivity to the drug.

Lifespan Considerations

Pediatric
When assessing the infant, look for ear pulling, grabbing, or tugging. Infants cannot tell you about pain, this behavior may be an indicator the child's ear hurts. Since infants do pull their ears for all kinds of reasons or for no reason at all, validate this behavior with the parent or caregiver. Additional signs include a change in behavior, crying, fussiness or irritability, or a fever.

NURSING DIAGNOSES

Drug-specific nursing diagnoses include the following:

- **Infection risk** (superinfection) related to prolonged use of the anti-infective otic drug
- **Anxiety** related to ear pain or discomfort, changes in hearing, diagnosis, or other factors

Nursing diagnoses related to drug administration are discussed in Chapter 4.

PLANNING
The expected outcomes of the client depend on the reason for administering the drug and may include an optimal response to the drug, support of client needs related to the management of adverse reactions, a reduction in anxiety, and confidence in understanding the application and use of an otic preparation.

IMPLEMENTATION

Promoting an Optimal Response to Therapy
Ear disorders may result in symptoms such as pain, a feeling of fullness in the ear, tinnitus, dizziness, or a change in hearing. Some of these same sensations may be felt by the client from the solutions used for treatment. Before instilling an otic solution, tell the client that a feeling of fullness may be felt in the ear and that hearing in the treated ear may be impaired while the solution remains in the ear canal.

Before instillation of otic preparations, hold the container in your hand for a few minutes to warm it to body temperature. Cold and too warm (above body temperature) preparations may cause dizziness or other sensations after being instilled into the ear.

! NURSING ALERT
Only preparations labeled as "otic" are instilled in the ear. Check the label of the preparation carefully for the name of the drug and a statement indicating that the preparation is for *otic use*.

Typically, the nurse will teach the client or caregiver the method to instill ear drops. To keep solutions in the ear when instilling ear drops, have the client lie on their side with the affected ear up toward the ceiling. If the client wishes to remain in an upright position, tilt the head toward the untreated side with the ear toward the ceiling. When administering an otic drug, the ear canal should be straightened. To achieve this in adults and children age 3 years and older, gently pull up and back the cartilaginous portion of the outer ear. Be particularly gentle, because some conditions make the ear canal very sensitive. Drop the solution into the ear canal; never insert the dropper or applicator tip into the ear canal.

Pediatric

In children younger than 3 years of age, the ear canal is straighter and needs less manipulation. Gently pull the outer ear down (instead of up) and back (Fig. 53.2).

The client is kept lying on the untreated side after the medication is instilled for approximately 5 minutes to facilitate the penetration of the drops into the ear canal. If medication is needed in the other ear, it is best to wait at least 10 minutes after instillation of the first ear drops before administering drops to the other ear. Once the client is upright, the solution running out of the ear may be gently removed with gauze. A piece of cotton can be loosely inserted into the ear canal to prevent the medication from flowing out. The cotton is not inserted too deeply because it may cause increased pressure within the ear canal.

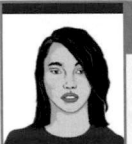

PHARMACOLOGY IN PRACTICE

INTERVENTIONS

Prior to instillation of an otic anti-infective preparation at home, the nurse teaches the client to hold the container in the hand for a few minutes. What is the reason for doing this?

1. To observe the number of drops in the applicator
2. To confirm if the drug was kept refrigerated
3. To observe if the drug is in suspension form
4. To prevent dizziness after being instilled

Cerumen is a natural product of the ear and is produced by modified sweat glands in the auditory canal. Ear wax is typically yellow to brown in color. If it is black, consider a fungal infection may be present and should be evaluated. Sometimes too much cerumen is produced, particularly in older adults. Drugs that loosen cerumen, such as Cerumenex, work by softening the dried ear wax inside the ear canal. Cerumenex is available by prescription and is not allowed to stay in the ear canal for more than 30 minutes before irrigation. When Cerumenex is administered, the ear canal is filled with the solution and a cotton plug is inserted. The drug is allowed to remain in the ear for 15–30 minutes, and then the ear is flushed with warm water using a soft rubber bulb ear syringe.

Gerontology

Cerumen is thicker in the older adult, making the accumulation of excess wax more likely. When hearing loss is suspected in the older adult, mentally impaired, or debilitated client, the ear should be checked for excess cerumen.

Monitoring and Managing Client Needs

Infection Risk

When using the otic antibiotics there is a danger of a superinfection, or another infection on top of the original one, from prolonged use of the drug (see Chapter 9 for a discussion of superinfection). If after administering the drops as directed for 1 week, and the infection does not improve, the primary health care provider should be notified.

Anxiety

Clients with an ear disorder or injury usually have great concern over the effect the problem will have on their hearing. Reassure the client that every effort is being made to treat the disorder and relieve the symptoms.

Pediatric

Because some children are prone to recurrent attacks of acute otitis media, parents should be taught to identify early signs and symptoms of otitis media and seek medical attention when their child exhibits these symptoms.

Educating the Client and Family

Provide the client or a family member written instructions or a demonstration of the installation technique of an otic preparation.

The following information may be given to the client when an ear ointment or solution is prescribed:

- Wash the hands thoroughly before cleansing the area around the ear (when necessary) and instilling ear drops or ointment.
- If the solution is cool or cold, warm it to room temperature by holding the solution in the hand for 1–2 minutes before administering.
- Instill the prescribed number of drops in the ear. Do not put the applicator or dropper tip in the ear or allow the tip to become contaminated from the fingers or other sources.

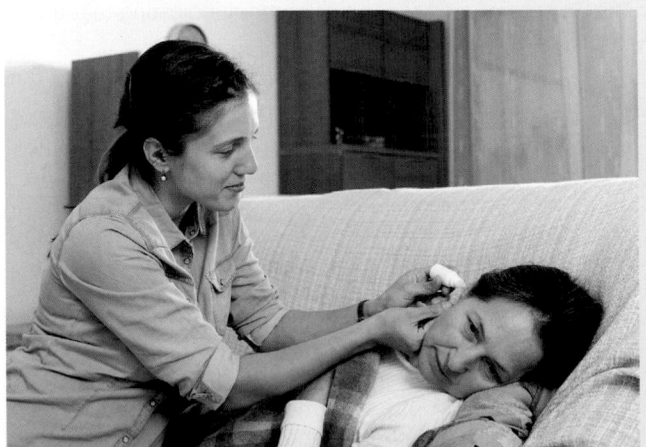

FIGURE 53.2 Instilling ear drops. With the affected ear up, the ear lobe is pulled to better visualize the auditory canal.

- Immediately after use, replace the cap or dropper and refrigerate the solution if so stated on the label.
- If the drops are in a suspension form, shake the container well for 10 seconds before using.
- Keep the head tilted or lie on the untreated side for approximately 5 minutes to allow the solution to remain in contact with the ear. Excess solution and solution running out of the ear can be wiped off with a tissue.
- Do not insert anything into the ear canal before or after applying the prescribed drug unless advised to do so by the primary health care provider. At times, a soft cotton plug may be inserted into the affected ear.
- Complete a full course of treatment with the prescribed drug to achieve satisfactory results.
- Do not use nonprescription ear products during or after treatment unless such use has been approved by the primary health care provider.
- Remember that temporary changes in hearing or a feeling of fullness in the ear may occur for a short time after the drug has been instilled.
- Notify the primary health care provider if symptoms do not improve or become worse.

Drugs Used to Remove Cerumen
- Do not put anything in the ear canal such as a Q-tip.
- Do not use a drug to remove cerumen if ear drainage, discharge, pain, or irritation occurs.
- Do not use for more than 4 days. If excessive cerumen remains, consult the primary health care provider.

- Any wax remaining after the treatment may be removed by gently flushing the ear with warm water using a soft rubber bulb ear syringe.
- If dizziness occurs, consult the primary health care provider.

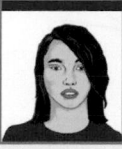

PHARMACOLOGY IN PRACTICE

MANAGING NEEDS

A client needs to administer otic preparations in both of the ears, how long should they wait to place drops in the second ear?
1. At least 30 seconds
2. At least 1 minutes
3. At least 5 minutes
4. At least 3 minutes

EVALUATION
- Therapeutic effect is achieved.
- Adverse reactions are identified, reported to the primary health care provider, and managed successfully with appropriate nursing interventions:
  - No evidence of infection is seen.
  - Anxiety is managed successfully.
- Client and family express confidence and demonstrate an understanding of the drug regimen.

OPHTHALMIC PREPARATIONS

Various types of preparations are used for treating **ophthalmic** (eye) disorders such as glaucoma, to lower the IOP (the pressure within the eye), macular degeneration, and to treat bacterial or viral infections of the eye, inflammatory conditions, and symptoms of allergy related to the eye.

GLAUCOMA

Glaucoma is a condition of the eye in which there is an increase in the IOP, causing progressive atrophy of the optic nerve with deterioration of vision and, if untreated, blindness. This condition is typically treated with eye drops and surgical procedures are held off until the medications no longer work.

The eye's lens, iris, and cornea are continuously bathed and nourished by a fluid called *aqueous humor*. As aqueous humor is produced, excess fluid normally flows out through a complex network of tissue called the *canal of Schlemm*. An angle is formed where the canal of Schlemm and iris meet. This forms a filtration angle that maintains the normal

pressure within the eye by allowing excess aqueous humor to leave the anterior chamber of the eye (Fig. 53.3).

There are two types of glaucoma: angle-closure glaucoma and open-angle, or chronic, glaucoma. Open-angle glaucoma is shown in the top portion of Figure 53.4. The illustration shows how the angle where aqueous humor drains is normal but does not function properly and excess

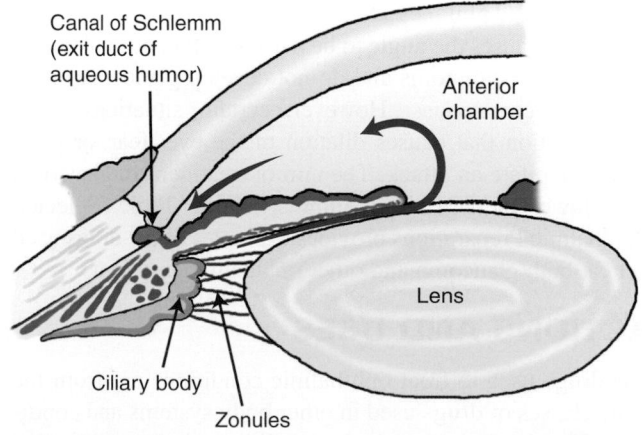

FIGURE 53.3 Flow of aqueous humor in the normal eye.

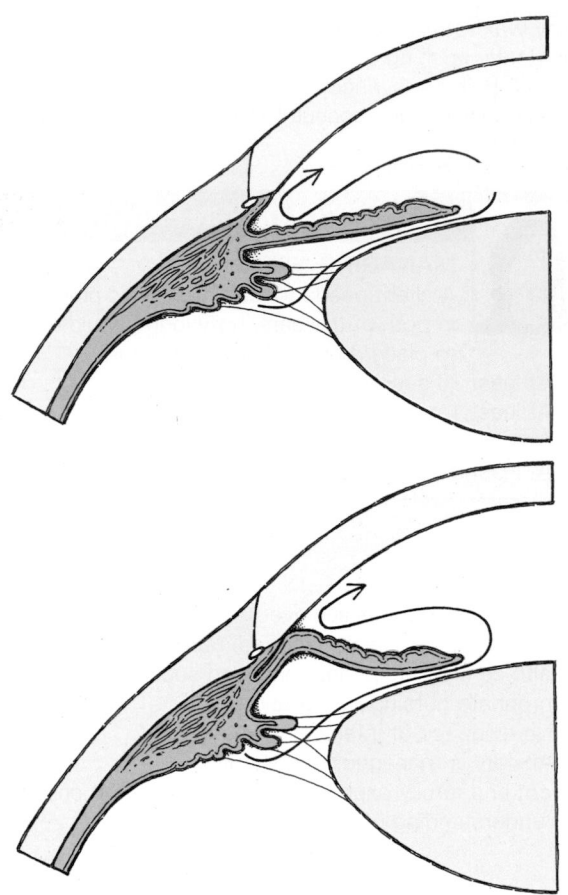

FIGURE 53.4 Two examples of glaucoma; the top shows normal angle in open-angle glaucoma, the bottom shows how the iris blocks the canal in angle-closure glaucoma.

fluid cannot leave the anterior chamber. In angle-closure glaucoma (the bottom picture in Fig. 53.4), the iris is bent at an angle and blocks the canal, limiting the flow of aqueous humor from the anterior chamber of the eye. The limitation of outflow in both types of glaucoma causes an accumulation of intraocular fluid, followed by increased IOP. As a result, the higher the IOP, the greater the risk of optic nerve damage, visual loss, and blindness. Some individuals have an anatomic defect that causes the angle to be narrower than normal but do not have any symptoms and do not develop glaucoma under normal circumstances. However, certain situations, such as medication that causes dilation of the eye, fear, or pain, may precipitate an attack. The aim of treatment in glaucoma is to lower the IOP. The Summary Drug Table: Selected Ophthalmic Preparations provides examples of the drugs used to treat both glaucoma and other ophthalmic problems.

ACTIONS AND USES

The drugs used to treat ophthalmic conditions are from the same classes of drugs used in other body systems and conditions. The drugs are grouped according to their active ingredients. Systemic effects are rare because only small amounts of these preparations may be absorbed systemically.

Agents Used to Treat Glaucoma

Prostaglandin Agonists

Prostaglandin agonists are used to lower IOP in clients with open-angle glaucoma and ocular hypertension. These drugs act to lower IOP by increasing the outflow of aqueous humor through the trabecular meshwork.

Beta-Adrenergic Blocking Drugs

The beta-adrenergic blocking drugs decrease the rate of production of aqueous humor and thereby lower the IOP. These drugs may be less expensive than the prostaglandin agonists, so some places may use them more frequently for clients.

Alpha$_2$-Adrenergic Drugs

Brimonidine is an alpha$_2$-adrenergic (α_2-adrenergic) receptor agonist used to lower IOP in clients with open-angle glaucoma or ocular hypertension. This drug acts to reduce production of aqueous humor and increase the outflow of aqueous humor.

Carbonic Anhydrase Inhibitors

Carbonic anhydrase is an enzyme found in many tissues of the body, including the eye. Inhibition of carbonic anhydrase in the eye decreases aqueous humor secretion, resulting in a decrease of IOP. These drugs are used in the treatment of elevated IOP seen in open-angle glaucoma. Except for dorzolamide and brinzolamide, carbonic anhydrase inhibitors are administered systemically.

Rho Kinase Inhibitors

Ripasudil works by acting directly on the trabecular meshwork and Schlemm canal cells to increase their permeability and decreasing the obstruction to aqueous humor outflow.

Other Drugs Used to Treat Glaucoma

Miotics (direct and cholinesterase inhibitors) contract the pupil of the eye (miosis), resulting in an increase in the space through which the aqueous humor flows, decreasing IOP. The miotics were, for a number of years, the drug of choice for glaucoma. These drugs are used less frequently now, having lost first-choice treatment status to the prostaglandin analogs and beta-adrenergic blocking drugs. Apraclonidine (a sympathomimetic) is used to control or prevent postoperative elevations in IOP. Dapiprazole acts by blocking the alpha-adrenergic receptor in smooth muscle and causes miosis (constriction of the pupil) through an effect on the dilator muscle of the iris. The drug is used primarily after ophthalmic examinations to reverse the diagnostic mydriasis (dilation of the pupil).

Mast Cell Stabilizers

Mast cell stabilizers are used to prevent itching of the eyes caused by allergic conjunctivitis. Mast cell stabilizers inhibit the antigen-induced release of inflammatory mediators (e.g., histamine) from human mast cells.

Nonsteroidal Anti-Inflammatory Drugs

Nonsteroidal anti-inflammatory drugs (NSAIDs) inhibit prostaglandin synthesis (see Chapter 14 for a discussion of the NSAIDs), thereby exerting anti-inflammatory action.

These drugs are used to treat postoperative pain and inflammation after cataract surgery, for the relief of itching of the eyes caused by seasonal allergies, and during eye surgery to prevent miosis.

Corticosteroids

These drugs possess anti-inflammatory activity and are used for inflammatory conditions, such as allergic conjunctivitis, keratitis, herpes zoster keratitis, and inflammation of the iris. Corticosteroids also may be used after injury to the cornea or after corneal transplantation to prevent rejection.

Antibiotics and Sulfonamides

Antibiotics possess antibacterial activity and are used in the treatment of eye infections. Sulfonamides possess a bacteriostatic effect against a wide range of gram-positive and gram-negative microorganisms. They are used in treating conjunctivitis, corneal ulcer, and other superficial infections of the eye. Ophthalmic tetracycline and erythromycin are used to prevent gonorrheal ophthalmia neonatorum (gonorrheal infection of the newborn's eyes).

Antiviral Drugs

Antiviral drugs interfere with viral reproduction by altering DNA synthesis. These drugs are used in the treatment of herpes simplex infections of the eye, in the treatment of immunocompromised clients with cytomegalovirus (CMV) retinitis, and for the prevention of CMV retinitis in clients undergoing transplantation.

Antifungal Drugs

Natamycin is the only ophthalmic antifungal in use. This drug possesses antifungal activity against a variety of yeast and other fungi.

Vasoconstrictors/Mydriatics

Mydriatics are drugs that dilate the pupil (mydriasis), constrict superficial blood vessels of the sclera, and decrease the formation of aqueous humor. These drugs are used to treat the redness of the eye and are available over the counter in pharmacies.

Cycloplegic Mydriatics

Cycloplegic mydriatics cause mydriasis and cycloplegia (paralysis of the ciliary muscle, resulting in an inability to focus the eye). These drugs are used in the treatment of inflammatory conditions of the iris and uveal tract of the eye and for examination of the eye.

VEGFR Inhibitors

Wet macular degeneration is an age-related vision loss that occurs over time. Vision change starts with distortion, leading to blurring and may present as visual hallucinations. Currently, there is no treatments to prevent the condition. Yet, a number of drugs called vascular endothelial growth factor receptor (VEGFR) inhibitors are being used to decrease new blood capillary formation—a leading issue in wet macular degeneration vision loss. The drug is injected directly into the fluid-filled eyeball.

ADVERSE REACTIONS

Although adverse reactions are rare, these drugs can cause visual impairment such as blurring of vision and local irritation and burning. These reactions are most often self-limiting and resolve if the client waits a few minutes. Visual impairment that does not clear within 30 minutes after therapy should be reported to the primary health care provider.

Drugs to Treat Glaucoma

Drugs used to treat glaucoma may cause transient local reactions and systemic reactions. Although side effects are usually mild they may include:

- Locally in or near the eye—burning and stinging, headache, visual blurring, tearing, foreign body sensation, ocular allergic reactions, and ocular itching
- Systemic effects—fatigue and drowsiness, palpations, nausea
- Prostaglandin analogs—slight iris color change, growth of eyelashes, drooping eyelids
- Carbonic anhydrase inhibitors—stomach upset, frequent urination
- Rho kinase inhibitors—reddened eyes, corneal deposits

Corticosteroids

Local adverse reactions associated with administration of the corticosteroid ophthalmic preparations include elevated IOP with optic nerve damage, loss of visual acuity, cataract formation, delayed wound healing, secondary ocular infection, exacerbation of corneal infections, dry eyes, ptosis, blurred vision, discharge, ocular pain, foreign body sensation, and pruritus.

Antibiotics, and Sulfonamides

Antibiotic and sulfonamide ophthalmic preparations are usually well tolerated, and few adverse reactions are seen. Local adverse reactions include occasional transient irritation, burning, itching, stinging, inflammation, and blurred vision. With prolonged or repeated use a superinfection may occur.

Antiviral Drugs

Administration of the antiviral ophthalmic preparations may cause local reactions such as irritation, pain, pruritus, inflammation, edema of the eyes or eyelids, foreign body sensation, and corneal clouding. Systemic reactions include photophobia and allergic reactions.

Antifungal Drugs

Adverse reactions are rare. Occasional local irritation to the eye may occur.

VEGFR Inhibitors

Adverse effects of the VEGFR inhibitors include increased IOP, hemorrhage, eye pain, cataract formation, vitreous detachment, and floaters. Retinal vasculitis has been reported with the use of these drugs.

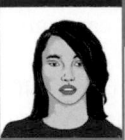

PHARMACOLOGY IN PRACTICE

ADVERSE REACTIONS

A client with glaucoma is being prescribed travoprost for the reduction of increased IOP. The nurse teaches the client which of the following may be a local adverse reaction?
1. Unpleasant taste
2. Eyelid discomfort
3. Asthma
4. Cold/flu symptoms

CONTRAINDICATIONS, PRECAUTIONS, AND INTERACTIONS

Drugs Used to Treat Glaucoma

These drugs are contraindicated in clients with hypersensitivity to the drug or any component of the drug. Clients wearing soft contact lenses should be cautioned, because the preservative in the drug may be absorbed by soft contact lenses and discoloration of the lenses may occur. Beta-adrenergic blocking drugs are in pregnancy category C (dapiprazole is pregnancy category B) and are used cautiously during pregnancy and lactation and in clients with cardiovascular disease, diabetes (may mask the symptoms of hypoglycemia), and hyperthyroidism (may mask symptoms of hyperthyroidism). The client taking beta-adrenergic blocking drugs for ophthalmic reasons may experience increased or additive effects when the drugs are administered with the oral beta-adrenergic blockers. Coadministration of timolol and calcium antagonists may cause hypotension, left ventricular failure, and condition disturbances within the heart. There is a potential additive hypotensive effect when the beta-adrenergic blocking ophthalmic drugs are administered with the phenothiazines.

Cholinesterase inhibitors are used cautiously in clients with myasthenia gravis (may cause additive adverse effects), before and after surgery, and in clients with chronic angle-closure (narrow-angle) glaucoma or those with anatomically narrow angles (may cause papillary block and increase the angle blockage). When cholinesterase inhibitors are administered with systemic anticholinesterase drugs, there is a risk for additive effects. Individuals such as farmers, warehouse workers, or gardeners working with carbamate–organophosphate insecticides or pesticides are at risk for systemic effects of cholinesterase inhibitors from absorption of the pesticide or insecticide through the respiratory tract or the skin. Individuals working with pesticides or insecticides containing carbamate–organophosphate and taking a cholinesterase inhibitor should be advised to wear respiratory masks, change clothes frequently, and wash exposed clothes thoroughly.

These drugs are used cautiously during pregnancy (epinephrine, pregnancy category B; apraclonidine, pregnancy category C) and lactation and in clients with cardiovascular disease, depression, cerebral or coronary insufficiency, hypertension, diabetes, hyperthyroidism, or Raynaud phenomenon. When brimonidine is used with central nervous system (CNS) depressants, such as alcohol, barbiturates, opiates, sedatives, or anesthetics, there is a risk for an additive CNS-depressant effect. Use the drugs cautiously in combination with antihypertensive drugs and cardiac glycosides because a synergistic effect may occur.

Adrenergic-blocking drugs are contraindicated in clients with bronchial asthma, obstructive pulmonary disease, sinus bradycardia, heart block, cardiac failure, or cardiogenic shock, and in clients with hypersensitivity to the drug or any components of the drug. These drugs should not be used in conditions in which pupil constriction is not desirable, such as in acute iritis (inflammation of the iris), and in the treatment of IOP in open-angle glaucoma.

Miotic drugs are contraindicated in clients with hypersensitivity to the drug or any component of the drug and in conditions where constriction is undesirable (e.g., iritis, uveitis, and acute inflammatory disease of the anterior chamber). The drugs are used cautiously in clients with corneal abrasion, pregnancy (pregnancy category C), lactation, cardiac failure, bronchial asthma, peptic ulcer, hyperthyroidism, gastrointestinal spasm, urinary tract infection, Parkinson disease, renal or hepatic impairment, recent myocardial infarction, hypotension, or hypertension. These drugs are also used cautiously in clients with angle-closure glaucoma, because miotics occasionally can precipitate angle-closure glaucoma by increasing the resistance to aqueous flow from posterior to anterior chamber.

Drugs Used to Treat Inflammation

These drugs are contraindicated in clients with hypersensitivity to the drug or any component of the drug. The mast cell stabilizers are used cautiously in clients who wear contact lenses (preservative may be absorbed by the soft contact lenses). NSAIDs are used cautiously in clients with bleeding tendencies. When used topically, there is less risk of interactions with drugs or other substances. There is a possibility of a cross-sensitivity reaction when NSAIDs are administered to clients allergic to salicylates. Corticosteroids and antibiotics are used cautiously in clients with sulfite sensitivity because an allergic-type reaction may result. The corticosteroid ophthalmic preparations are used cautiously in clients with infectious conditions of the eye. Prolonged use of corticosteroids may result in elevated IOP and optic nerve damage. Antibiotic and sulfonamide ophthalmic preparations are contraindicated in clients with epithelial herpes simplex keratitis, varicella, mycobacterial infection of the eye, and fungal diseases of the eye. These drugs are pregnancy category B or C drugs and are used cautiously during pregnancy and lactation.

LASA ALERT

The following drugs may sound alike; be sure to clarify when they are ordered:

Drug Name	*Sounds Like*
brolucizumab	Bevacizumab
carteolol	Carvedilol
dexAMETHasone	desoximetasone, dexMEDEtomidine, dextroamphetamine
ganciclovir	acyclovir, valGANciclovir
Iopidine	indapamide, iodine, Lodine
levoFLOXacin	levETIRAcetam, levodopa, levothyroxine
metipranolol	Metaproterenol
natacyn	Naprosyn
pegaptanib	PAZOPanib, peginesatide, pegaspargase, pegfilgrastim, peginterferon, pegvisomant, PONATinib
prednisoLONE	predniSONE
ranibizumab	bevacizumab, ramucirumab
Viroptic	Timoptic

Drugs that look alike are noted in the Summary Drug Tables of each chapter.

 H e r b a l   C o n s i d e r a t i o n s

Bilberry, also known as whortleberry, blueberry, and huckleberry, is a shrub with bluish flowers that appear in early spring and ripen in July and August. Its use appears to be beneficial in promoting healthy eyes. Other benefits reportedly include improved visual acuity, improved night vision, prevention of free radical damage, and promotion of capillary blood flow in the eyes, hands, and feet. Bilberry extract has been used in treating nonspecific, mild diarrhea and as a mouthwash or gargle for inflammation of the mouth and throat. Bilberry fruit is a safe substance with no known adverse reactions or toxicity. There are no known contraindications to its use as directed unless the individual has an allergy to bilberry. The dosage of standard extract is 80–160 mg/day (DerMarderosian & Beutler, 2003).

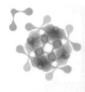 **NURSING PROCESS: STEPS TO BUILDING CLINICAL JUDGMENT**
Client Receiving an Ophthalmic Preparation

ASSESSMENT

Preadministration Assessment

The primary health care provider or eye specialist examines the eye and external structures surrounding the eye and prescribes the drug indicated to treat the disorder.

Data gathering suggestions before administering an ophthalmic drug include:

Objective data

- Snelling eye test
- Examination of the eye for irritation, redness, and the presence of any exudate

Subjective data

- Complaints of pruritus (itching)
- Description of vision changes and how it impacts activities of daily living
- Medication history, specifically looking at drugs taken systemically that may be used in eye drops

Ongoing Assessment

During the ongoing assessment, observe for a therapeutic drug response and report any increase in symptoms and the presence of any redness, irritation, or pain in the eye.

Clients admitted for treatment of acute glaucoma should be assessed every 2 hours for relief of pain. Pain in the eye may indicate increased IOP.

NURSING DIAGNOSES

Drug-specific nursing diagnoses include the following:

- **Injury risk** related to adverse reactions to drug therapy (blurring of the vision)
- **Acute pain** related to eye disorder or adverse reaction to medication
- **Anxiety** related to eye pain or discomfort, diagnosis, other factors

Nursing diagnoses related to drug administration are discussed in Chapter 4.

PLANNING

The expected outcomes of the client depend on the reason for administration but may include an optimal response to therapy, support of client needs related to the management of adverse reactions, minimized anxiety, and confidence in an understanding of the application and use of an ophthalmic preparation (see the Client Teaching for Improved Outcomes: Instilling an Ophthalmic Preparation).

IMPLEMENTATION

Promoting an Optimal Response to Therapy

> ⓘ **NURSING ALERT**
>
> Only preparations labeled as "ophthalmic" are instilled in the eye. Check the label of the preparation carefully for the name of the drug, the percentage of the preparation, and a statement indicating that the preparation is for ophthalmic use.

Many clients will self-administer ophthalmic preparations. In some instances when hospitalized, the client may have been using an ophthalmic preparation for a long time and the primary health care provider may allow the client to instill their own eye drops. When this is stated on the client's orders, consult with the pharmacy about leaving the drug at the client's bedside. Even though the drug is self-administered, check the client at intervals to be sure that the drug is instilled at the prescribed time using the correct technique for ophthalmic instillation. Always review basic administration steps with the client no matter whether the medication is given by you or the client. Steps to be reviewed include:

- The drug label must indicate that the preparation is for ophthalmic use.
- Check the medication to make sure the solution is clear and not discolored.
- Ophthalmic ointments are applied to the eyelids or dropped into the lower conjunctival sac; ophthalmic solutions are dropped into the middle of the lower conjunctival sac, not directly on the eyeball (Fig. 53.5).
- Avoid touching the eye with the tip of the dropper or container to prevent contamination of the product.
- When eye solutions are instilled, apply gentle pressure on the inner canthus to delay drainage of the drug down the tear duct, this is called **punctal occlusion**. This prevents the drug from being absorbed systemically.

Consult the primary health care provider regarding use of this technique before the first dose is instilled, because this technique can be potentially dangerous in some eye conditions, for example, after recent eye surgery. When two eye drops are prescribed for use at the same time, wait at least 5 minutes before instilling the second drug. This helps prevent dilution of the drug and loss of some therapeutic effect from tearing.

When a client is scheduled for eye surgery, it is most important that the eye drops ordered by the primary health care provider are instilled at the correct time. This is especially important when the purpose of the drug is to change the size of the pupil (dilate the pupil).

Monitoring and Managing Client Needs

Injury Risk

When the ophthalmic drugs produce blurring of vision, this can result in falls and other injuries. Keeping the client's room dimly lit at night is helpful, because night vision may be decreased. Obstacles that may hinder ambulation or result in falls, such as slippers, chairs, and tables, are placed out of the way, especially during the night. Warn clients to exercise care when getting out of bed when the vision is impaired by these drugs. If needed, provide assistance with ambulation to prevent injury from falls.

Acute Pain

Pain can occur with eye conditions such as glaucoma and eye infections. Clients with acute glaucoma are assessed for relief of pain. Pain in the eye may indicate increased IOP and should be reported to the primary health care provider. Pain associated with infection should decrease with administration of medication. Any increase in pain or no decrease in the symptoms after 1–2 days of treatment should be reported to the primary health care provider. Headache and brow ache are associated with adverse reactions of some of the ophthalmic agents and are usually self-limiting.

Anxiety

Eye injuries and some eye infections are very painful. Other eye conditions may result in discomfort or a loss of or change in vision. The client with an eye disorder or injury usually has great concern about the effect the problem will have on their vision. Reassure the client that every effort is being made to treat the disorder.

Educating the Client and Family

The client or a family member will require instruction in the technique of instilling an ophthalmic preparation (see Client Teaching for Improved Outcomes: Instilling an Ophthalmic Preparation). In addition, give the following information to the client and family member when an eye ointment or solution is prescribed:

- Eye preparations may cause a momentary stinging or burning sensation; this is normal.
- Temporary blurring of vision may occur. Avoid activities requiring visual acuity until vision returns to normal.
- If more than one topical ophthalmic drug is being used, administer the drugs at least 5–10 minutes apart or as directed by the physician.
- Complete a full course of treatment with the prescribed drug to achieve satisfactory results.
- Do not rub the eyes, and keep hands away from the eyes.

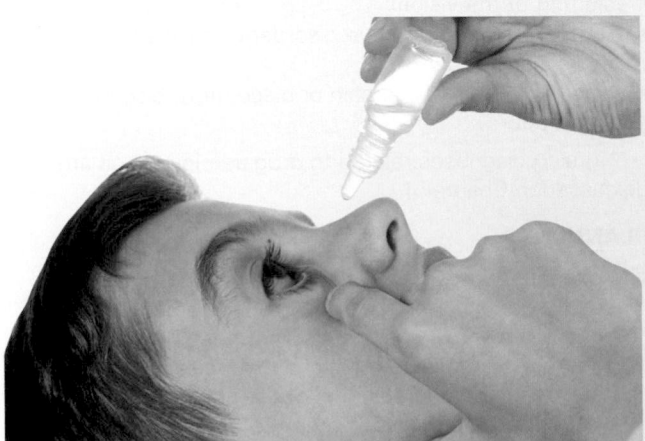

FIGURE 53.5 Instilling eye medication. While the client looks upward, gently pull the lower lid down and instill the correct number of drops into the lower conjunctival sac.

Client Teaching for Improved Outcomes

Instilling an Ophthalmic Preparation

Many eye surgeries are performed in ambulatory clinics, requiring the client to instill eye drops or ointment at home. If the client is unable to do so, a family member or friend may have to instill the preparation. Teaching the steps of preparation and administration are important for good outcomes. Discuss, demonstrate, and watch a "teach-back" from the client on the procedure before this becomes a self-administered task. Be sure the client understands the following:

✔ Wash hands thoroughly before beginning the process.
✔ Look at the solution each time; if discolored or unclear, do not use it!
✔ Hold bottle (drops) or tube (ointment) in hand for a few minutes before using to warm the solution.
✔ Cleanse the area around the eye of any secretions.
✔ Squeeze the eyedropper bulb to release and then refill the dropper, squeeze the bottle to fill the drop chamber, or squeeze ointment to tip of the tube.
✔ Tilt head slightly backward and toward the eye to be treated.
✔ Pull affected lower lid down.
✔ Position dropper, bottle, or tube over lower conjunctival sac.
✔ Steady hand by resting fingers against cheek or by resting base of hand on cheek.
✔ Look up at ceiling and squeeze dropper, bottle, or tube.
✔ Drop ordered number of drops into the middle of lower conjunctival sac; instill prescribed amount of ointment to eyelid or lower conjunctival sac.
✔ Close eye briefly and gently and release lower lid (do not squeeze eyes shut after instilling the drug).
✔ Place finger on inner canthus to avoid absorption through the tear duct (when instilling drops and only if ordered).
✔ Repeat procedure with other eye (if ordered).
✔ If more than one type of ophthalmic preparation is being instilled, wait the recommended time before instilling the second drug (usually 5 minutes for drops and 10–15 minutes for ointment).
✔ Replace the cap of the eye preparation immediately after instilling the eye drops or ointment. Do not touch the tip of the dropper, bottle, or tube.

• Do not use nonprescription eye products during or after treatment unless such use has been approved by the primary health care provider.
• Some of these preparations cause sensitivity (photophobia) to light; to minimize this, wear sunglasses.
• Notify the primary health care provider if symptoms do not improve or if they worsen.

Drugs to Treat Glaucoma
• The eye preparation may sting on instillation, especially the first few doses.
• Do not use if solution is brown or contains a precipitate.
• Do not use while wearing soft contact lenses.
• Headache or brow ache may occur.
• Report any decrease in visual acuity. Use caution when driving at night or performing activities in poor illumination.
• If more than one ophthalmic drug is being used, administer the drugs 5 minutes apart.
• Changes may occur to the lashes—length, thickness, pigmentation, and number—in the eye being treated.
• The color of the iris may change because of an increase in the brown pigment. This may be more noticeable in clients with blue, green, gray-brown, or other light-colored eyes. This discoloration may be permanent.

Drugs to Treat Inflammation
• If improvement in the condition being treated does not occur within 2 days, or pain, redness, itching, or swelling of the eye occurs, notify the primary health care provider.

EVALUATION

• Therapeutic effect is achieved.
• Adverse reactions are identified, reported to the primary health care provider, and managed successfully with appropriate nursing interventions:
  • No evidence of injury is seen.
  • Client has minimal to no pain.
  • Anxiety is reduced.
• Client and family express confidence and demonstrate an understanding of the drug regimen.

PHARMACOLOGY IN PRACTICE

USING CLINICAL REASONING

The primary health care provider has prescribed eye drops. Janna is fidgety and tells you she just cannot put those drops in her eyes. Design an age-appropriate teaching plan for this individual.

KEY POINTS

■ Otitis media is one of the most common middle ear conditions consisting of fluid buildup that may or may not be infected. Otic preparations are topical solutions used to treat the outer and middle ear conditions. The categories of otic preparations include antibiotics, antibiotic/steroid combinations, and different miscellaneous solutions.

■ Minimal drug enters the systemic circulation when administered properly; therefore, local adverse reactions predominate—irritation, itching, or a burning sensation. It is important never to touch the ear canal with an implement, even when administering ear medicines.

■ Glaucoma is one of the common ophthalmic conditions requiring medications. Ophthalmic solutions may also treat infections, inflammation, or allergies in the eye.

■ The drugs used to treat ophthalmic conditions are from the same classes of drugs used in other body systems and conditions. Systemic effects are rare because only small amounts of these preparations may be absorbed systemically. Local adverse reactions consist of irritation, a burning sensation, and temporary blurriness.

■ Take time to check solutions: *Otic* preparations are for ears, whereas *ophthalmic* preparations are for eyes.

SUMMARY DRUG TABLE
Selected Otic Preparations

Generic Combinations	Trade Name	Uses	Adverse Reactions	Dosage Ranges
Otic Antibiotic				
ciprofloxacin (otic) *sip-roe-FLOKS-a-sin*	Cetraxal, Otiprio	Otitis external, acute otitis media	Local irritation, itching, burning, earache	Multi/single dose instillation of 0.5/12 mg
ofloxacin (otic) *oh-FLOKS-a-sin*		Otitis external, chronic suppurative otitis media, acute otitis media	Local irritation, itching, burning, earache	Ages 1–12 years: 5 gtt BID into affected ear for 10 days Ages 12 years and older: 10 gtt BID into affected ear for 10–14 days
Otic Corticosteroid				
fluocinolone *floo-oh-SIN-oh-lone*	DermOtic, Flac	Eczematous external otitis	Local irritation, itching, burning, acne eruption	Up to 5 gtts daily into affected ear for 7–14 days
Corticosteroid and Antibiotic Combinations, Solutions				
ciprofloxacin, hydrocortisone	Cipro HC Otic	Bacterial external otitis	Ear irritation, burning, or itching	4 gtt instilled TID or QID
ciprofloxacin, dexamethasone	Ciprodex	Bacterial acute and external otitis	Ear irritation, burning, or itching	4 gtt instilled BID into affected ear for 7 days
ciprofloxacin, fluocinolone	Otovel	Bacterial acute and external otitis (with tubes)	Ear irritation, burning, or itching	0.25 mg instilled BID into affected ear for 7 days
hydrocortisone, neomycin, polymyxin B		Bacterial infections of the external auditory canal	Few; can cause ear irritation, burning, or itching; when used for prolonged periods there is a danger of a superinfection	4 gtt instilled TID or QID

SUMMARY DRUG TABLE
Selected Ophthalmic Preparations

Generic Name	Trade Name	Uses	Dosage Ranges
Drugs used to treat Glaucoma			
Prostaglandin Agonists			
bimatoprost *bi-MAT-oh-prost*	Lumigan, Latisse, Durysta	IOP reduction in open-angle glaucoma	1 gtt in affected eye(s) daily in the evening
latanoprostene bunod *la-tan-oh-PROS-teen BU-nod*	Vyzulta	IOP reduction in open-angle glaucoma	1 gtt in affected eye(s) daily
latanoprost *la-TA-noe-prost*	Xalatan, Xelpros	First-line treatment of open-angle glaucoma, ocular hypertension	1 gtt in affected eye(s) daily in the evening
tafluprost *TA-floo-prost*	Ziopan	IOP reduction in open-angle glaucoma, ocular hypertension	1 gtt in affected eye(s) daily
travoprost *TRA-voe-prost*	Travatan Z	Reduction of increased IOP in clients with glaucoma who do not respond to or cannot take other drugs to lower IOP	1 gtt in affected eye(s) daily in the evening

Generic Name	Trade Name	Uses	Dosage Ranges
Beta-Adrenergic Blocking Drugs			
betaxolol *be-TAKS-oh-lo*	Betoptic S	Chronic open-angle glaucoma, ocular hypertension	1–2 gtt in the affected eye(s) BID
carteolol *KAR-tee-oh-lol*		Same as betaxolol	1 gtt in affected eye(s) TID
levobunolol *lee-voe-BYOO-noe-lol*	AKBeta, Liquifilm	Same as betaxolol	0.5% Solution: 1–2 gtt in affected eye(s) daily 0.25% Solution: 1–2 gtt in affected eye(s) BID
metipranolol *met-i-PRAN-oh-lol*		Treatment of elevated IOP in clients with ocular hypertension or open-angle glaucoma	1 gtt in affected eye(s) BID
timolol *TIM-oh-lol*	Betimol, Timoptic, Timoptic-XE	Reduces IOP in ocular hypertension or open-angle glaucoma	1 gtt in affected eye(s) daily or BID Gel: invert the closed container and shake once before each use; administer 1 gtt/day
Alpha₂-Adrenergic Agonist			
brimonidine *bri-MOE-ni-deen*	Alphagan-P, Lumify	Lowers IOP in clients with open-angle (chronic) glaucoma	1 gtt in affected eye(s) TID
Carbonic Anhydrase Inhibitors			
brinzolamide *brin-ZOH-la-mide*	Azopt	Open-angle glaucoma, ocular hypertension	1 gtt in affected eye(s) TID
dorzolamide *dor-ZOLE-a-mide*	Trusopt	Open-angle glaucoma, ocular hypertension	1 gtt in affected eye(s) TID
Rho Kinase Inhibitor			
netarsudil *ne-TAR-soo-dil*	Rhopressa	Elevated IOP of hypertension or open-angle glaucoma	1 gtt in affected eye(s) daily
Combinations Used to Treat Glaucoma			
brimonidine/timolol	Combigan	Glaucoma	1 gtt in the affected eye(s) 2 times daily
dorzolamide/timolol	Cosopt	Open-angle glaucoma and ocular hypertension	1 gtt into the affected eye(s) BID
Miscellaneous Agents used to Treat Eyes			
Sympathomimetics and Alpha-Adrenergic Blocking Drugs			
apraclonidine *a-pra-KLOE-ni-deen*	Iopidine	1% Solution: control or prevention of postoperative elevations in IOP 0.5% Solution: short-term therapy in clients receiving maximal medical therapy who require additional IOP reduction	1% Solution: 1 gtt in operative eye 1 hour before surgery and 1 gtt immediately after surgery 0.5% Solution: 1–2 gtt in the affected eye(s) TID
dapiprazole *dap-ih-pray'-zoll*	Rev-Eyes	Reverse diagnostic mydriasis after ophthalmic examination	2 gtt into the conjunctiva of each eye, followed 5 minutes later by an additional 2 gtt
Miotics, Direct Acting, and Cholinesterase Inhibitors			
carbachol *KAR-ba-kole*	Miostat	Glaucoma	1–2 gtt up to TID
pilocarpine *pye-loe-KAR-peen*	Isopto Carpine	Glaucoma, preoperative and postoperative intraocular hypertension	Solution: 1–2 gtt in affected eye(s) Gel: apply a 0.5-in. ribbon in the lower conjunctival sac of affected eye(s) daily at bedtime
echothiophate iodide *ek-oh-THYE-oh-fate* *EYE-oh-dide*	Phospholine Iodide	Chronic open-angle glaucoma, accommodative esotropia (cross-eye)	Esotropia: 1 gtt daily Glaucoma: 2 doses/day in the morning and at bedtime or 1 dose every other day

Continued

SUMMARY DRUG TABLE (continued)
Selected Ophthalmic Preparations

Generic Name	Trade Name	Uses	Dosage Ranges
Mast Cell Stabilizers			
lodoxamide *loe-DOKS-a-mide*	Alomide	Allergic conjunctivitis	1–2 gtt in each eye QID
nedocromil *ne-doe-KROE-mil*	Alocril	Allergic conjunctivitis	1–2 gtt in each eye BID
NSAIDs			
bromfenac *BROME-fen-ak*	Prolensa	Postoperative pain and inflammation after cataract surgery	1 gtt BID
diclofenac *dye-KLOE-fen-ak*		Postoperative inflammation after cataract surgery	1 gtt QID
flurbiprofen *flure-BI-proe-fen*		Inhibition of intraoperative miosis	1 gtt q30min beginning 2 hours before surgery (total of 4 gtt)
ketorolac *KEE-toe-role-ak*	Acular	Relief of ocular itching caused by seasonal allergies, pain after corneal refractive surgery	Allergies: 1 drop QID Postoperative pain: 1 gtt in operated eye
nepafenac *ne-pa-FEN-ak*	Ilevro, Nevanac	Postoperative pain and inflammation after cataract surgery	1 gtt TID
Corticosteroids			
dexAMETHasone *deks-a-METH-a-sone*	Dextenza Maxidex	Treatment of inflammatory conditions of the conjunctiva, eyelid, cornea, anterior segment of the eye	Solution: 1–2 gtt qhr during the day and q2hr at night, reduced to 1 gtt q4hr when response noted, then 1 gtt TID or QID Ointment: thin coating in lower conjunctival sac TID or QID
difluprednate *dye-floo-PRED-nate*	Durezol	Treatment of eye swelling and pain following surgical procedures	Solution: 24 hours after surgery, 1–2 gtt 4 times daily for 2 weeks, then 2 times daily for 1 week
fluocinolone *floo-oh-SIN-oh-lone*	Iluvien, Retisert, Yutiq	Diabetic macular edema, treatment of inflammatory of the eye,	Implants used over 3 years
fluorometholone *flure-oh-METH-oh-lone*	Flarex, Fluor-Op	Treatment of inflammatory conditions of the conjunctiva, lid, cornea, anterior segment of the eye	Suspension: 1–2 gtt BID–QID, may increase to 2 gtt q2hr Ointment: thin coating in lower conjunctival sac 1–3 times daily (up to 1 application q4hr)
loteprednol *loe-te-PRED-nol*	Alrex, Lotemax	Allergic conjunctivitis	1–2 gtt QID
prednisoLONE *pred-NISS-oh-lonean*	Pred Forte, Pred Mild, Blephamide	Treatment of inflammatory conditions of the conjunctiva, lid, cornea, anterior segment of the eye	1–2 gtt/hr during the day and q2hr at night, reduced to 1 gtt q4hr, then 1 gtt TID or QID Suspensions: 1–2 gtt BID–QID
Antibiotics			
azithromycin *az-ith-roe-MYE-sin*	AzaSite	Treatment of eye infections	See package insert
bacitracin *bas-i-TRAY-sin*		Same as azithromycin	See package insert
besifloxacin *be-si-FLOX-a-sin*	Besivance	Same as azithromycin	See package insert
ciprofloxacin *sip-roe-FLOKS-a-sin*	Ciloxan	Same as azithromycin	See package insert
erythromycin *er-ith-roe-MYE-sin*		Same as azithromycin, neonatal ocular prophylaxis at birth	See package insert
gatifloxacin *gat-i-FLOKS-a-sin*	Zymaxid	Same as azithromycin	Days 1 and 2: instill 1 gtt in affected eye(s) q2hr while awake, up to 8 times daily Days 3–7: instill 1 gtt in affected eye up to QID while awake

Generic Name	Trade Name	Uses	Dosage Ranges
gentamicin jen-ta-MYE-sin	Gentak	Same as azithromycin	See package insert
levoFLOXacin lee-voe-FLOKS-ah-sin		Same as azithromycin	Days 1 and 2: instill 1–2 gtt in affected eye(s) q2hr while awake, up to 8 times daily Days 3–7: instill 1–2 gtt in affected eye up to QID while awake
moxifloxacin moxs-i-FLOKS-a-sin	Moxeza, Vigamox	Same as azithromycin	Adults and children at least 1 yr of age: 1 drop in affected eye TID for 7 days
ofloxacin oh-FLOKS-a-sin	Ocuflox	Same as azithromycin, corneal ulcers	Bacterial conjunctivitis: days 1 and 2: 1–2 gtt q2–4hr in the affected eye(s); days 3–7: 1–2 gtt QID Bacterial corneal ulcer: days 1 and 2: 1–2 gtt into the affected eye q30min while awake; awaken approximately q4–6hr and instill 1–2 gtt; days 3 through 7–9: instill 1–2 drops QID
tobramycin toe-bra-MYE-sin	Tobrex	Same as azithromycin	See package insert
sulfacetamide sul-fa-SEE-ta-mide	Bleph-10, Blephamide	Ocular infections, trachoma	Ocular infections: 1–2 gtt q1–4hr Trachoma: 2 gtt q2hr Ointments: 0.5 in into lower conjunctival sac TID or QID
Antiviral Drugs			
acyclovir ay-SYE-kloe-veer	Avaclyr	Herpes simplex keratitis	Apply ointment up to 5 times daily until ulcer heals
ganciclovir gan-SYE-kloe-veer	Zirgan	CMV retinitis, herpes keratitis	1 gtt up to 5 times daily
trifluridine trye-FLURE-i-deen	Viroptic	Keratoconjunctivitis keratitis, epithelial keratitis	Adults and children older than 6 years: 1 gtt onto the corners of affected eye(s) while awake Maximum daily dose: 9 gtt until corneal ulcer has completely re-epithelialized, treat for an additional 7 days with 1 gtt q4hr for a maximum of 5 gtt/day
Antifungal Drug			
natamycin na-ta-MYE-sin	Natacyn	Fungal infections of the eye	1 gtt q1–2hr
Vasoconstrictors/Mydriatics			
tetrahydrozoline tet-ra-hye-DROZ-a-leen	Murine Plus Eye Drops	Relief of eye redness caused by minor irritation	1–2 gtt up to QID
Cycloplegics/Mydriatics			
atropine A-troe-peen	Isopto-Atropine	Mydriasis/cycloplegia	1–2 gtt up to TID
cyclopentolate sye-kloe-PEN-toe-late	Cyclogy	Mydriasis/cycloplegia	1–2 gtt
homatropine hydrobromide hoe-MA-troe-peen	Isopto Homatropine	Mydriasis/cycloplegia	1–2 gtt q3–4hr
VEGFR Inhibitors			
aflibercept a-FLIB-er-sept	Eylea	Macular degeneration, diabetic macular edema/retinopathy	Intravitreal injection monthly/bimonthly
brolucizumab BROE-lue-SIZ-ue-mab	Beovu	Macular degeneration - wet	Intravitreal injection monthly for 3 months
Pegaptanib peg-AP-ta-nib	Macugen	Macular degeneration - wet	Intravitreal injection every 6 weeks
ranibizumab ra-ni-BIZ-oo-mab	Lucentis	Macular degeneration, diabetic macular edema/retinopathy	Intravitreal injection monthly

CHAPTER REVIEW

Know Your Drugs

Clients sometimes know a medication by the brand (or trade) name and not the generic name. To help you recognize both names, match the brand name with the generic name of the same medication.

Generic	Brand
1. ciprofloxin otic	A. Ocuflox
2. ranibizumab	B. Alocril
3. ofloxacin ophthalmic	C. Cetraxal
4. nedocromil	D. Lucentis

Calculate Medication Dosages

1. The primary health care provider orders 0.5 mL of Burow solution for ear pain. If the dropper used delivers 0.1 mL/drop, how many drops should be instilled into the ear?
2. If the ophthalmic drug Latisse comes in a 3-mL container and each drop is 0.05 mL, how many doses are there in the container?

Prepare for the NCLEX

RECALL THE FACTS

1. The cochlea and ossicles are in which segment of the ear?
   1. Inner ear
   2. Middle ear
   3. Outer ear
2. In glaucoma, IOP builds because _____.
   1. the client has a headache
   2. the drainage of the anterior eye chamber is blocked
   3. hypertension causes increased pressure
   4. the sinus cavities drain into the eye
3. When administering an otic solution, the drug is instilled into the _____.
   1. inner canthus
   2. auditory canal
   3. canal of Schlemm
   4. upper canthus
4. Which of the following adverse reactions would the nurse suspect in a client receiving prolonged treatment with an antibiotic otic drug?
   1. Congestive heart failure
   2. Superinfection
   3. Anemia
   4. Hypersensitivity reactions

5. When administering an ophthalmic solution, the drug is instilled into the _____.
   1. inner canthus
   2. upper conjunctival sac
   3. lower conjunctival sac
   4. upper canthus
6. Which of the following instructions would be included in a teaching plan for the client prescribed an ophthalmic solution?
   1. Squeeze the eyes tightly after the solution is instilled.
   2. Immediately wipe the eye using pressure to squeeze out excess medication.
   3. After the drug is instilled, remain upright with the head bent slightly forward for about 2 minutes.
   4. A temporary stinging or burning may be felt at the time the drug is instilled.

ANALYZE THE FACTS

7. What is the rationale for warming an otic solution that has been refrigerated before instilling the drops into the client's ear?
   1. The drug becomes thick when refrigerated, and warming liquefies the solution.
   2. It helps to prevent dizziness on instillation.
   3. A cold solution could significantly increase the client's blood pressure.
   4. A cold solution could damage the tympanic membrane.
8. *The client has vision problems, yet has been instilling their own eye solutions for years. The client brings medication to the hospital, and the nurse sees that the half-used bottle is yellow and cloudy. What is the *first* intervention the nurse should perform?
   1. Contact the primary health care provider immediately
   2. Set the solution out for the client to use
   3. Ask the client when they last used this specific container
   4. Throw it away and get a new bottle of solution

ALTERNATE-FORMAT QUESTIONS

9. Which sections of the ear are typically treated with topical preparations? **Select all that apply.**
   1. Inner ear
   2. Middle ear
   3. Outer ear
   4. The eye

To check your answers, see Appendix F.

*Indicates the question is directly linked to the NCLEX-PN test plan in Appendix G.

WANT TO KNOW MORE? A wide variety of resources are available to enhance your learning and understanding of this chapter.

- Visit the**Point** for resources such as:
  - NCLEX-Style Student Review Questions
  - Journal Articles
  - Dosage Calculations
  - Drug Monographs
  - Watch and Learn Videos
  - Concepts in Action Animations
- The *Study Guide to Accompany Introductory Clinical Pharmacology,* 12th edition, sold separately, will help you review and apply essential content.
- ✓**PrepU** is available to help students prepare for the NCLEX-PN examination.

54

Fluids, Electrolytes, and Parenteral Therapy

Key Terms

electrolyte electrically charged substance essential to the normal functioning of all cells

equal-analgesic conversion a chart to compare doses of opioids against one another to maintain the same level of pain control

extravasation escape of fluid from a blood vessel into surrounding tissue

fluid overload condition in which the body's fluid requirements are met and the administration of fluid occurs at a rate that is greater than the rate at which the body can use or eliminate the fluid; also called *circulatory overload*

infiltration collection of fluid into tissue

lock (saline or heparin) an IV access line that is not attached to a running bag of fluid; the equipment consisting of an adapter and tubing introduced into a vein to maintain access to the venous circulatory system

parenteral administration of a substance, such as a drug, by any route other than through the gastrointestinal (GI) system (e.g., oral or rectal route)

total parenteral nutrition (TPN) complex admixture of nutrients combined in a single container and administered to the body by an IV route

Learning Objectives

On completion of this chapter, the student will:

1. List the types and uses of solutions used in the parenteral management of body fluids.
2. Define the steps involved in the intravenous (IV) administration of a solution or electrolyte used in the management of body fluids.
3. Describe the calculations used to establish IV flow rates.
4. Compare and contrast the types and uses of electrolytes used in the management of electrolyte imbalances.
5. Explain the more common signs and symptoms of electrolyte imbalance.
6. Distinguish preadministration and ongoing assessment activities the nurse should perform with the client administered an electrolyte or an IV solution to manage body fluids.
7. List nursing diagnoses particular to a client receiving an electrolyte or a solution to manage body fluids.
8. Examine ways to promote an optimal response to therapy and important points to keep in mind when educating clients about the use of an electrolyte or a solution to manage body fluids.

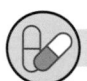 **Drug Classes**

Electrolytes
- Calcium
- Magnesium

- Potassium
- Sodium
Alkaline/acidifying agents.

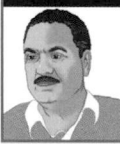 **PHARMACOLOGY IN PRACTICE**

Alfredo Garcia is a 55-year-old man being seen in the clinic for an upper respiratory infection. During the intake assessment, you find that his blood pressure is high and he continues to complain of "heartburn." Mr. Garcia attempted to use home remedies (e.g., drinking cream to coat the stomach) to decrease acid production. You have taught him about ulcer treatment, yet his heartburn persists. He continues to rely on home remedies, which are causing other problems. Mr. Garcia's weight is up, and looking at his legs, you note +2 pitting edema bilaterally. While reading the chapter, you will learn about some of the problems that can happen with electrolyte imbalances. How would you intervene in this scenario based on the information you learn?

Facility policies, state laws, and nurse practice acts govern your involvement in fluid and electrolyte management. No matter what your practice setting—whether it be acute care, ambulatory clinic, long-term care, or the community—it is important for you to have a

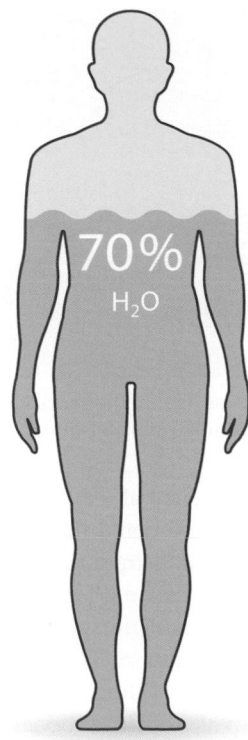

FIGURE 54.1 The majority of the human body is composed of fluid.

basic understanding of fluid management. This chapter offers information about our body fluids and electrolytes as well as basics on parenteral therapy. It is expected that you will build upon these basic concepts as you advance your practice.

Fluid makes up a major portion of our body tissues. Over 70% of our body is made up of fluid (Fig. 54.1). It gives our cells shape (intracellular), acts as a cushion by filling the void between cells (interstitial), and travels throughout our bodies with elements to help cells work or eliminate waste (plasma).

When individuals become ill, they may lose excess amounts of fluid or not feel well enough to maintain the daily intake of fluid needed for basic survival. Without fluids, the body's ability to transport oxygen and nutrients to the various tissues is compromised. Individual cells or organs are not able to function and the person becomes even more ill. Various solutions are used in the management of body fluids. These solutions are used when the body cannot sustain the fluid or electrolyte balance needed for normal functioning.

PARENTERAL MANAGEMENT OF BODY FLUIDS

Parenteral administration includes the injecting of drugs or solutions directly into the circulatory system. In the acute care or urgent care setting, solutions used to manage body fluids are usually administered intravenously (IV). The clinical setting where nurses work determines the role you will play in IV therapy. Who starts the IV, monitors it, and accesses the line for medication administration is different in each setting. No matter where you practice nursing, it

is important to understand the basic concepts of fluid and electrolyte balance.

IV replacement solutions are used for the following:

- As a parenteral source of electrolytes, calories, or water for hydration
- To facilitate nutrition and maintain electrolyte balance when the client cannot eat
- As a method to deliver drugs when a less invasive method is not suitable because of drug pharmacokinetics or client status

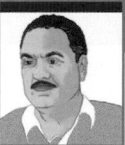

PHARMACOLOGY IN PRACTICE

SAFE ADMINISTRATION
A nurse is assigned to care for a client who is to have an IV started. Who is responsible for determining which nurse will start the IV infusion?
1. American Nurses Association
2. The school the nurse graduated from
3. Policies of the clinical setting
4. Each nurse gauges how responsible they choose to be in starting IVs

Establishing IV Access

All facilities have specific policies and procedures for cleaning, access, and stabilization of IV sites. No matter the facility, there are some basic guidelines you should be aware of regarding IV access.

Basic Guidelines

- The nondominant arm is typically chosen when selecting a vein for IV access.
- Sites are often chosen starting at the most distal point of the arm.
- Larger, more proximal veins may be selected, depending on the need for the IV therapy.
- IVs are never started on the same extremity as renal dialysis access device or mastectomy, ask about extremity restrictions.
- Ask if providers have remarked or noted issues before such as a bifurcated vein.

Following these guidelines can save time and reduce the pain of an unsuccessful attempt when the client's knowledge of previous care is considered.

Equipment

Selection of equipment will depend upon use of the IV access line. Larger gauge needles are used with rapid infusions or large amounts of fluid or blood products are anticipated. Indwelling devices are used when a longer duration is anticipated compared to only a few doses. Tubing selection will be dictated by whether the IV will run fluids continually or occasional access over the period of a day.

Technique

The tool used for venous access is called a short peripheral catheter (SPC), consisting of a metal needle and silicone

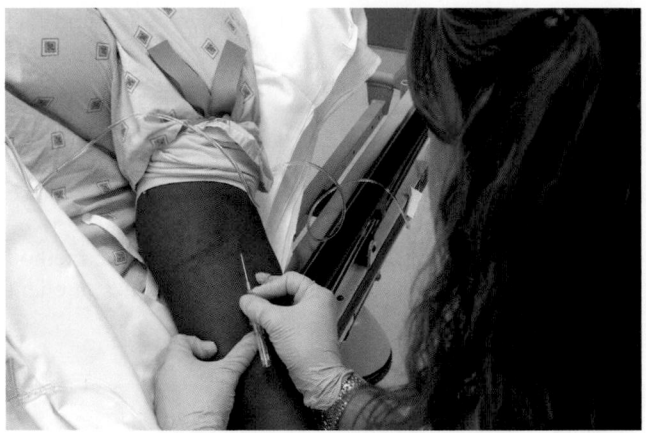

FIGURE 54.2 Confidence in IV placement comes with practice.

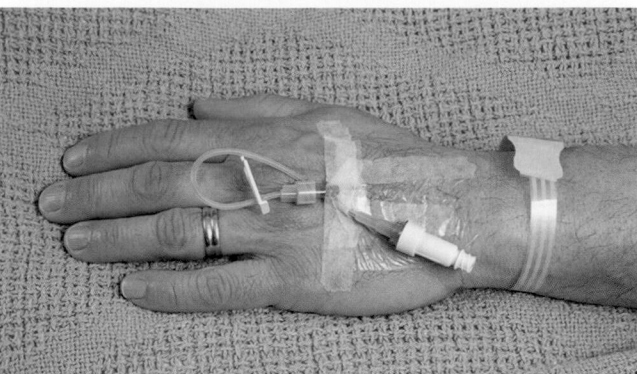

FIGURE 54.3 IV access (saline/heparin lock) for intermittent infusions or direct administration of drugs.

catheter. With this device, the needle is then removed, and a flexible cannula remains in the vein. When a site has been selected for venipuncture, place a tourniquet above the selected vein. It is important to tighten the tourniquet so that venous blood flow is blocked but arterial blood flow is not. Cleanse the site according to facility policy. The vein fills (distends) and then the skin is pulled taut (to anchor the vein and the skin) and the SPC is inserted into the vein with the needle bevel up and at a low angle to the skin (Fig. 54.2). Blood should immediately flow into the syringe if the needle is properly inserted into the vein. The needle is removed and the catheter is left in place and secured. The SPC device is ready for attachment to an IV line for continuous infusion or capping device for direct administration of drugs or fluids.

Performing a venipuncture requires practice. A suitable vein for venipuncture may be hard to find, and some veins are difficult to enter. Never repeatedly attempt an unsuccessful venipuncture. Depending on clinical judgment, two unsuccessful attempts on the same client warrant having a more skilled individual attempt the procedure (INS guidelines, 2020). Check facility policy regarding the number of times you can unsuccessfully attempt an IV start before you begin. Most agencies have training arms to learn and practice venous access; find out the policy for practicing and attend classes if you are interested in becoming proficient at starting IV access lines.

Maintaining IV Access

Fluids, electrolytes, and drugs are given by direct IV push, intermittent infusion, or continuous infusion. Direct push is not covered in this textbook, consult the clinical pharmacist for accurate information.

Intermittent IV Access

When the direct IV push method or intermittent infusion is used, the cannula that stays in the vein, an adapter, and small tubing with a cap are used. This is called a **lock**, and it is secured to the arm (Fig. 54.3). The device allows for a dose to be given directly into a vein or via intermittent IV administration without having to maintain a constant IV infusion. A lock also gives the client the ability to move about more freely without cumbersome IV lines or machines to impede activities such as ambulation.

To maintain the patency of the lock, a solution of saline or dilute heparin may be ordered for injection into the lock before and after the administration of a drug administered via the IV route. This is called a *lock flush*. The flush solution aids in preventing small clots from obstructing the cannula of the IV administration set. Clients may hear providers refer to the device as both a saline or a heparin lock. The primary health care provider or institutional policy dictates the use and strength of an IV lock flush solution. It is important to know the policies of your institution to be sure that you access the device with the appropriate solution. Should the policy of your institution be the use of heparin, be sure to prevent incompatibility of heparin with other drugs, and flush with sterile normal saline solution before and after any drug is given through the IV line.

Concern regarding dilution of IV push medications has been studied extensively by the Institute for Safe Medication Practices (ISMP, 2018). Deutsch (2020) found nurses will open and dilute prepackaged IV single-use drugs because they worry about client comfort during the IV push procedure. ISMP cautions providers that this can cause infection and the clinical pharmacist should be consulted. Multiple IV medications should not be mixed in a syringe (e.g., benzodiazepines and furosemide) without consulting the clinical pharmacist about compatibility. When injecting multiple drugs sequentially, always flush thoroughly and monitor the IV site for phlebitis and/or thrombosis.

Continuous Infusion Access

Continuous infusion involves a continual flow of fluid into a vein for replacement purposes and continuous or frequent drug administration, see Box 54.1 for solution selection. Electronic infusion devices monitor the rate and flow of IV fluids (Fig. 54.4). The purpose of the device is to monitor the flow of the IV solution. An alarm is set to sound if the rate of infusion is more or less than the preset rate. These machines are classified as either infusion controllers or infusion pumps. The primary difference between the two is that an infusion pump adds pressure to the infusion, whereas an infusion controller does not.

When any problem is detected by the device, an alarm is activated to alert the nurse. Controllers and pumps have detectors and alarms that sound when various problems

BOX 54.1 Preferred IV Fluid Solutions

The primary health care provider specifically orders the IV fluid solution, yet it is good for you to understand and anticipate why certain IV solutions are chosen over other fluids.

- Lactated Ringer's—burns, trauma, obstetric (OB) procedures where significant blood loss occurs
- Normal Saline (0.9% NaCl)—compatible with blood products; clients with kidney disease or HF
- ½ Normal Saline (0.45% NaCl)—hypernatremia or excessive edema
- Plasma-Lyte A—used in place of LR, is compatible with blood products
- Dextrose in Water—dehydration or to reduce potassium or sodium blood levels

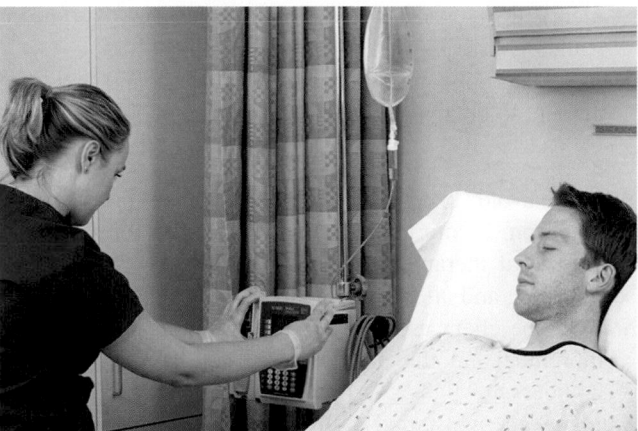

FIGURE 54.4 The nurse sets the electronic IV device to deliver a specific amount of IV fluid.

occur, such as air in the line, an occlusion, low battery, completion of an infusion, or an inability to deliver the preset rate.

! NURSING ALERT

Use of an infusion pump or controller still requires nursing supervision and frequent monitoring of the IV infusion.

It is important to monitor frequently for signs of **infiltration** (the collection of fluid into tissues), such as edema or redness at the site. Infiltration can progress rapidly because with the increased pressure the infusion will not slow until considerable edema has occurred. Careful monitoring of the pump or controller is also necessary to make sure the flow rate is correct.

When the client needs fluid replacement and at the same time drugs are to be administered, a secondary line is established using a connection called "Y" tubing. The drug solution will infuse in one arm of the "Y" while another solution is being given on a continuous basis in the other line of the "Y" tube. When this method is used, depending on the infusion machine you may have to clamp off the IV

fluid given on a continuous basis while the drug is allowed to infuse, or the two solutions may infuse at the same time.

Calculating IV Flow Rates

When fluid replacement is indicated, the amount (or volume) of fluid to be administered is ordered over a specified time period, such as 125 mL/hour or 1000 mL over 8 hours. Many infusion machines work by setting the volume of fluid to be infused over a specific time period. If the IV is not infused through a machine or if the machine monitors the drip rate, then the IV flow rate must be calculated.

The IV flow rate is obtained by counting the number of drops in the drip chamber and using the amount of fluid in each drop to calculate the volume. Drip chambers on the various types of IV fluid administration sets vary. Some deliver 15 drops/mL and others deliver more or less than this number. This is called the *drop factor*. The drop factor (number of drops/mL) is given on the package containing the drip chamber and IV tubing.

Below are three methods for calculating the IV infusion rate. Methods 1 and 2 can be used when the known factors are the total amount of solution, the drop factor, and the number of hours over which the solution is to be infused.

Method 1

Step 1. Total amount of solution ÷ number of hours = number of mL/hr.
Step 2. mL/hr ÷ 60 min/hr = number of mL/min.
Step 3. mL/min × drop factor = number of drops/min.

Example

1000 mL of an IV solution is to infuse over a period of 8 hours. The drop factor is 15.
Step 1. 1000 mL ÷ 8 hr = 125 mL/hr.
Step 2. 125 mL ÷ 60 min = 2.08 mL/min.
Step 3. 2.08 × 15 = 31.2 or (31–32) drops/min.

Method 2

Step 1. Total amount of solution ÷ number of hours = number of mL/hr.
Step 2. mL/hr × drop factor ÷ 60 = number of drops/min.

Example

1000 mL of an IV solution is to infuse over a period of 6 hours. The drop factor is 10.
Step 1. 1000 mL ÷ 6 hr = 166.6 mL/hr.
Step 2. 166.6 × 10 ÷ 60 = 26.66 or (26–27) drops/min.

Method 3

This method may be used when the desired amount of solution to be infused in 1 hour is known or written as a physician's order.

$$\frac{drops/mL \ of \ given \ set \ (drop \ factor)}{60 \times (minutes \ in \ an \ hour)} \times total \ hourly \ volume = drops/min$$

Example
If a set delivers 15 drops/min and 240 mL is to be infused in 1 hour:

$$\frac{15}{60} \times 240 = \frac{1}{4} \times 240 = 60 \, \text{drops/min}$$

Fluid Overload
One problem commonly associated with all solutions administered by the parenteral route is fluid overload, that is, the administration of more fluid than the body is able to handle.

The term **fluid overload** (also *circulatory overload*) describes a condition when the body's fluid requirements are met and the administration of fluid occurs at a rate that is greater than the rate at which the body can use or eliminate the fluid. Thus, the amount of fluid and the rate of administration of fluid that will cause fluid overload depend on several factors, such as the client's cardiac status and adequacy of renal function. The signs and symptoms of fluid overload are listed in Box 54.2.

Equal-Analgesic Conversions
Following surgical procedures, or when a client has severe, acute pain such as with kidney stones, IV opiate pain medication is frequently used. Sometimes when the client is ready for discharge and cannot take home the IV pain medication, the drug and dose will be changed to an oral form. Also, when a client has unrelieved pain and the drug form (IV, oral, dermal) is changed, you, as the nurse, want to be sure an equivalent dose is provided to support pain management. In these situations an equal-analgesic conversion chart is useful; converting opiate pain relievers to a different form or type of drug knowing you are giving something that is equivalent, not too high or low compared to the pain relief experienced.

Calculations for conversion use a chart to determine the amount of one drug compared to another drug. The drugs in the chart are all equal in strength to each other. By looking at the conversion box (Box 54.3) you will see that taking 30 mg of oral morphine is the equivalent to taking 10 mg of morphine by injection or 30 mg of oral morphine is the equivalent to 7.5 mg of oral hydromorphone.

Method
The following steps are used to convert opiate medications (Kishner & Schraga, 2016).

Step 1. Determine the total dose of the pain medication used during the last 24-hour period.

Step 2. Using the chart in Box 54.3, find the drug (in its current form) and convert it to an equivalent morphine dose.

Step 3. Convert the morphine dose to the new drug/form.

Step 4. Reduce the drug 50% (for elders/kidney impairment), 25%–50% (if good pain control), 0% (uncontrolled pain).

Step 5. Determine appropriate time intervals and divide up amount to be given over 1-day time frame.

Example
A 42-year-old knee replacement client is preparing to change from IV morphine to oral Vicoprofen for discharge. His physical therapy is rigorous and reports 7–8/10 pain scale during and after treatments.

Step 1. The client used patient-controlled analgesia (PCA) morphine and the dose was 20 mg IV over the last 24 hours.

Step 2. Since we started with morphine, we do not need to convert the drug. We determine the equivalent factor.

$$20 \, \text{mg IV} \div 10 \, \text{mg IV} = 2$$

Step 3. Vicoprofen (hydrocodone 7.5 mg/ibuprofen 200 mg in each tablet) is the new form. For this example, we are using just the opiate component. Find the equivalent (morphine 10 mg IV = hydrocodone 30–45 mg oral), then multiply by the factor of 2 (step 2), for this example, we will use the lower dose of hydrocodone.

BOX 54.2	Signs and Symptoms of Fluid Overload

- Headache
- Weakness
- Blurred vision
- Behavioral changes (confusion, disorientation, delirium, drowsiness)
- Weight gain
- Isolated muscle twitching
- Hyponatremia
- Rapid breathing
- Wheezing
- Coughing
- Rise in blood pressure
- Distended neck veins
- Elevated central venous pressure
- Convulsions

BOX 54.3	Equal-Analgesic Conversion

All drugs noted are equivalent strength.

Drug	Parenteral Dose (IV, Subcut, IM)	Oral
Morphine	10 mg	30 mg
Hydromorphone	1.5 mg	7.5 mg
Oxycodone	—	15–20 mg
Hydrocodone	—	30–45 mg
Oxymorphone	1 mg	10 mg
Fentanyl	0.2 mg	—

Kishner, S., & Schraga, E. (2016). *Opioid equivalents and conversions.* Medscape. Accessed March 1, 2017. http://emedicine.medscape.com/article/2138678-overview

$$30 \text{ mg} \times 2 = 60 \text{ mg}$$

Step 4. Looking at the client, no reduction for age or good pain control.

60 mg of hydrocodone to be given in a 24-hr period.

Step 5. Determine appropriate time intervals and divide up amount to be given over a 1-day time frame.

$$60 \text{ mg} \div 7.5 \text{ mg} = 8 \text{ tablets of vicoprofen}$$

Given every 6 hours (4 times daily) = 2 tablets of
vicoprofen each dose

Therefore, the client will need to take 2 tablets of Vicoprofen every 6 hours to maintain the pain relief of the 24-hr total dose of 20 mg IV morphine from the PCA infusion.

SOLUTIONS USED IN THE MANAGEMENT OF BODY FLUIDS

The next section gives a brief overview of the following IV replacement solutions: electrolytes, blood products and expanders, and **total parenteral nutrition**.

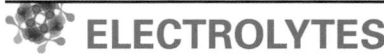 ELECTROLYTES

One of the primary purposes of administering an IV solution is to provide proper electrolyte balance in the body. An **electrolyte** is an electrically charged particle essential to the normal functioning of all cells. Intracellular and extracellular fluids have specific chemical compositions of electrolytes. Major electrolytes in intracellular fluid include:

- Potassium
- Magnesium

Major electrolytes in extracellular fluid include:

- Sodium
- Calcium

ELECTROLYTE IMBALANCES

Electrolytes circulate in the blood at specific levels, where they are available for use when needed by the cells. An electrolyte imbalance occurs when the concentration of an electrolyte in the blood is either too high or too low. In some instances, an electrolyte imbalance may be present without an appreciable disturbance in fluid balance. An electrolyte imbalance can profoundly affect a client's physiologic functioning, the body's water distribution, neuromuscular activity, and acid–base balance.

An electrolyte imbalance can occur from any disorder that alters electrolyte levels in the body's fluid compartments. An imbalance can also occur from vomiting, surgery, diagnostic tests, or drug administration. For example, a client taking a diuretic is typically able to maintain fluid balance by

an adequate oral intake of water, which replaces the water lost through diuresis. However, most clients are unable to replace by diet alone, the potassium that is also lost during diuresis.

When the potassium concentration in the blood is too low, as may occur with the administration of a diuretic, an imbalance may occur that requires the supplement of potassium. Electrolyte supplement (or replacement) drugs are inorganic or organic salts that increase deficient electrolyte levels that help to maintain homeostasis. Commonly used electrolyte replacement drugs are listed in the Summary Drug Table: Electrolytes.

INTRACELLULAR ELECTROLYTES

Action and Uses
Potassium (K⁺)

Potassium is the major electrolyte in intracellular fluid and must be consumed daily because it cannot be stored. It is necessary for the transmission of impulses; the contraction of smooth, cardiac, and skeletal muscles; and other important physiologic processes. Potassium may be given to correct hypokalemia (low blood potassium) resulting from increased potassium excretion or depletion. Examples of causes of hypokalemia are a marked loss of GI fluids (severe vomiting, diarrhea, nasogastric suction, draining intestinal fistulas), diabetic acidosis, marked diuresis, severe malnutrition, use of a potassium-depleting diuretic, excess antidiuretic hormone, and excessive urination. Potassium as a drug is available as potassium chloride (KCl) and potassium gluconate and is measured in milliequivalents (mEq)—for example, 40 mEq in 20 mL or 8-mEq controlled-release tablet.

Magnesium (Mg⁺⁺)

Magnesium plays an important role in the transmission of nerve impulses. It is also important in the activity of many enzyme reactions, such as carbohydrate metabolism. Magnesium sulfate is used as replacement therapy in hypomagnesemia. Magnesium is also used in the prevention and control of seizures in obstetric clients with pregnancy-induced hypertension (PIH; also referred to as *eclampsia* and *preeclampsia*). It may also be added to TPN mixtures.

> **! NURSING ALERT**
>
> The form of magnesium known as magnesium *citrate* is a laxative. The product label should be read carefully when administering to be sure a laxative is not given in place of supplement drug.

Adverse Reactions, Contraindications, Precautions, and Interactions
Potassium (K⁺)

Nausea, vomiting, diarrhea, abdominal pain, and phlebitis have been seen with oral and IV administration of potassium. Adverse reactions related to hypokalemia or hyperkalemia are listed in Box 54.4.

BOX 54.4 Signs and Symptoms of Electrolyte Imbalances

Calcium
Normal laboratory values: 4.5–5.3 mEq/L or 9–11 mg/dL[a]

Hypocalcemia
Hyperactive reflexes, carpopedal spasm, perioral paresthesias, positive Trousseau sign, positive Chvostek sign, muscle twitching, muscle cramps, tetany (numbness, tingling, and muscular twitching usually of the extremities), laryngospasm, cardiac arrhythmias, nausea, vomiting, anxiety, confusion, emotional lability, convulsions.

Hypercalcemia
Anorexia, nausea, vomiting, lethargy, bone tenderness or pain, polyuria, polydipsia, constipation, dehydration, muscle weakness and atrophy, stupor, coma, cardiac arrest.

Magnesium
Normal laboratory values: 1.5–2.5 mEq/L or 1.8–3.0 mg/dL[a]

Hypomagnesemia
Leg and foot cramps, hypertension, tachycardia, neuromuscular irritability, tremor, hyperactive deep tendon reflexes, confusion, disorientation, visual or auditory hallucinations, painful paresthesias, positive Trousseau sign, positive Chvostek sign, convulsions.

Hypermagnesemia
Lethargy, drowsiness, impaired respiration, flushing, sweating, hypotension, weak to absent deep tendon reflexes.

Potassium
Normal laboratory values: 3.5–5.0 mEq/L[a]

Hypokalemia
Anorexia, nausea, vomiting, mental depression, confusion, delayed or impaired thought processes, drowsiness, abdominal distention, decreased bowel sounds, paralytic ileus, muscle weakness or fatigue, flaccid paralysis, absent or diminished deep tendon reflexes, weak and irregular pulse, paresthesias, leg cramps, electrocardiographic changes.

Hyperkalemia
Irritability, anxiety, listlessness, mental confusion, nausea, diarrhea, abdominal distress, GI hyperactivity, paresthesias, weakness and heaviness of the legs, flaccid paralysis, hypotension, cardiac arrhythmias, electrocardiographic changes.

Sodium
Normal laboratory values: 132–145 mEq/L[a]

Hyponatremia
Cold and clammy skin, decreased skin turgor, apprehension, confusion, irritability, anxiety, hypotension, postural hypotension, tachycardia, headache, tremors, convulsions, abdominal cramps, nausea, vomiting, diarrhea.

Hypernatremia
Fever; hot, dry skin; dry, sticky mucous membranes; rough, dry tongue; edema; weight gain; intense thirst; excitement; restlessness; agitation; oliguria or anuria.

[a]Normal laboratory values ranges vary according to equipment used. This is a general range of electrolyte normalcy. The specific facility policy manual or laboratory values sheet should be consulted for the normal ranges of all laboratory tests.

Potassium is contraindicated in clients who are at risk for hyperkalemia, such as those with renal failure, oliguria, azotemia (the presence of nitrogen-containing compounds in the blood), anuria, severe hemolytic reactions, untreated Addison disease, acute dehydration, heat cramps, and any form of hyperkalemia. Potassium is used cautiously in clients with renal impairment or adrenal insufficiency, heart disease, metabolic acidosis, or prolonged or severe diarrhea.

Concurrent use of potassium with angiotensin-converting enzyme (ACE) inhibitors may result in an elevated serum potassium level. Potassium-sparing diuretics and salt substitutes used with potassium can produce severe hyperkalemia. The use of digitalis with potassium increases the risk of digoxin toxicity.

Magnesium (Mg++)
Adverse reactions from magnesium administration are most likely related to overdose and may include flushing, sweating, hypotension, depressed reflexes, muscle weakness, respiratory failure, and circulatory collapse (see Box 54.4). Magnesium is contraindicated in clients with heart block or myocardial damage and in women with PIH during the 2 hours before delivery. Magnesium is a pregnancy category A drug, and there is no increased risk of fetal abnormalities if the agent is used during pregnancy. Nevertheless, caution is used when administering magnesium during pregnancy.

Magnesium is used with caution in clients with renal function impairment. When magnesium is used with alcohol, antidepressants, antipsychotics, barbiturates, hypnotics, general anesthetics, and opioids, an increase in central nervous system depression may occur. Prolonged respiratory depression and apnea may occur when magnesium is administered with the neuromuscular-blocking agents. When magnesium is used with digoxin, heart block may occur.

EXTRACELLULAR ELECTROLYTES

Action and Uses
Sodium (Na+)
Sodium is a major electrolyte in extracellular fluid and is important in maintaining acid–base balance and normal heart action, and in the regulation of osmotic pressure in body cells (water balance). Sodium is administered for hyponatremia (low blood sodium). Examples of causes of hyponatremia are excessive diaphoresis, severe vomiting or

diarrhea, excessive diuresis, diuretic use, wound drainage, and draining intestinal fistulas.

Sodium, as sodium chloride (NaCl), may be given IV. A solution containing 0.9% NaCl is called *normal saline,* and a solution containing 0.45% NaCl is called half-normal saline. Sodium also is available combined with dextrose, such as dextrose 5% and sodium chloride 0.9% (D5NS).

Calcium (Ca⁺⁺)

Calcium is necessary for the functioning of nerves and muscles, the clotting of blood, the building of bones and teeth, and other physiologic processes. Examples of calcium salts are calcium gluconate and calcium carbonate. Calcium may be given for the treatment of hypocalcemia (low blood calcium), which may be seen in those with parathyroid disease or after accidental removal of the parathyroid glands during surgery of the thyroid gland. Calcium may also be given during cardiopulmonary resuscitation, particularly after open-heart surgery, when epinephrine fails to improve weak or ineffective myocardial contractions. Calcium may also be recommended for those eating a diet low in calcium or as a dietary supplement when there is an increased need for calcium, such as during pregnancy.

Combined Electrolyte Solutions

Combined electrolyte solutions are available for oral and IV administration. The IV solutions contain various electrolytes and dextrose. The amount of electrolytes, given as milliequivalents per liter (mEq/L), also varies. The IV solutions are used to replace fluid and electrolytes that have been lost and to provide calories through their carbohydrate content. Examples of IV electrolyte solutions are dextrose 5% with 0.9% NaCl, lactated Ringer (LR), and Plasma-Lyte. The primary health care provider selects the type of combined electrolyte solution that will meet the client's needs.

Oral electrolyte solutions contain a carbohydrate and various electrolytes. Examples of combined oral electrolyte solutions are Pedialyte and Rehydralyte. Oral electrolyte solutions are most often used to replace lost electrolytes and fluids in conditions such as severe vomiting or diarrhea.

Adverse Reactions, Contraindications, Precautions, and Interactions

Sodium (Na⁺)

Sodium as the salt (i.e., NaCl) has no adverse reactions except those related to overdose (see Box 54.4). In some instances, excessive oral use may produce nausea and vomiting.

Sodium is contraindicated in clients with hypernatremia or fluid retention and when the administration of sodium or chloride could be detrimental. Sodium is used cautiously in surgical clients and those with circulatory insufficiency, hypoproteinemia, urinary tract obstruction, heart failure (HF), edema, or renal impairment. Sodium is a pregnancy category C drug and is used cautiously during pregnancy.

Calcium (Ca⁺⁺)

Irritation of the vein used for administration, tingling, a metallic or chalky taste, and "heat waves" may occur when calcium is given IV. Rapid IV administration (calcium gluconate) may result in bradycardia, vasodilation, decreased blood pressure, cardiac arrhythmias, and cardiac arrest. Oral administration may result in GI disturbances. Administration of calcium chloride may cause peripheral vasodilation, a temporary fall in blood pressure, and local burning. Box 54.4 lists adverse reactions associated with hypercalcemia and hypocalcemia.

BLOOD PRODUCTS AND EXPANDERS

ACTIONS AND USES

Blood Plasma

Blood plasma is the liquid part of blood, containing water, sugar, electrolytes, fats, gases, proteins, bile pigment, and clotting factors. Human plasma, also called human pooled plasma, is obtained from donated blood. Although whole blood must be typed and crossmatched, plasma does not. This is because it lacks the red blood cells which determine blood type and Rh factors. Therefore, plasma can be given in acute emergencies before typing and crossmatching happens.

Plasma-administered IV is used to increase blood volume when severe hemorrhage has occurred, and it is necessary partially to restore blood volume while waiting for whole blood to be typed and crossmatched or when plasma alone has been lost, as may be seen in severe burns.

Plasma Protein Fractions

Plasma protein fractions include human plasma protein fraction 5% and normal serum albumin 5% (Albuminar-5, Buminate 5%) and normal serum albumin 25% (Albuminar-25, Buminate 25%). Plasma protein fraction 5% is an IV solution containing 5% human plasma proteins. Serum albumin is obtained from donated whole blood and is a protein found in plasma. The albumin fraction of human blood acts to maintain plasma colloid osmotic pressure and as a carrier of intermediate metabolites in the transport and exchange of tissue products. It is critical in regulating the volume of circulating blood. When blood is lost from shock, such as in hemorrhage, there is a reduced plasma volume. When blood volume is reduced, albumin quickly restores the volume in most situations.

Plasma protein fractions are used to treat hypovolemic (low blood volume) shock that occurs as a result of burns, trauma, surgery, and infections, or in conditions where shock is not currently present but likely to occur. As with human pooled plasma, blood type and crossmatch are not needed when plasma protein fractions are given. Adverse reactions are rare when plasma protein fractions are administered, but nausea, chills, fever, urticaria, and hypotensive episodes may occasionally be seen. Plasma proteins are contraindicated in those with a history of allergic reactions to albumin, severe anemia, or cardiac failure; in the presence of normal or increased intravascular volume; and in clients on cardiopulmonary bypass. Plasma protein fractions are used cautiously in clients who are in shock or dehydrated and in those with HF or hepatic or renal failure.

"Convalescent plasma" is a term used for plasma drawn from a client with a specific disease. Once a person has survived viral illness like Ebola or COVID-19, their plasma is full of antibodies to the virus. In efforts to treat clients of a specific viral infection like those above, plasma from an illness survivor (or a convalescent client) is collected and infused into clients with the disease in an effort to build antibody protection (Rubin, 2020).

Most of these solutions should not be combined with any other solutions or drugs but should be administered alone. Consult the drug insert or other appropriate sources before combining any drug with any plasma protein fraction. Solutions used in the management of body fluids are contraindicated in clients with hypersensitivity to any component of the solution. All solutions used to manage body fluids discussed in this chapter are pregnancy category C drugs and are used cautiously during pregnancy and lactation. No interactions have been reported.

Plasma Expanders

The IV solutions of plasma expanders include hetastarch (Hespan), low-molecular-weight dextran (Dextran 40), and high-molecular-weight dextran (Dextran 70, Dextran 75).

Plasma expanders are used to expand plasma volume when shock is caused by burns, hemorrhage, surgery, and other trauma or for prophylaxis of venous thrombosis and thromboembolism. When used in the treatment of shock, plasma expanders are not a substitute for whole blood or plasma but they are of value as emergency measures until the latter substances can be used.

Administration of hetastarch, a plasma expander, may be accompanied by vomiting, a mild temperature elevation, itching, and allergic reactions. Allergic reactions are evidenced by wheezing, swelling around the eyes (periorbital edema), and urticaria. Other plasma expanders may result in mild cutaneous eruptions, generalized urticaria, hypotension, nausea, vomiting, headache, dyspnea, fever, tightness of the chest, bronchospasm, wheezing, and, rarely, anaphylactic shock.

Plasma expanders are contraindicated in clients with hypersensitivity to any component of the solution and those with severe bleeding disorders, severe cardiac failure, renal failure with oliguria, or anuria. Plasma expanders are used cautiously in clients with renal disease, HF, pulmonary edema, and severe bleeding disorders. Plasma expanders are pregnancy category C drugs and are used cautiously during pregnancy and lactation. Consult the drug insert or other appropriate sources before combining a plasma expander with another drug for IV administration.

TOTAL PARENTERAL NUTRITION

When normal enteral feeding is not possible or is inadequate to meet an individual's nutritional needs, IV nutritional therapy or TPN is required. TPN is a method of administering nutrients to the body by an IV route. TPN uses a complex admixture of chemicals combined in a single container. The components of the TPN mixture may include proteins (amino acids), fats, glucose, electrolytes, vitamins, minerals, and sterile water. Products used to meet the IV nutritional requirements of the client include protein substrates (amino acids), energy substrates (dextrose and fat emulsions), fluids, electrolytes, and trace minerals.

TPN is used to prevent nitrogen and weight loss or to treat negative nitrogen balance (a situation in which more nitrogen is used by the body than is taken in) in the following situations:

- When oral, gastrostomy, or jejunostomy route cannot or should not be used.
- GI absorption of protein is impaired by obstruction.
- Inflammatory disease or antineoplastic therapy prevents normal GI functioning.
- Bowel rest is needed (e.g., after bowel surgery).
- Metabolic requirements for protein are significantly increased (e.g., in hypermetabolic states such as serious burns, infections, or trauma).
- Morbidity and mortality may be reduced by replacing amino acids lost from tissue breakdown (e.g., renal failure).
- Tube feeding alone cannot provide adequate nutrition.

RATIONALE

If a client's intake of protein nutrients is significantly less than is required by the body to meet energy expenditures, a state of negative nitrogen balance occurs. The body begins to convert protein from the muscle into carbohydrate for energy to be used by the body. This results in weight loss and muscle wasting. In these situations, traditional IV fluids do not provide sufficient calories or nitrogen to meet the body's daily requirements.

DELIVERY

TPN may be administered through a peripheral vein or a central venous catheter in a highly concentrated form to improve nutritional status, establish a positive nitrogen balance, and enhance the healing process. Peripheral TPN is used for relatively short periods (no more than 5–7 days) and when the central venous route is not possible or necessary. An example of a solution used in TPN is amino acids with electrolytes. These solutions may be used alone or combined with dextrose (5% or 10%) solutions.

TPN through a central vein is indicated to promote protein synthesis in clients who are severely hypercatabolic or severely depleted of nutrients, or who require long-term parenteral nutrition. For example, amino acids combined with hypertonic dextrose and IV fat emulsions (IVFEs) are infused through a central venous catheter to promote protein synthesis. Vitamins, trace minerals, and electrolytes may be added to the TPN mixture to meet the client's individual needs. The daily dose depends on the client's daily protein requirement and their metabolic state and clinical responses.

TPN is delivered via an infusion pump. The pump infuses a small amount (0.1–10 mL/hour) continuously to keep the vein open. Feeding schedules vary; one example is administration of the feeding continuously over a few hours, leveling off the rate for several hours, and then increasing the rate of administration for several hours to simulate a normal set of meal times.

HYPER/HYPOGLYCEMIA

Hyperglycemia is a metabolic complication seen with TPN infusions. If an infusion of TPN is given too rapidly it may result in hyperglycemia, glycosuria, mental confusion, and loss of consciousness. The use of fat emulsions (see below) helps to deliver calories without raising the level of glucose in TPN preparations (Spray, 2016). Blood glucose levels are monitored every 4–6 hours to identify hyperglycemia. To minimize these complications, the primary health care provider may decrease the rate of administration, reduce the dextrose concentration, or order administration of insulin.

Because TPN contains a concentrated dose of dextrose, the sudden withdrawal of the infusion can result in a rebound hypoglycemic reaction. To prevent this, the rate of administration is slowly reduced or the concentration of dextrose gradually decreased.

If TPN must be abruptly withdrawn, a solution of 5% or 10% dextrose is hung in its place to reduce gradually the amount of dextrose administered. The primary health care provider is notified if the client exhibits symptoms of hypoglycemia, including weakness, tremors, diaphoresis, headache, hunger, and apprehension. Other complications of TPN include bacterial infection, sepsis, embolism, metabolic problems, and hemothorax or pneumothorax.

FAT EMULSIONS

An important source of both calories and essential fatty acids is an IVFE. The body needs fat (or lipids) to aid in metabolism and to help cells function (Spray, 2016). Made from soybean or safflower oil and a mixture of natural triglycerides, it is used in the prevention and treatment of essential fatty acid deficiency. It also provides nonprotein calories for those receiving TPN when calorie requirements cannot be met by glucose alone. Examples of IVFE include Intralipid, Nutrilipid, and Liposyn III. Fat emulsion is used for clients requiring parenteral nutrition for extended periods (usually more than 5 days). No more than 60% of the client's total caloric intake should come from

fat emulsion, with carbohydrates and amino acids making up the remaining 40% or more of caloric intake.

The most common adverse reaction associated with the administration of fat emulsion is sepsis caused by administration equipment and thrombophlebitis caused by venous irritation from concurrently administering hypertonic solutions. Less frequent adverse reactions include dyspnea, cyanosis, hyperlipidemia, hypercoagulability, nausea, vomiting, headache, flushing, increased body temperature, sweating, sleepiness, chest and back pain, slight pressure over the eyes, and dizziness. IVFEs are contraindicated in conditions that interfere with normal fat metabolism (e.g., acute pancreatitis) and in clients allergic to eggs. IVFEs are used with caution in those with severe liver impairment, pulmonary disease, anemia, and blood coagulation disorders. These solutions are pregnancy category C drugs and are used cautiously during pregnancy and lactation.

PRACTICE CONSIDERATIONS

Fat emulsions can be used to prevent systemic absorption of a local anesthetic. In the condition of local anesthetic systemic toxicity (LAST), the anesthetic accidently gets into the systemic circulation. The lipid infusion works as an antidote pulling the anesthetic drug out of tissues (Spray, 2016).

Fat emulsions are attached to the TPN IV line distal to the client to allow the fluids to mix before entering the body. In general, fat emulsions should not be combined with any other solutions or drugs except when the drug is already combined in TPN. Consult appropriate sources before combining any drug with a fat emulsion.

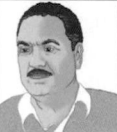

PHARMACOLOGY IN PRACTICE

SAFE DRUG ADMINISTRATION
A nurse is caring for a client who is being administered TPN. What percentage of the client's total caloric intake should be from a lipid infusion?
1. Less than 10%
2. A 50/50 ratio
3. No more than 60%
4. Approximately 85%

ALKALINIZING AND ACIDIFYING DRUGS

Acid-base imbalances involve the pH level in the blood plasma. A low blood pH means the body is in an acidic condition, and a high blood pH indicates an alkaline condition. Alkalinizing and acidifying drugs are used to correct an acid–base imbalance in the blood. The acid–base imbalances are:

- Metabolic acidosis—decrease in the blood pH (below 7.35) caused by an excess of hydrogen ions in the extracellular fluid (treated with alkalinizing drugs)
- Metabolic alkalosis—increase in the blood pH (above 7.45) caused by an excess of bicarbonate in the extracellular fluid (treated with acidifying drugs)

ALKALINIZING DRUG: BICARBONATE (HCO_3^-)

Correcting Metabolic Acidosis

When the blood plasma pH is below 7.35, this is an acidic condition and the plasma needs to be brought back into the normal range (7.35–7.45). Bicarbonate (HCO_3^-) plays a vital role in the acid–base balance of the body. Alkalinizing drugs are used to treat metabolic acidosis and to increase blood pH. Sodium bicarbonate, an alkalinizing drug, separates in the blood and the bicarbonate functions as a buffer to decrease the hydrogen ion concentration and raise the blood pH.

Sodium bicarbonate ($NaHCO_3$) may be given IV in the treatment of metabolic acidosis, a state of imbalance that may be seen in diseases or conditions such as severe shock, diabetic acidosis, severe diarrhea, extracorporeal circulation of blood, severe renal disease, and cardiac arrest. Oral sodium bicarbonate is used as a gastric and urinary alkalinizer. It may be used as a single drug or may be found as one of the ingredients in some antacid preparations. It is also useful in treating severe diarrhea accompanied by bicarbonate loss.

Adverse Reactions, Contraindications, Precautions, and Interactions

In some instances, excessive oral use of bicarbonate may produce nausea and vomiting. Some individuals may use sodium bicarbonate (baking soda) for the relief of GI disturbances such as pain, discomfort, symptoms of indigestion, and gas. Prolonged use of oral sodium bicarbonate or excessive doses of IV sodium bicarbonate may result in systemic alkalosis.

Bicarbonate is contraindicated in clients losing chloride by continuous GI suction or through vomiting; in clients with metabolic or respiratory alkalosis, hypocalcemia, renal failure, or severe abdominal pain of unknown cause; and in those on sodium-restricted diets.

Bicarbonate is used cautiously in clients with HF or renal impairment and those receiving glucocorticoid therapy. Bicarbonate is a pregnancy category C drug and is used cautiously during pregnancy.

Oral administration of bicarbonate may decrease the absorption of ketoconazole. Increased blood levels of quinidine, flecainide, or sympathomimetics may occur when these agents are administered with bicarbonate. There is an increased risk of crystalluria when bicarbonate is administered with the fluoroquinolones. Possible decreased effects of lithium, methotrexate, chlorpropamide, salicylates, and tetracyclines may occur when these drugs are administered with sodium bicarbonate. Sodium bicarbonate is not administered within 2 hours of enteric-coated drugs because the protective enteric coating may disintegrate before the drug reaches the intestine.

ACIDIFYING DRUG: AMMONIUM CHLORIDE

Correcting Metabolic Alkalosis

Metabolic alkalosis occurs when the body loses too much acid. This can happen with excessive vomiting, over use of diuretics, too much alcohol or antacid use. Ammonium chloride lowers the blood pH by being metabolized first into urea, then to hydrochloric acid, which is further metabolized to hydrogen ions to acidify the blood.

Adverse Reactions and Interactions

Adverse reactions to ammonium chloride include metabolic acidosis and loss of electrolytes, especially potassium. Use of ammonium chloride and spironolactone may increase systemic acidosis.

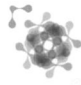

NURSING PROCESS: STEPS TO BUILDING CLINICAL JUDGMENT
Client Receiving a Solution for Management of Body Fluids

ASSESSMENT

Preadministration Assessment

Data gathering suggestions before administering an IV solution include:
Objective data

- Description of client's general status
- Vital signs (temperature, pulse, respirations, and blood pressure)
- Review of recent laboratory results (renal and hepatic function tests, complete blood count, and urinalysis if client has impaired function)
- Client weight
- Assess for signs of electrolyte imbalance (see Box 54.4)

- Assess site for IV insertion or IV site and line if existing
Subjective data

- Current symptoms resulting in need for fluids or electrolytes
- Allergy history, particularly a drug allergy

Ongoing Assessment

During the ongoing assessment of an IV line, site inspection is typically dictated by type of infusion and acuity of the client. A general guideline is as follows:

- Infusion of nonirritating fluids to alert/oriented adults—at least every 4 hours
- Infusion in a critical client, those unable to notify the nurse—every 1–2 hours

- Infusion into a neonatal or pediatric client—every hour
- Infusion of vesicant or vasoconstrictive solutions—every 5–15 minutes

The needle site is inspected for signs of **extravasation** (escape of fluid from a blood vessel into surrounding tissues) or infiltration (the collection of fluid into tissues). If signs of extravasation or infiltration are apparent, restart the infusion in another vein.

When the client is in a critical condition, a central venous pressure line may be inserted to monitor the client's response to therapy. Central venous pressure readings are taken as ordered. During administration of fluids and electrolytes in the critical setting, the blood pressure, pulse, and respiratory rate are continuously monitored. For example, a client in shock and receiving a plasma expander is monitored continuously, whereas the client with a saline lock 3 days after surgery may require monitoring only once or twice a shift.

During therapy, serum electrolyte or bicarbonate studies are drawn to monitor therapy.

Potassium

Clients receiving oral potassium should have their blood pressure and pulse monitored frequently, especially during early therapy. Observe the client for signs of hyperkalemia (see Box 54.4), which would indicate that the dose of potassium is too high. Signs of hypokalemia may also occur during therapy and may indicate that the dose of potassium is too low and must be increased. If signs of hypokalemia or hyperkalemia are apparent or suspected, contact the primary health care provider. In some instances, frequent laboratory monitoring of the serum potassium may be ordered.

Potassium is irritating to the tissues. When infusing potassium, inspect the IV needle site every 5–15 minutes for signs of extravasation. If extravasation occurs, discontinue the IV immediately and notify the primary health care provider. Best to check your facility's extravasation treatment protocol before therapy is initiated and have supplies readily available to treat the tissues, delaying further tissue damage.

The acutely ill client and the client with severe hypokalemia require ongoing cardiac monitoring during the IV infusion. Measure and record the intake and output every 8 hours. The infusion rate is slowed to keep the vein open, and the primary health care provider is notified if an irregular pulse is noted.

Calcium

Before, during, and after the administration of IV calcium, monitor the blood pressure, pulse, and respiratory rate every 5–15 minutes until the client's condition has stabilized. After administration of calcium, observe the client for signs of hypercalcemia (see Box 54.4).

⚠ NURSING ALERT

Overloading of calcium ions in the systemic circulation results in acute hypercalcemic syndrome. Symptoms of hypercalcemic syndrome include elevated plasma calcium, weakness, lethargy, severe nausea and vomiting, coma, and, if left untreated, death. Report signs of hypercalcemic syndrome immediately to the primary health care provider.

To combat hypercalcemic syndrome, the primary health care provider may prescribe IV sodium chloride and a potent IV diuretic such as furosemide. When used together, these two drugs markedly increase calcium renal clearance and reduce hypercalcemia.

Sodium

When NaCl is administered by IV infusion, observe the client during and after administration for signs of hypernatremia (see Box 54.4). Check the rate of IV infusion as ordered by the primary health care provider, usually every 5–15 minutes. To minimize venous irritation during administration of sodium or any electrolyte solution, use a small-bore needle placed well within the lumen of a large vein.

Clients receiving a 3% or 5% NaCl solution by IV infusion are observed closely for signs of pulmonary edema (i.e., dyspnea, cough, restlessness, bradycardia). If any one or more of these symptoms occurs, the IV infusion is slowed to keep the vein open and the primary health care provider is contacted immediately. Clients receiving NaCl by the IV route have their intake and output measured every 8 hours. Observe the client for signs of hypernatremia every 3–4 hours and contact the primary health care provider if this condition is suspected.

Magnesium

When magnesium is ordered to treat convulsions or severe hypomagnesemia, the client requires constant observation. Obtain the client's blood pressure, pulse, and respiratory rate immediately before the drug is administered, as well as place the client on a device for continuous monitoring. Continue monitoring these vital signs at frequent intervals until the client's condition has stabilized. Because magnesium is eliminated by the kidneys, it is used with caution in clients with renal impairment. Monitor the urine output to verify an output of at least 100 mL every 4 hours. Voiding less than 100 mL of urine every 4 hours is reported to the primary health care provider.

Bicarbonate

When given for the treatment of metabolic acidosis, the drug may be added to the IV fluid or given as a prepared IV sodium bicarbonate solution. Frequent laboratory monitoring of the blood pH and blood gases is usually ordered because dosage and length of therapy depend on test results. Observe frequently for signs of clinical improvement and monitor the blood pressure, pulse, and respiratory rate every 15–30 minutes or as ordered by the primary health care provider. Extravasation of the drug requires selection of another needle site because the drug is irritating to the tissues.

Fat Emulsions

When a fat emulsion is administered, monitor the client's ability to eliminate the infused fat from the circulation, because the lipidemia must clear between daily infusions. Additionally, monitor for lipidemia by assessing the results of the following laboratory examinations: hemogram, blood coagulation, liver function tests, plasma lipid profile, and platelet count. Report an increase in the results of any of these laboratory examinations as abnormal.

NURSING DIAGNOSES

Drug-specific nursing diagnoses include the following:

- **Fluid overload** related to adverse effects resulting from too rapid IV infusion
- **Hypovolemia** related to inability to take oral fluids, abnormal fluid loss, other factors (specify cause of hypovolemia)
- **Malnutrition risk** related to anorexia caused by opioids
- **Injury risk** related to adverse drug effects (muscular weakness)
- **Acute confusion** related to adverse drug effects
- **Decreased cardiac output risk** related to adverse drug effects (cardiac arrhythmias)

Nursing diagnoses related to drug administration are discussed in Chapter 4.

PLANNING

The expected outcomes of the client depend on the specific drug, dose, route of administration, and reason for administration of an electrolyte or fluid but may include an optimal response to therapy, supporting the client needs related to the management of adverse reactions, and confidence in an understanding of the treatment regimen.

IMPLEMENTATION

Promoting an Optimal Response to Therapy

The extremity used for administration should be made comfortable and supported, as needed, by a small pillow or other device. An IV infusion pump may be ordered for the administration of these solutions. Set the alarm of the infusion pump and check the functioning of the unit at frequent intervals.

NURSING ALERT

Administer all IV solutions with great care. At no time should any IV solution be infused at a rapid rate, unless there is a specific written order to do so.

Unless otherwise directed, the IV solution should be administered at room temperature. If the solution is refrigerated, allow the solution to warm by exposing it to room temperature 30–45 minutes before use. The average length of time for infusion of 1000 mL of an IV solution is 4–8 hours. One exception is when there is a written or verbal order by the primary health care provider to give the solution at a rapid rate because of an emergency. In this instance, the order must specifically state the rate of administration as drops per minute, milliliters per minute, or the period of time over which a specific amount of fluid is to be infused (e.g., 125 mL/hour or 1000 mL in 8 hours).

In some situations, electrolytes are administered when an electrolyte imbalance may potentially occur. For example, the client with nasogastric suction is prescribed one or more electrolytes added to an IV solution, such as 5% dextrose or a combined electrolyte solution, to be given IV to make up for the electrolytes that are lost through nasogastric suction. In other instances, electrolytes are given to replace those already lost, such as the client admitted to the hospital with severe vomiting and diarrhea of several days' duration.

When electrolytes are administered parenterally, the dosage is expressed in milliequivalents (mEq)—for example, calcium gluconate 7 mEq IV. When administered orally, sodium bicarbonate, calcium, and magnesium dosages are expressed in milligrams (mg). Potassium liquids and effervescent tablet dosages are expressed in milliequivalents; capsule or tablet dosages may be expressed as milliequivalents or milligrams.

Electrolyte disturbances can cause varying degrees of confusion, muscular weakness, nausea, vomiting, and cardiac irregularities (see Box 54.4 for specific symptoms). Serum electrolyte blood levels have a very narrow therapeutic range. Careful monitoring is needed to determine if blood levels fall above or below normal. Normal values may vary with the laboratory, but a general range of normal values for each electrolyte is found in Box 54.4. Adverse reactions are usually controlled by maintaining blood levels of the various electrolytes within the normal range.

Administering Potassium

When given orally, potassium may cause GI distress. Therefore, it is given immediately after meals or with food and a full glass of water. Oral potassium must not be crushed or chewed. If the client has difficulty swallowing, consult the primary health care provider regarding the use of a solution or an effervescent tablet, which fizzes and dissolves on contact with water. Potassium in the form of effervescent tablets, powder, or liquid must be thoroughly mixed with 4–8 ounces of cold water, juice, or other beverage. Effervescent tablets must stop fizzing before the solution is sipped slowly during a period of 5–15 minutes. Oral liquids and soluble powders that have been mixed and dissolved in cold water or juice are also sipped slowly over a period of 5–15 minutes. Advise clients that liquid potassium solutions have a salty taste. Some of these products are flavored to make the solution more palatable.

NURSING ALERT

Concentrated potassium solutions are for IV mixtures only and should never be used undiluted. Direct IV injection of potassium could result in sudden death. When potassium is given IV, it is always diluted in 500–1000 mL of an IV solution. The maximum recommended concentration of potassium is 80 mEq in 1000 mL of IV solution (although in acute emergency situations, a higher concentration of potassium may be required).

Administering Magnesium

Magnesium may be ordered intramuscularly (IM), IV, or by IV infusion diluted in a specified type and amount of IV solution. When ordered to be given IM, this drug is given undiluted as a 50% solution for adults and a 20% solution for children. Magnesium is given deep IM in a large muscle mass, such as the gluteus muscle.

Lifespan Considerations

Gerontology
Older adults may need a reduced dosage of magnesium because of decreased renal function. Closely monitor serum magnesium levels when magnesium is administered to older adults.

Monitor the client for early signs of hypermagnesemia (see Box 54.4) and contact the primary health care provider immediately if this imbalance is suspected. Frequent plasma magnesium levels are usually ordered. Contact the primary health care provider if the magnesium level is higher or lower than the normal range.

⚠ NURSING ALERT
As serum magnesium levels rise above 4 mEq/L, the deep tendon reflexes are first decreased and then disappear as the serum levels reach 10 mEq/L. The knee-jerk reflex is tested before each dose of magnesium. If the reflex is absent or a slow response is obtained, the nurse withholds the dosage and notifies the primary health care provider. IV calcium is kept available to reverse the respiratory depression and heart block that may occur with magnesium overdose.

Total Parenteral Nutrition
A microscopic filter is attached to the IV line when TPN solutions are administered. The filter prevents microscopic aggregates (particles that may form in the IV bag) from entering the bloodstream, where they could cause massive emboli.

Lipid Solutions
Fat solutions (emulsions) should be handled with care to decrease the risk of separation or "breaking out of the oil." Separation can be identified by yellowish streaking or the accumulation of yellowish droplets in the emulsion. Fat solutions are administered to adults at a rate no greater than 1–2 mL/minutes.

⚠ NURSING ALERT
During the first 30 minutes of infusion of a fat solution, carefully observe the client for difficulty in breathing, headache, flushing, nausea, vomiting, or signs of a hypersensitivity reaction. If any of these reactions occur, discontinue the infusion, keep the IV line open with fluid running, and immediately notify the primary health care provider.

Administering Bicarbonate
Give oral sodium bicarbonate tablets with a full glass of water; the powdered form is dissolved in a full glass of water. If oral sodium bicarbonate is used to alkalinize the urine, check the urine pH two or three times a day or as ordered by the primary health care provider. If the urine remains acidic, contact the primary health care provider, because an increase in the dose of the drug may be necessary. IV sodium bicarbonate is given in emergency situations, such as metabolic acidosis or certain types of drug overdose, when alkalinization of the urine is necessary to hasten drug elimination.

Monitoring and Managing Client Needs
When electrolyte solutions are administered, adverse reactions are most often related to overdose. Correcting the imbalance by decreasing the dosage or discontinuing the solution usually works, and the adverse reactions subside quickly. Frequent serum electrolyte levels are used to monitor blood levels.

Fluid Overload
Monitor clients receiving IV solutions at frequent intervals for signs of fluid overload. If signs of fluid overload (see Box 54.2) are observed, slow the IV infusion rate and immediately contact the primary health care provider.

Lifespan Considerations

Gerontology
Older adults are at increased risk of being fluid overloaded because of the increased incidence of cardiac disease and decreased renal function that may accompany old age. Careful monitoring for signs and symptoms of fluid overload is extremely important when administering fluids to older adults.

Hypovolemia and Malnutrition Risk
Often, the solutions used in the management of body fluids are given to correct a fluid volume deficit and to supply carbohydrates (nutrition). Review the client's record for a full understanding of the rationale for administration of the specific solution.

Electrolyte imbalances may cause nausea, vomiting, and other GI disturbances. If GI disturbances occur from oral administration, taking the drug with meals may decrease the nausea. Offering smaller, more frequent meals may help to stabilize nutritional status. Correcting the electrolyte imbalance usually solves the problem of nausea and vomiting.

Injury Risk
The client is at increased risk of falling because of weakness or muscular cramping. Frequent observation and quickly answering the call light help to maintain the client's safety. If weakness or muscular cramping occurs, assist the client when ambulating to prevent falls or other injury.

Acute Confusion
The client with an electrolyte imbalance may be confused or disoriented. Always identify yourself. Calling the client by name, tell the client where they are and approach the client in a calm and nurturing manner. Gently reorient or redirect the individual and explain any procedures carefully before performing any procedures with the client. Reassure the client that these symptoms are part of the imbalance but can recede as the imbalance improves (if applicable).

Decreased Cardiac Output Risk
Some electrolytes may cause cardiac irregularities. Check the pulse rate at regular intervals, telemetry or continual monitoring may be initiated if an irregularity in the heart rate is observed. For example, when potassium is administered to a client with cardiac

disease, a cardiac monitor is needed to monitor the heart rate and rhythm continuously during therapy.

NURSING ALERT

Mild (5.5–6.5 mEq/L) to moderate (6.5–8.0 mEq/L) potassium blood level increases may be asymptomatic and manifested only by increased serum potassium concentrations and characteristic electrocardiographic changes, such as disappearance of P waves or spreading (widening) of the QRS complex.

PHARMACOLOGY IN PRACTICE

MANAGING NEEDS

A nurse is caring for an 85-year-old client who needs to be administered IV fluids. What priority intervention should the nurse perform when monitoring and managing client needs?

1. Carefully monitor the client for signs and symptoms of fluid overload.
2. Carefully observe the client for difficulty in breathing, headache, or flushing.
3. Report any signs of hypercalcemic syndrome immediately to the primary health care provider.
4. Test the client's knee-jerk reflex before each dose to be administered.

Educating the Client and Family

When IV therapy is started, give the client or family a brief explanation of the reason for and the method of administration of an IV solution. Be sure and tell the client and family to notify you if the IV machine should alarm. Sometimes, when alarms go off, clients and families may feel the staff is too busy to respond and tamper with or adjust the rate of flow of IV administration sets. Emphasize the importance of calling for your help if there appears to be a problem with the IV site or the IV administration set or the equipment.

To ensure accurate adherence to the prescribed drug regimen, carefully explain the dose and time intervals to the client or a family member. Because overdose (which can be serious) may occur if the client does not adhere to the prescribed dosage and schedule, it is most important that the client completely understands how much and when to take the drug. Stress the importance of adhering to the prescribed dosage schedule during client teaching.

The primary health care provider may order periodic laboratory and diagnostic tests for some clients receiving oral electrolytes. Encourage the client to keep all appointments for these tests, as well as primary health care provider or clinic visits. Persons with a history of using sodium bicarbonate (baking soda) as an antacid are warned that overuse can result in alkalosis and could disguise a more serious problem.

EVALUATION

- Therapeutic response is achieved; fluid and electrolyte imbalances are corrected.
- Adverse reactions are identified, reported to the primary health care provider, and managed successfully with appropriate nursing interventions:
  - Client maintains an adequate fluid volume.
  - Client maintains an adequate nutritional status.
  - No evidence of injury is seen.
  - Orientation and mentation remain intact.
  - Cardiac output is maintained.
- Client and family express confidence and demonstrate an understanding of the drug regimen.

PHARMACOLOGY IN PRACTICE

USING CLINICAL REASONING

Mr. Garcia tells you that he has not deviated from the sodium-restricted diet that he was given. He cannot figure out why he has gained weight. He states that, with his heartburn, he knows he has been eating less. He also mentions that the soda bicarbonate he uses does little to relieve the heartburn. Describe how you would teach him about the side effects he is experiencing from the sodium bicarbonate.

KEY POINTS

- Fluids and electrolytes make up a major component of our bodies. Without fluids, the body's ability to transport oxygen and nutrients to the various tissues is compromised.

- Solutions used to manage body fluids are frequently delivered parenterally. Electrolytes, calories, or water is supplemented IV.

- IV access policies are written by each institution and include who may start lines, access them for administration, and monitor them.

- Venous access is typically initiated on a distal limb. Any provider should attempt venous access no more than two times before requesting assistance.

- IV sites should be routinely monitored no matter whether used for intermittent or continuous fluid.

- Solutions frequently infused include electrolytes, blood products, blood expanders, and TPN.

- Electrolytes circulate in the blood at specific levels, where they are available for use when needed by the cells. An electrolyte imbalance occurs when the concentration of an electrolyte in the blood is either too high or too low. An imbalance can also occur from vomiting, surgery, diagnostic tests, or drug administration.

- Blood products are used to increase blood volume from conditions such as hemorrhage or shock.

- TPN is used when the body cannot take in nutrients via the GI system.

- Conditions of acid–base imbalance can be corrected using drugs such as sodium bicarbonate.

SUMMARY DRUG TABLE
Electrolytes

Generic Name	Trade Name (Example)	Uses	Adverse Reactions	Dosage Ranges
calcium acetate	Phoslyra	Control of hyperphosphatemia in end-stage renal failure	See Box 54.4	3–4 tablets orally with each meal
calcium carbonate, citrate, gluconate, lactate	Tums, Citracal, Cal-Glu, Cal-lac	Dietary supplement for prevention or treatment of calcium deficiency, antacid	Rare; see Box 54.4 for signs of hypercalcemia	500–2000 mg/day orally
magnesium gluconate, L-aspartate, oxide	Slow-Mag	Dietary supplement, hypomagnesemia	Rare; see Box 54.4 for signs of hypermagnesemia	54–483 mg/day orally
magnesium sulfate (parenteral)		Mild to severe hypomagnesemia, seizures	Toxicity, weak or absent deep tendon reflexes, flaccid paralysis, drowsiness, stupor, weak pulse, arrhythmias, hypotension, circulatory collapse, respiratory paralysis	Hypomagnesemia: 2–5 g IV in 1 L of solution; 4–5 g over 3 hours Seizures: 4–5 g magnesium sulfate in 250 mL D_5W; simultaneously give 4–5 g magnesium sulfate (undiluted) IM to each buttock for initial dose of 10–14 g; followed by 1–2 g/hour IV infusion until seizure controlled
magnesium citrate	Citroma	Laxative for bowel constipation	Diarrhea	As noted on product label
oral electrolyte mixtures	Infalyte Oral Solution, NaturaLyte, Pedialyte, Pedialyte Oral Electrolyte, Pedialyte Freezer Pops, Rehydralyte, Resol Solution	Maintenance of water and electrolytes after corrective parenteral therapy of severe diarrhea; maintenance to replace mild to moderate fluid losses when food and liquid intake are discontinued, to restore fluid and minerals lost in diarrhea and vomiting in infants and children	Rare	Individualize dosage following the guidelines on the product labeling
potassium replacements	CereSport, Klor-Con	Hypokalemia, supplement for possible depletion—diuretic use	most common: nausea, vomiting, diarrhea, flatulence, abdominal discomfort, skin rash	40–100 mEq/day orally
sodium chloride	Slo-Salt	Prevention or treatment of extracellular volume depletion, dehydration, sodium depletion, aid in the prevention of heat prostration	Nausea, vomiting, diarrhea, abdominal cramps, edema, irritability, restlessness, weakness, hypertension, tachycardia, fluid accumulation, pulmonary edema, respiratory arrest (see Box 54.2)	Individualize dosage

Continued

SUMMARY DRUG TABLE (continued)
Antibacterial Drugs That Disrupt Bacterial Cell Wall Synthesis

Generic Name	Trade Name	Uses	Adverse Reactions	Dosage Ranges
Alkalinizing Drugs				
bicarbonate		Metabolic acidosis, cardiac arrest, systemic and urinary alkalinization	Tetany, edema, gastric distention, flatulence, belching, hypokalemia, metabolic alkalosis	Metabolic acidosis and cardiac arrest: dosage varies depending on laboratory results and client's condition
				Urinary alkalinization: 4 g orally initially, followed by 1–2 g orally q6hr
Acidifying Drug				
ammonium chloride		Metabolic alkalosis	Loss of electrolytes, especially potassium, metabolic acidosis	Varies depending on client's tolerance and condition

CHAPTER REVIEW

Calculate Medication Dosages

1. The client is to receive 1000 mL of 5% dextrose in water during a period of 10 hours. Calculate how many milliliters should be infused each hour.
2. The client is prescribed potassium 40 mEq orally. The drug is available from the pharmacy in a solution of 20 mEq/15 mL. The nurse administers _____.

Prepare for the NCLEX

RECALL THE FACTS

1. Fluid and electrolytes make up what percentage of the body?
   1. 10%
   2. 33%
   3. 70%
   4. 99%
2. Parenteral therapy is initiated _____.
   1. because client is too tired to eat
   2. for provider ease
   3. because of inability to handle GI nutrition/fluid
   4. because of better outcomes
3. Which of the following is a symptom of fluid overload?
   1. Tinnitus
   2. Hypotension
   3. Decreased body temperature
   4. Behavioral changes
4. Which of the following symptoms would indicate hypocalcemia?
   1. Tetany
   2. Constipation
   3. Muscle weakness
   4. Hypertension

5. Which of the following potassium serum concentration laboratory results would the nurse report immediately to the primary health care provider?
   1. 3 mEq/L
   2. 3.5 mEq/L
   3. 4.5 mEq/L
   4. 6 mEq/mL
6. Which of the following symptoms would most likely indicate hypernatremia?
   1. Fever, increased thirst
   2. Cold, clammy skin
   3. Decreased skin turgor
   4. Hypotension
7. Which of the following is a common metabolic complication of TPN?
   1. Hypomagnesemia
   2. Hypermagnesemia
   3. Hypoglycemia
   4. Hyperglycemia

ANALYZE THE FACTS

8. *When monitoring a client with an IV line, the nurse observes that the area around the needle insertion site is swollen and red. The first action of the nurse is to _____.
   1. check the client's blood pressure and pulse
   2. check further for possible extravasation
   3. ask the client if the IV site has been accidently injured
   4. immediately notify the primary health care provider

9. Which of the the following IV solutions must be typed and crossmatched for administration?
   1. Lipid solutions
   2. Platelets
   3. Whole blood
   4. Normal saline

ALTERNATE-FORMAT QUESTIONS

10. Order the steps used to start an IV access in a client.
   1. Apply tourniquet about intended puncture site.
   2. Inspect the limb.
   3. Cleanse the site for puncture.
   4. Ask the client about previous IV sites.
   5. Pull the skin taut for access.

To check your answers, see Appendix F.

---

*Indicates the question is directly linked to the NCLEX-PN test plan in Appendix G.

WANT TO KNOW MORE? A wide variety of resources are available to enhance your learning and understanding of this chapter.
- Visit thePoint for resources such as:
  • NCLEX-Style Student Review Questions
  • Journal Articles
  • Dosage Calculations
  • Drug Monographs
  • Watch and Learn Videos
  • Concepts in Action Animations
- The *Study Guide to Accompany Introductory Clinical Pharmacology,* 12th edition, sold separately, will help you review and apply essential content.
- ✓*PrepU* is available to help students prepare for the NCLEX-PN examination.

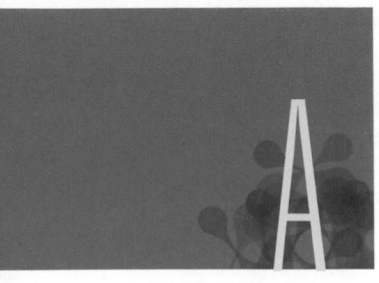

Drug Categories: Controlled Substances and Outgoing FDA Pregnancy Risk

Schedules of Controlled Substances

Schedule I (C-I)
- High abuse, severe dependence potential
- Lack of accepted safety, not approved for medical use in the United States
- Examples: heroin, cannabis (marijuana),[1] ecstasy (MDMA), peyote

Schedule II (C-II)
- Potential for high abuse with severe physical or psychological dependence
- Approved for medical use in the United States (and all categories below)
- Examples: opioids such as fentanyl, meperidine, methadone, morphine, oxycodone, hydrocodone alone or in any form such as with codeine compounded with a nonsteroidal anti-inflammatory drug (Vicodin), amphetamines (Adderall, Ritalin), cocaine, diet drug (Desoxyn)

Schedule III (C-III)
- Less abuse potential than schedule II drugs
- Potential for moderate or low physical or psychological dependence
- Examples: anabolic steroids, testosterone, ketamine, diet drug (Bontril), Marinol (synthetic THC), products with less than 90 mg of codeine (Tylenol with codeine)

Schedule IV (C-IV)
- Less abuse potential than schedule III drugs
- Limited dependence potential
- Examples: benzodiazepines, some sedatives (Ambien) and anxiety agents (Valium, Ativan), nonopioid analgesics (tramadol), diet drug (Belviq)

Schedule V (C-V)[2]
- Limited abuse potential
- Examples: small amounts of opioid (codeine) used as antitussives or antidiarrheals (Lomotil), pregabalin (Lyrica)

FDA Pregnancy (Fetal) Risk Categories[3]

Pregnancy Category A
- Adequate, well-controlled studies in pregnant women have not shown an increased risk of fetal abnormalities to the fetus in any trimester of pregnancy.

Pregnancy Category B
- Animal studies have revealed no evidence of harm to the fetus; however, there are no adequate and well-controlled studies in pregnant women.

OR

- Animal studies have shown an adverse effect, but adequate and well-controlled studies in pregnant women have failed to demonstrate a risk to the fetus in any trimester.

Pregnancy Category C
- Animal studies have shown an adverse effect and there are no adequate and well-controlled studies in pregnant women.

OR

- No animal studies have been conducted and there are no adequate and well-controlled studies in pregnant women.

Pregnancy Category D
- Adequate well-controlled or observational studies in pregnant women have demonstrated a risk to the fetus.
- However, potential benefits may outweigh the risk to the fetus. If needed in a life-threatening situation or a serious disease, the drug may be acceptable if safer drugs cannot be used or are ineffective.

Pregnancy Category X
- Adequate well-controlled or observational studies in animals or pregnant women have demonstrated positive evidence of fetal abnormalities or risks.
- The use of the product is contraindicated in women who are or may become pregnant.

Pregnancy Category N
- The drug is not classified by the FDA.

Regardless of the pregnancy category or the presumed safety of the drug, no drug should be administered during pregnancy unless it is clearly needed and the potential benefits outweigh the potential harm to the fetus.

---

[1]Thirty-three states and the District of Columbia allow marijuana for medicinal purposes. Eleven of these states have legalized marijuana for recreational use, too (1/21). State-specific requirements determine how a person applies for permission to purchase and use the product.
[2]Under federal law, limited quantities of certain schedule V drugs may be purchased without a prescription directly from a pharmacist if allowed under state law. The purchaser must be aged at least 18 years and must furnish identification. All such transactions must be recorded by the dispensing pharmacist.
Security of controlled substances is dependent upon the facility. When automated drug storage units are available, these controlled substances are kept and accounted for within the storage unit. Alarms for accounting discrepancies alert the clinical or pharmacy staff to manually account for the controlled substances in the unit compared to the computerized count. In facilities that are not automated, written ledgers may still be in use where two licensed staff members are required to visualize and manually count drug use versus remaining stock on hand when shifts are completed.

---

[3]This classification system was eliminated as of June 29, 2018, and phased out for all newly approved drugs started in 2015. Exception to this ruling is for drugs approved before June 29, 2001. Therefore, this listing is provided for your understanding when presented in the textbook or questioned by a client.

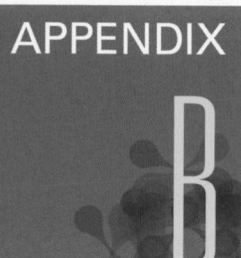
FDA and ISMP Lists of Look-Alike Drug Names with Recommended Tall Man Letters

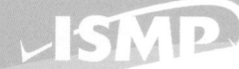

Institute for Safe Medication Practices

FDA and **ISMP** Lists of
Look-Alike Drug Names with Recommended Tall Man Letters

Since 2008, ISMP has maintained a list of drug name pairs and trios with recommended, **bolded** tall man (uppercase) letters to help draw attention to the dissimilarities in look-alike drug names. The list includes mostly generic-generic drug name pairs, although a few brand-brand or brand-generic name pairs are included. The US Food and Drug Administration (FDA) list of drug names with recommended tall man letters was initiated in 2001 with the agency's Name Differentiation Project (www.ismp.org/sc?id=520).

While numerous studies between 2000 and 2016 have demonstrated the ability of tall man letters alone or in conjunction with other text enhancements to improve the accuracy of drug name perception and reduce errors due to drug name similarity,[1-9] some studies have suggested that the strategy is ineffective.[10-12] The evidence is mixed due in large part to methodological differences and significant study limitations. Nevertheless, while gaps still exist in our full understanding of the role of tall man lettering in the clinical setting, there is sufficient evidence to suggest that this simple and straightforward technique is worth implementing as one among numerous strategies to mitigate the risk of errors due to similar drug names. To await irrefutable, scientific proof of effectiveness minimizes and undervalues the study findings and anecdotal evidence available today[13] that support this important risk-reduction strategy. As such, the use of tall man letters has been endorsed by ISMP, The Joint Commission (recommended but not required), the US Food and Drug Administration (as part of its Name Differentiation Project), as well as other national and international organizations, including the World Health Organization and the International Medication Safety Network (IMSN).[14]

Table 1 provides an alphabetized list of FDA-approved established drug names with recommended tall man letters.

Table 2 provides an alphabetized list of additional drug names with recommendations from ISMP regarding the use and placement of tall man letters. This is not an official list approved by FDA. It is intended for voluntary use by healthcare practitioners, drug information vendors, and medication technology vendors. Any product label changes by manufacturers require FDA approval.

To promote standardization regarding which letters to present in uppercase, ISMP follows a tested methodology whenever possible called the CD3 rule.[15] The methodology suggests working from the left of the drug name first by capitalizing all the characters to the right once 2 or more dissimilar letters are encountered, and then, working from the right, returning 2 or more letters common to both words to lowercase letters. When the rule cannot be applied because there are no common letters on the right side of the name, the methodology suggests capitalizing the central part of the word only. When application of this rule fails to lead to the best tall man lettering option (e.g., makes names appear too similar, makes names hard to read based on pronunciation), an alternative option is considered.

ISMP suggests that the **bolded**, tall man lettering scheme provided by FDA and ISMP for the drug name pairs listed in **Tables 1** and **2** be followed to promote consistency. continued on next page >

Table 1. FDA-Approved List of Generic Drug Names with Tall Man Letters	
Drug Name With Tall Man Letters	Confused With
aceta**ZOLAMIDE**	aceto**HEXAMIDE**
aceto**HEXAMIDE**	aceta**ZOLAMIDE**
bu**PROP**ion	bus**PIR**one
bus**PIR**one	bu**PROP**ion
chlorpro**MAZINE**	chlorpro**PAMIDE**
chlorpro**PAMIDE**	chlorpro**MAZINE**
clomi**PHENE**	clomi**PRAMINE**
clomi**PRAMINE**	clomi**PHENE**
cyclo**SERINE**	cyclo**SPORINE**
cyclo**SPORINE**	cyclo**SERINE**
DAUNOrubicin	**DOXO**rubicin
dimenhy**DRINATE**	diphenhydr**AMINE**
diphenhydr**AMINE**	dimenhy**DRINATE**
DOBUTamine	**DOP**amine
DOPamine	**DOBUT**amine
DOXOrubicin	**DAUNO**rubicin

continued on next page >

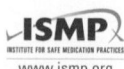

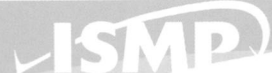

Institute for Safe Medication Practices

FDA and ISMP Lists of Look-Alike Drug Names with Recommended Tall Man Letters

Table 1. FDA–Approved List of Generic Drug Names with Tall Man Letters (continued)

Drug Name With Tall Man Letters	Confused With
glipiZIDE	glyBURIDE
glyBURIDE	glipiZIDE
hydrALAZINE	hydrOXYzine – HYDROmorphone
HYDROmorphone	hydrOXYzine – hydrALAZINE
hydrOXYzine	hydrALAZINE – HYDROmorphone
medroxyPROGESTERone	methylPREDNISolone - methylTESTOSTERone
methylPREDNISolone	medroxyPROGESTERone - methylTESTOSTERone
methylTESTOSTERone	medroxyPROGESTERone - methylPREDNISolone
mitoXANTRONE	Not specified
niCARdipine	NIFEdipine
NIFEdipine	niCARdipine
prednisoLONE	predniSONE
predniSONE	prednisoLONE
risperiDONE	rOPINIRole
rOPINIRole	risperiDONE
sulfADIAZINE	sulfiSOXAZOLE
sulfiSOXAZOLE	sulfADIAZINE
TOLAZamide	TOLBUTamide
TOLBUTamide	TOLAZamide
vinBLAStine	vinCRIStine
vinCRIStine	vinBLAStine

Table 2. ISMP List of Additional Drug Names with Tall Man Letters*

Drug Name With Tall Man Letters	Confused With
ALPRAZolam	LORazepam – clonazePAM
aMILoride	amLODIPine
amLODIPine	aMILoride
ARIPiprazole	RABEprazole
AVINza*	INVanz*
azaCITIDine	azaTHIOprine
azaTHIOprine	azaCITIDine
carBAMazepine	OXcarbazepine
CARBOplatin	CISplatin
ceFAZolin	cefoTEtan – cefOXitin – cefTAZidime – cefTRIAXone
cefoTEtan	ceFAZolin – cefOXitin – cefTAZidime – cefTRIAXone
cefOXitin	ceFAZolin – cefoTEtan – cefTAZidime – cefTRIAXone
cefTAZidime	ceFAZolin – cefoTEtan – cefOXitin – cefTRIAXone
cefTRIAXone	ceFAZolin - cefoTEtan – cefOXitin – cefTAZidime
CeleBREX*	CeleXA*
CeleXA*	CeleBREX*
chlordiazePOXIDE	chlorproMAZINE**

continued on next page >

* *Brand names always start with an uppercase letter. Some brand names incorporate tall man letters in initial characters and may not be readily recognized as brand names. An asterisk follows all brand names on the ISMP list.*
** *These drug names are also on the FDA list.*
*** *The ISMP list is not an official list approved by FDA. It is intended for voluntary use by healthcare practitioners and drug information and technology vendors. Any manufacturers' product label changes require FDA approval.*

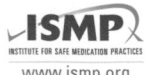

INSTITUTE FOR SAFE MEDICATION PRACTICES

www.ismp.org

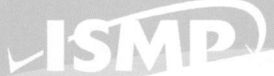

Institute for Safe Medication Practices

FDA and ISMP Lists of Look-Alike Drug Names with Recommended Tall Man Letters

Table 2. ISMP List of Additional Drug Names with Tall Man Letters*** (continued)	
Drug Name With Tall Man Letters	**Confused With**
chlorpro**MAZINE****	chlordiaze**POXIDE**
CISplatin	**CARBO**platin
clo**BAZ**am	clonaze**PAM**
clonaze**PAM**	clo**NID**ine – clo**ZAP**ine – clo**BAZ**am – **LOR**azepam
clo**NID**ine	clonaze**PAM** – clo**ZAP**ine – Klono**PIN***
clo**ZAP**ine	clonaze**PAM** – clo**NID**ine
DACTINomycin	**DAPTO**mycin
DAPTOmycin	**DACTIN**omycin
DEPO-Medrol*	**SOLU**-Medrol*
diaze**PAM**	dil**TIAZ**em
dil**TIAZ**em	diaze**PAM**
DOCEtaxel	**PACL**itaxel
DOXOrubicin**	**IDA**rubicin
DULoxetine	**FLU**oxetine – **PAR**oxetine
e**PHED**rine	**EPINEPH**rine
EPINEPHrine	e**PHED**rine
epi**RUB**icin	eri**BUL**in
eri**BUL**in	epi**RUB**icin
fenta**NYL**	**SUF**entanil
flavox**ATE**	fluvoxa**MINE**
FLUoxetine	**DUL**oxetine – **PAR**oxetine
flu**PHENAZ**ine	fluvoxa**MINE**
fluvoxa**MINE**	flu**PHENAZ**ine - flavox**ATE**
guai**FEN**esin	guan**FACINE**
guan**FACINE**	guai**FEN**esin
Huma**LOG***	Humu**LIN***
Humu**LIN***	Huma**LOG***
hydr**ALAZINE****	hydro**CHLORO**thiazide – hydr**OXY**zine**
hydro**CHLORO**thiazide	hydr**OXY**zine** – hydr**ALAZINE****
HYDROcodone	oxy**CODONE**
HYDROmorphone**	morphine – oxy**MOR**phone
HYDROXYprogesterone	medroxy**PROGESTER**one**
hydr**OXY**zine**	hydr**ALAZINE**** – hydro**CHLORO**thiazide
IDArubicin	**DOXO**rubicin** – idaru**CIZU**mab
idaru**CIZU**mab	**IDA**rubicin
in**FLIX**imab	ri**TUX**imab
INVanz*	**AVIN**za*
ISOtretinoin	tretinoin
Klono**PIN***	clo**NID**ine
La**MIC**tal*	Lam**ISIL***
Lam**ISIL***	La**MIC**tal*

continued on next page >

* *Brand names always start with an uppercase letter. Some brand names incorporate tall man letters in initial characters and may not be readily recognized as brand names. An asterisk follows all brand names on the ISMP list.*
** *These drug names are also on the FDA list.*
*** *The ISMP list is not an official list approved by FDA. It is intended for voluntary use by healthcare practitioners and drug information and technology vendors. Any manufacturers' product label changes require FDA approval.*

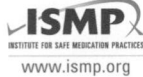

INSTITUTE FOR SAFE MEDICATION PRACTICES

www.ismp.org

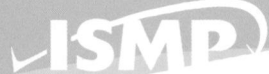

FDA and ISMP Lists of Look-Alike Drug Names with Recommended Tall Man Letters

Table 2. ISMP List of Additional Drug Names with Tall Man Letters*** (continued)	
Drug Name With Tall Man Letters	**Confused With**
lamiVUDine	lamoTRIgine
lamoTRIgine	lamiVUDine
levETIRAcetam	levOCARNitine – levoFLOXacin
levOCARNitine	levETIRAcetam
levoFLOXacin	levETIRAcetam
LEVOleucovorin	leucovorin
LORazepam	ALPRAZolam – clonazePAM
medroxyPROGESTERone**	HYDROXYprogesterone
metFORMIN	metroNIDAZOLE
methazolAMIDE	methIMAzole – metOLazone
methIMAzole	metOLazone – methazolAMIDE
metOLazone	methIMAzole – methazolAMIDE
metroNIDAZOLE	metFORMIN
metyraPONE	metyroSINE
metyroSINE	metyraPONE
miFEPRIStone	miSOPROStol
miSOPROStol	miFEPRIStone
mitoMYcin	mitoXANTRONE**
mitoXANTRONE**	mitoMYcin
NexAVAR*	NexIUM*
NexIUM*	NexAVAR*
niCARdipine**	niMODipine – NIFEdipine**
NIFEdipine**	niMODipine – niCARdipine**
niMODipine	NIFEdipine** – niCARdipine**
NovoLIN*	NovoLOG*
NovoLOG*	NovoLIN*
OLANZapine	QUEtiapine
OXcarbazepine	carBAMazepine
oxyCODONE	HYDROcodone – OxyCONTIN*– oxyMORphone
OxyCONTIN*	oxyCODONE – oxyMORphone
oxyMORphone	HYDROmorphone** – oxyCODONE – OxyCONTIN*
PACLitaxel	DOCEtaxel
PARoxetine	FLUoxetine – DULoxetine
PAZOPanib	PONATinib
PEMEtrexed	PRALAtrexate
penicillAMINE	penicillin
PENTobarbital	PHENobarbital
PHENobarbital	PENTobarbital
PONATinib	PAZOPanib
PRALAtrexate	PEMEtrexed
PriLOSEC*	PROzac*

* Brand names always start with an uppercase letter. Some brand names incorporate tall man letters in initial characters and may not be readily recognized as brand names. An asterisk follows all brand names on the ISMP list.

** These drug names are also on the FDA list.

*** The ISMP list is not an official list approved by FDA. It is intended for voluntary use by healthcare practitioners and drug information and technology vendors. Any manufacturers' product label changes require FDA approval.

continued on next page >

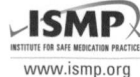

www.ismp.org

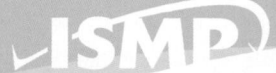

Institute for Safe Medication Practices

FDA and ISMP Lists of Look-Alike Drug Names with Recommended Tall Man Letters

Table 2. ISMP List of Additional Drug Names with Tall Man Letters* (continued)

Drug Name With Tall Man Letters	Confused With
PROzac*	PriLOSEC*
QUEtiapine	OLANZapine
quiNIDine	quiNINE
quiNINE	quiNIDine
RABEprazole	ARIPiprazole
raNITIdine	riMANTAdine
rifAMPin	rifAXIMin
rifAXIMin	rifAMPin
riMANTAdine	raNITIdine
RisperDAL*	rOPINIRole**
risperiDONE**	rOPINIRole**
riTUXimab	inFLIXimab
romiDEPsin	romiPLOStim
romiPLOStim	romiDEPsin
rOPINIRole**	RisperDAL*– risperiDONE**
SandIMMUNE*	SandoSTATIN*
SandoSTATIN*	SandIMMUNE*
sAXagliptin	SITagliptin
SEROquel*	SINEquan*
SINEquan*	SEROquel*
SITagliptin	sAXagliptin – SUMAtriptan
Solu-CORTEF*	SOLU-Medrol*
SOLU-Medrol*	Solu-CORTEF* – DEPO-Medrol*
SORAfenib	SUNItinib
SUFentanil	fentaNYL
sulfADIAZINE**	sulfaSALAzine
sulfaSALAzine	sulfADIAZINE**
SUMAtriptan	SITagliptin – ZOLMitriptan
SUNItinib	SORAfenib
TEGretol*	TRENtal*
tiaGABine	tiZANidine
tiZANidine	tiaGABine
traMADol	traZODone
traZODone	traMADol
TRENtal*	TEGretol*
valACYclovir	valGANciclovir
valGANciclovir	valACYclovir
ZOLMitriptan	SUMAtriptan
ZyPREXA*	ZyrTEC*
ZyrTEC*	ZyPREXA*

* Brand names always start with an uppercase letter. Some brand names incorporate tall man letters in initial characters and may not be readily recognized as brand names. An asterisk follows all brand names on the ISMP list.
** These drug names are also on the FDA list.
*** The ISMP list is not an official list approved by FDA. It is intended for voluntary use by healthcare practitioners and drug information and technology vendors. Any manufacturers' product label changes require FDA approval.

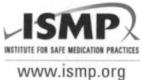

INSTITUTE FOR SAFE MEDICATION PRACTICES
www.ismp.org

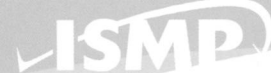

FDA and ISMP Lists of Look-Alike Drug Names with Recommended Tall Man Letters

References

1) DeHenau C, Becker MW, Bello NM, Liu S, Bix L. Tallman lettering as a strategy for differentiation in look-alike, sound-alike drug names: the role of familiarity in differentiating drug doppelgangers. *Appl Ergon.* 2016;52:77-84.

2) Filik R, Purdy K, Gale A, Gerrett D. Drug name confusion: evaluating the effectiveness of capital ("tall man") letters using eye movement data. *Soc Sci Med.* 2004;59(12):2597-601.

3) Filik R, Purdy K, Gale A, Gerrett D. Labeling of medicines and patient safety: evaluating methods of reducing drug name confusion. *Hum Factors.* 2006;48(1):39-47.

4) Grasha A. Cognitive systems perspective on human performance in the pharmacy: implications for accuracy, effectiveness, and job satisfaction (Report No. 062100). Alexandria (VA): NACDS. 2000.

5) Darker IT, Gerret D, Filik R, Purdy KJ, Gale AG. The influence of 'tall man' lettering on errors of visual perception in the recognition of written drug names. *Ergonomics.* 2011;54(1):21–33.

6) Or CK, Chan AH. Effects of text enhancements on the differentiation performance of orthographically similar drug names. *Work.* 2014;48(4):521–8.

7) Or CK, Wang H. A comparison of the effects of different typographical methods on the recognizability of printed drug names. *Drug Saf.* 2014;37(5):351–9.

8) Filik R, Price J, Darker I, Gerrett D, Purdy K, Gale A. The influence of tall man lettering on drug name confusion: a laboratory-based investigation in the UK using younger and older adults and healthcare practitioners. *Drug Saf.* 2010;33(8):677–87.

9) Gabriele S. The role of typography in differentiating look-alike/sound-alike drug names. *Healthc Q.* 2006; 9(Spec No):88-95.

10) Schell KL. Using enhanced text to facilitate recognition of drug names: evidence from two experimental studies. *Appl Ergon.* 2009;40(1):82–90.

11) Irwin A, Mearns K, Watson M, Urquhart J. The effect of proximity, tall man lettering, and time pressure on accurate visual perception of drug names. *Hum Factors.* 2013;55(2):253–66.

12) Zhong W, Feinstein JA, Patel NS, Dai D, Feudtner C. Tall man lettering and potential prescription errors: a time series analysis of 42 children's hospitals in the USA over 9 years. *BMJ Qual Saf.* Published Online First: November 3, 2015.

13) Leape LL, Berwick MB, Bates DW. What practices will most improve safety? Evidence-based medicine meets patient safety. *JAMA.* 2002;288(4):501-7.

14) Position statement on improving the safety of international non-proprietary names of medicines (INNs). Horsham (PA): International Medication Safety Network; November 2011.

15) Gerrett D, Gale AG, Darker IT, Filik R, Purdy KJ. Tall man lettering. Final report of the use of tall man lettering to minimise selection errors of medicine names in computer prescribing and dispensing systems. Loughborough University Enterprises Ltd; 2009.

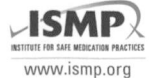

Typical Immunization Schedules

The ever-increasing list of preventable diseases is due in part to vaccination. Because it would be impossible to remember all this information on our own, the Centers for Disease Control and Prevention (CDC) updates and publishes immunization schedules annually.

Included below are the abbreviated, easy-to-read typical immunization schedules for all children (from birth to 18 years) and adults current for the year of publication. This document is produced yearly with current schedules, lists of medical conditions that may impact immunizations, and more. Access the entire document at https://www.cdc.gov/vaccines/schedules/

These schedules present information for provider documentation as well as helpful reminders to clients so that schedules are followed and immunity is maintained.

Recommended Child and Adolescent Immunization Schedule for ages 18 years or younger, United States, 2021

These recommendations must be read with the notes that follow. For those who fall behind or start late, provide catch-up vaccination at the earliest opportunity as indicated by the green bars. To determine minimum intervals between doses, see the catch-up schedule (Table 2). School entry and adolescent vaccine age groups are shaded in gray.

Vaccine	Birth	1 mo	2 mos	4 mos	6 mos	9 mos	12 mos	15 mos	18 mos	19–23 mos	2–3 yrs	4–6 yrs	7–10 yrs	11–12 yrs	13–15 yrs	16 yrs	17–18 yrs
Hepatitis B (HepB)	1st dose	←2nd dose→			←——————————— 3rd dose ———————————→												
Rotavirus (RV): RV1 (2-dose series), RV5 (3-dose series)			1st dose	2nd dose	See Notes												
Diphtheria, tetanus, acellular pertussis (DTaP <7 yrs)			1st dose	2nd dose	3rd dose			←————— 4th dose —————→				5th dose					
Haemophilus influenzae type b (Hib)			1st dose	2nd dose	See Notes		3rd or 4th dose, See Notes										
Pneumococcal conjugate (PCV13)			1st dose	2nd dose	3rd dose		←—— 4th dose ——→										
Inactivated poliovirus (IPV <18 yrs)			1st dose	2nd dose	←——————————— 3rd dose ———————————→							4th dose					
Influenza (IIV)										Annual vaccination 1 or 2 doses				Annual vaccination 1 dose only			
Influenza (LAIV4)											Annual vaccination 1 or 2 doses			Annual vaccination 1 dose only			
Measles, mumps, rubella (MMR)					See Notes		←——— 1st dose ———→					2nd dose					
Varicella (VAR)					See Notes		←——— 1st dose ———→					2nd dose					
Hepatitis A (HepA)							2-dose series, See Notes				See Notes						
Tetanus, diphtheria, acellular pertussis (Tdap ≥7 yrs)														Tdap			
Human papillomavirus (HPV)													See Notes *	See Notes			
Meningococcal (MenACWY-D ≥9 mos, MenACWY-CRM ≥2 mos, MenACWY-TT ≥2 years)														1st dose		2nd dose	
Meningococcal B															See Notes		
Pneumococcal polysaccharide (PPSV23)														See Notes			

Legend:
- Range of recommended ages for all children
- Range of recommended ages for catch-up immunization
- Range of recommended ages for certain high-risk groups
- Recommended based on shared clinical decision-making or *can be used in this age group
- No recommendation/not applicable

Recommended Adult Immunization Schedule by Age Group, United States, 2021

Vaccine	19–26 years	27–49 years	50–64 years	≥65 years
Influenza inactivated (IIV) or Influenza recombinant (RIV4)	1 dose annually			
or				
Influenza live, attenuated (LAIV4)	1 dose annually			
Tetanus, diphtheria, pertussis (Tdap or Td)	1 dose Tdap each pregnancy; 1 dose Td/Tdap for wound management (see notes)			
	1 dose Tdap, then Td or Tdap booster every 10 years			
Measles, mumps, rubella (MMR)	1 or 2 doses depending on indication (if born in 1957 or later)			
Varicella (VAR)	2 doses (if born in 1980 or later)		2 doses	
Zoster recombinant (RZV)			2 doses	
Human papillomavirus (HPV)	2 or 3 doses depending on age at initial vaccination or condition	27 through 45 years		
Pneumococcal conjugate (PCV13)	1 dose			1 dose
Pneumococcal polysaccharide (PPSV23)	1 or 2 doses depending on indication			1 dose
Hepatitis A (HepA)	2 or 3 doses depending on vaccine			
Hepatitis B (HepB)	2 or 3 doses depending on vaccine			
Meningococcal A, C, W, Y (MenACWY)	1 or 2 doses depending on indication, see notes for booster recommendations			
Meningococcal B (MenB)	19 through 23 years	2 or 3 doses depending on vaccine and indication, see notes for booster recommendations		
***Haemophilus influenzae* type b (Hib)**	1 or 3 doses depending on indication			

Legend:
- Recommended vaccination for adults who meet age requirement, lack documentation of vaccination, or lack evidence of past infection
- Recommended vaccination for adults with an additional risk factor or another indication
- Recommended vaccination based on shared clinical decision-making
- No recommendation/Not applicable

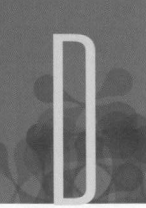

Select Herbs and Natural Products Used for Medicinal Purposes

Common Name(s)	Scientific Name	Uses	Adverse Reactions	Significant Considerations
Aloe vera	*Aloe vera*	To inhibit infection and promote healing of minor burns and wounds; as a laxative	None significant if used as directed; may cause burning sensation in wound	Rare reports of delayed healing when used in the gel form on a wound. If taken internally as a laxative, do not take longer than 1–3 wks without consulting primary health care provider. Decrease dosage if cramping occurs
Bilberry	*Vaccinium myrtillus*	For vision enhancement and eye health, microcirculation, spider veins and varicose veins, and capillary strengthening before surgery	No adverse effects reported in clinical studies	None
Black cohosh (black snakeroot, squawroot)	*Actaea racemosa*	For management of some symptoms of menopause and as an alternative to hormone replacement therapy; may be beneficial for hypercholesterolemia or peripheral vascular disease	Overdose causes nausea, dizziness, nervous system and visual disturbances, decreased pulse rate, and increased perspiration	Should not be used during pregnancy. Possible interactions with hormone therapy. Liver toxic if taken with other hepatotoxic drugs
Capsicum (hot peppers)	*Capsicum frutescens*	For neuralgic pain relief, bladder pain, and hyperreflexia; as an antipruritic for psoriasis	Burning sensation upon application	Creams should be applied with gloves and hands washed thoroughly before touching face or eyes
Chamomile	*Matricaria chamomilla*	Drunk as an infusion for gastrointestinal (GI) disturbances (e.g., diarrhea, flatulence, stomatitis); as a sedative and as an anti-inflammatory agent	Possible contact dermatitis and, in rare instances, anaphylaxis	Chamomile is a member of the ragweed family and those allergic to ragweed should not take the herb. Avoid use during pregnancy. May enhance anticoagulant effect when administered with anticoagulants. Do not administer to a child without checking with primary health care provider
Chondroitin	Chondroitin sulfate, chondroitin sulfuric acid, chonsurid	For arthritis—particularly osteoarthritis	None significant if used as directed	Because chondroitin is concentrated in cartilage, theoretically it produces no toxic or teratogenic effects
Cranberry	*Vaccinium macrocarpon*	To prevent urinary tract infection (UTI) by acidifying the urine; lower pH also reduces the ammonia odor of urinary incontinence	Large doses can produce GI symptoms (e.g., diarrhea)	None. Safe for use during pregnancy and while breastfeeding. Inform client that sugar-free cranberry juice or supplements are available if the client has diabetes mellitus. Antibiotic is usually needed to treat active UTI

Common Name(s)	Scientific Name	Uses	Adverse Reactions	Significant Considerations
Eucalyptus oil	*Eucalyptus globulus* Labillardiere	As a decongestant, expectorant for respiratory conditions; topically for antimicrobial effect	Pain, nausea, vomiting; individuals with acute intermittent porphyria should not take	Used in mouthwashes for antimicrobial properties. Adverse reactions of slowing the central nervous system (CNS), drowsiness, seizures, and coma when taken orally. Blood sugar levels may decrease with use
Feverfew	*Tanacetum parthenium*	As an antipyretic; for migraine headaches, asthma, arthritis, and relief of menstrual cramps	Most are mild; rash or contact dermatitis may indicate allergy and herb should be withdrawn	Possible interaction with anticoagulants. Client should be observed for abnormal bleeding. Do not use during pregnancy or lactation
Flaxseed	*Linum usitatissimum*	As a dietary fiber: for constipation	Abdominal cramping, constipation may worsen if not taken with ample fluids	If crushed, seed oil can be used as an emollient for inflammatory poultice
Garlic	*Allium sativum*	To lower blood glucose, cholesterol, and lipid levels; as topical antifungal	May cause abnormal blood glucose levels	Increased risk of bleeding in clients taking the warfarin, salicylates, or antiplatelet drugs. Can make protease inhibitors ineffective
Ginger (ginger root, black ginger)	*Zingiber officinale*	As antiemetic, cardiotonic, antithrombotic, antibacterial, antioxidant, antitussive, anti-inflammatory, and prophylaxis for nausea and vomiting; for GI disturbances, colic; to lower cholesterol	Excessive doses may cause CNS depression and interfere with cardiac functioning or anticoagulant activity	Theoretically, ginger could enhance the effects of the antiplatelet drugs, such as coumarin. Observe for excessive bleeding (e.g., nose bleeding, easy bruising). Consult primary health care provider for use during pregnancy
Ginkgo (maidenhair tree, kew tree)	*Ginkgo biloba*	For cerebral insufficiency dementias, circulatory problems, headaches, macular degeneration, diabetic retinopathy, and premenstrual syndrome	Rare if used as directed; possible effects include headache, dizziness, heart palpitations, GI effects, rash, and allergic dermatitis	Do not take with antidepressant drugs, such as the monoamine oxidase inhibitors, or antiplatelet drugs, such as coumarin, unless advised to do so by the primary health care provider. Discontinue use at least 2 wks before surgery
Goldenseal	*Hydrastis canadensis*	As antiseptic for skin (topical), astringent for mucous membranes (mouthwash), wash for inflamed eyes, and antidiarrheal	Large doses may cause dry or irritated mucous membranes and injury to the GI system	Should not be taken for more than 3–7 days. Contraindicated in pregnancy and hypertension
Glucosamine (chitosamine)	*2-Amino-2-deoxyglucose*	As antiarthritic in osteoarthritis	Usually well tolerated; mild adverse reactions such as heartburn, diarrhea, nausea, and itching have been reported	No direct toxic effects have been reported. Cautious use is recommended in diabetes because there is a potential for altering blood glucose levels
Green tea	*Camellia sinensis*	To reduce cancer risk, lower lipid levels, and help prevent dental caries; for antimicrobial and antioxidative effects	Well tolerated; contains caffeine (may cause mild stimulant effects such as anxiety, nervousness, heart irregularities, restlessness, insomnia, and digestive irritation)	No direct toxic effects have been reported. Contains caffeine and should be avoided during pregnancy and by individuals with hypertension, anxiety, eating disorders, insomnia, diabetes, and ulcers. Inform client to avoid taking green tea with iron supplements because green tea interferes with iron absorption

(Continued)

Common Name(s)	Scientific Name	Uses	Adverse Reactions	Significant Considerations
Hawthorne	*Crataegus oxyacantha*	For regulation of blood pressure and heart rhythm; to treat atherosclerosis and angina pectoris; as a sedative	Hypotension and sedation (in high doses)	May interfere with serum digoxin effects. Notify primary health care provider and pharmacist if taking the herb
Kava (kawa, kava-kava, awa, yaqona)	*Piper methysticum*	For mild to moderate anxiety; as a sedative	Scaly skin rash; disturbances in visual accommodation, habituation	Limit use to no more than 3 mo
Licorice	*Helichrysum petiolare*	For GI disturbances (heartburn, irritable bowel syndrome, cholesterol, and stomach ulcers)	Weakness, elevated blood pressure, and hypokalemia, confusion	Excessive amounts of licorice candy consumption (4 sticks daily for 9 mo) demonstrated muscle weakness and decreased reflexes
Marijuana, controlled substance not available in all states	*Cannabis*	For pain, muscle spasms, and other conditions not relieved by standard treatment or medications	Anxiety, panic reaction, psychotic symptoms, increased heart rate, and blood pressure changes	Smoking may produce an effect in 10 min, whereas ingestion requires at least 30–60 min. Because of this lag in time for edible products, people may feel they have not taken enough for effect and may ingest more resulting in a dangerous overdose
Melatonin	*Melatonin*	For insomnia; topically to protect against ultraviolet light	Headache, depression, and possible additive effects when taken with alcohol	Avoid hazardous activities until CNS effects of supplement are known. Do not take for prolonged periods because effects of prolonged use are not known. May interfere with conception
Prevagen	*Apoaequorin*	Memory enhancement	None described	Based on the idea that brain cells die due to lack of calcium in the brain, independent studies have not been able to replicate findings
Red yeast	*Monascus purpureus*	To reduce cholesterol levels in healthy people, gastric and circulation health	Same reactions as statin drugs; headache, dizziness, nausea, and constipation	Should not be taken with other antihyperlipidemia drugs
Saw palmetto (cabbage palm, fan palm, scrub palm)	*Serenoa repens*	For symptoms of benign prostatic hypertrophy	Generally well tolerated; occasional GI effects	May interact with hormones such as oral contraceptive drugs and hormone replacement therapy
St. John's wort (Klamath weed, goat weed, rosin rose)	*Hypericum perforatum*	As an antibacterial, antidepressant, or antiviral	Usually mild; may cause dry mouth, dizziness, constipation, other GI symptoms, and photosensitivity	May decrease efficacy of antiretrovirals, theophylline, warfarin, and digoxin; use with other antidepressant prescriptions is not recommended
Tea tree oil	*Melaleuca alternifolia*	As topical antimicrobial, antifungal	Contact dermatitis	For topical use only; do not take orally
Turmeric	*Curcuma longa*	For antioxidant effects in multiple conditions	Rare if used as directed	May lower testosterone levels and sperm motility in men
Valerian	*Valeriana officinalis*	For restlessness, sleep disorders	Rare if used as directed	May interact with benzodiazepines (e.g., diazepam), opioids (e.g., morphine), and barbiturates (e.g., phenobarbital)
Willow bark (weidenrinde, white willow, purple osier willow, crack willow)	*Salix alba, Sarracenia purpurea, Salix fragilis*	As an analgesic	Adverse reactions are those associated with the salicylates	Do not use with aspirin or other nonsteroidal anti-inflammatory drugs. Do not use in clients with peptic ulcers and other medical conditions in which the salicylates are contraindicated

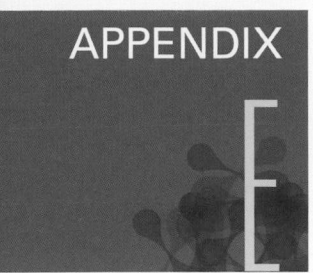

APPENDIX E Less Frequently Used Calculations, Measurements, and Basic Mathematical Review

Body Surface Area Nomograms

Nomogram for Estimating Body Surface Area of Infants and Young Children

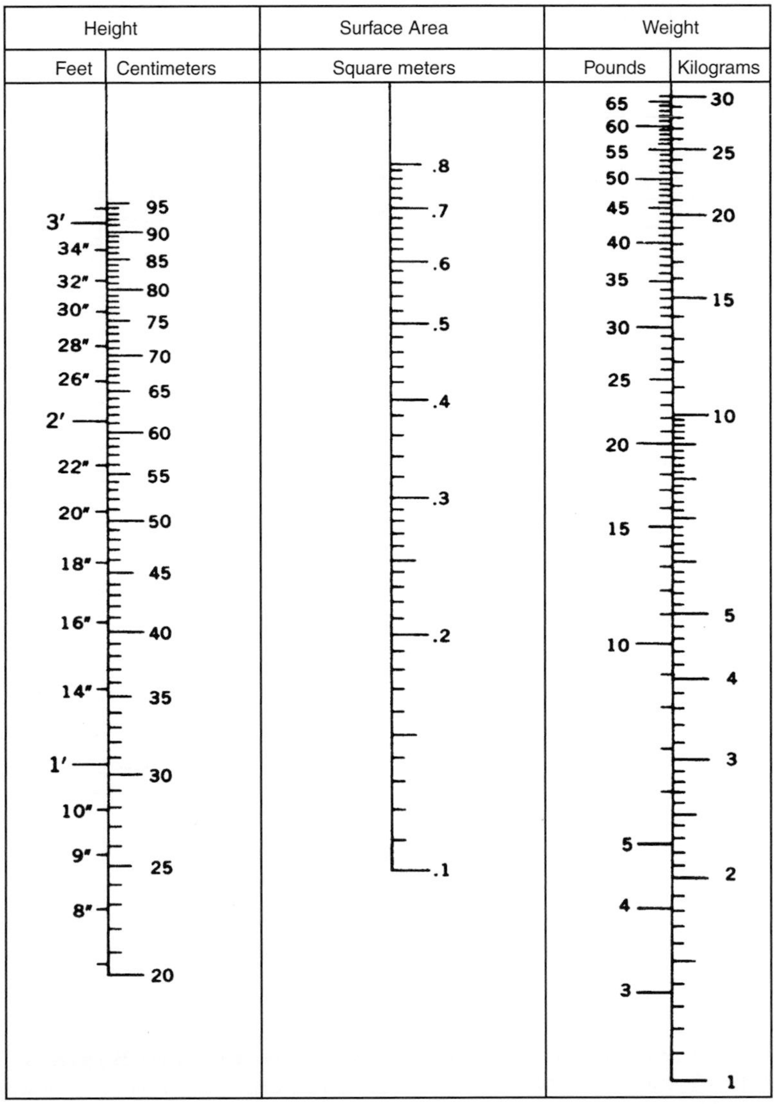

Height
Feet
Centimeters
Surface Area
Square meters
Weight
Pounds
Kilograms
3'
34"
32"
30"
28"
26"
2'
22"
20"
18"
16"
14"
1'
10"
9"
8"
95
90
85
80
75
70
65
60
55
50
45
40
35
30
25
20
.8
.7
.6
.5
.4
.3
.2
.1
65
60
55
50
45
40
35
30
25
20
15
10
5
4
3
30
25
20
15
10
5
4
3
2
1

Nomogram for Estimating Body Surface Area of Older Children and Adults

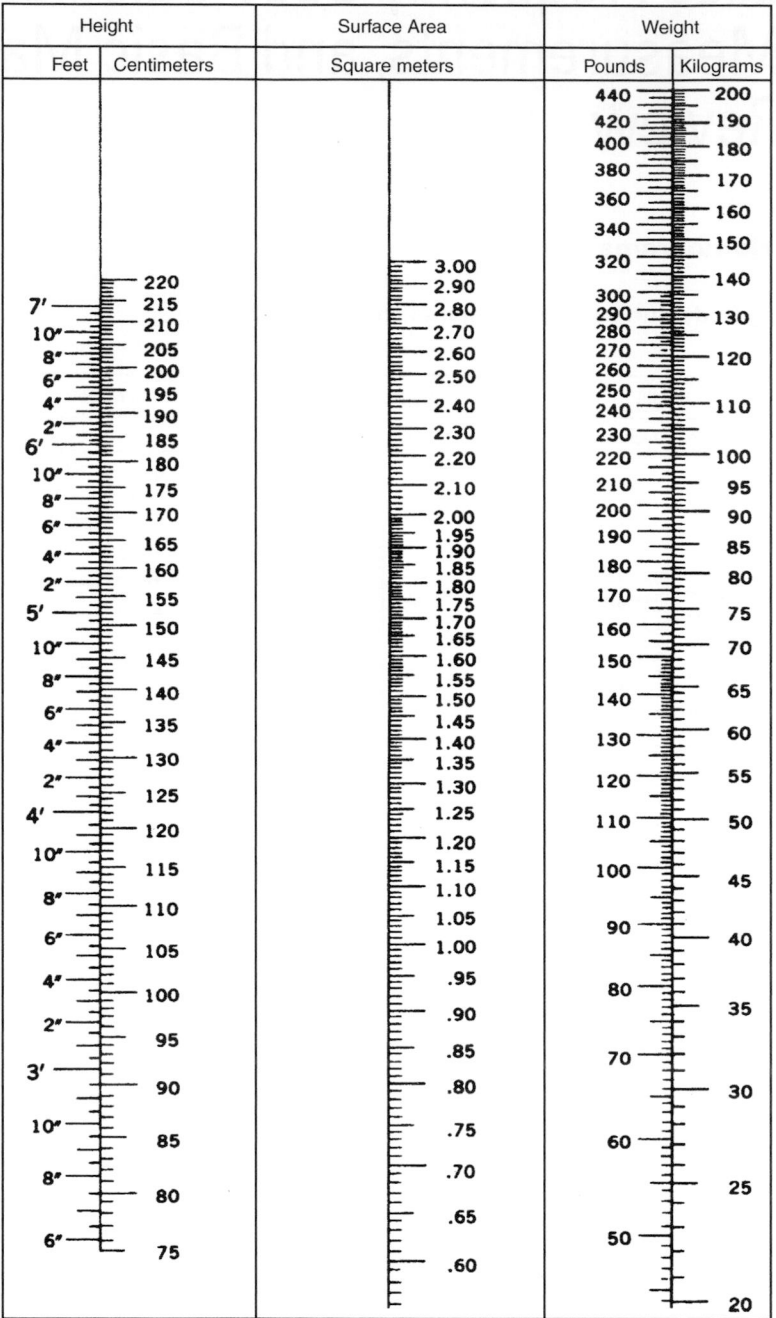

To determine the surface area of the client, draw a straight line between the point representing their height on the left vertical scale and the point representing the client's weight on the right vertical scale. The point at which this line intersects the middle vertical scale represents the client's surface area in square meters.

The Apothecary System

The apothecary system is an older, less accurate system of measurement than the metric system. Whenever possible, it is preferable to use the metric system. In 1994, the *United States Pharmacopeia* responded to errors stemming from confusion caused by the apothecary system of measurement by eliminating an apothecary system conversion table from its national formulary.

Approximate Equivalents of Systems of Measurement

Metric	Apothecary	Household
Weight		
0.1 mg	gr 1/600	
0.15 mg	gr 1/400	
0.2 mg	gr 1/300	
0.3 mg	gr 1/200	
0.4 mg	gr 1/150	
0.6 mg	gr 1/100	
1 mg	gr 1/60	
2 mg	gr 1/30	
4 mg	gr 1/15	
6 mg	gr 1/10	
8 mg	gr 1/8	
10 mg	gr 1/6	
15 mg	gr 1/4	
20 mg	gr 1/3	
30 mg	gr ss (1/2)	
60 mg	gr 1	
100 mg	gr i ss (1 1/2)	
120 mg	gr ii	
1 g (1000 mg)	gr xv	
Volume		
0.06 mL	min i	
1 mL	min xv or xvi	
4 mL	fluid dram i	1 teaspoon
15 mL	fluid drams iv	1/2 ounce
30 mL	fluid ounce i	1 ounce
500 mL	1 pint	1 pint
1000 mL (1 L)	1 quart	1 quart

In 2002, the Joint Commission adopted recommendations from the Institute for Safe Medication Practices' list of error-prone medication abbreviations, symbols, and dose designations for use in its National Patient Safety Goals. It has proven very difficult to convince practitioners of all types to relinquish use of the apothecary system. In keeping with current healthcare standards, this information is provided for situations in which conversion is necessary.

Mathematical Review
This section of Appendix E provides a review of basic math concepts. Should the drug dosage calculations in Chapter 3 cause confusion or if they are hard to understand, look here to find out how to perform the basic math before adding drug names or amounts.

Fractions
The two parts of a fraction are the numerator and the denominator.

$$\frac{2}{3} \leftarrow \text{numerator} \atop \leftarrow \text{denominator}$$

A proper fraction may be defined as a part of a whole or any number less than a whole number. An improper fraction is a fraction having a numerator the same as or larger than the denominator. For example,

proper fraction $\frac{1}{2}$

improper fraction $\frac{7}{3}$

The numerator and the denominator must be of *like entities or terms,* that is:

Correct (like terms)	Incorrect (unlike terms)
$\frac{2\,\text{acres}}{3\,\text{acres}}$	$\frac{2\,\text{acres}}{3\,\text{miles}}$
$\frac{2\,\text{g}}{3\,\text{g}}$	$\frac{2\,\text{g}}{5\,\text{mL}}$

Mixed Numbers and Improper Fractions
A mixed number is a whole number and a proper fraction. A whole number is a number that stands alone; 3, 25, and 117 are examples of whole numbers. A proper fraction is a fraction whose numerator is *smaller than* the denominator; 1/8, 2/5, and 3/7 are examples of proper fractions.

These are mixed numbers:

2 2/3   2 is the whole number and 2/3 is the proper fraction
3 1/4   3 is the whole number and 1/4 is the proper fraction

When doing certain calculations, it is sometimes necessary to change a mixed number to an improper fraction or change an improper fraction to a mixed number. An improper fraction is a fraction whose numerator is *larger than* the denominator; 5/2, 16/3, and 12 3/2 are examples of improper fractions.

To change a *mixed number* to an *improper fraction*, multiply the denominator of the fraction by the whole number, add the numerator, and place the sum over the denominator.

EXAMPLE: Mixed number 3 3/5

1. Multiply the denominator of the fraction (5) by the whole number (3), or 5 × 3 = 15:

$$3 \times \frac{3}{5}$$

2. Add the result of multiplying the denominator of the fraction (15) to the numerator (3), or 15 + 3 = 18:

$$\frac{15}{5} + \frac{3}{5}$$

3. Then place the sum (18) over the denominator of the fraction:

$$\frac{18}{5}$$

To change an *improper fraction to a mixed number*, divide the denominator into the numerator. The quotient (the result of the division of these two numbers) is the whole number. Then place the remainder over the denominator of the improper fraction.

EXAMPLE: Improper fraction 15/4

$$\frac{15}{4} \leftarrow \text{numerator}$$
$$\leftarrow \text{denominator}$$

1. Divide the denominator (4) into the numerator (15), or 15 divided by 4 (15 ÷ 4):

$$4\overline{)15} \begin{array}{l} 3 \leftarrow \text{quotient} \end{array}$$

$$\frac{12}{3} \leftarrow \text{remainder}$$

2. The quotient (3) becomes the whole number:

$$3$$

3. The remainder (3) now becomes the numerator of the fraction of the mixed number:

$$3\frac{3}{}$$

4. And the denominator of the improper fraction (4) now becomes the denominator of the fraction of the mixed number:

$$3\frac{3}{4}$$

Adding Fractions With Like Denominators

When the denominators are the *same*, fractions can be added by adding the numerators and placing the sum of the numerators over the denominator.

EXAMPLES

$$2/7 + 3/7 = 5/7$$
$$1/10 + 3/10 = 4/10$$
$$2/9 + 1/9 + 4/9 = 7/9$$
$$1/12 + 5/12 + 3/12 = 9/12$$
$$2/13 + 1/13 + 3/13 + 5/13 = 11/13$$

When giving a final answer, fractions are *always* reduced to the lowest possible terms. In the examples above, the answers of 5/7, 7/9, and 11/13 cannot be reduced. The answers of 4/10 and 9/12 can be reduced to 2/5 and 3/4.

To reduce a fraction to the lowest possible terms, determine if any number, which always must be the same, can be divided into both the numerator and the denominator.

4/10: the numerator *and* the denominator can be divided by 2.
9/12: the numerator *and* the denominator can be divided by 3.
For example:

$$\frac{4 \div 2 = 2}{10 \div 5 = 5}$$

If when adding fractions the answer is an improper fraction, it may then be changed to a mixed number.

$$2/5 + 4/5 = 6/5 \text{ (improper fraction)}$$
$$6/5 \text{ changed to a mixed number is } 1 \quad 1/5.$$

Adding Fractions With Unlike Denominators

Fractions with *unlike denominators* cannot be added until the denominators are changed to like numbers or numbers that are the same. The first step is to find the *lowest common denominator,* which is the lowest number divisible by (or that can be divided by) all the denominators.

EXAMPLE: Add 2/3 and 1/4

$$\frac{2}{3}$$
$$\frac{1}{4}$$

The lowest number that can be divided by these two denominators is 12; therefore, 12 is the lowest common denominator.

1. Divide the lowest common denominator (which in this example is 12) by each of the denominators in the fractions (in this example 3 and 4):

$$\frac{2}{3} = \frac{}{12} \quad (12 \div 3 = 4)$$
$$\frac{1}{4} = \frac{}{12} \quad (12 \div 4 = 3)$$

2. Multiply the results of the divisions by the numerator of the fractions (12 ÷ 3 = 4 × the numerator 2 = 8 and 12 ÷ 4 = 3 × the numerator 1 = 3) and place the results in the numerator:

$$\frac{2}{3} = \frac{}{12} \qquad \frac{8}{12}$$
$$\frac{1}{4} = \frac{}{12} \qquad \frac{3}{12}$$

3. Add the numerators (8 + 3) and place the result over the denominator (12):

$$\frac{11}{12}$$

Adding Mixed Numbers or Fractions With Mixed Numbers

When adding two or more mixed numbers or adding fractions and mixed numbers, the mixed number is first changed to an improper fraction.

EXAMPLE: Add 3 3/4 and 3 3/4

$$3\frac{3}{4} \quad \text{changed to an improper fraction} \rightarrow \frac{15}{4}$$

$$3\frac{3}{4} \quad \text{changed to an improper fraction} \rightarrow \frac{15}{4}$$

$$\text{The numerators are added} \rightarrow \frac{30}{4} = 7\,2/4 = 7\,1/2$$

The improper fraction (30/4) is changed to a mixed number (7 2/4) and the fraction of the mixed number (2/4) changed to the lowest possible terms (1/2).

EXAMPLE: Add 2 1/2 and 3 1/4

$$2\frac{1}{2} \quad \text{changed to an improper fraction} \quad \frac{5}{2}$$

$$3\frac{1}{4} \quad \text{changed to an improper fraction} \quad \frac{13}{4}$$

In the example above, 5/2 and 13/4 cannot be added because the denominators are not the same. It will be necessary to find the lowest common denominator first. For these two fractions, the lowest common denominator is 4.

$$\frac{5}{2} + \frac{13}{4} \quad \text{becomes} \quad \frac{10}{4} + \frac{13}{4}$$

$$\text{The numerators are added} \quad \frac{23}{4} \quad \text{changed to a mixed number} \quad 5\frac{3}{4}$$

Comparing Fractions

When fractions with *like* denominators are compared, the fraction with the *largest numerator* is the *largest* fraction.

EXAMPLES

Compare: 5/8 and 3/8   Answer: 5/8 is larger than 3/8.
Compare: 1/4 and 3/4   Answer: 3/4 is larger than 1/4.

When the denominators are *not* the same, for example, comparing 2/3 and 1/10, the lowest common denominator must first be determined. The same procedure is followed when adding fractions with unlike denominators (see above).

EXAMPLE: Compare 2/3 and 1/10 (fractions with unlike denominators)

$$\frac{2}{3} = \frac{20}{30}$$

$$\frac{1}{10} = \frac{3}{30} \quad \text{lowest common denominator}$$

The largest numerator in these two fractions is 20; therefore, 2/3 is larger than 1/10.

Multiplying Fractions

When fractions are multiplied, the numerators are multiplied *and* the denominators are multiplied.

EXAMPLES

$$\frac{1}{8} \times \frac{1}{4} = \frac{1}{32} \qquad \frac{1}{2} \times \frac{2}{3} = \frac{2}{6} = \frac{1}{3}$$

In the above examples, it was necessary to reduce one of the answers to its lowest possible terms.

Multiplying Whole Numbers and Fractions

When whole numbers are multiplied with fractions, the numerator is multiplied by the whole number and the product is placed over the denominator. When necessary, the fraction is reduced to its lowest possible terms. If the answer is an improper fraction, it may be changed to a mixed number.

EXAMPLES

$$2 \times \frac{1}{2} = \frac{2}{2} = 1 \, (\text{answer reduced to lowest possible terms})$$

$$2 \times \frac{3}{8} = \frac{6}{8} = \frac{3}{4} \, (\text{answer reduced to lowest possible terms})$$

$$4 \times \frac{2}{3} = \frac{8}{3} = 2\frac{2}{3} \, (\text{improper fraction changed to a mixed number})$$

Multiplying Mixed Numbers

To multiply mixed numbers, the mixed numbers are changed to *improper fractions* and then multiplied.

EXAMPLES

$$2\frac{1}{2} \times 3\frac{1}{4} = \frac{5}{2} \times \frac{13}{4} = \frac{65}{8} = 8\frac{1}{8}$$

$$3\frac{1}{3} \times 4\frac{1}{2} = \frac{10}{3} \times \frac{9}{2} = \frac{90}{6} = 15$$

Multiplying a Whole Number and a Mixed Number

To multiply a whole number and a mixed number, *both* numbers must be changed to improper fractions.

EXAMPLES

$$3 \times 2\frac{1}{2} = \frac{3}{1} \times \frac{5}{2} = \frac{15}{2} = 7\frac{1}{2}$$

$$2 \times 4\frac{1}{2} = \frac{2}{1} \times \frac{9}{2} = \frac{18}{2} = 9$$

A whole number is converted to an improper fraction by placing the whole number over 1. In the above examples, 3 becomes 3/1 and 2 becomes 2/1.

Dividing Fractions

When fractions are divided, the *second* fraction (the divisor) is inverted (turned upside down) and then the fractions are multiplied.

EXAMPLES

$$\frac{1}{3} \div \frac{3}{7} = \frac{1}{3} \times \frac{7}{3} = \frac{7}{9}$$

$$\frac{1}{8} \div \frac{1}{4} = \frac{1}{8} \times \frac{4}{1} = \frac{4}{8} = \frac{1}{2}$$

$$\frac{3}{2} \div \frac{1}{2} = \frac{3}{2} \times \frac{2}{1} = \frac{6}{4} = 1\frac{1}{2}$$

In the above examples, the second answer was reduced to its lowest possible terms and the third answer, which was an improper fraction, was changed to a mixed number.

Dividing Fractions and Mixed Numbers

Some problems of division may be expressed as (1) fractions and mixed numbers, (2) two mixed numbers, (3) whole numbers and fractions, or (4) whole numbers and mixed numbers.

Mixed Numbers and Fractions

When a mixed number is divided by a fraction, the whole number is first changed to a fraction.

EXAMPLES

$$2\frac{1}{3} \div \frac{1}{4} = \frac{7}{3} \div \frac{1}{4} = \frac{7}{3} \times \frac{4}{1} = \frac{28}{3} = 9\frac{1}{3}$$

$$2\frac{1}{2} \div \frac{1}{2} = \frac{5}{2} \div \frac{1}{2} = \frac{5}{2} \times \frac{2}{1} = \frac{10}{2} = 5$$

Mixed Numbers

When two mixed numbers are divided, they are both changed to improper fractions.

EXAMPLE

$$3\frac{3}{4} \div 1\frac{1}{2} = \frac{15}{4} \div \frac{3}{2} = \frac{15}{4} \times \frac{2}{3} = \frac{30}{12}$$

$$= 2\frac{6}{12} = 2\frac{1}{2}$$

Whole Numbers and Fractions

When a whole number is divided by a fraction, the whole number is changed to an improper fraction by placing the whole number over 1.

EXAMPLE

$$2 \div \frac{2}{3} = \frac{2}{1} \div \frac{2}{3} = \frac{2}{1} \times \frac{3}{2} = \frac{6}{2} = 3$$

Whole Numbers and Mixed Numbers

When whole numbers and mixed numbers are divided, the whole number is changed to an improper fraction and the mixed number is changed to an improper fraction.

EXAMPLE

$$4 \div 2\frac{2}{3} = \frac{4}{1} \div \frac{8}{3} = \frac{4}{1} \times \frac{3}{8} = \frac{12}{8} = 1\frac{4}{8} = 1\frac{1}{2}$$

Ratios

A ratio is a way of expressing *a part of a whole* or *the relation of one number to another*. For example, a ratio written as 1:10 means 1 in 10 parts, or 1 to 10. A ratio may also be written as a fraction; thus, 1:10 can also be expressed as 1/10.

EXAMPLES

1:1000 is 1 part in 1000 parts, or 1 to 1000, or 1/1000.

1:250 is 1 part in 250 parts, or 1 to 250, or 1/250.

Some drug solutions are expressed in ratios; for example, 1:100 or 1:500. These ratios mean that there is 1 part of a drug in 100 parts of solution or 1 part of the drug in 500 parts of solution.

Percentages

The term percentage or percent (%) means parts per hundred.

EXAMPLES

25% is 25 parts per hundred.

50% is 50 parts per hundred.

A percentage may also be expressed as a fraction.

EXAMPLES

25% is 25 parts per hundred or 25/100.

50% is 50 parts per hundred or 50/100.

30% is 30 parts per hundred or 30/100.

The above fractions may also be reduced to their lowest possible terms:

$$25/100 = 1/4, 50/100 = 1/2, 30/100 = 3/10.$$

Changing a Fraction to a Percentage

To change a fraction to a percentage, divide the denominator by the numerator and multiply the results (quotient) by 100 and then add a percent sign (%).

EXAMPLES

Change 4/5 to a percentage.

$$4 \div 5 = 0.8$$
$$0.8 \times 100 = 80\%$$

Change 2/3 to a percentage.

$$2 \div 3 = 0.666$$
$$0.666 \times 100 = 66.6\%$$

Changing a Ratio to a Percentage

To change a ratio to a percentage, the ratio is first expressed as a fraction with the first number or term of the ratio becoming the numerator and the second number or term becoming the denominator. For example, the ratio 1:500 when changed to a fraction becomes 1/500. This fraction is then changed to a percentage by the same method shown in the preceding section.

EXAMPLES

Change 1:125 to a percentage.

1:125 written as a fraction is 1/125.

$$1 \div 125 = 0.008$$
$$0.008 \times 100 = 0.8$$
$$\text{add the percent sign} = 0.8\%$$

Changing a Percentage to a Ratio

To change a percentage to a ratio, the percentage becomes the numerator and is placed over a denominator of 100.

EXAMPLES

Changing 5% and 10% to ratios

$$5\% \text{ is } \frac{5}{100} = \frac{1}{20} \text{ or } 1:20$$

$$10\% \text{ is } \frac{10}{100} = \frac{1}{10} \text{ or } 1:10$$

Proportions

A proportion is a method of expressing equality between two ratios. An example of two ratios expressed as a proportion is as follows: 3 is to 4 as 9 is to 12. This may also be written as:

$$3 : 4 \text{ as } 9{:}12$$

or

$$3{:}4{::}9{:}12$$

or

$$\frac{3}{4} = \frac{9}{12}$$

Proportions may be used to find an unknown quantity. The unknown quantity is assigned a letter, usually X. An example of a proportion with an unknown quantity is 5:10::15:X.

The first and last terms of the proportion are called the *extremes*. In the above expression, 5 and X are the extremes. The second and third terms of the proportion are called the *means*. In the above proportion, 10 and 15 are the means:

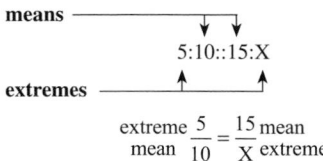

$$\text{means} \longrightarrow 5{:}10{::}15{:}X$$
$$\text{extremes} \longrightarrow$$

$$\begin{array}{c}\text{extreme} \\ \text{mean}\end{array} \frac{5}{10} = \frac{15}{X} \begin{array}{c}\text{mean} \\ \text{extreme}\end{array}$$

To solve for X:

1. Multiply the extremes and place the product (result) to the *left* of the equal sign.

$$\mathbf{5} : 10 :: 15 : \mathbf{X}$$
$$5X =$$

2. Multiply the means and place the product to the *right* of the equal sign.

$$5 : \mathbf{10} :: \mathbf{15} X$$
$$5X = 150$$

3. Solve for X by dividing the number to the right of the equal sign by the number to the left of the equal sign (150 ÷ 5).

$$5X = 150$$
$$X = 30$$

4. To prove the answer is correct, substitute the answer (30) for X in the equation.

$$5 : 10 :: 15 : X$$
$$5 : 10 :: 15 : 30$$

Then multiply the means and place the product to the left of the equal sign. Then multiply the extremes and place the product to the right of the equal sign.

$$5 : 10 :: 15 : 30$$
$$150 = 150$$

If the numbers are the same on both sides of the equal sign, the equation has been solved correctly.

If the proportion has been set up as a fraction, cross-multiply and solve for X.

$$\frac{5}{10} = \frac{15}{X}$$
$$5 \text{ times } X = 5X \text{ and } 10 \text{ times } 15 = 150$$
$$5X = 150$$
$$X = 30$$

To set up a proportion, remember that a sequence *must* be followed. If a sequence is not followed, the proportion will be stated incorrectly.

EXAMPLES

If a man can walk 6 *miles* in 2 *hours*, how many *miles* can he walk in 3 *hours?*

miles is to *hours* and *miles* is to *hours*
or
miles:hours::miles:hours
or

$$\frac{\text{miles}}{\text{hours}} = \frac{\text{miles}}{\text{hours}}$$

The unknown fact is the number of miles walked in 3 hours:

$$6 \text{ miles} : 2 \text{ hours} :: X \text{ miles} : 3 \text{ hours}$$
$$2X = 18$$
$$X = 9 \text{ miles (he can walk 9 miles in 3 hours)}$$

If there are 15 *grains* in 1 *gram*, 30 *grains* equals how many *grams?*

$$15 \text{ grains} : 1 \text{ gram} :: 30 \text{ grains} : X \text{ grams}$$
$$15X = 30$$
$$X = 2 \text{ grams (30 grains equals 2 grams)}$$

Decimals

Decimals are used in the metric system. A decimal is a fraction in which the denominator is 10 or some power of 10. For example, 2/10 (read as two tenths) is a fraction with a denominator of 10; 1/100 (read as one one hundredth) is an example of a fraction with a denominator that is a power of 10 (i.e., 100).

A power (or multiple) of 10 is the *number 1 followed by one or more zeros.* Therefore, 100, 1000, 10,000, and so on are powers of 10 because the number 1 is followed by two, three, and four zeros, respectively. Fractions whose denominators are 10 or a power of 10 are often expressed in decimal form.

Parts of a Decimal

There are three parts to a decimal:

	1.25	
number(s)	**d**	number(s)
to the	**e**	to the
left of	**c**	right of
the	**i**	the
decimal	**m**	decimal
	a	
	l	

Types of Decimals

A decimal may consist only of numbers to the right of the decimal point. This is called a decimal fraction. Examples of decimal fractions are 0.05, 0.6, and 0.002.

A decimal may also have numbers to the left *and* right of the decimal point. This is called a mixed decimal fraction. Examples of mixed decimal fractions are 1.25, 2.5, and 7.5.

Reading Decimals
To read a decimal, the position of the number to the left or right of the decimal point indicates how the decimal is to be expressed.

0 hundred thousands
0 ten thousands
0 thousands
0 hundreds
0 tens
0 units

Decimal Point
0 tenths
0 hundredths
0 thousandths
0 ten thousandths
0 hundred thousandths

Adding Decimals
When adding decimals, place the numbers in a column so that the whole numbers are aligned to the left of the decimal and the decimal fractions are aligned to the right of the decimal.

EXAMPLE

$20.45 + 2.56$	$2 + 0.25$
is written as :	is written as :
20.45	2.00
+2.56	+0.25
23.01	2.25

Subtracting Decimals
When subtracting decimals, the numbers are aligned to the left and right of the decimal in the same manner as for the addition of decimals.

EXAMPLE

$20.45 - 2.56$	$9.74 - 0.45$
is written as :	is written as :
20.45	9.74
−2.56	−0.45
17.89	9.29

Multiplying a Whole Number by a Decimal
To multiply a whole number by a decimal, move the decimal point of the product (answer) as many places to the left as there are places to the right of the decimal point.

EXAMPLES

500	there are two places to the right
×.05 ←	of the decimal
2500.	the decimal point is moved two places to the left

After moving the decimal point, the answer reads 25.

250	there is one place to the right
×0.3 ←	of the decimal
750.	the decimal point is moved one place to the left

After moving the decimal point, the answer reads 75.

Multiplying a Decimal by a Decimal
To multiply a decimal by a decimal, move the decimal point of the product (answer) as many places to the left as there are places to the right in *both* decimals.

EXAMPLE

	there are two places to the right
2.75 ←	of the decimal
×0.5 ←	plus two places to the right of the decimal, move the
1375.	decimal point four places to the left

After moving the decimal point, the answer reads 0.1375.

Dividing Decimals
The divisor is a number that is divided into the dividend.

EXAMPLE

$$0.69 \div 0.3 \qquad 0.3 \overline{)0.69}$$

dividend divisor   divisor dividend

This may be written or spoken as 0.69 divided by 0.3. To divide decimals:

1. The *divisor* is changed to a whole number. In this example, the decimal point is moved one place to the right so that 0.3 now becomes 3, which is a whole number.

$$3\overline{)0.69}$$

2. The decimal point in the *dividend* is now moved the *same number of places* to the right. In this example, the decimal point is moved one place to the right, the same number of places the decimal point in the divisor was moved.

$$3\overline{)6.9}$$

3. The numbers are now divided.

$$\begin{array}{r} 2.3 \\ 3\overline{)6.9} \end{array}$$

When only the dividend is a decimal, the decimal point is carried to the quotient (answer) in the same position.

EXAMPLES

$$\begin{array}{r} 0.375 \\ 2\overline{)0.750} \end{array} \qquad \begin{array}{r} 1.736 \\ 2\overline{)3.472} \end{array}$$

To divide when only the divisor is a decimal, for example,

$$0.3\overline{)66}$$

1. The divisor is changed to a whole number. In this example, the decimal point is moved one place to the right.

$$3\overline{)66}$$

2. The decimal point in the dividend must also be moved one place to the right.

$$3\overline{)6.6}$$

3. The numbers are now divided.

$$3\overline{)6.6}^{\,2.2}$$

Whenever the decimal point is moved in the dividend, it must *also* be moved in the divisor, and whenever the decimal point in the divisor is moved, it must *also* be moved in the dividend.

Changing a Fraction to a Decimal
To change a fraction to a decimal, divide the numerator by the denominator.

EXAMPLES

$$\frac{1}{5}=5\overline{)1.0}^{\,0.2}\quad \frac{3}{4}=4\overline{)3.00}^{\,0.75}\quad \frac{1}{6}=6\overline{)1.000}^{\,0.166}$$

Changing a Decimal to a Fraction
To change a decimal to a fraction:

1. Remove the decimal point and make the resulting whole number the numerator: 0.2 = 2.
2. The denominator is stated as 10 or a power of 10. In this example, 0.2 is read as two tenths, and therefore the denominator is 10.

$$0.2 = \frac{2}{10}\text{ reduced to the lowest possible number is }\frac{1}{5}$$

ADDITIONAL EXAMPLES

$$0.75 = \frac{75}{100} = \frac{3}{4} \qquad 0.025 = \frac{25}{1000} = \frac{1}{40}$$

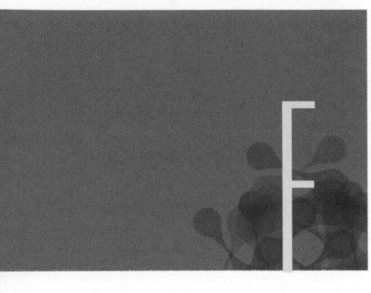

Answers to Review Questions and Medication Dosage Problems

Unit 1. Nursing Foundation of Clinical Pharmacology

Chapter 1. General Principles of Pharmacology
Review Questions: Prepare for the NCLEX
1. 3
2. 3
3. 2
4. 2
5. 4
6. 1
7. 1
8. 4
9. 1, 2, 4, 3
10. 1, 3, 4

Chapter 2. Administration of Drugs
Review Questions: Prepare for the NCLEX
1. 3
2. 4
3. 3
4. 2
5. 4
6. 2
7. 3
8. 2
9. 2, 3, 4
10. 2, 3

Chapter 3. Making Drug Dosing Safer
Questions
1. Tagamet is the brand name; cimetidine is the generic name.
2. The form of the drug is a Tiltab tablet, and 400 mg is in each tablet of Tagamet.
3. Zyprexa (brand) and olanzapine (generic) are the names; it comes in tablet form, and the dose strength is 5 mg.
4. Lanoxin (brand) and digoxin (generic) are the names; it comes in tablet form, and the dose strength is 250 mcg or 0.25 mg.
5. Augmentin (brand) and amoxicillin/clavulanate potassium (generic) are the names; it comes in liquid form, and the dose strength is 250 mg in 5 mL.

Calculations
1. 1 tablet after breakfast
2. 2 tablets after every meal
3. 2 tablets daily
4. 2 tablets daily
5. 5 mL in each dose
6. Client's weight in kilograms: $142 \div 2.2 = 64.5$ kg; child's weight in kilograms: $43 \div 2.2 = 19.5$ kg

Review Questions: Prepare for the NCLEX
1. 2
2. 4
3. 4
4. 4
5. 3
6. 1
7. 3
8. 3
9. 2
10. 2

Chapter 4. The Nursing Process
Review Questions: Prepare for the NCLEX
1. 3
2. 4
3. 4
4. 3
5. 3
6. 1
7. 4
8. 4
9. 2, 1, 5, 4, 3
10. 1, 4

Chapter 5. Client and Family Teaching
Hints for Pharmacology in Practice: Using Clinical Reasoning
Reviewing the clients presented, look at Box 5.1. Are any of them potential high-risk clients? What should you refrain from asking when you question the clients to assess if they have limited health literacy? Make a list of questions you could use with any clients that you interact with in your daily practice.

Review Questions: Prepare for the NCLEX
1. 4
2. 4
3. 3
4. 1
5. 2
6. 2
7. 3
8. 2
9. 3, 2, 1, 4
10. 1, 3, 4

Unit 2. Drugs Used to Fight Infections

Chapter 6. Antibacterial Drugs: Sulfonamides

Hints for Pharmacology in Practice: Using Clinical Reasoning

What is the relationship between urinary tract infections, memory, and cognitive processes in older adults? What do you know about limited health literacy? Would Mrs. Moore be at high risk for problems? Check Chapter 5 for hints to help her remember to take the medication. When should you reassess her mental status?

Review Questions: Know Your Drugs
1. B
2. A

Calculate Medication Dosages
1. 10 mL
2. 2 tablets

Prepare for the NCLEX
1. 2
2. 4
3. 1
4. 3
5. 3
6. 2
7. 2
8. 3
9. 4, 2, 3, 1
10. 2, 3, 4

Chapter 7. Antibacterial Drugs That Disrupt the Cell Wall

Hints for Pharmacology in Practice: Using Clinical Reasoning

Review Chapter 5 for methods to assess health literacy and limited English proficiency. When you teach should you be using Mrs. Garcia for interpretation? Because Mr. Garcia is taking a cephalosporin, what do you need to tell him specifically about alcohol, and why?

Review Questions: Know Your Drugs
1. C
2. D
3. A
4. B

Calculate Medication Dosages
1. 1 teaspoon (t) = 5 mL, then 1 teaspoon = 250 mg of amoxicillin. The nurse will teach the caregiver to administer 2 teaspoons (t) or 10 mL of amoxicillin.
2. 1 g cefoxitin = 4 mL of solution; this would require two IM injections.

Prepare for the NCLEX
1. 1
2. 4
3. 2
4. 1
5. 1
6. 2
7. 4
8. 2
9. 4
10. 1, 2, 4

Chapter 8. Antibacterial Drugs That Interfere With Protein Synthesis

Hints for Pharmacology in Practice: Using Clinical Reasoning

Review the drug–drug interactions in this chapter. What may happen with the medication combinations that Mrs. Moore is taking? Look for teaching hints in Chapter 5.

Review Questions: Know Your Drugs
1. D
2. C
3. B
4. A

Calculate Medication Dosages
1. 2 mL
2. 20 mL

Prepare for the NCLEX
1. 3
2. 2
3. 4
4. 1
5. 2
6. 1
7. 2
8. 4
9. 1, 3, 4
10. Day 1 = 2 tablets, days 2 through 5 = 1 tablet daily

Chapter 9. Antibacterial Drugs That Interfere With DNA/RNA Synthesis

Hints for Pharmacology in Practice: Using Clinical Reasoning

Think about what diarrhea means when someone is taking an anti-infective. Look at the information in this chapter's Client Teaching for Improved Outcomes. What factors could be contributing to this condition? What assessment should be carried out?

Review Questions: Know Your Drugs
1. B
2. A
3. C

Calculate Medication Dosages
1. 1 tablet every 12 hr
2. 3 tablets each dose

Prepare for the NCLEX
1. 4
2. 3
3. 1
4. 1
5. 3
6. 1
7. 2
8. 4
9. 30 mL of solution
10. 2, 3, 4

Chapter 10. Antitubercular Drugs

Hints for Pharmacology in Practice: Using Clinical Reasoning

Think about the risk factors for TB and what Betty Peterson's perceptions of her living situation are in relation to those factors.

Review Questions: Know Your Drugs
1. A
2. B
3. C
4. D

Calculate Medication Dosages
1. 6 mL
2. 4 tablets

Prepare for the NCLEX
1. 4
2. 4
3. 2
4. 4
5. 1
6. 2
7. 1
8. 4
9. 1, 2, 4, 5
10. 2

Chapter 11. Antiviral Drugs

Hints for Pharmacology in Practice: Using Clinical Reasoning

Think about the mode of transmission of the herpes zoster (shingles) virus. What childhood disease would alert you to who (staff or residents) would be at risk to get the infection? Review information about the drug, and then think about drug interactions and the medications that Mr. Park is currently taking.

Review Questions: Know Your Drugs
1. D
2. A
3. B
4. C

Calculate Medication Dosages
1. 2 tablets
2. 10 mL

Prepare for the NCLEX
1. 2
2. 3
3. 1
4. 1
5. 1
6. 2
7. 3
8. 1
9. 2 dose inhalations total in 24 hr, which is 10 mg of zanamivir in 24 hr
10. 1 = C, 2 = E, 3 = A, 4 = B, 5 = D

Chapter 12. Antifungal and Antiparasitic Drugs

Hints for Pharmacology in Practice: Using Clinical Reasoning

Review information about collecting pinworm samples. Do you need face-to-face instruction or could you relay this information accurately over the telephone? Review client education for information to include about treating both the client and the entire household when infection is suspected.

Review Questions: Know Your Drugs
1. C
2. A
3. D
4. B

Calculate Medication Dosages
1. 2 tablets
2. 2 capsules

Prepare for the NCLEX
1. 2
2. 2
3. 3
4. 2
5. 4
6. 1
7. 1
8. 2
9. 1, 2, 3
10. 95.4 mg (140 lb = 63.6 kg) 1.5 mg/63.6 kg/day = 95.4 mg or 95 mg if rounding to the nearest whole number

Unit 3. Drugs Used to Manage Pain
Chapter 13. Nonopioid Analgesics: Salicylates and Nonsalicylates

Hints for Pharmacology in Practice: Using Clinical Reasoning

Review information on GI distress and the nonopioid analgesics. What problems could the aspirin product be causing? If Betty does switch to an acetaminophen product, what other drugs or foods should Betty avoid that might contain salicylates?

Review Questions: Know Your Drugs
1. A, D
2. B, C, E

Calculate Medication Dosages
1. 1.5 or 1½ mL
2. 2 tablets

Prepare for the NCLEX
1. 4
2. 3
3. 1
4. 3
5. 3
6. 2
7. 3
8. 4
9. 1, 4, 5
10. 12 tablets in 1 day (3900 mg); each tablet is 325 mg, maximum dose is 4000 mg (4 g) per day; using 3250 mg standard would equal 10 tablets in 1 day (3250 mg)

Chapter 14. Nonopioid Analgesics: Nonsteroidal Anti-Inflammatory Drugs (NSAIDs) and Migraine Headache Medications
Hints for Pharmacology in Practice: Using Clinical Reasoning
As you assess drug use, what are some of the adverse reactions to salicylate therapy? With regard to GI-related adverse reactions when using a COX-2 inhibitor, would you see a difference? Think about the daughter's concerns; what could be causing the hearing difficulty, and would that change with a change of medications?

Review Questions: Know Your Drugs
1. C
2. A
3. B
4. D

Calculate Medication Dosages
1. 10 mL
2. 2 tablets

Prepare for the NCLEX
1. 2
2. 4
3. 1
4. 1
5. 4
6. 2
7. 4
8. 3
9. 2, 3, 4
10. 1, 3, 4

Chapter 15. Opioid Analgesics and Antagonists
Hints for Pharmacology in Practice: Using Clinical Reasoning
Think about all components of a pain assessment; which ones were neglected in the client interview? What defines the opioid-naive client, and what steps should you take to facilitate breathing before administering an opioid antagonist?

Review Questions: Know Your Drugs
1. C
2. B
3. A
4. D

Calculate Medication Dosages
1. 1.2 mL
2. 0.8 mL

Prepare for the NCLEX
1. 4
2. 3
3. 3
4. 1
5. 4
6. 3
7. 2
8. 3, 4
9. Vicodin contains 300-mg acetaminophen in each tablet (Table 15.2), 6 tablets = 1800 mg
10. 4 injections; 0.4 mg + 0.2 mg + 0.2 mg + 0.2 mg = 1 mg

Practice: Using Clinical Reasoning

Chapter 16. Anesthetic Drugs
Hints for Pharmacology in Practice: Using Clinical Reasoning
Think about what you learned about the additive epinephrine in this chapter. When should it be used and when should it not be used?

Review Questions: Know Your Drugs
1. D
2. A
3. B
4. C

Calculate Medication Dosages
1. 1 mL

Prepare for the NCLEX
1. 3
2. 2
3. 3
4. 1
5. 2
6. 4
7. 4
8. 1 = C, 2 = A, 3 = D, 4 = B
9. 3, 2, 4, 1
10. 0.3 mg

Unit 4. Drugs That Affect the Central Nervous System

Chapter 17. Central Nervous System Stimulants
Hints for Pharmacology in Practice: Using Clinical Reasoning
Key assessment items would include inattention, hyperactivity, and impulsiveness. What is the importance of maintaining a specific weight to a gymnast? Could the mother be looking for an anorexiant to maintain Janna's weight for the gymnastics team?

Review Questions: Know Your Drugs
1. B
2. D
3. A
4. C

Calculate Medication Dosages
1. 2 capsules
2. 2 tablets

Prepare for the NCLEX
1. 3
2. 3
3. 1
4. 4
5. 4
6. 1
7. 2
8. 1
9. 1, 2, 4
10. 24 mg; yes, it is appropriate.

Chapter 18. Antidementia Drugs
Hints for Pharmacology in Practice: Using Clinical Reasoning
What are the primary adverse reactions of the cholinesterase inhibitors? Why would Mrs. Moore have on multiple patches?

Review Questions: Know Your Drugs
1. A
2. D
3. C
4. B

Calculate Medication Dosages
1. 3 mL
2. 2 tablets

Prepare for the NCLEX
1. 1
2. 2
3. 3
4. 1
5. 4
6. 3
7. 3
8. 2
9. 1, 2, 3, 5
10. 2, 3

Chapter 19. Antianxiety Drugs
Hints for Pharmacology in Practice: Using Clinical Reasoning
Do Mr. Garcia's vital signs indicate anxiety? What are the cultural implications to consider with this client if he is displaying anxiety? How will you interact when an interpreter is involved in client teaching?

Review Questions: Know Your Drugs
1. D
2. B
3. C
4. A

Calculate Medication Dosages
1. 1 mL
2. 2 tablets/dose

Prepare for the NCLEX
1. 2
2. 1
3. 4
4. 2
5. 3
6. 2
7. 2
8. 4
9. 1, 2, 3, 4, 5
10. 2 mL

Chapter 20. Sedatives and Hypnotics
Hints for Pharmacology in Practice: Using Clinical Reasoning
What reasons should hypnotics be used and for how long? Is Mr. Phillip's grief reaction an appropriate use of the drug? What other nonpharmacologic interventions could you recommend in place of using a hypnotic?

Review Questions: Know Your Drugs
1. C
2. D
3. A, B

Calculate Medication Dosages
1. 1 tablet
2. 2 tablets

Prepare for the NCLEX
1. 4
2. 2
3. 3
4. 1
5. 4
6. 3
7. 1
8. 2
9. 1, 3, 4
10. 1, 2, 3

Chapter 21. Antidepressant Drugs
Hints for Pharmacology in Practice: Using Clinical Reasoning
How long does it take for antidepressant medications to take effect? In Chapter 20, we learned that Mr. Phillip was prescribed a hypnotic for sleep. What are the drug interactions when using these medications together?

Review Questions: Know Your Drugs
1. C, D
2. A
3. B

Calculate Medication Dosages
1. 3 tablets
2. 25 mL

Prepare for the NCLEX
1. 4
2. 3
3. 2
4. 2
5. 3
6. 3
7. 2
8. 4
9. 1, 2, 3
10. 2, 3, 4

Chapter 22. Antipsychotic Drugs
Hints for Pharmacology in Practice: Using Clinical Reasoning
What type of symptoms does she have, positive or negative? Mrs. Moore had a UTI earlier; what is the relationship between UTI and cognition? Does she have a condition that contradicts the use of the medication? How would you present this information to the daughter?

Review Questions: Know Your Drugs
1. A
2. C
3. D
4. B

Calculate Medication Dosages
1. 2 tablets
2. 0.6 mL will be 3 mg of haloperidol

Prepare for the NCLEX
1. 2
2. 3
3. 3
4. 2
5. 4
6. 3
7. 3
8. 2
9. 1, 2, 3
10. 1 = B, 2 = A, C, D, E

Unit 5. Drugs That Affect the Peripheral Nervous System

Chapter 23. Adrenergic Drugs
Hints for Pharmacology in Practice: Using Clinical Reasoning
Review the client teaching for improved outcomes; how could you use this information to decrease Mrs. Wong's concerns? Check Chapter 5 for suggestions.

Review Questions: Know Your Drugs
1. C
2. B
3. A

Calculate Medication Dosages
1. 2 mL
2. 0.5 mL

Prepare for the NCLEX
1. 2
2. 3
3. 2
4. 1
5. 4
6. 4
7. 2
8. 4
9. 1, 3
10. 0.6 mg

Chapter 24. Adrenergic Blocking Drugs
Hints for Pharmacology in Practice: Using Clinical Reasoning
When are the blood levels of a drug taken daily the highest and the lowest? What items should Mr. Garcia be taught each time he changes position?

Review Questions: Know Your Drugs
1. C
2. B
3. A
4. D

Calculate Medication Dosages
1. 2 tablets
2. 1 capsule

Prepare for the NCLEX
1. 2
2. 4
3. 4
4. 1
5. 3
6. 2
7. 3
8. 2 (12 mL of propranolol oral solution + 30 mL of flush solution = 42 mL total)
9. 2, 3
10. 4 tablets

Chapter 25. Cholinergic Drugs
Hints for Pharmacology in Practice: Using Clinical Reasoning
In addition to considering the drugs to help stimulate the bladder to contract and produce urine, review Chapter 23 and apply the information learned to the situation with Mr. Park's bladder when the sympathetic system was activated by the stressful state of the initial hip fracture.

Review Questions: Know Your Drugs
1. A, C
2. B

Calculate Medication Dosages
1. 0.5 mL

Prepare for the NCLEX
1. 4
2. 4
3. 2
4. 3
5. 1, 2, 4
6. 10 tablets

Chapter 26. Cholinergic Blocking Drugs
Hints for Pharmacology in Practice: Using Clinical Reasoning
Review the side effects that can occur with the different cholinergic blocking drugs. What is the impact specifically on the bowels and mobility?

Review Questions: Know Your Drugs
1. A
2. D
3. B
4. C

Calculate Medication Dosages
1. 0.5 mL
2. 10 mL

Prepare for the NCLEX
1. 1
2. 2
3. 2
4. 4
5. 2
6. 3
7. 4
8. 3
9. 2, 4
10. 1, 3, 4, 5

Unit 6. Drugs That Affect the Neuromuscular System

Chapter 27. Antiparkinson Drugs

Hints for Pharmacology in Practice: Using Clinical Reasoning

What is the cluster of symptoms described in the case study? What are some of the adverse reactions to medications that Betty is currently using?

Review Questions: Know Your Drugs

1. D
2. B
3. C
4. A

Calculate Medication Dosages

1. One 500-mg tablet and one 250-mg tablet = 750 mg or 0.75 g
2. 3 tablets

Prepare for the NCLEX

1. 2
2. 1
3. 2
4. 3
5. 2
6. 4
7. 4
8. 2
9. 1, 3
10. 2, 4, 3, 1

Chapter 28. Antiepileptics

Hints for Pharmacology in Practice: Using Clinical Reasoning

What type of seizures do you think Ms. Chase had following her accident? What questions would you ask before you discuss your findings with the primary health care provider regarding Ms. Chase's intermittent use of the medications?

Review Questions: Know Your Drugs

1. C
2. D
3. A
4. B

Calculate Medication Dosages

1. 2 tablets
2. 10 mL

Prepare for the NCLEX

1. 3
2. 3
3. 1
4. 3
5. 1
6. 3
7. 2
8. 2
9. 2 mL
10. Dilantin

Chapter 29. Skeletal Muscle, Bone, and Joint Disorder Drugs

Hints for Pharmacology in Practice: Using Clinical Reasoning

Review the drug administration requirements and the fact that Mrs. Moore suffers from periodic confusion.

Review Questions: Know Your Drugs

1. C
2. D
3. A
4. B

Calculate Medication Dosages

1. 3 tablets
2. 3 tablets

Prepare for the NCLEX

1. 2
2. 1
3. 3
4. 4
5. 4
6. 1
7. 4
8. 4
9. 1, 2, 3, 4, 5
10. 252 mg

Unit 7. Drugs That Affect the Respiratory System

Chapter 30. Upper Respiratory System Drugs

Hints for Pharmacology in Practice: Using Clinical Reasoning

Janna Wong competes on her school's gymnastic team. How might her abilities be altered by the influence of either the antihistamine or nasal decongestant? Check earlier pain relief chapters; what do you need to discuss with teens independently taking medications?

Review Questions: Know Your Drugs

1. A
2. D
3. C
4. B

Calculate Medication Dosages

1. 5 mL
2. 2 tablets

Prepare for the NCLEX

1. 2
2. 1
3. 1
4. 2
5. 3
6. 4
7. 1
8. 1
9. 1
10. 2, 3, 4

Chapter 31. Lower Respiratory System Drugs

Hints for Pharmacology in Practice: Using Clinical Reasoning

Check the chapter for the medication taken. What medication did Mrs. Chase's mother use in the inhalation device, and how are Mrs. Chase's medications different?

Review Questions: Know Your Drugs

1. B
2. A
3. C
4. D

Calculate Medication Dosages
1. 0.25 mL
2. 2 tablets, 40 mg each day

Prepare for the NCLEX
 1. 2
 2. 3
 3. 4
 4. 1
 5. 1
 6. 4
 7. 2
 8. 3
 9. 1, 3
10. 1, 3

Unit 8. Drugs That Affect the Cardiovascular System

Chapter 32. Diuretics
Hints for Pharmacology in Practice: Using Clinical Reasoning
What are some recommendations you can make to facilitate correct use of the medication? Review Mrs. Moore's status in Chapters 6 and 22; what could be contributing to her urinary tract infections? Think about fluids.

Review Questions: Know Your Drugs
1. B
2. C
3. D
4. A

Calculate Medication Dosages
1. 2 tablets
2. 2.5 mL

Prepare for the NCLEX
 1. 4
 2. 4
 3. 4
 4. 3
 5. 4
 6. 4
 7. 2
 8. 2
 9. 1, 2, 3
10. 1 = C; 2 = B, E; 3 = D; 4 = A

Chapter 33. Antihyperlipidemic Drugs
Hints for Pharmacology in Practice: Using Clinical Reasoning
Review Chapter 5 and principles of adult learning. What information from the two sets of laboratory values and vital signs can be used to motivate adherence to Lillian's lifestyle changes? How can you plug this information into an online CV risk calculator? What information about her medications can help reduce constipation symptoms?

Review Questions: Know Your Drugs
1. B
2. C
3. A
4. D

Calculate Medication Dosages
1. 2 tablets
2. 40 mg, dose requirement = four 20-mg tablets or two 40-mg tablets; the 40-mg tablet size is less in number

Prepare for the NCLEX
 1. 3
 2. 2
 3. 3
 4. 1
 5. 2
 6. 1
 7. 3
 8. 4
 9. 1, 4, 5
10. Yes, 200 mg is an appropriate dosage. However, if the client requires 200 mg, it is preferable to give a 200-mg capsule rather than three 67-mg capsules. The nurse should notify the primary health care provider that only 67-mg capsules are available.

Chapter 34. Antihypertensive Drugs
Hints for Pharmacology in Practice: Using Clinical Reasoning
Where can you access information for clients with limited English proficiency (LEP)? What are some diet resources? What questions do you need to ask Mr. Garcia about flavor preferences?

Review Questions: Know Your Drugs
1. C
2. D
3. A
4. B

Calculate Medication Dosages
1. 2 tablets
2. 3 capsules

Prepare for the NCLEX
 1. 2
 2. 3
 3. 3
 4. 3
 5. 4
 6. 2
 7. 4
 8. 3
 9. 1, 3
10. 90-mg tablets and give 2 tablets

Chapter 35. Antianginal and Vasodilating Drugs
Hints for Pharmacology in Practice: Using Clinical Reasoning
A likely choice may be the transdermal system; check Chapter 18. Is this a good solution for Mrs. Moore? Is she able to remember when to replace patches, and what would happen if she forgot to remove an old one?

Review Questions: Know Your Drugs
1. B
2. A
3. C
4. D

Calculate Medication Dosages
1. 3 tablets
2. 2 tablets

Prepare for the NCLEX
1. 2
2. 1
3. 2
4. 2
5. 3
6. 2
7. 4
8. 4
9. 1, 2, 3
10. In 1 min, and then again in 5 more minutes

Chapter 36. Anticoagulant and Thrombolytic Drugs

Hints for Pharmacology in Practice: Using Clinical Reasoning

What could be the effect of taking a different strength of warfarin for each dose?

Review Questions: Know Your Drugs
1. D
2. C
3. A
4. B

Calculate Medication Dosages
1. 2 mL
2. 2 tablets

Prepare for the NCLEX
1. 3
2. 4
3. 4
4. 2
5. 1
6. 4
7. 2
8. 1
9. 1, 4, 5
10. 1 = C, 2 = A, 3 = B

Chapter 37. Cardiotonic and Antiarrhythmic Drugs

Hints for Pharmacology in Practice: Using Clinical Reasoning

Mr. Phillip has multiple medications and schedules. Review client teaching and medication administration. How can you help him safely self-administer the medications?

Review Questions: Know Your Drugs
1. D
2. C
3. A
4. B

Review Questions: Calculate Medication Dosages
1. 2 mL
2. 2 tablets

Prepare for the NCLEX
1. 4
2. 1
3. 1
4. 2
5. 1
6. 3
7. 3
8. 1
9. One 0.5-mg tablet and one 0.25-mg tablet
10. 2 tablets daily

Unit 9. Drugs That Affect the Gastrointestinal System

Chapter 38. Upper Gastrointestinal System Drugs

Hints for Pharmacology in Practice: Using Clinical Reasoning

Where can you access information for clients with LEP? Review in Chapter 5 how to handle what may be a longstanding cultural practice. Do antacids actually coat the stomach lining? What do they actually do? By examining the different elements, determine what a person should reduce in their diet when dealing with hypertensive disease. Which elements promote constipation?

Review Questions: Know Your Drugs
1. C
2. A
3. B
4. D

Calculate Medication Dosages
1. 2 capsules
2. 20 mL

Prepare for the NCLEX
1. 3
2. 4
3. 2
4. 3
5. 2
6. 2
7. 2
8. 1 = B, C; 2 = A, D
9. 10 mL
10. 1 tablet

Chapter 39. Lower Gastrointestinal System Drugs

Hints for Pharmacology in Practice: Using Clinical Reasoning

What do the medications listed do to the bowel? There are different preparations to add bulk, soften stool, and so forth. Which does Betty need based on the drugs she is currently taking?

Review Questions: Know Your Drugs
1. B
2. A
3. D
4. C

Calculate Medication Dosages
1. 3 capsules
2. 5 mg

Prepare for the NCLEX
1. 3
2. 3
3. 3
4. 1
5. 4
6. 4
7. 2
8. 3
9. 1, 3, 4
10. 3 hr (2.7, question asks in hours so round to within 3 hr)

Unit 10. Drugs That Affect the Endocrine System

Chapter 40. Antidiabetic Drugs
Hints for Pharmacology in Practice: Using Clinical Reasoning
Review strategies to promote client adherence to medication regimens. What skills can you sequence to provide a positive learning experience for Mr. Phillip?

Review Questions: Know Your Drugs
1. A
2. B
3. D
4. C

Calculate Medication Dosages
1. 4 tablets
2. 45 units

Prepare for the NCLEX
1. 2
2. 1
3. 3
4. 4
5. 3
6. 2
7. 3
8. C, B, D, A
9. 45 units; inject air into NPH vial, inject air into regular vial, draw out 5 units of regular insulin, then draw out 40 units NPH
10. 2 tablets per dose; total daily dose = 2000 mg

Chapter 41. Pituitary and Adrenocortical Hormones
Hints for Pharmacology in Practice: Using Clinical Reasoning
Desmopressin replaces which hormone made by the pituitary gland? What is the function of this hormone, and why would you want more in the system at night than in the daytime when you are more active?

Review Questions: Know Your Drugs
1. D
2. C
3. B
4. A

Calculate Medication Dosages
1. 2 tablets
2. 2 tablets

Prepare for the NCLEX
1. 3
2. 4
3. 2
4. 1
5. 3
6. 3
7. 2
8. 2
9. 1
10. 1 = A, B, D; 2 = C

Chapter 42. Thyroid and Antithyroid Drugs
Hints for Pharmacology in Practice: Using Clinical Reasoning
Be sure to assess why Betty believes there is danger before you work to educate her about the radioactive iodine. This will make it easier to clarify unrealistic beliefs.

Review Questions: Know Your Drugs
1. C
2. D
3. B
4. A

Calculate Medication Dosages
1. 4 tablets
2. 2 tablets

Prepare for the NCLEX
1. 3
2. 1
3. 2
4. 2
5. 3
6. 1
7. 3
8. 2
9. 1, 2
10. 1, 2, 4

Chapter 43. Male and Female Hormones
Hints for Pharmacology in Practice: Using Clinical Reasoning
Is Janna sexually active, or does she want to begin birth control for another reason? What is the best method for her to use? Are there any indications from previous chapters that would negate the use of any specific methods?

Review Questions: Know Your Drugs
1. B
2. C
3. D
4. A

Calculate Medication Dosages
1. 1.6 mL
2. 1 mL

Prepare for the NCLEX
1. 2
2. 3
3. 4
4. 3
5. 2
6. 1
7. 1
8. 3
9. 1, 2
10. 1, 2, 3, 4

Chapter 44. Uterine Drugs
Hints for Pharmacology in Practice: Using Clinical Reasoning
Be sure to assess Betty's health literacy regarding the birth process. How can you explain what oxytocin does to induce labor in terminology that is easy for her to understand?

Review Questions: Know Your Drugs
1. C
2. A
3. D
4. B

Calculate Medication Dosages
1. 0.5 mL
2. 1 mL

Prepare for the NCLEX
1. 4
2. 2
3. 4
4. 1
5. 1
6. 4
7. 4
8. 2
9. 5 mL/min
10. 1 = indomethacin, NSAID; 2 = nifedipine, calcium channel blocker; 3 = terbutaline, bronchodilator

Unit 11. Drugs That Affect the Urinary System

Chapter 45. Menopause and Andropause Drugs
Hints for Pharmacology in Practice: Using Clinical Reasoning
What happens to urinary structures when fluids are reduced, since that is contrary to recommended practices for treating urinary symptoms?

Review Questions: Know Your Drugs
1. D
2. C
3. A
4. B

Calculate Medication Dosages
1. 2 tablets
2. 2 tablets

Prepare for the NCLEX
1. 3
2. 4
3. 3
4. 2
5. 1
6. 2
7. 2
8. 2
9. 1, 3, 5
10. 2, 3, 4

Chapter 46. Urinary Tract Anti-Infectives and Other Urinary Drugs
Hints for Pharmacology in Practice: Using Clinical Reasoning
Review the Client Teaching for Improved Outcomes. What behaviors do you need to address?

Review Questions: Know Your Drugs
1. B
2. D
3. C
4. A

Calculate Medication Dosages
1. 2 tablets
2. 10 mL

Prepare for the NCLEX
1. 1
2. 3
3. 3
4. 4
5. 1 = A, 2 = C, 3 = B, 4 = D

Unit 12. Drugs That Affect the Immune System

Chapter 47. Vaccines
Hints for Pharmacology in Practice: Using Clinical Reasoning
Think about the consequences to the child should he acquire the illness in the timeframe of the delay in immunization.

Review Questions: Know Your Drugs
1. C
2. A
3. B
4. D

Calculate Medication Dosages
1. 6 vials of the FluLaval vaccine

Prepare for the NCLEX
1. 3
2. 3
3. 2
4. 1
5. 3
6. 1
7. 2
8. 2, 4, 5
9. 1, 3, 4

Chapter 48. Immune Stimulants
Hints for Pharmacology in Practice: Using Clinical Reasoning
What are the stipulations for use of erythropoiesis-stimulating agents (ESAs) in dialysis?

Review Questions: Know Your Drugs
1. D
2. C
3. A
4. B

Calculate Medication Dosages
1. 0.5 mL
2. 0.2 mL

Prepare for the NCLEX
1. 3
2. 4
3. 1
4. 1
5. 1
6. 1
7. 3
8. 2
9. 3 tablets day 1, 1 tablet day 5
10. 1 = C, 2 = B, 3 = A

Chapter 49. Immune Blockers
Hints for Pharmacology in Practice: Using Clinical Reasoning
Mr. Park's arthritic condition is osteoarthritis, not rheumatoid arthritis. Therefore, his condition is not inflammatory related.

Review Questions: Know Your Drugs
1. B
2. C
3. A
4. D

Calculate Medication Dosages
1. 152 mg in the infusion

Prepare for the NCLEX
 1. 2
 2. 3
 3. 4
 4. 2
 5. 3
 6. 2
 7. 3
 8. 3
 9. 2, 4, 3, 1
10. No; 76 pounds = 34.5 kg, dose for tofacitinib is 4 mg/kg = 138 mg; 172 mg is too high

Chapter 50. Traditional Chemotherapy
Hints for Pharmacology in Practice: Using Clinical Reasoning
Mr. Phillip is now ready to discuss his losses. What in addition to the medications prescribed should be recommended?

Review Questions: Know Your Drugs
1. B
2. C
3. A
4. D

Calculate Medication Dosages
1. 12.8 mg/day
2. 13.5 units

Prepare for the NCLEX
 1. 2
 2. 4
 3. 4
 4. 2
 5. 2
 6. 3
 7. 3
 8. 1
 9. 3
10. 1, 2, 3, 4

Chapter 51. Immunotherapy
Hints for Pharmacology in Practice: Using Clinical Reasoning
During Mrs. Phillip's immunotherapy she may have had the flu-like symptoms, putting on a warm jacket in the summer sounds like she experienced chills during her treatment with Herceptin.

Review Questions: Know Your Drugs
1. B
2. D
3. A
4. C

Calculate Medication Dosages
1. The infusion should be 15 min.

Prepare for the NCLEX
 1. 2
 2. 1
 3. 2
 4. 2
 5. 4
 6. 2
 7. 2
 8. 2
 9. 3
10. 1, 2, 4

Unit 14. Drugs That Affect Other Body Systems

Chapter 52. Skin Disorder Topical Drugs
Hints for Pharmacology in Practice: Using Clinical Reasoning
What are the differences in the treatment of herpes simplex virus (HSV) oral lesions and the varicella-zoster virus that presents on the skin?

Review Questions: Know Your Drugs
1. D
2. B
3. A
4. C

Prepare for the NCLEX
 1. 2
 2. 2
 3. 2
 4. 4
 5. 2
 6. 1
 7. 3
 8. 4
 9. Fissure
10. 30 mL

Chapter 53. Otic and Ophthalmic Preparations
Hints for Pharmacology in Practice: Using Clinical Reasoning
Appealing to principles of personal growth and development and using the concepts you learned about health literacy, what would be the best way to interact with and teach Janna?

Review Questions: Know Your Drugs
1. C
2. D
3. A
4. B

Calculate Medication Dosages
1. 5 (gtt) drops
2. 60 doses

Prepare for the NCLEX
1. 1
2. 2
3. 2
4. 2
5. 3
6. 4
7. 2
8. 3
9. 2, 3

Chapter 54. Fluids, Electrolytes, and Parenteral Therapy

Hints for Pharmacology in Practice: Using Clinical Reasoning

Describe what electrolyte imbalance is occurring as a result of taking sodium bicarbonate for stomach ailments.

Calculate Medication Dosages
1. 100 mL/hr
2. 30 mL

Prepare for the NCLEX
1. 3
2. 3
3. 4
4. 1
5. 4
6. 1
7. 4
8. 2
9. 3
10. 4, 2, 1, 3, 5

G

NCLEX-PN Prep

Introduction

At the end of each chapter in the section called Prepare for the NCLEX, you are provided approximately 10 questions to test your knowledge base and retention of pharmacology information.

The first section, Recall the Facts, provides questions about information and content retention.

In the section called Analyze the Facts, analysis and application questions that are designed using the 2020 NCLEX-PN Detailed Test Plan are provided.

An Alternate-Format Questions section gives you exposure to the different ways in which questions are presented in the examination.

To successfully pass the NCLEX-PN examination, it helps to understand how the test you take is constructed. Although the examination itself is adaptive—meaning it changes for each person who takes the test—it is initially constructed to test the same concepts for each participant. See the following pages for a pictorial diagram of how a sampling of the Prepare for the NCLEX review questions in each chapter is correlated with the most recent NCLEX-PN Test Plan.

The best way to use this diagram is to look at the selected questions in each chapter to get a feel for what information you know and understand. Correctly answering the selected questions, which are marked with an asterisk (*) in each chapter could indicate that you have mastered the concepts of a specific portion of the Test Plan. This means if you correctly answered question #10 in Chapter 3 and question #10 in Chapter 17, you probably understand how to use clinical decision making when calculating a drug dose. (Look at the diagram to find these two questions under the box called "Use clinical decision making when calculating doses" under the section **Dosage Calculation**.) This information will help you focus your study time in order to concentrate on learning concepts that are harder for you and, therefore, to be more successful on the NCLEX-PN examination.

Below, you will find how specific questions from each chapter correspond directly to the items on the Detailed Test Plan, Pharmacologic Therapies section. In this way, you can prepare for the NCLEX-PN examination by focusing on the areas you need to improve your understanding and by practicing with sample questions that are of the type used in the examination.

2020 NCLEX-PN Mapping for section: Pharmacological Therapies

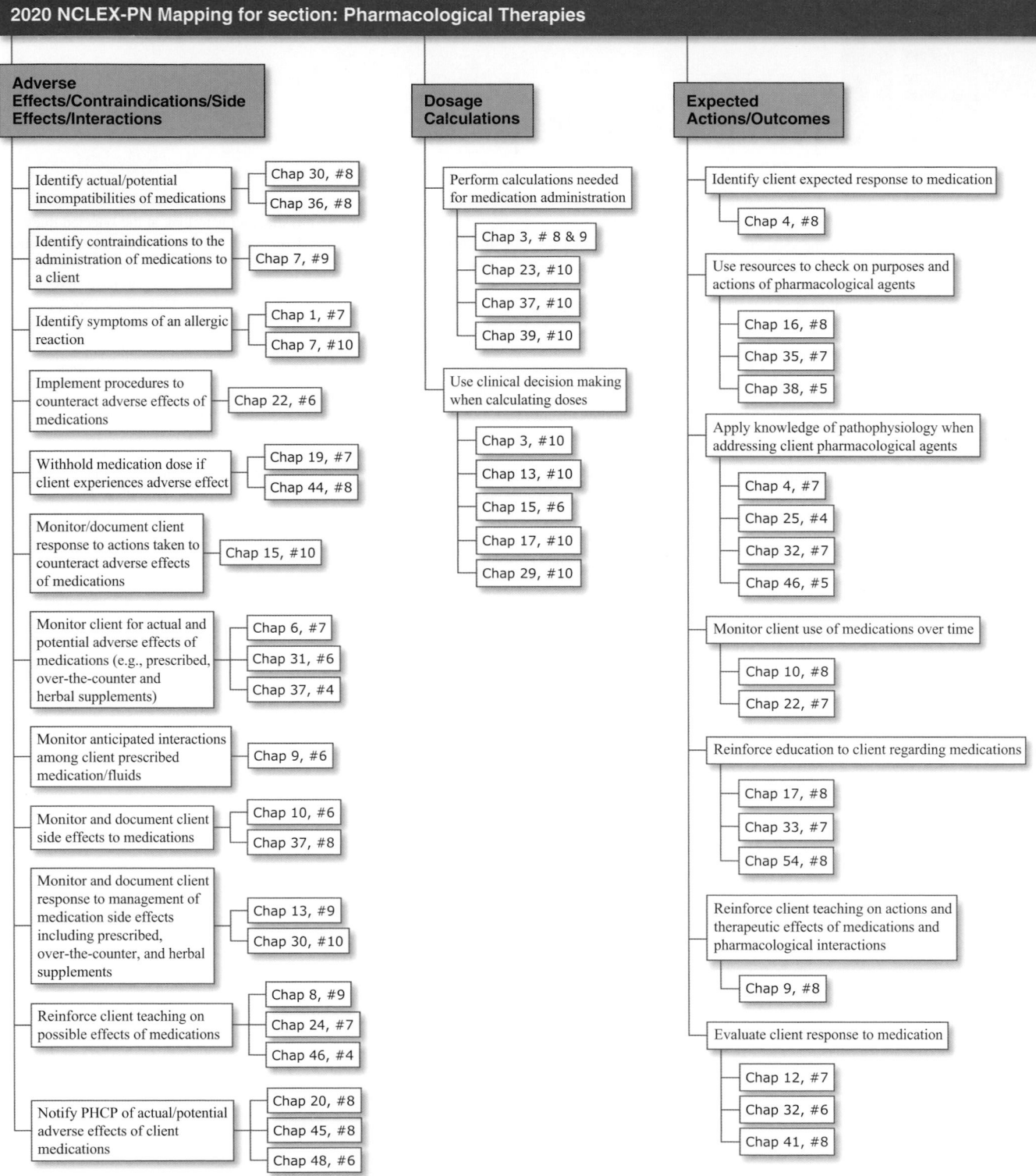

Adverse Effects/Contraindications/Side Effects/Interactions

Identify actual/potential incompatibilities of medications
- Chap 30, #8
- Chap 36, #8

Identify contraindications to the administration of medications to a client
- Chap 7, #9

Identify symptoms of an allergic reaction
- Chap 1, #7
- Chap 7, #10

Implement procedures to counteract adverse effects of medications
- Chap 22, #6

Withhold medication dose if client experiences adverse effect
- Chap 19, #7
- Chap 44, #8

Monitor/document client response to actions taken to counteract adverse effects of medications
- Chap 15, #10

Monitor client for actual and potential adverse effects of medications (e.g., prescribed, over-the-counter and herbal supplements)
- Chap 6, #7
- Chap 31, #6
- Chap 37, #4

Monitor anticipated interactions among client prescribed medication/fluids
- Chap 9, #6

Monitor and document client side effects to medications
- Chap 10, #6
- Chap 37, #8

Monitor and document client response to management of medication side effects including prescribed, over-the-counter, and herbal supplements
- Chap 13, #9
- Chap 30, #10

Reinforce client teaching on possible effects of medications
- Chap 8, #9
- Chap 24, #7
- Chap 46, #4

Notify PHCP of actual/potential adverse effects of client medications
- Chap 20, #8
- Chap 45, #8
- Chap 48, #6

Dosage Calculations

Perform calculations needed for medication administration
- Chap 3, # 8 & 9
- Chap 23, #10
- Chap 37, #10
- Chap 39, #10

Use clinical decision making when calculating doses
- Chap 3, #10
- Chap 13, #10
- Chap 15, #6
- Chap 17, #10
- Chap 29, #10

Expected Actions/Outcomes

Identify client expected response to medication
- Chap 4, #8

Use resources to check on purposes and actions of pharmacological agents
- Chap 16, #8
- Chap 35, #7
- Chap 38, #5

Apply knowledge of pathophysiology when addressing client pharmacological agents
- Chap 4, #7
- Chap 25, #4
- Chap 32, #7
- Chap 46, #5

Monitor client use of medications over time
- Chap 10, #8
- Chap 22, #7

Reinforce education to client regarding medications
- Chap 17, #8
- Chap 33, #7
- Chap 54, #8

Reinforce client teaching on actions and therapeutic effects of medications and pharmacological interactions
- Chap 9, #8

Evaluate client response to medication
- Chap 12, #7
- Chap 32, #6
- Chap 41, #8

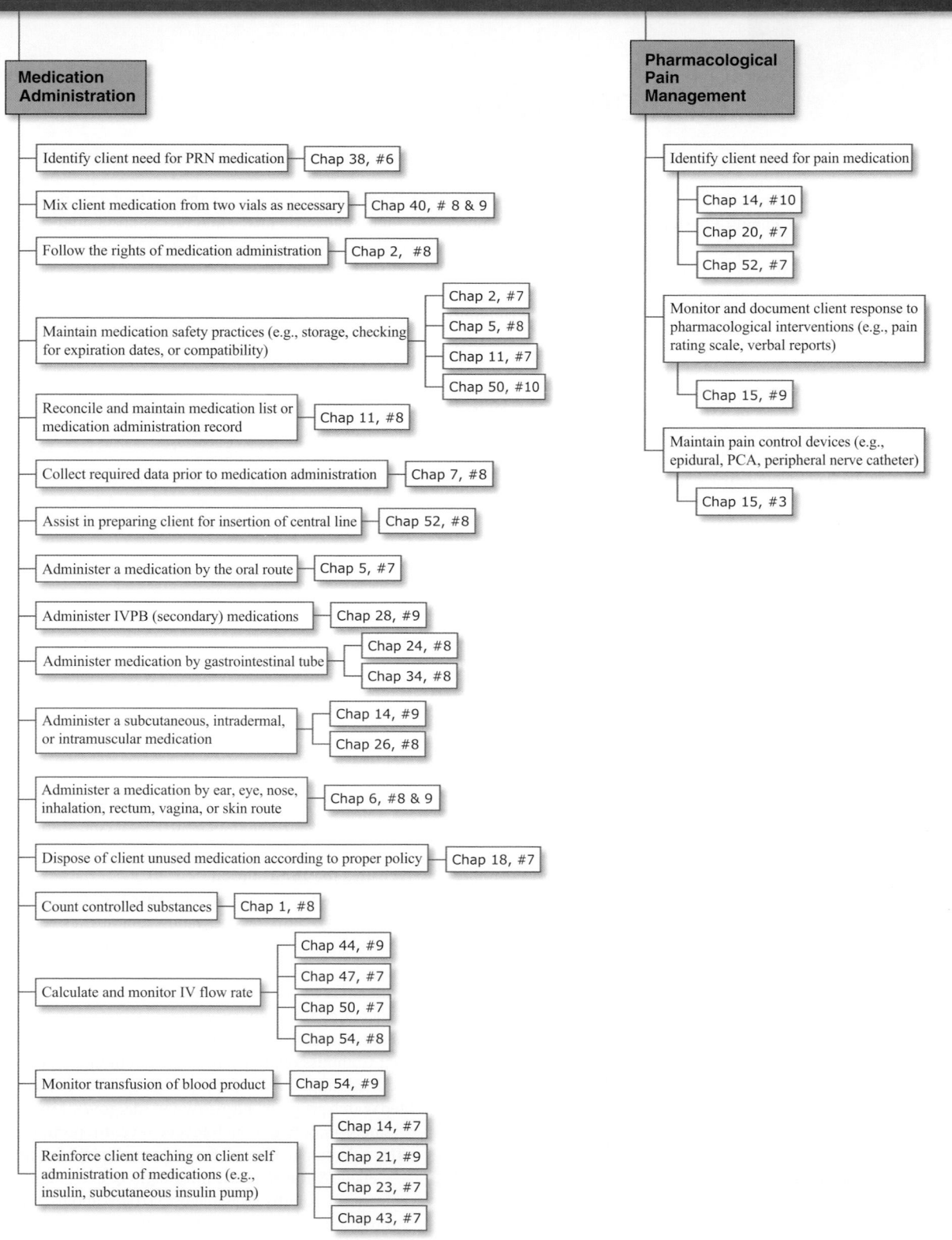

Medication Administration

Identify client need for PRN medication — Chap 38, #6

Mix client medication from two vials as necessary — Chap 40, # 8 & 9

Follow the rights of medication administration — Chap 2, #8

Maintain medication safety practices (e.g., storage, checking for expiration dates, or compatibility)
- Chap 2, #7
- Chap 5, #8
- Chap 11, #7
- Chap 50, #10

Reconcile and maintain medication list or medication administration record — Chap 11, #8

Collect required data prior to medication administration — Chap 7, #8

Assist in preparing client for insertion of central line — Chap 52, #8

Administer a medication by the oral route — Chap 5, #7

Administer IVPB (secondary) medications — Chap 28, #9

Administer medication by gastrointestinal tube
- Chap 24, #8
- Chap 34, #8

Administer a subcutaneous, intradermal, or intramuscular medication
- Chap 14, #9
- Chap 26, #8

Administer a medication by ear, eye, nose, inhalation, rectum, vagina, or skin route — Chap 6, #8 & 9

Dispose of client unused medication according to proper policy — Chap 18, #7

Count controlled substances — Chap 1, #8

Calculate and monitor IV flow rate
- Chap 44, #9
- Chap 47, #7
- Chap 50, #7
- Chap 54, #8

Monitor transfusion of blood product — Chap 54, #9

Reinforce client teaching on client self administration of medications (e.g., insulin, subcutaneous insulin pump)
- Chap 14, #7
- Chap 21, #9
- Chap 23, #7
- Chap 43, #7

Pharmacological Pain Management

Identify client need for pain medication
- Chap 14, #10
- Chap 20, #7
- Chap 52, #7

Monitor and document client response to pharmacological interventions (e.g., pain rating scale, verbal reports)
- Chap 15, #9

Maintain pain control devices (e.g., epidural, PCA, peripheral nerve catheter)
- Chap 15, #3

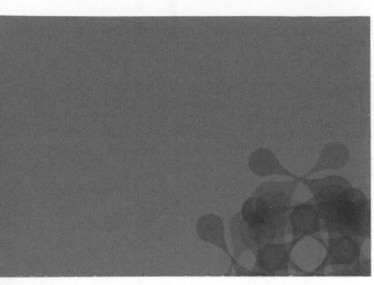

Bibliography

Unit 1

American Academy of Family Physicians. Herbal health products and supplements. FamilyDoctor.org. http://familydoctor.org/familydoctor/en/drugs-procedures-devices/over-the-counter/herbal-products-and-supplements.html

Beyea, S. (1999). Nursing diagnosis or patient problem? *Nursing Diagnosis, 10*(1), 32–34.

Bonsall, A., Mosby, A., Walz, M., & Wintermute, K. (2016). Health care professionals' knowledge of occupational therapy. *The American Journal of Occupational Therapy, 70.* https://doi.org/10.5014/ajot.2016.70S1-PO1060

Carlton, G., & Blegen, M. (2006). Medication-related errors: A literature review of incidence and antecedents. *Annual Review of Nursing Research, 24,* 19–38.

Carpenito-Moyet, L. (2006). *Nursing diagnosis: Application to clinical practice* (11th ed., pp. 473–480). Lippincott Williams & Wilkins.

Eisenhauer, L., Nichols, L., Spencer, R., & Bergan, F. (1998). *Clinical pharmacology and nursing management* (5th ed., p. 189). Lippincott-Raven.

Esposito, L. (2016). Living well with a feeding tube. *U.S. News and World Report.* https://health.usnews.com/wellness/articles/2016-12-21/life-with-a-feeding-tube

Fontaine, K. L. (2000). *Healing practices: Alternative therapies for nursing* (pp. 126–127). Prentice Hall.

Goossens, G. (2015). Flushing and locking of venous catheters: Available evidence and evidence deficit. *Nursing Research and Practice, 2015,* 985686. https://doi.org/10.1155/2015/985686

Health resources and services administration (HRSA) training course: Effective communication tools for healthcare professionals 101. (June 26, 2012).

Herdman, T. H., & Kamitsuru, S. (2014). *Nursing diagnoses: Definitions and classification 2015–2017* (10th ed.). Wiley Blackwell.

Hughes, R. G., & Blegen, M. A. (2008). Medication administration safety. In R. G. Hughes, (Ed.). *Patient safety and quality: An evidence-based handbook for nurses.* Agency for Healthcare Research and Quality. http://www.ncbi.nlm.nih.gov/books/NBK2656/

Institute of Medicine. (1999). *To err is human: Building a safer health system.* National Academy Press.

Just culture and its critical link to patient safety. (2012). *ISMP medication safety alert—acute care* (pp. 1–2). Institute for Safe Medication Practice (ISMP).

Kessels, R. P. (2003). Patients' memory for medical information. *Journal of the Royal Society of Medicine, 96*(5), 219–222.

Lim, S. (2019). *The process and costs of drug development.* https://theskepticalchemist.com/process-costs-drug-development/

London, F. (2016). *Using teach back in patient education.* http://NURSE.com

Lorig, K., Halstead, H., Sobel, D., Laurent, D., Gonzalez, V., & Minor, M. (2012). *Living a healthy life with chronic conditions* (4th ed., pp. 31–33). Bull Publishing.

Pape, T. M., Guerra, D. M., Muzquiz, M., Bryant, J. B., Ingram, M., Schranner, B., Alcala, A., Sharp, J., Bishop, D., Carreno, E., & Welker, J. (2005). Innovative approaches to reducing nurses' distractions during medication administration. *Journal of Continuing Education in Nursing, 36*(3), 108–116.

Saini, R., Saini, S., & Sugandha, R. (2010). Pharmacogenetics: The future medicine. *Journal of Advanced Pharmaceutical Technology & Research, 1*(4), 423–424. http://www.japtr.org

Scamman, K. (2018). *Interactive map of languages spoken in the United States.* https://telelanguage.com/interactive-map-of-languages-united-states/

Shahrokhi, A., Ebrahimpour, F., & Ghodousi, A. (2013). Factors effective on medication errors: A nursing view. *Journal of Research in Pharmacy Practice, 2*(1), 18–23.

Side tracks on the safety express, interruptions lead to errors and unfinished…wait what was I doing? (2012). *ISMP medication safety alert—acute care* (pp. 1–3). Institute for Safe Medication Practice (ISMP).

Solis-Moreira, J. (2020). *How did we develop a COVID-19 vaccine so quickly?* https://www.medicalnewstoday.com/articles/how-did-we-develop-a-covid-19-vaccine-so-quickly

Websites for Information

Administration on Aging (U.S. Department of Health and Human Services). http://acl.gov/sites/default/files/Aging%20and%20Disability%20in%20America/2018OlderAmericansProfile.pdf

Council for Responsible Nutrition. 2017 Consumer Survey. https://www.crnusa.org/newsroom/dietary-supplement-usage-increases-says-new-survey

Institute for Safe Medication Practices. http://www.ismp.org/

Joint Commission. http://www.jointcommission.org

LactMed. https://www.ncbi.nlm.nih.gov/books/NBK501922/

MedWatch program. https://www.fda.gov/safety/medwatch-fda-safety-information-and-adverse-event-reporting-program

NIH – National Center for Advancing Translational Sciences, Genetic & Rare Disease Information Center. https://rarediseases.info.nih.gov/diseases/pages/31/faqs-about-rare-diseasREMS program. http://www.proliahcp.com/risk-evaluation-mitigation-strategy/index.html

Hale, T. (2012). Breastfeeding Scale, Texas Tech University. http://www.infantrisk.com/

Unit 2

Brown, T. (2012). Protection against urinary tract infections seen with cranberry products. *Archives of Internal Medicine, 172*, 988–996.

Centers for Disease Control and Prevention. (2016). *STD treatment guidelines*. https://www.cdc.gov/std/tg2015/sexual-assault.htm

Centers for Disease Control and Prevention. (2019). *Healthcare-associated methicillin resistant Staphylococcus aureus (HA-MRSA)*. https://www.cdc.gov/hai/organisms/mrsa-infection.html

DerMarderosian, A., & Beutler, J., (Eds.). (2003). *Guide to popular natural products* (3rd ed.). Lippincott Williams & Wilkins.

Duplessis, C., & Crum-Cianflone, N. F. (2011). Ceftaroline: A new cephalosporin with activity against methicillin-resistant *Staphylococcus aureus* (MRSA). *Clinical Medicine Reviews in Therapeutics, 3*, a2466. https://doi.org/10.4137/CMRT.S1637

Gurley, B., Fifer, E., & Gardner, Z. (2012). Pharmacokinetic herb-drug interactions (part 2): Drug interactions involving popular botanical dietary supplements and their clinical relevance. *Planta Medica, 78*(13), 1490–1514.

Levy-Hara, G., Amábile-Cuevas, C. F., Gould, I., Hutchinson, J., Abbo, L., Saxynger, L., Vlieghe, E., Cardoso, F. L., Methar, S., Kanj, S., Ohmagari, N., Harbarth, S., & International Society of Chemotherapy Antimicrobial Stewardship Working Group. (2011). "Ten commandments" for the appropriate use of antibiotics by the practicing physician in an outpatient setting. *Frontiers in Microbiology, 2*, 230. https://doi.org/10.3389/fmicb.2011.00230

Li, G., Ma, X., Deng, L., Zhao, X., Wei, Y., Gao, Z., Jia, J., Xu, J., & Sun, C. (2015). Fresh garlic extract enhances the antimicrobial activities of antibiotics on resistant strains in vitro. *Jundishapur Journal of Microbiology, 8*(5), e14814. https://doi.org/10.5812/jjm.14814

Macy, E., & Contreras, R. (2013). Health care use and serious infection prevalence associated with penicillin 'allergy' in hospitalized patients: A cohort study. *The Journal of Allergy and Clinical Immunology, 133*(3), 790–796.

Munsiff, S., Kambili, C., & Ahuja, S. (2006). Rifapentine for the treatment of pulmonary tuberculosis. *Clinical Infectious Diseases, 43*(11), 1468–1475.

Neofytos, D., Fishman, J. A., Horn, D., Anaissie, E., Chang, C. H., Olyaei, A., Pfaller, M., Steinbach, W. J., Webster, K. M., & Marr, K. A. (2010). Epidemiology and outcome of invasive fungal infections in solid organ transplant recipients. *Transplant Infectious Disease, 12*, 220–229.

Padmapriyadarsini, C., Narendran, G., & Swaminathan, S. (2011). Diagnosis & treatment of tuberculosis in HIV co-infected patients. *The Indian Journal of Medical Research, 134*(6), 850–865. https://doi.org/10.4103/0971-5916.92630

Reports

Centers for Disease Control and Prevention. Core elements of Hospital Antibiotic Stewardship Programs. https://www.cdc.gov/antibiotic-use/core-elements/hospital.html

Dellit, T. H., Owens, R. C., McGowan, J. E., Jr., Gerding, D. N., Weinstein, R. A., Burke, J. P., Huskins, W. C., Paterson, D. L., Fishman, N. O., Carpenter, C. F., Brennan, P. J., Billeter, M., Hooton, T. M., Infectious Diseases Society of America, & Society for Healthcare Epidemiology of America. (2007). Infectious Diseases Society of America; Society for Healthcare Epidemiology of America. Infectious Diseases Society of America and the Society for Healthcare Epidemiology of America guidelines for developing an institutional program

to enhance antimicrobial stewardship. *Clinical Infectious Diseases, 44*, 159–177.

World Health Organization. Global tuberculosis report 2012. http://www.who.int/tb/publications/global_report/en/

World Health Organization. Malaria fact sheet. https://www.who.int/health-topics/malaria#tab=tab_1

Unit 3

Blayney, M. (2012). Procedural sedation for adult patients: An overview. *Continuing Education in Anaesthesia Critical Care & Pain, 12*(4), 176–180. https://doi.org/10.1093/bjaceaccp/mks016

DerMarderosian, A., & Beutler, J., (Eds.). (2003). *Guide to popular natural products* (3rd ed.). Lippincott Williams & Wilkins.

International Association for the Study of Pain. (1979). Subcommittee on taxonomy: Pain terms. A list with definitions and notes on usage. *Pain, 6*, 249.

ISMP. (2012). Label change for morphine injection. *ISMP Medication Safety Alert, 17*(25).

Kapur, J. (2015). *Medical marijuana: Clinical implications*. Women's Health Drug Therapy, sponsored by University of Washington School of Nursing.

Karakashian, A., & Caple, C. (2019). *Moderate conscious sedation: Caring for and monitoring the adult patient*. CINAHL Nursing Guide.

Ostling, P., Davidson, K. S., Anyama, B. O., Helander, E. M., Wyche, M. Q., & Kaye, A. D. (2018). America's opioid epidemic: A comprehensive review and look into the rising crisis. *Current Pain & Headache Reports, 22*, 32.

Painter, S. G. (2017). Opiate crisis and healthcare reform in America: A review for nurses. *The Online Journal of Issues in Nursing, 22*(2), manuscript 3.

Parikh, S. K., & Silberstein, S. D. (2019). Preventative treatment for episodic migraine. *Neurologic Clinics, 37*(4), 735–770.

Rivera, B. (2015). The current status of nurse-administered propofol sedation in endoscopy: An evidence-based practice nurse fellowship project. *Gastroenterology Nursing, 38*(4), 297–304.

Vargas-Schaffer, G. (2010). Is the WHO analgesic ladder still valid? Twenty-four years of experience. *Canadian Family Physician [Medecin de famille canadien], 56*(6), 514–e205.

Wilson, N., Kariisa, M., Seth, P., Smith IV, H., & Davis, N. L. (2020). Drug and opioid-involved overdose deaths—United States, 2017-2018. *Morbidity Mortality Weekly Report (MMWR), 69*, 290–297.

Websites for Information

Morphine Milligram Equivalent (MME) Calculator, NY city department of Health and Mental Hygiene. https://www1.nyc.gov/site/doh/providers/health-topics/mme-calculator.page

WONDER - wide-ranging online data for epidemiologic research. (2020). CDC, National Center for Health Statistics. http://wonder.cdc.gov

Reports

Centers for Disease Control and Prevention. (2020). *National Center for Injury Prevention and Control*.

Opioid Addiction Disease. (2015). *Facts and Figures, prepared by the American Society of Addiction Medicine*. http://www.asam.org/docs/default-source/advocacy/opioid-addiction-disease-facts-figures.pdf

A scientific review paper and recommendation statement from CDER's Acetaminophen Hepatotoxicity Working Group. (Finalized February 26, 2008).

Unit 4

Alzheimer's Association. (2020). *Alzheimer's disease facts and figures.* https://www.alz.org/alzheimers-dementia/facts-figures

Bedlack, R., & ALSUntangled Group, . (2013). ALSUntangled no. 18: Apoaequorin (Prevagen). *Amyotrophic Lateral Sclerosis & Frontotemporal Degeneration, 14*(1), 78–79. https://doi.org/10.3109/17482968.2012.727302

Billioti de Gage, S., Bégaud, B., Bazin, F., Verdoux, H., Dartigues, J. F., Pérès, K., Kurth, T., & Pariente, A. (2012). Benzodiazepine use and risk of dementia: Prospective population based study. *British Medicine Journal, 345,* 6231.

Boukhris, T., Sheehy, O., Mottron, L., & Bérard, A. (2015). Antidepressant use during pregnancy and the risk of autism spectrum disorder in children. *JAMA Pediatric, 170,* 117–124.

Cummings, D. (2020). *Health at any size/obesity.* Women's Health Drug Therapy, sponsored by University of Washington School of Nursing.

DerMarderosian, A., & Beutler, J., (Eds.). (2003). *Guide to popular natural products* (3rd ed.). Lippincott Williams & Wilkins.

Diagnostic criteria and guidelines for Alzheimer's disease. https://www.alz.org/research/diagnostic_criteria/

Food and Drug Administration. (2009). *Kava—FDA consumer advisory.* (Issued February 7, 2009).

Fuller, R. W., & Wong, D. T. (1985). Effects of antidepressants on uptake and receptor systems in the brain. *Progress in Neuropsychopharmacology, Biology, and Psychiatry, 9*(5–6), 485–490.

Gallagher, P. J., Castro, V., Fava, M., Weilburg, J. B., Murphy, S. N., Gainer, V. S., Churchill, S. E., Kohane, I. S., Iosifescu, D. V., Smoller, J. W., & Perlis, R. H. (2012). Antidepressant response in patients with major depression exposed to NSAIDs: A pharmacovigilance study. *American Journal of Psychiatry, 169*(10), 1065–1072.

Grigoriadis, S., Vonderporten, E. H., Mamisashvili, L., Tomlinson, G., Dennis, C. L., Koren, G., Steiner, M., Mousmanis, P., Cheung, A., & Ross, L. E. (2014). Prenatal exposure to antidepressants and persistent pulmonary hypertension of the newborn: Systematic review and meta-analysis. *British Medical Journal, 348,* f6932.

Jack, C. R., Jr., Albert, M. S., Knopman, D. S., McKhann, G. M., Sperling, R. A., Carrillo, M. C., Thies, B., & Phelps, C. H. (2011). Introduction to the recommendations from the national institute on aging—Alzheimer's association workgroups on diagnostic guidelines for Alzheimer's disease. *Alzheimer's & Dementia: The Journal of the Alzheimer's Association, 7*(3), 257–262.

Kishi, T., Sakuma, K., & Iwata, N. (2020). Efficacy and safety of psychostimulants for Alzheimer's disease: A systematic review and meta-analysis. *Pharmacopsychiatry, 53,* 109–114.

Llorente, M., & Urrutia, V. (2006). Diabetes, psychiatric disorders, and the metabolic effects of antipsychotic medications. *Clinical Diabetes, 24*(1), 18–24.

Manos, M. J., Tom-Revzon, C., Bukstein, O. G., & Crismon, M. L. (2007). Changes and challenges: Managing ADHD in a fast-paced world. *Journal of Managed Care Pharmacy, 13*(9), 2–13.

Martin, R. C. (2012). Calcium: A proven target in the war on alzheimer's disease and apoaequorin as a potential therapeutic. *Nutritional Perspectives: Journal of the Council on Nutrition, 35*(2), 22–24.

Pirschel, C. (February, 2018). *When counting sheep just doesn't work, sleep-wake disturbances in patients with cancer.* ONS Voice, pp 16–20.

Reisberg, B., Osorio, R., Khan, A., Torossian, C., Roy, K., Boksay, I., Thwin, O., Khanzada, N., Kumar, P., Shulman, M., & Lobach I. (2012). P1-043: Remission of pre-mild cognitive impairment (MCI), subjective cognitive impairment (SCI): a two-year prospective study of demographic and behavioral markers. *Alzheimer's & Dementia, 8,* 121–122. https://doi.org/10.1016/j.jalz.2012.05.318

Rojo, L. E., Gaspar, P. A., Silva, H., Risco, L., Arena, P., Cubillos-Robles, K., & Jara, B. (2015). Metabolic syndrome and obesity among users of second generation antipsychotics: A global challenge for modern psychopharmacology. *Pharmacological Research, 101,* 74–85. https://doi.org/10.1016/j.phrs.2015.07.022

Rothman, R., Baumann, M. H., Dersch, C. M., Romero, D. V., Rice, K. C., Carroll, F. I., & Partilla, J. S. (2001). Amphetamine-type central nervous system stimulants release norepinephrine more potently than they release dopamine and serotonin. *Synapse, 39*(1), 32–41. https://doi.org/10.1002/1098-2396(20010101)39:1%3C32::AID-SYN5%3E3.0.CO;2-3

Sakata, N., & Okumura, Y. (2018). Thyroid function tests before prescribing anti-dementia drugs: A retrospective observational study. *Clinical Interventions in Aging, 13,* 1219–1223. https://doi.org/10.2147/CIA.S168182

Snitz, B. E., O'meara, E. S., Carlson, M. C., Arnold, A. M., Ives, D. G., Rapp, S. R., Saxton, J., Lopez, O. L., Dunn, L. O., Sink, K. M., DeKosky, S. T., & Ginkgo Evaluation of Memory (GEM) Study Investigators, . (2009). Ginkgo biloba for preventing cognitive decline in older adults: A randomized trial. *Journal of the American Medical Association, 302*(24), 2663–2670.

University of Maryland Medical Center. (2011). *Facts on ginkgo biloba.* University of Maryland Center for Integrative Medicine.

Wang, S., Mosher, C., Gao, S., Kirk, K., Lasiter, S., Khan, S., Kheir, Y. N., Boustani, M., & Khan, B. (2017). Antidepressant use and depressive symptoms in Intensive Care Unit survivors. *Journal of Hospital Medicine, 12*(9), 731–734. https://doi.org/10.12788/jhm.2814

Zeller, S. L., & Citrome, L. (2016). Managing agitation associated with schizophrenia and bipolar disorder in the emergency setting. *Western Journal of Emergency Medicine: Integrating Emergency Care With Population Health, 17*(2). https://doi.org/10.5811/westjem.2015.12.28763. https://escholarship.org/uc/item/74w6d6vr

Websites for Information

National Sleep Foundation. http://www.sleepfoundation.org/

Unit 5

Buels, K. S., & Fryer, A. D. (2012). *Muscarinic receptor antagonists: Effects on pulmonary function. Handbook of experimental pharmacology,* (Vol. 208, pp. 317–341). https://doi.org/10.1007/978-3-642-23274-9_14

Chaudhry, R., Portnoy, J., & Purser, J. (2012). *Patients forget how to use EpiPens after 3 months.* Abstract 59. *Presented at the American College of Allergy, Asthma & Immunology (ACAAI) 2012 Annual Scientific Meeting, November 12, 2012.*

DerMarderosian, A., & Beutler, J., (Eds.). (2003). *Guide to popular natural products* (3rd ed.). Lippincott Williams & Wilkins.

Ferdinand, K., & Armani, A. (2007). The management of hypertension in African Americans. *Critical Pathways in Cardiology, 6*(2), 67–71.

Huang, H., & Fox, K. (2012). The impact of beta-blockers on mortality in stable angina: A meta-analysis. *Scottish Medical Journal, 57,* 69–75.

Magee, L., Elran, E., Bull, S. B., Logan, A., & Koren, G. (2000). Risks and benefits of beta-receptor blockers for pregnancy hypertension: Overview of the randomized trials. *European Journal of Obstetrics, Gynecology, and Reproductive Biology, 88*(1), 15–26.

Unit 6

Black, D., & Rosen, C. (2016). Postmenopausal osteoporosis. *New England Journal of Medicine, 374,* 254–262.

DerMarderosian, A., & Beutler, J., (Eds.). (2003). *Guide to popular natural products* (3rd ed.). Lippincott Williams & Wilkins.

Dias, R., Bateman, L. M., Farias, S. T., Li, C. S., Lin, T. C., Jorgensen, J., & Seyal, M. (2010). Depression in epilepsy is associated with lack of seizure control. *Epilepsy and Behavior, 19,* 445–447.

Fisher, R. S., Acevedo, C., Arzimanoglou, A., Bogacz, A., Cross, J. H., Elger, C. E., Engel, J., Jr., Forsgren, L., French, J. A., Glynn, M., Hesdorffer, DC., Lee, B. I., Mathern, G. W., Moshé, S. L., Perucca, E., Scheffer, I. E., Tomson, T., Watanabe, M., & Wiebe, S. (2014). A practical clinical definition of epilepsy. *Epilepsia, 55,* 475–482.

Kwan, P., & Brodie, M. J. (2000). Early identification of refractory epilepsy. *The New England Journal of Medicine, 342,* 314–319.

Li, F., Harmer, P., Fitzgerald, K., Eckstrom, E., Stock, R., Galver, J., Maddalozzo, G., & Batya, S. S. (2012). Tai Chi and postural stability in patients with Parkinson's disease. *The New England Journal of Medicine, 366,* 511–519.

McClung, M. (2013). Controversies in osteoporosis management: Concerns about BSP and when are 'drug holidays' required? *Clinical Obstetrics and Gynecology, 56*(4), 743–748.

Miller, J. W. (2008). Of race, ethnicity, and rash: The genetics of antiepileptic drug-induced skin reactions. *Epilepsy Currents, 8*(5), 120–121. https://doi.org/10.1111/j.1535-7511.2008.00263.x

Trivedi, B. S., Darji, N. H., Malhotra, S. D., & Patel, P. R. (2016). Antiepileptic drugs-induced stevens-johnson syndrome: A case series. *Journal of Basic and Clinical Pharmacy, 8*(1), 42–44. https://doi.org/10.4103/0976-0105.195130

Vacca, V. (2019). Parkinson disease: Enhance nursing knowledge. *Nursing, 49*(11), 24–32.

Websites for Information

International League Against Epilepsy. https://www.ilae.org/about-ilae

National Osteoporosis Foundations. https://www.nof.org/patients/what-is-osteoporosis/

North American AED Pregnancy Registry. http://www.aedpregnancyregistry.org/for-pregnant-women-introduction/

Parkinson's disease Foundation. https://www.parkinson.org/Understanding-Parkinsons/Statistics

Unit 7

DerMarderosian, A., & Beutler, J., (Eds.). (2003). *Guide to popular natural products* (3rd ed.). Lippincott Williams & Wilkins.

Forster, V. (2020). Teen dies after doing TikTok 'Benadryl Challenge' as doctors warn of dangers. *Forbes.*

Institute for Safe Medication Practices. (2007). *Seasonal mix-ups. ISMP medication safety alert—acute care* (p. 1). Institute for Safe Medication Practice (ISMP).

Klass, P. (2019, June 3). When social media is really problematic for adolescents. *New York Times.* https://www.nytimes.com/2019/06/03/well/family/teenagers-social-media.html

Lee, L. A., Sterling, R., Máspero, J., Clements, D., Ellsworth, A., & Pedersen, S. (2014). Growth velocity reduced with once-daily fluticasone furoate nasal spray in prepubescent children with perennial allergic rhinitis. *Journal of Allergy and Clinical Immunology, 2*(4), 421–427.

Prybys, K. (2017). *Triple C overdose. UMEM educational pearls.* https://em.umaryland.edu/educational_pearls/3236/

Simon, H. (2016, May 31). Chronic obstructive pulmonary disease. *New York Times.*

Websites for Information

Asthma Action Plan - NIH. http://www.nhlbi.nih.gov/BreatheBetter

Asthma Action Plan – State specific plans. https://www.cdc.gov/asthma/actionplan.html

National Center for Health statistics—Asthma. http://www.cdc.gov/asthma/most_recent_national_asthma_data.htm

Reports

NHLBI Asthma Action Plan. https://www.nhlbi.nih.gov/health-topics/all-publications-and-resources/asthma-action-plan-2020

NHLBI Guidelines Asthma Care Quick Reference Guide (with NAEPP 2012 revisions). https://www.nhlbi.nih.gov/files/docs/guidelines/asthma_qrg.pdf

U.S. Department of Health and Human Services, National Institutes of Health, National Heart, Lung, and Blood Institute. (2007). *The Expert Panel Report 3 (EPR–3) full report 2007: Guidelines for the diagnosis and management of asthma. Developed by an expert panel commissioned by the National Asthma Education and Prevention Program (NAEPP) Coordinating Committee (CC), coordinated by the National Heart, Lung, and Blood Institute (NHLBI) of the National Institutes of Health.*

Unit 8

Albert, N. (2012). Strategies in heart failure. *Critical Care Nurse, 32*(2), 20–34.

Allen, L. A., Fonarow, G. C., Grau-Sepulveda, M. V., Hernandez, A. F., Peterson, P. N., Partovian, C., Li, S. X., Heidenreich, P. A., Bhatt, D. L., Peterson, E. D., Krumholz, H. M., & American Heart Association's Get With the Guidelines Heart Failure Investigators, . (2014). Hospital variation in intravenous inotrope use for patients hospitalized with heart failure. *Circulation. Heart Failure, 7,* 251–260.

Arnett, D., Blumenthal, R. S., Albert, M. A., Buroker, A. B., Goldberger, Z. D., Hahn, E. J., Himmelfarb, C. D., Khera, A., Lloyd-Jones, D., McEvoy, J. W., Michos, E. D., Miedema, M. D., Muñoz, D., Smith, S. C., Jr., Virani, S. S., Williams, K. A., Sr., Yeboah, J., & Ziaeian, B. (2019). ACC/AHA guideline on the primary prevention of cardiovascular disease: A report of the American College of Cardiology/American Heart Association task force on clinical practice guidelines. *Circulation, 140*(11), e596–e646.

Ballestri, S., Capitelli, M., Fontana, M. C., Arioli, D., Romagnoli, E., Graziosi, C., Lonardo, A., Marietta, M., Dentali, F., & Cioni, G. (2020). Direct oral anticoagulants in patients with liver disease in the era of non-alcoholic fatty liver disease global epidemic: A narrative review. *Advances in Therapy, 37,* 1910–1932. https://doi.org/10.1007/s12325-020-01307-z

Butt, D., Mamdani, M., Austin, P. C., Tu, K., Gomes, T., & Glazier, R. H. (2012). The risk of hip fracture after initiating antihypertensive drugs in the elderly. *Archives of Internal Medicine, 172*(22), 1739–1744.

Chaudhry, R., Usama, S. M., & Babiker, H. M. (2020). *Physiology, coagulation pathways.* In *StatPearls* [Internet]. StatPearls Publishing. https://www.ncbi.nlm.nih.gov/books/NBK482253/

Couris, R., Tataronis, G., McCloskey, W., Oertel, L., Dallal, G., Dwyer, J., & Blumberg, J. B. (2006). Dietary vitamin K variability affects international normalized ration (INR) coagulation indices. *International Journal of Vitamin and Nutrition Research, 76*(2), 65–74.

DerMarderosian, A., & Beutler, J., (Eds.). (2003). *Guide to popular natural products* (3rd ed.). Lippincott Williams & Wilkins.

Duprez, D. (2012). Treatment of isolated systolic hypertension in the elderly. *Expert Review of Cardiovascular Therapy, 10*(11), 1367–1373.

Dykewicz, M. (2004). Cough and angioedema from angiotensin-converting enzyme inhibitors: New insights into mechanisms and management. *Current Opinion in Allergy and Clinical Immunology, 4*(4), 267–270.

Ehrlich, J. R., Nattel, S., & Hohnloser, S. H.. (2002). Atrial fibrillation and congestive heart failure: Specific considerations at the intersection of two common and important cardiac disease sets. *Journal of Cardiovascular Electrophysiology, 13*(4), 399–405. https://doi.org/10.1046/j.1540-8167.2002.00399.x. PMID: 12033360.

Fisher, A. D., & Maggi, M. (2015). Endocrine treatment of transsexual male-to-female persons. In C. Trombetta, G. Liguori, & M. Bertolotto, (Eds.). *Management of gender dysphoria: A multidisciplinary approach.* Springer.

Fogoros, R. (2020). *Beta blocker for treating patients with angina.* VeryWellHealth. https://www.verywellhealth.com/beta-blockers-for-angina-1745909

Freeman, J., Reynolds, K., Fang, M., Udaltsova, N., Steimle, A., Pomernacki, N. A., Borowsky, L. H., Harrison, T. N., Singer, D. E., & Go, A. S. (2015). Digoxin and risk of death in adults with atrial fibrillation: The ATRIA-CVRN study. *Circulation: Arrhythmia and Electrophysiology, 8*(1), 49–58.

Gómez-Outes, A., Suárez-Gea, M. L., Lecumberri, R., Terleira-Fernández, A. I., & Vargas-Castrillón, E. (2015). Direct-acting oral anticoagulants: pharmacology, indications, management, and future perspectives. *European Journal of Haematology, 95*(5), 389–404.

Hall, T. M., Shoptaw, S., & Reback, C. J. (2015). Sometimes poppers are not poppers: Huffing as an emergent health concern among MSM substance users. *Journal of Gay & Lesbian Mental Health, 19*(1), 118–121.

Hwang, R., Chuan, F., Peters, R., & Kuys, S. (2013). Frequency of urinary incontinence in people with chronic heart failure. *Heart and Lung, 42*(1), 26–31.

James, P. A., Oparil, S., Carter, B. L., Cushman, W. C., Dennison-Himmelfarb, C., Handler, J., Lackland, D. T., LeFevre, M. L., MacKenzie, T. D., Ogedegbe, O., Smith, S. C., Jr., Svetkey, L. P., Taler, S. J., Townsend, R. R., Wright, J. T., Jr., Narva, A. S., & Ortiz, E. (2014). 2014 evidence-based guideline for the management of high blood pressure in adults: Report from the panel members appointed to the eighth joint national committee (JNC 8). *The Journal of the American Medical Association, 311*(5), 507–520. https://doi.org/10.1001/jama.2013.284427. Erratum in: *JAMA.* 2014 May 7, 311(17), 1809. PMID: 24352797.

Januzzi, J., Silver, M., & Desai, A. (2016). Three new concepts in HF: What you need to know to improve outcomes. *Medscape.*

http://www.medscape.org/viewarticle/864375?src=mkmcmr_driv_invit_mscpedu

Johnson, J. A., Gong, L., Whirl-Carrillo, M., Gage, B. F., Scott, S. A., Stein, C. M., Anderson, J. L., Kimmel, S. E., Lee, M. T., Pirmohamed, M., Wadelius, M., Klein, T. E., Altman, R. B., & Clinical Pharmacogenetics Implementation Consortium,. (2011). Clinical Pharmacogenetics Implementation Consortium. Clinical Pharmacogenetics Implementation Consortium Guidelines for CYP2C9 and VKORC1 genotypes and warfarin dosing. *Clinical Pharmacology and Therapeutics, 90*(4), 625–629. https://doi.org/10.1038/clpt.2011.185. PMID: 21900891; PMCID: PMC3187550.

Khalesi, S., Irwin, C., & Schubert, M. (2015). Flaxseed consumption may reduce blood pressure: A systematic review and meta-analysis of controlled trials, *The Journal of Nutrition, 145*(4), 758–765. https://doi.org/10.3945/jn.114.205302

Lapi, F., Gallo, E., Bernasconi, S., Vietri, M., Menniti-Ippolito, F., Raschetti, R., Gori, L., Firenzuoli, F., Mugelli, A., & Vannacci, A. (2008). Myopathies associated with red yeast rice and liquorice: Spontaneous reports from the Italian Surveillance System of Natural Health Products. *British Journal of Clinical Pharmacology, 66*(4), 572–574. https://doi.org/10.1111/j.1365-2125.2008.03224.x

Mureebe, L. (2007). Direct thrombin inhibitors: Alternatives to heparin. *Vascular, 15*(6), 372–375.

Myerson, M. (2016, March 28). PCSK9 inhibitors: A brief primer. *Medscape.*

Naito, R., Miyauchi, K., & Daida, H. (2017). Racial differences in the cholesterol-lowering effect of statin. *Journal of Atherosclerosis and Thrombosis, 24*(1), 19–25.

Patel, T., & Shah, S. (2019, September 24). Blood pressure medication recall: What you need to know. *ABC News.*

Saleh, M. I. (2016). Clinical predictors associated with warfarin sensitivity. *American Journal of Therapeutics, 23*(6), e1690–e1694. https://doi.org/10.1097/MJT.0000000000000248. PMID: 25830869.

Santos, R. D., & Watts, G. F. (2015). Familial hypercholesterolaemia: PCSK9 inhibitors are coming. *The Lancet, 385*(9965), 307–310.

Santye, L. (2017, March 17). Is the $14K annual cost of Repatha worth it? *Contemporary Clinic.*

Sharma, A., Colvin-Adams, M., & Yancy, C. W. (2014). Heart failure in African Americans: Disparities can be overcome. *Cleveland Clinic Journal of Medicine, 81*(5), 301–311.

Siskey, J., & Deyo, Z. (2014, January 14). New therapies: Homozygous familial hypercholesterolemia. *Pharmacy Times.*

Uribe, L. P. M., & Oji, ODAF-B. (2018). Hypertension, isolated systolic. In D. Pravikoff, (Ed.), *CINAHL nursing guide.* http://search.ebscohost.com.proxy.heal-wa.org/login.aspx?direct=true&db=nup&AN=T703295&site=eds-live

Virani, S. S., Alonso, A., Benjamin, E. J., Bittencourt, M. S., Callaway, C. W., Carson, A. P., Chamberlain, A. M., Chang, A. R., Cheng, S., Delling, F. N., Djousse, L., Elkind, M. S. V., Ferguson, J. F., Fornage, M., Khan, S. S., Kissela, B. M., Knutson, K. L., Kwan, T. W., Lackland, D. T., …. Tsao, C. W. (2020). Heart disease and stroke statistics—2020 update: A report from the American Heart Association Circulation. *Circulation, 141*(9), e139–e596.

Wee, Y., Burns, K., & Bett, N. (2015). Medical management of chronic stable angina. *Australian Prescriber, 38*(4), 131–136. https://doi.org/10.18773/austprescr.2015.042

Wright, J. M., Musini, V. M., & Gill, R. (2018). First-line drugs for hypertension. *Cochrane Database Systematic Review, 4*(4), CD001841. https://doi.org/10.1002/14651858.CD001841.pub3. PMID: 29667175; PMCID: PMC6513559.

Xiao, Y.-F. (2011). Cardiac arrhythmia and heart failure: From bench to bedside. *Journal of Geriatric Cardiology, 8*, 131–132. https://doi.org/10.3724/SP.J.1263.2011.00131

York, M., & Farber, H. W. (2011). Pulmonary hypertension: Screening and evaluation in scleroderma. *Current Opinion in Rheumatology, 23*(6), 536–544.

Websites for Information

American Heart Association. http://www.heart.org

Mayo Clinic. https://www.mayoclinic.org/diseases-conditions/high-blood-pressure/in-depth/diuretics/art-20048129

My Food Data – free tools to understand what you eat (USDA Food Data Central). https://myfooddata.com/

National Organization for Rare Disorders (NORD). https://rarediseases.org/rare-diseases/pulmonary-arterial-hypertension/

Red Yeast Rice. http://nccam.nih.gov/health/redyeastrice

Unit 9

Bhattacharya, A., & Osterman, M. (2020). Biologic therapy for ulcerative colitis. *Gastroenterology Clinics of North America, 49*, 717–729. https://doi.org/10.1016/j.gtc.2020.08.002

DerMarderosian, A., & Beutler, J., (Eds.). (2003). *Guide to popular natural products* (3rd ed.). Lippincott Williams & Wilkins.

FDA. (2020). FDA requests removal of all ranitidine products (Zantac) from the market. *FDA News Release.* https://www.fda.gov/news-events/press-announcements/fda-requests-removal-all-ranitidine-products-zantac-market

Fisher, L., & Fisher, A. (2017). Acid-suppressive therapy and risk of infections: Pros and cons. *Clinical Drug Investigation, 37*(7), 587–624. https://doi.org/10.1007/s40261-017-0519-y. PMID: 28361440.

Manoguerra, A. S., & Cobaugh, D. J. (2005). Guideline on the use of ipecac syrup in the out-of-hospital management of ingested poisons. *Clinical Toxicology, 43*(1), 1–10.

Moukarbel, G. V., & Bhatt, D. L. (2012). Antiplatelet therapy and proton pump inhibition: Clinician update. *Circulation, 125*, 375–380.

National Institute of Health. (2012). Facts on IBS. https://www.niddk.nih.gov/health-information/digestive-diseases/irritable-bowel-syndrome/symptoms-causes

Olle, D. A. (2020). *Helicobacter pylori infection.* Salem Press Encyclopedia of Health. http://search.ebscohost.com.proxy.heal-wa.org/login.aspx?direct=true&db=ers&AN=94416926&site=eds-live

Websites for Information

Crohn's and Colitis Foundation of America. http://www.ccfa.org/

State Medical Marijuana Laws (National Conference of State Legislatures). http://www.ncsl.org/issues-research/health/state-medical-marijuana-laws.aspx

Unit 10

Agito, K., & Manni, A. (2015). Acute pancreatitis induced by methimazole in a patient with subclinical hyperthyroidism. *Journal of Investigative Medicine High Impact Case Reports, 3*(2), 2324709615592229. https://doi.org/10.1177/2324709615592229

Alfirevic, Z., Aflaifel, N., & Weeks, A. (2014). Oral misoprostol for induction of labour. *Cochrane Database of Systematic Reviews*, (6), CD001338. https://doi.org/10.1002/14651858.CD001338.pub3.

Barbieri, R. (2016). Stop using rectal misoprostol for the treatment of postpartum hemorrhage caused by uterine atony. *OBG Management, 28*(7), 8–10, 12.

Barusiban, A. (2006). An effective long-term treatment of oxytocin-induced preterm labor in nonhuman primates. *Biological Reproduction, 75*(5), 809–814.

Bonyata, K. (2016). *Prescription drugs used to increasing milk supply.* Kellymom.com. http://kellymom.com/bf/can-i-breastfeed/meds/prescript_galactagogue/

Casciotti, D., Zuckerman, D., Stebbins, J., & National Center for Health Research. (2015). *Are some birth control pills too risky?* http://www.center4research.org/birth-control-pills-risky/

Cowley, K. (2005). Psychogenic and pharmacologic induction of the let-down reflex can facilitate breastfeeding by tetraplegic women: A report of 3 cases. *Archives of Physical and Medical Rehabilitation, 86*(6), 1261–1264.

Craft, S., Baker, L. D., Montine, T. J., Minoshima, S., Watson, G. S., Claxton, A., Arbuckle, M., Callaghan, M., Tsai, E., Plymate, S. R., Green, P. S., Leverenz, J., Cross, D., & Gerton, B. (2012). Intranasal insulin therapy for Alzheimer disease and amnestic mild cognitive impairment: A pilot clinical trial. *Archives of Neurology, 69*(1), 29–38.

DerMarderosian, A., & Beutler, J., (Eds.). (2003). *Guide to popular natural products* (3rd ed.). Lippincott Williams & Wilkins.

Dinsmoor, R. (2014). *Insulin analog. Diabetes self-management.* http://www.diabetesselfmanagement.com/diabetes-resources/definitions/insulin-analog/

FDA. (2016). Drug Alert.

Fewtrell, M., Loh, K. L., Blake, A., Ridout, D. A., & Hawdon, J. (2006). Randomised, double blind trial of oxytocin nasal spray in mothers expressing breast milk for preterm infants. *Archives of Disease in Childhood: Fetal and Neonatal Edition, 91*, F169–F174.

Franklyn, J., & Boelaert, K. (2012). Thyrotoxicosis. *Lancet, 379*(9821), 1155–1166.

Garber, A. J., Handelsman, Y., Grunberger, G., Einhorn, D., Abrahamson, M. J., Barzilay, J. I., Blonde, L., Bush, M. A., DeFronzo, R. A., Garber, J. R., Garvey, W. T., Hirsch, I. B., Jellinger, P. S.,Jellinger, P. S., McGill, J. B., Mechanick, J. I., Perreault, L., Rosenblit, P. D., Samso, S., & Umpierrez, G. E. (2020). Consensus statement by the AACE and ACE on the comprehensive type 2 diabetes management algorithm – 2020 Executive Summary. *Endocrine Practice, 26*(1), 107–139.

Gebel, E. (2013). Making insulin, a behind the scenes look at producing a lifesaving medication. *Diabetes Forecast.* http://www.diabetesforecast.org/2013/jul/making-insulin.html

Golobof, A., & Kiley, J. (2016). The current status of oral contraceptives: Progress and recent innovations. *Seminars in Reproductive Medicine, 34*(3), 145–151.

Greenfield, M. F. (2010). Shellfish-iodine nexus is a myth. *The Journal of Family Practice, 59*(6), 314. http://search.ebscohost.com.proxy.heal-wa.org/login.aspx?direct=true&db=mdc&AN=20544062&site=eds-live

Gromko, L. (2020, May 14). *Transgender care: A basic introduction to transgender medicine. Sexual and reproductive health drug therapy conference.* Seattle, WA.

Hacking, S., Uppal, N. N., Khan, N., Ionescu, M., & Bijol, V. (2019). Systemic p-ANCA vasculitis with fatal outcome, arising in the setting of methimazole use. *Clinical Nephrology. Case Studies, 7*, 23–26. https://doi.org/10.5414/CNCS109759

Inzucchi, S. E., Bergenstal, R. M., Buse, J. B., Diamant, M., Ferrannini, E., Nauck, M., Peters, A. L., Tsapas, A., Wender, E., & Matthews, D. R. (2015). Management of hyperglycemia in type 2 diabetes, 2015: A patient-centered approach. Update to a position statement of the American diabetes association and the European association for the study of diabetes. *Diabetes Care, 38*, 140–149.

Kelbach, J. (2016). *Treatment of preterm labor: Terbutaline.* Healthline.com. http://www.healthline.com/health/pregnancy/preterm-labor-terbutaline#Overview1

Lower, A. (2003). Sliding scale insulin regimens demonstrate no added benefit for patients with type 2 diabetes mellitus. *Annals of Family Medicine.* http://www.aafp.org/online/annals/home/tips/05-29-03.html

Menke, A., Casagrande, S., Geiss, L., & Cowie, C. C. (2015). Prevalence of and trends in diabetes among adults in the United States, 1988–2012. *The Journal of the American Medical Association, 314*(10), 1021–1029.

Schabelman, E., & Witting, M. (2010). The relationship of radiocontrast, iodine, and seafood allergies: A medical myth exposed. *The Journal of Emergency Medicine, 39*(5), 701–707.

Valdés, E., Salinas, H., Toledo, V., Lattes, K., Cuellar, E., Perucca, E., Diaz, R., Montecinos, F., & Reyes, A. (2012). Nifedipine versus fenoterol in the management of preterm labor: A randomized, multicenter clinical study. *Gynecologic and Obstetric Investigation, 74*(2), 109–115.

Vann, M. (2009). *The link between gestational diabetes and Type 2.* https://www.everydayhealth.com/type-2-diabetes/gestational-diabetes-and-type-2.aspx

Young, D. C., Delaney, T., Armson, B. A., & Fanning, C. (2020). Oral misoprostol, low dose vaginal misoprostol, and vaginal dinoprostone for labor induction: Randomized controlled trial. *PLoS One, 15*(1), e0227245. https://doi.org/10.1371/journal.pone.0227245

Websites for Information

American Diabetes Association. http://www.diabetes.org/
American Thyroid Association. http://www.thyroid.org/
March of Dimes. http://www.marchofdimes.org/

Unit 11

Abbo, L. M., & Hooton, T. M. (2014). Antimicrobial stewardship and urinary tract infections. *Antibiotics (Basel, Switzerland), 3*(2), 174–192. https://doi.org/10.3390/antibiotics3020174

Bent, S., Kane, C., Shinohara, K., Neuhaus, J., Hudes, E. S., Goldberg, H., & Avins, A. L. (2006). Saw palmetto for benign prostate hyperplasia. *The New England Journal of Medicine, 354*(6), 557–566.

Brown, T. (2012). Protection against urinary tract infections seen with cranberry products. *Archives of Internal Medicine, 172*, 988–996.

DerMarderosian, A., & Beutler, J., (Eds.). (2003). *Guide to popular natural products* (3rd ed.). Lippincott Williams & Wilkins.

Dhingra, N., & Bhagwat, D. (2011). Benign prostate hyperplasia: An overview of existing treatment. *Indian Journal of Pharmacology, 43*(1), 6–12.

Goetsch, M., Lim, J., & Caughety, A. (2015). A practical solution for dyspareunia in breast cancer survivors: A randomized controlled trial. *Journal of Clinical Oncology, 33*, 3394–3400.

Maximov, P. Y., Lee, T. M., & Jordan, V. C. (2013). The discovery and development of selective estrogen receptor modulators (SERMs) for clinical practice. *Current Clinical Pharmacology, 8*(2), 135–155.

Pinkerton, M., Bongu, J., James, A., Lowder, J., & Durkin, M. (2020). A qualitative analysis of diagnostic testing, antibiotic selection, and quality improvement interventions for uncomplicated urinary tract infections. *PLoS One, 15*(9), e0238453. https://doi.org/10.1371/journal.pone.0238453

Pinkerton, J., & Thomas, S. (2014). Use of SERMs for treatment in postmenopausal women. *The Journal of Steroid Biochemistry and Molecular Biology, 142*, 142–154.

Shanahan, E. (2015). *Hormone replacement therapy: What women need to know.* http://www.everydayhealth.com/menopause/about-hormone-replacement.aspx

Solis-Moreira, J. (2020). *How did we develop a COVID-19 vaccine so quickly?* https://www.medicalnewstoday.com/articles/how-did-we-develop-a-covid-19-vaccine-so-quickly

Websites for Information

American Cancer Society. https://www.cancer.org/cancer/breast-cancer/understanding-a-breast-cancer-diagnosis/breast-cancer-hormone-receptor-status.html
American Urological Association. http://www.urologyhealth.org

Unit 12

Advisory Committee of Immunization Practices. (2012). Prevention and control of influenza with vaccines: Recommendations of the advisory committee of immunization practices (ACIP)–United States, 2012–13 influenza season. *Morbidity and Mortality Weekly Report, 61*(32), 613–618.

Auerbach, M., & Macdougall, I. C. (2014). Safety of intravenous iron formulations: Facts and folklore. *Blood Transfusion, 12*(3), 296–300. https://doi.org/10.2450/2014.0094-14. PMID: 25074787; PMCID: PMC4111808.

Barshes, N., Goodpastor, S., & Goss, J. (2004). Pharmacologic immunosuppression. *Frontiers in Bioscience, 1*(9), 411–420.

Basson, M. (2019). Ulcerative colitis medication. *Medscape.* https://emedicine.medscape.com/article/183084-medication#3

The Editors of Encyclopaedia Britannica. (2021). *Multiple sclerosis.* Encyclopedia Britannica. https://www.britannica.com/science/multiple-sclerosis

CDC. (2021). *Understanding and explaining mRNA COVID-19 vaccines.* https://www.cdc.gov/vaccines/covid-19/hcp/mrna-vaccine-basics.html#

College of Physicians of Philadelphia. (2016). *History of anti-vaccination movements.* http://www.historyofvaccines.org/content/articles/history-anti-vaccination-movements

DerMarderosian, A., & Beutler, J., (Eds.). (2003). *Guide to popular natural products* (3rd ed.).Lippincott Williams & Wilkins.

Dyson, B. (2016, August 31). Making sense of monoclonal antibodies. *Pharmacy Times.*

Filipi, M., & Jack, S. (2020). Interferons in the treatment of MS: A clinical efficacy, safety, and tolerability update. *International Journal of MS Care, 22*(4), 165–172.

Hale, T. (2012). Hale's breastfeeding safety ratings. http://www.womensmentalhealth.emory.edu/Blog/indexBreastfeeding%202011.10.28.html

Ionescu, A., Sharma, A., Kundnani, N. R., Mihăilescu, A., David, V. L., Bedreag, O., Săndesc, D., Dinu, A. R., Săndesc, M. A., Albulescu, N., & Drăgoi, R. G. (2020). Intravenous iron infusion as an alternative to minimize blood transfusion in peri-operative patients. *Scientific Reports, 10*(1), 18403. https://doi.org/10.1038/s41598-020-75535-2. PMID: 33110237; PMCID: PMC7591902.

Joseph, A. (2020). *'A huge experiment': How the world made so much progress on a covid-19 vaccine so fast*. Heath, Stat News. https://www.statnews.com/2020/07/30/a-huge-experiment-how-the-world-made-so-much-progress-on-a-covid-19-vaccine-so-fast/

Offit, P. A., Quarles, J., Gerber, M. A., Hackett, C. J., Marcuse, E. K., Kollman, T. R., Gellin, B. G., & Landry, S. (2002). Addressing parents' concerns: Do multiple vaccines overwhelm or weaken the infant's immune system? *Pediatrics, 109*(1), 124–129.

Ogbru, O., & Davis, C. (2021). *Monocolonal antibodies*. Medicinenet.com. https://www.medicinenet.com/monoclonal_antibodies/article.htm#what_are_human_monoclonal_antibodies

Patti, F., Zimatore, G. B., Morra, V. B., Aguglia, U., Bossio, R., Marziolo, R., Valentino, P., Chisari, C. G., Capacchione, A., Zappia, M., & on behalf of RELIEF Study Group, . (2020). Administration of subcutaneous interferon reducing flu like symptoms. *Journal of Neurology, 267*, 1812–1823. https://doi.org/10.1007/s00415-020-09771-x

Pullen, L. (2014). *T cells and autoimmune diseases*. The Rheumatologist. https://www.the-rheumatologist.org/article/t-cells-autoimmune-diseases/

Quarles, J., Gerber, M. A., Hackett, C. J., Marcuse, E. K., Kollman, T. R., Gellin, B. G., & Landry, S. (2002). Addressing parents' concerns: Do multiple vaccines overwhelm or weaken the infant's immune system? *Pediatrics, 109*(1), 124–129.

Scott, G. (August 19, 2016). Sorting through the confusion of biologic drug names. *Medscape Pharmacists.*

Stedman online dictionary. (2020). https://stedmansonline.com/content.aspx?id=mlrI1300002567&termtype=t

Stephenson, L. (2017). Monoclonal antibody therapy for asthma. *Clinical Pulmonary Medicine, 24*(6), 250–257. https://doi.org/10.1097/CPM.0000000000000234

Taddio, A., McMurtry, C. M., Shah, V., Riddell, R. P., Chambers, C. T., Noel, M., MacDonald, N. E., Rogers, J., Bucci, L. M., Mousmanis, P., Lang, E., Halperin, S. A., Bowles, S., Halpert, C., Ipp, M., Asmundson, G. J. G., Rieder, M. J., Robson, K., Uleryk, E., … Bleeker, E. V. (2015). Reducing pain during vaccine injections: Clinical practice guideline. *Canadian Medical Association Journal, 187*(13), 975–982.

Voge, N. V., & Alvarez, E. (2019). Monoclonal antibodies in multiple sclerosis: Present and future. *Biomedicines, 7*(1), 20. https://doi.org/10.3390/biomedicines7010020. PMID: 30875812; PMCID: PMC6466331.

Vogel, W. (2010). Infusion reactions: diagnosis, assessment, and management. *Clinical Journal of Oncology Nursing, 14*(2), E10–E21. https://doi.org/10.1188/10.CJON.E10-E21

Wujcik, D. (2018). *Targeted therapy*. In *Cancer nursing: Principles and practice* (8th ed.). Jones and Barlett Learning.

Reports

IOM childhood immunization schedule and safety. (2013). http://books.nap.edu/openbook.php?record_id=13563

Websites for Information
Immunization Action Coalition. http://www.immunize.org
National Vaccine Information Center. http://www.nvic.org

Unit 13

American Society of Clinical Oncology. (2020). *Understanding immunotherapy*. https://www.cancer.net/navigating-cancer-care/how-cancer-treated/immunotherapy-and-vaccines/understanding-immunotherapy

Brahmer, J., Lacchetti, C., Schneider, B. J., Atkins, M. B., Brassil, K. J., Caterino, J. M., Chau, I., Ernstoff, M. S., Gardner, J. M., Ginex, P., Hallmeyer, S., Holter Chakrabarty, J., Leighl, N. B., Mammen, J. S., McDermott, D. F., Naing, A., Nastoupil, L. J., Phillips, T., Porter, L. D., … National Comprehensive Cancer Network, . (2018). Management of immune-related adverse events in patients treated with immune checkpoint inhibitors therapy: ASCO clinical practice guideline. *Journal of Clinical Oncology, 36*(17), 1714–1768. https://doi.org/10.1200/JCO.2017.77.6385

Cai, J., Ma, H., Huang, F., Zhu, D., Bi, J., Ke, Y., & Zhang, T. (2013). Correlation of bevacizumab-induced hypertension and outcomes of metastatic colorectal cancer patients treated with bevacizumab: A systematic review and meta-analysis. *World Journal of Surgical Oncology, 11*, 306.

Ganguly, S. (2015). Immunotherapy and intracellular signaling inhibition in oncology. *Pharmacology Updates in Oncology Practice Mtg*, 9/26. Memphis, TN.

Hale, T. (2012). *Hale's breastfeeding safety ratings*. http://www.womensmentalhealth.emory.edu/Blog/indexBreastfeeding%202011.10.28.html

Houlihan, N., Tyson, L., & Wood, L., (2005). Targeted therapies in non-small cell lung cancer. *Cont. Ed Monograph Produced by OES.*

Kim, H. S., Kim, S. S., & Park, S. G. (2014). Bowel perforation associated sunitinib therapy for recurred gastric gastrointestinal stromal tumor. *Annals of Surgical Treatment and Research, 86*(4), 220–225.

King, S. E. (2004). Therapeutic cancer vaccines: An emerging treatment option. *Clinical Journal of Oncology Nursing, 8*, 271–278.

Knoop, T. (2015). Pharmacologic treatment of solid tumors. *Pharmacology Updates in Oncology Practice Mtg, 9/26*. Memphis, TN.

Kreidieh, F., Moukadem, H., & Saghir, N. (2016). Overview, prevention and management of chemotherapy extravasation. *World Journal of Clinical Oncology, 7*(1), 87–97.

Lamprecht, M., & Dansereau, C. (2019). Car T-cell therapy: Update on the state of the science. *Clinical Journal of Oncology Nursing, 23*(2), 6–12.

Mavroukakis, S., Muehlbauer, P. M., White, R. L., Jr., & Schwartzentruber, D. J. (2001). Clinical pathways for managing patients receiving Interleukin 2, *Clinical Journal of Oncology Nursing, 5*(5), 1–11.

Menonna-Quinn, D., Polovich, M., & Marshall, B. (2019). Personal protective equipment: Evaluating usage among inpatient and outpatient oncology nurses. *Clinical Journal of Oncology Nursing, 23*(3), 260–265.

Olsen, M., LeFebvre, K., & Brassil, K., (Eds.). (2018). *Chemotherapy and immunotherapy guidelines and recommendations for practice*. Oncology Nursing Society.

ONS Position Statement. (2016). Ensuring healthcare worker safety when handling hazardous drugs. https://www.ons.org/

make-difference/ons-center-advocacy-and-health-policy/position-statements/ensuring-healthcare

Petrelli, F., Borgonovo, K., Cabiddu, M., Lonati, V., & Barni, S. (2012). Relationship between skin rash and outcome in non-small-cell lung cancer patients treated with anti-EGFR tyrosine kinase inhibitors: A literature-based meta-analysis of 24 trials. *Lung Cancer, 78*(1), 8–15.

Polovich, M., (Ed.). (2011). *Safe handling of hazardous drugs* (2nd ed.). ONS Publisher.

Puksic, S., Mitrovic, J., Culo, M. I., Zivkovic, M., Orehovec, B., Bobek, D., & Morovic-Vergles, J. (2021). Effects of yoga in daily life program in rheumatoid arthritis: A randomized controlled trial. *Complementary Therapies in Medicine, 57*, 102639. https://doi.org/10.1016/j.ctim.2020.102639

Rubin, K. (2015). Understanding immune checkpoint inhibitors for effective patient care. *Clinical Journal of Oncology Nursing, 19*(6), 709–717.

Vogel, W. (2010). Infusion reactions: diagnosis, assessment, and management. *Clinical Journal of Oncology Nursing, 14*(2), E10–E21. https://doi.org/10.1188/10.CJON.E10-E21

Websites for Information

National Cancer Institute. https://www.cancer.gov/about-cancer/treatment/types/targeted-therapies/targeted-therapies-fact-sheet#r2

Unit 14

Bertolino, G., Pitassi, A., Tinelli, C., Staniscia, A., Guglielmana, B., Scudeller, L., & Luigi Balduini, C. (2012). Intermittent flushing with heparin versus saline for maintenance of peripheral intravenous catheters in a medical department: A pragmatic cluster-randomized controlled study. *Worldviews in Evidence-Based Nursing, 9*(4), 221–226.

DerMarderosian, A., & Beutler, J., (Eds.). (2003). *Guide to popular natural products* (3rd ed.). Lippincott Williams & Wilkins.

Deutsch, L. (2020). Dilution is no solution. *Nursing, 50*(5), 54–60. https://doi.org/10.1097/01.NURSE.0000659332.20270.6c

Goode, C., Kleiber, C., Titler, M., Small, S., Rakel, B., Steelman, V. M., Walker, J. B., & Buckwater, K. C. (1993). Improving practice through research: The case of heparin vs. saline for peripheral intermittent infusion devices. *Medsurg Nursing, 2*(1), 23–27.

Hadaway, L. (2007). Infiltration and extravasation, preventing a complication of IV catheterization. *American Journal of Nursing, 107*(8), 64–72.

Health Canada. (2019). Health Canada warns Canadians of potential cancer risk associated with gentian violet. *Recall and Safety Alerts.* https://healthycanadians.gc.ca/recall-alert-rappel-avis/hc-sc/2019/70179a-eng.php

ISMP. (2018). Part I: Survey results show unsafe practices persist with IV push medications. *ISMP Medication Safety Alert!, 11*(1).

Kishner, S., & Schraga, E. (2016). Opioid equivalents and conversions. *Medscape.* http://emedicine.medscape.com/article/2138678-overview

Rubin, R. (2020). Testing an old therapy against a new disease, convalescent plasma for COVID-19. *Journal of American Medical Association, 323*(21), 2114–2117. https://doi.org/10.1001/JAMA.2020.7456

Schallom, M., Prentice, D., Sona, C., Micek, S. T., & Skrupky, L. P. (2012). Heparin or 0.9% sodium chloride to maintain central venous catheter patency: A randomized trial. *Critical Care Medicine, 40*(6), 1820–1826.

Spray, J. W. (2016). Review of intravenous lipid emulsion therapy. *Journal of Infusion Nursing: The Official Publication of the Infusion Nurses Society, 39*(6), 377–380. https://doi.org/10.1097/NAN.0000000000000194

Websites for Information

https://www.ins1.org/

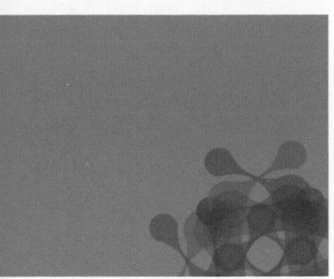

Index

Note: Page numbers followed by f, t, and d, indicate figures, tables, and display material respectively.